Contents

KU-079-068

Section 1   Principles of Emergency Medicine

Section 2   Primary Complaints

An Introduction to
Clinical Emergency Medicine

and interpret appropriate laboratory and graphic tests. This textbook also provides nt management and disposition strategies controversies presented, including pearls, ls, and myths for topics covered. Chapters written by nationally- and internationally-ected clinicians, educators, and researchers field of emergency medicine. An *Introduction nical Emergency Medicine* offers just the right bination of text, clinical images, and practi-nformation for students, residents, physician stants, nurse practitioners, and experienced cians in all medical disciplines. The over-ng goal of this textbook is to improve the ctitioner's understanding of emergency med-le principles and practice, directly benefiting tient care in a variety of emergency settings.

An Introduction to

Clinical Emergency Medicine

Swaminatha V. Mahadevan, MD, FACEP, FAAEM

Associate Chief, Division of Emergency Medicine
Assistant Professor of Surgery (Emergency Medicine)
Stanford University School of Medicine
Emergency Department Medical Director
Medical Student Clerkship Director
Stanford University Medical Center, Stanford, CA

Gus M. Garmel, MD, FACEP, FAAEM

Co-Program Director, Stanford/Kaiser Emergency Medicine Residency
Clinical Associate Professor of Surgery (Emergency Medicine)
Stanford University School of Medicine
Senior Staff Emergency Physician, The Permanente Medical Group
Clerkship Director for Medical Students and Rotating Interns
Kaiser Permanente Medical Center, Santa Clara, CA

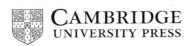

CAMBRIDGE
UNIVERSITY PRESS

CAMBRIDGE UNIVERSITY PRESS
Cambridge, New York, Melbourne, Madrid, Cape Town, Singapore, São Paulo

CAMBRIDGE UNIVERSITY PRESS
The Edinburgh Building, Cambridge CB2 2RU, UK

Published in the United States of America by Cambridge University Press,
New York

www.cambridge.org
Information on this title: www.cambridge.org/9780521542593

First published 2005

Printed in the United Kingdom at the University Press, Cambridge

A catalog record for this book is available from the British Library

Library of Congress Cataloging in Publication data

ISBN-13 978-0-521-54259-3 paperback
ISBN-10 0-521-54259-6 paperback

List of contributors

Kumar Alagappan, MD, FACEP, FAAEM
Associate Chairman, Emergency Medicine
Long Island Jewish Medical Center
New Hyde Park, NY
Associate Professor of Clinical Emergency
Medicine, Albert Einstein College of Medicine

Janet G. Alteveer, MD
Associate Prof. Emergency Medicine, Assistant
Director Emergency Department, Cooper
Hospital, Robert Wood Johnson Medical School
of UMDNJ, Camden, NJ

J. Michael Ballester, MD
Assistant Professor of Emergency Medicine
University of Cincinnati Department of
Emergency Medicine, Cincinnati, OH

Paul D. Biddinger, MD
Director of Prehospital Care and Disaster
Medicine, Massachusetts General Hospital
Department of Emergency Medicine
Instructor in Surgery, Harvard Medical School
Boston, MA

Victoria Brazil, MBBS, FACEM
Staff Specialist and Director of Emergency
Medicine Training, Royal Brisbane Hospital
Australia

Lance Brown, MD, MPH, FACEP
Chief, Division of Pediatric Emergency Medicine
Associate Professor of Emergency Medicine and
Pediatrics, Loma Linda University Medical
Center and Children's Hospital, Loma Linda
California

Andrew K. Chang, MD
Assistant Professor, Dept of Emergency
Medicine, Albert Einstein College of Medicine
Montefiore Medical Center, Bronx, NY

Robert L. Cloutier, MD, FAAEM, FAAP
Assistant Professor of Emergency Medicine
Adjunct Assistant Professor of Pediatrics
Oregon Health and Science University
Doernbecher Children's Hospital, Portland
Oregon

Wendy C. Coates, MD
Associate Professor of Medicine and Chair
Acute Care College, UCLA School of Medicine
Director, Medical Education, Harbor-UCLA
DEM, Torrance, CA

Jamie Collings, MD
Program Director, Department of Emergency
Medicine, Northwestern University Hospital
Assistant Professor of Emergency Medicine
Northwestern University Feinberg School of
Medicine, Chicago, IL

Jonathan E. Davis, MD
Associate Residency Program Director
Assistant Professor, Georgetown University
Hospital/Washington Hospital Center
Washington, D.C.

Peter M.C. DeBlieux, MD
LSUHSC Professor of Clinical Medicine
LSUHSC Charity Hospital, New Orleans
Louisiana

Pamela L. Dyne, MD
Associate Professor of Clinical Medicine/
Emergency Medicine, Olive View-UCLA
Department of Emergency Medicine, Sylmar, CA

Cemil M. Erdem, MD
Attending Physician, Holyoke Medical Center
Holyoke, Massachusetts

Gino A. Farina, MD, FACEP
Assistant Professor of Emergency Medicine
Albert Einstein College of Medicine-Long Island
Jewish Medical Center, New Hyde Park, NY

Robert Galli, MD, FACEP
Professor and Chair, University of Mississippi
Medical Center, Jackson, MS

Gus M. Garmel, MD, FACEP, FAAEM
Co-Program Director, Stanford/Kaiser
Emergency Medicine Residency
Clinical Associate Professor of Surgery
(Emergency Medicine), Stanford University
School of Medicine
Senior Staff Emergency Physician, The
Permanente Medical Group
Clerkship Director for Medical Students and
Rotating Interns, Kaiser Permanente Medical
Center, Santa Clara, CA

Dan Garza, MD
Sports Medicine Fellow, Department of
Orthopedic Surgery
Clinical Instructor, Division of Emergency
Medicine, Stanford University School of
Medicine, Stanford, CA

Gregory H. Gilbert, MD
Clinical Instructor, Division of Emergency
Medicine
Associate Medical Student Clerkship Director
Stanford University School of Medicine
Stanford, CA

Michael A. Gisondi, MD
Assistant Professor of Emergency Medicine
Associate Residency Director
Department of Emergency Medicine
Northwestern University, Chicago, IL

Steven Go, MD
Assistant Dean for Medical Education
University of Missouri-Kansas City School of
Medicine, Kansas City, Missouri

Steven M. Green, MD, FACEP
Professor of Emergency Medicine & Pediatrics
Loma Linda University, Loma Linda
California

Gregory Guldner, MD, MS, FACEP
Program Director, Emergency Medicine
Residency, Loma Linda University Medical
Center & Children's Hospital, Loma Linda, CA

Swaminatha V. Gurudevan, MD
Assistant Professor of Clinical Medicine
University of California, Irvine School of Medicine
Associate Director, Noninvasive Cardiac
Laboratories, UCI Medical Center

Glenn C. Hamilton, MD, MS
Professor and Chair
Department of Emergency Medicine
Wright State University School of Medicine
Dayton, Ohio

Stephen R. Hayden, MD, FACEP, FAAEM
Associate Professor of Clinical Medicine
Program Director Emergency Medicine
Residency, University of California
San Diego Medical Center, San Diego, CA

Gregory W. Hendey, MD, FACEP
Associate Clinical Professor of Medicine
UCSF Fresno Medical Education Program

Mel Herbert, MD, FACEP, FAAEM
Associate Professor of Clinical Emergency
Medicine, Keck USC School of Medicine

Michelle Huston, MD
Staff Emergency Physician,
Franklin Square Hospital Center
Baltimore, MD

Loretta Jackson-Williams, MD, PHD
Assistant Professor Emergency Medicine
Clinical Course Director for Students and
Residents
Director Basic Science Research
University of Mississippi Medical Center

Peter G. Kumasaka, MD
Assistant Professor of Clinical Medicine
University of Minnesota
Department of Emergency Medicine
Regions Hospital, St. Paul, MN

Melissa J. Lamberson, MD, FACEP
Assistant Professor, Dept of Emergency
Medicine
Emory University School of Medicine
Atlanta, GA

Mary Lanctot-Herbert, RN, MSN, FNP
Assistant Clinical Professor of Nursing, Acute
Care Division, UCLA School of Nursing

Amy Leinen, ESQ
Senior Attorney, Snell & Wilmer, LLP, Irvine, CA

Robert R. Leschke, MD
Assistant Professor, Associate Residency
Program Director, Director of Undergraduate
Medical Education, Medical College of
Wisconsin, Milwaukee, WI

Michelle Lin, MD
Assistant Clinical Professor of Medicine
UC San Francisco, San Francisco General
Hospital Emergency Services, San Francisco, CA

Douglas W. Lowery, MD
Associate Professor of Emergency Medicine
Emory University, Atlanta, Georgia

Sharon E. Mace, MD, FACEP, FAAP
Associate Professor, Department of Emergency
Medicine Ohio State University School of
Medicine Director Pediatric Education/ Quality
Improvement, Observation Unit, Cleveland
Clinic Foundation, Cleveland, Ohio

Swaminatha V. Mahadevan, MD, FACEP, FAAEM
Associate Chief, Division of Emergency
Medicine
Assistant Professor of Surgery (Emergency
Medicine), Stanford University School of
Medicine
Emergency Department Medical Director
Medical Student Clerkship Director
Stanford University Medical Center
Stanford CA

Diku Mandavia, MD, FACEP, FRCPC
Attending Staff Physician, Department of
Emergency Medicine, Cedars-Sinai Medical
Center
Clinical Associate Professor of Emergency
Medicine, Director of Emergency Ultrasound
Keck School of Medicine University of
Southern California, Los Angeles
California

David E. Manthey, MD, FAAEM, FACEP
Associate Professor, Director of Undergraduate
Medical Education, Wake Forest University
School of Medicine, Winston-Salem, NC

Amal Mattu, MD
Program Director, Emergency Medicine
Residency
University of Maryland School of Medicine
Baltimore, Maryland

Lynne McCullough, MD, FACEP
Assistant Professor of Medicine
David Geffen School of Medicine at UCLA
Associate Program Director UCLA/
Olive View-UCLA Emergency Medicine
UCLA Emergency Medicine Center
Los Angeles, CA

Steven A. McLaughlin, MD
Associate Professor, EM Residency Program
Director
University of New Mexico Albuquerque, NM

Tim Meyers, MD, MS
Emergency Medicine Physician
Boulder Community Hospital, Boulder, CO
Attending Physician, San Francisco General
Hospital, San Francisco, CA

Christopher R.H. Newton, MD
Assistant Program Director, Emergency
Medicine Residency, University of Michigan/
St Joseph Mercy Hospital, Ann Arbor, MI

Flavia Nobay, MD
Assistant Clinical Professor of Medicine
Division of Emergency Medicine
University of California at San Francisco
(UCSF)

Robert L. Norris, MD, FACEP
Associate Professor of Surgery
Chief of Emergency Medicine
Stanford University School of Medicine
Editor-in-Chief, *Wilderness and Environmental
Medicine*

Jennifer A. Oman, MD, FACEP, FAAEM
Program Director, Emergency Medicine
Assistant Clinical Professor of Emergency
Medicine
University of California, Irvine Medical Center

Rita Oregon, MD, FACOG
Assistant Clinical Professor
Department of Obstetrics and Gynecology
Olive View-UCLA Medical Center, Sylmar, CA

Tamas R. Peredy, MD, FACEP
Emergency Physician, Maine Medical Center
Medical Toxicology Fellow
University of Connecticut, Portland
Maine and Hartford Connecticut

Stephen J. Playe, MD, FACEP
Assistant Professor of Emergency Medicine
Tufts University School of Medicine
Residency Program Director, Dept of Emergency
Medicine, Baystate Medical Center
Springfield, MA

Susan B. Promes, MD, FACEP
Associate Clinical Professor, Program Director
Division of Emergency Medicine
Duke University, Durham, NC

Kristy Self Reynolds, MD
Attending Physician, INOVA Fair Oaks Hospital
Fairfax, Virginia

Carolyn J. Sachs, MD, MPH
Associate Professor, David Geffen School of
Medicine, Los Angeles, CA

Eric Savitsky, MD
Associate Professor of Medicine
UCLA Emergency Medicine Residency Program
Los Angeles, CA

Rawle A. Seupaul, MD
Assistant Professor of Clinical Emergency
Medicine, Indiana University School of
Medicine, Indianapolis, IN

Fred A. Severyn, MD, FACEP
Assistant Professor of Surgery/Emergency
Medicine, University of Colorado Health
Sciences Center, Denver, CO

Lee W. Shockley, MD, FACEP
Emergency Department Medical Director
Associate Professor, Associate Residency
Director, Denver Health Medical Center
Denver, Colorado

Robert J. Sigillito, MD
Assistant Clinical Professor of Medicine
Louisiana State University Health Sciences
Center, New Orleans, Louisiana

Barry Simon, MD
Associate Clinical Professor of Medicine
UCSF Chairman, Department of Emergency
Medicine, Highland General Hospital
Oakland, CA

Shannon Sovndal, MD
Emergency Medicine Physician, Boulder
Community Hospital, Boulder, CO

George Sternbach, MD, FACEP
Clinical Professor of Surgery, Stanford
University Medical Center, Stanford, CA

Eustacia (Jo) Su, MD
Associate Professor, Emergency Medicine and
Pediatrics, Oregon Health Sciences University
Portland, Oregon

Rita A. Sweeney, MD, MPH
Clinical Instructor, Alameda County Medical
Center, Highland Campus, Oakland, CA

Jeffrey A. Tabas, MD
San Francisco General Hospital Emergency
Services, Associate Professor of Medicine
University of California San Francisco, School of
Medicine, San Francisco, CA

J. Scott Taylor, MD
Clinical Instructor, University of Michigan
Hurley Hospital, Flint, MI

Brigham Temple, MD
Clinical Instructor, Northwestern University
Feinberg School of Medicine, Evanston-
Northwestern Healthcare, Evanston, IL

Stephen H. Thomas, MD, MPH
Assistant Professor of Surgery, Harvard
Medical School
Director of Undergraduate Emergency
Medicine Education, Massachusetts General
Hospital

R. Jason Thurman, MD
Assistant Professor of Emergency Medicine
Assistant Director, Residency Program
Department of Emergency Medicine
Vanderbilt University Medical Center
Co-Chairman, Operation Stroke Nashville

F.C. von Trampe, MD, MPH
Clinical Instructor of Medicine, David
Geffen-UCLA School of Medicine
Attending Staff, Harbor-UCLA Medical Center
Los Angeles, California, Attending Staff, Kaiser
Southbay, Los Angeles

Ken Zafren, MD, FACEP
Clinical Assistant Professor, Division of
Emergency Medicine, Stanford University
Medical Center, Stanford, CA
Staff Emergency Physician, Alaska Native
Medical Center, Anchorage, AK

Foreword

Emergency medicine represents the unique combination of rapid data gathering, simultaneous prioritization, and constant multi-tasking in a time-constrained fish bowl – with all decisions subject to second-guessing by others. It is a patient complaint-oriented specialty in which stabilization based on anticipation supersedes lengthy differentials and diagnostic precision.

In light of these unique aspects and attributes of clinical practice, one would expect the textbook-based literature supporting this specialty to be uniquely written and reflective of its singular approach. This has rarely been the case, a fact that has puzzled me for almost 30 years. It is true that sequential prose does not accurately represent the parallel processing necessary to practice effective and efficient emergency medicine. Still, it would seem the ideas of priority diagnoses, stabilization, initial assessment, prioritized differential diagnosis, and the rest that follows could be delineated and emphasized within the limitations of the printed word. I am pleased and delighted to find and convey to the reader that this text succeeds in translating this untraditional emergency medicine approach into a textbook format.

This text, edited by two academicians, Swaminatha V. Mahadevan, MD and Gus M. Garmel, MD from one of the nation's premier academic institutions and leading health care organizations, fulfills what I have long believed is the correct and necessary pathway to understanding the approach and thought processes that drive clinical decision-making in emergency medicine. The focus of the text is appropriately "presenting complaint-oriented," with a thorough coverage of the chief complaints responsible for the majority of emergency department visits. Each chapter is structured in a consistent manner that allows the experienced and uninitiated alike to clearly track the thought process needed to bring one to a successful prioritized conclusion of care, even when a specific diagnosis has not been made.

The range of authorship is excellent, reflecting the talents and capabilities of an entire new generation of emergency physicians trained in the specialty. These authors clearly understand emergency medicine's unique principles.

It is a rare gift to witness and participate in the passing of our unique specialty's visions onto the capable hands of those you have had the opportunity to train and know. Due to this textbook's organization and content, I am pleased to finally "rest in peace," at least academically. Drs. Garmel and Mahadevan demonstrate their clear understanding and literary virtuosity in conveying the truth about our specialty to others.

It is my pleasure to congratulate them on a successful venture, to warn them that having started on this path serial additions and subsequent editions will rule their life for as long as they, the publisher, and the sales last, and to express a personal sense of satisfaction and pride in their accomplishment. To the reader, I say enjoy yourself. Take much away from this text and welcome the truth as we currently know it, presented in a manner that accurately reflects the way we practice.

Glenn C. Hamilton, MD, MSM
Professor and Chair
Department of Emergency Medicine
Wright State University School of Medicine
Editor, *Emergency Medicine: An Approach to Clinical Problem-Solving*

Acknowledgments

Drs. Mahadevan and Garmel would like to express gratitude to Barbara Wada and Rachel Lauterbach for their invaluable administrative assistance. Dr. Kathryn Stevens was extremely generous with her time, providing radiographs and detailed captions. We are indebted to the following individuals at Cambridge University Press: Richard Barling, Peter Silver, Sue Tuck, Geoff Nuttal, Dominic Lewis and Heidi Lovette (formerly of CUP). Their confidence in our vision allowed our concept for a unique textbook to become a reality. We are also grateful for the outstanding work done by Geetha Williams and the staff at Charon Tec.

A special thank you goes to Dr. Glenn Hamilton for writing our preface and confidently "passing the torch" to us as medical educators. The diligent efforts by our contributors, who produced the most updated and comprehensive chapters possible, was astonishing. Several friends and colleagues assisted in reviewing chapters and should be recognized: Drs. George Sternbach, Greg Moran, Darius Moshfeghi, and Robert Norris. Drs. Amal Mattu, Steven Shpall, and R. Brooke Jeffrey contributed ECGs, dermatologic images, and radiographs, respectively, at our request. Other authors granted us permission to use images from their own textbooks: Drs. Lawrence Stack, Basil Zitelli, Diku Mandavia, and Ron Walls. Finally, we are grateful to Chris Gralapp, MA, CMI (Medical and Scientific Illustration, www.biolumina.com), whose original art is not only stunning but also certain to assist the readers' understanding of the challenging concepts presented in this textbook.

Dedication

Swaminatha V. Mahadevan, MD, FACEP, FAAEM

To my parents, Sarojini and M.S. Venkatesan, and my grandparents: thank you for your continual sacrifices for the sake of your children.

To my mentors: thank you for teaching me not to follow blindly but to ask, question, and discover.

To the residents and medical students: I am continually inspired by your genuine desire to learn, and marvel at your ideas, enthusiasm and accomplishments. It is a privilege to teach, advise, and befriend each one of you.

To Gus: without you, this book would have remained another good idea (and wasted opportunity).

To my wife Rema and my children, Aditya and Lavanya: thank you for allowing me to pursue and fulfill my goals and dreams, both in and out of medicine. You fill me with strength, hope and happiness.

Gus M. Garmel, MD, FACEP, FAAEM

To my parents, siblings, and extended family: thanks for your unconditional love and support.

To my friends and physician colleagues, who share my passion for life and emergency medicine.

To residents, medical students, and patients, past and present, who inspire me daily.

To the Permanente Medical Group, Kaiser Permanente Medical Center, Santa Clara, CA, and Stanford University, the institutions that support my clinical and academic pursuits. Also to the Stanford/Kaiser Emergency Medicine Residency Program, which affords me infinite joy and immeasurable pride.

To Maha, who, in collaboration, made this vision a reality.

And to Laura: my spouse, partner, and best friend. You are my oxygen.

Section 1

Principles of Emergency Medicine

1 Approach to the emergency patient

Gus M. Garmel, MD

The emergency department (ED) is a challenging environment for patients, families, and medical personnel. Many challenges result from our practice's principles: available at any time for any patient with any complaint. Patients who come to the ED are not familiar with us personally, yet must feel confident about our abilities to help them during their time of greatest concern. Their needs may be as straightforward as an excuse note for work or a prescription refill in the middle of the night, or as complex as an acute illness or injury, an exacerbation of a chronic condition, or a cry for help if depressed or suicidal. Even providing reassurance about a child's fever to a concerned parent is a critical function of emergency physicians (EPs).

Qualities successful EPs exhibit include intelligence, sensitivity, humility, insight, proficiency making decisions with and acting on limited information, and the ability to multi-task. Being skillful negotiators, working well with individuals having different backgrounds and ethnicities, and advocating strongly for patients at all times are essential qualities. In addition to these traits, EPs must be experts in trauma and medical resuscitation of adults and children, and in sharing news with patients and family members about the outcomes of these events.

The majority of patients use the ED infrequently. Many may be experiencing this setting for the first time. Patients' lack of familiarity with this environment, fear, stress, waiting times, painful procedures, and overall discomfort often preclude them from having a positive experience. These are only some of the issues that patients contend with in the ED.

EPs confront numerous challenges when taking care of patients presenting to the ED. Perhaps the greatest challenge is the spectrum of diseases which EPs must be able to identify. Rather than having to know only the first 15 minutes of an illness, EPs must be familiar with all stages of all illnesses, often presenting in atypical fashion. In addition, time pressures inherent to providing emergency care, the lack of existing relationships with patients, unfamiliarity with their medical history, and the inability to review patients' medical records challenge EPs daily. EPs must rapidly and simultaneously evaluate, diagnose and treat multiple patients with multiple conditions, often with limited information, without confusing subtle nuances between patients. They must be insightful, anticipatory, and prepared to act and react to prevent morbidity and, when possible, mortality. Considering worse case scenarios is fundamental to EM practice. Most importantly, EPs must be comfortable providing detailed, often devastating information in a concise yet understandable manner to patients and family members who may have different cultural backgrounds.

It is indeed a privilege to be in a position to offer care to patients during what is likely to be their time of greatest need. Approaching patients sensitively, recognizing their apprehension, pain, concerns, and perhaps shame is critical to our mission. This is true no matter how trivial a patient's problem may seem. Often, patients consult with EPs to seek approval about their desire to leave a spouse, to get an opinion regarding a physician's recommendation for surgery, or to receive confirmation that they are making the right decision about a parent, child, or loved one. Serving in this capacity, without judgment, is not only appropriate but also essential.

It is imperative that EPs approach each patient with an open mind, committed to identify and address not only the presenting problem but also any coexisting problems. For example, a patient with the history and presenting complaint of esophageal reflux may in fact have acute coronary syndrome (ACS). A patient with the apparent problem of insomnia may have an underlying concern about his or her safety, security, or mental wellness. The ability of an EP to evaluate each patient using history-taking and physical examination abilities, as well as laboratory or radiography interpretation skills, when appropriate, is only a portion of our armamentarium. An experienced EPs "sixth sense" is something that, over time, has become recognized and respected by non-EM colleagues.

Unfortunately, the ED environment is not always conducive to privacy. Despite the Health Insurance Portability and Accountability Act (HIPAA) of 1996 and Protected Health

Information (PHI) for patients, attempts to maintain patient confidentiality in the ED present a continuous challenge. Discussions about patient care issues between health care providers, staff, patients, and family members often take place behind nothing more than a curtain. Shared spaces, hallways, lack of private rooms or beds, and the demands of time-pressured discussions, often in open spaces, over the phone, or with consultants stretch efforts at maintaining patient confidentiality. The leadership role that EPs have in the ED affords them the opportunity to demonstrate respect for patient confidentiality and to remind others of the importance of upholding this principle.

Recently, there has been tremendous publicity regarding medical errors and patient safety. Human error may occur at any time, but is more likely during high patient volumes or when multiple complicated patients of high acuity present simultaneously. Error has been demonstrated to occur more frequently when provider fatigue is greatest (for example, at the end of a challenging shift or after being awake all night). Systems errors are even more likely to occur during these circumstances. Attention has been placed on reducing errors and improving patient safety, using the airline industry as an example. Airline pilots, however, are not required to fly more than one plane at the same time, while simulating take-off, landing, and changing course. The EM community should embrace the federal government's attention to medical systems and its role in medical error, as patient safety is a top priority. Hospital quality committees review errors of omission and commission, medication errors, errors in patient registration, and errors of judgment. Given the pace of the ED environment, it is remarkable that more errors do not occur. The rapid need for patient turnover, room changes, and test result reporting does not occur with such immediacy in most other areas of the hospital. Hospital administrators with limited insight about the uniqueness of EM practice should focus attention to, and provide support for, this essential aspect of patient care.

EPs must recognize that patients signed over to them at the end of a shift pose increased risk. These patients typically have laboratory or X-ray results pending, are being observed for continued improvement or worsening in their condition, or are waiting for consultants. They should have treatment and disposition plans in place, predetermined by the EP who initially evaluated them based on anticipated outcomes. However, it may

be these signed-over patients do not have well-established dispositions and need a new EP's perspective. In such cases, it is better to inform the receiving EP that a good understanding about what is going on with that patient does not exist than leave things vague or unclear. As long as patients present to EDs at any time, patients signed over at shift's end will continue to challenge our ability to provide safe care within our practice.

Scope of the problem

A landmark article by Schneider, et al. from the EM literature defines our specialty as one "... with the principle mission of evaluating, managing, treating and preventing unexpected illness and injury." As emergency medical care is an essential component of a comprehensive health care delivery system, it must be available 24 hours a day. EPs provide rapid assessment and treatment of any patient with a medical emergency. In addition, they are responsible for the initial assessment and care of any medical condition that a patient believes requires urgent attention. One key aspect of this commentary is that patients may believe they require urgent attention, when in fact they do not. It remains our mission to provide patients the opportunity to receive sensitive medical care and reassurance even under this circumstance. EPs also provide medical support for individuals who lack access to other avenues of care. As the number of uninsured and underinsured persons in the US increases, and growing numbers of health clinics close, many of these individuals will use the ED for their primary as well as emergency care. This has placed a tremendous burden on the safety net provided by the specialty of EM.

In 2000, ED visits climbed to 108 million, a 14% increase from 1997. In California, patients visiting EDs were found to be sicker than ever before, with an increase in critical emergency care visits by 59% between 1990 and 1999. Although there were just over 4,000 EDs in 2000, the number of EDs has decreased as hospitals and trauma centers are forced to close. The number of EPs in clinical practice reported by the American College of Emergency Physicians (ACEP) in 1999 was just under 32,000, a decrease from 1997. There has been an increase in the number of nurse practitioners and physician assistants trained to work in emergency care settings, and many hospitals are staffing urgent care and fast-track areas with these practitioners.

With decreased funding available for non-ED clinics, and increasing numbers of patients without health insurance who use the ED as their primary (or only) source of health care, the worsening of ED overcrowding is inevitable.

Hamilton describes the clinical practice of EM in his textbook as one that "... encompasses the initial evaluation, treatment, and disposition of any person at any time for any symptom, event, or disorder deemed by the person – or someone acting on his or her behalf – to require expeditious medical, surgical, or psychiatric attention." This philosophy creates tremendous challenges, as well as opportunities, unique to the specialty of EM. EDs must be fully staffed and always prepared while never entirely certain of patient needs at any given moment. Despite statistics on the number of patients presenting at different times on different days in different months, no one can predict the exact number of medical staff needed to care for even one emergency patient. Clearly, staffing an ED to be fully operational is an expensive proposition given this scenario.

Clinical scope of the problem

Table 1.1 provides the ten most common reasons for patients to visit the ED, according to a 2001 survey. Patients come to the ED due to only a few general categories of problems or complaints. These may be grouped as follows, listed in decreasing frequency.

Table 1.1 Top 10 reasons for an ED visit (2001, National Hospital Ambulatory Medical Care Survey – CDC-P)

1. abdominal pain (6,789,000)
2. chest pain (5,798,000)
3. fever (4,383,000)
4. headache (2,962,000)
5. shortness of breath (2,701,000)
6. back symptoms (2,595,000)
7. cough (2,592,000)
8. pain (2,335,000)
9. laceration (2,322,000)
10. throat symptoms (2,043,000)

CDC-P: Centers for Disease Control and Prevention.

Pain

Pain is the most likely reason for patients to seek medical care at an ED. It can be traumatic or atraumatic in nature. Chest, abdominal, head, extremity, low back, ear, throat, and eye pain are only a few examples.

Difficulty with ...

This can be difficulty with breathing, vision, urination, swallowing, concentration, thinking, balance, coordination, ambulation, or sensation. Difficulty controlling seizure activity would also fall into this broad category.

Fever

Fever is common in children, and of great concern to parents. It can be a presenting complaint in adults as well. Conditions causing fever include viral or bacterial infections, such as upper respiratory infection (URI), gastroenteritis, otitis media, urinary tract infection (UTI), cellulitis, pneumonia, and bronchitis. Surgical conditions (such as appendicitis, cholecystitis, atelectasis, and postoperative wound infections), obstetric-gynecologic problems (such as pelvic or cervical infections, mastitis, postpartum infections), deep venous thrombosis (DVT), drugs and drug interactions, cancer, tick-borne infections, malaria or other parasitic infections, vasculitis, and arthritis are other conditions causing fever.

Bleeding

Bleeding may be painful or painless, and may or may not have other associated symptoms. Examples include lacerations, vaginal bleeding (with or without pregnancy), gastrointestinal (GI) bleeding, epistaxis, and hematologic illnesses such as anemia, von Willebrand's disease, or hemophilia (often resulting in spontaneous bleeding).

Social concerns

Social issues for which patients come to the ED include an inability to care for oneself, a change in behavior (either organic or functional), drug and/or alcohol-related problems, homelessness, hunger, or concerns of family members that something might be wrong.

In EM, it is essential that care is *coordinative*, meaning that EPs should seek assistance with patient care, relying on more than just the patient to assess the situation. Family members often provide additional information about illness progression that patients fail to recognize or neglect to share. Prehospital care providers often have useful information about the patient's living situation and how appropriate it is. Psychosocial aspects of each patient must be considered when interpreting presenting complaints and determining patient dispositions, including the appropriate use of consultation. Involving a consultant who focuses solely on his or her area of expertise may result in a less optimal outcome, as he or she may overlook a combination of etiologies causing the problem. When the care of a particular patient is beyond the scope of EM practice, the EP must make certain that the "proper" consultants and the appropriate teams are involved. EPs must know how and where to access information, and to whom to turn in order to ensure patient beneficence. EPs often coordinate patient care behind the scenes, without always receiving the recognition they deserve.

Anatomic essentials

Anatomic essentials for the patient presenting to the ED are covered in detail throughout the text. Airway, Breathing, Circulation, Disability, and Exposure are crucial to the initial evaluation and management of emergency patients with emergent or urgent conditions. This may be true for conditions that do not seem emergent at the time, such as the *airway* of a talking patient recently exposed to intense heat (fire, smoke, or steam). The airway is essential not only for gas exchange, but for protection against aspiration. It may be used for the administration of certain medications. With conditions causing increased intracranial pressure (ICP), airway management with modest hyperventilation results in cerebral vasoconstriction, one aspect of therapy. *Breathing* is not only dependent on the lungs, but on the thoracic cavity, respiratory musculature, and central nervous system (CNS). *Circulation* may be compromised as a result of hemorrhage, dehydration, vascular catastrophe, cardiovascular collapse, or vasoconstriction or vasodilatation in response to shock. Evaluating *disability* includes a careful yet focused neurological exam, including an assessment of the level of consciousness, mini-mental status, and evaluation of motor, sensory, reflexes, cranial nerves, and cerebellar function as appropriate. A thorough understanding of neurovascular supply to extremities, especially following traumatic lacerations or injuries, helps identify limb threats or potential morbidity. Knowledge of dermatomes is also helpful when assessing

neurologic symptoms. The Alertness, Verbal response, Pain response, Unresponsive (AVPU) scale and the Glasgow Coma Scale (GCS) are two simple evaluation tools that can be recorded to describe general neurologic status of a patient, as well as follow neurologic change over time. *Exposure* is essential so injuries are not missed, as well as to consider possible environmental elements that may contribute to the presentation (e.g., heat, cold, water, toxins).

History

The patient's history has always been considered one of the most important elements in determining a final diagnosis. It is accepted that the history (and physical examination) can determine the diagnosis in up to 85% of patients. A patient's history should focus on the current problem(s), allowing room to identify additional information and determine its relevance. When patients present in extremis, the traditional approach to obtaining the patient's history must be abandoned. In this situation, history and physical examination information must be obtained concurrently. EPs are often forced to rely on clinical assessment and impression, and utilize many important diagnostic studies during their decision-making. Some studies that assist in establishing a final diagnosis, such as an electrocardiogram (ECG), glucose, urine dipstick, and other bedside tests can be obtained while gathering historical data. However, establishing a final diagnosis is not always possible during the course of the patient's evaluation in the ED. Fortunately, having a final diagnosis is not always necessary, as an appropriate disposition with follow-up evaluation and tests during hospitalization or as an outpatient may be of far greater importance.

When approaching any emergency patient, a brief introduction using the appropriate prefix (doctor or medical student) is preferred by patients. It is reasonable to include with this introduction relevant background information, such as your current level and specialty of training. A gentle yet professional touch, such as a handshake or touch of the wrist is a kind gesture. This gesture of reaching out to a patient is favorably received in general. Before questioning a patient about his or her present illness or medical history, sit down at the patient's bedside if the situation allows. This not only eliminates towering over a patient, but demonstrates that you are interested in what he or she has to say, and plan to be present and listen for a while (even if this time is short). Patients recall that the amount of time their physician spent with them was greater if their physician sat down during the interaction. After sitting down, *listen* to what the patient has to say. Physicians interrupt their patients early and often, and EPs are some of the biggest offenders. *Look* patients in the eye so they know you are present, listening, and care about their concerns. If you will be taking notes during the interview, do so following a short period of good eye contact. Demonstrate respect for a patient's well-being and privacy by offering a pillow, blanket, adjusting their bed, assisting with covering their person, or providing water (if appropriate). This can be done in a few seconds at the start of each patient interaction.

When possible, use open-ended questions to elicit historical information about a patient's condition. This allows patients to describe their concerns using their own terms. Certainly, some questions require yes or no answers ("Do you have diabetes?"). There will be times when directed questions are required, such as to a patient in extremis, or when a patient does not answer questions promptly or concisely. However, most patients will get to the point in a relatively short time.

The P-Q-R-S-T mnemonic assists with gathering important historical elements of a presenting complaint from a patient. Using the example of "pain," questions relating to the history of a painful condition include (Table 1.2):

Table 1.2 P-Q-R-S-T mnemonic for history

P	is for *provocative/palliative*, as in "What makes this pain worse or better?"
Q	is for the *quality* of pain, as in "Describe your pain?" or, "Is your pain sharp or dull?"
R	is for *region/radiation*, as in "What region of body does this pain occur?" and "Does it radiate, or move, to any other location(s)?"
S	is for *severity*, which may be communicated using a numeric scale from 0–10 or a happy-sad faces scale.
T	is for *timing/temporal* relationships associated with the pain. Questions might include "When did the pain start?", "How long did the pain last?", and "What were you doing when the pain started (eating, exertion, watching television, going to bed)?"

Additional historical information to learn may be obtained using the mnemonic A-M-P-L-T-O-E (Table 1.3).

Table 1.3 A-M-P-L-T-O-E mnemonic for additional history

A	is a reminder to discuss *allergies* to medications, latex, seasonal allergens, or other things.
M	is for *medications*, including prescription and non-prescription. Surprisingly, many patients do not consider acetaminophen, ibuprofen, oral contraceptives, insulin, or vitamins (including herbal remedies) to be medications, and do not offer this information.
P	is for *previous or past medical history*, which may provide a clue to the present condition. If this patient has had a similar illness before, he or she may have it again, or is at greater risk for it to recur.
L	is for *last meal*, perhaps the least helpful of these questions. Last meal does, however, relate to airway protection in the event of procedural sedation or a surgical procedure.
T	is for *tetanus* status, which should be updated every 5–10 years, depending on the type of wound and its likelihood for being tetanus-prone.
O	is for *other associated symptoms/operations*. Associated symptoms may assist in reaching a diagnosis, and may afford the opportunity to relieve discomfort. Some patients do not include previous surgeries in their medical history.
E	is for *events/EMS/environment*, which include the events leading up to the illness, the role of the emergency medical system (EMS) during transport (interventions, complications), if applicable, and any environmental influences on the presentation (heat, cold, rave or other party).

Information regarding a patient's family and social history should also be reviewed. Family members with similar illnesses or conditions who present similarly to this patient are important to identify. Examples include a strong family history of cardiac or thromboembolic disease, appendicitis, gallbladder disease, or cancer. Social history includes the patient's living situation, marital status, use or abuse of tobacco, alcohol, and/or drugs, occupation, and handedness (in the setting of neurologic disease or extremity trauma).

Several key questions might therefore include:

- How did the pain begin (sudden vs. gradual onset)?
- What were you doing when the pain began?
- What does the pain feel like?
- On a scale of 0–10, how severe is the pain?
- Where is your pain?
- Has it always been there?
- Does the pain radiate anywhere else?
- Does anything make the pain better or worse?
- Have you had this pain before?

- Have any family members had pain similar to this?
- What do you think is the cause of your pain?

Associated symptoms are important, as many diseases have a specific collection of symptoms associated with them. The concept of *parsimony* is an important one, in which a diagnosis has a higher likelihood of being correct if one disease can be used to explain the entire constellation of associated symptoms. This provides a more likely explanation than the coincidence of more than one disease being responsible. Additional caution should occur with patients at the extremes of age (newborn and elderly), as the likelihood of serious infections, decreased physiologic reserve, and comorbid or coexisting conditions increases in these patients. Some key associated symptoms are listed in Table 1.4. Warning signs in the history are provided in Table 1.5:

Table 1.4 Key associated symptoms

Cardiopulmonary symptoms
Cough, dyspnea, orthopnea, palpitations, dizziness, syncope, and chest pain.

Gastrointestinal symptoms
Abdominal pain, nausea, vomiting, anorexia, constipation, diarrhea, and bleeding.

Genitourinary symptoms
Dysuria, frequency, urgency, hematuria, and pneumaturia.

Obstetric/Gynecologic symptoms
Pregnancy, menses, age of menarche, contraception, fertility, sexual activity, sexually-transmitted infections, vaginal discharge or bleeding, dyspareunia, previous surgeries, recent procedures, and other pelvic infections.

Neurologic symptoms
Weakness, difficulty speaking, concentrating, swallowing, or thinking, imbalance, sensory changes, visual problems, and headache.

Physical examination

The physical examination should be complete enough to identify unexpected conditions, while focused on areas likely to be contributing to or responsible for disease. Unfortunately, many EPs are challenged for time and act quickly, performing abbreviated physical examinations while relying on laboratory and radiologic studies. In some circumstances, this may be necessary. However, it

Table 1.5 Warning signs in the history

---

1. Sudden onset of symptoms (especially first time)
2. Significant worsening of symptom(s) which had been stable
3. True loss of consciousness or alteration of consciousness
4. Cardiopulmonary symptoms (dyspnea, chest pain or pressure)
5. Extremes of age (newborn, elderly)
6. Immune compromise (HIV-positive, AIDS, cancer, diabetes, or on immunosuppressant therapy such as chemotherapy or chronic steroids)
7. Poor historian, including language barriers
8. Repeated visit(s) to a clinic or ED, especially recent
9. Incomplete immunizations
10. Patient signed over at the end of a shift

---

is best to do a detailed, problem-pertinent physical examination so that important findings are not missed. In addition, concentrating on associated organ systems that may have a role in the illness is recommended. These areas may provide clues to the etiology of the pain or illness. In fact, establishing a comprehensive differential diagnosis for that patient's complaint and examining areas of the body that may contribute to the condition allows EPs to prioritize the likelihood of other diagnoses causing the symptoms.

As this chapter describes the approach to the emergency patient, it will address only the general appearance, vital signs, and physical examination pearls in general. Other chapters provide greater detail for a particular condition or constellation of symptoms.

General appearance

This may be the most important element of the physical examination for EPs, as it assists with determining who is sick and who is not. Experienced EPs can look at patients and have a reasonably accurate idea of who needs to be hospitalized. This is one reason why EPs feel concern for patients in the waiting room, whom they have not yet visualized. General appearance is particularly important in the pediatric population, as social interaction, playfulness, physical activity (including strength of cry) and hydration status (amount of tears, for example) are significant findings that can be identified within moments. The younger the patient is, the more difficult it is for EPs to determine wellness based on general appearance alone. The fact that a patient's general appearance is less helpful to EPs at the extremes of age makes caring for these patients more challenging.

Vital signs

Vital signs are important for all emergency patients. A complete set of vital signs should be obtained and repeated during the emergency visit. Often, the vital signs are obtained in triage and not repeated until many hours later when patients are placed in examination rooms. Many EDs have policies that vital signs must be repeated for patients in the waiting room. This is a wise strategy, even though abnormal vital signs may not require action. EPs should at the very least review one complete set of appropriate vital signs on every patient, and address each abnormal vital sign (or consider why it is abnormal). At times, rechecking the vital signs is extremely important, such as the heart rate in a patient with ACS or acute myocardial infarction (AMI), the respiratory and heart rates in patients with breathing difficulty, or the temperature of a child who experienced a febrile seizure. It is of far greater importance to recheck the temperature of a previously afebrile patient with a possible surgical condition or serious bacterial infection than a febrile child's temperature following acetaminophen or ibuprofen if they are now well-appearing, playful, and at low risk for a febrile seizure. Orthostatic vital signs (heart rate and blood pressure in supine, sitting, and standing positions) are inherently time-consuming, unreliable, and nonspecific. However, if the situation suggests that these measurements would be in the patient's best interest, they may provide useful information (Table 1.6). It is good practice to recheck a patient's vital signs prior to discharge.

Table 1.6 12 Vital signs to consider

1. General appearance (perhaps the most important and underutilized vital sign)
2. Temperature (rectal temperature should be considered in newborns or infants, and the elderly who are hypothermic, tachypneic and mouth-breathing, or in patients with alterations of consciousness)
3. Heart rate (including strength, quality, and regularity)
4. Respiratory rate (often miscalculated due to multiplication error)
5. BP (consider orthostatic BP, although may be falsely negative; also consider BP measurements in each arm or upper and lower extremities in certain conditions)
6. Oxygen saturation (pulse oximetry)
7. Blood sugar (bedside glucose), which provides an immediate value for situations including an altered LOC, a diabetic with the likelihood of abnormally high or low glucose, or when glucose is the only blood test necessary
8. Pain score (from 0–10, or happy–sad faces scale), repeated frequently and after interventions as indicated
9. GCS (best eye opening, verbal, and motor responses) or other methods which measure LOC or mental status, such as AVPU or mini-mental status examination
10. Visual acuity (for patients with visual or neurologic complaints)
11. ETCO$_2$ for intubated patients
12. Fetal heart tones (for pregnant patients)

AVPU: alertness, verbal response, pain response, unresponsive.
BP: blood pressure.
ETCO$_2$: end-tidal carbon dioxide.
GCS: Glasgow Coma Scale.
LOC: level of consciousness.

Pearls specific to the physical

Be professional

A professional greeting and introduction should evoke warmth and kindness. Patients want to know that the EP they "have" (they did not "choose") is considerate, sensitive, thoughtful, competent, and listens well; in other words, a true professional. Most patients aren't interested in a joke or a discussion of current events when they are in the ED, at least not immediately. EPs should wear clean and appropriate clothing, be polite, well-mannered, well-groomed, and appear well-rested. A current hospital ID badge with name and photograph should be prominently displayed. A health care provider should never bring food or beverages into the examination room.

Go slowly

Try not to rush patients, or to seem rushed, despite how busy you may be. Speak slowly and clearly, with increased volume for elderly patients should they need it. Warm and clean hands are essential for patient comfort. If you are using gloves, tell patients that this is your practice for all patients. A well-lighted, warm room (if possible) is also preferred. Having a chaperone of the same gender as the patient present is always a good idea, especially during examination of private (genitals, breasts, pelvic and rectal) areas. Again, let patients know that this is your standard practice and you are doing it for their benefit (even if you are protecting yourself as well). Having translators or family members present (when appropriate) also makes patients more comfortable.

Be gentle

Do not proceed immediately to the area of pain, and do not palpate a tender area using more pressure than is absolutely necessary. If possible, try to distract patients while you examine a painful area. This is especially true for pediatric patients. Always examine the joints above and below an injured area, as other injuries may coexist due to transmitted forces. Remove all constricting jewelry and clothing distal to an injured area, as swelling due to dependent edema is likely to occur. Patients may not appreciate this gesture at the time, but it will be valuable in terms of patient safety and preventing damage to an item that may require removal later.

Be sensitive

Make patients aware that you are focused on them during your examination, not on other patients or problems. Furthermore, let patients briefly know what you find immediately following each phase of the examination. There is no reason to do your entire examination and then tell the patient that it was normal. Share with patients that their heart or lungs sound fine right after auscultation. If patients have abnormal findings, they may have been aware of these from a previous physician's examination. Ask if they had been aware of this finding, without accusing the physician of missing something if they had not been told. When appropriate, let them know immediately that it is not dangerous or worrisome if this is the case. There is no reason to increase their anxiety by telling them they have a heart murmur if it is inconsequential. Offering findings in this manner increases patients' confidence in your abilities, because you were able to identify a heart murmur (for example) that they already knew existed.

Be thorough

This is important so that critical findings or other clues to the patient's final diagnosis are not missed. For example, lacerations, contusions, rashes, or bruises might imply spouse abuse. If it may be relevant to the presenting complaint, expose the patient's skin during the examination of the body region. Rashes may be present which identify life-threatening infectious diseases or may eliminate the need for further diagnostic studies (e.g., meningococcemia or herpes zoster).

Be thoughtful

Use language that patients and family members understand. It does not impress patients when physicians use technical jargon to look smart. If patients are not familiar with abbreviations or terms that you have used, they may not be comfortable asking for their meaning. For example, despite the common use of the abbreviation "MI" for myocardial infarction, many people do not know what it means. You may tell a patient that he had an MI, only to be asked later if he suffered a heart attack. In children, consider efforts to involve parents with the examination, such as looking in a parent's throat or ear first. Other skills to use when examining children include letting the child touch your stethoscope or otoscope before using it. Involve older children in the examination by asking which ear they would prefer be examined first. Recognize that hospital gowns are not flattering; it is a kind gesture to assist a patient by offering to tie his or her gown, especially if they are going to leave their ED gurney.

Be efficient

An entire physical examination does not need to be done on every patient. For example, a funduscopic examination does not need to be performed on a patient presenting with an ankle injury. Furthermore, examine patients starting with the position they are in, rather than from head-to-toe, which can save time. For example, if the patient is supine in the gurney, consider examining their abdomen before their lungs.

Differential diagnosis

Following the history and physical examination, with careful review of the vital signs, a differential diagnosis should be established. This differential diagnosis should be as comprehensive as possible, as it suggests which diagnostic tests should be obtained, and in which order. This differential diagnosis also establishes which therapeutic approaches should be initiated, if they have not already begun.

Diagnostic testing

Diagnostic testing in the ED is performed to include ("rule in") or exclude ("rule out") conditions responsible for the patient's symptoms. As such, it is imperative that EPs have a sense of pretest probability, which includes disease prevalence, and the sensitivity, specificity, positive and negative predictive values, and accuracy of the tests they are ordering. It is important to be familiar with likelihood and odds ratios as well.

Laboratory studies

Because of the time pressures for patient dispositions, many tests have been or are being developed which can be done at the bedside, to decrease the turnaround time for results. Known as "point-of-care" testing, one classic example is the bedside glucose test. Numerous implications of this rising technology's role in EM have been studied. Current research using new bedside tests of cardiac markers and other tests of cardiac function is ongoing. Treadmill tests on low-risk cardiac patients have been performed from (or in) the ED to risk-stratify patients regarding their need for hospitalization. Bedside ultrasonography is a similar test being utilized by EPs with increased frequency to assist with patient diagnosis, treatment, and disposition. As more hospitals and EDs subscribe to these concepts, and more physicians gain skills in these areas, these tests will assume an even greater role in the evaluation and treatment of emergency patients. Unfortunately, regulations have removed many tests from the ED that were previously performed there, such as pregnancy tests and microscopic evaluation of vaginal flora. Having these tests done in a laboratory increases the time to receive results, if for no other reason than sample transport time. The implications of increased laboratory turnaround time are enormous given ED closures, lack of ED and hospital bed availability, and increased patient volumes in EDs across the US.

Some tests are being ordered or performed by certified nurses during the triage process, as patients register for evaluation by EPs. These tests include urine collection to screen for pregnancy, blood, or infection, ECGs to evaluate cardiac function, and radiographs. There has been extensive research to develop rules to assist health professionals with determining a patient's need for an X-ray. If these clinical criteria are met, trained nurses in many institutions may order X-rays from the triage area in an effort to streamline care and reduce overall patient time in the ED. Examples of some rules found in the literature include the Ottawa ankle, knee, and foot rules, the Pittsburgh knee rule, the Nexus rule for cervical spine radiographs, and several head computed tomography (CT) rules. Depending on

the situation, nurses generally use the extremity rules in their practice, while physicians apply the C-spine and head CT rules. Some EDs have a physician or nurse order necessary blood tests and send them to the lab from the triage area, in an effort to improve patient throughput.

Electrocardiography

With ECGs, it is a good idea to obtain old ECGs whenever possible to allow comparison with the new (current) ECG. This is of particular importance in patients with abnormal conduction, abnormal intervals, or abnormal ST and T wave segments. ECGs should be repeated in the ED if patients develop chest pain or if their chest pain resolves, whether spontaneously or following intervention. The importance of serial ECGs cannot be overemphasized in the setting of ACS, or if the possibility of a cardiac etiology for chest pain is entertained. ECGs are invaluable in patients with acute ST-segment elevation MI (STEMI), as the determination for thrombolysis or percutaneous coronary intervention (PCI) is time-sensitive from the time of the first diagnostic ECG. They also serve as useful adjuncts in the evaluation of several toxic ingestions or presenting symptoms such as weakness, dizziness, abdominal pain, back pain, confusion, or alterations of mental status.

Radiologic studies

Regarding the use of radiology in diagnostic testing, physicians seem to rely on imaging to a greater extent than they did years ago. This is due in part to the greater role imaging plays in patient care, the increased availability of CT scanners, the manner in which physicians are currently trained, and the increased concern over litigation. Nevertheless, obtaining radiologic imaging (especially CT) has become a standard that physicians must recognize, and that patients often demand. Not ordering radiologic studies to identify certain conditions may be indefensible, as these tests are sensitive, specific, and readily available 24 hours a day in nearly all EDs. The development of guidelines to help determine which patients require X-rays has provided physicians the ability to safely reduce the number of radiographs ordered. EPs use bedside ultrasonography as part of their physical examination skill set in many hospitals, often with the support of radiology. This situation arose out of the need for EPs to have ultrasound available to their patients on a 24-hour basis, to identify hemoperitoneum following abdominal trauma, gallbladder disease, cardiac tamponade, ectopic pregnancy, or other illnesses. EPs first used bedside ultrasonography for the focused assessment with sonography for trauma (FAST) exam. Tremendous success with this limited use encouraged EPs to incorporate ultrasound technology into other necessary areas of their clinical practice. It is important for both EPs and radiologists to work collaboratively in this area, keeping patient advocacy and safety the first priority at all times.

General treatment principles

When evaluating and treating patients presenting to the ED, it is imperative to address life-threats first. A tremendous amount of information can be obtained from the patient's general appearance, vital signs, and history of presenting illness (HPI). This is essentially a less than one minute assessment. Risk stratification into "sick" or "not sick," or "stable" or "unstable" is part of this process. Attention to the airway, breathing, and circulation (ABCs) is critical, as is having the correct personnel, equipment, and monitors available. Much of this process occurs simultaneously, often automatically, with more than one health care provider involved in a patient's care. While nurses are measuring vital signs, connecting patients to monitors, and starting peripheral intravenous (IV) catheters for blood draw and circulation access, physicians can be intervening with airway management and assessing breathing and circulation. In trauma patients, the mnemonic A-B-C-D-E-F-G is addressed in the primary and secondary surveys (Table 1.7).

Table 1.7 A-B-C-D-E-F-G mnemonic for trauma patients

A	Airway
B	Breathing
C	Circulation
D	Disability (neurologic)
E	Exposure
F	Foley (following inspection of the involved areas and rectal examination)
G	Gastric decompression (provided no contraindications exist)

Cervical spine immobilization and protection is part of this process. "F" also reminds us of the importance of family and friends. They may provide information about the circumstances leading up to the present condition, and should be kept updated as much as possible. When caring for pediatric patients, current literature demonstrates that family members' presence during resuscitation efforts or invasive procedures is extremely important to them, provided their presence does not interfere with medical care delivery.

At times, histories and physical examinations must be abbreviated and more focused than one might prefer. This is often a necessary part of EM practice. Treatment may need to be initiated based on limited information, previous episodes, physician experience, or physician speculation. In true emergencies, assessment and treatment occur simultaneously. It may be necessary to determine a patient's resuscitation status in an instant, which is extremely difficult for EPs. As quickly as possible, attempts should be made to learn this information from the patient, prehospital care providers, family members, nursing home or skilled facilities. Having a system in place with electronic medical records or a designated individual (social services, ED tech, or nurse) available to make calls may save precious minutes. When in doubt, always do what is medically indicated for the patient, rather than making assumptions that may be incorrect. Remember to do no harm, and always relieve pain, suffering, and anxiety.

Adequate pain control is an important element of EM practice. If a patient has a painful condition, it is good practice to address issues of pain control as early as possible. This is true not only for patients presenting with abdominal pain, but in patients with traumatic injuries who would benefit from adequate analgesia. Waiting to administer pain medication to a patient with a clinical fracture until after the X-ray is reviewed is inappropriate. As previously mentioned, reassess patients after each intervention, whether following intubation for airway control or the administration of analgesia. Continued reassessment of all patients, particularly the sickest or those at greatest risk for decompensation, is critical.

All patients should be treated sensitively, with attention paid to their fears and anxieties. Patients don't wish to be in the ED, where privacy concerns, noises, and discomfort predominate. They would much rather be at home, without pain, or in a familiar physician's office. In this sense, EPs and EDs start out with strikes against them. Add to this the long wait, the uncertainty, and the likelihood that someone will be less than pleasant results in an emergency experience rarely seen favorably by patients. Respectful treatment, without discrimination or condescension, should be integral to our approach towards all patients.

ACEP and other organizations have developed a number of clinical policies by consensus in an attempt to improve patient care and reduce medical error. Although many EPs feel that these policies might be used against them in litigation, or are an attempt to standardize patient care, these policies are established using research and opinion and are an excellent resource. This is especially true for challenging conditions or those with unclear or rapidly changing diagnostic and treatment approaches. These policies are generally available from these organizations at no charge. Many similar treatment guidelines may be found on-line to assist providers with an evidence-based medicine (EBM) approach to patient care.

Special patients

Elderly

Individuals over 85 years of age are the fastest growing segment of the population. With advances in medical care, and the increasing importance placed on disease prevention, diet and exercise, this portion of the population will continue to grow at a tremendous rate. The special needs of this group of patients are often significant. It has been repeatedly established that the majority of medical care expenses are spent on the geriatric population during their last few years of life. Geriatric patients are at risk for falls, functional decline, changes in cognition, as well as cardiac, pulmonary, and vascular emergencies. They have reduced physiologic reserve, and often are too ill, weak, or complicated to use medical offices for even routine care. As such, many rely on EDs for their overall health care, assuming they get any care at all. When geriatric patients present to the ED, they are far more likely to be admitted to the hospital than younger patients. They are also far more likely to require social services if discharged. The best solution is to integrate social services into the care of all geriatric patients. EPs should consider why social services should *not* be asked to see an elderly patient in the ED, as they can offer home safety checks, access to meals, transportation to medical appointments, and address social isolation, depression, financial security, and common feelings of being a burden to family members. Furthermore, elder neglect or abuse is far more prevalent than reported. From a social perspective, geriatric patients prefer being referred to as "young"

rather than "old" (as in 75 years young), and prefer being referred to as "older" rather than "old."

Many medical conditions in older patients do not present as they might in a younger or healthier patient. A UTI in an elderly patient often presents with confusion, as might ACS or a pulmonary infection. Many geriatric patients are not able to mount a febrile response to sepsis or infections. In fact, geriatric patients are often hypothermic when septic. As a result, rectal temperatures should be measured in this population. Geriatric patients commonly use over-the-counter medications, increasing their risk of adverse drug reactions. On average, elderly patients take 5 prescription medications daily. Polypharmacy is a frequent concern in the geriatric population, increasing the likelihood of drug–drug interactions. Primary providers are often unaware of all medications their elderly patients take, as physician colleagues, consultants, and urgent care providers may prescribe additional medications without them knowing. Prehospital personnel should be encouraged to bring all medication bottles with patients to the ED so they can be reviewed. This may help identify possible adverse drug reactions or interactions. Many drugs interact with warfarin, commonly prescribed in the geriatric population. Special ID bracelets should be provided to and worn by elderly patients, which should include select medical conditions, addresses, contacts, medications, and allergies.

Eyesight often fails in the geriatric population, so it is important to check this and consider outpatient referrals to optometry. Difficulties with eyesight may result in the inability to read food or medication instructions, especially insulin doses. Difficulty with vision in low light makes it nearly impossible for elderly patients to reliably comment on their stools turning darker (hematochezia or melena). Driving abilities may be impaired by visual difficulties or by neck arthritis (which makes it difficult to change lanes), muscle power (required for defensive maneuvers), or fine motor control and coordination. Driving is of vital importance for independence, and is therefore a skill that many elderly do not wish to relinquish.

Falls are more common in the elderly, not only because of visual difficulties but also because of their diminished ability to avoid objects, climb stairs, or maintain balance and posture. As financial issues are of great concern, medications may not be taken regularly or may be cut in half to decrease the cost. The same goes for food – soups are inexpensive and easy to cook, although many have high sodium contents. A dietician or nutritionist can discuss healthy eating habits with elderly patients. Plans for assisted living or skilled facilities should be addressed with geriatric patients before the need is imminent, as should advance directives and powers of attorney. Even a discussion of wills and plans for death should be addressed, although this is best done at a scheduled time in the primary care provider's office. Postal carriers and apartment managers are particularly important to the safety of the elderly population who live alone, as they can check to see that the mail is being picked up daily, make sure that the individual has eaten or gotten up that morning, or provide brief social contact. These resources can be investigated by social workers.

Pediatric

Pediatric patients often make up a high percentage of patient visits to an ED, especially at night when pediatric clinics are closed. Many EDs have separate patient care and waiting room areas for pediatric patients, so they are not as frightened during their visit. Some EDs have special pediatric rooms with colors and decorations to improve these patient's experience. Coloring books, stickers, and stuffed animals may be helpful as well. It is inadvisable to have a belligerent patient sharing a room with a child (or any patient, for that matter). This may not be possible, however, given the demands for ED space during times when patient volumes are increased and pediatric patients are most likely to present. EDs should have a resuscitation area especially for children, using colors for equipment storage matching those on the Broselow resuscitation tape.

Pediatric patients are generally evaluated with parents, which may help the evaluation or make it more difficult. It is important to observe the manner in which children interact with their parents. Physical, emotional, and sexual abuse or neglect should be considered in *all* pediatric visits, especially cases of traumatic injury, genitourinary complaints, or failure to thrive. At times, therefore, it may be necessary to have a discussion with a pediatric patient without a parent present. If this situation is necessary, it is advisable to have a second health care professional, preferably of the same gender as the patient, in the room with you. Every attempt should be made to minimize a child's time away from his or her parent or guardian unless this separation is warranted. Parents are often concerned about

their child's fever, but their true concern may be meningitis or some other serious infection. With as much certainty as possible, these concerns should be addressed. Pediatric patients with ventriculoperitoneal (VP) shunts, leukemias, cancers, cardiac or lung disease, transplants, seizure disorders, or other specialized conditions are generally closely followed by their pediatricians or pediatric specialists, who should be included in or informed of care decisions. As younger pediatric patients are at risk for serious bacterial illness (SBI) and have less reserve than older children or adults, close follow-up of patients and cultures (if obtained) should be encouraged according to hospital practices, as patients in this age group can become extremely sick or dehydrated quickly.

Drug-seekers

The practice of EM has a set of unique patients who use and abuse the ED. Patients who seek drugs, whether they are drug-addicted, drug-dependent, or in constant pain are common patients seen after clinic hours or when primary physicians are unavailable. Some of these patients may simply have decreased abilities to tolerate pain. Many hospitals and EDs have policies about providing narcotic medication to drug-seeking patients, or patients who have abused the system. It is far easier for administrators to write policies for such patients than for EPs to apply them in clinical practice. Whatever the outcome, it is always the best practice to be sensitive to that patient's condition. There have been several situations in which denying narcotics to a patient demanding them resulted in injury to or even death of health care providers. Referrals to pain clinics, psychiatry, narcotics anonymous, and social services are always appropriate but rarely helpful.

Difficult patients

Patients with personality disorders, malingerers, manipulators, litigious patients, and patients with behavioral problems often use the ED for their health care, as they may not have insurance or may not be able to access clinics. These patients are particularly challenging to the staff's patience. Federal law prohibits EDs from turning away patients, without at least preforming a medical screening examination (MSE) to evaluate for any emergency medical condition (EMC). At times, security personnel or the police may need to be involved with these challenging patients. In our role as health care's safety net physicians, we must interact with these unique and challenging patients on a regular basis given the ED's open-door policy. An EP's goal is to treat these patients with respect, set strict limits, refer aggressively, and recognize other factors that may be influencing their behavior. Conditions such as reflex sympathetic dystrophy, fibromyalgia, post-herpetic neuralgia, claudication, or psychosocial conditions such as abuse may not have been considered by other physicians during past visits.

Frequent flyers

Patients labeled as "frequent flyers" may or may not have addictions to narcotics or psychiatric illnesses, although they often do. However, isolation, homelessness, boredom, mental illness, or searching for attention and care may be reasons for repeat visits. Despite overutilizing the ED, these individuals should be treated respectfully. Many medical staff fear that nice treatment will encourage repeat visits, but providing a meal or a warm place to sit for a short time may be necessary regardless of the number of visits. Abuse of the prehospital care system is even more upsetting to many emergency medical personnel, as the number of available ambulances and prehospital providers decrease during attention to these individuals. However, it is always possible that frequent flyers have or will have real illness. It may be necessary to focus evaluations and minimize testing, although studies often are performed despite the high likelihood of being negative. The use of derisive or condescending language to individuals who abuse the medical system is never acceptable. Respectfully addressing their abuse of the system and its impact on others is certainly warranted. When possible, ED or hospital administrators should be notified of these abuses using mechanisms in place.

Police custody

Sadly, patients in police custody who need medical attention for evaluation and treatment have no place to go other than the ED (occasionally, some urgent care centers have contractual agreements for this). Often, police bring patients to the ED for medical clearance. This requires an EP to attempt to determine whether or not the patient's actions can be explained by a medical (or psychiatric) condition. Patients often come to the ED in police custody with injuries following an altercation, often with a police officer or officers. This establishes a difficult context for EPs because officers may have injured certain patients in response to their aggressive behavior. If the EP feels safe, he or she should interview patients outside of police presence. It is always difficult to feel comfortable evaluating patients handcuffed to gurneys, with or without police present. However, a thorough yet cautious evaluation for injuries, including contusions, bruises, marks, scratches, abrasions, and bites must be performed and documented. Patients may be placed into police custody from the ED if they are violent, abusive, stealing supplies, or exhibiting inappropriate behavior. Police must be notified about all violent injuries, and may place patients in custody or take them from the ED to jail. Police often deliver intoxicated patients to an ED so they can sober before going to jail. Patients who are intoxicated may have additional reasons for combative behavior or altered mental status, including traumatic brain injury or other medical conditions, thus mandating a thorough evaluation. Intoxicated patients may be released to the care of the EP and medical staff if they have cooperated with the police and are not under arrest. When this occurs, careful observation until daylight hours, a meal if possible, and careful plans for disposition, follow-up, and referral should be discussed with a non-intoxicated family member or friend. Clearly, a close working relationship between fire, police, and emergency personnel is crucial to our safety and success.

Disposition
Consultation

Dealing with consultants is an art that is often difficult. Consultants respect straightforward, focused, and well-planned presentations with a direct question or goal being clearly stated. They may not appreciate being told what to do, such as "this patient needs to go to the operating room." Any ED consultation is unplanned work for a consultant. Reimbursement issues may negatively impact consultants to a far greater extent than most EPs recognize. Despite such issues, EPs must serve as their patient's advocate at all times. EPs should never do something that makes them uncomfortable, even if a consultant recommends it. This is especially true if a consultant does not formally evaluate the patient. Disagreements about the best plan of action for patients are common. These may be due to financial, time, or hospital pressures. In general, consultants do not wish to hospitalize patients who, in their opinion, do not need admission. Since EPs do not wish to send patients home who, in their opinion, should not be discharged, conflict may be inherent to this interaction. As always, keep the patient's best interests in mind. Consider alternate options such as holding patients in the ED until the next consultant comes on duty, finding a different service to admit the patient, enlisting the assistance of social services, admitting the patient to an observation unit (either in the ED or the hospital), or recognizing that it may be safe to send that particular patient home despite your initial impression. If absolutely needed, EPs can always contact the chief of service, administrator on call, or chief of staff for truly unacceptable situations. When possible, notifying a patient's primary physician or specialist with information about his or her visit, evaluation, laboratory results, and treatment plan is uniformly appreciated, and is in the patient's best interest. Not only does this serve as an opportunity for continued care, it also assists in transferring care for that patient. Follow-up notification by EPs to patient's physicians earns additional respect for our specialty, and is a fantastic way to let other physicians know that we care about their (our) patients. If interested, request follow-up from these physicians to learn about patient care outcomes.

Serial evaluation

Repeat evaluation of patients is an important aspect of emergency care, as a patient's condition may change over a period of time. Many presentations warrant repeat evaluation, including head or traumatic injuries, seizures, hypoglycemic episodes, abdominal pain, shortness of breath, and chest pain, to list a few. Time alone may allow a diagnosis to become more apparent or declare itself, or may lead to the resolution of symptoms. It is critical that patients who are impaired (drug or alcohol intoxication, altered mental status, or confused) or are restrained (chemical, physical, or both) have frequent and repeated evaluations by both physicians and nurses. Serial evaluation is necessary following interventions, such as the administration of nitroglycerin (NTG), analgesics, bronchodilators, or anxiolytics. This is important not only to determine the patient's response to that intervention, as many interventions are diagnostic as well as therapeutic, but also helps determine if an additional or different intervention is needed. Documentation of this response to therapy is important, as it records the patient's ED course. Repeat evaluations of patients after important laboratory or X-ray results become available, and/or before they are discharged is recommended, although the extent of this reevaluation differs with each clinical scenario.

Admission/discharge

The decision to admit or discharge patients from the ED is perhaps the most challenging part of EM practice. Multiple factors must be considered in this decision, including psychosocial, biological, medicolegal, and, unfortunately, financial. When possible, a patient's wishes should be included in this decision. With the advent of more aggressive outpatient strategies (low-molecular-weight heparin for DVT, longer-acting antibiotics with greater potency) and research suggesting similar outcomes in selected patients, many patients previously hospitalized are now being safely treated as outpatients with close follow-up. Many disposition differences exist between hospitals for certain conditions; it is a good idea for EPs to familiarize themselves with hospital or community practices. In smaller hospitals, EPs may be responsible for writing admission orders for patients. Although EM organizations discourage this practice, it still occurs. Admission orders written by EPs should clearly transfer care to the admitting physician upon the patient's arrival to the floor. The nurses should be instructed to notify the admitting physician upon the patient's arrival, if the patient has any special needs, or for any change in vital signs, including pain. Unstable or particularly complex patients should remain in the ED until the admitting physician has the opportunity to evaluate them. In some hospitals, EPs on duty are responsible to respond to in-hospital medical emergencies. Hospital or ED policies should set guidelines to define the circumstances under which the EP can (and cannot) respond to acute medical care situations within the hospital. Similarly, hospital policies should address acceptable time standards for admitting physicians to evaluate their patients so they are not held in the ED for extended periods.

For patients being discharged, clear and legible discharge instructions should encourage patients to return if their symptoms get worse, change, or don't improve. All discharge instructions should include 4 categories of instructions: (1) what to do, (2) what not to do, (3) when (and where) to follow-up, and (4) reasons to return to the ED. *What to do* includes instructions such as rest, ice, compression, and elevation for an ankle injury. *What not to do* instructions might include don't smoke, don't drive, don't stop your antibiotics until completed or instructed by your physician. *When (and where) to follow-up* for re-evaluation, and with whom, is beneficial information for discharged patients. The time frame for follow-up should directly relate to the certainty of the diagnosis and the likelihood of the illness or injury degenerating to a critical condition. Close follow-up is important for all patients with high-risk medical conditions. The ideal situation is to schedule a follow-up appointment for the patient at the time of his or her discharge. Give the patient this follow-up physician's name, the date and time of the appointment, and the address with directions to the clinic. Perhaps the most important discharge instruction is the list of *reasons to return to the ED.* These might include but are not limited to any increase in pain, new or different pain, worsening of symptoms, inability to take medications or fluids, allergic reactions to any medications, fever, vomiting, bleeding, or any other concerns or fears. Pre-printed discharge instruction sheets are helpful if they are written in a language that the patient can understand. These may allow EPs to be more efficient. However, patients deserve personalized instructions as well, as each patient is an individual, not a disease or set of symptoms.

Assisting patients with filling their prescriptions at discharge is important, although this does not ensure compliance. If this is not possible, discharging patients with one day's supply of medication is a reasonable gesture. Testing a patient's gait prior to discharge helps determine their balance, coordination, and likelihood of success at home. If a patient walked in to the ED, or "should be able to walk," then this patient should be able to walk at discharge. Patients should be discharged to a safe environment, preferably in the company of a responsible adult who also understands the discharge instructions. If they have been in the ED for an extended period, providing a meal is appropriate, as they may be too ill or tired to prepare one for themselves upon returning home. Wheelchairs may be used to assist patients to their cars. Patients should not drive if they might be distracted, were given medication that may interfere with driving, or presented with a lapse of consciousness that may recur without warning. In this last situation, a report must be filed with the appropriate

authorities, and the patient needs to be informed that this has occurred. They should not drive until an appropriate physician and the proper authorities approve this at a follow-up appointment. Rides home, often paid for by the ED or hospital, may be necessary, as might a clean or warm set of clothes. Clothing donated by the medical staff or other sources for patients to use is one option if the hospital budget does not allow for this.

Pearls, pitfalls, and myths

Always address life-threats first, including patient and staff safety.

An exact diagnosis is not always possible in EM, and not always necessary. Often, an appropriate disposition, such as admission to a monitored bed, intensive care unit (ICU), operating room, skilled nursing facility, or discharge home with close follow-up is the best that can be expected.

Always attempt to get the appropriate service or consultant involved. Make every effort to inform a patient's primary care provider about the circumstances leading up to the patient's ED visit, the care provided while there, laboratory and X-ray results, and a suggested follow-up plan.

Not all is what is seems; expect the unexpected, or you won't find it. Consider alternative diagnoses and the possibility of lab error or false negative (or positive) test results if things don't seem as expected. Repeat tests if the original test result doesn't "fit" with what you expected. Be wary about the wrong test results being placed on the wrong patient's chart, or a laboratory specimen or radiograph being mislabeled, improperly marked, or incorrectly collected.

People with psychiatric illness may have medical illnesses too. Consider ingestions, or cardiac, metabolic, infectious, and CNS derangements as well.

Many elderly patients have uncommon presentations for common conditions, such as ACS or sepsis. Furthermore, polypharmacy and drug–drug interactions should be considered, along with elder abuse, neglect, and depression (including suicidal gesture or attempt). Consider the safety of an elderly patient being discharged, and always remain his or her advocate.

Never rush a patient out of the ED with a condition that may recur, such as asthma, seizures, chest pain, breathing difficulty, or alteration of consciousness (following head trauma or intoxicants).

Be sensitive, sit with patients, make good eye contact, and listen well for apparent as well as hidden issues. Hidden issues may not be the ones initially offered by patients, as they may wait to gain your trust before sharing.

Review nursing and EMS notes on all patients. Look for hidden clues that the patient may not offer or tell you. Enlist the assistance of others to help you with patient care, including nursing, family, EMS, social services, consultants, or a patient's primary care physician. Poison centers and on-line resources may be extremely valuable as well.

Use caution in patients with language or cultural barriers. Translators and family members may not provide complete or accurate information, details which you might have been able to elicit if these barriers did not exist. This is especially true for patients who are deaf or have speech impediments.

Think about abuse or neglect in *every* case. If you aren't thinking about it, you will not uncover it.

Document clear and appropriate findings in the medical record, including repeat examinations, laboratory results and radiograph interpretations, discussions with consultants or primary providers, and discharge instructions. Documenting the time and consultant's name with whom you spoke is always helpful.

Consider dangerous outcomes or the worst-case scenario in every patient. Minimize the likelihood of these outcomes with appropriately focused histories, physical examinations, laboratory and radiograph ordering and interpretation, and disposition. Never do something you are not comfortable with, despite a consultant's recommendation.

Enjoy the privilege of providing emergency care to all patients.

References

1. American Hospital Association. Hospital Statistics. 2002 edition. Chicago, IL: Health Forum, LLC;2002.

2. Dailey RH. Approach to the patient in the Emergency Department. Emergency Medicine: Concepts and Clinical Practice, 4th ed., Rosen P (ed), St. Louis: Mosby, 1998, pp. 137–150.

3. Finkel MA, Adams JG. Professionalism in emergency medicine. *Emerg Clinics NA.* 1999;17:443–450.

4. Fontanarosa PB. An evidence based approach to diagnostic testing in emergency medicine. *Emerg Clinics NA.* 1999;17:1–8.

5. Hamilton GC, Sanders AB, Strange GR, Trott AT: Emergency Medicine: An Approach to Clinical Problem-Solving, 2nd ed., WB Saunders. 2003.

6. Hockberger RS, La Duca A, Orr NA, Reinhart MA, Sklar DP. Creating the model of a clinical practice: The case of emergency medicine. *Acad Emerg Med.* 2003;10:161–168.

7. Holliman CJ. The art of dealing with consultants. *J Emerg Med.* 1993;11:633–640.

8. http://www.acep.org/1,381,0.html (ACEP website link). *Accessed 1/30/05.*

9. Lambe S, Washington DL, Fink A, et al. Trends in the use and capacity of California's emergency departments, 1990–1999. *Ann Emerg Med.* 2002;39:389–396.

10. Oslin DW: Prescription and Over-the-Counter Drug Misuse Among the Elderly. *Geriatric Times*, vol. 1; May/June 2000.

11. Schenkel S. Promoting patient safety and preventing medical error in emergency departments. *Acad Emerg Med.* 2000;7: 1204–1222.

12. Schneider SM, Hamilton GC, Moyer P, Stapczynski JS: Definition of Emergency Medicine. *Acad Emerg Med.* 1998;5:348–351.

2 Airway management

S.V. Mahadevan, MD and Shannon Sovndal, MD

Scope of the problem

Airway management is arguably the single most important skill taught to and possessed by emergency physicians. It represents the "A" of the mnemonic ABC (Airway, Breathing, Circulation), which forms the foundation for the resuscitation of critically ill and injured patients. Airway management encompasses the assessment, establishment and protection of the airway in combination with effective oxygenation and ventilation. Timely effective airway management can mean the difference between life and death, and takes precedence over all other clinical considerations with the sole exception of immediate defibrillation of the patient in cardiac arrest due to ventricular fibrillation.

This chapter reviews airway anatomy and assessment, approaches for noninvasive airway management, and indications and techniques for definitive airway management. The approach to the challenging patient with a difficult or failed airway will also be explored, as well as specialized devices, techniques and medications employed in these challenging clinical situations.

Anatomic essentials

A clear understanding of airway anatomy is requisite for advanced airway management. Internally, the airway is made up of many structures and well-defined spaces. It originates at the nasal and oral cavities (Figure 2.1). The *nasal cavity* extends from the nostrils to the posterior nares or choana. The *nasopharynx* extends from the end of the nasal cavity to the level of the soft palate. The *oral cavity* is bounded by the teeth anteriorly, hard and soft palate superiorly and the tongue inferiorly. The *oropharynx*, which communicates with the oral cavity and nasopharynx, extends from the soft palate to the tip of the epiglottis. The oropharynx continues as the *laryngopharynx (hypopharynx)*, which extends from the

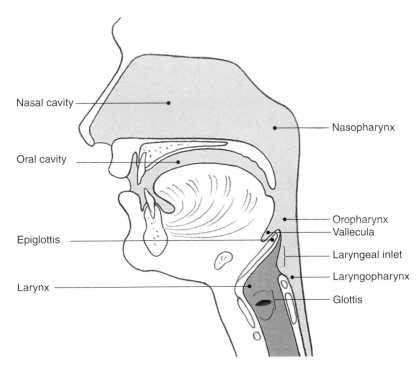

Figure 2.1
Lateral view of airway anatomy.

Nasal cavity

Oral cavity

Epiglottis

Larynx

Nasopharynx

Oropharynx
Vallecula

Laryngeal inlet

Laryngopharynx

Glottis

epiglottis to the upper border of the cricoid cartilage (level of the C6 vertebral body). The *larynx* lies between the laryngopharynx and trachea.

The flexible *epiglottis*, which originates from the hyoid bone and the base of the tongue, covers the glottis during swallowing and protects the airway from aspiration. During laryngoscopy, the epiglottis serves as an important landmark for airway identification and laryngoscope positioning (Figure 2.2). The *vallecula* is the space at the base of the tongue formed posteriorly by the epiglottis and anteriorly by the anterior pharyngeal

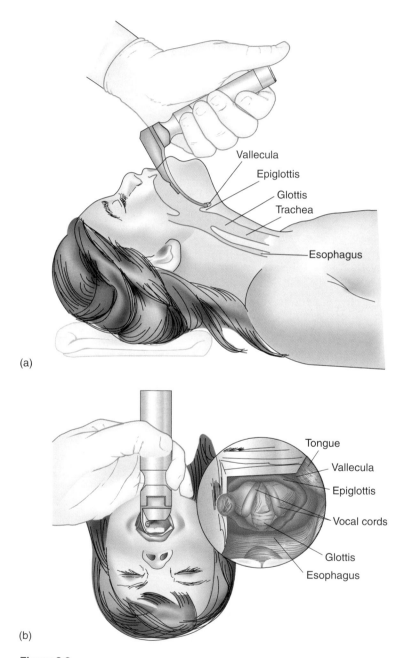

(a)

(b)

Figure 2.2
(a) Position of laryngoscope blade when using a curved blade (b) Operator's view of anatomy. Reproduced with permission, PALS Provider Manual, © 2002, Copyright American Heart Association.

wall. The *laryngeal inlet* is the opening to the larynx bounded by the epiglottis, aryepiglottic folds and arytenoid cartilages. The *glottis* is the vocal apparatus, including the true and false vocal cords and the glottic opening. The *glottic opening* is the opening into the trachea (as seen from above) through the vocal cords, and lies inferior and posterior to the epiglottis.

Externally, specific identifiable landmarks are important to airway assessment and management (Figure 2.3). The *mentum* is the anterior aspect of the mandible and represents the tip of the chin. The *hyoid bone* forms the base of the floor of the mouth. The *thyroid cartilage* forms the laryngeal prominence ("Adam's apple") and thyroid notch. The *cricoid cartilage*, lying inferior to the thyroid cartilage, forms a complete ring that provides structural support to the lower airway. The *cricothyroid membrane* lies between the thyroid and cricoid cartilage, and serves as an important site for surgical airway management.

Initial airway assessment

The initial assessment of airway patency and respiratory function focuses on determining:

1. whether the airway is open and protected;
2. if breathing is present and adequate.

This is carefully achieved through inspection, auscultation and palpation.

The patient should be observed for objective signs of airway compromise. Agitation may represent hypoxia, obtundation suggests hypercarbia, and cyanosis indicates hypoxemia.

The patient's respiratory rate and pattern are important. Bradypnea or tachypnea may be signs of impending respiratory compromise. Respiratory muscle fatigue may result in the recruitment of accessory muscles of respiration, clinically manifested as suprasternal, supraclavicular or intercostal retractions. Look for a symmetrical rise and fall of the chest. A significant traumatic injury to the chest may result in paradoxical or discordant chest wall movement.

The presence or absence and quality of speech may be used to identify airway abnormalities. A normal voice suggests that the airway is adequate for the moment. *Stridor*, a high-pitched inspiratory sound, may be associated with partial airway obstruction at the level of the larynx (inspiratory stridor) or the trachea (expiratory stridor). Snoring usually indicates partial airway obstruction at the pharyngeal level, while hoarseness suggests a laryngeal process. *Aphonia* in the conscious patient is an extremely worrisome sign; a patient who is too short of breath to speak is in grave danger of impending respiratory collapse.

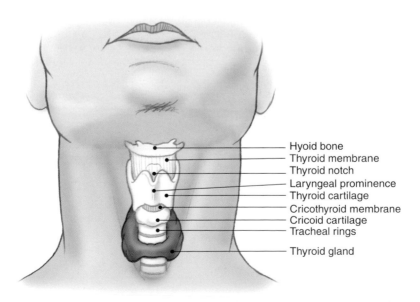

Hyoid bone
Thyroid membrane
Thyroid notch
Laryngeal prominence
Thyroid cartilage
Cricothyroid membrane
Cricoid cartilage
Tracheal rings

Thyroid gland

Figure 2.3
External airway anatomy.

The central face and mandible should be inspected and palpated for structural integrity; injuries to these structures may lead to airway distortion or loss. The anterior neck should be carefully inspected for penetrating wounds, asymmetry or swelling that may herald impending airway compromise. The palpation of subcutaneous air suggests a direct airway injury.

Feel for air movement at the mouth and nose. Open the mouth and inspect the upper airway, taking care not to extend or rotate the neck. Look for and remove any vomitus, blood or other foreign material. Identify swelling of the tongue or uvula, sites of bleeding, or other visible abnormalities of the oropharynx. Gentle use of a tongue blade may facilitate this task. The patient's ability to spontaneously swallow and handle secretions is an important indicator of intact protective airway mechanisms. In the unconscious patient, the absence of a gag reflex has traditionally been associated with loss of protective airway reflexes.

Auscultation should demonstrate clear and equal breath sounds. Diminished breath sounds may be the result of pneumothorax, hemothorax or pleural effusion. Wheezing and dyspnea imply lower airway obstruction.

In pediatric patients, visual signs of possible airway and respiratory compromise include tachypnea, cyanosis, drooling, nasal flaring and intercostal retractions. A child with severe upper airway obstruction may get in to the "sniffing position" to straighten the airway and reduce occlusion. A child with severe lower airway obstruction may assume the "tripod" posture – sitting up and leaning forward on outstretched arms – to augment accessory muscle function.

Noninvasive airway management

Opening the airway

Ensuring airway patency is essential for adequate oxygenation and ventilation, and is the first priority in airway control. The conscious patient uses the musculature of the upper airway to maintain patency, and protective reflexes to protect against aspiration of foreign substances, gastric contents or secretions. In the severely ill, compromised or unconscious patient, these protective airway mechanisms may be impaired or lost.

Upper airway obstruction in the unconscious patient is most commonly the result of posterior displacement of the tongue and epiglottis at the level of the pharynx and larynx. This occlusion results directly from loss of submandibular muscle tone, which provides direct support to the tongue and indirect support to the epiglottis.

Simple bedside maneuvers can correct this occlusion and reestablish airway patency and airflow. The *head tilt with chin lift* (Figure 2.4) is a simple, effective technique for opening the airway, but should be avoided in any patient with a potentially unstable cervical spine. The *jaw thrust without head tilt* (Figure 2.5), however, can be performed while maintaining cervical spine alignment. Although these techniques work well, they require the continuous involvement of a single provider to maintain airway patency.

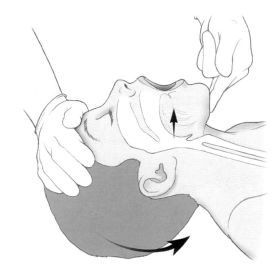

Figure 2.4
Head tilt with chin lift.

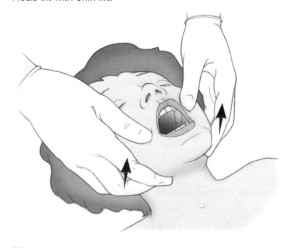

Figure 2.5
Jaw thrust without head tilt.

Several airway adjuncts have been developed to maintain airway patency while freeing the health care provider to perform other duties. The *oropharyngeal airway* (OPA) is an S-shaped device designed to hold the tongue off the posterior pharyngeal wall while providing an air channel and suction conduit through the mouth (Figure 2.6). It is most effective in patients who are spontaneously breathing but lack a gag or cough reflex. The use of an OPA in a patient with a gag or cough reflex is contraindicated as it may stimulate vomiting or laryngospasm. The OPA comes in various sizes to accommodate children through large adults. The proper OPA size is estimated by placing the OPA's flange at the corner of the mouth; the distal tip of the device should reach the angle of the jaw.

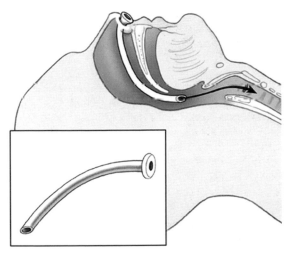

Figure 2.7
Nasopharyngeal airway.

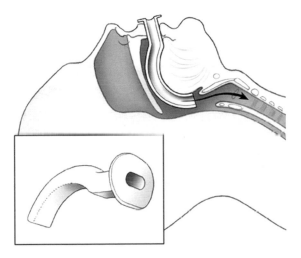

Figure 2.6
Oropharyngeal airway.

The *nasopharyngeal airway* (NPA) is an uncuffed trumpet-like tube made of soft rubber or plastic that provides a conduit for airflow between the nares and pharynx (Figure 2.7). It is commonly used in intoxicated or semiconscious patients who do not tolerate an OPA. It is also effective when trauma, trismus ("clenched teeth") or another obstacle (e.g., wiring of the teeth) preclude the placement of an OPA. Proper NPA length is determined by measuring the distance from the tip of the nose to the tragus of the ear. Though OPAs and NPAs help establish artificial airways, they do not provide definitive airway protection from aspiration.

Supplemental oxygen

Oxygen (O_2) should be administered to all seriously ill or injured patients with cardiac disease, respiratory distress, shock or trauma, even if their measured arterial O_2 tension is normal. A variety of O_2 delivery techniques may be employed depending on the desired O_2 concentration and clinical circumstance (Table 2.1). Administration should begin at a high level and then be titrated downward. Though O_2 should never be withheld from a hypoxic patient with respiratory distress, care should be exercised when treating patients with chronic hypercarbia, such as patients with chronic obstructive pulmonary disease (COPD). Unmonitored treatment of these patients with high O_2 concentrations can result in respiratory depression from loss of their hypoxic ventilatory drive.

Ventilation

Despite an open airway and supplemental O_2, a patient who is not adequately ventilating cannot conduct meaningful gas exchange. Adequate ventilation implies inhalation of enough air to deliver O_2 to the alveoli and exhalation of enough air to facilitate the removal of carbon dioxide (CO_2).

The sequence of interventions for the inadequately-ventilating patient is opening the airway followed by bag-valve-mask (BVM) ventilation. The self-inflating ventilation bag with face mask provides an emergent means of ventilation. It is equipped with several valves that allow for coordinated flow of air into and out of the patient. This includes a non-rebreathing valve that allows exhaled CO_2 to escape into the atmosphere without being entrained back into the lungs. When

Table 2.1 Oxygen delivery techniques

O$_2$ delivery technique	Flow rate (L/minute)	Concentration delivered (%)	Other
Nasal cannula	1–6	24–44	Inspired O$_2$ concentration depends on flow rate and patient's tidal volume
Simple face mask	6–10	35–60	May promote CO$_2$ retention at lower flow rates
Venturi mask	2–12	24–60	Accurately controls proportion of inspired O$_2$ Use in patients with chronic hypercarbia (i.e., COPD)
Face mask with O$_2$ reservoir	12–15	60–90	Provides high inspired O$_2$ concentration
Bag-valve-mask	15	100	Provides the highest inspired O$_2$ concentration
Blow-by	6–10	Varies	For infant or young child who will not tolerate face mask or cannula

COPD: chronic obstructive pulmonary disease; O$_2$: oxygen.

attached to a high-flow O$_2$ source (10–15 L/minute), the BVM can supply an O$_2$ concentration of nearly 100%. The adapter for the face mask is interchangeable with an endotracheal tube (ETT), so the same bag can be used post-intubation.

The use of the BVM is a vital emergency skill. Competence with the BVM is a prerequisite for using paralytic agents to intubate a patient. Substantial proficiency is required to use one hand to maintain an adequate mask seal, position the patient's head, and assure airway patency, while using the other hand to ventilate. Although mastery of solo BVM technique is imperative, recruitment of another individual allows one person to perform a jaw thrust and ensure a good mask seal with both hands while the second individual squeezes the bag.

The effectiveness of BVM ventilation can be determined by watching the chest rise and fall, feeling the resistance in the bag and monitoring the patient's O$_2$ saturation.

Indications for definitive airway management

A definitive airway implies "patency and protection." This requires an ETT in the trachea secured in place, with the cuff inflated, and attached to an O$_2$-rich ventilation device. The inability or failure to secure a definitive airway in a timely manner can have disastrous consequences for the patient.

Though the ultimate decision to intubate a patient is often complicated and may depend on a variety of clinical factors, there are five fundamental reasons that patients require definitive airway management:

1. Failure of ventilation or oxygenation
2. Inability to maintain or protect the airway
3. Potential for deterioration based on the patient's clinical presentation
4. Delivery of treatment
5. Patient saftey and protection

Failure to ventilate or oxygenate

The patient who is inadequately ventilating despite maximal clinical therapy or remains severely hypoxemic despite supplemental O$_2$ may need intubation. The decision to intubate these patients is based on a combination of clinical findings including general appearance, perfusion status, work of breathing, O$_2$ saturation and clinical course. Intubation allows for the delivery of higher concentrations of O$_2$ as well as positive-pressure ventilation which tends to improve most circumstances of hypoxia and ventilatory failure.

Inability to maintain or protect the airway

An open airway is required for adequate oxygenation and ventilation. Patients who are unable to swallow spontaneously and handle their secretions, or lack a gag reflex, are at risk for aspiration.

Though repositioning maneuvers (chin lift, jaw thrust) or airway adjuncts (OPA, NPA) may serve as temporizing measures, they do not provide definitive airway protection from aspiration, which carries a significant associated morbidity and mortality. Therefore, patients who are unable to maintain or protect their own airway need intubation. The exception to this rule is the patient with a rapidly reversible condition, such as a narcotic overdose or dysrhythmia.

Potential for deterioration based on the patient's clinical presentation

Anticipating airway compromise before it occurs is one of the most challenging aspects of emergency airway management. Certain conditions mandate the need for definitive airway management even in the absence of specific airway, ventilatory or oxygenation failure. This decision to intubate is based on anticipated anatomic or physiologic airway deterioration or ventilatory compromise. For example, the decision to intubate an awake, talking patient with a suspected thermal injury to the airway may be difficult but necessary to avoid future airway occlusion and compromise. Delaying definitive airway management in this patient could allow for the interval development of significant airway edema, making endotracheal intubation extremely difficult if not impossible. Other patients in whom early airway management should be considered include those with significant facial fractures, penetrating neck trauma, tracheal or laryngeal injuries, severe head injury, multiple trauma, sustained seizure activity or certain overdoses (e.g., tricyclic antidepressant).

Delivery of treatment

The ETT may also provide a route for lifesaving medications or therapy (e.g., rewarming) to a critical patient. In the patient with unobtainable or delayed intravenous (IV) access, an often overlooked method of medication administration is ETT delivery. Narcan, Atropine, Versed (Midazolam), Epinephrine and Lidocaine can be administered through the ETT, and can be remembered by the mnemonic *NAVEL*. The absorption and extent of medication delivery via ETT is typically reduced; therefore, tracheal doses should be 2–4 times the IV dose. Additionally, a hypothermic patient can be gradually rewarmed via heated, humidified O_2 continuously delivered via the ETT.

Patient safety and protection

Agitated, combative or confused patients may harm themselves in certain clinical situations, making them candidates for prophylactic intubation. For an agitated multiple trauma patient with an unstable cervical spine injury, sedation and intubation may be the only safe way to adequately immobilize and protect the patient during the initial assessment, diagnosis and treatment.

Definitive airway management
Immediate "crash" intubation

Patients with respiratory arrest, agonal respirations or deep unresponsiveness require immediate intubation without the use of supplemental medications. The advantages of this approach are technical ease and immediacy. Disadvantages include the potential for increased intracranial pressure (ICP) from the stress of intubation, as well as possible emesis and aspiration.

Rapid sequence intubation

Rapid sequence intubation (RSI) is a series of defined steps intended to allow for rapid oral intubation of a patient without BVM ventilation. Given that most patients requiring emergent intubation have not fasted and may have full stomachs, BVM ventilation may inadvertently lead to gastric distention and increase the risk of aspiration. To avoid this complication, the patient is first pre-oxygenated with 100% supplemental O_2 to allow for a period of apnea without assisted ventilation. This is followed by the sequential administration of an induction agent and a rapidly-acting neuromuscular blocking agent (NMBA) to induce a state of unconsciousness and paralysis, respectively. The patient may then be intubated without the need for BVM ventilation.

The steps making up RSI can be thought of as nine "Ps" (Table 2.2).

Possibility of success

The patient should be carefully evaluated for a potentially difficult airway, and assessed for ease of BVM ventilation should the intubation prove difficult or impossible.

Table 2.2 The nine P's of Rapid Sequence Intubation

Time	Action
0 − 10 minutes	Possibility of success
0 − 10 minutes	Preparation
0 − 5 minutes	Pre-oxygenation
0 − 3 minutes	Pretreatment
Time zero	Paralysis (with induction)
0 + 20–30 seconds	Protection and positioning
0 + 45 seconds	Placement
0 + 45 seconds	Proof
0 + 1 minute	Post-intubation management

Anticipating the difficult airway

When evaluating a patient for ease of intubation and ventilation, it is important to use a consistent approach. A logical easily-remembered approach to identifying the difficult airway is the *LEMON* law (Look externally, Evaluate the 3-3-2 rule, Mallampati, Obstruction, Neck mobility).

Look externally

A brief and targeted exam of the jaw, mouth, neck and internal airway may help identify features that predict a difficult airway. Initial inspection should identify anatomic features such as morbid obesity, abnormal facial shape, facial or neck trauma, large or abnormal teeth, protruding tongue or the presence of facial hair that may pose a challenge to intubation, ventilation or both. An abnormal facial shape, extreme cachexia, a "toothless" mouth with sunken cheeks, trauma to the lower face or facial hair may prevent an adequate seal for effective BVM ventilation. Large buckteeth or central incisors, a receding mandible or short bull-neck may provide anatomic barriers to oral intubation. Obesity generally makes intubation and ventilation more challenging. Some of these features may also be remembered by the mnemonic *BONES* (Beard, Obese, No teeth, Elderly, Sleep apnea/snoring.)

Evaluate the 3-3-2 rule

The 3-3-2 rule describes the ideal dimensions of the airway that facilitate direct visualization of the larynx. It is easily remembered as three (of the patient's) fingers in the mouth, three fingers under the chin and two fingers at the top of the neck. The ability to accommodate three fingers in the mouth indicates an adequate mouth opening. Three fingers from the tip of the chin (mentum) to the floor of the mouth (hyoid bone) indicate the patient's mandible is large enough to accommodate a normally-sized tongue. A small mandible and large tongue may obstruct access to the larynx during intubation. Finally, two finger's breadth from the floor of the mouth (hyoid bone) to the thyroid cartilage indicates an adequate neck length and laryngeal position. A high or anteriorly-placed larynx may be very difficult to visualize during laryngoscopy.

Mallampati

The Mallampati classification is a scale (I–IV) used to predict the ability of a patient's mouth to accommodate both the laryngoscope and ETT. To determine a patient's classification, ask the patient to extend their neck, open their mouth as widely as possible and stick out their tongue without phonating. The degree to which the base of the tongue, faucial pillars, uvula and posterior pharynx are visible determines the Mallampati class (Figure 2.8). Class I and II predict greater oral access for the laryngoscope and superior laryngeal exposure, thereby portending a greater likelihood of successful intubation. In the case of Class III and IV scores, the tongue is large in relation to the oral cavity, signifying limited oral access, a limited view and higher intubation failure rates.

Obstruction of the airway

Upper airway obstruction can make intubation and ventilation difficult if not impossible. When time allows, patients should be screened for the presence of upper airway infections (epiglottitis, peritonsillar abscess, preverterbral abscess), laryngeal masses or tumors, or any other upper airway conditions that may complicate laryngoscopy and BVM ventilation. Foreign bodies, extrinsic airway compression and direct airway trauma (including the possibility of airway disruption) should be considered strong evidence of an obstruction that could hinder or preclude intubation and ventilation.

Neck mobility

Proper mobility and alignment of the head and neck can facilitate laryngoscopy and intubation. Certain conditions such as cervical spine immobilization and degenerative arthritis may limit mobility and complicate intubation.

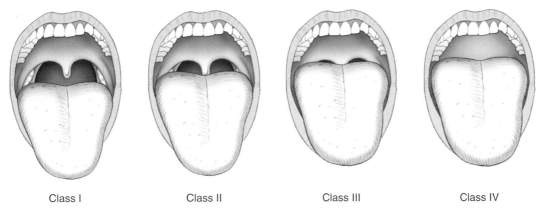

| Class I | Class II | Class III | Class IV |

Figure 2.8
Mallampati classification. The classification of tongue size relative to the size of the oral cavity as described by Mallampati and colleagues. Class I: faucial pillars, soft palate, and uvula visualized. Class II: faucial pillars and soft palate visualized, but the uvula is masked by the base of the tongue. Class III: only the base of the uvula can be visualized. Class IV: none of the three structures can be visualized.

Preparation

Prior to initiating RSI, careful preparation is essential to achieving success. This point cannot be emphasized enough. The *SOAP ME* mnemonic is used to summarize the necessary preparatory steps.

SOAP ME

Suction
Suction should be tested and available at the bedside.

Oxygen
A high flow O_2 mask and BVM ventilation device should be ready for use.

Airway equipment
At least two functioning laryngoscope handles and the appropriately-sized and shaped laryngoscope blades should be available. The anticipated blade of choice should be clicked into position to ensure that the light functions properly. An ETT should be chosen based on the patient's anatomy, and one smaller size should be prepared as well. The typical adult male will accept a 7.5- or 8.0-size ETT, the typical adult female a 7.0- or 7.5-size ETT. In children, the ETT size may be estimated by the formula ETT size = 4 + (age in years/4). The ETT cuff should be inflated to test for an air leak. A stylet should be inserted within the ETT to shape it into a configuration that will facilitate insertion into the airway. This configuration varies between physicians, although most prefer a gentle curve at the distal portion to a near 45-degree angle. Care must be taken to ensure that the tip of the stylet does not protrude from the end of the ETT or through the small distal side port (Murphy's eye). Preparation of the ETT with the stylet inserted is recommended, as it is easier to remove a stylet (if not needed) than to add one during RSI.

Pharmacy
The patient should have at least one IV line, and patency should be ensured. The specific RSI medications, proper dosing and sequence of administration should be determined, and the agents drawn up and labeled.

Monitoring Equipment
Cardiac blood pressure and pulse oximetry monitoring are mandatory for all patients. If available, an end-tidal CO_2 (ETCO$_2$) monitor should be prepared as well.

Respiratory therapy should be at the bedside, as they play a crucial role in assisting with airway management, including securing the ETT and post-intubation care. When dealing with a complicated airway, anesthesiology or ear, nose and throat (ENT) specialists should be called in to assist with airway management.

Pre-oxygenation

During RSI, the process of direct laryngoscopy and ETT placement precludes the delivery of O_2 to the paralyzed apneic patient, which could lead to arterial O_2 desaturation (<90%). Pre-oxygenation establishes an O_2 reservoir within the patient's lungs and body tissues that allows for a period of prolonged apnea without detrimental arterial O_2 desaturation. This is accomplished through the

Table 2.3 Pretreatment medications: LOAD

Drug	Indication	Mechanism	Adult dose (IV)	Pediatric dose (IV)	Notes
Lidocaine	↑ICP, RAD	↓ intracranial response to intubation, mitigates bronchospasm in RAD	1.5 mg/kg	1.5 mg/kg	
Opioid (fentanyl)	↑ICP, ischemic heart disease, aortic dissection	Blunts sympathetic response to laryngoscopy	3–6 mcg/kg	1–3 mcg/kg	Use with caution in young children
Atropine	Children SP < 10 years Adults receiving a second dose of SCh	Mitigates bradycardic response to SCh	2.0 mg	0.02 mg/kg (minimum dose 0.1 mg)	
Defasciculation (pancuronium, vecuronium)	↑ICP or globe injury	Defasiculates and mitigates ICP response to SCh	0.01 mg/kg	0.01 mg/kg	Only for adults and children >20 kg

ICP: intracranial pressure; LOAD: lidocaine, opioid, atropine, defasciculation; RAD: reactive airway disease; SCh: succinylcholine.

administration of 100% O_2 to the patient for 5 minutes prior to paralysis, effectively leading to "nitrogen washout." This replaces room air (80% nitrogen, 20% O_2) in the lung with nearly 100% O_2.

The time to desaturation following pre-oxygenation is determined by the duration of pre-oxygenation as well as the patient's age and body habitus. Children and obese adults tend to desaturate more rapidly than typical adults.

A non-rebreather O_2 mask delivers O_2 concentrations in the range of 70–75%. A ventilation bag and mask placed over the patient's mouth and nose (without actively bagging) delivers 100% O_2 to the patient. In circumstances where time is limited, a patient can be quickly pre-oxygenated by taking eight vital capacity (the largest possible) breaths in rapid succession from a 100% O_2 source.

Pretreatment

During RSI, the use of succinylcholine (SCh), a depolarizing NMBA, and the act of intubation can lead to a number of adverse effects including increased ICP, increased intraocular pressure, increased intragastric pressure, bronchospasm in patients with reactive airway disease, increased sympathetic discharge and bradycardia (especially in children).

Selected pretreatment medications may be given to mitigate these adverse effects; they may be remembered using the mnemonic LOAD (Lidocaine, Opioid, Atropine, Defasciculation). These medications, their indications, mechanisms of action and doses are summarized in Table 2.3.

Paralysis (with induction)

The next step in RSI is the rapid IV administration of an induction agent followed immediately by an NMBA to induce complete motor paralysis.

Induction agents

All patients with few exceptions (i.e., benzodiazepine overdose) should receive an induction agent prior to neuromuscular blockade. Induction agents induce complete loss of consciousness prior to NMBA-induced paralysis. Paralysis without sedation can lead to detrimental physiologic and undesirable psychologic sequelae. When combined with NMBAs, induction agents also enhance muscle relaxation, thereby creating improved intubating conditions.

There is no single induction agent of choice for RSI in the ED. The choice of an induction agent is based on the patient's clinical circumstance and the agent's attributes. The most commonly used induction agents are discussed below and summarized in Table 2.4.

Etomidate

Etomidate is a non-barbiturate sedative-hypnotic agent. For most ED patients, it is the induction agent of choice for RSI. It has a rapid onset, brief duration of action and causes minimal respiratory and myocardial depression. Etomidate is the

Table 2.4 Induction agents

Induction agents	Induction dose (IV)	Onset of action	Duration of action	Benefits	Precautions
Barbiturates					
Thiopental	3–6 mg/kg (adult) 1–3 mg/kg (elderly)	<30 sec	5–10 min	↓ ICP	↓ BP Laryngospasm
Methohexital	1–3 mg/kg	<30 sec	5–10 min	↓ ICP Short duration	↓ BP Laryngospasm Seizures
Benzodiazepines					
Midazolam	0.2–0.3 mg/kg	30–60 sec	15–30 min	Reversible Amnestic Anticonvulsant	Apnea No analgesia Variable dosing
Etomidate	0.3 mg/kg	15–45 sec	3–12 min	↓ ICP Rarely ↓ BP	Myoclonic jerks Vomiting No analgesia
Ketamine	1–2 mg/kg	45–60 sec	10–20 min	↑ BP Bronchodilator Dissociative amnesia	↑ Secretions ↑ ICP Emergence phenomenon
Propofol	1.5–3 mg/kg	15–45 sec	5–10 min		

BP: blood pressure; ICP: intracranial pressure; IOP: intraocular pressure.

most hemodynamically stable of the currently available induction agents. Even so, the dose should be reduced by 50% to 0.15 mg/kg in unstable patients. Etomidate reduces cerebral blood flow and cerebral metabolic O_2 demand without adversely affecting cerebral perfusion pressure. Due to such cerebroprotective effects and its unique hemodynamic stability, etomidate is considered the induction agent of choice in patients with elevated ICP. Side effects of etomidate include vomiting, pain at the injection site, myoclonic movements and hiccups. Adverse effects from cortisol suppression have not been reported with one-time use in the ED.

Ketamine
Ketamine is a dissociative anesthetic derived from phencyclidine (PCP) that induces a cataleptic state rather than true unconsciousness. It results in analgesia, amnesia and anesthesia. Ketamine stimulates the endogenous release of catecholamines causing a rise in heart rate, blood pressure, myocardial consumption and bronchodilation. For this reason, it is the induction agent of choice for hypotensive, hypovolemic or bronchospastic patients requiring intubation. Care should be taken in patients with ischemic

heart disease. As ketamine increases ICP, cerebral blood flow, and cerebral metabolic rate, it is generally avoided in patients with potentially increased ICP. Ketamine is known to enhance laryngeal reflexes, increase airway secretions and precipitate laryngospasm. For this reason, atropine 0.02 mg/kg IV may be given in conjunction with ketamine to promote a drying effect. Ketamine may produce an unpleasant emergence phenomenon, including hallucinations or frightening dreams in the first 3 hours after awakening. Such reactions are more common in adults than children and can be reduced through the concomitant administration of a benzodiazepine such as lorezepam (0.05 mg/kg) or diazepam (0.2 mg/kg) after intubation.

Thiopental and methohexital
The barbiturates thiopental and methohexital are short-acting sedative-hypnotic agents that provide no analgesia. The benefits of these agents are their short onset of action and rapid depression of central nervous system (CNS) activity. These agents also reduce ICP by reducing cerebral blood flow, and provide cerebroprotective effects through reductions in cerebral metabolic O_2 consumption (while still maintaining cerebral

perfusion pressure). Their major disadvantage is their propensity to induce significant hypotension from myocardial depression and venodilation. For this reason, these agents are best avoided in hypotensive patients. Other side effects of thiopental include central respiratory depression, histamine release (avoid use in asthmatic patients), tissue injury and necrosis with extravasation. It is contraindicated in patients with porphyria. Methohexital is shorter-acting and more potent than thiopental, and not surprisingly associated with more profound hypotension and respiratory depression.

Propofol

Propofol is an alkylphenol derivative with hypnotic properties. It is rapid acting and has a short duration of action. Although it blunts the potential rise in ICP associated with intubation, it adversely reduces cerebral perfusion pressure as well as systemic blood pressure. As a result, propofol is uncommonly used for induction in the ED.

Midazolam

Midazolam and other benzodiazepines cause amnesia, anxiolysis, central muscle relaxation, sedation, and hypnosis. They also have anticonvulsant effects. As induction agents, their primary indications are to promote sedation and amnesia, their greatest asset. A drawback to their use is their great dosing variability, depending on the patient's gender and age. Midazolam is a myocardial depressant and reduces systemic vascular resistance. It should be used with caution in elderly patients and those with hemodynamic compromise. Though midazolam may be used as the primary induction or adjunctive agent during RSI, it is more commonly utilized for sedation in combination with an analgesic agent in patients who are intubated.

Neuromuscular blockade

NMBAs do not provide analgesia, sedation or amnesia; they are used to paralyze the patient, facilitating rapid endotracheal intubation. The ideal NMBA would have a rapid onset, a short duration of action and few adverse side-effects.

SCh, a *depolarizing* NMBA, comes closest to meeting all of these traits and is the most commonly used NMBA in the ED. At the neuromuscular junction, SCh binds tightly to acetylcholine receptors, causing depolarization of the motor endplate and muscle contraction. Clinically, this initially manifests as muscle fasciculations followed by paralysis. IV administration of SCh results in muscle fasciculations within 10–15 seconds followed by complete paralysis after 45–60 seconds. Because of its short duration of action, patients may begin spontaneously breathing within 3–5 minutes.

The dose of SCh is 1.5 mg/kg rapid IV push in adults. In children <10 years of age, the recommended dose is 2 mg/kg rapid IV push. In newborns, use 3 mg/kg rapid IV push. There is little harm to giving too much SCh; however, giving too little SCh can result in an inadequately paralyzed patient and affect one's ability to successfully intubate.

The main drawback to SCh are its side effects, including muscle fasciculations, bradycardia, hyperkalemia, prolonged neuromuscular blockade, trismus (masseter spasm) and malignant hyperthermia. The muscle fasciculations are associated with rises in ICP, intragastric and intraocular pressure, and can be inhibited through the use of a defasciculating dose of a non-depolarizing NMBA. The bradycardia that follows the administration of SCh most commonly occurs in children and can be avoided by pretreatment with atropine (0.02 mg/kg). Under usual circumstances, SCh induces a small but clinically insignificant rise in serum potassium of 0.5 mEq/L. However, in large burns, crush injuries, denervation or neuromuscular disorders, the administration of SCh may lead to an exaggerated rise in potassium levels of 5–10 mEq/L and result in hyperkalemic dysrhythmias or cardiac arrest. Fortunately, the hyperkalemia risk is not immediate in these patients but occurs typically 2–7 days post-event, depending on the injury or underlying process.

Non-depolarizing NMBAs such as rocuronium compete with acetylcholine for receptors at the neuromuscular junction, thereby causing paralysis. Although these agents are commonly used as defasciculating agents or for post-intubation patient management, they may also be used as the primary RSI paralytic agent in specific patient populations or in patients who have a contraindication to SCh. They have much fewer side effects than SCh but are generally less effective for intubation because of their delayed time to paralysis, prolonged duration of action, or both.

Specific attributes of the depolarizing and non-depolarizing NMBAs are listed in the Table 2.5.

Protection

Following the administration of induction and paralytic agents, the patient will predictably lose consciousness and become apneic. Sellick's

Table 2.5 Neuromuscular blocking agents

Neuromuscular blocking agent	Intubating dose (IV)	Onset	Duration
Depolarizing agent			
Succinylcholine	1.5 mg/kg (adult) 2 mg/kg (child) 3 mg/kg (infant)	45–60 sec	6–12 min
Non-depolarizing			
Rocuronium	1.0 mg/kg	50–70 sec	30–60 min
Vecuronium	0.15 mg/kg	90–120 sec	60–75 min
Pancuronium	0.1 mg/kg	100–150 sec	120–150 min

maneuver (cricoid pressure) should be applied by an assistant just as the patient is noted to lose consciousness. This application of firm pressure (10 lb) to the cricoid cartilage compresses the esophagus and prevents passive regurgitation of gastric contents (Figure 2.9). Sellick's maneuver should be maintained until the ETT has been placed, its position verified, and the cuff inflated.

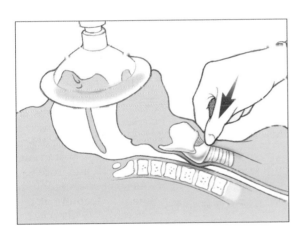

Figure 2.9
Cricoid pressure (Sellick's maneuver).

If Sellick's maneuver is applied too early, the patient may find it uncomfortable or vomit. This maneuver should be discontinued if the patient is actively vomiting because of the risk of esophageal rupture.

Positioning

Based on the patient's age, anatomy and other conditions (cervical arthritis, cervical spine precautions), the patient should be carefully positioned in the manner that increases the odds of successful intubation.

The airway can be thought of as having three separate axes: the oral, pharyngeal and laryngeal. Proper positioning prior to laryngoscopy helps align these axes and improve visualization of the glottis. In the neutral position, these axes are misaligned (Figure 2.10).

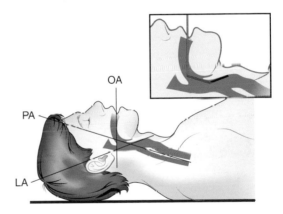

Figure 2.10
Head on bed, neutral position. PA: pharyngeal axis; OA: oral axis; LA: laryngeal axis. Reproduced with permission from Walls RM et al, Manual of Emergency Airway Management, 2nd ed. and Companion Manual to the Airway Course (www.theairwaysite.com), Lippincott Williams & Wilkins, 2004.

Placing a small pillow under the patient's occiput flexes the lower cervical spine relative to the torso and aligns the pharyngeal and laryngeal axes (Figure 2.11). Positioning the patient in the "sniffing" position with extension of the head on the neck aligns all the three axes (Figure 2.12).

Patients with possible cervical spine injury should be maintained in the neutral position.

Placement

After the administration of SCh, the patient will predictably have muscle fasciculations followed

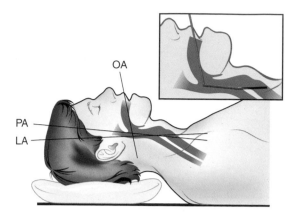

Figure 2.11
Head elevated on pad, neutral position. PA: pharyngeal axis; OA: oral axis; LA: laryngeal axis. Reproduced with permission from Walls RM et al, Manual of Emergency Airway Management, 2nd ed. and Companion Manual to the Airway Course (www.theairwaysite.com), Lippincott Williams & Wilkins, 2004.

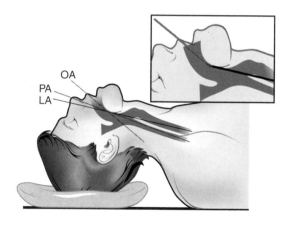

Figure 2.12
Head elevated on pad, head extended on neck. PA: pharyngeal axis; OA: oral axis; LA: laryngeal axis. Reproduced with permission from Walls RM et al, Manual of Emergency Airway Management, 2nd ed. and Companion Manual to the Airway Course (www. theairwaysite.com), Lippincott Williams & Wilkins, 2004.

by paralysis and apnea. If the patient has been adequately pre-oxygenated, arterial O_2 saturations will remain normal despite apnea. Complete muscular paralysis can be confirmed by gently grasping the patient's mandible and checking for flaccidity. It is important to wait until the patient is completely paralyzed before proceeding with intubation.

With the laryngoscope in the left hand, the mouth is opened with the right hand. The laryngoscope is gently inserted into the right side of

the patient's mouth, and the tongue is displaced to the left. The curved (Macintosh) blade is slid into the vallecula; the straight (Miller) blade is positioned below the epiglottis. The laryngoscope handle is advanced along the axis of the blade at an angle of 45° to the patient's body. Care should be taken not to use the teeth as a fulcrum for the laryngoscope.

If the glottic aperture is not readily visible, the intubator or an assistant may perform the BURP (Backward, Upward, Rightward Pressure) maneuver. The hand is placed on the thyroid cartilage followed by the application of BURP to help bring the glottis into the intubator's view (Figure 2.13). The resulting displacement of the thyroid cartilage backwards against the cervical vertebrae, upward or as superiorly as possible, and laterally to the right has been found to significantly improve the view of the glottis during laryngoscopy.

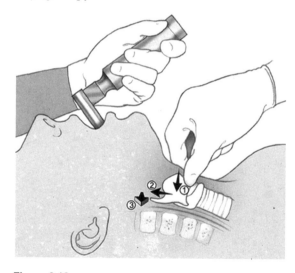

Figure 2.13
BURP maneuver: Backward, upward, rightward pressure.

With a clear view of the glottis, the right hand gently inserts the ETT until the cuff is about 2–3 cm past the vocal cords. In the adult male, the 23 cm marker of the ETT will be located at the corner of the mouth (21 cm in women). Once in place, the stylet should be removed and the cuff inflated until there is no audible air leak with BVM ventilation.

Adequate pre-oxygenation will allow the laryngoscopist several attempts at intubation before arterial O_2 desaturation occurs. A dedicated team member should be focused on the patient's cardiac rhythm, blood pressure and O_2 saturation during laryngoscopy, and should alert the intubator to any abnormalities. After any unsuccessful attempt, always recheck the patient's position and make needed adjustments. Consider changing the size or type of laryngoscope blade. It is important to change "something" prior to a second look to ensure the same problem is not encountered.

Proof: confirmation of endotracheal tube placement

As inadvertent intubation of the esophagus can occur during airway management, proper placement of the ETT within the trachea needs to be confirmed after every intubation. Sellick's maneuver should not be released until confirmation of correct ETT placement. Failure to recognize an esophageal intubation can be disastrous.

Methods used to confirm correct ETT placement include clinical assessment, pulse oximetry, ETCO$_2$ detection and aspiration techniques. Chest radiography can be used to assess ETT position but does not confirm ETT placement within the trachea. Since the esophagus lies directly behind the trachea, an ETT placed in the esophagus may appear to be within the trachea on an AP chest X-ray (CXR).

Clinical assessment

Classically, a combination of clinical observations has been used to confirm correct ETT placement. These include:

1. The laryngoscopist observing the ETT pass through the vocal cords during intubation
2. Auscultation of clear and equal breath sounds over both lung fields
3. Absence of breath sounds when auscultating over the epigastrium
4. Observation of symmetrical chest rise during ventilation
5. Observation of condensation ("fogging") of the ETT during ventilation.

Though these clinical findings should be assessed in every intubated patient, they are prone to error as the sole means for confirming ETT placement.

Pulse oximetry

Continuous noninvasive pulse oximetry should be standard for every patient being intubated. A drop in the measured O$_2$ saturation following intubation is worrisome for an esophageal intubation; however, this drop may be delayed for several minutes if the patient was adequately pre-oxygenated, giving health care providers a false sense of security. In certain patients (i.e., hypotensive), O$_2$ saturation measurements may be unreliable or difficult to detect. Although pulse oximetry is important, it should not be the primary indicator of successful ETT placement.

End-tidal carbon dioxide (ETCO$_2$) detection

Detection and measurement of exhaled CO$_2$ is a highly reliable method for detecting proper placement of the ETT within the trachea. It is achieved through one of the three approaches:

Colorometric ETCO$_2$ detector is a small disposable device that connects between the bag and the ETT. When the device detects ETCO$_2$, its colorometric indicator changes from purple to yellow; the absence of this color change indicates the tube is incorrectly placed in the esophagus. A false positive color change may occur if the tube is placed just above the glottis. A false negative color change may occur (even with correct ETT placement) in some cases of cardiac arrest and profound circulatory collapse, as CO$_2$ production and delivery to the lungs abruptly declines.

Qualitative ETCO$_2$ detection devices use a light indicator with an audible alert, as opposed to a color change, to indicate the presence of exhaled CO$_2$. Many of these devices have alarms that sound if the detection of ETCO$_2$ ceases.

Quantitative ETCO$_2$ detectors perform capnography, the graphic display of CO$_2$ concentrations seen as a wave form on the monitor, or capnometry, the measurement and display of CO$_2$ concentrations.

Aspiration devices

Aspiration devices may also be used for confirmation of ETT placement. These work based on the principle that the trachea is a rigid air-filled structure, whereas the esophagus has collapsible walls. Attempts to draw air through an ETT placed in the esophagus will meet resistance from collapse of the esophageal wall around the distal ETT. Air will freely flow when drawn through an ETT in the trachea.

The two commonly used aspiration appliances are the *bulb aspiration* and the *syringe aspiration* devices. The bulb aspiration device is a round compressible plastic globe ("turkey baster") which is compressed and deflated before placement in the ETT, and then released. If the bulb reexpands rapidly, the ETT is likely in the trachea. Failure to reexpand or delayed reexpansion suggests that the ETT is in the esophagus. Syringe aspiration devices are large syringes (usually 30 ml) which are inserted into the ETT. The syringe plunger is then drawn back rapidly to allow the brisk aspiration of a large amount of air. The rapid easy flow of air suggests tracheal intubation, whereas meeting resistance suggests an esophageal intubation. Though these aspiration techniques are easy to perform, they are not as reliable as ETCO$_2$ detection.

Post-intubation management

After correct placement of the ETT in the trachea has been verified, a few "housekeeping" issues must be addressed. The tube should be secured in place (taped or tied) to ensure it does not move. The patient's blood pressure and other vitals should be repeated frequently. Bradycardia following intubation should be assumed due to esophageal intubation and resulting hypoxia. Hypertension post-intubation suggests inadequate sedation. Hypotension may be the result of a tension pneumothorax, decreased venous return, a cardiac cause, or the induction agent.

A mechanical ventilator should be configured according to the patient's size and needs. A CXR should be taken to assess the ETT position (depth of placement) and the condition of the patient's lungs. Proper tube depth is generally 2–3 cm above the carina. Insertion of the ETT into the right main stem bronchus is a common complication (Figure 2.14).

Following intubation, consideration should be given to long-term sedation and paralysis using a benzodiazepine and NMBA. Diazepam (0.2 mg/kg) may be given initially for sedation and repeated for any signs of awareness. Lorazepam (0.05–0.1 mg/kg) is a perfectly acceptable alternative. Pancuronium (0.1 mg/kg) or vecuronium (0.1 mg/kg) may be used for long-term paralysis; a repeat dose (one-third the initial dose) may be given after 45–60 minutes if motor activity is detected. An opioid agent such as morphine sulfate (0.2 mg/kg) may also be administered for additional patient comfort.

Awake oral intubation

Awake oral intubation is a technique utilizing liberal topical airway anesthesia and mild IV

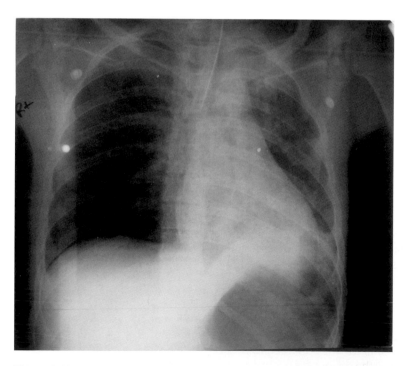

Figure 2.14
Right main stem bronchus intubation. AP supine chest radiograph on a trauma board showing an endotracheal tube in the right main stem bronchus, hyperinflation of the right lung and marked loss of volume in the left lung.

sedation prior to inspection or intubation of an "awake" patient's airway. The approach conveniently allows for the preservation of the patient's airway reflexes and spontaneous breathing while the laryngoscopist takes a gentle look at the glottis, vocal cords and internal airway anatomy. Whether to intubate the patient immediately or defer for a controlled RSI depends on the potential for progressively increased airway difficulty or compromise. One might elect to immediately intubate a patient with an airway burn or anaphylaxis with progressive swelling.

The classic scenario for employing this technique is the patient with distorted upper airway anatomy, such as that resulting from blunt or penetrating anterior neck trauma. Under these circumstances, intubation by RSI may be unsuccessful or impossible and subsequent BVM ventilation may allow air to enter the neck via the airway injury, complicating further management. Disadvantages of the awake oral intubation technique include oversedation, discomfort and stress, and potential for deleterious effects in patients with cardiac disorders or increased ICP.

Blind nasotracheal intubation

Although commonly employed previously, blind nasotracheal intubation (BNTI) has lost ground to other more effective airway approaches. When compared with RSI, BNTI consumes more time, fails more often, involves the passage of a smaller ETT, and results in a higher number of complications.

There are certain clinical circumstances (spontaneously breathing patient presenting with a difficult airway) where RSI is not advisable and BNTI may be the preferred route of intubation. In the patient with anatomic features that may pose a challenge to RSI and BVM ventilation, awake BNTI can be performed while preserving the patient's spontaneous respirations.

The procedure for BNTI begins with proper mucosal preparation to minimize epistaxis. Both nares should be sprayed with generous amounts of a topical vasoconstrictor anesthestic agent such as cocaine or the combination phenylephrine–lidocaine. Select a cuffed ETT size 0.5–1.0 mm smaller than would be used for oral intubation. The tube should be lubricated with KY jelly or another water-soluble lubricant to facilitate passage. The balloon at the distal portion of the ETT should be completely deflated. The bed may be reclined or left in the upright position, preferred by most patients and physicians. While standing to the side of the patient, the tube is inserted into the more patent of the two nares. The right side is preferable because the tube bevel will face the septum, thus avoiding Kiesselbach's plexus. If going through the left naris consider inserting the tube "upside down," then rotating it such that the curve follows the posterior nasopharynx once the turbinates are passed. Direct the tube straight back along the nasal floor toward the occiput, rotating it 15–30° with advancement. Once the tube has neared the glottis, listen for airflow within the tube and watch the chest rise with each breath. When maximal airflow is heard, quickly and gently advance the tube on inhalation. A cough will likely be heard with the passage of the tube into the trachea. The tube should be advanced to 32 cm at the naris in the adult male and 27–28 cm in the adult female. As the tube is placed blindly, it may also be misdirected into the esophagus, piriform sinus or vallecula (rare). When this occurs, withdraw the tube slightly, redirect and retry. If the tube becomes caught on the vocal cords, rotate the tube slightly to realign the bevel with the cords. Occasionally, external manipulation of the larynx posteriorly or laterally with one's nondominant hand will facilitate successful passage.

BNTI is contraindicated in the apneic patient, since air movement is essential to tube placement. BNTI is also contraindicated in patients with the possibility of cribriform plate injury, basilar skull or midface fracture out of concern that the tube may enter the cranial vault. Patients with bleeding disorders or coagulopathy may develop massive epistaxis from BNTI. A complete list of contraindications to BNTI is listed in Table 2.6.

Table 2.6 Contraindications to blind nasotracheal intubation

- Apnea
- Cribriform plate injury, basilar skull fracture, midface fracture
- Combative patients
- Increased intracranial pressure
- Coagulopathy or bleeding disorders
- Neck hematoma
- Upper airway obstruction or anatomic alteration from trauma, edema or infection
- Any patient requiring immediate airway management

Epistaxis and nasal turbinate injury from the procedure can be greatly reduced by prior administration of vasoconstrictor agents and proper technique. Long-term complications such as sinusitis or turbinate destruction are uncommon and result from multiple intubation attempts or prolonged intubation.

The difficult airway

It has been estimated that between 1–3% of patients present with a "difficulty airway," defined as difficulty securing the airway under direct laryngoscopic vision. Before administering NMBAs, the emergency physician should always assess the likelihood of a difficult intubation and the probability for success. Every intubation should be assumed difficult, especially in the pediatric population, and a back-up plan should be formulated prior to proceeding. Success or failure is often directly related to the airway

manager's ability to anticipate problems, prepare for the worst-case scenario and address failure (Figure 2.15).

The failed airway

The failed airway may be clinically defined in two manners:

1. The *"cannot intubate, can oxygenate"* scenario occurs when a skilled airway manager fails to intubate on three attempts but can successfully BVM ventilate the patient.
2. The *"cannot intubate, cannot oxygenate"* scenario arises when the failure to intubate, regardless of the number of attempts, occurs in the face of O_2 saturations that cannot be maintained above 90% or higher using a BVM.

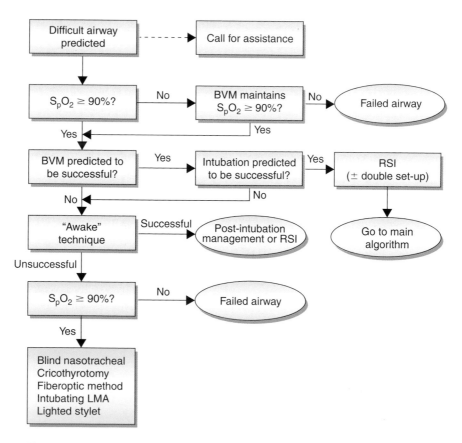

Figure 2.15
Algorithm for the difficult airway. LMA: laryngeal mask airway; BVM: bag-valve-mask; RSI: rapid sequence intubation; S_pO_2: saturated pressure of oxygen measured with pulse oximetry. Reproduced with permission from Walls RM et al, Manual of Emergency Airway Management, 2nd ed. and Companion Manual to the Airway Course (www.theairwaysite.com), Lippincott Williams & Wilkins, 2004.

The management of the failed airway is dictated by whether or not the patient can be oxygenated (Figure 2.16).

Devices and techniques for the difficult or failed intubation

This section briefly describes some of the devices and techniques that may be employed in the event of a difficult or failed intubation.

Lighted stylet intubation

The use of a lighted stylet apparatus utilizes transillumination of the soft tissues of the neck to signify correct ETT placement within the trachea. Due to the anterior location of the trachea relative to the esophagus, a well-defined, circumscribed glow can readily be seen in the anterior neck when the ETT and light enter the glottic opening. If the tip of the tube is placed in the esophagus, the light glow is diffuse and not well seen.

Retrograde intubation

Retrograde intubation involves needle puncture of the cricothyroid membrane followed by threading a guidewire retrograde through the vocal cords and out the mouth or nose. The wire is then used to guide the ETT through the glottis before it is removed.

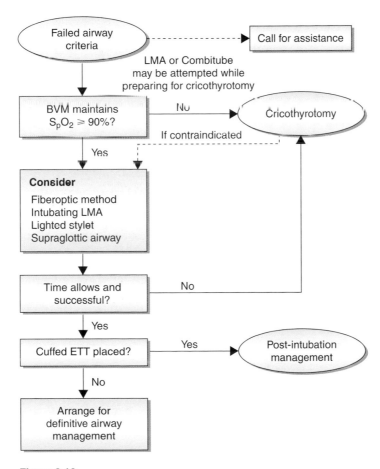

Figure 2.16
Algorithm for the failed airway. ETT: endotracheal tube; BVM: bag-valve mask; S_pO_2: saturated pressure of oxygen measured with pulse oximetry. LMA: laryngeal mask airway. Reproduced with permission from Walls RM et al, Manual of Emergency Airway Management, 2nd ed. and Companion Manual to the Airway Course (www.theairwaysite.com), Lippincott Williams & Wilkins, 2004.

Digital intubation

Digital intubation is a technique in which the index and long fingers of the nondominant hand are used to identify the epiglottis and then manually direct an ETT into the larynx. This requires a profoundly unresponsive patient.

Laryngeal mask airway

The laryngeal mask airway (LMA) is a modified ETT with an inflatable, oval collar ("laryngeal mask") at its base. The LMA is blindly inserted into the pharynx where it covers the glottic opening. Inflation of the collar provides a seal that allows tracheal ventilation. Though these devices are relatively easy to use, they do not provide a definitive airway since the supraglottic cuff does not prevent aspiration.

An updated version of the original LMA, known as the intubating LMA, facilitates blind endotracheal intubation by allowing passage of an ETT through the device and into the trachea with a high degree of success.

Combitube™

The Combitube™ is a dual-lumen, dual-cuffed esophageal/tracheal airway; one lumen functions as an esophageal airway while the other performs as a tracheal airway. Though the Combitube is blindly inserted and typically enters the esophagus, the presence of dual lumens allows ventilation even if it inadvertently enters the trachea.

Fiberoptic intubation

Fiberoptic techniques for endotracheal intubation have emerged as invaluable tools for the management of the difficult airway. These include the use of fiberoptic intubating bronchoscopes, rigid fiberoptic laryngoscopes, and ETTs with embedded fiberoptic bundles. These devices require considerable technical skill and repeated practice to maintain speed and success.

Surgical airways

Surgical airway management, unlike conventional airway management, entails the creation of an opening into the trachea to provide oxygenation and ventilation. Proficiency with surgical airway techniques can mean the difference between life and death.

Cricothyrotomy

Cricothyrotomy is the creation of a surgical opening through the cricothyroid membrane to allow placement of an ETT or cuffed tracheostomy tube (Figure 2.17). The proximal ends of these tubes can be hooked up to a BVM for oxygenation and ventilation. A primary indication for cricothyrotomy is the need for a definitive airway in the patient in whom orotracheal or BNTI has failed, is contraindicated or is extremely difficult. A classic example is the patient with severe facial trauma in whom conventional airway management is extremely complicated or unfeasible.

The primary contraindication to cricothyrotomy is young age. Due to anatomic considerations, the procedure is extremely difficult in children <10–12 years of age and therefore generally avoided in this population. Other contraindications to cricothyrotomy include preexisting tracheal or laryngeal pathology, anatomic obliteration of the landmarks (i.e., hematoma), coagulopathy and operator inexperience with the procedure. Complications of cricothyrotomy include incorrect airway placement, hemorrhage, tracheal or laryngeal injury, infection, pneumomediastinum, subglottic stenosis and voice change.

Transtracheal jet ventilation (TTJV)

An alternative surgical airway procedure is needle cricothyrotomy with percutaneous TTJV (Figure 2.18). In this technique, a transtracheal catheter is inserted through the cricothyroid membrane into the trachea and connected to a jet ventilation system which includes high-pressure tubing, an oxygen source at 50 psi, and an in-line one-way valve for intermittent administration of oxygen. 100% oxygen is then delivered at 12–20 bursts per minute. The inspiratory phase should last 1 second while the expiratory phase lasts 2–4 seconds.

Advantages of this technique include its simplicity, safety and speed. There is typically less bleeding when compared with cricothyrotomy, and age is not a contraindication, making it the preferred surgical airway in children <12 years.

During TTJV, the upper airway must be free of obstruction to allow for complete exhalation, or the patient is at risk of barotrauma from air stacking. All patients receiving TTJV should have an oral and nasal airway placed. Unlike cricothyrotomy, TTJV does not provide complete airway protection. Therefore, it should be considered a temporizing measure until a definitive airway can be established.

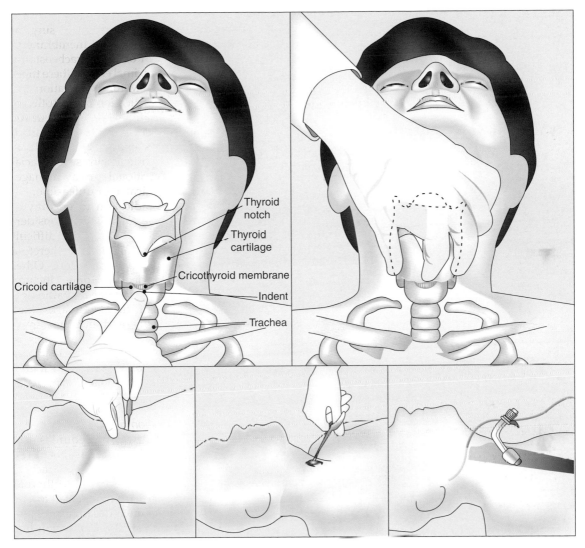

Figure 2.17
Surgical cricothyrotomy. Used with permission from American College of Surgeons' Committee on Trauma, *Advanced Trauma Life Support © for Doctors, Student Course Manual*, 6th ed., Chicago, American College of Surgeons, 1997, page 85.

Special patients

Pediatric

Though the principles of airway management in adults and children are the same, a number of age-related differences must be accounted for when managing the pediatric airway. Specific anatomic differences between adults and children and their clinical significance in airway management are summarized in Table 2.7 and Figure 2.19.

Physiologically, pediatric patients have a higher rate of O_2 consumption and smaller functional residual capacity; therefore, they tend to desaturate more rapidly than adults. Compared with adults, children tend to have a shortened period of protection from hypoxia following pre-oxygenation, and infants and small children may require BVM ventilation during RSI to avoid hypoxia.

Airway equipment selection is also based on the child's weight and length (Table 2.8). A child's ETT size can be estimated by the size of their external naris, the diameter of their little finger, or the formula ETT size = 4 + (age in years/4). The depth of ETT placement may be remembered as approximately three times ETT size or (age in years/2) + 12.

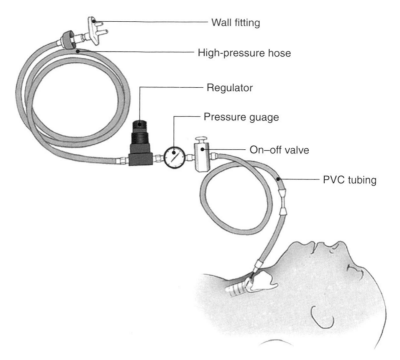

Figure 2.18
Transtracheal jet ventilation. PVC: polyvinyl chloride.

Table 2.7 Anatomic airway differences between children and adults. Reproduced with permission from Walls RM et al, Manual of Emergency Airway Management, 2nd ed. and Companion Manual to the Airway Course (www.theairwaysite.com), Lippincott Williams & Wilkins, 2004

Anatomy	Clinical significance
Large intraoral tongue occupying relatively large portion of the oral cavity High tracheal opening: C1 in infancy versus C3–4 at age 7, C4–5 in the adult	1. High anterior airway position of the glottic opening compared with that in adults 2. Straight blade preferred over curved to push distensible anatomy out of the way to visualize the larynx
Large occiput that may cause flexion of the airway, large tongue that easily collapses against the posterior pharynx	Sniffing position is preferred. The large occiput actually elevates the head into the sniffing position in most infants and children. A towel may be required under shoulders to elevate torso relative to head in small infants
Cricoid ring narrowest portion of the trachea as compared with the vocal cords in the adult	1. Uncuffed tubes provide adequate seal as they fit snugly at the level of the cricoid ring 2. Correct tube size essential since variable expansion cuffed tubes not used
Consistent anatomic variations with age with fewer abnormal variations related to body habitus, arthritis, chronic disease	<2 years, high anterior 2 to 8, transition >8, small adult
Large tonsils and adenoids may bleed. More acute angle between epiglottis and laryngeal opening results in nasotracheal intubation attempt failures	Blind nasotracheal intubation not indicated in children Nasotracheal intubation failure
Small cricothyroid membrane	Needle cricothyroidotomy difficult, surgical cricothyroidotomy impossible in infants and small children

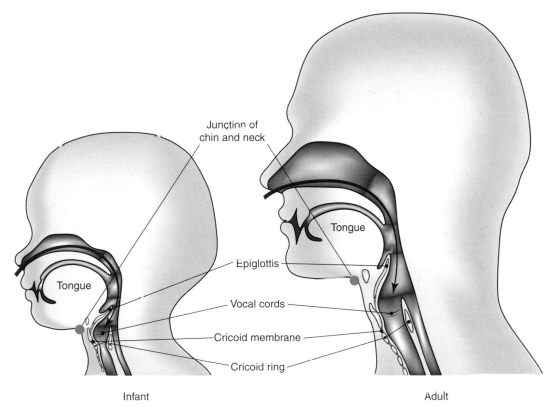

Junction of
chin and neck

Tongue

Epiglottis

Tongue

Vocal cords

Cricoid membrane

Cricoid ring

Infant

Adult

Figure 2.19
Anatomic airway differences between children and adults. The anatomic differences particular to children include: 1. Higher, more anterior position for the glottic opening. (Note the relationship of the vocal cords to the chin/neck junction). 2. Relatively larger tongue in the infant, which lies between the mouth and glottic opening. 3. Relatively larger and more floppy epiglottis in the child. 4. Cricoid ring is the narrowest portion of the pediatric airway; in adults, it is the vocal cords. 5. Position and size of the cricothyroid membrane in the infant. 6. Sharper, more difficult angle for blind nasotracheal intubation. 7. Larger relative size of the occiput in the infant. Reproduced with permission from Walls RM et al, Manual of Emergency Airway Management, 2nd ed. and Companion Manual to the Airway Course (www.theairwaysite.com), Lippincott Williams & Wilkins, 2004.

Drug dosing in children and the choice of medications for RSI is based on a child's age and weight. Of note, the dose of SCh is higher in children (2 mg/kg) and infants (3 mg/kg) than in adults. Children younger than 5 years are not given a defasciculating dose of a nondepolarizing NMBA but are treated with atropine to prevent bradycardia from airway manipulation. Atropine should also be administered to all children <10 years of age receiving SCh to prevent bradycardia. Fentanyl should be used with caution in infants and small children, as it may lead to respiratory depression or hypotension.

Status asthmaticus

Managing the sick asthma patient in the ED can present a tremendous challenge. Fatigue from prolonged respiratory effort in the face of severe small airway resistance commonly results in respiratory failure; approximately 1–3% of asthma exacerbations require intubation. In general, these patients are extremely difficult to pre-oxygenate due to a reduced functional residual capacity, and may be very difficult to ventilate with a BVM as a result of severe airway obstruction.

The single most important intervention in the patient with status asthmaticus and respiratory failure is early control of the airway. RSI is the method of choice (performed by the most experienced laryngoscopist) along with preparation for rescue cricothyrotomy. When compared with RSI, BNTI is more time-consuming, results in greater O_2 desaturation, and has a higher rate of complication or failure.

Table 2.8 Pediatric airway equipment selection. Reproduced with permission from Walls et al, Manual of Emergency Airway Management, 2nd ed. and Companion Manual to the Airway Course (www.theairwaysite.com), Lippincott Williams & Wilkins, 2004

Length (cm) and weight (kg) based pediatric equipment chart

	Pink 6–7	Red 8–9	Purple 10–11	Yellow 12–14	White 15–18	Blue 19–23	Orange 23–31	Green 31–41
Weight (kg)								
Length (cm)	60.75–67.75	67.75–75.25	75.25–85	85–98.25	98.25–110.75	110.75–122.5	122.5–137.5	137.5–155
ETT size (mm)	3.5	3.5	4.0	4.5	5.0	5.5	6.0 cuff	6.5 cuff
Lip-tip length (mm)	10.5	10.5	12.0	13.5	15.0	16.5	18.0	19.5
Laryngoscope	1 Straight	1 Straight	1 Straight	2 Straight	2 Straight	2 Straight or curved	2 Straight or curved	3 Straight or curved
Suction catheter	8F	8F	8F	8–10F	10F	10F	10F	12F
Stylet	6F	6F	6F	6F	6F	14F	14F	14F
Oral airway	50 mm	50 mm	60 mm	60 mm	60 mm	70 mm	80 mm	80 mm
Nasopharyngeal airway	14F	14F	18F	20F	22F	24F	26F	30F
Bag-valve device	Infant	Infant	Child	Child	Child	Child	Child/adult	Adult
Oxygen mask	Newborn	Newborn	Pediatric	Pediatric	Pediatric	Pediatric	Adult	Adult
Vascular access	22–24/23–25	22–24/23–25	20–22/23–25	18–22/21–23	18–22/21–23	18–20/21–23	18–20/21–22	16–20/18–21
Catheter/butterfly	intraosseous	intraosseous	intraosseous	intraosseous	intraosseous	intraosseous		
Nasogastric tube	5–8F	5–8F	8–10F	10F	10–12F	12–14F	14–18F	18F
Urinary catheter	5–8F	5–8F	8–10F	10F	10–12F	10–12F	12F	12F
Chest tube	10–12F	10–12F	16–20F	20–24F	20–24F	24–32F	24–32F	32–40F
Blood pressure cuff	Newborn/infant	Newborn/infant	Infant/child	Child	Child	Child	Child/adult	Adult
LMA[†]	1.5	1.5	2	2	2	2–2.5	2.5	3

Directions for use: 1. Measure patient length with centimeter tape, or with a Broselow tape; 2. Using measured length in centimeters or Broselow tape measurement, access appropriate equipment column; 3. For endotracheal tubes, oral and nasopharyngeal airways, and laryngeal mask airways (LMAs), always select one size smaller and one size larger than the recommended size, in addition to the recommended size.

[†]Based on manufacturer's weight-based guidelines.

Mask size: 1 1.5 2 2.5 3

Patient size (kg): up to 5 5–10 10–20 20–30 Over 30

Permission to reproduce with modification from Lutten RC, Wears RL, Broselow J, et al. *Ann Emerg Med* 1992;21:900–904.

If the patient is most comfortable sitting upright, allow him to maintain that position. All patients should be pretreated with lidocaine 1.5 mg/kg which suppresses coughing, improves ETT tolerance and reduces bronchospasm. Ketamine 1.5 mg/kg is the induction agent of choice in status asthmaticus as it stimulates the release of catecholamines and produces bronchodilation.

Upon loss of consciousness, the patient should be laid supine and intubated. The largest possible ETT should be used to allow for aggressive pulmonary toilet. The intubated asthmatic patient should then be paralyzed and sedated to facilitate oxygenation and ventilation. The patient's clinical condition may worsen after intubation if the patient proves to be difficult to ventilate, develops a tension pneumothorax or develops hypotension; caution is warranted.

Increased intracranial pressure

The presence or suspicion of increased ICP directly affects the approach to RSI, as the techniques and medications used during RSI may further increase the patient's ICP. There is a reflex sympathetic response to laryngoscopy that results in a systemic release of catecholamines and increased ICP. This response can be blunted through the administration of fentanyl (3 mcg/kg), which is given over 30–60 seconds during the pretreatment phase of RSI. Laryngoscopy or any laryngeal stimulation (i.e., suctioning) may also increase ICP by a direct reflex mechanism unrelated to this catecholamine surge. The administration of lidocaine (1.5 mg/kg) during the pretreatment phase effectively blunts this response and may also reduce ICP.

Unlike nondepolarizing NMBAs, SCh administration increases ICP. However, the administration of a small "defasciculating dose" (about one-tenth the paralyzing dose) of a competitive neuromuscular blocker given during the pretreatment phase mitigates this response. Pancuronium (0.01 mg/kg) or vecuronium (0.01 mg/kg) administered 3 minutes before the administration of SCh effectively blunts the rise in ICP.

The ideal induction agent should reduce ICP, maintain cerebral perfusion and provide some cerebral protective effect. Sodium thiopental effectively reduces ICP by decreasing cerebral blood flow, and confers a cerebroprotective effect by lowering O_2 utilization within the brain. However, thiopental is a potent venodilator and negative inotrope which can lead to hypotension,

a factor associated with significantly increased mortality in head-injured patients. Etomidate has emerged as the induction agent of choice in patients with increased ICP. It reduces ICP and confers cerebroprotection in a manner similar to thiopental but provides remarkable hemodynamic stability.

Suspected cervical spine injury

All patients with significant blunt trauma are assumed to be at risk for cervical spine injury. Inadvertent movement of the neck of a patient with an unstable cervical spine injury can lead to permanent neurologic disability or death. Accordingly, many trauma patients are transported to the ED in a stiff cervical collar and immobilized to a backboard. Though providing protection of the cervical spine, immobilization places the patient at risk for aspiration and ventilatory compromise.

If the patient requires airway management, precious time should not be wasted obtaining a single lateral radiograph of the cervical spine to exclude cervical spine injury. This approach delays definitive airway management and provides a false sense of security, as a single view is inadequate to exclude injury to the cervical spine.

Numerous studies have shown that the proper approach to managing these patients is RSI with in-line immobilization (Figure 2.20). Paralyzing

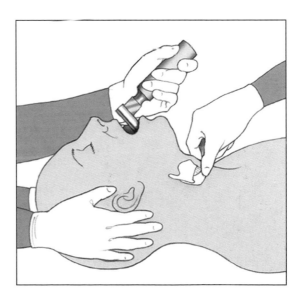

Figure 2.20
In-line immoblilization of the cervical spine.

the patient reduces the risk of patient movement during intubation. A second individual maintaining immobilization of the head and neck in the neutral position throughout the procedure prevents neck hyperextension during laryngoscopy.

Pearls, pitfalls, and myths

- Learn to recognize objective signs of impending airway compromise.
- Though bedside maneuvers or airway adjuncts can reestablish airway patency, they do not provide definitive airway protection.
- A definitive airway requires an ETT in the trachea secured in place with the cuff inflated and attached to an O_2-rich ventilation device.
- Competence with the bag-valve-mask is required for airway management.
- Lifesaving medications may be given via the ETT.
- Learn the 9 P's of Rapid Sequence Intubation
- Prior to initiating RSI, prepare for intubation using the mnemonic *SOAP ME*.
- Adequate preoxygenation may allow the larygnoscopist several attempts for successful intubation prior to arterial O_2 desaturation.
- Select your pretreatment (LOAD) medications to mitigate the adverse effects of SCh and the act of intubation.
- NBMAs do not provide analgesia, sedation or amnesia, so always provide an induction agent prior to neuromuscular blockade.
- After any unsuccessful intubation attempt, change "something" prior to the next attempt.
- Proper ETT placement needs to be confirmed after every intubation; do not rely on only one approach as the sole means for confirming ETT placement.
- Following confirmation of ETT placement, secure the ETT, check vital signs, order a chest X-ray and provide long-term sedation and paralysis (if appropriate).
- Not every patient needs RSI. Learn the indications and techniques for awake oral intubation and BNTI.
- Every intubation should be assumed difficult, and a back-up plan should be formulated prior to proceeding.

- Be familiar with the algorithms, devices, and techniques used for the failed airway.
- Airway equipment selection and drug dosing is based on a child's age, weight and length. A child's ETT size = 4 + (age in years/4).
- Use RSI with in-line immobilization for airway management of any patient with potential cervical spine injury.

References

1. *ATLS: Advanced Trauma Life Support for Doctors*. American College of Surgeons. 1997.
2. Cummins RO (ed.). *ACLS Provider Manual*. American Heart Association. 2002.
3. Danzl DF. Tracheal intubation and mechanical ventilation. In: Tintinalli JE (ed.). *Emergency Medicine: A Comprehensive Study Guide*, 5th ed., McGraw Hill, 2000.
4. Dieckmann R (ed.). *Pediatric Education for Prehospital Providers*. American Academy of Pediatrics, 2000.
5. Doak SA. Airway management. In: Hamilton G (ed.). *Emergency Medicine: An Approach to Clinical Problem-Solving*, 2nd ed., W.B. Saunders, 2003.
6. Hazinski MF (ed.). *PALS Provider Manual*. American Heart Association, 2002.
7. Kaide CG, Hollingsworth JH. *Current Strategies for Airway Management in the Trauma Patient*, Parts 1 and 2. *Traum Rep* 2003, 4(1&2).
8. McGill JW, Cliinton JE. Tracheal intubation. In: Roberts JR, Hedges JR (eds). *Clinical Procedures in Emergency Medicine*, 3rd ed., 1998.
9. Parr MJA, et al. Airway management. In: Skinner D, Swain A, Peyton R, Robertson C (eds). *Cambridge Textbook of Accident and Emergency Medicine*, 5th ed., Cambridge University Press, 1997.
10. Roman AM. Non-invasive airway management. In: Tintinalli JE (ed.). *Emergency Medicine: A Comprehensive Study Guide*, 5th ed., McGraw Hill, 2000.
11. Rubin M, Sadovnikoff N. Pediatric airway management. In: Tintinalli JE (ed.). *Emergency Medicine: A Comprehensive Study Guide*, 5th ed., McGraw Hill, 2000.
12. Vanstrum GS. Airway. In: Vanstrum GS (ed.). *Anesthesia in Emergency Medicine*. Little, Brown and Company, 1989.

13. Walls R (ed.). *Manual of Emergency Airway Management*. Philadelphia: Lippincott Williams & Wilkins, 2000.

14. Walls RM. Airway. In: Marx JA (ed.). *Rosen's Emergency Medicine: Concepts and Clinical Practice*, 5th ed., St. Louis: Mosby, 2002.

15. Ward KR. Trauma airway management. In: Harwood-Nuss A (ed.). *The Clinical Practice of Emergency Medicine*, 3rd ed., Philadelphia: Lippincott Williams & Wilkins, 2001.

3 Cardiopulmonary and cerebral resuscitation

Robert R. Leschke, MD

Introduction

One of the defining characteristics of emergency physicians is their ability to recognize and manage the undifferentiated patient in cardiac or respiratory arrest. Emergency practitioners must be experts in understanding the pathophysiology of cardiopulmonary arrest and the principles behind the resuscitation of these patients.

Modern cardiopulmonary resuscitation (CPR) began in the late 1950s with the rediscovery of closed chest cardiac massage and mouth-to-mouth ventilation. Advances in external defibrillation and other non-invasive techniques improved success rates of resuscitation and increased the number of individuals who could be adequately trained to immediately provide these interventions. The highest potential survival rate from cardiac arrest can be achieved when there is recognition of early warning signs, activation of the emergency medical system (EMS), rapid initiation of basic CPR, rapid defibrillation and Advanced Cardiovascular Life Support (ACLS), including definitive airway management and intravenous (IV) medications. These steps are known as the "chain of survival."

While many factors determine survival from cardiac arrest, initiation of early CPR has been scientifically shown to save lives. Data from Seattle demonstrated successful outcome in 27% of patients if ACLS is started within 8 minutes of cardiac arrest. The *Journal of the American Medical Association* reported that for patients who have CPR started within 4 minutes of arrest and ACLS within 8 minutes, successful resuscitation is increased to 43%.

Pathophysiology

Sudden cardiac death due to unexpected cardiac arrest claims the lives of an estimated 250,000 adult Americans each year. Most of these events will occur outside of the hospital. The majority of these patients are men between the ages of 50 and 75 years, who have significant atherosclerotic heart disease. Underlying disease and co-morbid factors significantly affect the metabolic state of cells before the onset of cardiac ischemia and alter the ability of cells to recover from a prolonged ischemic event. Hypoxia or hypotension prior to arrest, even if brief, creates tissue acidosis in diseased cells, making them more resistant to resuscitative efforts.

Cardiac arrest results in cessation of blood flow throughout the body. Anaerobic metabolism begins almost immediately. A cascade of metabolic events is created, including calcium release, generation of free radicals, and activation of catabolic enzymes that further injure the body's cells. The brain is most susceptible to the absence of circulation and traditionally suffers irreversible damage after 5 minutes in an arrest state. Restoration of pre-arrest neurologic function rarely occurs in patients with untreated cardiac arrest of longer than 10 minutes duration. The heart is the second most susceptible organ. Patients who suffer cardiac arrest from a non-cardiac cause remain at risk for secondary cardiac ischemia in the post-resuscitation period.

CPR, even utilizing maximal chest compressions, can only generate 30% of baseline cardiac output. The resuscitation period, therefore, still contributes to ongoing global ischemia. The goal of CPR is to preferentially direct blood flow to the heart and brain in order to adequately restore organized myocardial electrical activity while minimizing ischemic brain injury. There are two main theories to explain how this happens. In the *cardiac compression model*, the heart is squeezed between the sternum and the thoracic spine creating a pressure gradient between the ventricles and the great vessels. This causes blood to flow into the systemic and pulmonary arterial circulation. In the *thoracic pump model*, chest compressions cause a rise in the intrathoracic pressure that creates a pressure gradient between the intrathoracic vascular bed and the extrathoracic arterial bed, which causes blood to flow down the pressure gradient.

The primary survey

Emergency personnel need a systematic approach to resuscitation. The simplest and most familiar approach follows the concept of the primary and secondary surveys, and utilizes the ABCs (Airway, Breathing, Circulation) as a reminder (Figure 3.1).

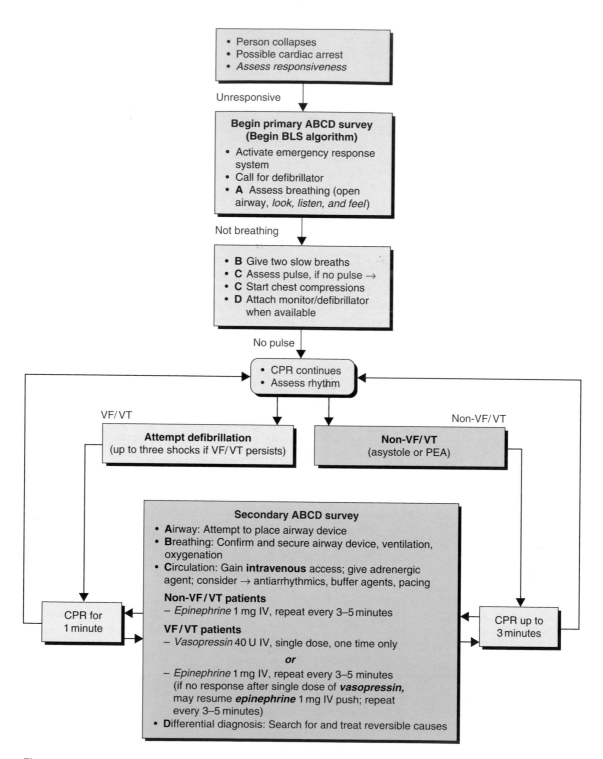

Figure 3.1
Comprehensive emergency cardiovascular care algorithm. ABCD: Airway, Breathing, Circulation, Defibrillation; CPR: cardiopulmonary resuscitation; VF: ventricular fibrillation; VT: ventricular tachycardia; PEA: pulseless electrical activity; BLS: Basic Life Support. Reproduced with permission, ACLS Provider Manual, © 2001, Copyright American Heart Association.

In the primary survey, the focus is on basic CPR and defibrillation:

Airway: Open the airway
Breathing: Provide positive-pressure ventilation
Circulation: Give chest compressions
Defibrillation: Identify and shock ventricular fibrillation (VF) and ventricular tachycardia (VT)

Airway

The first step to assessing the patient's airway is to look for respiratory activity, listen for breathing, and feel for air exchange at the patient's nose and mouth. If these are present, assess the patient's ability to protect the airway by asking them to speak. If the patient can speak, immediate definitive airway management is not likely needed. If the patient does not respond to questions, the absence of a strong gag reflex confirms the inadequacy of protective airway mechanisms. Once you have established that the patient is not breathing or unable to protect the airway, steps must be taken to provide airway support. If you are alone in the room, immediately call for assistance and then place the patient in a supine position. One must be careful in a patient who is suspected of having neck trauma to maintain in-line stabilization of the cervical spine. This is performed by keeping one hand behind the head and neck while the other hand rolls the patient toward you.

Once the patient is correctly positioned on his/her back, open the airway. An unresponsive or unconscious patient will have decreased muscle tone, allowing the tongue and epiglottis to fall back and obstruct the pharynx and larynx. In order to correctly position the head and open the airway of the patient without suspected traumatic injury, use the *head tilt-chin lift maneuver* (Figure 2.4). If standing on the patient's right side, place the left hand on the patient's forehead and the fingers of the right hand under the bony part of the chin. Simultaneously apply firm backward pressure on the forehead tilting the head back and lifting the chin up and forward. Open the patient's mouth to prepare for ventilation. If there is visible foreign material in the airway, it should be removed or suctioned away.

If there is the possibility of neck trauma, the head tilt-chin lift maneuver could cause cervical spine injury if the neck is hyper-extended. In such cases, the *jaw thrust maneuver* (Figure 2.5)

should be utilized. To perform this maneuver, position yourself at the patient's head. Place your thumbs on the zygomatic arches on either side of the face. Grasp the angles of the victim's lower jaw with your remaining fingers, and lift the lower jaw up and forward. Visible foreign material in the airway should be removed or suctioned away.

Breathing

Most victims suffering from cardiopulmonary arrest will not breathe spontaneously. After positioning the head and opening the airway, one should quickly assess for chest excursion and the presence of exhalation. If the patient is not breathing or has inadequate respirations, assist the patient with artificial respiration. In the emergency department (ED) setting, a bag-valve-mask device should be readily available. Utilizing the same technique as the jaw thrust maneuver for opening the airway, squeeze the mask between your thumbs and your remaining fingers as you lift the jaw. This will create an airtight seal while another rescuer provides rescue breathing through compression of the bag. If you are alone, apply the mask to the patient's face. Place the middle, ring, and little fingers of one hand along the bony portion of the mandible, and place the thumb and index finger of the same hand on the mask. Squeeze the mask between your fingers on to the patient's face to create an airtight seal. Compress the bag with your other hand. Provide rescue breaths of 2 seconds duration while watching for chest rise.

If you do not see the chest rise or find it difficult to compress air from the bag into the patient's airway, reposition the head and mask and try again. If subsequent attempts to ventilate the patient are unsuccessful, the patient may have an obstructed airway. Open the patient's mouth by grasping both the tongue and the lower jaw between the thumb and fingers, and then lift the mandible. If you see obstructing material, use a McGill forceps or clamp to remove it. If this equipment is not available, slide your index finger down the inside of the cheek to the base of the tongue and dislodge any foreign bodies using a hooking action. Use caution to avoid pushing any obstructing material further down the airway.

If you still cannot effectively administer rescue breathing and suspect an obstructed airway, perform abdominal thrusts. These abdominal thrusts elevate the diaphragm and increase airway pressure. The resulting air escape from the lungs can effectively dislodge an obstructing foreign body from the upper airway. To perform this maneuver, place the heel of one hand against the patient's abdomen just above the navel and well below the xiphoid process. Place your other hand on top of the first. Press both hands into the abdomen five times in a quick upward-thrusting motion maintaining a midline position. Then, reattempt ventilation.

Circulation

In the patient with suspected cardiopulmonary arrest, one should check for a carotid pulse, as this is the most central of the peripheral arteries. A carotid pulse may persist even in the presence of poor perfusion. If no pulse is present, chest compressions should be initiated and the patient should be placed on a cardiac monitor. To adequately perform chest compressions, the heel of one hand should be placed in the midline on the lower part of the sternum (just above the notch where the ribs meet the lower sternum). The other hand is placed on top of the first hand and the fingers interlocked and kept off of the chest. Position your shoulders directly over your hands and lock your elbows. Depress the sternum about 1.5–2 inches approximately 100 times per minute, while allowing another member of the team to give rescue breathing after every five compressions. Properly performed compressions can produce a systolic blood pressure of 60 mmHg.

Defibrillation

Cardiac arrest from a primary cardiac etiology typically presents as ventricular fibrillation (VF) or less often as pulseless ventricular tachycardia (VT). Both are treated identically. Early defibrillation is the one intervention that has been shown to increase survival for patients in VF or pulseless

VT. When defibrillation can be successfully performed within the first minute or two, as many as 90% of patients return to their pre-arrest neurologic status. The longer the patient remains in cardiac arrest, the more likely that defibrillation and resuscitation will be unsuccessful. Survival rates are <10% when defibrillation is delayed 10 minutes or more after a patient's collapse.

The term automatic external defibrillator (AED) refers to a sophisticated computerized device that incorporates a rhythm analysis system and a shock advisory system. AEDs are designed to recognize VF or VT and advise the user to deliver an electric shock to convert the non-perfusing rhythm to a perfusing one. Placing AEDs in public access areas like airports, sports stadiums, or restaurants allows quicker access to life-saving defibrillation. When police officers in Rochester, Minnesota were equipped with an AED, survival from out-of-hospital VF averaged 50% with a median time from collapse to defibrillation of 5 minutes. Similar statistics have been reported in public access trials in other states. These survival rates are twice those previously reported for the most effective emergency medical systems (EMS).

Since survival from VF or pulseless VT is so time-sensitive, defibrillation in witnessed VF or pulseless VT should preclude any other type of evaluation. Defibrillation should be attempted with up to three shocks as soon as the diagnosis is made (Figure 3.2). Using gel or defibrillation pads, one paddle should be placed to the right of the sternum below the right clavicle and the other in the midaxillary line at the level of the nipple. Firm pressure of approximately 25 lb should be applied to each paddle. Alternatively, "hands off" defibrillator pads can be used that are placed on the chest and the back, sandwiching the heart.

Successful defibrillation depends on the amount of current transmitted across the heart. This is proportional to the energy output of the defibrillator and inversely proportional to the

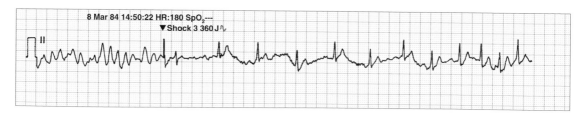

Figure 3.2
Rhythm strip of a patient with pulseless ventricular tachycardia (VT). Following the third defibrillation attempt at 360 J, the patient returned to sinus rhythm. HR: heart rate; J: joules; SpO₂: saturated pressure of oxygen. *Courtesy*: S.V. Mahadevan, MD.

transthoracic impedance, which depends on chest size, phase of respiration, and other variables. Current defibrillators are monophasic and do not adjust for the transthoracic impedance. The first biphasic waveform defibrillator was approved in 1996. While not used in all EDs worldwide, the biphasic waveform adjusts for differences in transthoracic impedance, allowing less energy requirements for successful defibrillation. Animal studies showed their superiority over monophasic defibrillation for the termination of VF and pulseless VT. Early clinical experience with 150 J biphasic waveform defibrillation for treatment of VF was very positive. Evidence to date suggests that non-progressive impedance-adjusted low-energy biphasic countershock (150 J three times) is safe, acceptable, and clinically effective.

The secondary survey

The secondary survey uses the same mnemonic as the primary survey; however, the interventions are more involved and aggressive:

Airway: Definitive airway management
Breathing: Confirmation of adequate ventilation
Circulation: Intravenous access, ACLS medications, fluids
Defibrillation: Continued rhythm analysis and treatment

Airway

Endotracheal intubation is the most effective method of ensuring adequate ventilation, oxygenation, and airway protection against aspiration during cardiac arrest. In addition, it is an additional route of entry for some resuscitation medications, such as atropine, epinephrine, and lidocaine. Refer to Chapter 2 for a detailed discussion of the preparation and performance of definitive airway management.

Breathing

If the patient has been intubated in the pre-hospital setting, the adequacy of intubation should be checked by auscultating the chest for equal bilateral breath sounds, identifying fog in the endotracheal tube on exhalation, and monitoring end-tidal CO_2 (using colorimetry or capnography). The presence of exhaled CO_2 on a monitor indicates proper

tracheal tube placement and can detect subsequent tube dislodgement. False readings can occur if CO_2 delivery is low in cardiac arrest patients due to low blood flow to the lungs. False readings have also been reported in patients who ingested carbonated liquids prior to intubation. A chest X-ray can help determine the location of the tip of the endotracheal tube in relation to the carina. The patient should be placed on a ventilator for positive-pressure ventilation. Continuous high flow oxygen and pulse oximetry should be maintained.

Circulation

Intravenous (IV) access should be obtained, preferably with a central venous catheter in the internal jugular, subclavian, or femoral vein. Two large bore peripheral lines may be acceptable and IV fluids should be infused. The patient's rhythm should be identified and appropriate interventions instituted based on accepted ACLS guidelines (see Figures 3.1, 3.3–3.5).

Ventricular fibrillation (VF) or pulseless ventricular tachycardia (VT)

VF and pulseless VT remain the most common underlying rhythms of cardiac arrest (Figure 3.3). The therapeutic goal is to convert these nonperfusing rhythms into perfusing ones. Early defibrillation has been shown to be the most effective intervention, which is why recognition of VF/VT and defibrillation are addressed in the primary survey. If VF or pulseless VT is refractory to three initial attempts at defibrillation, vasopressor therapy in the form of epinephrine or vasopressin should be administered. These agents have been shown to improve the success rate of subsequent defibrillation attempts as well as improve myocardial and cerebral perfusion during CPR. Antiarrhythmic agents such as amiodarone, lidocaine and procainamide raise the fibrillation threshold. Administration of these agents should always be followed by repeated countershocks. The patient's cardiac rhythm should be monitored for changes between interventions, with resuscitation strategies modified based on any changes in rhythm or perfusion.

Asystole and bradycardia

Bradycardia leading to asystole uniformly has a poor prognosis. The goal of therapy is to increase the heart rate to provide a perfusing blood pressure or, in the case of asystole, to re-establish a spontaneous rhythm (Figure 3.4). Primary brady-cardia occurs when the heart's intrinsic electrical system fails to generate an adequate heart rate. Secondary bradycardia occurs when factors other than the heart's own electrical system cause a slow rate, such as hypoxia, stroke, or cardiodepressant medications (beta blockers, calcium channel blockers, or opiates). Atropine and epinephrine are two medications that have demonstrated benefit in this setting. Atropine has a vagolytic effect by antagonizing the parasympathetic system. Epinephrine improves myocardial and cerebral blood flow during CPR. Though early transcutaneous pacing should be considered for bradycardia, routine transcutaneous pacing for asystole has not been shown to improve survival. As some

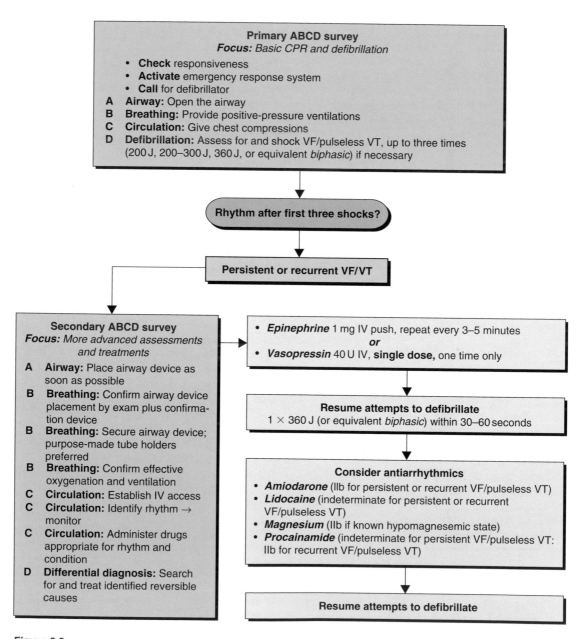

Figure 3.3
Ventricular fibrillation or pulseless ventricular tachycardia algorithm. VF: ventricular fibrillation; VT: ventricular tachycardia; ABCD: Airway, Breathing, Circulation, Defibrillation; CPR: cardiopulmonary resuscitation.
Reproduced with permission, ACLS Provider Manual, © 2001, Copyright American Heart Association.

patients with asystole are actually in fine VF, two or more cardiac leads should be checked before determining that the patient is truly in asystole. A recent large randomized study from Europe comparing epinephrine with vasopressin for patients in asystole demonstrated that vasopressin was superior to epinephrine, suggesting that vasopressin followed by epinephrine may be more effective than epinephrine alone in the treatment of refractory cardiac arrest.

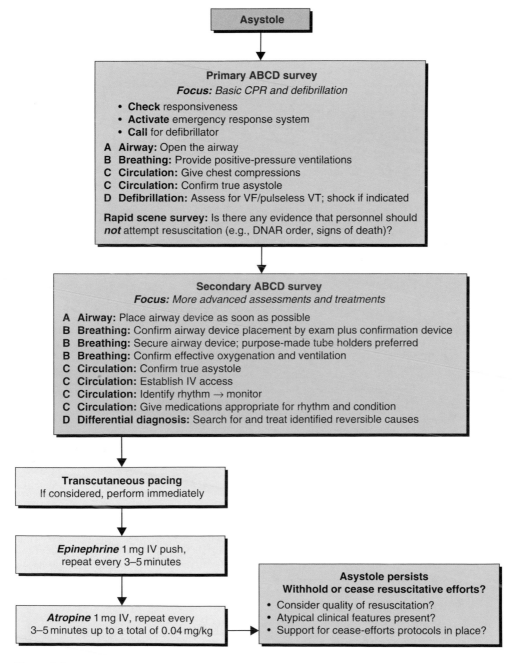

Figure 3.4
Asystole: The silent heart algorithm. ABCD: Airway, Breathing, Circulation, Defibrillation; CPR: cardiopulmonary resuscitation; VF: ventricular fibrillation; VT: ventricular tachycardia; DNAR: do-not-attempt resuscitation. Reproduced with permission, ACLS Provider Manual, © 2001, Copyright American Heart Association.

Pulseless electrical activity

Pulseless electrical activity (PEA), formerly known as electromechanical dissociation (EMD), is defined as cardiac electrical activity without associated mechanical pumping. These patients will have a rhythm but no pulse. Successful resuscitation of patients with PEA should focus on determining and reversing the cause (Figure 3.5). The most common causes include severe hypovolemia (usually related to significant blood loss), hypoxia, acidosis, pericardial tamponade, tension pneumothorax, large pulmonary embolus, myocardial infarction, hypothermia, or drug overdose. A patient identified as having

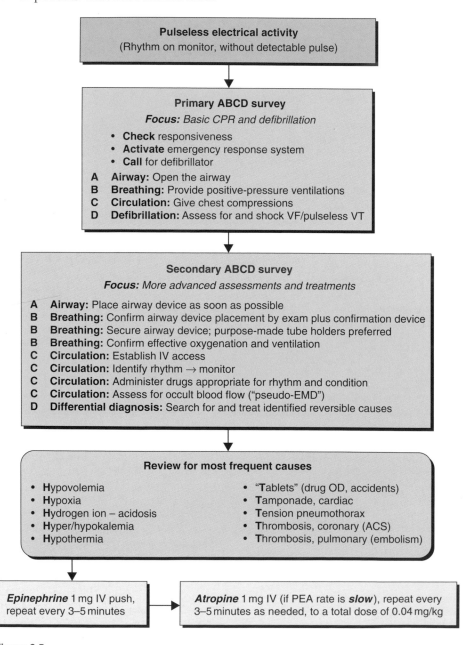

Figure 3.5
Pulseless electrical activity algorithm. ABCD: Airway, Breathing, Circulation, Defibrillation; CPR: cardiopulmonary resuscitation; VF: ventricular fibrillation; VT: ventricular tachycardia; EMD: electromechanical dissociation; ACS: acute coronary syndrome; OD: overdose; PEA: pulseless electrical activity. Reproduced with permission, ACLS Provider Manual, © 2001, Copyright American Heart Association.

PEA should be intubated to provide adequate oxygenation and given a rapid IV infusion of crystalloid. If the patient has a treatable rhythm, appropriate rhythm-specific ACLS algorithms should be utilized. If the situation warrants, pericardiocentesis or needle thoracostomy should be performed. If no reversible cause can be determined, the patient should be given epinephrine every 3–5 minutes. If the PEA rate is slow, atropine can also be given. Unless a reversible cause is discovered, the prognosis of PEA is poor, with only 1–4% of patients surviving to hospital discharge.

Tachycardias

Tachycardias may be common in patients prior to hemodynamic collapse. There are numerous reasons for patients to have tachycardia, not all of which cause hemodynamic compromise. The key issue in patients with tachycardia is whether or not the patient tolerates their heart rate. In other words, is the patient stable and able to support a reasonable blood pressure that provides perfusion to the brain at that heart rate. Using the heart rate alone to determine hemodynamic stability is inappropriate. Other issues to investigate include whether or not the tachycardia is causing the patient's symptoms, whether it is regular or irregular, has narrow or wide complexes, and what might be the underlying cause (or causes). The diagnosis and management of brady-arrhythmias and tachyarrhythmias is discussed in greater detail in Chapter 4.

History

Obtaining historical information about a patient in cardiac arrest can be difficult. Utilizing other resources becomes paramount. Information must be gathered from pre-hospital providers, family, previous medical records, medication lists, or primary care physicians. Clues on the patient's body (wallet, ID bracelet, traumatic injuries, needle marks, scars, dialysis shunts) may be identified. An attempt to learn the following information should be made:

What were the events surrounding the arrest?

Determine whether the patient had a witnessed arrest or was found unconscious. What was the approximate duration of time prior to initiation of CPR (downtime)? Patients with shorter downtimes have a better chance of recovery. Ask whether the patient was having any concerning symptoms prior to the arrest like chest pain, palpitations, or shortness of breath.

What has been the extent of the resuscitation thus far?

Determine the patient's initial cardiac rhythm and any subsequent changes in rhythm throughout the resuscitation. Find out which interventions have been made including defibrillation, airway intervention, and medications, and the patient's response to these interventions.

What is the patient's past medical history?

Concentrate on the patient's cardiac history and risk factors for coronary artery disease. Heart disease is the most common cause of dysrhythmias and sudden cardiac death. Knowing the patient's prior medical problems or medications can point to other possible causes of the cardiac arrest.

This information is likely to be obtained while the patient is being resuscitated or stabilized. Another member of the health care team may search for it if the physician cannot leave the bedside. Much of this information may be obtained from family members. It is important to ask questions in a concise but sensitive manner. Communicate the critical nature of the situation while providing reassurance that care is being provided and that the patient is not suffering. If appropriate, it is also important to reassure the family that they did not cause or contribute to the situation.

Physical examination

Following the secondary survey, the physical examination should focus on vital systems and additional clues that might point to the cause of the arrest. The physician should begin with the baseline rhythm and vital signs (if they are present). A quick cardiopulmonary examination will determine cardiac activity, pulses, and the presence or absence of breath sounds. If the patient is already intubated, the adequacy of the airway should be rechecked. A quick head to toe survey, including the skin and neurologic examination may provide further clues. Subsequent examinations should focus on assessing the response to interventions. After every intervention, vital signs and rhythm should be reassessed for any change. A focused examination should be repeated after each procedure to assess for possible complications (Table 3.1).

Table 3.1 Physical examination findings indicating potential cause of cardiac arrest and complications of therapy

Physical examination	Abnormalities	Potential causes
General	Pallor	Hemorrhage
	Cold	Hypothermia
Airway	Secretions, vomitus, or blood	Aspiration Airway obstruction
	Resistance to positive-pressure ventilation	Tension pneumothorax Airway obstruction Bronchospasm
Neck	Jugular venous distention	Tension pneumothorax Cardiac tamponade Pulmonary embolus
	Tracheal deviation	Tension pneumothorax
Chest	Median sternotomy scar	Underlying cardiac disease
Lungs	Unilateral breath sounds	Tension pneumothorax Right mainstem intubation Aspiration
	Distant or no breath sounds, or no chest expansion	Esophageal intubation Airway obstruction Severe bronchospasm
	Wheezing	Aspiration Bronchospasm Pulmonary edema
	Rales	Aspiration Pulmonary edema Pneumonia
Heart	Audible heart tones	Hypovolemia Cardiac tamponade Tension pneumothorax Pulmonary embolus
Abdomen	Distended and dull	Ruptured abdominal aortic aneurysm or ruptured ectopic pregnancy
	Distended, tympanitic	Esophageal intubation Gastric insufflation
Rectal	Blood, melena	Gastrointestinal hemorrhage
Extremities	Asymmetric pulses	Aortic dissection
	Arteriovenous shunt or fistula	Hyperkalemia
Skin	Needle tracts or abscesses	Intravenous drug abuse
	Burns	Smoke inhalation Electrocution

Source: From Marx J (ed.). *Rosen's Emergency Medicine Concepts and Clinical Practice*. St. Louis: Mosby, Inc, 2002.

Diagnostic studies

Given that more than half of cardiopulmonary arrests in the adult US population are cardiac in origin, the most important diagnostic studies include the 12-lead electrocardiogram (ECG) and continuous cardiac monitoring. The physician should look for ST-segment elevation consistent with an acute myocardial infarction, T-wave changes consistent with hyperkalemia, or ECG changes consistent with various toxin exposures.

Arterial blood gas (ABG) measurements may offer insight into the patient's acid–base status by providing the patient's pH and bicarbonate levels. Blood gas measurements can also assist the practitioner with optimizing a patient's ventilator settings if the patient is intubated. In the patient who is spontaneously breathing, blood gases can help the physician determine whether mechanical ventilation would improve the patient's oxygenation and ventilation.

Serum electrolytes should be measured to identify the presence of life-threatening hyperkalemia and renal failure. A glucose measurement should be done initially during the resuscitation, as profound or protracted hypoglycemia can lead to cardiac arrest.

If the historical data, clinical picture, and physical examination suggest the possibility of a toxicologic cause for the arrest, the patient's serum and urine should be sent for analysis. Levels of prescription or over-the-counter drugs that can contribute to arrest should be measured. Treatment may be required based on the suspicion of toxicity, as levels may not be back promptly.

A chest X-ray is a mandatory diagnostic study that may help establish a definitive diagnosis in a patient with cardiopulmonary arrest, especially if the precipitating cause was pulmonary in origin. The chest radiograph can also confirm correct placement of the endotracheal tube, central access catheters, and nasogastric (NG) tube.

The use of bedside ultrasonography in patient's with cardiac arrest has become more widespread, in an attempt to identify any cardiac activity in the pulseless patient. It can differentiate asystole from VF and confirm PEA. Pericardial effusions resulting in tamponade can also be identified. Transesophageal ultrasound or echocardiography may be used to look for the presence of embolus in the pulmonary vasculature.

Post-resuscitation care

More often than not, patients who have been resuscitated following cardiac arrest are hemodynamically unstable, ventilator-dependent and comatose. Aggressive management post-resuscitation is essential to maximize their chances for recovery.

The immediate goals for post-resuscitation care include the following list:

1. Provide cardiorespiratory support to optimize tissue perfusion, especially to the brain.
2. Transport the patient to an appropriate intensive or critical care unit (ICU or CCU). If one is not available, the patient should be transferred to a tertiary institution that can provide critical care.
3. Continue efforts to identify the precipitating causes of the arrest.
4. Institute measures to prevent recurrence, including but not limited to maintenance of antiarrhythmic drips when appropriate.

All patients require a repeat thorough physical examination. Particular attention should be paid to the patient's cardiopulmonary status. A chest X-ray should be reviewed or obtained to confirm endotracheal tube position. Ventilator settings should be adjusted to the necessary level of mechanical support as determined by arterial blood gas values and the patient's spontaneous efforts. A 12-lead ECG should be repeated and compared to previous tracings. Continuous cardiac monitoring must be maintained. In the hemodynamically unstable patient, assess circulating fluid volume, urine output, and ventricular function to determine the need for additional crystalloid replacement or vasopressor infusion. Invasive hemodynamic monitoring, such as arterial lines and Swan Ganz catheters, should be considered, although controversy exists regarding the necessity of such monitoring in the ED. Laboratory evaluations of electrolytes, cardiac markers, or drug levels should be reviewed, including the reassessment of the patient's acid–base status. All patients resuscitated from VF or VT should receive antiarrhythmic therapy during the first 24 hours post-resuscitation.

A significant amount of brain damage can occur when blood flow to the brain is re-established after resuscitation. This reperfusion injury involves many physiologic processes and is not completely understood. It is important to maintain blood pressure, acid–base status, oxygenation, and adequate sedation during the post-resuscitation period in order to improve long-term neurologic outcome.

Termination of efforts

Despite our best efforts, some patients cannot be resuscitated. The decision to terminate efforts at saving a life can be a difficult one. Many factors need to be considered, including time to the initiation of CPR, time to defibrillation, co-morbid disease, age of the patient, initial rhythm, quality of life prior to the arrest, and expected quality of life if resuscitated. The most important prognostic factor is the duration of cardiac arrest. The chance of being discharged from the hospital alive and neurologically intact diminishes as resuscitation time increases. Available scientific studies have shown that prolonged resuscitation efforts are unlikely to be successful if there is no return of spontaneous circulation at any time during 30 minutes of cumulative ACLS. Reversible causes of cardiac arrest such as drug overdose, electrolyte abnormalities, or profound hypothermia should be taken into account when considering termination of efforts. Treatment of these causes may improve the efficacy of the resuscitation effort and the patient's chances of survival.

Hypothermia (core body temperature of <30°C/86°F) is associated with marked depression of cerebral blood flow, oxygen requirement, cardiac output, and arterial pressure. Hypothermia may exert a protective effect on the brain and other organs in cardiac arrest. Although rare, full resuscitation with intact neurologic recovery may be possible after prolonged hypothermic cardiac arrest. Research is ongoing to determine the role of induced hypothermia in cardiac arrest.

When all Basic Life Support (BLS) or ACLS measures have been reasonably attempted and the likelihood of survival is minimal, resuscitation efforts should be discontinued. Informing family members of the death of a loved one is a very difficult responsibility faced by emergency physicians. Prior to such a disclosure, family members should be gathered in a quiet and private area. Social service personnel and nursing staff should be asked to assist. It is best to be honest and straightforward using language that is appropriate for the family's education level and culture. Briefly relate the circumstances regarding the resuscitation efforts ending with the news that their loved one is dead. Avoid terminology such as "passed away" or "is gone," which may lead to confusion. Family will often want to know what, if anything, they could have done to change the outcome. It is important to reassure them that they did nothing wrong if this is appropriate. Enlist the support of social services, clergy, or other culturally-appropriate personnel to assist you with some of the associated issues, such as autopsy, organ donation, and viewing the body. Express your sympathy and make sure that there is reasonable social support before leaving.

Special patients

The evaluation and treatment of cardiopulmonary arrest is particularly challenging in the pediatric population. Unlike adults, pediatric cardiac arrests are most commonly the result of respiratory causes. Reduced familiarity with procedures as well as anatomic issues (i.e., decreased size of structures) make definitive airway management and vascular access more challenging in pediatric patients. In addition, psychosocial issues are generally more complex in these patients. Neonatal Advanced Life Support (NALS), Pediatric

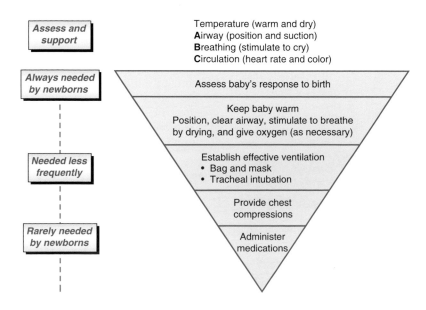

Figure 3.6
Neonatal resuscitation inverted pyramid. Reproduced with permission, PALS Provider Manual, © 2002, Copyright American Heart Association.

Advanced Life Support (PALS), and Advanced Pediatric Life Support (APLS) courses exist to teach these differences. The cardiopulmonary arrest algorithms are similar between children and adults, although the energy of defibrillation and medication dosing are weight-based. The Broselow tape which bases a neonate's or child's weight on the length is an essential piece of equipment for pediatric resuscitation. It has the appropriate medication doses, equipment sizes, and defibrillation energies listed for the appropriate length (weight), and is color coded. Many EDs arrange the pediatric resuscitation equipment by these colors, in order to make the appropriate equipment more readily accessible during resuscitation.

The algorithms for neonatal and pediatric resuscitations are included (Figures 3.6–3.9). Detailed discussions of these scenarios are beyond the scope of this chapter. There no longer seems to be controversy regarding parents or family members witnessing resuscitation attempts. This offers family members the chance to see the health care team doing their best under difficult circumstances, and affords family members the opportunity to more readily accept any outcomes. Again, support staff should be made available during these difficult situations. It is recommended that debriefing opportunities for the emergency health care team be arranged in a timely manner, for as many providers as possible. These are best lead by

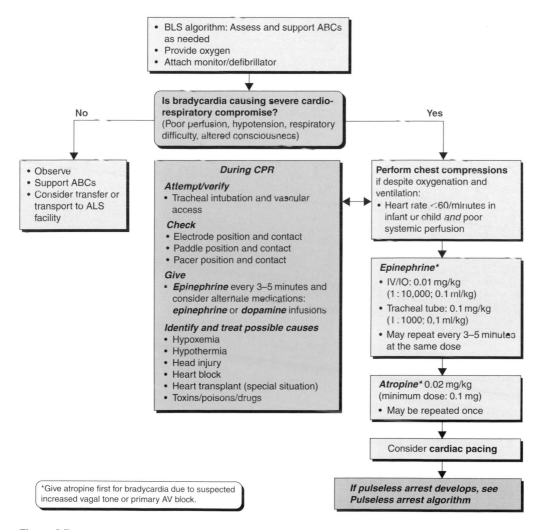

Figure 3.7
Pediatric Advanced Life Support pulseless arrest. CPR: cardiopulmonary resuscitation; ALS: Advanced Life Support; BLS: Basic Life Support; IO: intraosseous. Reproduced with permission, PALS Provider Manual, © 2002, Copyright American Heart Association.

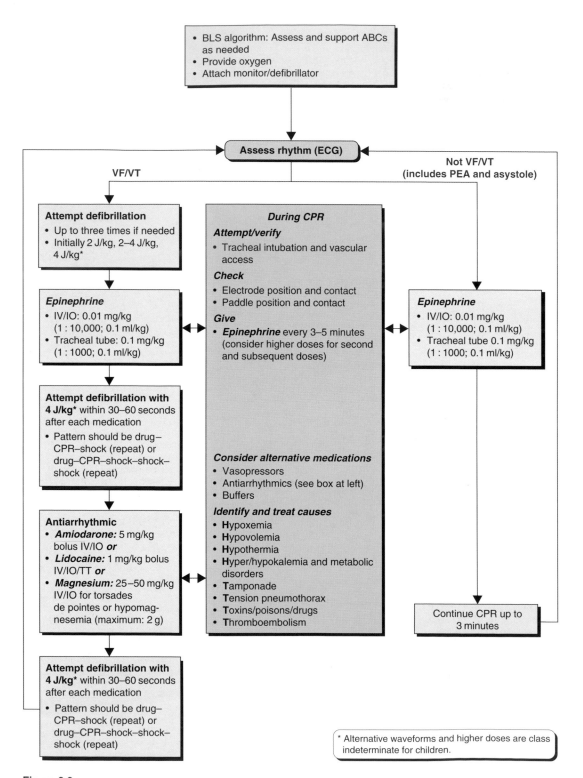

Figure 3.8
Pediatric Advanced Life Support bradycardia. CPR: cardiopulmonary resuscitation; VF: ventricular fibrillation;
VT: ventricular tachycardia; IO: intraosseous; PEA: pulseless electrical activity; TT: Tracheal tube; BLS: Basic Life
Support. Reproduced with permission, PALS Provider Manual, © 2002, Copyright American Heart Association.

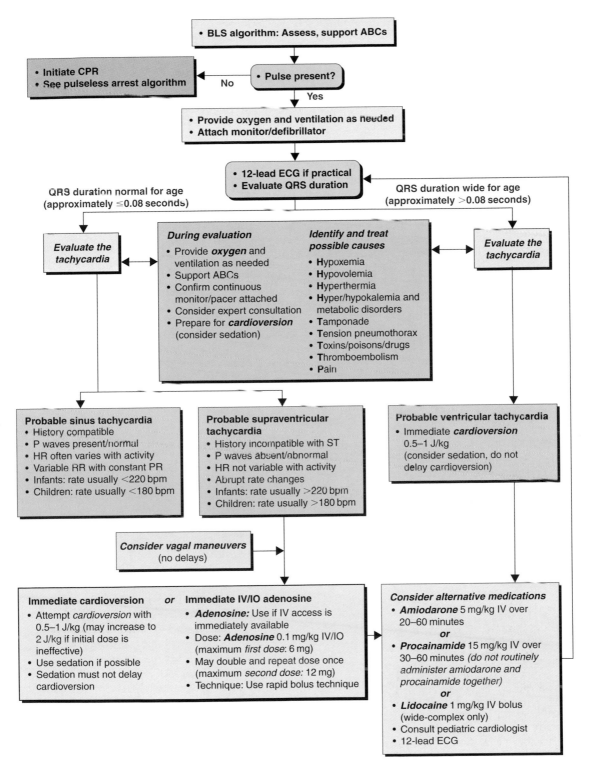

Figure 3.9
Pediatric Advanced Life Support tachycardia poor perfusion. CPR: cardiopulmonary resuscitation; HR: heart rate; ST: sinus tachycardia; RR: R-R interval; PR: P-R interval; IO: intraosseous; BLS: Basic Life Support. Reproduced with permission, PALS Provider Manual, © 2002, Copyright American Heart Association.

personnel specifically trained in psychology, psychiatry, or critical debriefing.

Pearls and summary points

- The highest potential survival rate from cardiac arrest can be achieved when following the "chain of survival."
- The brain and heart are the two organs most susceptible to damage from cardiac arrest.
- VF and pulseless VT remain the most common underlying rhythms of adult cardiac arrest.
- Many factors must be considered when deciding whether to continue a resuscitation. Prolonged resuscitation efforts are unlikely to be successful if there is no return of spontaneous circulation at any time during 30 minutes of cumulative ACLS.
- Aggressive post-resuscitation care can limit further cardiac and cerebral damage.
- In the pediatric population, arrest is due primarily to respiratory causes.
- All family members and loved ones of patients experiencing cardiac arrest should be treated with extreme sensitivity, honesty, and respect. Whenever possible, trained support personnel should assist family members and emergency providers with the challenges of death notification, grieving, acceptance, and final arrangements.

References

1. American Heart Association (AHA). Low energy biphasic waveform defibrillation: evidenced based review applied to emergency cardiovascular care guidelines. www.americanheart.org/scientific/statements, 1998.
2. Del Guercio LRM, et al. Comparison of blood flow during external and internal cardiac massage in man. *Circulation* 1965;31/32(suppl. I):171.
3. Eisenberg MS, et al. Cardiac resuscitation in the community: importance of rapid provision and implications for program planning. *J Am Med Assoc* 1979;241:1905.
4. Eisenberg MS, et al. Cardiac arrest and resuscitation: a tale of 29 cities. *Ann Emerg Med* 1990;19:179–186.
5. *Guidelines 2000* for *Cardiopulmonary Resuscitation and Emergency Cardiovascular Care, International Consensus on Science.*
6. Halperin HR. Mechanisms of forward flow during CPR. In: Paradis N, Nowak R, Halperin H (eds). *Cardiac Arrest: The Science and Practice of Resuscitation Medicine.* Baltimore: Williams & Wilkins, 1996.
7. Hamilton GC. Sudden death in the emergency department: telling the living. *Ann Emerg Med* 1988;17:382.
8. Janz T. Cardiopulmonary cerebral resuscitation. In: Hamilton GC (ed.). *Emergency Medicine: An Approach to Clinical Problem Solving.* Philadelphia, PA: WB Saunders, 2003.
9. Neumar RW, Ward KR. Adult resuscitation. In: Marx J (ed.). *Rosen's Emergency Medicine Concepts and Clinical Practice.* St. Louis: Mosby, Inc, 2002.
10. Ornato JP. Sudden cardiac death. In: Tintinalli J, Kelen G, Stapczynski J (eds). *Emergency Medicine: A Comprehensive Study Guide.* New York: McGraw-Hill, 2000.
11. Sanders AB. Cardiac arrest and resuscitation. In: Harwood-Nuss A (ed.). *The Clinical Practice of Emergency Medicine.* Philadelphia: Lippincott Williams & Wilkins, 2001.
12. Schneider SM. Hypothermia: from recognition to rewarming. *Emerg Med Rep* 1992;13:1–20.
13. Sirbaugh PE, et al. A prospective population based study of the demographics, epidemiology, management, and outcome of out-of-hospital pediatric cardiopulmonary arrest. *Ann Emerg Med* 1999;33:174–184.
14. Standards and guidelines for cardiopulmonary resuscitation and emergency cardiac care. *J Am Med Assoc* 1992;268:2171.
15. Sterz F, et al. Mild hypothermic cardiopulmonary resuscitation improves outcome after prolonged cardiac arrest in dogs. *Crit Care Med* 1991;19:493–498.
16. Stults KR, et al. Self adhesive monitor/defibrillator pads improve prehospital defibrillator success. *Ann Emerg Med* 1987;16:872–877.
17. Wenzel V, Krimsmer AC, Arntz R, et al. A comparison of vasopressin and epinephrine for out-of-hospital cardiopulmonary resuscitation. *New Engl J Med* 2004;350:105–112.
18. White RD. Early out-of-hospital experience with an impedance-compensating low-energy biphasic waveform automatic external defibrillator. *J Interv Card Electrophysiol* 1997;1:203–208.

4 Cardiac dysrhythmias

Swaminatha V. Gurudevan, MD

Scope of the problem

Cardiac dysrhythmias are an important first manifestation of cardiovascular disease. Coronary heart disease is the leading single cause of death in the US, accounting for 21% of all deaths. In the year 2000, approximately 681,000 Americans died of coronary heart disease, amounting to one death every 60 seconds. Even more striking was the fact that nearly half of these deaths occured before the patient reached a hospital. Most of these were sudden deaths, usually resulting from ventricular fibrillation. In fact, an estimated 491,000 deaths in 2000 had cardiac dysrhythmias mentioned as a contributing factor. Despite the strong link between cardiac dysrhythmias and cardiovascular disease, rhythm disturbances may also occur in the absence of structural heart disease or as a result of generalized systemic illness.

Proper identification of cardiac dysrhythmias is a vital skill for emergency providers. A critical aspect is the differentiation of benign from malignant dysrhythmias. The appropriate identification of the rhythm disturbance and a solid understanding of the underlying disease process are critical to the appropriate short- and long-term management of the patient. Dysrhythmias can be broadly divided into three categories: tachydysrhythmias, bradydysrhythmias, and disorders of conduction. The recently updated Advanced Cardiovascular Life Support (ACLS) guidelines place a great emphasis not only on identification of the rhythm disturbance, but also on recognition of patients with left ventricular (LV) systolic dysfunction, as these patients are known to have a significantly higher mortality from each dysrhythmia.

Anatomic essentials

The sinoatrial node

Normal cardiac conduction is initiated by the dominant pacemaker of the heart, the sinoatrial (SA) node (Figure 4.1). The SA node is located at

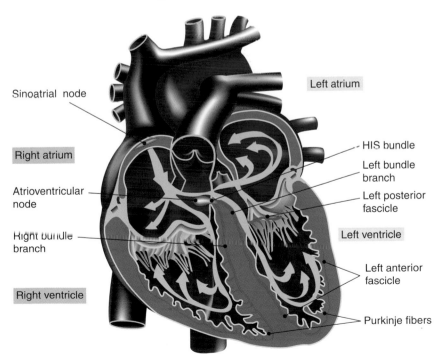

Left atrium

Sinoatrial node

HIS bundle

Left bundle branch

Right atrium

Left posterior fascicle

Atrioventricular node

Left ventricle

Right bundle branch

Left anterior fascicle

Right ventricle

Purkinje fibers

Figure 4.1
The cardiac conduction system. Copyright © 2000, General Electric.

the junction of the right atrium and superior vena cava, and its vascular supply is from the SA nodal artery, which originates from the right coronary artery in 55% of patients and the left circumflex artery in the remaining 45% of patients. The SA node is innervated by parasympathetic fibers from the vagus nerve and sympathetic fibers from the thoracic sympathetic trunk. Its normal discharge rate is between 60 and 100 times per minute.

The atrioventricular node

In the normal heart, conduction proceeds through the atrial fibers to the atrioventricular (AV) node, which is located beneath the right atrial endocardium directly above the insertion of the septal leaflet of the tricuspid valve. On the electrocardiogram (ECG), atrial depolarization is represented by the P wave (Figure 4.2). The AV nodal artery provides the blood supply for the AV node, arising in the majority of cases (90%) from the right coronary artery. In patients with a left-dominant or co-dominant coronary circulation (10%), the AV nodal artery may arise from the left circumflex. Physiologically, the AV node slows conduction velocity to allow greater time for ventricular filling during diastole. In addition, its long refractory period protects the ventricles from excessively rapid stimulation which could cause

inadequate diastolic filling time and acute cardiac failure. The AV node is innervated by the same parasympathetic and sympathetic fibers as the SA node. On the ECG, the PR interval represents the time between the onset of depolarization in the atria and the onset of depolarization in the ventricles, and is used as an estimation of AV nodal conduction time. The normal PR interval is between 0.12 and 0.20 seconds. Prolongation of the PR interval may occur as a result of excessive vagal stimulation, drugs affecting the AV node, AV nodal ischemia, or underlying conduction system disease.

The His–Purkinje system

Depolarization proceeds from the AV node to the bundle of His, which is composed of rapidly conducting Purkinje fibers. The bundle divides in the muscular interventricular septum into two major branches: the left and right bundle branches, which innervate the left and right ventricle (LV and RV), respectively. The left bundle branch divides into the left anterior and left posterior fascicles. Ventricular conduction and depolarization through the His–Purkinje system are represented on the surface ECG by the QRS complex. Normal QRS width is 0.06–0.10 seconds. Widening of the QRS complex beyond 0.12 seconds represents ventricular conduction delay, which can occur as

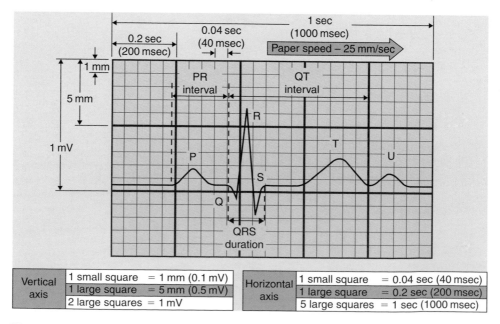

Figure 4.2
Components of the electrocardiogram. Copyright © 2000, General Electric.

a result of bundle branch blocks, aberrant conduction, electrolyte abnormalities, drugs affecting the myocardium, or rhythms that originate in the ventricular myocardium.

Ventricular repolarization

Repolarization of the ventricular myocardium is represented by the T-wave. Mechanical contraction typically follows depolarization through excitation–contraction coupling and fractional shortening of cardiac myocytes. The QT interval, which represents ventricular depolarization and repolarization time, is dependent to some extent on heart rate. A corrected QT interval (QT_c) is obtained by dividing the measured QT interval by the square root of the RR interval. A normal QT_c is less than 0.47 seconds. Prolongation of the QT interval can occur secondary to drug effects, electrolyte abnormalities, and congenital abnormalities; a prolonged repolarization period increases the "vulnerable period" of the ventricle, during which premature ventricular contraction can trigger a reentrant ventricular tachydysrhythmia.

Tachycardias and bradycardias

The normal range of heart rates in a healthy adult with an intact sinus node is 60–100 beats per minute. *Bradycardia* is defined as a heart rate less than 60 beats per minute, while *tachycardia* is defined as a heart rate greater than 100 beats per minute.

History

The history is the most important component in the evaluation of a patient with a cardiac dysrhythmia. Patients with cardiac dysrhythmias may complain of palpitations, or the sensation of a rapid or irregular heart rhythm. They may not notice the abnormal heart rhythm, and may instead complain of chest pain, shortness of breath, lightheadedness, fatigue, presyncope, syncope, or convulsions.

Do you have chest pain or shortness of breath?

Chest pain or shortness of breath may reflect underlying cardiac ischemia. Patients with underlying coronary artery disease (CAD) can experience symptoms of demand-related ischemia during a tachydysrhythmia or a bradydysrhythmia. Alternatively, ischemia can cause both tachydysrhythmias and bradydysrhythmias. In fact, sudden death from unstable tachydysrhythmias such as ventricular fibrillation (VF) and ventricular tachycardia (VT) represent the leading cause of out-of-hospital death from cardiac causes. A history of exertional or rest angina may provide clues to an acute coronary syndrome. Similarly, a history of orthopnea, paroxysmal nocturnal dyspnea, or lower extremity edema may suggest underlying LV dysfunction, which would increase the risk of sudden death from ventricular tachydysrhythmias.

Did you feel lightheaded, dizzy, or lose consciousness?

Syncope is an important finding, as it portends a poorer prognosis in patients with either tachydysrhythmias or bradydysrhythmias, mandating an aggressive workup to exclude an dysrhythmogenic cause of syncope. Cerebral hypoperfusion from lack of cardiac output is the mechanism of cardiogenic syncope; cerebral hypoperfusion can also manifest as a seizure or an alteration in level of consciousness.

When did your symptoms begin, and if they are episodic, how often do they occur and how long do they last?

If the patient complains of chest pain or palpitations, it is crucial to know how long these symptoms last when they occur (seconds, minutes, or hours). How many times a day or week do they occur? During the workup of a cardiac dysrhythmia, it is important to correlate the presence of the dysrhythmia with concomitant clinical symptoms – chest pain, shortness of breath, or presyncope/syncope. The frequency of symptom occurrence may dictate the type of monitoring device (Holter or event monitor) to use when planning an outpatient workup.

Do you have a previous history of coronary artery disease (CAD), congestive heart failure (CHF), dysrhythmias, or valvular heart disease? Have you had prior cardiac surgery?

Given that CAD, CHF, and primary dysrhythmias are recurrent illnesses, it is important to identify those patients with a prior history of CAD or CHF, as these patients may be more likely to manifest certain dysrhythmias. Valvular heart diseases such as mitral stenosis and mitral regurgitation can predispose to atrial tachydysrhythmias. Atrial fibrillation, AV nodal reentrant tachydysrhythmias, and ventricular tachydysrhythmias can have a relapsing and remitting course, and often recur. Certain dysrhythmias, especially atrial fibrillation and VT, can occur following cardiac surgery. These rhythm disturbances have a different management and prognosis in this setting.

Do you have a pacemaker or implanted defibrillator?

Pacemakers are typically implanted for symptomatic bradydysrhythmias such as sinus bradycardia, sick sinus syndrome, or high-degree AV block. A four- or five-letter code assigned to each type of pacemaker describes the chamber paced, the chamber sensed, the response to sensing, and the rate adaptation programmability of the pacemaker. For example, a VVIR pacemaker is a single-chamber pacemaker that paces the ventricle (V), senses the ventricle (V), inhibits pacing (I) if a native beat is sensed, and has rate modulation programmability (R). A DDDR pacemaker is a dual-chamber pacemaker that paces both the atrium and the ventricle (D), senses both the atrium and the ventricle (D), either inhibits pacing of or triggers pacing of both the atrium and the ventricle (D) in response to sensing, and is rate modulation programmable (R). Newer biventricular pacemakers have a third lead in the coronary sinus that allows for synchronized pacing of the LV and RV.

Implantable cardioverter defibrillators (ICDs) are more common today given recent clinical trials demonstrating their effectiveness in preventing sudden death in certain patients. These include patients with CAD and LV dysfunction or patients with prior episodes of VT or resuscitated ventricular fibrillation arrest (termed sudden cardiac death). They are almost always dual-chamber devices and also function as pacemakers.

Both pacemakers and ICDs have a stored memory that can be interrogated by the pacemaker company representative or, in many cases, a skilled cardiologist. This information can be extremely helpful in the analysis of a current or recent dysrhythmia and can serve as a "continuous telemetry box" for the patient. The patient typically carries a card with the pacemaker company and the model, and a company representative is generally available 24 hours a day to interrogate the pacemaker if necessary.

Ask for a complete list of medications, including cardiac medications, non-prescription medications, herbal, and alternative medicines. Ask about illicit substance abuse.

Medications and drug interactions are an important cause of bradydysrhythmias, tachydysrhythmias, and conduction system disorders. Beta-blockers (atenolol, metoprolol, carvedilol) and calcium channel blockers (verapamil, diltiazem) can be negatively chronotropic and contribute to bradydysrhythmias and conduction system disorders. Digoxin toxicity can be responsible for bradydysrhythmias, conduction system disorders, and tachydysrhythmias by increasing the parasympathetic tone at the SA and AV nodes and by increasing automaticity in the ventricular myocardium. Antihistamines, neuroleptics, and gastrointestinal (GI) medications such as metoclopramide can prolong the QT interval and thereby predispose to ventricular tachydysrhythmias. Herbal medications such as ephedra (Ma Huang) or jimsonweed tea can have sympathomimetic or anticholinergic effects, respectively. Excessive caffeine intake can have a sympathomimetic effect, and can shorten the refractory period in the slow pathway of the AV node, predisposing one to AV nodal reentrant tachycardia (AVNRT). Sympathomimetic drug abuse (cocaine, crystal methamphetamine) usually causes tachydysrhythmias. Injection drug use can contribute to the development of infectious endocarditis, which may manifest as heart block.

Do you have any other medical problems, such as chronic obstructive pulmonary disease, renal failure, or thyroid disease?

Chronic pulmonary diseases can predispose patients to atrial tachydysrhythmias, especially multifocal atrial tachycardia (MAT). Inhaled beta-agonists and anticholinergic agents used to treat chronic obstructive pulmonary disease (COPD) and asthma can contribute to tachydysrhythmias as well. Renal failure can contribute to hyperkalemia, which may cause heart blocks and bradydysrhythmias, and worsens digoxin toxicity. Hypocalcemia from chronic renal failure can cause prolongation of the QT interval. Hypothyroidism can present with significant sinus bradycardia. Thyrotoxicosis can present with sinus tachycardia and is an important cause of atrial fibrillation.

Is there a family history of dilated cardiomyopathy, sudden cardiac death, or early coronary artery disease?

Patients with a strong family history have a higher risk of similar diseases and carry a poorer prognosis. Dilated cardiomyopathy is known to be an X-linked genetic disease. Certain hereditary conditions such as Brugada syndrome predispose individuals to VT and sudden cardiac death. A history of a first-degree relative with CAD before the age of 50 years is an independent risk factor for coronary events.

Physical examination

General appearance

This is perhaps the most important part of the physical examination in terms of guiding the management of a cardiac dysrhythmia. Does the patient appear ill? Is the patient clinically stable or unstable? A patient is clinically unstable if they have evidence of end-organ hypoperfusion as a direct result of the dysrhythmia. This may be manifested as severe chest pain, hypotension due to myocardial ischemia, or respiratory failure with pulmonary edema. Patients who are clinically unstable require immediate aggressive, focused management of their dysrhythmia including medications, cardioversion, defibrillation, or pacing according to ACLS guidelines. Patients who are clinically stable can be evaluated and treated in a more methodical fashion.

Vital signs

Is the patient hypertensive or hypotensive? The absolute blood pressure may be deceiving, and comparing the current blood pressure with previous normal blood pressures should be done. For example, a blood pressure of 100/50 mmHg in an elderly patient with hypertension and CAD whose normal blood pressure is 160/90 mmHg may be more significant than a blood pressure of 85/50 mmHg in a young, healthy female without prior history of cardiac disease. Assess the heart rate as well as the caliber and regularity of the pulses. Atrial fibrillation typically presents with an irregularly irregular pulse.

Skin

Inspect the skin for pallor, cyanosis, or duskiness which reflects tissue hypoperfusion. Palpate the skin to assess the temperature and moisture. In thyrotoxicosis, the skin is typically warm and moist; cool or clammy skin suggests hypoperfusion.

Head, eyes, ears, nose, and throat

Look for exophthalmos, which may be a physical finding of Graves' disease. Look for nasal flaring which may reflect acute respiratory distress and air hunger. Examination of the oral mucous membranes provides clues towards the patient's hydration status. Look for perioral cyanosis, another sign of tissue hypoperfusion.

Neck

Inspect the level of the jugular venous pulsations to assess the patient's volume status. Press below the costal margin to assess for hepatojugular reflux. When seen, cannon A waves in the jugular venous pulse suggest AV dissociation, which can occur in third-degree heart block and VT. The cannon A waves reflect atrial contraction against a closed tricuspid valve. Inspect the thyroid gland for a goiter, thyroidectomy scar, or any nodularity.

Cardiovascular

Inspect the chest wall for the point of maximal impulse (PMI). Palpate the PMI and note any displacement. The normal position of the PMI is the 5th intercostal space in the midclavicular line. Inferior and lateral displacement of the PMI to the anterior axillary line or midaxillary line can occur with progressive LV dilation and failure. Palpate for an RV parasternal heave which can reflect RV failure. Next, auscultate the heart, listening for the regularity of rhythm, the loudness and splitting of S1 and S2, and for systolic or diastolic murmurs. Atrial fibrillation is most commonly associated with an irregularly irregular rhythm. A left bundle branch block can cause S2 to be paradoxically split (A2 will come after P2 and inspiration will cause the split to come together). A right bundle branch block can cause wider splitting of S2. Listen for an S3 gallop which reflects LV failure. Finally, assess the quality of the pulses and evaluate capillary refill.

Chest and lungs

Look for a midline sternotomy scar that may reflect prior cardiac surgery. Inspect for accessory muscle use for breathing. Pulmonary rales or wheezes may reflect volume overload and LV failure. Percuss the chest wall for dullness and listen for decreased breath sounds; these findings may suggest a pleural effusion and volume overload.

Abdomen

Inspect for any evidence of abdominal distention or ascites. Palpate the liver edge; a pulsatile liver may reflect pulmonary hypertension with significant tricuspid regurgitation.

Extremities

Inspect the extremities for their degree of warmth. The presence of cyanosis or clubbing may indicate chronic pulmonary disease. Pitting edema may reflect volume overload.

Neurologic

Assess the level of consciousness. Is the patient's mental status different from baseline? Is there a focal neurologic deficit that warrants investigation of a cerebrovascular accident related to the dysrhythmia?

Diagnostic testing

Electrocardiogram with rhythm strip

A 12-lead ECG is an essential part of the initial evaluation of a patient with a cardiac rhythm disturbance. All patients with a cardiac dysrhythmia should be on continuous telemetry monitoring and have a 12-lead ECG performed on arrival to the emergency department.

Radiologic studies

All patients should have a portable chest X-ray performed to evaluate the cardiac silhouette, assess for pulmonary vascular congestion, and confirm the appropriate placement of pacemaker or defibrillator leads, if present. Pacemaker lead fractures, although difficult to identify, may be a cause for pacemaker malfunction or failure.

Laboratory studies

Cardiac enzymes

Serum creatine kinase (CK), CK-MB, and troponin I should be ordered in all patients in whom myocardial ischemia is suspected. CK-MB begins to rise 4 hours after myocardial injury, but is not always specific for myocardial injury. Troponin I rises 6 hours after myocardial injury, and remains elevated for several days following the injury. It is nearly 100% specific for myocardial injury, and can establish that myocardial necrosis has occurred so that appropriate disposition and treatment of the patient can be carried out. In addition, troponin I helps to risk stratify patients presenting with a cardiac dysrhythmia, as those with elevated troponin Is are likely to have myocardial damage.

Electrolytes

A stat serum electrolyte panel should be obtained in every patient with a new cardiac dysrhythmia. In particular, serum potassium, calcium, and magnesium should be evaluated. If the patient is clinically unstable, some of these tests can be ordered as part of an arterial blood gas analysis, with the results available more rapidly. Hyperkalemia predisposes the patient to bradydysrhythmias and heart block. It causes flattening of the P wave, peaking of the T-wave, and widening of the QRS complex. Conversely, hypokalemia may predispose individuals to ventricular tachydysrhythmias. Severe hypokalemia results in a more prominent P wave, a flattened T-wave, and a prominent U-wave seen following the T-wave on the surface ECG. Hypocalcemia may prolong the QT interval, while hypercalcemia can result in shortening of the QT interval. Serum magnesium levels are also important, as levels influence the body's potassium homeostasis. Hypomagnesemia can cause prolongation of the QT interval and predispose a patient to torsades de pointes.

Thyroid function tests

A serum thyroid-stimulating hormone (TSH) should be obtained in patients with new onset atrial fibrillation or inappropriate sinus tachycardia. If the TSH is abnormal, a complete thyroid panel should also be obtained. Similarly, patients with unexplained sinus bradycardia should have a TSH drawn to rule out significant hypothyroidism. Although these results are rarely available during a patient's emergency department course, they are of use to the physician who admits the patient or sees the patient in follow-up.

Drug levels

A digoxin level should be obtained in patients taking this medication. Digoxin toxicity should be suspected if the patient presents with symptomatic bradycardia, high-grade AV block, atrial tachycardias with block, or bidirectional VT. A urine toxicology screen should also be obtained, especially from those patients in whom illicit sympathomimetic substance abuse is suspected.

Management of bradydysrhythmias

General management

After assessing and securing (if necessary) the airway, breathing, and circulation, obtaining intravenous (IV) access, and placing the patient on a cardiac monitor, a 12-lead ECG should be obtained. Stat bloodwork should be ordered as discussed.

First, assess for the presence of serious signs or symptoms due to the bradydysrhythmia. These include hypotension, impaired tissue perfusion, or any alteration in sensorium. If present, treatment should be initiated immediately.

IV fluids should be started if there is no overt evidence of CHF. Atropine should be given as it is effective in reversing supranodal causes of bradycardia and may reverse functional AV nodal conduction block. Two milligrams of atropine causes complete vagal blockade, so it is unlikely that doses higher than this will contribute to improvement. However, research is ongoing about the appropriate maximum dose. ACLS guidelines recommend a maximum dose of 0.04 mg/kg for symptomatic bradycardia.

If symptomatic bradycardia persists, the next medication to administer is IV dopamine at the beta-receptor dosing range of 5–20 mcg/kg/minute. Dopamine is both positively chronotropic and ionotropic, and may assist with hypotension. It should be given through a central line if possible to avoid dopamine-induced skin necrosis. Other medications that may be useful are IV epinephrine, a beta-predominant sympathomimetic agent, and isoproterenol, a pure sympathomimetic beta-agonist (Figure 4.3).

If serious signs and symptoms of bradycardia persist despite appropriate medical therapy, transcutaneous pacing should be initiated with preparations for urgent temporary transvenous pacemaker placement.

Management of specific bradydysrhythmias

Sinus bradycardia

Sinus rates of less than 60 beats per minute are termed sinus bradycardia. Sinus bradycardia is commonly observed in individuals with a high resting vagal tone (athletes) or patients on negatively chronotropic medications (beta-blockers, calcium channel blockers, digoxin, amiodarone, and clonidine). Sinus bradycardia can also be seen early in the course of an acute inferior wall myocardial infarction, triggered by parasympathetic stimulation, known as the Bezold–Jarisch reflex.

Sinus bradycardia should only be treated if there are associated symptoms. Elimination of reversible aggravating factors is an essential first step in management. This includes discontinuing negatively chronotropic medications and considering administration of reversal agents (IV glucagon for beta-blockers, IV calcium gluconate for calcium channel blockers, and Digibind™ for digoxin). If the symptoms persist despite discontinuation of all bradycardia-aggravating medications or if the medications are essential to the patient's overall management, permanent pacemaker placement is indicated. Patients with an inappropriate sinus bradycardia should be investigated to rule out myocardial ischemia, significant hypothyroidism, adrenal insufficiency, overmedication, or certain uncommon infectious diseases.

Ectopic atrial rhythm or wandering atrial pacemaker

This dysrhythmia is caused by an ectopic atrial focus distinct from the sinus node that represents the dominant sinus rhythm. On the ECG, ectopic P waves are recognized as being different from those in the patient's usual rhythm, and the PR interval may vary from the patient's baseline PR interval, depending on the location of the ectopic atrial focus. If three or more different atrial foci are seen, the rhythm is termed a wandering atrial pacemaker. These rhythms do not have clinical significance, and no specific treatment is required unless warranted by symptoms.

Sinoatrial block (sinus exit block)

Sinoatrial (SA) block is characterized by the absence of atrial depolarization. This can occur due to the SA node's failure to generate an impulse or failure of the SA nodal impulse to conduct to the atria. On the ECG, P waves are typically absent. The most common factors that predispose to SA block are ischemia, hyperkalemia, excessive vagal tone or negative chronotropic drugs.

Typically, an alternate region of myocardium becomes the dominant pacemaker and manifests an escape rhythm. Junctional escape rhythms are

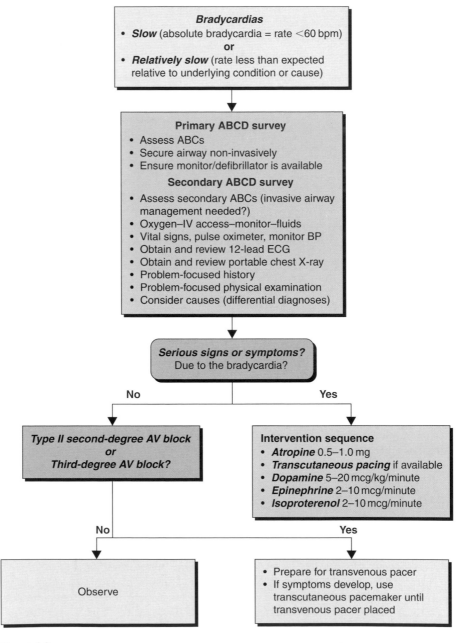

Figure 4.3
Bradycardias. bpm: beats per minute; ABCD: Airway, Breathing, Circulation, Defibrillation. Reproduced with permission, ACLS Provider Manual, © 2001, Copyright American Heart Association.

usually narrow-complex rhythms at 45–60 beats per minute, while escape rhythms originating from the His–Purkinje system are wide-complex with a rate of 30–45 beats per minute. Treatment of SA block with escape rhythms is indicated based on the patient's symptoms.

Sick sinus syndrome

Sick sinus syndrome is a syndrome of abnormalities in cardiac impulse formation and AV conduction that manifest as combinations of tachydysrhythmias and bradydysrhythmias. It is also referred to as *tachy–brady syndrome*. Most patients present to the emergency department with symptomatic bradydysrhythmias and a history of episodic palpitations. The ECG manifestations include SA block, sinus or atrial bradycardia with bursts of an atrial tachydysrhythmia (usually atrial fibrillation). Treatment of this syndrome is directed towards the specific manifestation of the syndrome – either augmentation of rate with atropine if the patient has bradycardia or rate control of an atrial tachydysrhythmia with a beta-blocker, calcium channel blocker, or digoxin. One must exercise caution with these agents, as they may lead to excessive tachycardia or bradycardia. In the long term, most patients require a permanent pacemaker for support during excessive sinus bradycardia and an antidysrhythmic medication to suppress tachydysrhythmias

First-degree atrioventricular block

AV block is divided into three grades, based on the ECG characteristics and the degree of the block. AV block is the result of impaired conduction through the atria, AV node, or His–Purkinje system.

First-degree AV block is defined as prolonged AV conduction without loss of conduction of any single atrial impulse. On the ECG, it is manifested by a PR interval greater than 0.20 seconds. In first-degree AV block, the ventricular rate is not slow unless there is concomitant sinus bradycardia. No specific treatment is indicated. Negatively chronotropic medications should be used with caution in these patients.

Second-degree atrioventricular block

In second-degree AV block, most but not all atrial impulses are conducted to the ventricles. It is divided into two subtypes based on the ECG appearance and the underlying pathophysiology.

Type I second-degree

Type I second-degree AV block (referred to as the Wenckebach phenomenon or Mobitz Type I block) is caused by a conduction defect within the AV node itself (Figure 4.4). On the ECG there is progressive lengthening of the PR interval on successive cardiac cycles until eventually a P wave is not conducted ("dropped"). This results in an irregular rhythm with "grouped beating," usually in pairs or triplets, but occasionally larger groups. Progressive lengthening of the PR intervals occurs because each successive atrial impulse arrives earlier and earlier in the refractory period of the AV node, and therefore takes longer and longer to conduct to the ventricle. Another feature is a progressive shortening of the RR interval in the grouped beats preceding the dropped beat. Type I second-degree AV block can occur following inferior wall myocardial infarction, and occasionally requires temporary pacing in this setting. In the majority of cases, however, it is asymptomatic and requires no treatment.

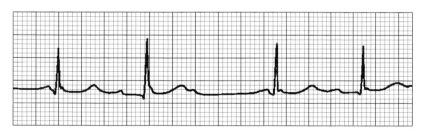

Figure 4.4
Second-degree AV block, Mobitz Type I. From Da Costa D, Brady WJ, Edhouse J. Bradycardias and atrioventricular conduction block. *Br Med J* 2002;324(7336): 535–538. Printed with permission.

Type II second-degree

Type II second-degree AV block (or Mobitz Type II block) suggests a conduction block below the level of the AV node (Figure 4.5). This finding is much more ominous than Type I block, as there is a significant risk of progression to complete heart block. It is caused by degenerative disease of the conduction system, termed *Lev* or *Lenegre disease*. On the ECG there is preservation of a constant PR interval on conducted beats with sudden loss of P wave conduction. There is often a concomitant bundle branch block or baseline first-degree AV block reflecting underlying conduction system disease. Patients with this form of AV block can present with symptomatic bradydysrhythmias or syncope. As parasympathetic innervation is absent below the level of the AV node, atropine is not effective in treating bradycardia associated with this type of conduction block. Permanent pacemaker placement is indicated.

2 : 1 block

A third type of AV block exists that cannot be definitively classified as Type I or Type II. It is termed as 2 : 1 block and is characterized by two P waves for every QRS complex. The location of the block cannot be determined with certainty based on the ECG alone, as it may represent a 2 : 1 Mobitz Type I block or high-grade conduction system disease. This type of conduction block can occur with digoxin toxicity or AV nodal ischemia. Further invasive electrophysiologic (EP) testing involving measurement of H–V conduction times is necessary to clarify the location of the block and determine further treatment.

Third-degree atrioventricular block

Third-degree AV block occurs when there is absolutely no conduction of atrial impulses to the ventricle (Figure 4.6). Atrial and ventricular impulses may be present, but each occur independent of the other. This phenomenon is also termed *AV dissociation*. With third-degree AV block, a secondary pacemaker below the AV node assumes control and produces an escape rhythm. This escape pacemaker can originate from low in the AV node or from the His–Purkinje system. This is usually evident from the width of the QRS complex. On the ECG, there are visible P waves with a constant PP interval that continuously

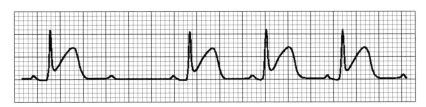

Figure 4.5
Second-degree AV block, Mobitz Type II. From Da Costa D, Brady WJ, Edhouse J. Bradycardias and atrioventricular conduction block. *Br Med J* 2002;324(7336): 535–538. Printed with permission.

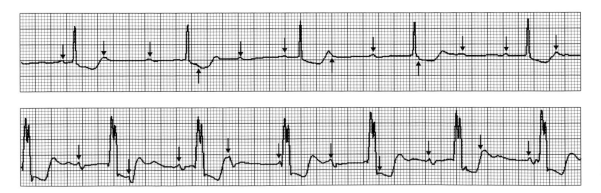

Figure 4.6
Third-degree AV Block. From Da Costa D, Brady WJ, Edhouse J. Bradycardias and atrioventricular conduction block. *Br Med J* 2002;324(7336):535–538. Printed with permission.

marches through the strip. In addition, there are visible QRS complexes with a constant RR interval that also marches through. As there is AV dissociation, and the atria and ventricles beat independent of each other, the PR interval is variable. In some instances, it may be difficult to identify AV dissociation as the atrial and ventricular rates may be similar (termed isorhythmic AV dissociation), and longer rhythm strips may be necessary.

Management of third-degree AV block depends on the patient's clinical status. Drugs that can cause AV nodal block should be reversed. If there is evidence of significant hemodynamic compromise, transcutaneous or transvenous pacemaker placement is indicated. Unless a clearly reversible cause of third-degree block is present, most patients will require permanent pacemaker placement. With all forms of AV block, the patient should be questioned regarding risk factors for Lyme disease, myocarditis, endocarditis, or lupus erythematosus, as these systemic illnesses can contribute to disease of the cardiac conduction system.

Management of tachydysrhythmias

General management

As with bradydysrhythmias, assessment and stabilization of the airway, breathing, and circulation should occur rapidly. IV access should be obtained, the patient should be placed immediately on a cardiac monitor, and a 12-lead ECG should be performed and reviewed. Stat serum electrolytes should be ordered as dictated.

First, assess for the presence of serious signs or symptoms due to the tachydysrhythmia. These include hypotension, impaired tissue perfusion, chest pain, hypoxemia, other signs of worsening myocardial ischemia, or altered sensorium. If there are serious signs and symptoms, treatment should be initiated immediately, as determined by ACLS guidelines (Figure 4.7).

Management of specific tachydysrhythmias

Tachydysrhythmias can be best understood by grouping them broadly into two categories: *narrow-complex tachydysrhythmias* (defined as those with a QRS duration less than 120 milliseconds), and *wide-complex tachydysrhythmias* (QRS

duration greater than 120 milliseconds). Narrow-complex tachydysrhythmias are best understood when grouped into those that are *regular,* with a relatively constant RR interval, and those that are *irregular*, with a highly variable, RR interval. The regular narrow-complex tachydysrhythmias include sinus tachycardia, paroxysmal atrial tachycardia (PAT), AV nodal reentrant tachycardia (AVNRT), AV reentrant tachycardia (AVRT) and non-paroxysmal junctional tachycardia. Irregular narrow-complex tachycardias are those in which the RR interval is irregular. These include atrial fibrillation, atrial flutter, and multifocal atrial tachycardia (MAT). Atrial flutter can present with either an irregular or regular ventricular response rate (or both).

Sinus tachycardia

In sinus tachycardia, a P wave precedes each QRS complex with a relatively uniform morphology and constant PR interval. The heart rate usually ranges from 100 to 160 beats per minute. Small variations in PR interval may be present, related to physiologic sinus dysrhythmia.

As a general rule, sinus tachycardia is not a disease in itself; rather, it is a response to an extracardiac stimulus. As such, the rate itself does not require treatment; rather, the underlying cause should be addressed. An important exception to this rule is sinus tachycardia that occurs in the setting of acute myocardial ischemia. In this setting, reducing the heart rate with beta-blockade is indicated, in order to reduce myocardial oxygen demand and improve mortality. Systemic causes of sinus tachycardia include pain, hypovolemia, anemia, fever, hypoxemia, anxiety, sympathomimetic drugs, pregnancy, and pulmonary embolism.

Sinus tachycardia can be mistaken for other causes of regular narrow-complex tachycardia, especially in children and young adults. Sinus tachycardia that is near 150 beats per minute should be re-examined closely to ensure that it is not atrial flutter with 2:1 block.

Paroxysmal atrial tachycardia (PAT)

PAT is associated with a reentrant ectopic atrial focus distinct from the sinus node. It is characterized by a heart rate from 100 to 160 beats per minute, having a different P wave morphology from the patient's normal P wave. There may be 1:1 conduction or variable degrees of AV block present.

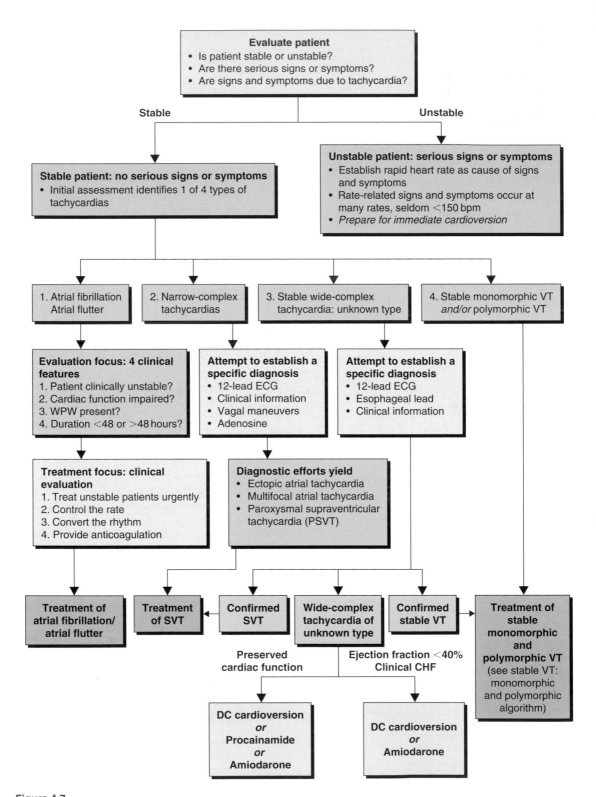

Figure 4.7
Tachycardias: overview algorithm. bpm: beats per minute; WPW: Wolff–Parkinson–White syndrome; CHF: congestive heart failure; SVT: supraventricular tachycardia; VT: ventricular tachycardia. Reproduced with permission, ACLS Provider Manual, © 2001, Copyright American Heart Association.

No specific therapy is indicated for PAT. It occurs in association with underlying electrolyte disturbances, drug toxicity, hypoxemia, and fever. Digoxin toxicity should be investigated in any patient presenting with PAT with 2:1 block or complete AV block, as these are classic dysrhythmias of digoxin toxicity.

Atrioventricular nodal reentrant tachycardia (AVNRT)

AVNRT is a reentrant tachydysrhythmia that involves a micro-reentrant circuit within the AV node (Figure 4.8). There are typically two anatomic pathways for transit of atrial impulses through the AV node, a fast pathway (through which sinus impulses normally travel) and a slow pathway (which is typically blocked due to a long inherent refractory period). AVNRT is triggered when a premature atrial impulse passes through one of the pathways then travels retrograde up the other pathway, causing depolarization of the atrium. The impulse returns to the AV node and the cycle repeats.

In the majority of cases, the impulse travels down the fast pathway and up the slow pathway ("fast–slow" AVNRT), while in the remainder of cases, the impulse travels down the slow pathway and up the fast pathway ("slow–fast" AVNRT). On the ECG, a regular narrow-complex tachycardia is present. Due to the timing of atrial depolarization, the P waves are usually buried within the QRS complexes and are therefore not visible. With the slow–fast AVNRT, inverted P waves may be present before the QRS complex.

Treatment of AVNRT is predicated on temporarily interrupting the reentrant circuit, or converting the unidirectional block to a bidirectional block. This can be accomplished through vagal maneuvers or through drugs that prolong the AV nodal refractory period, such as adenosine, beta-blockers or calcium channel blockers. AVNRT may also be corrected through radiofrequency catheter ablation of the slow pathway.

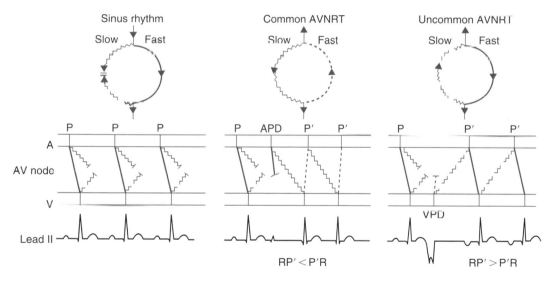

Figure 4.8
Ladder diagrams showing normal sinus conduction pattern through AV node, conduction pattern with slow–fast atrioventricular nodal reentrant tachycardia (AVNRT), and conduction pattern with fast–slow AVNRT. Corresponding ECG tracings are shown below. Each panel shows the AV node (top), a Lewis diagram (middle), and a surface ECG lead (bottom). Solid lines indicate anterograde AV nodal conduction, and broken lines retrograde conduction; straight lines indicate conduction over the fast pathway, and wavy lines conduction over the slow pathway. P denotes sinus P wave. P', atrial echoes resulting from AV nodal reentry; APD, atrial premature depolarization; VPD, ventricular premature depolarization, and R, R waves. During sinus rhythm the presence of the slow pathway is concealed because the impulse traveling over the fast pathway turns around after traversing the AV node and retrogradely penetrates the slow pathway, colliding with the oncoming impulse moving anterogradely over the slow pathway. Note the simultaneous registration of P' waves and QRS complexes during common AVNRT, with RP' < P'R. Retrograde P' waves result in the appearance of pseudo waves in the inferior ECG leads. During uncommon AVNRT, inverted P' waves are visible, with RP' < P'R. Diagram from Ganz LI, Friedman PL. Supraventricular tachycardia. *New Engl J Med* 1995;332(3):162–173. Printed with permission.

Atrioventricular reentrant tachycardia (AVRT)

AVRT involves a macro-reentrant circuit including the AV node and a coexistent accessory pathway of conduction from the atria to the ventricles (Figure 4.9). In 90% of cases, the impulse starts in the atria and travels antegrade down the AV node, then retrograde up the accessory pathway (referred to as *orthodromic* AVRT) before depolarizing the atrium again. In the remaining 10% of cases, the impulse travels antegrade down the accessory pathway, then retrograde through the His–Purkinje system and the AV node (referred to as *antidromic* AVRT) before depolarizing the atria. On the ECG, orthodromic AVRT appears as a regular narrow-complex tachycardia with inverted retrograde P waves appearing after the QRS complex. Antidromic AVRT, however, appears as a wide-complex tachycardia given the antegrade conduction down the accessory pathway. Retrograde P waves are sometimes visible, so this dysrhythmia may be mistaken for VT. AVRT can also be treated with adenosine or calcium channel blockers which block conduction through the AV node and break the macro-reentrant circuit.

Extreme caution should be used if calcium channel blockers are given to individuals with wide-complex tachycardias.

Non-paroxysmal junctional tachycardia

Junctional tachycardia occurs when there is increased automaticity of the AV node and a coexistent AV block. This results in a narrow- or wide-complex tachycardia, depending on where in the AV node the impulse originates. It can occur in the setting of digoxin toxicity, inferior myocardial infarction, or acute rheumatic fever. Treatment is supportive. In a patient with chronic atrial fibrillation on digoxin therapy, the finding of a *regular* ventricular response rate despite underlying atrial fibrillation should raise the suspicion of digoxin toxicity causing complete AV block with a junctional escape pacemaker.

Atrial fibrillation

Atrial fibrillation is characterized by chaotic, disorganized depolarization of the atria with

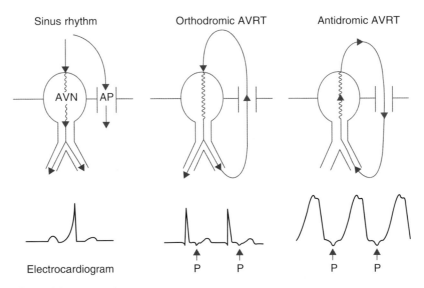

Figure 4.9
Ladder diagrams showing conduction pattern with sinus rhythm and Wolff–Parkinson–White syndrome (WPW), orthodromic and antidromic AVRT (atrioventricular reentrant tachycardia). Corresponding ECG tracings are shown below. During sinus rhythm, the slurred initial portion of the QRS delta wave is due to early activation of part of the ventricles through rapid anterograde conduction over the AP (accessory pathway). During orthodromic AVT (atrioventricular tachycardia), no delta wave is seen because all anterograde conduction is over the AV node (AVN) and through the normal His–Purkinje system. Retrograde P waves are visible shortly after each QRS. During antidromic AVT, there is maximal pre-excitation with wide, bizarre QRS complexes, because ventricular activation results entirely from anterograde conduction over the AP. Diagram from Ganz LI, Friedman PL. Supraventricular tachycardia. *New Engl J Med* 1995;332(3):162–173. Printed with permission.

multiple impulses from the atrial tissue (Figure 4.10). Mechanically, there is no effective contraction of the atria, only a quivering of the atrial muscle. The atrial impulses travel to the AV node, where the majority are blocked and the remainder are conducted to the ventricles. This produces a heart rate from 100 to 180 beats per minute in patients with a healthy AV node. On the ECG, the hallmark is the absence of definitive atrial activity with either coarse or fine atrial fibrillatory waves. The ventricular response rate is almost always irregular.

Atrial fibrillation usually occurs in the setting of underlying heart disease, with systemic hypertension being the most common coexistent condition. Other associated conditions include valvular heart disease (especially mitral stenosis) and ischemic heart disease. It can be triggered by extracardiac conditions as well, including thyrotoxicosis, underlying infection, or pulmonary embolism. The immediate hemodynamic consequence of atrial fibrillation is the loss of the atrial contribution (termed the atrial kick) to diastolic filling of the LV. This should not significantly affect individuals with a normal heart, as diastolic filling in a normal ventricle results predominantly from relaxation of the ventricular myocardium. However, some patients with systolic or diastolic CHF depend on the atrial kick for a large part of diastolic filling. In these patients, atrial fibrillation can result in hypotension or pulmonary edema, especially if there is a rapid ventricular response that limits time for passive diastolic ventricular filling.

In clinically stable patients, the treatment of atrial fibrillation is predicated on slowing the ventricular response rate, which allows more time for diastolic filling. This can be accomplished with beta-blockers, calcium channel blockers, or digoxin. However, if atrial fibrillation with pre-excitation is suspected, these agents are contraindicated. In such cases, they can accentuate conduction through the accessory pathway by prolonging the AV nodal refractory period. In clinically unstable patients manifesting hypotension, worsening cardiac ischemia, acute pulmonary edema, or alteration in sensorium, the treatment of choice is immediate synchronized direct current (DC) cardioversion.

Due to the disorganized atrial contraction associated with this dysrhythmia, atrial fibrillation predisposes individuals to thrombus formation in the left atrial appendage. Accordingly, atrial fibrillation carries an increased risk of thromboembolic stroke. The risk is greatest during the first 48 hours following DC cardioversion. Anticoagulation with adjusted dose warfarin can reduce the risk of thromboembolism. Stable patients should be anticoagulated for at least 3 weeks before undergoing elective DC cardioversion. If atrial fibrillation has been present for less than 48 hours, DC cardioversion or chemical cardioversion (with agents such as amiodarone, procainamide or ibutilide) can be performed without anticoagulation, provided that post-cardioversion anticoagulation is given. An alternative approach is to screen patients for thrombus with transesophageal echocardiography (TEE). If the TEE shows no evidence of thrombus, cardioversion can be performed without anticoagulation. All patients with atrial fibrillation should be referred for elective echocardiography to evaluate their left atrial size and LV systolic function, and should have a TSH level drawn to exclude underlying thyrotoxicosis.

Atrial flutter

Atrial flutter is characterized by a macro-reentrant dysrhythmia involving the atria with "flutter waves" being generated at 280–320 beats per minute (Figure 4.11). It typically presents with 2:1 block and can be mistaken for sinus tachycardia. It can also present with 4:1 or variable AV block. On the ECG, flutter waves are best seen in lead II as an inverted sawtooth pattern, but may be concealed within T waves or QRS complexes.

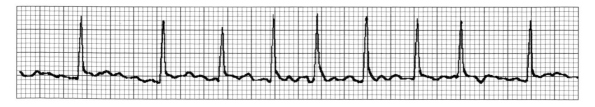

Figure 4.10
Atrial fibrillation. From Edhouse J, Morris F. ABC of clinical electrocardiography: broad complex tachycardia – Part II. *Br Med J* 2002;324(7340):776–779. Printed with permission.

Atrial flutter is commonly associated with underlying heart disease, such as ischemic heart disease or dilated cardiomyopathy. It is considered to have the same pathologic spectrum as atrial fibrillation, and patients with atrial flutter often have concomitant atrial fibrillation. Less commonly it is associated with myocarditis, blunt chest trauma, or pulmonary embolism.

The treatment of atrial flutter in stable patients is rate control with a beta-blocker or calcium channel blocker. In unstable patients or patients with refractory atrial flutter, synchronized DC cardioversion with 50 joules of energy often converts atrial flutter to sinus rhythm. Ibutilide, amiodarone, or procainamide can also be used to convert atrial flutter to sinus rhythm. Ibutilide should be used with caution in patients with structural heart disease or hypomagnesemia, as there is a higher risk of torsades de pointes in these patients. Atrial flutter carries with it a lower risk of thromboembolism than atrial fibrillation, but anticoagulation should be considered in patients with coexistent atrial fibrillation, patients greater than 70 years of age, patients with prior thromboembolism, or patients with structurally abnormal hearts. Atrial flutter is curable through radiofrequency catheter ablation, so these patients should be referred to a cardiologist for further evaluation.

Multifocal atrial tachycardia (MAT)

MAT occurs when there are numerous ectopic atrial foci that simultaneously depolarize, producing at least three different P wave morphologies, a narrow QRS complex (unless a coexistent bundle branch block is present), variable PR intervals, and a heart rate between 100 and 180 beats per minute (Figure 4.12). It is commonly associated with chronic lung disease and can be a manifestation of theophylline toxicity. Fortunately, it is seldom life-threatening. Treatment should be directed primarily at the underlying chronic lung disease, although judicious use of calcium channel blockers may provide symptomatic relief through rate control. Electrical cardioversion is not effective given the numerous sites of atrial ectopy present.

Ventricular tachycardia (VT)

VT is defined as three or more consecutive QRS complexes originating from the ventricles and occurring at a rapid rate. It may develop in a sporadic, intermittent fashion that interrupts the patient's underlying sinus rhythm (non-sustained VT), or as a consistent, uninterrupted wide-complex rhythm (sustained VT). It is typically regular or only slightly irregular. VT is almost always associated with underlying structural heart disease, and is therefore more common in older patients. It can have a single reentrant focus as the nidus for the dysrhythmia (*monomorphic* VT) or multiple reentrant foci (*polymorphic* VT), especially in the setting of ischemia (Figure 4.13). The most common underlying causes of VT are chronic ischemic heart disease and acute myocardial infarction. VT is important to recognize and treat as it has the potential to degenerate into ventricular fibrillation. All patients with VT require an aggressive workup for possible cardiac ischemia and admission to a coronary care unit.

Perhaps the most challenging aspect of cardiac rhythm analysis is the differentiation of VT from supraventricular tachycardia (SVT) with aberrant conduction. While no set of criteria will absolutely differentiate the two, several criteria have been developed to assist clinicians. There are several characteristics on the 12-lead ECG that strongly suggest the diagnosis of VT rather

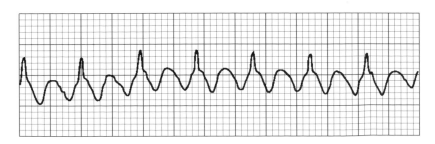

Figure 4.11
Atrial flutter. From Goodacre S, Irons R. ABC of clinical electrocardiograpy: atrial dysrhythmias. *Br Med J* 2002;324(7337):594–597. Printed with permission.

than another cause of wide-complex tachycardia. These include the following:

1. *QRS-complex duration greater than 140 milliseconds*: If the QRS complex is greater than 140 milliseconds, this strongly suggests that the rhythm is ventricular in origin. An important exception to this rule would be a patient with a baseline bundle branch block in whom the baseline QRS duration for normal sinus beats is 140 milliseconds or greater. This is a rare scenario, however.

2. *Precordial QRS concordance*: When the initial deflection in all of the ventricular complexes from V1 through V6 are either positive or negative, this strongly suggests VT. This is very specific for VT but not very sensitive. Negative precordial QRS concordance suggests the origin of the tachycardia is the posterior wall of the LV and always connotes VT. Positive precordial QRS concordance suggests an origin from the anterior wall of the LV and may connote VT.

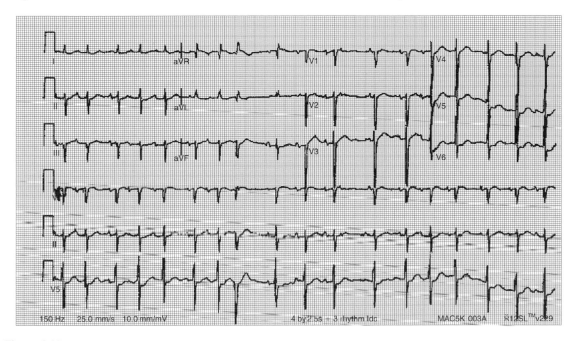

Figure 4.12
Multifocal atrial tachycardia. Note three different P wave morphologies. From Pollack ML, Brady WJ, Chan TC. Electrocardiographic manifestations: narrow QRS complex tachycardias. *J Emerg Med* 2003;24(1):35–43. Printed with permission.

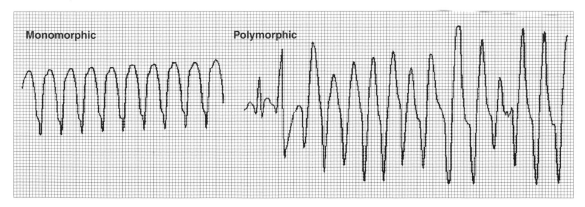

Figure 4.13
Monomorphic and polymorphic ventricular tachycardia. From Edhouse J, Morris F. Broad complex tachycardia – Part I. *Br Med J* 2002;324(7339):719–722. Printed with permission.

3. *Presence of AV dissociation*: Given that VT is caused by an independent pacemaker within the ventricle, there is no relation of the atrial rhythm to the faster ventricular rhythm. Therefore, P waves and unrelated wide QRS complexes can often be seen in the same rhythm strip. Clinically, intermittent cannon A waves may be present in the patient's jugular venous pulse; these represent right atrial contraction against a closed tricuspid valve. This clinical finding is a hallmark of AV dissociation.

4. *Presence of capture beats and/or fusion beats*: These beats represent interruptions of the underlying ventricular rhythm by atrial impulses that depolarize the ventricle, and strongly suggest VT. A *capture beat* (Figure 4.14) occurs when a P wave arrives before a ventricular impulse and results in a normal-appearing narrow-complex QRS in the midst of a group of wide-complex ventricular beats. The P wave temporarily "captures" the ventricle, but the underlying wide-complex rhythm eventually takes over. A *fusion beat* (Figure 4.15) occurs when a P wave arrives at the same time as the ventricular impulse. The result is a QRS complex which is a hybrid between the normal narrow-complex and the wide-complex QRS of the ventricular rhythm.

Neither the rate alone nor the clinical scenario determines whether the rhythm is VT. However, a useful general principle is to treat any wide-complex QRS rhythm as VT until proven otherwise, especially if the patient is clinically unstable, has known structural heart disease, or a previous MI.

Treatment of VT depends on the stability of the patient. Unstable patients require immediate DC cardioversion. Pulseless VT is treated as ventricular fibrillation, with immediate defibrillation. Stable patients can be treated with IV antidysrhythmic medications such as amiodarone, procainamide, or lidocaine (Figure 4.16). Serum electrolytes should be drawn in all patients, and hypokalemia and hypomagnesemia should be corrected if present.

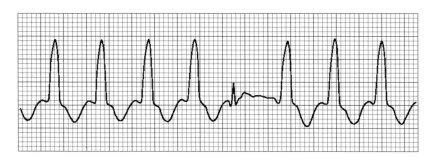

Figure 4.14
Capture beat. From Edhouse J, Morris F. Broad complex tachycardia – Part I. *Br Med J* 2002;324(7339):719–722. Printed with permission.

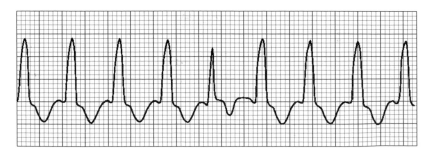

Figure 4.15
Fusion beat. From Edhouse J, Morris F. Broad complex tachycardia – Part I. *Br Med J* 2002;324(7339):719–722. Printed with permission.

Supraventricular tachycardia (SVT) with aberrant conduction

Any of the previously discussed narrow-complex tachydysrhythmias can be accompanied by aberrant conduction (Figure 4.17). This can be either a left or right bundle branch block pattern. The following criteria suggest a supraventricular rhythm with aberrancy rather than VT:

1. A bundle branch morphology identical to that of the previous 12-lead ECG.
2. An ectopic P wave that precedes the QRS complex.
3. Variable coupling intervals between beats.
4. Response to adenosine or carotid sinus massage. SVT with aberrancy will usually respond with a slowing of the heart rate and possible termination of the dysrhythmia, while VT does not typically.

When in doubt, it is safest and most appropriate to assume the rhythm disturbance is VT and treat accordingly. The treatment for all unstable patients is synchronized electrical cardioversion.

Torsades de pointes

Torsades de pointes ("twisting of the points") is a special type of polymorphic VT that arises in patients with pre-existing prolongation of the QT interval (Figure 4.18). It is a wide-complex tachycardia with an undulating amplitude that varies

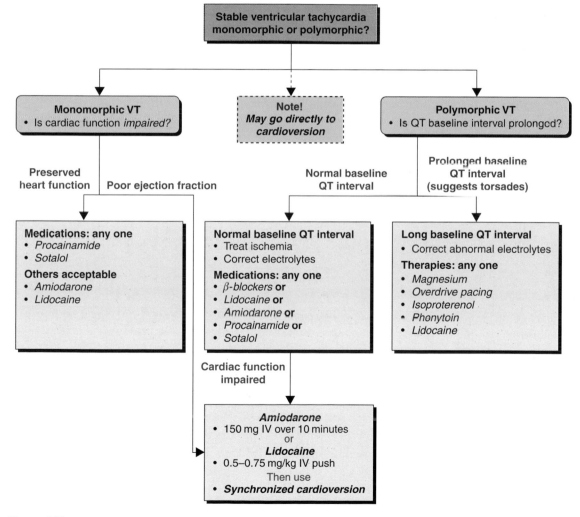

Figure 4.16
Stable ventricular tachycardia (VT). Reproduced with permission, ACLS Provider Manual, © 2001, Copyright American Heart Association.

above and below the baseline. Its rate varies from 180 to 250 beats per minute. Prolongation of the QT interval can occur as a result of the prodysrhythmic effects of numerous drugs, including quinidine, procainamide, ibutilide, amiodarone, sotalol, phenothiazines, certain antihistamines, and tricyclic antidepressants. Electrolyte abnormalities such as hypomagnesemia, hypokalemia, and hypocalcemia can cause prolongation of the QT interval as well.

Treatment of torsades de pointes is aimed at interrupting the ventricular rhythm and restoring sinus rhythm. As the majority of patients with this dysrhythmia are clinically unstable, DC cardioversion is the treatment of choice. Electrolyte abnormalities such as hypokalemia, hypocalcemia, and hypomagnesemia should be aggressively corrected. In more stable patients, other treatment options include IV isoproterenol and overdrive pacing of the ventricle. Some clinicians empirically administer IV magnesium sulfate to treat this condition.

Atrial fibrillation with pre-excitation

This is a special case of atrial fibrillation where conduction occurs antegrade down a pre-existing bypass tract (Figure 4.19). As there is no inherent refractory period in bypass tract tissue unlike in the AV node, ventricular response rates are usually much higher. On the ECG, there is a wide-complex, irregular tachycardia with a rate ranging from 150 to 300 beats per minute. Delta waves (which may be seen on previous ECGs), a previous history of Wolff–Parkinson–White (WPW) syndrome, or irregular R-R intervals which may be as fast as 300 are major clues to this diagnosis.

Conventional treatment of atrial fibrillation with AV nodal blocking agents is contraindicated in the presence of a bypass tract. Instead, stable patients should receive IV procainamide which attempts to chemically cardiovert the patient to sinus rhythm without slowing conduction through the AV node. Unstable patients should undergo synchronized electrical cardioversion. Patients who manifest this rhythm should be referred to a cardiologist for radiofrequency catheter ablation of the bypass tract to prevent recurrences.

Accelerated idioventricular rhythm (AIVR)

Accelerated idioventricular rhythm (AIVR) is a wide-complex dysrhythmia of ventricular origin

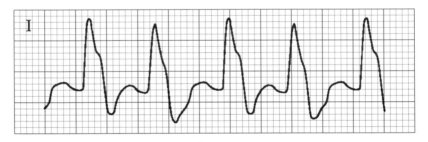

Figure 4.17
Supraventricular tachycardia (SVT) with aberrant conduction. From Edhouse J, Morris F. ABC of clinical electrocardiography: broad complex tachycardia – Part II. *Br Med J* 2002;324(7340):776–779. Printed with permission.

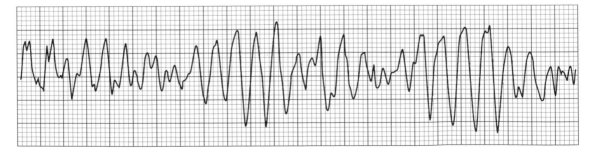

Figure 4.18
Torsades de Pointes. From Edhouse J, Morris F. ABC of clinical electrocardiography: broad complex tachycardia – Part II. *Br Med J* 2002; 324(7340): 776–779. Printed with permission.

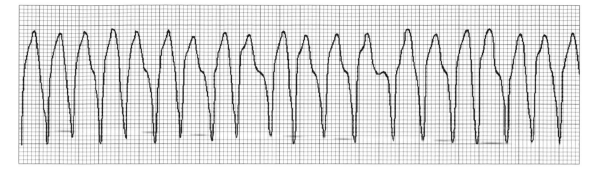

Figure 4.19
Atrial fibrillation with pre-excitation. From Edhousie J, Morris F. ABC of clinical electrocardiography: broad complex tachycardia. Part II. *Br Med J* 2002;324(7340):776–779. Printed with permission.

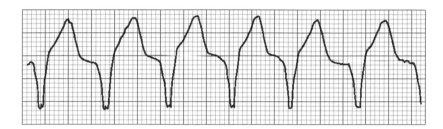

Figure 4.20
Accelerated idioventricular rhythm. From Edhouse J, Morris F. Broad complex tachycardia – Part I. *Br Med J* 2002;324(7339):719–722. Printed with permission.

which occurs at a rate of 40–100 beats per minute (Figure 4.20). It is characterized by regular, wide QRS complexes that are not preceded by P waves. It is commonly seen following acute myocardial infarction, and is known as a "reperfusion dysrhythmia." AIVR is a stable rhythm that usually produces no symptoms and therefore requires no treatment. In some instances, the ventricular pacemaker may be the only functioning pacemaker in the heart, and suppressing it with antidysrhythmics such as lidocaine can lead to asystole.

Pearls, pitfall and myths

- Consider the etiology of the cardiac dysrhythmia, not just the rhythm itself.
- Certain medications and electrolyte abnormalities may predispose the patient to serious dysrhythmias.
- Learn to distinguish benign from malignant dysrhythmias.
- The patient's clinical (hemodynamic) stability is integral to the appropriate evaluation and management of dysrhythmias.

- Treat the patient, not the rhythm.
- Err on the side of caution, especially with regard to medication choices or rhythm interpretation.
- Serial administration of medications is generally safer than a single large bolus.
- When in doubt about the etiology of a wide-complex tachycardia, treat as ventricular tachycardia until proven otherwise.
- Before semi-elective cardioversion of atrial fibrillation, consider the risk of thromboembolic stroke and the need for anticoagulation.
- Beware of atrial fibrillation in the setting of pre-excitation, as treatment with AV nodal blockade can lead to ventricular fibrillation.

References

1. Braunwald E, Libby P, Zipes D. *Heart Disease: A Textbook of Cardiovascular Medicine*, 6th ed., ISBN 0721685617, WB Saunders, 2001.

2. Da Costa D, Brady WJ, Edhouse J. Bradycardias and atrioventricular conduction block. *Br Med J* 2002;324(7336):535–538.
3. Edhouse J, Morris F. Broad complex tachycardia – Part I. *Br Med J* 2002;324(7339):719–722.
4. Edhouse J, Morris F. ABC of clinical electrocardiography: broad complex tachycardia – Part II. *Br Med J* 2002;324(7340):776–779.
5. Fuster V, O'Rourke RA, Alexander RW. *Hurst's The Heart*, 10th ed., ISBN 00713556940, McGraw Hill Publishers, 2000.
6. Ganz LI, Friedman PL. Supraventricular tachycardia. *New Engl J Med* 1995;332(3):162–173.
7. Goodacre S, Irons R. ABC of clinical electrocardiography: atrial dysrhythmias. *Br Med J* 2002;324(7337):594–597.
8. Morady F. Radio-frequency ablation as treatment for cardiac dysrhythmias. *New Engl J Med* 1999;340(7):534–544.
9. Pollack ML, Brady WJ, Chan TC. Electrocardiographic manifestations: narrow QRS complex tachycardias. *J Emerg Med* 2003;24(1):35–43.
10. Wagner GS. *Marriott's Practical Electrocardiography*, 10th ed., ISBN 0683307460, Williams and Wilkins, 1999.

5 Shock

Robert J. Sigillito, MD and Peter M.C. DeBlieux, MD

Scope of the problem

Shock is a state in which the oxygen (O_2) and metabolic demands of the body are not met by the cardiac output. When this process occurs in a single organ, rather than throughout the body, organ ischemia and infarction ensue. When shock occurs on a more global level, multiorgan dysfunction and failure are the consequence, ultimately leading to death if not corrected. Shock is most often accompanied by hypotension, termed *decompensated shock*. However, shock may also occur with normal or elevated blood pressure. Examples include hypertensive emergency with compromised cardiac output, or carbon monoxide intoxication with the inability to deliver O_2 despite normal hemodynamics. The approach to the patient in shock must proceed with the same urgency as the patient suffering from an acute myocardial infarction or cerebral vascular accident.

Classification

Shock states are classified according to the underlying physiologic derangement. Table 5.1 lists the most commonly used classification system. *Hypovolemic shock* is defined by decreased circulating blood volume, either due to blood or fluid loss, such that cardiac output is compromised. Impaired cardiac performance characterizes *cardiogenic shock*. Loss of vasomotor tone with hypotension is the hallmark of *distributive shock*, as in sepsis, anaphylaxis, or certain intoxications. Anatomic interruption of sympathetic output, usually secondary to spinal cord injury with disruption of the cervical sympathetic chain, leads to bradycardia and hypotension in *neurogenic shock*. Obstruction of blood flow through the cardiopulmonary circuit is the etiology of *obstructive shock*, as in tension pneumothorax, cardiac tamponade, or massive pulmonary embolus. Finally, a few patients present with a *mixed syndrome*, such as a patient with sepsis who develops gastrointestinal (GI) hemorrhage, or who suffers a concomitant myocardial infarction.

General approach to the patient in shock

If shock is defined by impaired global organ perfusion, then it follows that signs of shock are derived from impaired organ function. Hypotension is an obvious sign of decompensated hemodynamics associated with shock. Alteration in mental status, chest pain, signs of cardiac failure, difficulty breathing, abdominal pain from intestinal ischemia, low urinary output, and mottled skin all suggest shock.

In a proportion of patients, the etiology of the shock state remains in question after initial evaluation. Often, therapeutic intervention must be initiated without a firm diagnosis. The core principle in treatment of such patients is that O_2 delivery to the vital organs must be optimized.

History

Obtaining an accurate history is essential to approaching undifferentiated patients in shock.

Table 5.1 Classification of shock states

Hypovolemic shock Hemorrhage Fluid loss/dehydration
Cardiogenic shock Pump failure Valvular disorders Cardiac dysrhythmia
Distributive shock Sepsis Anaphylaxis Intoxications
Neurogenic shock[b] Spinal cord injury
Obstructive shock Tension pneumothorax Pericardial tamponade/constrictive pericarditis[a] Massive pulmonary embolus Severe pulmonary hypertension Severe valvular stenosis
[a] Classified by some as cardiogenic shock. [b] Classified by some as distributive shock.

Deficiencies in the historical database lead to poor treatment choices and increase patient morbidity and mortality. Unfortunately, many patients in shock states are not up to the task of providing an accurate and complete history. Medical records, family members, and friends are invaluable resources in these situations. Time course and progression of illness provide important information regarding the rapidity of decline and may help narrow the differential diagnosis. Pre-existing conditions, particularly limitations of the cardiopulmonary system and immune deficiencies, predispose patients to poor outcomes.

Obtaining a patient's complete medication list is vital in addressing the needs of the patient in shock. Medications that impair normal cardiac compensation in shock states, such as beta blockers, calcium channel blockers, or digitalis, may alter patient presentations in profound shock. Likewise, immunosuppressant agents, such as prednisone and chemotherapeutic drugs, may impair host immune response and mask serious or life-threatening infections. Lastly, social historical data focusing on alcohol, illicit drug use, work history, and psychosocial support systems may offer insight into these complex patients.

Physical examination

Physical examination and rapid assessment of the patient in shock follow the basic tenants of emergency medicine. Airway, breathing, circulation, disability, and exposure (ABCDE) are vital in the initial evaluation of the most complex patient presentations. If the impairment of shock is the inability to adequately provide O_2 at the end organ, then the first critical appraisal must be airway, quickly followed by breathing and circulation. These first three steps comprise the critical care concept of "cardiopulmonary reserve." Cardiopulmonary reserve refers to the interdependence of the heart, lungs, and O_2-carrying capacity of any given patient. Those patients with an impaired cardiac pump, pre-existing pulmonary disease, or abnormalities in hemoglobin may require a more immediate intervention for possibly milder shock states when compared to patients with normal physiology. Normal lungs, heart, and hemoglobin permit a degree of physiologic reserve that allows patients to compensate for any given cardiopulmonary insult.

One of the first steps in determining cardiopulmonary reserve is vital sign assessment. In evaluating and treating patients in shock, the goal is to maintain adequate oxygenation and organ perfusion. Pulse oximetry is a rapid bedside tool that can be utilized as an initial screening tool to determine the adequacy of oxygenation. Goal saturations during resuscitation and treatment should be maintained above 90%, although outcome data does not exist for this universally-accepted goal. The use of O_2 delivery devices may be required to reach the goal of 90%; if adequate O_2 saturations are not obtained with 100% non-rebreather mask, then patients should be endotracheally intubated and placed on mechanical ventilation.

Once oxygenation has been addressed, the focus should be placed firmly on maintaining adequate cerebral and coronary perfusion pressures to prevent injury to these vital organs. Vital organ perfusion pressure is a function of mean arterial blood pressure (MABP). The critical nature of diastolic blood pressure (DBP) can be seen, as it is the main component of that calculation:

$$MABP = DBP + \tfrac{1}{3}(SBP - DBP)$$

where SBP = systolic blood pressure.

Goals for resuscitation and maintenance in the majority of shock states should attempt to get MABP in the 70–80 mmHg range to offer adequate cerebral and coronary perfusion.

MABP can be better understood as it relates to preload and afterload. Physiologically, *preload* is defined as the left ventricular end diastolic wall tension. Clinically, several measures can be used to estimate whether the preload is low, normal, or high. The clinical situation may strongly suggest a patient's volume status. Actively bleeding patients, trauma victims, or chronically dehydrated patients are virtually certain to have a low preload. The edematous patient with congestive heart failure (CHF) is likely to be volume overloaded. Estimation of the jugular venous pressure (JVP) on physical examination can be rapidly performed; however, the accuracy of this technique is not high, even in the hands of an experienced clinician. Auscultation of the heart and lungs is sensitive for detecting signs of volume overload (S3, crackles, and rales), but does not distinguish the hypovolemic state. Assessment of skin turgor, capillary refill, and the mucous membranes can likewise be misleading.

Afterload is the force that the heart must generate in order to eject blood into the arterial compartment. Since MABP is proportional to the product of systemic vascular resistance (SVR) and the cardiac output (CO), SVR is one of the main determinants of afterload. A comprehensive review of the technique for insertion, calibration, and collection of data from a pulmonary artery (PA) catheter is beyond the scope of this chapter.

It is essential to note that excessive heart rate (HR) increases myocardial O_2 consumption and may further compromise at-risk myocardium. Additionally, patients with normal vital signs can be in profound shock states despite calculated MABP, central venous pressure (CVP), HR, and O_2 saturation that are considered within normal ranges.

After the assessment of the cardiopulmonary reserve, a rapid neurological assessment is performed followed by complete exposure of the patient. Next, a comprehensive head-to-toe physical examination is performed to identify evidence of decreased organ perfusion and to search for the etiology of the presenting complaint. Altered mental status, cyanosis, delayed capillary refill, and skin mottling may be early signs of decreased oxygenation and perfusion.

Differential diagnosis

Physical examination and right heart catheterization are useful in the determination of the etiology of the various shock states, but the latter is rarely immediately available in the emergency department (ED). Table 5.2 outlines the physiologic parameters that characterize each shock state.

Hypovolemic shock

Hypovolemic shock is defined by the loss of intravascular volume. CVP, pulmonary artery occlusion pressure (PAOP), and cardiac output are low, while SVR is elevated. In the early compensated stages, the pulse pressure is narrowed due to vasoconstriction, but ultimately hypotension occurs with decompensation. The initial treatment of hypovolemic shock is aggressive volume expansion with crystalloid solution. Transfusion of blood products may be required if hemorrhage is the cause of hypovolemia.

Cardiogenic shock

The most common cause of cardiogenic shock is acute myocardial infarction, accounting for nearly half the cases. Low cardiac output and high SVR characterize cardiogenic shock. CVP and PAOP are most often elevated during acute exacerbations of CHF, but may be normal if the patient has

Table 5.2 Physiologic parameters in shock states

	CVP	PAOP	SVR/ SVRI	CO/ CI
Hypovolemic	↓	↓	↑	↓
Cardiogenic	↑	↑	↑	↓
Distributive				
Sepsis	↔↓	↔↓	↓	↕
Anaphylaxis	↔↓	↔↓	↓	↑
Neurogenic	↔	↔	↓	↔↑
Obstructive				
Tamponade	↑	↑	↑	↓
Tension PTX	↑a	↑a	↑	↓
Massive PE	↑	↑b	↑	↓

CVP: central venous pressure
PAOP: pulmonary artery occlusion pressure
SVR: systemic vascular resistance
SVRI: systemic vascular resistance index
CO/CI: cardiac output/cardiac index
PTX: pneumothorax
PE: pulmonary embolism.

[a] True CVP and PAOP are diminished due to impaired venous return. Measured pressure is falsely elevated, reflecting pleural pressure rather than vascular pressure.

[b] True left atrial pressure is low due to obstruction of flow through the pulmonary vasculature. Measured pressure may be falsely elevated, reflecting pulmonary vascular resistance rather than left heart filling pressure.

received adequate diuresis. Suggested cardiac parameters for the diagnosis of cardiogenic shock include cardiac index (CI) $< 1.8\,\text{L}/\text{min}/\text{m}^2$, SBP $< 80\,\text{mmHg}$, and PAOP $> 18\,\text{cmH}_2\text{O}$. The initial treatment of CHF includes preload and afterload reduction. When shock is present, addition of a cardiotonic vasopressor is required. Strong evidence supporting selection of one vasopressor over another does not exist. Consensus committee (ACC/AHA) has recommended the use of dobutamine if SBP is greater than 90, dopamine if SBP is less than 90, and norepinephrine if hypotension is severe or refractory to dopamine infusion. An intra-aortic balloon pump (IABP) should be considered for patients who do not respond to vasopressor therapy. This technique employs placing an intra-aortic balloon that inflates during diastole, augmenting MABP and systemic perfusion, and deflates during systole, effectively diminishing afterload and improving cardiac output. Percutaneous coronary angioplasty and/or coronary artery bypass grafting should be strongly considered in patients with acute coronary ischemia complicated by shock.

Distributive shock

In early sepsis, SVR is elevated. However, as septic shock progresses, SVR drops precipitously. Cardiac output is increased in most cases, but a cytokine known as myocardial depressant factor is believed to be released from the pancreas, and may impair systolic function in later stages. Impaired cardiac perfusion will also adversely affect cardiac output. Vascular permeability is increased. Fluid shifts and increased insensible losses may lead to intravascular volume depletion and low CVP and PAOP. Early broad-spectrum antibiotic therapy and emergent surgical drainage or debridement, when indicated, are the cornerstones of treatment. Volume replacement should be guided by invasive monitoring of either CVP or PAOP. Norepinephrine is the vasoactive agent of choice. Recently introduced to the US, activated protein C complex (Xigris®) may improve survival.

Anaphylactic shock is accompanied by the massive release of cytokines in an inflammatory cascade, with loss of vasomotor tone and increased vascular permeability. Epinephrine, steroids, and antihistamines are initial therapies. Persistent hypotension requires infusion of an agent that supports vasomotor tone. Again, norepinephrine makes the most sense physiologically.

Neurogenic shock

Neurogenic shock, classified by some as a type of distributive shock, is a consequence of injury to the sympathetic ganglion chain. Neurogenic shock characteristically manifests as hypotension and bradycardia. Since spinal cord injury is most prevalent in the young population, this entity usually occurs in patients with normal cardiac function. It is of the utmost importance to rule out occult hemorrhage, and to use signs of organ perfusion to guide the initiation of pharmacologic therapy. Many of these patients perfuse their organs well at below-normal MABP. If signs of hypoperfusion develop, then selection of an agent that supports SVR (norepinephrine or neosynephrine) makes the most sense physiologically.

Obstructive shock

Two causes of obstructive shock, tension pneumothorax and cardiac tamponade, are reversible by surgical intervention. Support of the patient by volume loading is temporizing at best. Massive pulmonary embolus causes the release of vasoactive cytokines from the pulmonary vascular bed, obstruction of flow, and acute right ventricular dysfunction, collectively impairing left ventricular filling. Thrombectomy or thrombolysis can be life-saving interventions. Support of cardiac function with volume infusions and dobutamine may be a bridge to these interventions. Chronic pulmonary hypertension may also limit flow through the pulmonary vascular bed. The onset of shock is an end-stage, pre-terminal event. Treatment with potent pulmonary vasodilators is hazardous in this shock state since hypotension from peripheral arterial dilation is a frequent side effect, mandating use of a pulmonary artery catheter.

Diagnostic testing

Rapid bedside screening is the hallmark of the initial approach to screening and assessment of the undifferentiated patient in shock. Vital signs, pulse oximetry, and continuous monitoring are the standard testing. Following a head-to-toe assessment, a Foley catheter should be placed with an urometer to assess adequate hourly urinary output (0.5ml/kg/hour). Initial screening studies for the undifferentiated patient include: bedside blood sugar analysis, arterial blood gas analysis, chest radiography, and an electrocardiogram. A comprehensive metabolic profile, urinalysis, and complete blood count are required on each patient. Consideration for toxicologic studies, blood and urine cultures, cardiac profiles, and endocrinologic screening should be made on a case-by-case basis. Serum lactate levels can be used to guide therapy, and may have prognostic value. An argument can be made to perform a quick, bedside echocardiogram to exclude cases of cardiac tamponade and global cardiac hypokinesis, but controlled trials supporting this approach have not been published. Additional radiographic studies of the head, chest, abdomen, pelvis, and extremities are second-tier studies and should only be obtained once the patient has been clinically stabilized.

General treatment principles
Oxygenation

Whenever a shock state is present, O_2 supplementation is required. O_2 may be delivered via facial delivery devices, non-invasive mechanical ventilation, or by conventional mechanical ventilation.

Simple means of delivering supplemental O_2 include the use of a nasal cannula, venturi mask, or O_2-reservoir non-rebreathing apparatus. O_2 delivered via nasal cannula is appropriate only when low O_2 flow is required. It is impossible to determine the fraction of inspired O_2 (FiO_2) delivered to any given patient because it varies with respiratory rate, the degree of nasal versus mouth breathing, and the O_2 flow rate. In general, if more than 5 L/min of O_2 flow is required with a nasal cannula, then an alternative device should be employed.

A venturi mask uses various O_2 flow rates combined with various venturi apertures to produce increasing O_2 supplementation, generally higher than can be delivered by nasal cannula. Although each mask lists specific FiO_2 ratings from 0.28 to 0.50, these are rough estimates at best. If the listed flow rate with the smallest aperture does not provide enough supplemental O_2, then an alternative device is required.

A non-rebreathing apparatus combines a collapsible bag reservoir with high-flow O_2 and an exhalation valve so that high FiO_2 can be delivered. When used optimally, the FiO_2 range may approach 0.6–0.8.

The current literature supports the use of non-invasive positive pressure ventilation (NPPV) in patients without hemodynamic compromise, cardiac dysrhythmias, or altered mental status. Therefore, NPPV use in the management of shock should be limited to patients with respiratory failure without hemodynamic instability. This literature strongly supports the use of NPPV in patients with hypercapneic hypoxemic respiratory failure, such as those with exacerbation of chronic obstructive pulmonary disease (COPD). Data from descriptive studies regarding its use in selected cases of hypoxemic respiratory failure, such as acute respiratory distress syndrome (ARDS), is available, but prospective randomized trials are lacking. Prospective trials investigating NPPV use in CHF with pulmonary edema suggest that continuous positive airway pressure (CPAP) is beneficial. Studies utilizing bilevel positive airway pressure (BiPAP) have been small and did not demonstrate benefit.

Early generations of non-invasive ventilators bled O_2 into the ventilator tubing, so FiO_2 was not tightly controlled. O_2 flow was increased until the patient's arterial O_2 saturation (SaO_2) was optimized. In newer models, the FiO_2 can be more precisely set with a mixture valve, and adjusted as needed based on saturation monitoring.

Invasive mechanical ventilation should be considered for any patient who does not achieve adequate SaO_2 despite maximal non-invasive O_2 supplementation. All patients who are placed on invasive ventilation should initially receive an FiO_2 of 1.0 because the switch from spontaneous breathing (negative pressure) to assisted ventilation (positive pressure) causes unpredictable alterations in pulmonary blood flow and ventilation–perfusion mismatch. FiO_2 can then be decreased as the patient's SaO_2 allows. Patients with pulmonary edema, particularly those with ARDS, may require the addition of positive end-expiratory pressure (PEEP) to optimize oxygenation. Although many factors must be considered in determining the optimal level of PEEP, most authors recommend starting at 3–5 cmH$_2$O. Thereafter, PEEP is incrementally increased by 2–3 cmH$_2$O, allowing 15–30 minutes after each increase for alveolar recruitment. PEEP is increased until SaO_2 reaches a minimum 88–90%. Further increases in PEEP may then be required to allow the FiO_2 to be decreased to 0.6. As PEEP is increased, the mean intrathoracic pressure increases. A critical point is reached when venous return to the heart is compromised due to increased intrathoracic pressure, impairing cardiac output. PEEP should not be increased beyond the point where hemodynamic compromise occurs.

Cardiac intervention

Pathologic rhythms may be a cause or consequence of a shock state. In either scenario, the goal of therapy should be to convert this to a perfusing rhythm. Bradycardic rhythms should be sped up either pharmacologically or with electrical transthoracic or transvenous pacing. Atropine is considered the first-line agent in patients with a pulse. It should be considered a temporary measure, and preparation for pacing should be rapidly accomplished. In contrast, a bradycardiac patient without a pulse should receive CPR and alternating doses of epinephrine and atropine while preparing to initiate electrical pacing.

The principles for electrically pacing the heart are the same for transthoracic and transvenous techniques. In both modes, the initial HR is set between 80 and 100 beats per minute. In the pulseless patient, the output is set at maximum, and dialed downward after the heart demonstrates capture. In contrast, the output is set at a minimum in the patient with a pulse, and dialed upward until capture is achieved.

In both scenarios, the final output should be set at 10–20% above the threshold for capture. The causes of failure to capture include malposition of the pacing leads, hypothermia, hypoglycemia, hypoxemia, acidosis, and electrolyte disturbance.

Sinus tachycardia in the shock state is compensatory. Except in some types of intoxication (sympathomimetic or anticholinergic overdose), acute ischemic coronary syndromes, and other unusual circumstances, measures directed at slowing the HR should be limited to correcting the underlying cause. All other tachycardias are pathologic, and may be the etiology for the shock state. These should be converted to a perfusing rhythm by the most rapid means, usually electrical cardioversion. The exception to this rule is atrial fibrillation (Afib). Acute Afib, defined as Afib of less than 48 hours duration, may be treated with cardioversion. Patients with chronic Afib, defined as Afib of greater than 48 hours duration, have an increased risk of systemic embolization of an atrial thrombus. Such patients, or those in whom the duration of Afib is unknown, should receive anticoagulation or undergo transesophageal echocardiography before attempts at cardioversion are undertaken. The decision to cardiovert such a patient should be made in consultation with a cardiologist.

Volume intervention

Following initial assessment of the preload, either fluid or diuretic therapy should be instituted. The size of an initial fluid bolus is a matter of clinical judgment. A previously healthy young adult with acute hemorrhage may safely receive rapid infusion of several liters of a crystalloid solution. In contrast, a frail, elderly patient with a history of CHF may require boluses of only a few hundred milliliters at a time. The crucial step is reassessment after each intervention to decide whether further volume expansion is indicated.

A patient who is volume overloaded requires diuresis. Loop diuretics, such as furosemide, torsemide, and bumetadine, are the most commonly used first-line agents. Frequent reassessment of the response in urinary output is mandatory to guide subsequent therapy. Other interventions that may be employed to lower preload include the administration of B-type natriuretic peptide (nesiritide), nitrates, opiates, rotating tourniquets, and dialysis. Opiates should be used with caution as they are associated with worse outcomes in acute CHF.

Blood transfusion intervention

The effect of raising the hemoglobin (Hgb) on O_2 delivery is profound. The administration of 2 units of packed red blood cells (RBCs) to increase the Hgb by 25% (e.g., an increase of hematocrit from 20% to 25%) will also increase the calculated O_2 delivery by 25%. For this reason, administration of blood should be considered in patients with shock and anemia. Rapid estimation of Hgb is available in most centers by commercially-available analyzers, blood gas machines, or centrifuge techniques.

The threshold for administration of blood has been dictated by practice habit, and not by the evidence in the medical literature. It is generally recommended that adult trauma victims unresponsive to initial volume expansion with 2 L of crystalloid receive blood transfusion. Patients with coronary artery disease or CHF should be transfused with a goal of keeping the hematocrit above 30%. Other patients may benefit from blood therapy if the hematocrit falls below 20–24%. Of note, blood therapy has not been demonstrated to improve survival, decrease the duration of mechanical ventilation, or decrease the need for vasopressors. Controversy also exists because transfused allogenic RBCs may impair host immune response, and are less efficient at carrying O_2 than native RBCs.

Vasoactive agent intervention

Treatment of abnormalities in contractility and afterload should follow correction of preload, particularly in hypovolemic states. Use of vasoconstricting agents in the setting of volume depletion will further compromise organ perfusion, causing organ ischemia and infarction. Many of the vasoactive medications used to treat shock affect both myocardial contractility and SVR. A thorough knowledge of the action of adrenergic receptor physiology and the action of the vasoactive agents on these receptors is necessary to guide selection of a vasoactive agent.

Alpha-1 (α-1) receptors are found in arterial smooth muscle and in the conduction system of the heart. The physiologic effect of α-1 stimulation is increased cardiac excitation/conduction and arterial vasoconstriction (including coronary, cerebral, renal, and splanchnic arterial beds). Beta-1 (β-1) receptors are found in the myocardium and the conduction system. β-1 stimulation results in increased contractility and cardiac excitation. Beta-2 (β-2) receptors are found in arterial and bronchial smooth muscle. β-2 stimulation results in arterial vasodilation.

Vasopressors

The vasopressors are listed in Table 5.3, as first- and second-line agents. Table 5.4 provides the relative affinity of the first-line agents at the α and β receptors. Table 5.5 lists the suggested dose ranges.

Table 5.3 Vasoactive medications and initial dose

First-line agents
Norepinephrine 1 mcg/minute
Dopamine 3 mcg/kg/minute
Dobutamine 3 mcg/kg/minute
Phenylephrine 20 mcg/minute

Second-line agents
Amrinone 1 mcg/kg bolus, then 2 mcg/kg/minute
Milrinone 50 mcg/kg load, then 0.375 mcg/kg/minute
Epinephrine 1 mcg/minute
Vasopressin 0.03 international units/minute

Table 5.4 Receptor affinity and hemodynamic effects

	α-1[a]	β-1[b]	β-1[c]	β-2[d]
Dopamine				
Low dose	0	2+	2+	2+
High dose	3+	2 l	2+	2+[e]
Dobutamine				
Low dose	0	4+	1+	1–2+
High dose	1–2+	4+	1+	1–2+
Norepinephrine	4+	2+	2+	0
Epinephrine	4+	4+	4+	3+
Phenylephrine	4+	0	0	0

a: vasoconstriction; b: inotropic; c: chronotropic;
d: vasodilation; e: effect lost.
Modified from: Khalaf S, DeBlieux P. *J Crit Illness*
June 1, 2001.

Table 5.5 Dose ranges of vasoactive agents in adults

Dopamine and dobutamine
Low dose   3–8 mcg/kg/minute
High dose   8–20 mcg/kg/minute

Norepinephrine and epinephrine
1–10 mcg/minute

Phenylephrine
20–200 mcg/minute

Norepinephrine is predominately an α-1 agonist, although it has non-selective β activity as well. At low doses, it raises cardiac output and SVR proportionately, but the potential to raise cardiac output is limited. As the infusion rate increases, its effect is essentially limited to an increase in SVR and HR. The primary role of norepinephrine is in the treatment of septic shock with hypotension attributable to low SVR. A consensus committee has previously recommended norepinephrine as the agent of choice in cardiogenic shock with SBP below 70 mmHg.

Dopamine activates β receptors at moderate dose range (3–8 mcg/kg/minute) and both α and β receptors at higher infusion rates (>8 mcg/kg/minute). Clinically, SVR is decreased and cardiac output is increased at low doses. At higher doses, SVR increases, blunting further rises in cardiac output. Dopamine has been recommended as the agent of choice in patients with cardiogenic shock and SBP between 70–90 mmHg. Dopamine may cause pulmonary vasoconstriction, with resultant rise in PAOP, limiting its value as an index of left heart preload. Tachyphylaxis to dopamine infusion may also occur.

Dobutamine activates β receptors throughout its dose range, and is a more potent cardiac stimulant than dopamine. It has weaker α receptor activity than dopamine. The balance of the effect of increased cardiac output and decreased SVR can have a variable effect on MABP. Those patients with large increases in contractility tend to experience a rise in MABP, while those with a weak increase in cardiac output in response to dobutamine tend to have no change in or diminished MABP. It is impossible to predict which patients will respond with increased cardiac output; however, younger patients tend to be more responsive than the elderly. In contrast to dopamine, dobutamine tends to cause pulmonary vasodilation.

Epinephrine is a potent α and β agonist, roughly 500 times more potent than dopamine or dobutamine. It is arrhythmogenic, increases myocardial O_2 consumption, and causes tachycardia. Its use is limited to cardiac arrest, refractory life-threatening bradycardia, and anaphylactic shock.

Phenylephrine is a pure α-1 agonist. It may be useful in the management of vasomotor collapse, as in distributive or neurogenic shock. However, because it is less well studied than the other vasopressors, its routine use is not advocated at present.

Isoproterenol is a potent β agonist. It causes a marked increase in HR and myocardial O_2

consumption. Its only role is in the treatment of life-threatening bradycardia. Its use should therefore be limited to failure of electrical cardiac pacing.

Amrinone and milrinone are not adrenergic receptor agonists. Instead, they inhibit phosphodiesterase, producing an effect similar to β agonists. These are second-line agents for the treatment of CHF, and may be additive in effect to dobutamine.

Vasopressin is an endogenous peptide hormone that has vasoconstrictive and antidiuretic effects via receptors in the vascular smooth muscle and the kidneys. It has undergone preliminary investigation as an agent for use in septic shock. However, its routine use cannot be advocated until prospective randomized trials are completed.

Pitfalls

- Failure to recognize early signs of shock, before hypotension develops.
- Failure to provide early ventilatory support to the hemodynamically-compromised patient.
- Inadequate fluid resuscitation of the volume-depleted patient before initiating vasoactive infusion.
- Delay in administration of empiric broad-spectrum antibiotics in septic shock.
- Failure to continuously monitor hemodynamic parameters (Table 5.6) as a guide to titration of fluid therapy and vasoactive infusions.
- Improper selection of vasoactive agents.
- Reliance on pulse oximetry as an index of SaO_2 during periods of hypoperfusion, severe hypoxemia, or when a hemoglobinopathy is present.

Table 5.6 Normal values of hemodynamic parameters

CVP	2–6 cmH$_2$O
PAOP	8–12 cmH$_2$O
CO	3.8–7.5 L/min (approximate for normal size adult)
CI	2.4–4.0 L/min/m^2
SVR	800–1400 dyne/s/cm^5 (approximate for normal size adult)
SVRI	1600–2400 dyne/s/m^2/cm^5

CVP: central venous pressure
PAOP: pulmonary artery occlusion pressure
CO: cardiac output
CI: cardiac index
SVR: systemic vascular resistance
SVRI: systemic vascular resistance index

References

1. ACC/AHA Guidelines for the Management of Patients with Acute Myocardial Infarction 1999 Updated Guideline, Web Version (www.acc.org).
2. Bernard GR, Vincent JL, Laterre PF, et al. Efficacy and safety of recombinant human activated protein C for severe sepsis. *New Engl J Med* 2001;344(10):699–709.
3. Chakko S, Woska D, Martinez H, et al. Clinical, radiographic, and hemodynamic correlations in chronic congestive heart failure: conflicting results may lead to inappropriate care. *Am J Med* 1991;90:353–359.
4. Cook D. Clinical assessment of central venous pressure in the critically ill. *Am J Med Sci* 1990;299(3):175–178.
5. ECC Guidelines. *Circulation.* 2000;102 (suppl. 1).
6. Fuster et al. ACC/AHA/ESC Guidelines for the management of patients with atrial fibrillation. *J Am Coll Cardiol* 2001;38:1231–1266 (www.acc.org).
7. Holmes CL, Patel BM, Russell JA, Walley KR. Physiology of vasopressin relevant to management of septic shock. *Chest* 2001;120(3):989–1002.
8. Khalaf S, DeBlieux PMC. Managing shock: the role of vasoactive agents, part one. *J Crit Illness* 2001;16(6):281–287.
9. Khalaf S, DeBlieux PMC. Managing shock: the role of vasoactive agents, part two. *J Crit Illness* 2001;16(7):334–342.
10. Practice Guidelines for Blood Component Therapy Anesthesiology 1996;84:732–747.
11. The Acute Respiratory Distress Syndrome Network Authors. Ventilation with lower tidal volumes as compared with traditional tidal volumes for acute lung injury and the acute respiratory distress syndrome. *New Engl J Med* 2000;342:1301–1308.

6 Traumatic injuries

David E. Manthey, MD

Scope of the problem

Traumatic injuries account for about 37% of emergency department (ED) visits. In 2000, EDs in the US evaluated and treated more than 29.5 million people for injuries. More than 148,000 of these people died as a result of traumatic injuries. Of these deaths, 43,354 were the result of motor vehicle crashes, 16,765 from homicide, and 13,322 from falls. Each year, approximately 7000 fatalities occur in pedestrians struck by automobiles. Falls are the number one cause of non-fatal trauma and the second leading cause of brain injury. According to a 1999 study (using 1993 data), the treatment and long-term care of injuries cost $69 billion, approximately 12% of medical care expenditures.

Patients with severe or life-threatening traumatic injuries may present to the ED at any time of day, either immediately following their injury or in a delayed fashion. They may arrive by ambulance having benefited from pre-hospital care and advanced notification, or be "dropped off" by a friend or family member. Emergency physicians must be skilled at the initial evaluation and treatment of these patients.

Peaks of death

Death from traumatic injury tends to occur during one of three distinct time frames following the injury. The first "peak of death" occurs within seconds to minutes of the injury, typically resulting from devastating injuries to the central nervous system, heart, or major vessels. Very few of these patients can be saved.

The second "peak of death" occurs minutes to hours following the injury. Deaths during this period occur as a result of major head, chest, abdominal or pelvic injuries, as well as injuries associated with significant blood loss. During the "golden hour" of trauma care, the rapid transportation, identification, and resuscitation of these injuries is essential to preserving life. These injuries require emergent stabilization and generally surgical intervention.

The third "peak of death" occurs days to weeks after the original injury. This is most often the result of sepsis or multiorgan failure.

Primary survey

Initial evaluation of the trauma patient begins with the primary survey:

- Airway with cervical spine control
- Breathing
- Circulation with hemorrhage control
- Disability
- Exposure and environmental control

This is a systematic approach to the assessment and simultaneous treatment of life-threatening traumatic injuries.

It is essential that traumatic life- or limb-threatening injuries are treated at the time they are identified, not after the entire examination is completed. Obtaining a detailed patient history and evaluation for secondary (non-life threatening) injuries are deferred until the secondary survey. This is often difficult because some secondary injuries are very dramatic, and human nature draws us to them.

Airway with cervical spine control

Assessment

The airway should be assessed immediately to make certain that it is both patent and protected. If there is a risk that the patient will not be able to maintain his or her airway, early intervention must be considered. Establishment of a secure airway takes precedence over the remainder of the trauma evaluation.

Listen for stridor and/or dysphonia, as both serve as indicators that the trachea or surrounding structures have been injured. When either of these findings is present, rapid intervention is required.

Assess the patient for agitation, obtundation, and cyanosis. These findings may be indirect signs that the patient is not adequately oxygenating or ventilating, resulting in hypoxia or hypercarbia.

Examine the patient for the presence of facial fractures that may lead to bleeding or airway obstruction. Carefully remove the front of the cervical collar (while providing spinal stabilization) to look for evidence of penetrating injuries, subcutaneous emphysema, or an expanding hematoma of the anterior neck. Determine if the trachea is midline. Deviation of the trachea may be associated with a local hematoma or tension pneumothorax.

Open the patient's mouth carefully to identify abnormalities such as bleeding or swelling. The gentle use of a tongue blade may facilitate this task. Can the patient swallow and handle secretions?

Some trauma patients arrive at the ED after intubation in the field. Do not assume that the airway is secure. Correct endotracheal (ET) tube placement may be confirmed by the direct visualization of the ET tube passing through the vocal cords, the presence of a normal oxygen saturation, and the detection of end-tidal carbon dioxide (CO_2). Other measures to assess ET tube placement include auscultation of symmetric breath sounds over the chest, the absence of breath sounds over the epigastrium, fogging within the ET tube, symmetric chest rise with ventilation, and the esophageal bulb detection device. However, these methods are not as reassuring as direct visualization and the detection of end-tidal CO_2.

Assume injury to the cervical spine in any patient with the following findings:

- multi-system or major trauma;
- altered level of consciousness;
- blunt injury above the clavicles;
- appropriate mechanism of injury;
- neck pain, ecchymosis or deformity;
- neurologic deficits.

Treatment

All trauma patients should receive supplemental oxygen regardless of their oxygen saturation. Oxygenation may be monitored with a pulse oximeter if an appropriate waveform can be identified.

The tongue remains the most common reason for airway obstruction. When a patient is supine or unconscious, the tongue can be raised by maneuvers such as the chin lift or jaw thrust, or with devices such as the nasopharyngeal or oropharyngeal airway. The neck should neither be flexed nor extended if a cervical spine injury is suspected or the patient is unconscious (Figure 6.1). The airway should remain clear of debris and vomit by a manual sweep or a suction device.

A trauma patient should be intubated for any of the following reasons:

- apnea or inadequate ventilation;
- protection from aspiration;
- impending or suspected airway compromise;
- hypoxia despite supplemental oxygen;
- closed head injury with Glasgow Coma Scale (GCS) <9.

A complete approach to controlling a patient's airway is described in Chapter 2. An organized approach in a stepwise pattern should utilize one or more of the following methods:

(a) *Chin lift/jaw thrust/nasopharyngeal airway/oropharyngeal airway:* The use of adjunctive airways and simple maneuvers to lift the tongue out of the pharynx often allows ventilation of the patient until a definitive airway can be established.

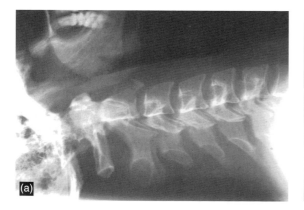 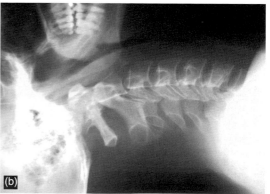

Figure 6.1
(a) A patient with an extension teardrop fracture of the vertebral body of C2. (b) Inadvertent hyperextension of the patient's neck could lead to subluxation of the vertebral bodies and injury to the spinal cord. *Courtesy*: Michael Zucker, MD.

(b) *Bag-valve mask (BVM):* Every clinician should be skilled at ventilating a patient using a BVM, which allows ventilation of an apneic patient or patient with respiratory distress until a definitive airway can be established. Providing a good mask seal and ensuring that the tongue does not obstruct the pharynx are essential for effective BVM ventilation.

(c) *Intubation:* ET intubation can be performed by direct laryngoscopy, over an endoscope or guidewire, or through a laryngeal mask airway (LMA). Direct laryngoscopy is safe in the trauma patient when performed with in-line immobilization to protect the cervical spine. Rapid sequence intubation (RSI) may facilitate intubation of a patient without requiring bag-valve mask ventilation. However, prior to paralyzing the patient, it is important to assess for a difficult airway and ensure that the patient can be effectively BVM-ventilated should the intubation prove difficult or impossible.

(d) *Transtracheal jet ventilation:* When intubation fails, ventilation using a needle placed through the cricothyroid membrane will temporarily allow oxygenation of the patient.

(e) *Surgical cricothyroidotomy.* This surgical airway may be necessary when ET intubation either fails or is not feasible. It involves incising the cricothyroid membrane to allow placement of an ET or tracheostomy tube directly into the trachea (Figure 6.2).

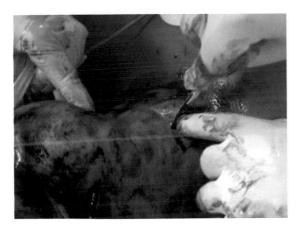

Figure 6.2
Surgical cricothyroidotomy. *Courtesy:* Mel Herbert, MD.

Breathing

Assessment

Evaluation of the patient's breathing determines how well the patient is oxygenating and ventilating. Employ a pulse oximeter to assess oxygenation and, if available, a quantitative end-tidal CO_2 monitor to assess ventilation. An arterial blood gas will assess both oxygenation and ventilation, and provides the patient's acid–base status, which is often related to the adequacy of resuscitation efforts.

Auscultate the lungs for bilateral symmetric breath sounds. The lack of breath sounds on one side may indicate a pneumothorax or hemothorax. The clinician should search for signs of a tension pneumothorax, such as a deviated trachea away from the affected side, distended neck veins, decreased breath sounds on the affected side, and hypotension (Figure 6.3).

Percussion of the chest may help differentiate a pneumothorax from a hemothorax. However, this technique may be of limited utility during a noisy trauma resuscitation.

Observe the chest wall for symmetric rise as well as for any paradoxical movement suggestive of a flail chest (Figure 6.4). Flail chest is caused by the fracture of two or more ribs at two or more segments, causing a free-floating segment that moves inward with inspiration due to negative pressure generated.

Palpate the entire thorax (anterior and posterior) for crepitus and rib tenderness. Crepitus suggests an underlying pneumothorax, while rib tenderness alerts the physician to a possible rib fracture and underlying pulmonary contusion.

Look for an open (sucking) chest wound. If the chest wound is two-thirds the size of the patient's trachea or larger, air can preferentially enter the thoracic cavity through this chest wall injury, resulting in a tension or open pneumothorax.

Treatment

When evaluating a trauma patient's respiratory status, one must keep in mind life-threatening conditions that must be addressed. These include hypoxia, tension pneumothorax, open pneumothorax, massive hemothorax, tracheo-bronchial tree disruption, and flail segment.

Hypoxia should be treated with supplemental oxygen. Intubation should be performed if necessary. A diligent search for reversible causes of impaired ventilation should occur.

Emergent treatment of a tension pneumothorax converts it to a simple pneumothorax. This can be accomplished by needle decompression (needle thoracostomy) using a 14-G catheter over needle (Figure 6.5). Insertion of the needle over the third rib (second intercostal space) in the midclavicular line results in a release of intrapleural air and the subsequent reversal of adverse hemodynamic effects. The catheter is left in place until a 36-French chest tube is promptly placed at the 4th intercostal space in the mid-axillary line (chest tube thoracostomy).

An open pneumothorax allows air to preferentially enter the thoracic cavity through the defect rather than the trachea. This results in significant hypoxia, increased work of breathing, and hypercarbia. This wound should be treated with an air occlusive dressing (such as a defibrillator pad or

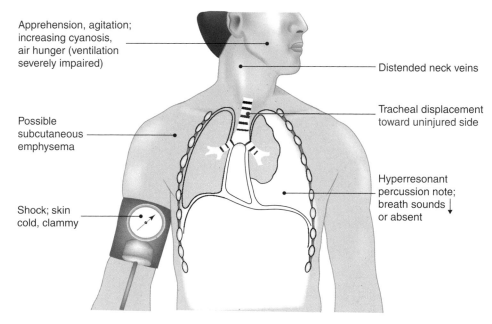

Apprehension, agitation; increasing cyanosis, air hunger (ventilation severely impaired)

Possible subcutaneous emphysema

Shock; skin cold, clammy

Distended neck veins

Tracheal displacement toward uninjured side

Hyperresonant percussion note; breath sounds ↓ or absent

Figure 6.3
Tension pneumothorax. Campbell, John E., Basic Trauma Life Support for Advanced Providers, 5th ed., Copyright 2004. Reprinted by permission of Pearson Education, Inc., Upper Saddle River, NJ.

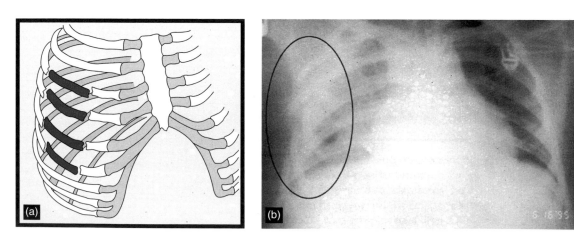

Figure 6.4
(a) Illustration of flail chest. (b) Chest X-ray showing flail chest with an underlying lung contusion. Reproduced from D. Mandavia et al, *Color Atlas of Emergency Trauma*, Cambridge, Cambridge University Press, 2003.

Vaseline gauze) taped on three sides to produce a flutter valve (Figure 6.6). This type of dressing will prevent the entrance of air into the pleural space during inhalation but allow the escape of intrapleural air during exhalation.

A massive hemothorax (Figure 6.7) is identified by more than 1500 ml of blood within the thoracic cavity. It is initially treated and diagnosed with a tube thoracostomy. The use of an auto-transfuser with the pleuravac will allow this blood to be infused back to the patient. Continued

bleeding (the drainage of >200 ml of blood per hour for 2–4 hours), blood transfusions, or the patient's hemodynamic status dictate the need for operative intervention (thoracotomy).

A flail segment occurs when two or more contiguous ribs are broken in two or more places. The paradoxical movement of this segment, the restricted chest wall movement due to pain, and the underlying pulmonary contusion lead to hypoxia and ineffective ventilation. Prevention of over hydration in this clinical situation may

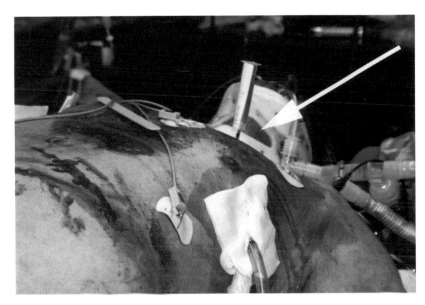

Figure 6.5
Needle thoracostomy for tension pneumothorax. Reproduced from D. Mandavia et al, *Color Atlas of Emergency Trauma*, Cambridge, Cambridge University Press, 2003.

On inspiration, dressing seals wound, preventing air entry

Dressing allows trapped air to escape through untaped section of dressing on expiration

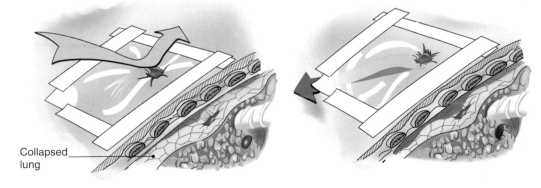

Collapsed lung

Figure 6.6
Treatment of an open pneumothorax. Campbell, John E., Basic Trauma Life Support for Advanced Providers, 5th ed., Copyright 2004. Reprinted by permission of Pearson Education, Inc., Upper Saddle River, NJ.

avert fluid overload of the injured lung. Intubation with positive pressure ventilation is often required to treat this injury.

Circulation

Assessment

Shock is defined by inadequate organ perfusion and tissue oxygenation, not by a specific blood pressure measurement. A patient with a low blood pressure may continue to perfuse well, as evidenced by normal mentation, skin temperature, and color. Alternatively, a "normal" measured blood pressure may be found in a patient who is not adequately perfusing his or her vital organs.

Hypovolemia, typically from hemorrhage, is the most common cause of shock in trauma patients. Most preventable trauma deaths result from the failure to recognize and adequately treat hemorrhagic shock. Always assume that hypovolemic shock is present, and treat it until proven otherwise. Familiarity with the classes of hypovolemic shock is important, as they correlate with blood loss and help guide therapy (Table 6.1). Other causes of shock in the trauma patient include neurogenic shock (from spinal cord injury), obstructive shock (from cardiac tamponade), and distributive shock (from sepsis). Cardiogenic shock may be the initial cause of a traumatic injury, but is rarely the result of one.

Evaluation of a patient's circulatory status can be difficult. Use all available options when assessing a trauma patient for the presence of shock. Assess the patient's mental status. Confusion, restlessness, combativeness or unconsciousness may all result from shock. Other causes of altered mental status in the trauma patient include head injury or intoxication.

Check and re-check the patient's vital signs. The presence of hypotension suggests a significant shock state. However, children and healthy adults can maintain their blood pressure in the face of severe blood loss, although other signs of shock will usually be apparent.

Calculate the pulse pressure, which is the difference between the systolic and diastolic blood pressure. A narrowed pulse pressure may reflect peripheral vasoconstriction occuring in order to maintain cardiac output.

The patient's pulse may be elevated due to hypovolemia, or secondary to pain and stress. The earliest manifestations of shock include tachycardia and cutaneous vasoconstriction. The pulse may also be misleadingly normal due to the inability to develop tachycardia secondary to age,

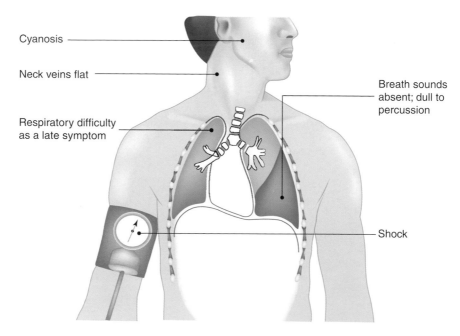

Cyanosis

Neck veins flat

Breath sounds absent; dull to percussion

Respiratory difficulty as a late symptom

Shock

Figure 6.7
Massive hemothorax. Campbell, John E., Basic Trauma Life Support for Advanced Providers, 5th ed., Copyright 2004. Reprinted by permission of Pearson Education, Inc., Upper Saddle River, NJ.

medications (such as beta- or calcium channel blockers), or a vagotonic response to hemoperitoneum.

Examine the patient's extremities. Delayed capillary refill time (>2 seconds) may reflect decreased peripheral perfusion. Cool, moist, or pale extremities suggest shock.

Always compare peripheral and central pulses. If the central pulses are markedly stronger than the peripheral pulses, this may be a sign of peripheral vasoconstriction in order to preserve preload and maintain cardiac output.

Evaluate the patient's jugular veins. Flat jugular veins suggest hypovolemia. Full neck veins are normal in the recumbent patient. Distended jugular veins suggest an obstructive process. When combined with impending shock, this finding suggests cardiac tamponade (Figure 6.8), tension pneumothorax, or cardiogenic shock in the trauma patient.

Assess the patient's urinary output. It should be at least 0.5 ml/kg/hour in the adult patient, 1 ml/kg/hour in the pediatric patient and 2 ml/kg/hour in children <1 year of age. Decreased urine output may reflect poor renal perfusion secondary to continued hypovolemia and under-resuscitation.

The assessment of a patient's circulatory status is an ongoing process. When resuscitating the patient with the crystalloid, it is important to determine how the patient responds to each fluid challenge.

Treatment

During the assessment of the patient's circulation, one must stop all obvious external bleeding. Direct pressure or a compression bandage accomplishes this in most instances. In some cases, placing a hemostatic figure-of-eight stitch over the bleeding area may be required. Blind probing or clamping deep within a wound should be avoided.

Venous access is required in all trauma patients for the administration of isotonic fluids and blood (if necessary). Two large-bore intravenous (IV) catheters (16 G or larger) are preferred. Short, large-caliber peripheral IVs allow the rapid infusion of large volumes of fluid. If the patient's condition prevents placement of peripheral IVs, a central venous catheter may be placed

Table 6.1 Estimated blood loss, signs and treatment for classes of shock

Class of shock	Blood loss	Signs	Treatment
Class I	0–750 ml (up to 15% of blood volume)	Tachycardia	PO fluids (if not NPO), IV crystalloid fluids
Class II	750–1500 ml (15–30% of blood volume)	Tachycardia Tachypnea Pulse pressure narrows	IV crystalloid fluids
Class III	1500–2000 ml (30–40% of blood volume)	Tachycardia (>120) Tachypnea (30–40) Narrowed pulse pressure Decreased systolic blood pressure Decreased urinary output Decreased mental status Decreased capillary refill	IV crystalloid fluids, packed RBCs
Class IV	>2000 ml (>40% blood volume)	Tachycardia (>140) Tachypnea (>35) Absent pulse pressure Markedly decreased systolic blood pressure No urinary output Confused to lethargic Markedly decreased capillary refill	IV crystalloid fluids with packed RBCs

NPO: nil per os; RBCs: red blood cells. *Source*: Committee on Trauma, American College of Surgeons. *Advanced Trauma Life Support Instructor Manual*, 5th ed., Chicago: American College of Surgeons, 1997.

in the subclavian, internal jugular, or femoral vein. A peripheral venous cutdown may be performed on the saphenous vein. In children <8 years of age, intraosseous placement of a needle may provide rapid vascular access as the primary approach or if peripheral IV access fails.

Fluid resuscitation should be given rapidly, up to a predetermined amount. The patient's hemodynamic response should be evaluated after this initial bolus. Patients who respond quickly may not need further fluids or blood, as they may have limited blood loss. Patients who respond only transiently are likely to have ongoing blood loss, requiring further resuscitation with fluids and likely blood products. These patients require a rapid search for the cause of their blood loss. Patients who do not respond to the initial bolus require additional resuscitation with blood and fluids. An emergent trip to the operating room (OR) may be required to diagnose the source of bleeding, as well as control it. Finally, consider other causes for hemodynamic compromise, such as neurogenic or cardiogenic shock, which require alternate therapeutic approaches.

Blood products should be used for patients who remain hemodynamically unstable or who have ongoing blood loss requiring replacement. When there is no time to type and screen a patient, type O blood should be utilized. Administer Rh-negative blood to women of childbearing age. When it is available, administer ABO type-specific and Rh-compatible blood. This blood can be ready approximately 15 minutes after the blood bank receives the type and screen specimen. Type and crossmatched blood is the best source to avoid incompatibility reactions, but requires over an hour to obtain.

Depending on the etiology of the shock state, the physician may utilize other procedures such as:

1. needle decompression followed by tube thoracostomy for tension pneumothorax;
2. needle pericardiocentesis or pericardial window for cardiac tamponade;
3. circumferential pelvic binding, external fixation, or pelvic angiography with embolization of bleeding vessels for the treatment of displaced pelvic fractures.

An ED thoracotomy is indicated for a penetrating chest trauma patient who loses vital signs within a few minutes of arriving at or within the ED. This procedure should only be performed if the hospital has the facilities and staff to address the injury. A thoracotomy allows for definitive treatment of pericardial tamponade, repair of a cardiac laceration, cross-clamping the aorta to prevent ongoing blood loss, and clamping the pulmonary arteries.

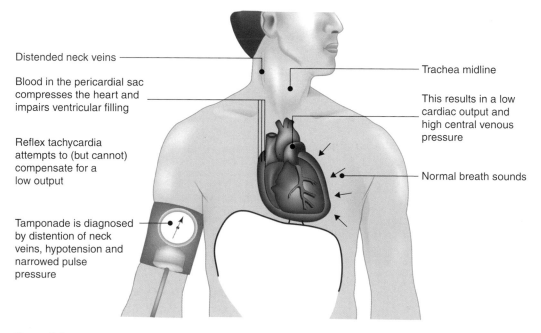

Figure 6.8
Cardiac tamponade. Campbell, John E., Basic Trauma Life Support for Advanced Providers, 5th ed., Copyright 2004. Reprinted by permission of Pearson Education, Inc., Upper Saddle River, NJ.

Often the patient may leave the ED for the OR during the circulation assessment portion of the primary resuscitation. This may be necessary to obtain control of active bleeding within the chest or abdominal cavity.

Disability

Assessment

Assessment of the patient's disability during the primary survey should be brief and directed to the following three areas: level of consciousness, pupillary examination, and movement of extremities. It is always important to assess neurologic function prior to paralysis of the patient as part of rapid sequence intubation (RSI).

Assess the level of consciousness with the AVPU approach or the Glasgow Coma Scale (GCS). AVPU relates to the patient's level of response: the patient may be Alert, respond to Voice or Pain, or remain Unresponsive.

The GCS (Table 6.2) is used to follow the patient's status, guide therapy, and communicate with consultants. Scores range from a minimum of 3 to a maximum of 12, with a score of 8 or less indicating coma. A GCS drop of two is considered deterioration, while a drop of three is considered a catastrophic change.

The pupil examination should look for pupil symmetry and reactivity to light. A dilated,

unreactive ("blown") pupil in a comatose patient suggests transtentorial intracranial herniation leading to unilateral compression of the third cranial nerve. Disconjugate gaze may be associated with various etiologies of coma.

Assessment of movement in all extremities is a gross evaluation of spinal cord function, not peripheral nerve function. It is more important to judge symmetry and strength in all extremities than isolated peripheral nerve function.

Treatment

The two most dangerous insults to the traumatized brain, hypoxia and hypotension, should be addressed during the initial evaluation and resuscitation. ET intubation is indicated in any patient with a GCS <9.

In cases of neurologic deterioration or lateralizing neurologic signs, mannitol and controlled hyperventilation to a partial pressure of carbon dioxide (PCO_2) between 30 and 35 mmHg may be employed as temporizing measures to reduce intracranial pressure. Other therapies to consider in the severely brain injured patient include anticonvulsants, deep sedation, and elevating the head of the bed to 30°. Neurosurgical procedures such as operative craniotomy, skull trephination with burr hole placement (Figures 6.9a and b), or intraventricular pressure monitor placement are often required.

Table 6.2 Glasgow Coma Scale

Eye opening		
Spontaneous	4	Reticular activating system intact (though patient may not be aware)
To verbal command	3	Opens eyes when told to do so
To pain	2	Opens eyes in response to pain
None	1	Does not open eyes to any stimuli
Verbal response		
Oriented – converses	5	Aware of self and environment; oriented to person, place and time
Disoriented – converses	4	Organized and well articulated, but disoriented to person, place or time
Inappropriate words	3	Random exclamatory recognizable words
Incomprehensible	2	Moaning, no recognizable words
No response	1	No response or intubated
Motor response		
Obeys verbal commands	6	Readily moves limbs when told to do so
Localizes to painful stimuli	5	Moves limb in an effort to remove painful stimulus
Flexion withdrawal	4	Pulls away from pain in flexion
Abnormal flexion	3	Decorticate rigidity
Extension	2	Decerebrate rigidity
No response	1	Hypotonic, flaccid; suggests loss of medullary function or concomitant spinal cord injury

Adapted from Marx JA (ed). *Rosen's Emergency Medicine: Concepts and Clinical Practice*, 5th ed., St. Louis: Mosby, 2002.

The cervical collar should be maintained until a cervical spine injury has been excluded. However, once the stability of the spine has been assessed, the patient may be carefully log rolled off the spine board to prevent skin breakdown and minimize patient discomfort.

For patients with acute spinal cord injuries, rapid IV administration of high-dose steroids has been recommended, although this treatment remains controversial. Early discussion with neurosurgical consultants is recommended.

Exposure and environmental control

Assessment

Fully undress the victim from "head to toe" to allow a complete assessment. Look under collars and splints, in the axilla and under skin folds, and log roll the patient to examine the back and buttocks. Identify and treat any active sites of bleeding. Failure to completely expose the patient may result in missing a significant traumatic injury, such as a gunshot or stab wound (Figure 6.10).

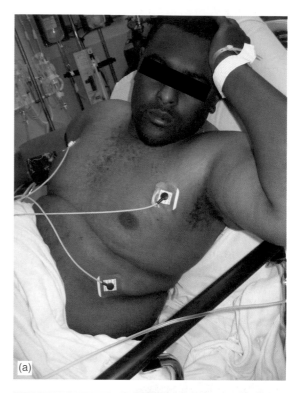
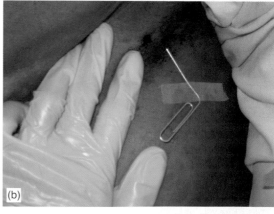

Figure 6.10
(a) A patient with a suspected gunshot wound. The initial physical examination did not reveal the injury, delaying definitive treatment. (b) The gunshot wound was later located under the patient's skin fold. *Courtesy*: Clement Yeh, MD.

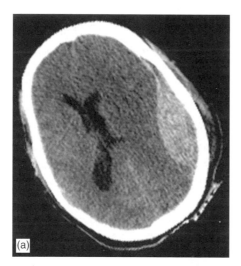
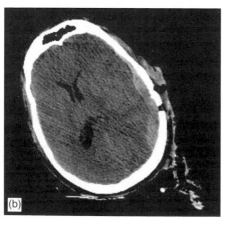

Figure 6.9
(a) Epidural hematoma. (b) Evacuation of the epidural hematoma following burr hole placement in the ED. *Courtesy*: Damon Kuehl, MD.

Treatment

Remove all wet or contaminated clothing. If the patient has been in an industrial or chemical accident, decontamination is critical for patient care. It is also critical that the medical staff protect themselves from exposure, morbidity, and incapacitation.

Keep the patient warm by raising the temperature of the resuscitation room, applying warm blankets, ventilating with warm humidified air, and administering warmed IV fluids. Hypothermia in trauma patients is associated with increased mortality, and should be prevented. The patient's chance of survival may drop with every degree drop in core temperature.

Secondary survey

This detailed head to toe examination is initiated only after life-threatening injuries have been evaluated and treated during the primary survey. At that time, multiple other evaluations may occur, including trauma radiographs and laboratory studies. Although there are a multitude of items to address in each anatomical area, what follows is a review of items specific to trauma.

1. Head, eyes, ears, nose, and throat (HEENT)
   (a) Assess for evidence of a basilar skull fracture by identifying the presence of Battle's sign (ecchymosis over the mastoid) (Figure 6.11), Raccoon eyes (ecchymosis around the eyes) (Figure 6.12) or hemotympanum (blood behind the eardrum) (Figure 6.13). Look for a cerebrospinal fluid (CSF) leak manifested by rhinorrhea or otorrhea.
   (b) Assess for depressed skull fractures by careful palpation. Impaled foreign bodies and bone fragments should not be manipulated.
   (c) Assess for facial injury and stability by palpating the facial bones. Severe facial fractures can lead to airway compromise and may alter the approach to the airway. Malocclusion of the teeth may indicate a mandible fracture (Figure 6.14).
   (d) Look for lacerations that will require repair. Unattended scalp lacerations can bleed vigorously.

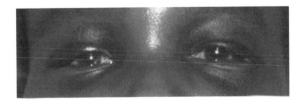

Figure 6.12
Raccoon eyes due to a frontobasilar skull fracture. Reproduced from D. Mandavia et al, *Color Atlas of Emergency Trauma*, Cambridge, Cambridge University Press, 2003.

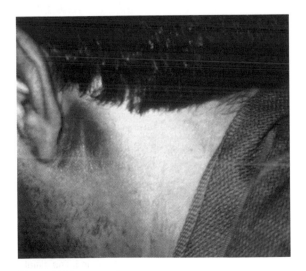

Figure 6.11
Battle's sign. Reproduced from D. Mandavia et al, *Color Atlas of Emergency Trauma*, Cambridge, Cambridge University Press, 2003.

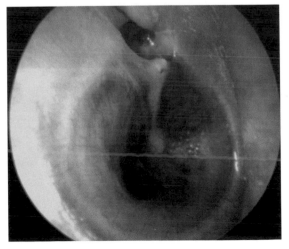

Figure 6.13
Hemotympanum. Reproduced from D. Mandavia et al, *Color Atlas of Emergency Trauma*, Cambridge, Cambridge University Press, 2003.

(e) Determine visual acuity and assess pupillary size and function. Assess the eye for globe injury and signs of internal damage, such as hyphema.

(f) Examine the nasal septum for a hematoma, which, if untreated, may lead to an abscess or nasal cartilage necrosis.

2. Cervical spine/neck

(a) Palpate the cervical spine and identify areas of tenderness, swelling or step-off deformity.

(b) Look for penetrating injuries within the three separate zones of the neck.

(c) Evaluate for subcutaneous emphysema, which may be associated with laryngotracheal injury or pneumothorax.

3. Chest

(a) Palpate the sternum, clavicles, and ribs for tenderness or crepitus. The presence of subcutaneous emphysema suggests an underlying pneumothorax.

(b) Look for bruising or deformity to suggest an injury to the underlying lung.

4. Abdomen

(a) Assess for any distention, tenderness, rebound or guarding. Two common sources of blood loss in patients with abdominal trauma are injuries to the liver and spleen.

(b) Flank ecchymosis may suggest a retroperitoneal bleed.

(c) The presence of a "seat belt sign" is correlated with an eight-fold higher relative risk of intraperitoneal injury (Figure 6.15).

(d) Reliable assessment of the abdomen may be compromised by the presence of altered mental status, intoxication with alcohol or illicit drugs, or the presence of painful distracting injuries.

5. Back

(a) Log roll the patient with assistance while maintaining spinal alignment. Palpate the entire spine for any spinous process tenderness.

(b) Assess for hidden wounds in the axilla, under the cervical collar, and in the gluteal region.

6. Pelvis

(a) In order to assess the stability of the pelvis, the physician may *gently* employ anterior–posterior compression of the anterior superior iliac spines, lateral compression of iliac crests, and cranial–caudal distraction of opposite iliac crests. This should be performed one time only, as vigorous manipulation of the bony pelvis may exacerbate bleeding from a pelvic fracture or the venous plexus.

(b) Palpate the symphysis pubis for pain, crepitus, or widening.

(c) Pelvic fractures can be responsible for as much as 4–6 L of occult blood loss.

7. Perineum

(a) Evaluate the perineum for ecchymosis, suggestive of a pelvic fracture or urethral disruption.

8. Urethra

(a) Look for blood at the urethral meatus to assess for possible urethral disruption before placing a urinary catheter.

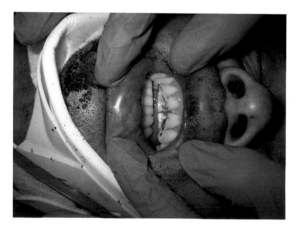

Figure 6.14
Malocclusion associated with a mandible fracture.
Courtesy: S.V. Mahadevan, MD.

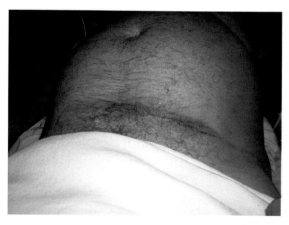

Figure 6.15
Seat belt sign. *Courtesy*: Jo Feldman, MD.

9. Rectum
   (a) A rectal examination is required to assess sphincter tone during the neurological examination.
   (b) A high-riding prostate suggests disruption of the membranous urethra. A urinary catheter should not be placed in this circumstance.
   (c) A pelvic fracture may cause a rectal wall laceration and rectal bleeding.
   (d) Gross blood on digital rectal examination suggests a bowel injury.
10. Vagina
   (a) A vaginal examination should be performed in female patients to assess for palpable fractures, vaginal lacerations, and blood within the vaginal vault.
11. Extremity examination
   (a) Re-check the vascular status of each extremity, including pulses, color, capillary refill, and temperature.
   (b) Inspect every inch, palpate every bone, and check the range of motion of all joints. Assess for deformity, crepitus, tenderness, swelling, and lacerations.
   (c) Unstable fractures or those associated with neurovascular compromise should be reduced immediately. Splinting of fractured bones can provide hemostasis, prevent further injury, and enhance patient comfort.
   (d) Femur fractures can result in as much as 2 units of occult blood loss.
12. Neurologic
   (a) At this time, a complete neurologic examination should be done. This includes a repeat GCS score, re-evaluation of the pupils, a cranial nerve examination, a complete sensory and motor examination, testing of the deep tendon reflexes, and an assessment of the response to plantar stimulation.

History

Where and how were you injured (shot, struck)? Where are you hurting?

An understanding of the mechanism of injury may provide clues to the type(s) of injuries seen in trauma patients (Table 6.3). Significant injuries may occur without obvious external evidence of trauma. The cervical spine is a classic example.

Did you lose consciousness?

Although many argue about the significance of the duration of unconsciousness, most agree that its presence should increase concern for an intra-cranial injury.

Table 6.3 Mechanisms of traumatic injury and associated injuries

Mechanism	Possible traumatic injury
Steering column damage	Myocardial or pulmonary contusion
Sudden deceleration (fall, MVC)	Traumatic aortic disruption, immobile C7-T1 junction injury
Windshield star	Subdural hematoma, epidural hematoma, cervical spine injury
Rear impact, head turned to side	Jumped cervical facet
Side impact	Fractured hip
Seat belt sign, stab wound below the nipple or scapular tip	Intra-abdominal injury
Fall, landing on heels	Tibial plateau fracture, lumbar spine fracture, calcaneal fracture
Direct blow to head	Coup and contre-coup brain injuries
Blast injury	Air-containing body cavities most vulnerable
High kinetic energy missile (bullet)	Injury extends beyond bullet wound
MVC: motor vehicle collision.	

What amount of blood loss occurred at the scene/en route?

Quantifying this amount may be difficult, but recognizing that the patient has already lost a significant amount of blood will guide therapy.

What was the temperature at the scene?

Assesses the potential for hypothermia or hyperthermia.

What was the direction of impact?

This allows clinicians to ascertain the forces imposed upon the body and identify associated injuries, such as a jumped facet in the cervical spine.

What was the appearance of the vehicle?

This includes damage to the steering wheel, starring of the windshield, and intrusion of the door into the passenger compartment. Report of this information, or a photo allows an estimation of the amount of kinetic energy delivered to the patient (Figure 6.16).

What was your position in the car?

Knowledge of both damage to the car and the patient's position in the car allow the clinician to better ascertain what the patient's injuries might be.

What was the speed of the vehicle (if isolated collision) or vehicles? What type of vehicle(s) were involved?

Remember that energy equals mass times velocity squared, so you need to know the mass and velocity to determine the amount of force transmitted. Larger cars, sport utility vehicles (SUVs), and trucks that ride higher off the ground generally protect the passenger more than small, light vehicles.

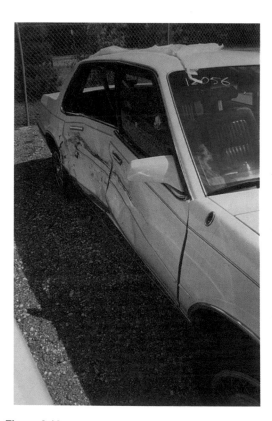
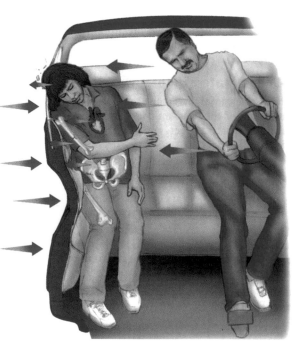

Figure 6.16
Side impact motor vehicle collision with passenger space intrusion. Campbell, John E., Basic Trauma Life Support for Advanced Providers, 5th ed., Copyright 2004. Reprinted by permission of Pearson Education, Inc., Upper Saddle River, NJ.

Did you use restraining devices?

Ask about the use of seat belts (including shoulder and lap, or lap-only restraints) and the deployment of air bags.

Did their vehicle roll over? Was there a fatality at the scene?

Affirmative answers to any of these questions raise the likelihood of serious injury.

Were you wearing a helmet?

For patients of motorcycle or bicycle crashes, this information is important given the amount of protection that helmets afford the brain. Evaluation of the helmet is also important to determine the amount of force distributed to the head.

How far did you fall and what did you land on?

Both the height of the fall and the hardness of the surface the patient struck are important in determining the likelihood of injury and the body parts injured.

What caused the fall?

Did the patient have a seizure or syncope which caused the fall? Was the fall preceded by chest pain or difficulty breathing? Was alcohol involved? Was this a suicide attempt?

Did an explosion occur?

What was the patient's distance from the blast? Blast injuries may occur from the primary blast force, secondary missiles, or due to tertiary impact against a hard surface (Figure 6.17).

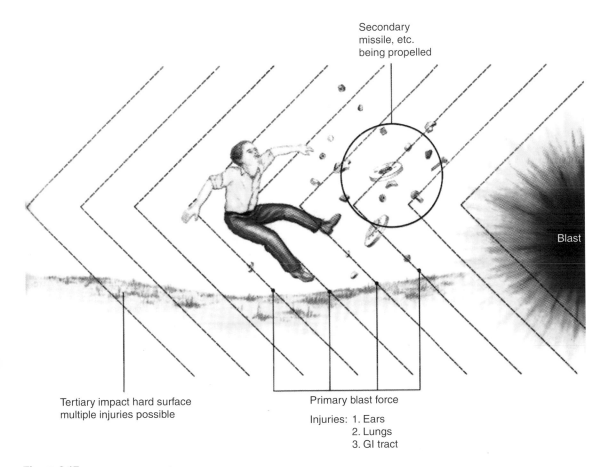

Secondary missile, etc. being propelled

Blast

Tertiary impact hard surface multiple injuries possible

Primary blast force

Injuries: 1. Ears
2. Lungs
3. GI tract

Figure 6.17
Blast injury. Explosions can cause injury with the initial blast, when the victim is struck by debris, or by the victim being thrown against the ground or other fixed objects by the blast. Campbell, John E., Basic Trauma Life Support for Advanced Providers, 5th ed., Copyright 2004. Reprinted by permission of Pearson Education, Inc., Upper Saddle River, NJ.

How many shots were fired?

This question may help determine if you are missing an injury or if the wounds may represent two separate entrance wounds rather than a single wound (entrance and exit).

Do you know what type of weapon was used?

Although this is notoriously unreliable, knowledge of the type of weapon and the bullet's velocity may help determine the injury pattern. The length and width of the blade in a stab wound may also assist with patient evaluation. Additionally, for stab wounds, the hand dominance and gender of the attacker may provide useful information if it is known.

What were you struck with?

Being struck with a bat or pipe versus a fist implies a greater magnitude of force applied to the tissue, suggesting the possibility of a larger amount of external and internal damage.

Was this a crush injury?

If so, ascertain the weight and force of the object that struck the patient.

Were there any drugs (including alcohol) at the scene?

Ask this question of emergency medical system (EMS) providers in addition to querying the patient about his or her use of drugs. This is important in the assessment of mental status and establishing the patient's reliability.

Associated symptoms

Did you experience any symptoms (chest pain, seizure, abdominal pain, headache, etc.) before the collision?

It is possible that the patient may have had a collision resulting from a medical problem. Always give consideration to these conditions as a possible cause of the incident. Furthermore, these conditions may be exacerbated by the stress of the incident.

Past medical

Can you tell me your AMPLE history?

Always take an "AMPLE" history from the patient or EMS providers. This information will help clinicians if the patient subsequently becomes non-communicative:

A	Allergies
M	Medications
P	Past surgical and medical history
L	Last meal
E	Events surrounding trauma/environment

When was your last tetanus?

As almost all trauma patients have some degree of injury to skin coupled with contamination (tetanus-prone), it is important to inquire about the patient's immunization status. This question can wait until the end of the evaluation. Tetanus status should be updated according to accepted guidelines.

Do you have a bleeding disorder or are you taking anticoagulant medication?

Patients with bleeding disorders or taking anticoagulant medication (Coumadin) may bleed significantly following even minor trauma; the threshold to search for occult bleeding is lower. It is important to get this information early on to allow timely administration of whatever factor or product is needed for correcting any abnormalities.

Are you taking any medication that would limit your cardiovascular response?

Patients taking certain medications (i.e., beta blockers or calcium channel blockers), and patients with pacemakers may present with a "relative bradycardia" (a normal heart rate despite significant blood loss).

Differential diagnosis

Although not an exhaustive list, injuries that can be elusive or determined by physical examination have been included (Table 6.4).

Diagnostic testing

Laboratory studies

Type and crossmatch

A type and cross should be obtained immediately on all significant trauma patients. This allows for

Table 6.4 Traumatic injuries

Diagnosis	Symptoms	Signs	Workup	Treatment
Airway obstruction/ esophageal intubation	Altered mental status, combativeness.	Hypoxia, gastric breath sounds, abdominal distention, inability to BVM ventilate.	Check ET tube placement and oxygen supply.	Replace ET tube.
Cardiac tamponade	Shortness of breath, shock.	Beck's triad: shock, muffled heart tones, and JVD.	Ultrasound (echocardiography).	Pericardiocentesis, pericardial window, open thoracotomy.
Flail chest	Shortness of breath, chest pain.	Rib fractures, paradoxical movement of ribs, hypoxia.	CXR may show pulmonary contusion as well as fractures.	Pain control, positive pressure ventilation.
Head injury (subdural, epidural, impending herniation)	Altered mental status, headache, combativeness.	Focal neurologic examination, asymmetric pupils, Cushing's triad (HTN, bradycardia, and irregular respirations).	Brain CT scan will define emergent intracranial injuries.	OR or ICU management, intracranial pressure monitor.
Hemothorax	Shortness of breath, chest pain.	Decreased breath sounds, percussion dullness.	CXR may reveal opacification of the affected side due to supine position.	Tube thoracostomy, consider cell-saver device and auto-transfusion.
Neurogenic shock	Paralysis, shock.	Hypotension, bradycardia, paralysis, absence of sweating, wide pulse pressure.	Clinical examination, CVP monitoring, exclude other causes.	Fluids, atropine, dopamine/ norepinephrine, phenylephrine.
Open pneumothorax	Open defect in chest wall at least two-thirds the diameter of the trachea.	"Sucking" chest wound.	Detect on clinical examination, CXR.	Occlude wound on three sides to create one-way valve, tube thoracostomy.
Pneumothorax	Shortness of breath, chest pain.	Decreased breath sounds, percussion tympany.	CXR may demonstrate lung line.	Tube thoracostomy.
Pulmonary contusion	Shortness of breath, chest pain.	Decreased breath sounds.	CXR, pulmonary infiltrates; ABG for A-a gradient, PaO_2	Intubation if necessary and pain control.
Tension pneumothorax	Shortness of breath, shock.	Hypotension, unilateral decreased breath sounds, tracheal deviation, JVD.	Detect on clinical examination, not by CXR.	Needle decompression followed by tube thoracostomy.
Tracheo-bronchial tree disruption	Shortness of breath.	Decreased breath sounds, persistent air leak with chest tube.	CXR, CT scan.	Open thoracotomy and repair.
Traumatic aortic disruption	Chest pain radiating to back, between scapulae.	Limited findings externally.	CXR: widened mediastinum CT angiography: periaortic hematoma, aortography.	Fluid and blood resuscitation, emergent operative repair.

BVM: bag-valve mask; ET: endotracheal tube; JVD: jugular venous distension; CXR: chest X-ray; ABG: arterial blood gas; CVP: central venous pressure; HTN: hypertension; OR: operating room; ICU: intensive care unit.

the shortest time to obtain type and screened blood during the initial resuscitation.

Complete blood count

A complete blood count (CBC) may be misleading. The white blood cell (WBC) is often elevated due to demargination of WBCs during the stress response and is unlikely due to infection. A hemoglobin concentration of less than $10\,g/dl$ in a trauma patient indicates clinically significant anemia. Conversely, a normal initial hemoglobin level does not exclude significant hemorrhage. A patient's hemoglobin value is not a real-time indicator of his or her intravascular blood volume. It takes many minutes to hours before hemoglobin value accurately reflects the degree of blood loss in trauma patients. Following the trend of serial hemoglobin measurements every 15 to 30 minutes can provide useful information regarding ongoing blood loss.

Coagulation studies

Although these are often normal early in the treatment of a trauma patient, early identification and aggressive treatment of the inability to clot is important, especially in patients receiving anticoagulants.

Electrolytes and renal function

Routine assessment of electrolyte status and kidney function is important, as patients are likely to receive contrast for imaging studies or may have baseline renal insufficiency. Serious electrolyte imbalances should be recognized and treated depending on their role and risk to the patient.

Arterial blood gas

An arterial blood gas assesses both oxygenation (PaO_2 – partial pressure of oxygen in arterial blood) and ventilation ($PaCO_2$ – partial pressure of carbon dioxide in arterial blood) of a patient. Many trauma surgeons utilize the *base deficit* to assess the patient's response to resuscitation efforts. The presence of an increased base deficit (≥ 6) or decreased serum bicarbonate may signify a metabolic acidosis resulting from acute blood loss and under-resuscitation.

Lactate

The body produces lactate during anaerobic glycolysis which occurs during a shock state. A lactate may be followed to identify the adequacy of resuscitation.

Drug screen

Many institutions routinely obtain a urine drug screen on all trauma patients. This policy has limited utility, as most illicit drugs do not have specific antidotes (with the exception of opiates) and only require supportive care. Additionally, by the time the levels return, the condition as it relates to the traumatic injury should have already been identified and treated.

Pregnancy

The presence of a first trimester pregnancy does little to change the evaluation of a trauma patient. However, a positive pregnancy test may influence the selection of medication and the use of radiographic studies.

Urinalysis

Hypotension with microscopic hematuria requires an assessment of the renal system. In most cases, however, this will have already occurred before the formal urinalysis result returns.

Electrocardiogram

The electrocardiogram (ECG) has limited utility in the trauma patient. An ECG should be obtained if a myocardial infarction is suspected or dysrhythmia is present, or as an aid to identifying the cause of trauma. An ECG and cardiac monitoring are recommended in cases of suspected traumatic cardiac injury, although the evaluation of this diagnostic entity remains controversial.

Radiologic studies

Trauma radiographs should include an anteroposterior (AP) chest, AP pelvis, and cervical spine series.

Chest X-ray

A chest radiograph is useful to assess for pneumothorax, hemothorax, pulmonary contusion, and rib fractures (Figures 6.18a and b). It also allows for the early nonspecific assessment of an aortic injury by demonstrating a widened mediastinum or blurring of aortic knob (Figure 6.19).

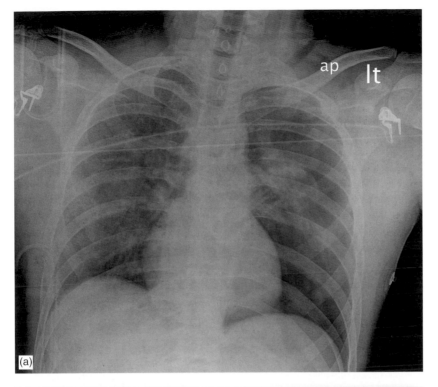

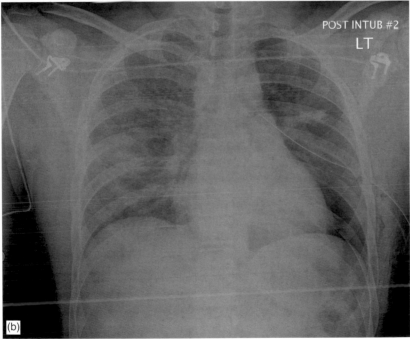

Figure 6.18
(a) Supine chest radiograph on a trauma board demonstrating a fracture of the left 7th rib posteriorly. A large left-sided pneumothorax is present, with deepening of the costophrenic sulcus, and partial collapse of the underlying lung. There are also fractures of the right posterior 5th, 6th, and 7th ribs, with no obvious pneumothorax on the right. (b) Anteroposterior (AP) chest radiograph following chest tube placement, with almost complete resolution of the pneumothorax and re-expansion of the left lung. Band atelectasis is present in the left mid-zone. *Courtesy*: S.V. Mahadevan, MD.

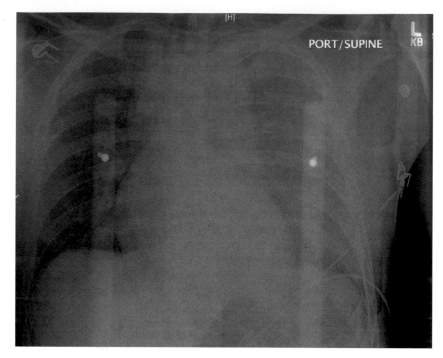

Figure 6.19
AP supine chest radiograph demonstrating widening of the superior mediastinum, with a poorly-defined aortic contour, and apical pleural capping suggestive of an underlying aortic injury. There is also a layering hemothorax on the left, with mediastinal shift to the right. *Courtesy*: S.V. Mahadevan, MD.

Pelvis X-ray

An AP plain radiograph of the pelvis will identify the majority of pelvic fractures. It allows for early identification of serious pelvic injuries that may be a source of blood loss, and may also detect proximal femur fractures and hip dislocations.

Cervical spine X-ray

Most trauma centers obtain at least a three-view plain film series of the cervical spine to assess for fracture, subluxation, and dislocation.

The NEXUS cervical spine criteria identify low-risk trauma patients who do not require cervical spine radiography. Patients who meet all of the following five clinical criteria are at extremely low risk for cervical spine injury:

1. normal level of consciousness,
2. no painful distracting injuries,
3. no evidence of intoxication,
4. no posterior midline cervical tenderness,
5. no focal neurologic deficits.

Ultrasound

The Focused Assessment with Sonography in Trauma (FAST) examination has become a widely utilized tool in the evaluation of the trauma patient. The FAST exam has the advantages of being quick, non-invasive, and performed concurrently with the trauma resuscitation. The purpose of the FAST examination is the rapid identification of free fluid (presumably blood) in the peritoneal cavity or pericardial space. The FAST examination may be repeated as many times as necessary. In skilled hands, the FAST examination provides an attractive alternative to diagnostic peritoneal lavage (DPL) in unstable trauma patients. A detailed description of the FAST examination can be found in Appendix E.

Computed tomography

Computed tomography (CT) is an essential diagnostic tool for the evaluation of hemodynamically stable trauma patients. CT scanning is commonly performed of the head, cervical spine, chest, abdomen, and pelvis. The advent of helical (spiral) CT scanners has improved both the speed and accuracy of CT imaging. The use of reformatted CT images aids in the detection and characterization of subtle traumatic injuries. However, since most CT scanners are located outside of the ED, the decision to send a patient to the CT scanner should be made only after careful assessment of a patient's clinical condition (i.e., hemodynamic status) and the likelihood of hemodynamic decline.

Angiography

Many specialty centers have angiography suites designed for treatment of certain traumatic vascular injuries. In skilled hands, with the right staff, embolization of bleeding vessels can control or stop hemorrhage from pelvic fractures or other vascular sources with success rates approaching or surpassing those from surgery. It is important that the ED staff, trauma team, and angiography staff work together regarding the management of these challenging patients.

Additional therapies

A nasogastric tube may decompress the stomach and decrease the risk of aspiration. However, nasogastric tube insertion is contraindicated in the presence of midface fractures. This may result in the inadvertent insertion of the nasogastric tube through a fractured cribriform plate into the cranial vault (Figure 6.20). An orogastric tube can still be placed in this circumstance if done carefully.

A transurethral bladder (Foley) catheter monitors urine output, a sensitive indicator of renal perfusion and volume status. The Foley catheter is contraindicated if a urethral injury is suspected as suggested by the following clinical findings:

1. perineal ecchymoses,
2. blood at the urethral meatus,
3. high-riding or non-palpable prostate, or
4. scrotal hematoma.

With any of these findings, a retrograde urethrogram may be necessary to exclude urethral injury prior to Foley catheter insertion.

Consider IV antibiotics and tetanus administration for traumatic wounds. In patients with open fractures, empiric prophylactic antibiotics should be administered as soon as possible after the injury.

Remember to treat pain early. It is important to frequently reassess the patient's need for additional pain medications.

Special patients

Pediatric

Pediatric trauma patients require specialized management with respect to almost all portions of care. Physicians experienced in managing pediatric trauma and post-trauma care at centers experienced in pediatrics should assume this responsibility.

Airway management of a child may be more difficult than an adult due to anatomical differences, such as a larger head, more prominent tongue, anterior larynx, and floppy epiglottis. Children commonly develop shock due to respiratory compromise rather than cardiac causes, so airway and breathing must be assessed and addressed rapidly and repeatedly.

Children may maintain their blood pressure until impending hemodynamic collapse. Hypotension in a child is a dangerous and often premorbid condition. Vascular access in children is commonly difficult. The use of an intraosseous

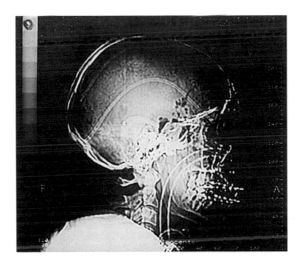

Figure 6.20
Computed tomography scout film reveals intracranial placement of a nasogastric tube in a patient with severe craniofacial trauma. Reprinted from Oral Surgery, Oral Medicine, Oral Pathology, Oral Radiology, and Endodontology, Vol. 90, Ferreras J, Junquera LM, Garcia-Consuegra L, Intracranial placement of a nasogastric tube after severe craniofacial trauma, 564–566, © 2000 Mosby, with permission from Elsevier. Image courtesy of LM Junquera, Universidad de Oviedo, Spain.

needle in patients <8 years old should be considered if peripheral access is not obtained within 3 minutes. Isotonic crystalloid fluid boluses should be given in 20 ml/kg amounts, with blood given in 10 ml/kg aliquots to patients not responding to crystalloid.

As the ribs are more pliable in children, significant injury to the lungs may occur without external evidence of injury. Identification of rib fractures in young children suggests a massive energy transfer and the possibility of severe underlying organ injury. The liver often protrudes below the protective rib margin, and is therefore at greater risk for injury.

Head injuries in children are often devastating, as little room exists for brain swelling. Damage to the spinal cord and resulting neurologic injury may occur without evidence of spinal column fracture. This condition is known as SCIWORA (Spinal Cord Injury Without Radiographic Abnormality). The GCS is modified for pediatrics by altering the pediatric verbal score for children <4 years of age (Table 6.5).

Due to the increased body surface area-to-volume ratio of children, they are prone to develop hypothermia more quickly than adults. Prevention of heat loss is of tremendous importance in pediatric trauma patients.

Elderly

The elderly population is extremely prone to falls and subsequent injury. Decreased coordination,

Table 6.5 Modified Glasgow Coma Scale for preverbal children

Eye opening	
Spontaneous	4
To verbal command	3
To pain	2
None	1
Verbal response	
Coos, babbles	5
Cries, consolable	4
Persistently irritable (cries)	3
Restless, agitated (moans)	2
No response	1
Motor response	
Spontaneous	6
Withdraws to voice	5
Withdraws to pain	4
Abnormal flexion	3
Abnormal extension	2
No response	1

muscle strength, vision, and fine motor skills needed for driving place the elderly population at greater risk of injury. The evaluation of elderly patients may be more challenging due to changes in their anatomy and physiology. These patients often lack the cardiovascular reserve necessary to respond to hypovolemia, and may not develop tachycardia. Decreased sensitivity of the peritoneal cavity due to aging allows these patients to have a benign abdominal examination despite catastrophic disease. As the brain atrophies, it is displaced from the inner skull, which creates a space spanned by bridging vessels. These vessels are more prone to injury during impact, and this additional space may hide clinical signs of intracranial bleeding for an unspecified period of time.

Pregnant

Advanced Trauma Life Support (ATLS) suggests that a qualified trauma surgeon and obstetrician should be consulted early in the evaluation of the pregnant trauma patient. However, the initial evaluation and management priorities of a pregnant woman remain unchanged. The best care for the fetus is to provide optimal care to the mother, with early assessment of the fetus. This includes adequate fluid resuscitation, prevention of maternal hypoxia or hypercarbia, and understanding the physiologic changes that occur in pregnancy.

After approximately the 10th week, pregnant women develop both an increased cardiac output and plasma volume. This cardiac output can be markedly decreased if the uterus sits on the inferior vena cava when the patient is supine after 20 weeks gestation. This *supine hypotension syndrome* may occur in a pregnant patient immobilized on a backboard. It is important to elevate the right side of the board or manually displace the gravid uterus to the left to relieve this pressure.

This alteration in physiology means that the pregnant trauma patient may sustain a larger amount of blood loss before showing clinical signs. Accordingly, the fetus may be in shock even though the mother appears stable. Direct evaluation of the fetus is accomplished by cardiotocography for a minimum of 4 hours, to evaluate uterine contractions and fetal cardiac activity.

The pregnant patient should be assessed for vaginal bleeding or leakage of amniotic fluid. Although the uterus and pelvis provides an additional cushion for the fetus, lack of abdominal injury to the mother does not exclude the possibility of significant injury to the fetus, uterus, or placenta.

A Kleihauer–Betke (KB) acid elution test on maternal blood should be performed to assess for fetomaternal hemorrhage. Its purpose in the ED is to screen Rh-negative woman at risk for large fetomaternal hemorrhage that exceeds the efficacy of the 300 mcg dose of Rhogam. Rh immunoglobulin (RhIG) can effectively prevent Rh isoimmunization if administered within 72 hours of exposure to the Rh antigen. All Rh-negative pregnant trauma patients should be considered for RhIG therapy. Remember to administer O negative blood if a type and cross-match is not feasible.

As a rule, all pregnant women who sustain trauma of any type should be considered as victims of intimate partner violence (IPV). Pregnant patients are far too often assaulted, kicked, or pushed during arguments, without being considered as victims. In fact, many abused pregnant women do not consider themselves victims of violence. It is common for women in this situation to be afraid to describe the details of their injury. Also, it is common that their injuries do not fit the mechanism they describe. Fear of being alone, intimidation, subsequent acts of violence, or losing financial support are only a few reasons for not reporting IPV. Social services, police involvement, housing assistance and emotional support should be provided under such circumstances.

Disposition

Although most EMS providers have established guidelines for transporting trauma patients to specific trauma centers, every ED should be prepared to handle patients who sustain traumatic injuries. Patients who require subspecialty care not available at your institution should be considered for transfer. The transfer process should be started as soon as a need for transfer is identified. Most trauma centers prefer to receive the patient earlier in the course of care, following initial stabilization with less evaluation, rather than later. All life-threatening injuries should be evaluated and addressed prior to transfer.

Trauma patients with evidence of airway, breathing, or circulatory compromise require the consultation of a trauma surgeon. This should be done while providing necessary stabilization and appropriate treatment. Waiting on the arrival of the surgeon before performing life-saving procedures should not occur.

Institutions have specific criteria to notify the trauma or surgical service of a trauma patient's arrival. Familiarity with an institution's criteria is extremely important to patient care. Often emergency physicians perform the primary and secondary surveys prior to the arrival of a trauma surgeon or team, with consultation directed by the injuries identified. Most of the time, however, a trauma surgeon will be involved in the initial evaluation of the trauma patient, and will assist with admission and disposition decisions after the initial resuscitation. Emergency physicians have the primary responsibility for trauma patients while they remain in the ED.

Disposition options for each trauma patient include discharge to home, admission to an observation unit, ward or intensive care unit (ICU), a trip to the OR, or transfer to another facility. Admission decisions should not be delayed until completion of an exhaustive evaluation. Rather, disposition options should be considered early and repeatedly throughout the evaluation.

Pearls, pitfalls, and myths

- Remember the ABCs. Always start with airway, followed by breathing, circulation, and disability. Exposure is important during the evaluation. Attention should not be drawn to grotesque injuries, which may result in missing life-threatening ones. If things start to deteriorate, return to the ABCs.
- Be suspicious of injuries based on the mechanism of injury. Maintain a high level of suspicion for injuries even if the patient looks well initially. The examination of the trauma patient should be thorough and systematic.
- Be quick but thorough. Managing the resuscitation of the trauma patient in the first (golden) hour often determines the patient's outcome. Being idle or not attending to detail can prove devastating.
- Work collaboratively with your trauma consultants. Clearly established roles for physicians involved in trauma resuscitation result in the best care, and benefit everyone.
- Keep all trauma patients warm. Exposure and IV fluids can cause hypothermia, which may lead to coagulopathy and worsening prognosis.

References

1. Campbell JE (ed.). *Basic Trauma Life Support*, 5th ed., Pearson Prentice Hall, 2004.
2. Committee on Trauma, American College of Surgeons. *Advanced Trauma Life Support Instructor Manual*, 5th ed., Chicago: American College of Surgeons, 1997.
3. Hamilton GC (ed.). *Emergency Medicine: An Approach to Clinical Problem-Solving*, 2nd ed., Philadelphia: W.B. Saunders, 2002.
4. Harwood-Nuss A (ed.). *The Clinical Practice of Emergency Medicine*, 3rd ed., Philadelphia: Lippincott Williams & Wilkins, 2001.
5. Howell JM (ed.). *Emergency Medicine*, 1st ed., Philadelphia: W.B. Saunders, 1998.
6. Ferrera (ed.). *Trauma Management: An Emergency Medicine Approach*, 1st ed., St. Louis: Mosby, 2001.
7. Marx JA (ed.). *Rosen's Emergency Medicine: Concepts and Clinical Practice*, 5th ed., St. Louis: Mosby, 2002.
8. Tintinalli JE (ed.). *Emergency Medicine: A Comprehensive Study Guide*, 3rd ed., McGraw Hill, 2000.

Paul D. Biddinger, MD and Stephen H. Thomas, MD

History of emergency medical services

Over the past four decades, prehospital care and emergency medical services (EMS) in the US have evolved rapidly from near nonexistence into key links in the chain of survival for patients with acute injury or illness. Beginning in the mid-1960s, after a landmark report titled *Accidental Death and Disability: The Neglected Disease of Modern Society* detailed serious deficiencies in out-of-hospital trauma management, state and federal lawmakers began to enact new standards for training, equipment, and oversight in EMS systems. The resulting translation into the field of formerly hospital-limited therapies for life threats, such as the unstable airway, respiratory failure, hemodynamic collapse, and dysrhythmias, in addition to traumatic injuries, has resulted in countless numbers of lives saved. With further advances in research, technology, and education, today's prehospital care providers are continually becoming more sophisticated in the diagnosis and treatment of acute injury and illness. Understanding the structure and capabilities of EMS is a critical component of emergency medicine, as the collaboration between prehospital and hospital-based providers determines the quality of emergency medical care delivered to the community.

Prehospital systems

Each municipality or rural area has several options with regard to the administration of their EMS. When government-run, EMS can be administered either as a stand-alone agency or under the command of the fire department. Alternatively, prehospital care can be provided by a local hospital or private ambulance company under contract to the city or county. In rural areas, EMS can be provided by volunteers on call from home. Regional coordination of EMS care, especially at the Advanced Life Support (ALS) level, can optimize response times and maximize system resource utilization. The ideal structure of an emergency medical system is frequently debated, but must vary depending on the setting. The key factors that influence the choice of system include population size and density, municipal budget, and political concerns. Air medical systems are typically administered by a hospital (or hospital consortium) or state agency to provide care for a large geographic region.

EMS personnel and qualifications

There are generally three broad categories of EMS personnel: first responders, basic emergency medical technicians (EMTs) (also known as EMT-basic or EMT-B), and paramedics (or EMT-P).

First responders are trained in basic first aid measures such as bandaging, splinting, hemorrhage control, and cardiopulmonary resuscitation (CPR). Generally, these are police, firefighters, and other volunteers who may be the first to arrive at an accident scene. First responders usually do not transport patients.

EMT-Bs are trained to assess signs and symptoms, safely extricate, immobilize, and transport the patient, and administer certain non-invasive therapies such as oxygen. Though not trained in cardiac rhythm interpretation, many EMTs can defibrillate through the use of automatic external defibrillators (AEDs). Care by EMT-Bs is termed basic life support (BLS). Most EMT-B courses consist of approximately 120 to 160 hours of clinical instruction and several hours of observation in emergency departments and obstetric units. The EMT-intermediate (EMT-I) is an extension of the EMT-B with additional training to obtain intravenous (IV) access, administer IV fluids, and use airway adjuncts such as the laryngeal mask airway (LMA) or pharyngotracheal lumen airway (PTLA). The EMT-I generally does not administer medications. Many systems that employ EMT-Is are in rural areas that cannot afford or recruit full paramedic coverage.

EMT-Ps are trained in advanced airway management, including endotracheal intubation, cardiac rhythm interpretation and defibrillation, and parenteral medication administration. Additionally, many paramedics are trained in cricothyrotomy and needle chest decompression when state and regional protocols allow. Prehospital care by paramedics is termed ALS. Paramedic training programs consist of at least 500 hours of classroom instruction as well as mandatory supervised hospital and field internships.

With increasing regionalization of specialized medical and surgical services, critical care transport (either by air or ground) is increasingly recognized as a unique area of expertise. Many states now allow for paramedics with specialized additional training and supervision to function at a level beyond standard protocols. Additional personnel beyond the EMT-Ps are also frequently used both in air and ground-based critical care transport. Physicians are standard members of the air medical crew in most non-US settings, but in the US, non-physicians staff over 90% of most crews. One exception to this rule in the US is where emergency medicine residencies provide physician coverage. Nurses staffing critical care transport units generally have experience in both emergency and critical care settings, with additional experience (pediatric or obstetric) depending on the characteristics of the program's patient population. Other crewmembers, such as neonatal nurse practitioners or balloon pump specialists, may be used depending on local preferences and specific patient needs. At this time, consistent national standards for critical care transport do not exist, but at least one non-governmental accreditation agency (the Commission on Accreditation of Medical Transport Systems) has recognized that the level of care, rather than the transport vehicle, should be a prime focus for the evaluation of critical care transport services.

EMS response

911 system

Approximately 96% of the US population currently have access to emergency care via the 911-telephone system. Enhanced 911 systems use computer databases to display the address of the caller, activating the 911 system in the event the caller is unable to speak. Although many mobile phones cannot be precisely located, there are emerging technologies that may help dispatchers approximate the location of a cellular phone. Global Positioning System (GPS) software is now available in mobile phones so that callers may be located if they are lost or unable to speak. Many EMS systems train their dispatchers to follow a careful script of questions when they are called

for help in a medical emergency. The answers to these questions determine the priority of the call and allow for the nearest available ambulance to be dispatched to the patient with the highest priority complaint.

Arrival on scene

The first priority of rescuers in any emergency is to ensure scene safety. Rescuers have a duty to themselves and the people they have been sent to assist. They should be able to care for and transport patients and not become patients themselves. Violent crimes often occur in scenes that remain unsafe after the initial injury. Despite the usual temptation to aid the victim as soon as possible, rescuers must not enter a violent crime scene until the police or detectives have first secured it. Rescuers are also at risk on the scene of motor vehicle collisions. When approaching an accident, the rescuers must survey the scene for potential hazards such as passing traffic, hazardous materials, or electrical wires. In accidents involving hazardous materials, rescuers must position themselves at a safe distance uphill and upwind, and the materials should be identified before personnel enter the scene. Specialized teams may need to be activated before the patient may be reached. In all cases, victims and EMS providers must be adequately decontaminated before arrival at the hospital to avoid further spread of toxins to other patients and health care providers. Certain other circumstances require mobilization of additional resources before the patient may be safely reached. These include water rescue, trench and confined space rescue, and high-angle (high-elevation) rescue. These situations may be beyond the training of local authorities, and additional personnel and resources may need to be summoned from larger community units in the state or surrounding area.

Extrication

Extrication is the technique of safely removing the patient from his or her environment and reaching the transport vehicle. This may be especially difficult with tight spaces, obese patients, rough terrain, and trauma. Extrication in trauma may involve displacing debris that entraps the patient. Since significant force using hydraulic or air pressure often must be employed to manipulate the debris, carefully trained rescuers are critical to minimize the risk of further injury to the patient either from the debris or from unnecessary movement. While certain therapies such as oxygen administration, IV therapy, parenteral analgesia, needle decompression of the thorax, and occasionally definitive airway management may be started before the patient is free of the entrapment, delay in transport to a hospital while extrication occurs is generally associated with worse outcome. Prolonged extrication time (more than 20 minutes) is considered a marker for potentially severe injury, and warrants triage directly to a trauma center when possible.

Clinical capabilities of EMS

Airway management

There are multiple devices designed to assist in the prehospital management of the patient's airway and breathing. Rescuers at all levels are trained in the use of the bag-valve-mask (BVM) device and both the nasopharyngeal airway (NPA) and oropharyngeal airway (OPA). The NPA and OPA are curved pieces of plastic that are inserted blindly, provided there are no contraindications. They are used chiefly to maintain airway patency.

Rescuers either not trained in endotracheal intubation or unable to achieve tracheal intubation with direct laryngoscopy may use the PTLA (Figure 7.1) or Combitube (Figure 7.2) for a patient

with airway compromise. The PTLA and Combitube are similar devices (with multiple tubes bound together) designed for blind insertion into the patient's airway. Their success depends on the operator being able to correctly identify which of the blindly-inserted tubes ends up in the esophagus, and which tube can adequately ventilate the trachea. The LMA (Figure 7.3) was first introduced in the operative setting in the late 1980s as an alternative to endotracheal intubation for selected patients, but has increasingly been used as an alternative when endotracheal intubation cannot be achieved. The device consists of an inflatable V-shaped diaphragm at the end of a large-bore tube that is placed blindly into the larynx. It is relatively easy to use and minimizes the risk of gastric insufflation during assisted ventilation. It does not, however, protect the trachea from aspiration of blood or vomitus.

Endotracheal intubation (ETI) remains the gold standard for airway protection, though this technique is most dependent on operator skill and patient factors. Many factors common in prehospital care can make oral ETI difficult or impossible: operator's inexperience, inadequate patient sedation or relaxation, blood or vomitus in the airway, and anatomic variables such as an anterior larynx or expanding neck hematoma. Outside of investigational protocols, oral ETI is attempted in the prehospital setting only by rescuers with paramedic training or above. Blind nasotracheal intubation (BNTI) may be attempted for patients

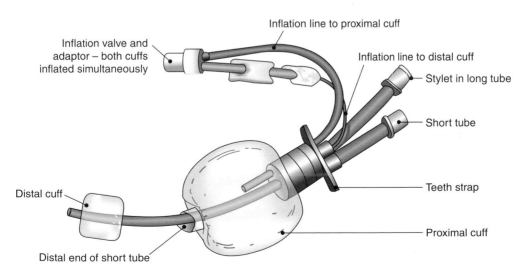

Figure 7.1
Pharyngotracheal lumen airway (PTLA). Reproduced from D. Skinner et al, *Cambridge Textbook of Accident and Emergency Medicine*, Cambridge, Cambridge University Press, 1997.

Inflation line to proximal cuff

Inflation valve and adaptor – both cuffs inflated simultaneously

Inflation line to distal cuff

Stylet in long tube

Short tube

Teeth strap

Proximal cuff

Distal cuff

Distal end of short tube

who still have spontaneous respiratory effort but need definitive airway control. This technique is of greatest use when orotracheal intubation is either not possible or very unlikely to succeed due to anatomic or traumatic reasons. The BNTI technique, uncommonly utilized at receiving trauma centers, is employed more frequently in the prehospital setting when neuromuscular blockade is not available, and jaw clenching prevents oral intubation. BNTI is contraindicated in patients with significant facial trauma. While neuromuscular-blocking agents (paralytics) are an integral component of rapid sequence intubation (RSI) in the hospital, historical concerns exist about their use by prehospital personnel. These providers may only infrequently intubate and, if unable to intubate or ventilate a previously spontaneously-breathing patient, have severely limited access to rescue techniques. Many helicopter transport services have reported high rates of successful intubations (>96%) using paralytics, but in general they employ a very select and experienced group of practitioners. Some ground transport services have also reported high success rates (>94%) using paralytics, but most frequently this is in high-volume urban areas under very close medical direction. At the current time, the use of paralytics (and concomitant induction agents) to facilitate

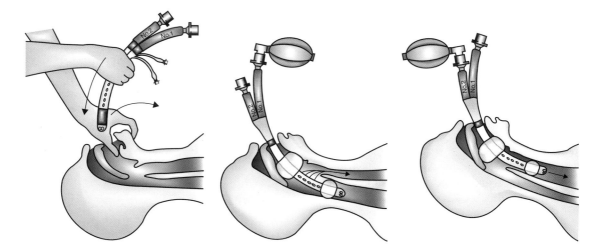

Figure 7.2
The Combitube. Reproduced from D. Skinner et al, *Cambridge Textbook of Accident and Emergency Medicine*, Cambridge, Cambridge University Press, 1997.

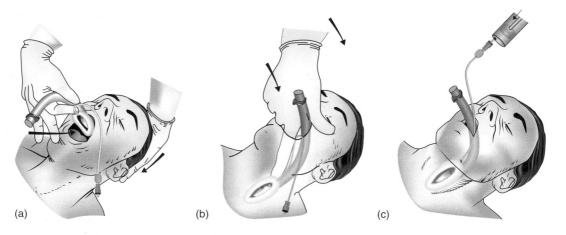

(a)   (b)   (c)

Figure 7.3
Laryngeal Mask Airway. (a) LMA in place with cuff overlying larynx. (b) LMA placement into the pharynx. (c) LMA placement using the index finger as a guide. Reprinted from Clinical Procedures in Emergency Medicine, 4th ed., Eds Roberts JR, Hedges J, page 62, Copyright 2003, with permission from Elsevier.

intubation should only be allowed in systems with highly-trained and experienced providers operating under tight medical control; sufficient backup and rescue techniques must be available in the event of failed ETI.

Approximately 70% of US ground paramedics and all air medical paramedics are allowed to perform some form of surgical airway access if needed. Skills range from needle cricothyrotomy with jet ventilation, to the use of percutaneous kits that employ the Seldinger technique (such as the Melker kit), to open cricothyrotomy. The need for cricothyrotomy in the field is fortunately infrequent. Surprisingly, given the lack of experience, reported success rates in the field are high (82–100%). All systems employing the use of paralytics must equip and train their providers to perform a surgical airway in the event of failed intubation and ventilation.

Intravenous access and fluid administration

Paramedics and EMT-Is should attempt IV access on all unstable or potentially unstable patients in the field. Many life-saving medications are most effective, or only available, when administered IV. Furthermore, IV crystalloid infusion remains the cornerstone of management of hypotension in the field. When possible, every trauma patient should have two large-bore (e.g., 14- or 16-gauge) IV catheters placed in the field. However, attempts at cannulation have been reported to add as much as 12 minutes to on-scene times. Rescuers must not delay transport when adequate access has not been obtained. For most patients, the appropriate rule of thumb is two attempts per provider, ideally during transport of the patient. In 1994, a prominent Houston study reported that aggressive prehospital fluid resuscitation of hypotensive victims of penetrating trauma did not improve survival and actually increased total blood loss when compared with delayed resuscitation in the hospital. The results of this study and its applicability to other settings are still debated. However, this remains an area of ongoing research interest, so prehospital providers and physicians developing EMS protocols should be cognizant of the need to avoid over-resuscitation (with concomitant risk of increased hemorrhage) and under-resuscitation (with attendant risk of hypoperfusion). Transport time and time to definitive control of suspected hemorrhage are important factors to consider when choosing to begin prehospital fluid resuscitation. Not all parameters will consistently be improved by fluid administration (e.g., altered mental status in the head-injured patient), and providers must exercise judgment as to the adequacy and appropriateness of their resuscitation.

Cardiac monitoring and defibrillation

Early defibrillation is critically important for patients with non-perfusing ventricular tachycardia or ventricular fibrillation, since survival for these patients decreases by 10% per minute. With the advent of AEDs, most first responders and EMT-Bs who arrive on scene before paramedics can now defibrillate pulseless patients in ventricular fibrillation or ventricular tachycardia. However, rhythm interpretation and the decision to cardiovert borderline perfusing rhythms remain solely within the scope of ALS. Many paramedics are now trained to perform and interpret 12-lead electrocardiograms (ECG); some have the capability of radio transmission of the ECG to the hospital. Multiple studies have demonstrated that well-trained paramedics have excellent accuracy for both rhythm recognition and detection of ST-segment elevation in acute coronary syndromes. Such skills are critical for proper application of the American Heart Association's Advanced Cardiovascular Life Support (ACLS) guidelines.

Medication administration

Although certain states allow EMT-Bs to administer one or two selected life saving medications such as glucose, epinephrine, or albuterol, most BLS providers cannot administer medications. In general, only paramedics may administer medications. Paramedics are equipped with medicines to treat pain, selected overdoses, hypoglycemia, bronchospasm, allergic reactions, hypotension and cardiac ischemia, and follow all ACLS protocols. Certain ALS systems may carry paralytic agents to facilitate intubation at the discretion of the state and local medical directors. Field medication use, especially with controlled substances and with potentially pro-arrhythmic agents, must be tightly monitored and subject to regular quality assurance by the medical director.

Needle decompression

Most paramedics are permitted to perform chest decompression in the patient with suspected tension pneumothorax. Signs suggestive of tension pneumothorax include tachypnea, hypoxia, unilateral decreased or hyper-resonant breath sounds, jugular venous distention, and deviation of the trachea away from the affected side. Needle decompression is indicated for a patient in severe distress with the above signs or in cardiac arrest following trauma.

Immobilization

All EMS personnel are trained in the proper technique for spinal immobilization of patients (Figure 7.4). An appropriately-sized, rigid cervical collar should be placed on every victim of trauma with potential for spinal injury, including

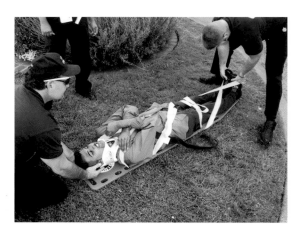

Figure 7.4
Spinal immobilization. *Courtesy*: S.V. Mahadevan, MD.

patients with pain, tenderness, or a suspicious mechanism of injury. However, since the cervical collar alone does not provide adequate immobilization for transport, patients should also be stabilized with a rigid backboard and some form of lateral stabilization (such as foam blocks) secured with straps or tape. Special steps, such as the use of a towel roll under the shoulders, may need to be taken to maximize head position (i.e., prevent flexion) in pediatric patients. Pregnant patients should have the right side of the backboard elevated 30° to keep the uterus off the inferior vena cava. This is done to avoid hypotension and fetal hypoperfusion. Patients with gunshot wounds to the neck, thorax, or abdomen not meeting the criteria above are not at increased risk for occult spinal injury and therefore do not need full immobilization on a backboard. Placement of a patient on a backboard is not innocuous; studies have shown that pressure-mediated skin damage can begin to develop after as little as 30 minutes on a backboard.

The Kendrick extrication device (KED) is made up of a series of parallel splints longitudinally bound together in a vest-like device that provides assistance with spinal stabilization during the extrication of a trauma patient from an enclosed space, such as a motor vehicle. It does not provide full spinal immobilization, and therefore cannot be used in lieu of a backboard for adults. Due to its wrap-around nature, however, it may be useful for pediatric patients who cannot or will not lie still on a standard backboard.

Patients with unstable vital signs should have only the injured extremities immobilized which have the potential to cause further hemorrhage if moved (i.e., pelvis and long bones, especially suspected femur fractures). Angulated extremity fractures should be carefully evaluated for distal neurovascular status. Currently, most prehospital jurisdictions call for traction splinting of suspected femur fractures, but this is subject to debate. These devices require time for application, are of debatable benefit in the field, and have contraindications (e.g., pelvic fracture) which may be unapparent. Any patient with an angulated fracture of any extremity with absent distal pulses should have in-line traction applied and be splinted. All other suspected fractures should be immobilized in the position of greatest comfort for transport.

Pneumatic anti-shock garment/military anti-shock trousers

Developed during the Vietnam War to treat soldiers exsanguinating in the field, the pneumatic anti-shock garment (PASG) was a mainstay of prehospital trauma care for nearly 20 years until its use was called into question by two outcome studies in the 1990s. Formerly known as the military anti-shock trousers (MAST), this device consists of a set of nylon pants with separately inflatable leg and abdominal sections that attach to a manual pump with a pressure gauge. Currently, the literature does not support the use of the PASG in penetrating trauma. There is some reason to believe that the PASG may be a useful immobilization device for pelvic fractures and/or femur fractures. Use in blunt trauma patients with severe hypotension is still debated, but it is used in some regions for this indication. The PASG is contraindicated in patients who are pregnant or who have pulmonary edema, evisceration of abdominal organs, cardiac tamponade, or cardiogenic shock.

Wound care

All EMS providers are trained to control external hemorrhage with direct pressure and elevation of the injury above the heart. Bandages that become soaked with blood are not removed, but rather reinforced with further gauze. Tourniquets are only placed in cases of life-threatening limb hemorrhage that cannot be controlled with continuous direct pressure, elevation, and bandaging. If tourniquets are applied in the field, they should not be removed by EMS providers.

Pediatrics

Although EMS personnel at all levels are trained to evaluate, treat, and transport pediatric patients, many prehospital providers are uncomfortable when caring for acutely ill children. Such patients are relatively rare, and most cases evoke much more than the usual stress for those involved. In general, the most significant differences between acutely ill adult and pediatric patients are:

1. vital sign abnormalities indicating significant injury or illness may be delayed compared with adult patients;
2. the age-specific nature of normal pediatric vital signs may lead practitioners to misinterpret absolute vital signs;
3. procedures, including IV access and intubation, are technically more challenging in children; and
4. children may be unable to give adequate histories or cooperate with procedures such as immobilization, and may require additional restraint for safe transport.

Recent data demonstrate that well-trained paramedics can deliver high-quality care to both adult and pediatric patients in nearly all arenas, but such care requires intensive education and regular review of skills. One very important exception to this rule is that pediatric patients should rarely be intubated in the field, even in cases of respiratory failure. Published data show that, in contrast with adults, morbidity and mortality are increased when prehospital care providers attempt to intubate apneic or hypoventilating pediatric patients. In general, prehospital pediatric intubation should only be attempted when effective BVM ventilation cannot be achieved.

Mass casualty incidents/disaster

A mass casualty incident (MCI) is any event that produces multiple casualties (injuries or illness). A disaster is any event that overwhelms the capabilities of the local emergency response system

and facilities. Although the two concepts are different, the principles of triage and care often overlap. Rescuers must be able to perform a brief (less than 60 seconds) evaluation of each patient in an MCI, focusing on ventilation, perfusion, and mental status, and triage each patient according to severity of injury. In large mass casualty incidents, a color-coded tag is attached to each victim to aid in efficient triage and transport. A sample medical emergency triage tag (METTAG) system is shown in Figure 7.5 and Table 7.1.

Incident command

Incident command is the system used for overall management of the disaster event, and is generally the responsibility of the ranking fire service officer on scene. EMS officials and occasionally an on-site physician experienced in disaster management are responsible for coordinating the medical activities and care with the incident commander.

Community-wide disaster systems

Planning and preparation prior to a disaster and/ or MCI is critical for a successful response. Preparation should include plans for field response, hazardous materials, staging and transportation, documentation of available local hospital resources, communication plans and backup systems, documentation, and debriefing and counseling after the events and recovery. Regular practice and drills are vital to train rescuers and test the system.

Medical direction

All care delivered by EMS personnel is provided under protocols and authority given to them by a physician medical director. The responsibility a physician assumes for the care delivered in an EMS system is called medical direction or medical control. Most of the real-time medical care delivered by prehospital providers is done following prewritten standing orders ("off-line" medical control). This does not require direct communication with a physician during the patient encounter. In these cases, patient care is reviewed retrospectively through standard processes, known as continuous quality improvement (CQI). This "off-line" component of education, training, and continuing care review is the largest and the most important part of medical direction in EMS. In certain instances, however,

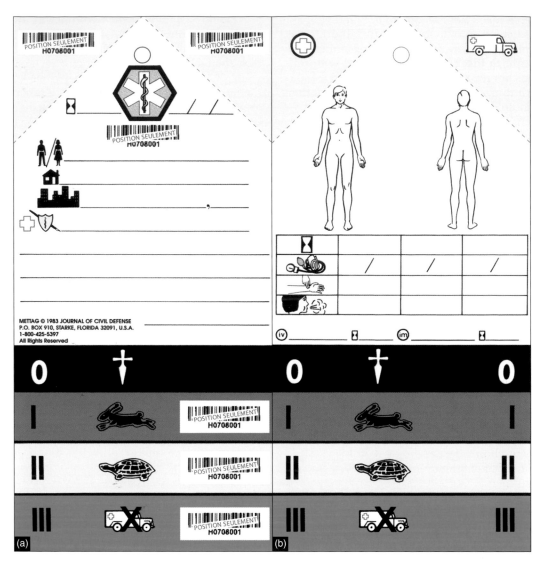

Figure 7.5
METTAG: Medical Emergency Field Triage Tag.

Table 7.1 Medical emergency triage tag system of field triage in a mass casuality incident

A suggested approach to treatment prioritization of victims is that found in the medical emergency triage tag system. The treatment priorities are defined as:

Zero priority (black): Deceased or live patients with obvious fatal and non-resuscitatable injuries.

First priority (red): Severely injured patients requiring immediate care and transport (e.g., respiratory distress, thoracoabdominal injury, severe head or maxillofacial injuries, shock or severe bleeding, severe burns).

Second priority (yellow): Patients with injuries that are determined not to be immediately life-threatening (e.g., abdominal injury without shock, thoracic injury without respiratory compromise, major fractures without shock, head injury/cervical spine injury, and minor burns).

Third priority (green): Patients with minor injuries that do not require immediate stabilization (e.g., soft tissue injuries, extremity fractures and dislocations, maxillofacial injuries without airway compromise, and psychological emergencies).

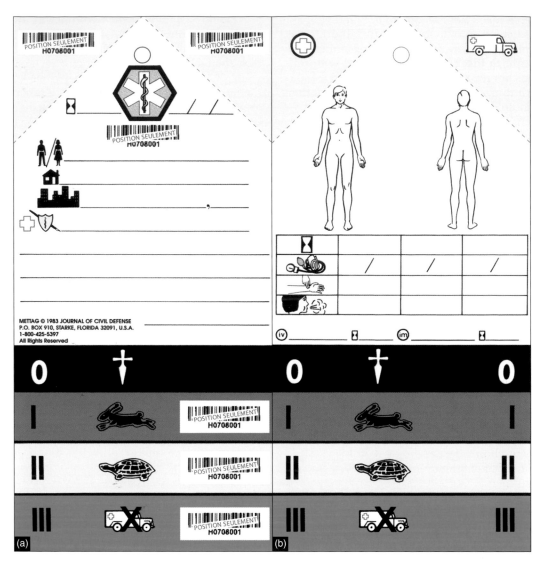

such as the administration of IV opiates in some jurisdictions, paramedics must contact a physician directly by radio or phone for "on-line" medical control. In those cases, the orders given by the physician must still conform to the state protocols and not exceed the paramedic's scope of practice. Rescuers may also use the on-line system to obtain a "field-consultation" from a physician when necessary, as in cases of a patient's refusal of transport or for other questions.

Patient transport

Vehicles

Standard ambulances come in various types, characterized by different vehicle designs. Type I ambulances are conventional box-type vehicles which lack a passageway between the driver and patient care compartments. Type II vehicles are van-type trucks. Type III vehicles are larger units with a forward cab and a walk-through passageway to the patient care area. Some units may require special equipment in order to provide electrical power to medical devices.

Many types of helicopters are used for patient transport. Depending on the resources and needs of a particular region, helicopters of particular sizes, speeds, costs, and physical characteristics may be chosen. Most helicopters in use in the US are twin-engine models, which have improved safety margins due to the redundancy afforded by the extra engine. Helicopter transports usually involve one patient only. For less acute patients, two-patient transports can be performed (if the helicopter allows). There is great variation between helicopter models with respect to size and speed; slower aircraft travel at little over 100–110 meters per hour, whereas other helicopters cruise nearly twice as fast.

Fixed-wing aircraft (airplanes) vary just as helicopters do, with a myriad of propeller- and jet-powered vehicles in use. In general, jet aircraft provide a smoother ride, faster speed, and are more likely to be able to pressurize to sea level, especially when flying at higher altitudes. Due to the relative isolation of patient care in a fixed-wing aircraft, patients should be reasonably stable before fixed-wing transport is undertaken.

Emergency warning devices

While the use of warning lights and siren (L&S) is standard among emergency vehicles, it is not without risk and controversy. Each year, rescuers, patients, and bystanders are injured or killed in collisions during the use of L&S. In general, when operating with L&S, rescuers must exercise "due regard" for other vehicles; in all cases, the use of L&S must be based upon standardized protocols that account for the severity of the complaint or the acuity of illness.

Patient transfer

It is not uncommon for IV catheters or endotracheal tubes (ETTs) to become dislodged during patient transport. Every possible precaution should be taken to secure medical access devices following their placement, and transfer patients slowly and deliberately. Optimally, one prehospital provider should have as his or her sole responsibility the assurance of maintaining ETT position during patient transfers. Additionally, re-confirmation of ETT position is warranted each time an intubated patient is moved from one surface to another.

Communication

Communication between prehospital providers and hospital personnel most commonly occurs via simplex (one-way) radio systems using either ultra high frequency (UHF) or very high frequency (VHF). Advancing technology is increasingly allowing EMS providers to receive dispatch and scene information by computer and converse with dispatch or hospital personnel in a duplex (two-way) fashion, either with paired radio frequencies or cellular phones. Whenever possible, prehospital personnel should have backup systems to their primary means of communication.

Destination criteria

Severely injured victims of trauma should be transported directly to a designated Level I or II trauma center, bypassing smaller hospitals when transport times are not excessive. One study revealed that patients who must be transferred secondarily from a local hospital to a trauma center had a 30% increased risk of mortality compared with those who were transported directly to the trauma center from the scene. Furthermore, for similarly injured patients, the risk of dying in a Level I trauma center was 54% lower than in Level II centers and 75% lower than in hospitals that are not trauma centers. Rescuers should follow state protocols regarding indications for transport directly to a trauma center, but most protocols are similar to the American College of Surgeon's Field Triage Algorithm (Table 7.2). The patient in cardiac arrest should be transported directly to the nearest available emergency department, even in cases of trauma. Victims of trauma who arrest in the field have a dismal prognosis but warrant the immediate application of hospital resources to treat potentially reversible causes of death.

As with victims of major trauma, significantly burned patients meeting appropriate triage criteria should be transported directly to a designated burn center when feasible (Table 7.3).

Currently, nationally-recognized point-of-entry (POE) criteria, which allow EMS personnel to bypass a nearby hospital for one farther away with specialty services, only exist for the transport of patients with severe trauma or burns. Expanded POE criteria are being instituted in several communities for selected disease processes, such as ST-elevation myocardial infarction (MI) or acute stroke, but are not yet the standard of care.

Special considerations in air transport

The decision of when a helicopter should respond to the scene of injury or illness remains an inexact science. The best sources acknowledge that the judgment of the prehospital personnel at the scene is of primary importance, but the decision to use helicopter transport can be bolstered by criteria listed below and in Table 7.4:

1. Mechanism of injury
2. Physiologic variables
3. Anatomic variables
4. Time and logistics.

Space constraints are the major issue in providing care in any aircraft. Both the actual space (cubic feet) and the arrangement of the space (cabin configuration) can have profound effects on the ability of the air medical crew to perform interventions such as intubation. This translates into the need for the air medical crew to sometimes adjust the care provided accordingly. One example would be intubating patients prior to flight if there is a significant chance of airway deterioration while en route. Crewmembers should be cross-trained to allow either crewmember to provide indicated medical interventions during flight. Some interventions, such as provision of

chest compressions, are extremely difficult to provide effectively in the air medical setting.

Noise is of a sufficient degree to preclude reliable auscultation and monitoring of aural alarms (e.g., on a ventilator). The flight crew must learn to use other means of patient assessment and equipment monitoring.

Vibration is a theoretical problem for the patient, and high-frequency vibrations have been shown to induce fatigue in caregivers. In general, however, the ride in a helicopter or fixed-wing aircraft can often be much smoother than a ride in a ground ambulance.

Lighting in an aircraft, and to a lesser extent in a ground ambulance, differs from that which is normally available in a well-lit hospital resuscitation area. Some helicopters, for instance, have patient care cabins which are contiguous with (and not separated from) the pilot seat; in such situations the medical crew must work in red, blue, and/or dimmed lighting at night.

Altitude issues relate to hypoxemia, pressure–volume changes, temperature, and humidity. Altitude-related hypoxemia is not usually an issue due to the fact that patients receive oxygen therapy and the altitude is usually not sufficiently high for the crew to require supplemental oxygen. Exceptions to this general rule occur, however, with both patients (e.g., premature neonates with narrow therapeutic windows for oxygen administration) and crew (e.g., crew in programs based at higher altitudes, who wear oxygen masks for prevention of hypoxemic symptoms). Boyle's law describes the inverse relationship between ambient pressure and gas volume. This is a factor with respect to both equipment (e.g., ventilator, intra-aortic balloon pump, Minnesota tubes for upper gastrointestinal hemorrhage tamponade) and patients (e.g., need for pre-flight placement of a gastric tube to prevent vomiting in unconscious patients). High altitude is associated with decreased ambient temperature. Especially in colder climates where the patient may be hypothermic before being loaded onto the aircraft, and in aircraft with suboptimal heating systems, hypothermia is a risk of helicopter transport. Higher altitude and lower temperature are associated with decreased humidity. This can result in hardening of secretions, such as in the ETT, which the air medical crew should monitor (and suction) as indicated. Helicopters generally transport patients at altitudes of 500–2000 feet above ground level. Therefore, unless transports occur at geographic locations where ground level is significantly elevated, altitude issues are of

Table 7.2 American College of Surgeons' (ACS) Field Triage Algorithm

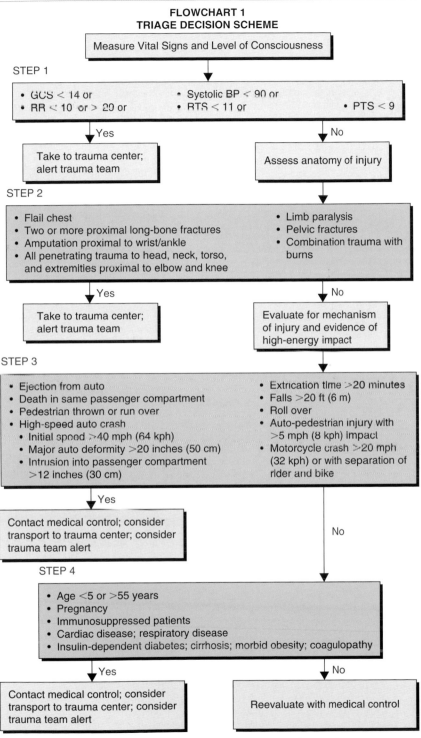

FLOWCHART 1
TRIAGE DECISION SCHEME

Measure Vital Signs and Level of Consciousness

STEP 1

- GCS < 14 or
- RR < 10 or > 29 or
- Systolic BP < 90 or
- RTS < 11 or
- PTS < 9

Yes → Take to trauma center; alert trauma team

No → Assess anatomy of injury

STEP 2

- Flail chest
- Two or more proximal long-bone fractures
- Amputation proximal to wrist/ankle
- All penetrating trauma to head, neck, torso, and extremities proximal to elbow and knee
- Limb paralysis
- Pelvic fractures
- Combination trauma with burns

Yes → Take to trauma center; alert trauma team

No → Evaluate for mechanism of injury and evidence of high-energy impact

STEP 3

- Ejection from auto
- Death in same passenger compartment
- Pedestrian thrown or run over
- High-speed auto crash
  - Initial speed >40 mph (64 kph)
  - Major auto deformity >20 inches (50 cm)
  - Intrusion into passenger compartment >12 inches (30 cm)
- Extrication time >20 minutes
- Falls >20 ft (6 m)
- Roll over
- Auto-pedestrian injury with >5 mph (8 kph) impact
- Motorcycle crash >20 mph (32 kph) or with separation of rider and bike

Yes → Contact medical control; consider transport to trauma center; consider trauma team alert

No

STEP 4

- Age <5 or >55 years
- Pregnancy
- Immunosuppressed patients
- Cardiac disease; respiratory disease
- Insulin-dependent diabetes; cirrhosis; morbid obesity; coagulopathy

Yes → Contact medical control; consider transport to trauma center; consider trauma team alert

No → Reevaluate with medical control

When in Doubt, Take to a Trauma Center!

BP: blood pressure; GCS: glasgow coma scale; PTS: pediatric trauma score; RR: respiratory rate; RTS: revised trauma score.

Table 7.3 Criteria for transport directly to a designated burn center

1. Partial thickness burns >10% (total body surface area)
2. Burns that involve the face, hands, feet, genitalia, perineum, or major joints
3. Third-degree burns in any age group
4. Electrical burns, including lightning injury
5. Chemical burns
6. Inhalation injury
7. Burn injury in patients with pre-existing medical disorders that could complicate management, prolong recovery, or affect mortality. Burns in any patients with concomitant trauma (such as fractures) in which the burn injury poses the greatest risk of morbidity or mortality. In such cases, if the trauma poses a greater immediate risk than the burns, it may be necessary to stabilize the patient in a trauma center before being transferred to a burn unit. Physician judgment is necessary in such situations and should be in concert with the regional medical control plan and triage protocols
8. Burns in children being cared for in hospitals without qualified personnel or equipment for the care of children
9. Burn injury in patients who will require special social, emotional, or long-term rehabilitative intervention

Table 7.4 National Association of Emergency Medical Service Physicians guidelines for dispatching a helicopter to an emergency scene

Clinical
1. General
   (a) Trauma victims need to delivered as soon as possible to a regional trauma center
   (b) Stable patients who are accessible to ground vehicles probably are best transported by ground
2. Specific
   Patients with critical injuries resulting in unstable vital signs require the fastest and most direct route of transport to a regional trauma center in a vehicle staffed with a team capable of offering critical care enroute. Often this is the case in the following situations:
   (a) Trauma score <12
   (b) Glasgow coma scale score <10
   (c) Penetrating trauma to the abdomen, pelvis, chest, neck, or head
   (d) Spinal cord or spinal column injury, or any injury producing paralysis of any extremity if any lateralizing signs
   (e) Partial of total amputation of an extremity (excluding digits)
   (f) Two of more long bone fractures or a major pelvic fracture
   (g) Crushing injuries to the abdomen, chest, or head
   (h) Major burns of the body surface area, or burns involving the face, hands, feet or perineum, or burns with significant respiratory involvement or major electrical or chemical burns
   (i) Patients involved in a serious traumatic event who are <12 or >55 years of age
   (j) Patients with near-drowning injuries, with or without existing hypothermia
   (k) Adult trauma patients with any of the following vital sign abnormalities:
      (i) systolic blood pressure <90 mmHg
      (ii) respiratory rate <10 or >35/minute
      (iii) heart rate <60 or >120/minute
      (iv) unresponsive to verbal stimuli

Operational situations in which helicopter use should be considered:
1. Mechanism of injury:
   (a) Vehicle roll-over with unbelted passengers
   (b) Vehicle striking pedestrian at >10 miles per hour
   (c) Falls from >15 feet
   (d) Motorcycle victim ejected at >20 miles per hour
   (e) Multiple victims
2. Difficult access situations:
   (a) Wilderness rescue
   (b) Ambulance egress or access impeded at the scene by road conditions, weather, or traffic
3. Time/distance factors:
   (a) Transportation time to the trauma center >15 minutes by ground ambulance
   (b) Transport time to local hospital by ground greater than transport time to trauma center by helicopter
   (c) Patient extrication time >20 minutes
   (d) Utilization of local ground ambulance leaves local community without ground ambulance coverage

relatively minor concern for the majority of helicopter transports. On the other hand, fixed-wing transports occur at much higher altitudes, which brings into play issues of cabin pressurization and risks of sudden decompression.

Safety is the paramount consideration for any air transport service. At any time, in any mission, the pilot or medical crew should be empowered to halt the transport if safety considerations become a concern. Direct comparison between air and ground vehicle safety is difficult, since crashes involving medical helicopters (or less commonly, fixed-wing aircraft) are more reliably tracked and more widely publicized than crashes of ground vehicles. Sometimes, considerable judgment must be exercised in determining whether to perform a critical procedure (e.g., intubation) before or after transport commences. Except in cases where a fixed-wing aircraft is used solely because critical patients cannot be evacuated by air (e.g., fog precludes helicopter operations but a fixed-wing aircraft can safely operate in a remote area), patients transported by airplane typically have lesser acuity and greater stability than those transported by ground.

References

1. Cone DC, Wydro GC, Mininger CM. Current practice in clinical cervical spinal clearance: implication for EMS. *Prehosp Emerg Care* 1999;3:42–46.
2. Clawson J, Forbuss R, Hauert S, Hurtado F, Kuehl A, Maningas P, Ryan J, Sharpe D. Use of warning lights and siren in emergency medical vehicle response and patient transport. *Prehosp Disaster Med* 1994.
3. Dieckmann RA, Athey J, Bailey B, Michael J. A pediatric survey for the National Highway Traffic Safety Administration: emergency medical services system re-assessments. *Prehosp Emerg Care* 2001;5:231–236.
4. Domeier RM. Indications for prehospital spinal immobilization. National Association of EMS Physicians Standards and Clinical Practice Committee. *Prehosp Emerg Care* 1999;3:251–253.
5. Eckstein M, Chan L, Schneir A, Palmer R. Effect of prehospital advanced life support on outcomes of major trauma patients. *J Trauma* 2000;48(4):643–648.
6. Fowler R, Pepe PE. Prehospital care of the patient with major trauma. *Emerg Med Clin of North Am* 2002;20(4):953–974.
7. Gerich TG, Schmidt U, Hubrich V, Lobenhoffer HP, Tscherne H. Prehospital airway management in the acutely injured patient: the role of surgical cricothyrotomy revisited. *J Trauma* 1998;45:312–314.
8. Karch S, Lewis T, Young S, Hales D, Ho C. Field intubation of trauma patients: complications, indications and outcomes. *Am J Em Med* 1996;14:617–620.
9. Kuehl A. *Prehospital Systems and Medical Oversight.* Kendall-Hunt Publishing, 2002.
10. Lockey DJ. Prehospital trauma management. *Resuscitation* 2001;48:5–15.
11. Novak L, Shackford SR, Bourguignon P, Nichols P, Buckingham S, Osler T, Sartorelli K. Comparison of standard and alternative prehospital resuscitation in uncontrolled hemorrhagic shock and head injury. *J Trauma* 1999;47:834–844.
12. O'Connor R, Domeier R. Use of the Pneumatic Antishock Garment (PASG). *Prehosp Emerg Care* 1997; Jan/March.
13. Paul TR, Marias M, Pons PT, Pons KA, Moore EE. Adult versus pediatric prehospital trauma care: is there a difference? *J Trauma* 1999;47:455–459.
14. Pepe PE, Mosesso Jr VN, Falk JL. Prehospital fluid resuscitation of the patient with major trauma. *Prehosp Emerg Care* 2002;6(1):81–91.
15. Sampalis J, Denis R, Frechette P, Brown R, Fleiszer D and Mulder D. Direct transport to tertiary trauma centers versus transfer from lower level facilities: impact on mortality and morbidity among patients with major trauma. *J Trauma* 1997;43:228–296.
16. Thomas SH, Harrison TH, Buras WR, et al. Helicopter transport and blunt trauma outcome. *J Trauma* 2002;52:136–145.
17. Thomas SH, Harrison T, Wedel SK. Flight crew airway management in four settings: A six-year review. *Prehosp Emerg Care* 1999;3:310–315.
18. Thomas SH, Cheema F, Wedel SK, Thomson D. Helicopter EMS trauma transport: annotated review of selected outcomes-related literature. *Prehosp Emerg Care* 2002;5 (In press).
19. Wayne MA, Friedland E. Prehospital use of succinylcholine – a 20-year review. *Prehosp Emerg Care* 1999;3(2):107–109.

8 Pain management

Eustacia (Jo) Su, MD

Scope of the problem

Acute pain is the most common complaint of patients presenting to the emergency department (ED), comprising 60% of presenting complaints in one study. Recognition and acknowledgment of a patient's pain, adequate treatment, and timely reassessment are essential to acute pain management in the ED. Unfortunately, it has been demonstrated that many physicians fail to treat pain promptly or adequately in both inpatient and outpatient settings.

Pain

Pain is whatever the experiencing person says it is, existing whenever he or she says it does. The International Association for the Study of Pain defines pain as "an unpleasant sensory and emotional experience associated with actual or potential tissue damage, or described in terms of such damage," "always subjective," and "learned through experiences related to injury in early life." Pain includes behavioral and physical indicators, in addition to self-report. Thus, preverbal, nonverbal, or cognitively-impaired individuals who experience pain can benefit from objective pain assessment. Fear and anxiety increase the perception of physical pain – the unfamiliar and frequently unfriendly ED environment does little to ameliorate a patient's pain.

Acute pain is a symptom of injury or illness, which serves the biologic purpose of warning an individual of a problem and limiting activities that might exacerbate it. Acute pain is usually associated with identifiable pathology and causes anxiety. By convention, it is present for less than 6 months.

Chronic, malignant pain is associated with a terminal disease, such as cancer or acquired immune deficiency syndrome (AIDS). These patients are usually under the care of a multidisciplinary team that directs their analgesia regimen and comfort care.

Chronic, nonmalignant pain is a complex problem, defined as pain being present for greater than 6 months. In general, it is not associated with a readily treatable, or sometimes even identifiable, cause. It is generally associated with depression rather than anxiety. Patients may have a well-defined cause (e.g., tic douloureux) or no objectively confirmed cause (e.g., reflex sympathetic dystrophy). These patients frequently arouse animosity amongst ED staff because they can be quite demanding, and at times manipulative. The staff often senses that acute interventions will generally fail to help these patients for any length of time.

There are patients who feign pain to acquire opioids, either for their own use or to sell on the streets. These individuals may be difficult to distinguish from the group previously defined.

Analgesia

Analgesia is the "loss of sensitivity to pain." In the ED, this means the reduction of pain through therapy. The therapy is not solely pharmacologic in nature – psychologic and social support, as well as physical positioning for maximum comfort help reduce perceived pain. These interventions reassure the patient that the provider is aware of his or her pain and is making attempts to relieve it. Child life therapists, when available, provide psychologic support to children as well as distraction from painful procedures, such as starting an intravenous (IV) line.

Oligoanalgesia

Inadequately or poorly treated acute pain may result in negative physiologic outcomes. Poorly treated acute pain may exacerbate the underlying pathophysiology of many illnesses and injuries, and may result in the development of chronic pain.

The failure of physicians to treat pain has been documented in the ED as well as in the inpatient setting. Children receive fewer doses of analgesia, in general, and opiates, in particular, than adults with equivalent diagnoses or undergoing equally painful procedures.

Wilson and Pendleton reported in 1989 that in one academic ED, 56% of patients presenting with painful conditions received no analgesics. Furthermore, only 14% received any analgesia within the first hour of their ED stay. In this study, meperidine was the medication used most commonly. Findings included inadequate doses 55% of the time, and 60% of agents were given by intramuscular (IM) injection, despite the known disadvantages of this route of administration. In this study, only 31% of patients with an acute myocardial infarction and persistent chest pain received IV opioids. Lewis and Sasater studied eight EDs and found that only 30% of patients with acute fractures received opioids while in the ED.

Assessment and measurement of pain
Goals and challenges

It is imperative for physicians to detect and measure pain rapidly so that they can institute prompt treatment and assess its effect. Even though a patient may not appear to be in pain, he or she may actually be in severe pain. Careful listening, observation, and repeated solicitation may be necessary to fully elicit an admission of pain. Assessment must be both qualitative (is pain present?) and quantitative (how much does it hurt?). "Has the pain improved following treatment?" is an important reassessment question. Early reassessment must follow the initial treatment to ensure its adequacy and that repeated medication doses are given promptly to prevent pain recurrence.

There are no reliable objective or physiologic signs of pain. Normal vital signs may persist despite severe pain. Medication, a personal or cultural tendency to stoicism, or adaptive mechanisms, such as joking, may mask the presentation

of pain. Language and cultural barriers also interfere with the patient's ability to communicate his or her pain to the physician and health care team. Preverbal children, especially toddlers, may only be able to express an "owie." Neonates and young infants cannot verbalize at all; interpreting their cries requires time, experience, and motivation to understand and treat their pain.

Self-report assessment

The most reliable approach to assessing pain severity is patient self-report. Self-report tools are the mainstay of pain management research, but require that patients have cognitive and communication skills. The ideal self-report tool should be easy to use and applicable across language, cultural, age, and gender differences. It should also be valid and reliable between observers. Table 8.1 describes several commonly used tools for pain assessment in the ED.

Most of the tools are numerical. The Adjectival Rating Scale features six phrases describing pain intensity in ascending order. These are arrayed on a 10-cm baseline. They offer the same information as the numerical tools but with the numbers removed, an advantage for those patients who cannot describe their pain numerically.

The Numerical Rating Scale is the most commonly used pain scale. It involves asking the patient to rate his or her pain on a scale from 0 to 10. In this scale, 0 is equivalent to no pain, 1 is equivalent to barely perceptible pain, and 10 represents the greatest pain that the patient has ever experienced or could imagine. Even adults who are native speakers of the same language as

Table 8.1 Self-report assessments for pain

Adjectival	None	Mild	Moderate	Severe	Very severe	Worst possible	Comments
Numerical	0		5			10	Routine bedside evaluation
Visual analog scale (VAS) (10 cm baseline)	None					Worst imaginable	When hard copy needed
Hurt thermometer	White		Blue			Red	Bedside
Pictorial (faces)	😀	🙂	😐	🙁	😣	😫	>6 years old
Pieces of Hurt (poker chips)	0	1	2	3		4	>3 years old
Thumb-to-index finger distance							Some toddlers

the care providers have difficulty with this concept. Adults conversing in their second or non-native language may not be able to understand this scale or be able to express their pain adequately. Most children do not understand this at all: "big hurt," as opposed to "little hurt" may be the most that they can manage verbally.

The Visual Analog Scale (VAS) is the most widely used scale for clinical research. This is a 100 mm scale that has "no pain" on the left end and "maximum possible pain" on the right. Patients indicate a point on the scale to correspond to their level of pain. Visual, manual, and some conceptual skills are required for patients to be able to do this. Patients seem able to reliably indicate a point to describe the level of their pain, and to shift this point in an expected direction after therapy. The major limitation of the VAS is that the distance that constitutes a significant clinical change has not been validated. Most studies indicate that a change of 13 mm constitutes a statistically significant change, but this does not necessarily correlate with clinical significance.

The Faces scale (Figure 8.1) seems to work well for younger school-age children. The scale is self-explanatory and has strong agreement among children about the severity of pain reflected in the faces. The scale has also demonstrated adequate test–retest reliability.

The Hurt thermometer scale has faces superimposed on a scale on which the left end is white and represents no pain. From left to right, the color progresses from blue to red, with the bright-red end at the right representing maximal pain. This probably has no advantage in the assessment of pain in children, but may help assess pain in patients whose primary language differs from members of the health care team.

The Poker Chip Tool or Pieces of Hurt scale works well for preschool children. The child gives between one and four poker chips to the care provider to indicate the "size" of pain the child is currently experiencing. For even younger children, the thumb-to-index-finger measurement offers another modality of pain communication. The child indicates the severity of his or her pain by spreading the thumb from the index finger. Children seem able to grasp subunit quantity when expressed as a change in the relationship of body parts at a much younger age than they can with objects such as building blocks.

Nonself-report assessment

Infants, toddlers, cognitively-impaired patients, and those who do not speak the language of the health care team cannot effectively communicate their pain by the usual self-report scales. The physician is reduced to careful searching for cues that suggest the presence of pain. Soliciting comments from caregivers may help with the assessment of the patient's pain and the effectiveness of treatment.

Neonates have a limited repertoire of expression, and their ability to show body posturing is even further limited by the prevailing fashion of wrapping or swaddling. Evaluation of neonatal facial expressions provides the best estimate of their level of pain, even when their face is partially obscured by a nipple or pacifier. Of 10 possible facial actions in neonates, three provide the most reliable indicators of pain: the furrowed brow, the forehead bulge (just above the eyebrows), and squeezing of the eyes. Other facial actions include the nasolabial furrow, which can be obscured by a pacifier, open lips, horizontal and vertical mouth stretch, taut tongue, chin quiver, lip purse, and tongue protrusion. The cry in response to pain tends to be more high-pitched and drawn out than the usual cry for food or diaper changing. Caregivers are often able to describe how the current cry differs from the usual cry, and whether or not the baby is more difficult to console. Moaning or whimpering is not normal for a neonate.

The FLACC scale (face, legs, activity, cry, and consolability) is sometimes useful in infants

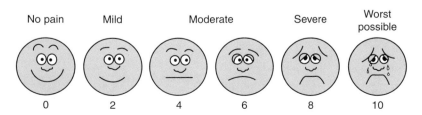

No pain	Mild	Moderate	Severe	Worst possible
0	2	4	6	8	10

Figure 8.1
Faces scale.

Table 8.2 FLACC pain scale (each category is scored from 0 to 2, totals up to 10)

Categories	0	1	2
Face	Smile or no expression	Occasional grimace or frown; withdrawn	Quivering chin, clenched jaw
Legs	Normal position or relaxed	Uneasy, tense, restless	Kicking, legs drawn up
Activity	Lying quietly, moves easily	Squirming, tense shifting back and forth	Arched, rigid, jerking
Cry	No cry	Moans or whimpers; occasional complaints	Crying, screaming, frequent complaints
Consolability	Content, relaxed	Reassured by occasional touch, hug, or talk; distractible	Difficult to console or comfort

(Table 8.2). Facial distortions due to pain are described above. The limbs are assessed for rigidity and muscle tone. In the infant with severe cerebral palsy or known spasticity, this may not prove helpful in the assessment of pain. Crying and consolability are assessed with the help of the caregivers.

Assessment of pain in patients with limited communication skills is very challenging. Patients with developmental disabilities or cognitive impairment are often unable to express pain. It is unclear whether their neurologic impairment means that these patients do not actually experience pain, or if the pain experience is diminished for them. There are no valid or reliable tools for assessment of pain in patients with significant neurologic impairment. As much as possible, the clinician should keep caregivers at hand to assist with communication and management, maintain typical means of communication (e.g., patient's laptop), maintain typical means of comfort and mobility (e.g., wheelchair, form board), and remember that improved function may not mean that the pain has completely abated.

Treatment of pain

Expediting relief

Patients generally wait too long for their pain to be treated. Untreated pain has physiologic consequences and must be mitigated as soon as possible. Treatment should begin *even before* a definitive diagnosis has been established. Multiple studies have shown that patients who have undifferentiated abdominal pain, even children, can safely receive analgesics without a worse outcome.

The need for informed consent in the immediate future is often given as a reason for withholding pain therapy. The concern that analgesics may compromise a patient's competency (ability to understand and sign an informed consent form for a procedure) is unfounded. Analgesia can be titrated so that the patient's consciousness is not clouded. Additionally, if absolutely necessary, an opioid antagonist can be administered. Pain itself can alter mood and thought. Furthermore, the patient may detect an element of coercion if he or she is told that pain medication will only be given after the consent is signed.

Safety, speed of onset, and ease of pain medication administration are key elements to pain relief in the ED setting. First, the patient must be monitored, and safety measures (such as putting up the gurney's side rails) must be instituted. The agent and route of administration must ensure rapid onset of adequate analgesia. In general, IV or inhalational routes ensure the fastest onset of action. Sophisticated techniques exist for delivering analgesia to specific sites. Many of these, such as intrathecal opioids, are too complicated and cumbersome for use in the ED environment. Sometimes, establishing an IV can be extremely difficult, especially in toddlers or chronically-ill patients with friable or scarred veins. Transmucosal absorption of drugs (fentanyl) may provide relief of pain and may help the patient cooperate better during attempts at IV access. Intranasal administration of ketamine, midazolam, and sufentanil offers another alternative.

Nonpharmacologic modalities

Physical and psychologic comfort measures can set the tone for an ED visit, and help relieve pain and anxiety while preparations are under way for delivery of pharmacologic analgesia. Physical comfort measures include positioning the patient to minimize discomfort (e.g., in patients with musculoskeletal back pain); adjusting the lighting of the room (e.g., for the patient with photophobia from migraine headache); ensuring that the patient is warm enough (providing blankets); or immobilizing, elevating and supporting injured extremities, and placing ice packs on the site of injury.

Fear and anxiety exacerbate a patient's pain and suffering. The ED environment is unfamiliar to most patients, and the patients feel dependent on strangers for help. Patients may also fear that their injury may result in permanent disability, or that their pain may be due to cancer. Young children often fear that their pain is punishment for perceived misdeeds, and often believe that the body part that hurts will be amputated. Anxiety and anger on the part of family members may also heighten a patient's pain. Early reassurance that the patient and his or her family and friends will be treated with respect and compassion helps decrease suffering and ameliorate pain. Offering a patient choices whenever possible (e.g., where the IV will be placed) lessens the feeling of loss of control. Letting the patient know approximately how long it will take to obtain the medication, before the medication begins working, and whether to expect relief to be partial or full are important as well.

For pediatric patients, music, storytelling, blowing bubbles, and other verbal or imagery techniques can distract the child from a painful procedure as well as reduce anxiety (Table 8.3). The Child Life Department, if available, can be invaluable in providing positive interactions with children and caregivers.

Pharmacologic therapy

Pharmacologic therapy can be either curative or palliative. Relief of cardiac chest pain by the vasodilatory effect of nitroglycerin is an example of curative therapy. This chapter deals primarily with palliative therapy; once a diagnosis has been established, curative therapy is preferred over palliation alone if possible.

Non-opioid agents

Non-opioid agents are listed in Table 8.4.

Acetaminophen

Acetaminophen is an effective analgesic for mild to moderate pain. Its mechanism of action is

Table 8.3 Analgesic modalities and their mechanisms of action

Distraction	Cognitive focus away from pain
Music	Cognitive focus away from pain and decreased anxiety
Hypnosis	Cognitive reinterpretation of painful stimuli
Biofeedback	Decreases muscle tension
Placebo	Activates descending pain inhibitory pathways. May involve endorphins
TENS	Interferes with transmission in dorsal horn ganglia. Possibly stimulates endorphins
Acupuncture	Probably similar to TENS
Local anesthesia	Blocks transmission of afferent nerve impulses
NSAIDs	Block production of prostaglandins
Opioids	Bind to opiate receptors in central nervous system (CNS) and possibly in peripheral nerves
Nitrous oxide	Blunts emotional reaction to pain; possible role of endogenous opioids

NSAIDs: non-steroidal anti-inflammatory drugs;
TENS: transcutaneous electrical nerve stimulation.

unclear, yet it seems to act centrally. Acetaminophen has little anti-inflammatory effect and few gastrointestinal side effects. It does not affect platelet aggregation. Significant hepatotoxicity is known to occur with large overdoses.

Non-steroidal anti-inflammatory drugs

The mechanism of action of NSAIDs is thought to be due to inhibition of prostaglandin, and possibly leukotriene production. Alone, prostaglandins do not cause pain, but sensitize nerve endings to perceive an ordinary, non-painful stimulus as painful. NSAIDs are widely used for their antipyretic and anti-inflammatory properties, in addition to their analgesic properties. They are effective for mild to moderate pain, and their lack of respiratory depression and abuse potential makes them an attractive choice. There is a "ceiling effect" beyond which no further analgesia can be produced, even when a different NSAID is added. Their major side effects include

Table 8.4 Non-opioid analgesics

Generic (proprietary)	Dose	Pediatric dose	Toxic dose	Maximum dose
Acetaminophen (APAP)	650–1000 mg PO q4–6 h 1 g PR q6 h 1–2 g PR q12 h	10–20 mg/kg PO 20–40 mg/kg PR q4 h	Not an NSAID. Exact mechanism unknown. Liver toxicity possible when above 150 mg/kg is taken in 24 hour	100 mg/kg/day
Aspirin (ASA)	650–975 mg PO q4 h	10–15 mg/kg PO	Reye's syndrome in children who subsequently get flu or chickenpox. Tinnitus Toxic dose 150 mg/kg	60 mg/kg/day
Ibuprofen	600 mg PO q6–8 h	10 mg/kg PO q6–8 h	GI irritation Platelet dysfunction Renal dysfunction Bronchospasm	40 mg/kg/day
Naproxen	250 mg PO q6–8 h 500–100 PR q12 h	5–7 mg/kg PO q12 h	Interacts with protein-bound drugs	20 mg/kg/day
Indomethacin	25–50 mg PO q12 h 100 mg PR q24 h	N/A	As for naproxen	3 mg/kg/day
Ketorolac	60 mg IM/dose 30 mg IV/dose	0.5 mg/kg IV q6 h Max 120 mg/d	Same as IB. Decrease dose by one-half in elderly.	
Rofecoxib (Vioxx)	12.5–50 mg PO qd	Available as liquid	Selective COX-2 inhibitor. Withdrawn due to increased risk of serious cardiovascular events	
Celecoxib	200 PO bid	Not approved	Not available as liquid; contraindicated in sulfa allergy. May increase risk of serious cardiovascular events	
Valdecoxib	10 mg PO qd	Not approved	No renal elimination; should not be given to sulfa-allergic patients. May increase risk of serious cardiovascular events	
Tramadol	50–100 mg PO	Not approved	May precipitate serotonin syndrome in SSRI patients (no actual pediatric indications, but studies support safety and efficacy in children)	

COX: cyclooxygenase; GI: gastrointestinal; IB: ibuprofen; IM: intramuscular; IV: intravenous; NSAID: non-steroidal anti-inflammatory drug; PO: per os; PR: per rectum; SSRI: selective serotonin reuptake inhibitors.

gastrointestinal bleeding, renal failure, anaphylaxis, and platelet dysfunction. The same analgesics that are effective in adults can be safely administered to children greater than 2 months of age. In children, the margin of safety of these drugs approximately equals that in adults.

Aspirin

Aspirin may cause Reye's syndrome in children who contract influenza or chickenpox. Aspirin is now seldom used in children, except to treat autoimmune diseases such as juvenile rheumatoid arthritis.

Ketorolac tromethamine

Ketorolac is the first non-opioid analgesic agent available for parenteral use in the US. For acute musculoskeletal pain, 60 mg ketorolac administered IM has been shown approximately equivalent in analgesic efficacy to 800 mg of oral ibuprofen. Ketorolac inhibits prostaglandin synthesis, so its onset is no faster than that of an equivalent agent given orally. Ketorolac is considered to be most useful in the context of renal colic because decreased prostaglandin synthesis results in decreased ureteral peristalsis. In theory, opioids increase smooth muscle spasm and peristalsis; nonetheless, opioids have proven to be effective analgesics in renal colic and should be considered as standard therapy. Ketorolac is approximately 10–35 times more expensive than morphine.

Cyclooxygenase-2 specific inhibitors

Cyclooxygenase-1 (COX-1) serves as a "clean-up" or reparative agent and is not inducible with stimulation from inflammation or injury. COX-2 is present in lower levels and is inducible, showing increases that are closely related to the inflammatory response to injury or inflammation. Most traditional NSAIDs block both COX-1 and COX-2. The selective COX-2 inhibitors rofecoxib and celecoxib provide anti-inflammatory effects and moderate analgesia with a lower incidence of gastrointestinal side effects. Both are eliminated by the liver, and share similar drug interactions with standard NSAIDs. They may precipitate anaphylaxis in patients with aspirin allergy. Celecoxib is metabolized by the cytochrome P450 system and may cross-react in patients who have a sulfonamide allergy. Rofecoxib (Vioxx) has been taken off the market because of its association with an increased incidence of myocardial infarction.

General guidelines for choosing non-opioid analgesic agents

1. Use cautiously in the elderly, who are at greater risk of developing gastrointestinal bleeding, renal toxicity and renal failure.
2. Patients who are dehydrated or hypovolemic are at high risk of acute renal impairment.
3. All have the potential for gastrointestinal side effects.
4. They may interfere with the effects of many antihypertensives.
5. There is little clinical evidence of individual superiority of one particular agent over another.
6. Newer agents may cost as much as fifty times more than older ones.

Opioid analgesic agents

Opioid analgesics are the mainstay of pharmacologic management of acute, moderate to severe pain (Table 8.5). The beneficial physiologic and psychologic effects of opium have been well documented for centuries; so have its toxicity and potential for abuse. Fear of inducing addiction has led to the underuse of opioids by many physicians. However, many studies have shown that short-term use of opioid analgesics for acute pain syndromes is not associated with future dependence.

There are multiple opioid receptors, each affected by opioids in different ways. The most commonly used opioids are μ-agonists: morphine, meperidine, methadone, codeine, oxycodone, and the fentanyls. An agonist acts as a neurotransmitter – when the receptor recognizes the agonist, it causes alterations within the cell. An antagonist blocks the receptor by occupying it without initiating transduction. Partial agonists produce a partial response with decreased intrinsic activity. By binding the receptor site, they also block access of full agonists and function as partial antagonists.

Morphine

Morphine is the gold standard opioid agent. In standard dosage, it produces analgesia without loss of consciousness. Relief of tension, anxiety, and pain then results in drowsiness and sleep. Nausea, vomiting, pruritus, and miosis are the most common side effects. Vasodilatation and venous pooling from morphine do not cause significant hemodynamic effects in normovolemic patients, but can cause significant hypotension in hypovolemic patients. Morphine causes dose-dependent depression of ventilation, reducing the respiratory rate and then tidal volume. Morphine increases sphincter tone at the pylorus, ileo-cecal junction, and the sphincter of Oddi, and decreases peristalsis, resulting in constipation.

Fentanyl

Fentanyl's advantages over morphine include a rapid onset (<1 minute) and brief duration of action (30–45 minutes). It is 50–100 times more potent than morphine and has little hypnotic or sedative effect. Fentanyl's main disadvantage is the glottic and chest wall rigidity that may develop after rapid infusion of higher doses

Table 8.5 Opioid analgesics

Generic (proprietary)	Oral equipotent dose	Parenteral	Duration (in hours)	Comments	Precautions
Morphine	30–60 mg (0.5 mg/kg)	10 mg (0.1 mg/kg)	3–5	Standard for comparison	Respiratory depression Hypotension Sedation Histamine release
Codeine	30–100 mg (2 mg/kg)	30–100 mg (0.5 mg/kg)	4	Poor analgesic Good cough suppressant	Constipation, nausea and vomiting, abuse potential
Hydromorphone (Dilaudid)	2–6 mg (0.02–0.1 mg/kg)	1–2 mg (0.015 mg/kg)	2–4	Available as suppository	Euphoria
Hydrocodone (Vicodin, Lortab)	5–10 mg	N/A	3–4	Good cough suppressant Fewer side effects than codeine and greater potency	Greater abuse potential
Oxycodone (Percocet, Tylox)	5–10 mg	N/A	3	Parenteral form not available in the US. Very effective analgesic	Euphoria, abuse potential
Meperidine (Demerol)	250–300 mg (1.5–2.0 mg/kg)	75–125 mg (1.0 mg/kg)	2–3	Toxicity from metabolite normeperidine	Avoid with MAOI. Caution in renal or hepatic failure
Fentanyl	N/A	0.1–0.2 mg (0.001 mg/kg)	1–2	No histamine release. Transcutaneous and transmucosal absorption	For IV administration, push and flush slowly to avoid "rigid chest" syndrome
Alfentanil	N/A	1 mg/kg (0.01 mg/kg)	1.5	Shortest half-life, minimal cardiovascular side effects	Muscular rigidity if administered too quickly; expensive

MAOI: monoamine oxidase inhibitor; IV: intravenous.

(>5 mcg/kg). The mechanism of the "rigid chest" syndrome is unclear, but can be life-threatening, since assisted ventilation may be impossible without muscle relaxants.

Hydromorphone

Hydromorphone is a derivative of morphine, and has greater selectivity for μ-opioid receptors. It has a rapid onset of action and lasts 4–6 hours. Hydromorphone is five times more potent and ten times more lipid soluble than morphine, yet less sedating. It also produces less nausea.

Opioid drug selection

The idea that some opioids are weak and ineffective in severe pain is outdated. In equipotent doses, opioid agents can achieve the same effect as other opioids, but differ in their side effects and half-life. Factors affecting drug selection include: the intensity of the pain, coexisting disease, potential drug interactions, treatment history, physician preference, patient preference, and proposed route of administration.

Choice of route of administration

Injectable

The IV route results in the shortest time to onset of pain relief. There is no "maximal" dose of opioid; induction of undesired side effects usually signals the limit of the patient's ability to tolerate the drug. Patient-controlled analgesia (PCA) is commonly used in the inpatient setting for severe pain that is expected to last for hours or days. In general, PCA does not have a role in the

ED setting, but may be beneficial to patients in observation units or for those whose ED stay is prolonged due to lack of inpatient beds.

The IM route has multiple disadvantages. Among them, the pain of the injection limits the physician's ability to titrate the drug effect. Furthermore, drug uptake is variable, depending on the patient's peripheral circulation.

Oral

First-pass hepatic metabolism may inactivate as much as 80% of an oral opioid dose. Patients who will require general anesthesia cannot take anything by mouth. Patients who are vomiting will not be able to retain the drug long enough for absorption to occur. Time to onset of analgesia is much longer and titration is more difficult. Outpatient pain control after discharge is the main reason to use oral opioids.

Rectal

The rectal route has the advantages of transmucosal absorption without the first-pass effect. Additionally, it does not rely on gastric motility. Absorption, however, is variable. Patients may object to this route of administration. Hydromorphone is the only opioid available as a suppository. The IV form can also be given rectally.

Transmucosal

Fentanyl lollipops are the most common form of opioid using the transmucosal route. This is especially helpful in children, but requires patient cooperation.

Combination therapy

The combination of a non-opioid analgesic and an opioid agent produces significantly greater pain relief than either agent alone.

Use of adjuvant agents

Adjuvant agents are used in combination with opioids for various reasons: to provide synergy; to decrease side effects; to decrease anxiety; and to relax muscles, especially in acute musculoskeletal pain. The phenothiazines and hydroxyzine are most commonly used. There is no evidence, however, for analgesic synergy with these agents.

Phenothiazines do not potentiate analgesia, as previously believed, and may actually diminish the analgesic effect of the simultaneously administered opioid. Hydroxyzine not only requires an additional injection, but also increases respiratory depression. In severe musculoskeletal pain associated with muscle spasm, the addition of a muscle relaxant may provide more relief than an opioid alone. In this scenario, respiratory status must be monitored closely. In general, adjuvant agents provide little additional analgesia and may potentiate or add side effects to the clinical picture.

Special patients
Undifferentiated abdominal pain

Fear of masking the clinical findings and missing the diagnosis has long prevented physicians from giving opioids to patients with undifferentiated abdominal pain, leaving them to suffer for hours while establishing a diagnosis and definitive treatment. This practice was first promulgated by Cope, from his 1921 text *The Early Diagnosis of Abdominal Pain*. "If morphine be administered, it is possible to die happy in the belief that he is on the road to recovery, and in some cases, the medical attendant may for a time be induced to share the same delusive hope." Newer diagnostic techniques, better monitoring, and more accurate opioid titration have made his dire warning obsolete. In fact, the most recent edition of Cope's textbook retracts this myth. Several studies have documented that early pain relief in patients with acute abdominal pain is safe and does not result in worse outcomes, even in children.

Migraine headaches

There have been many studies comparing the effectiveness of non-opioid agents to opioids in the management of migraine headaches. The phenothiazines have shown success rates as high as 95%. Sumatriptan and dihydroergotamine have been associated with recurrence rates as high as 50%, especially in patients with persisting headache at the time of discharge from the ED. Many other drugs (metoclopramide, haloperidol, droperidol, NSAIDs, and narcotics) have been studied. The relative benefit of any of these drugs or any combinations has not been established. Opioids have not been shown to perform better in clinical trials and have the potential to be associated with subsequent drug-seeking behavior.

Chronic pain

The patient with a terminal illness and chronic pain should receive generous amounts of opioids while the physician searches for a new process that might have caused increased pain. These patients will have great tolerance for the analgesic effects of opioids, but not necessarily for their side effects. Patients who have chronic pain with a non-terminal illness should be under the care of a primary care provider who has a plan for managing this pain. Close consultation with that primary care provider, or the pain management team, if applicable, will optimize the patient's care and reduce dependency and abuse.

Suspected drug-seeker

Some patients will feign pain or claim pain syndrome diagnoses in order to receive opioids, either for their own use or to sell. Suspected drug-seeking behavior should be documented and will become evident as the number of ED visits increase. In general, it is better to err on the side of humane treatment than to deprive a patient of needed pain relief. Diligence in checking the history and physical for inconsistencies, communicating with the patient's primary care provider, and checking the medical records will help identify drug seekers and drug-seeking behavior. Non-narcotic medications should be substituted when possible. Prescriptions should be written for only small amounts of medication, in matching alphabetic and numeric formats. Communication between the primary care provider and ED personnel will serve not only to confirm the physician's suspicions, but can also provide the basis for a consistent care plan for future visits. Documentation of findings and discussions are necessary parts of the medical record.

Pearls and pitfalls

Pearls

- Treat pain early and often; anticipate pain prior to its recurrence.
- Reassess patients frequently.
- Use enough agent to achieve the desired effect, or until an undesirable side effect occurs. Switch to a different agent if side effects occur and pain persists, or if the initial agent is not effective.
- Select the route of administration that allows the fastest relief for the patient but neither

delays definitive care nor causes unnecessary, additional discomfort.

Pitfalls

- *Wrong agent*: Most opioids can achieve the desired degree of analgesia. A major exception is oral codeine. Codeine is a weak agonist with a high incidence of nausea, vomiting, and constipation; it has not been shown to be more effective than acetaminophen alone.
- *Wrong dosage*: Titrate the dosage to achieve the desired degree of analgesia. There is no "maximal" dose of any opioid.
- *Wrong route*: The IM route has several disadvantages: pain, delayed onset of action, unpredictable uptake, difficult and painful titration, and complications such as hematoma formation or damage to structures in the path of the injection.
- *Wrong frequency*: Preventing pain from recurring by earlier readministration of opioid will result in less opioid use overall than the retreatment of pain that has had time to reestablish itself.
- *Incorrect use of adjuvant agents*: Adjuvant agents do not reduce the dosage of opioid needed. Antiemetics may be used if nausea and vomiting persist after adequate analgesia has been achieved. The sedation or respiratory depression that occurs with most of the commonly-used adjuvant agents is undesirable.

References

1. Acute Pain Management Guideline Panel. *Acute Pain Management: Operative or Medical Procedures and Trauma.* Guideline Report. AHCPR. Pub. No. 92-002. Rockville, MD; Agency for Health Care Policy and Research, Public Health Service, U.S. Department of Health and Human Services, 1993.
2. Brewster GS, Herbert ME, Hoffman JR. Medical myth: analgesia should not be given to patients with an acute abdomen because it obscures the diagnosis. *West J Med* 2000;172:209–210.
3. Ducharme J. Acute pain in pain control: state of the art. *Ann Emerg Med* 2000;35:592–603.

4. Franck LS, Greenberg CS, Stevens B. Pain assessment in infants and children. *Pediatr Clin North Am* 2000;47(3).

5. Gaffney A, McGrath PJ, Dick B. Measuring pain in children: developmental and instrument issues. In: Schechter N (ed.). *Pain in Infants, Children and Adolescents*, 2nd ed., Philadelphia, PA: Lippincott Williams & Wilkins, 2003.

6. Glazier HS. Potentiation of pain relief with hydroxyzine: a therapeutic myth? *Ann Pharmacother* 1990;24:484.

7. Graber MA. Informed consent and general surgeons' attitudes toward the use of pain medication in the acute abdomen. *Am J Emerg Med* 1999;17(2):113–116.

8. Kim MK, Strait RT, Sato TT, et al. A randomized clinical trial of analgesia in children with acute abdominal pain. *Acad Emerg Med* 2002;9(4):281–287.

9. Koltzenburg M. Stability and plasticity of nociceptor function.

10. Lewis LM, Sasater LC, Brooks CB. Are emergency physicians too stingy with analgesics? *South Med J* 1994;87:7.

11. Liebelt E, Levick N: Acute pain management, analgesia and anxiolysis in the adult patient. In: Tintinalli JE (ed.). *Emergency Medicine: A Comprehensive Study Guide*, 5th ed., New York: McGraw-Hill, 1995.

12. Marks RD, Sachar EJ. Undertreatment of medical inpatients with narcotic analgesics. *Ann Int Med* 1973;78:173.

13. Paris PM, Yealy DM. Pain management. In: Marx JA, editor-in-chief. *Rosen's Emergency Medicine: Concepts and Clinical Practice*, 5th ed., St Louis: Mosby, 2003.

14. Patt RB, Proper G, Reddy S. The neuroleptics as adjuvant analgesics. *J Pain Symptom Management* 1994;9:446.

15. Ready LB, Edwards WT. *Management of Acute Pain: A Practical Guide*. International Association for the Study of Pain, Seattle. IASP Publications, 1992.

16. Rosenzweig S, Mines D. Acute pain management. In: Harwood-Nuss A (ed.). *The Clinical Practice of Emergency Medicine*, 3rd ed., Philadelphia, PA: Lippincott Williams & Wilkins, 2001.

17. Thomas SH, Silen W. Effect on diagnostic efficiency of analgesia for undifferentiated abdominal pain. *Br J Surg* 2003;90(1):5–9.

18. Todd KJ. Clinical versus statistical significance in the assessment of pain relief. *Amm Emerg Med* 1996; 27:439.

19. Turturro MA, Paris PM, Seaburg DC. Intramuscular ketorolac versus oral ibuprofen in acute musculoskeletal pain. *Ann Emerg Med* 1995;26:117.

20. Weisman SJ, Schechter NL. The management of pain in children. *Pediatr Rev* 1991;12:237.

21. Wilson JE, Pendleton JM. Oligoanalgesia in the emergency department. *Am J Emerg Med* 1989;7:620–623.

Section 2

Primary Complaints

9 Abdominal pain

S.V. Mahadevan, MD

Scope of the problem

Evaluation of the patient with acute abdominal pain is one of the most challenging aspects of emergency medicine. Abdominal pain is the presenting complaint in as many as 10% of emergency department (ED) patients. Diagnostic possibilities range from immediately life-threatening conditions (e.g., ruptured abdominal aortic aneurysm (AAA)), to self-limiting (e.g., abdominal wall strain), and from common (e.g., gastroenteritis) to unusual (e.g., black widow spider bite). Though the etiology of pain is initially undetermined in as high as 30–40% of patients, recognition of surgical or life-threatening causes is more important than establishing a firm diagnosis.

Anatomic essentials

Abdominal pain is typically derived from one or more of three distinct pain pathways: visceral, parietal (somatic) and referred.

Visceral abdominal pain

Visceral abdominal pain is usually caused by distention of hollow organs or capsular stretching of solid organs. Less commonly, it is caused by ischemia or inflammation when tissue congestion sensitizes nerve endings of visceral pain fibers and lowers the threshold for stimulus. Often the earliest manifestation of a particular disease process, visceral pain may vary from a steady ache or vague discomfort to excruciating or colicky pain. If the involved organ is affected by peristalsis, the pain is often described as intermittent, crampy, or colicky in nature.

Since the visceral pain fibers are bilateral, unmyelinated, and enter the spinal cord at multiple levels, visceral abdominal pain is usually dull, poorly localized and experienced in the midline. Visceral pain is perceived from the abdominal region corresponding to the diseased organ's embryonic origin. Foregut structures, such as the stomach, duodenum, liver, biliary tract and pancreas produce upper abdominal pain, often in the epigastric region. Midgut structures, such as the small bowel, appendix and proximal colon cause periumbilical pain. Hindgut structures, such as the distal colon and genitourinary system cause lower abdominal pain.

Parietal (somatic) abdominal pain

Parietal or somatic abdominal pain results from ischemia, inflammation or stretching of the parietal peritoneum. Myelinated afferent fibers transmit the painful stimulus to specific dorsal root ganglia on the same side and dermatomal level as the origin of the pain. For this reason, parietal pain, in contrast to visceral pain, often can be localized to the region of the painful stimulus. This pain is typically sharp, knife-like and constant; coughing and moving are likely to aggravate it. Conditions resulting in parietal pain often account for physical examination findings of tenderness to palpation, guarding, rebound and rigidity.

The classic presentation of appendicitis involves both visceral and somatic pain. The pain of early appendicitis is often periumbilical (visceral) but localizes to the right lower quadrant (RLQ) when the inflammation extends to the peritoneum (parietal).

Referred pain

Referred pain is defined as pain felt at a distance from the diseased organ. It results from shared central pathways for afferent neurons from different locations. For instance, a patient with pneumonia may present with abdominal pain because the T9 distribution of neurons is shared by the lung and abdomen. Other examples of referred pain include epigastric pain associated with myocardial infarction (MI), shoulder pain associated with diaphragmatic irritation (e.g., ruptured spleen), right infrascapular pain associated with biliary disease, and testicular pain associated with acute ureteral obstruction.

History

In patients with abdominal pain, a careful and focused history is the key to uncovering the etiology of most cases.

Where is your pain? Has it always been there?

The location of abdominal pain often corresponds to specific disease entities and is very important for the development of an initial differential diagnosis (Figure 9.1). Keep in mind that the location of abdominal pain may vary with time, especially as the underlying disease evolves and the pain progresses from visceral to somatic. Periumbilical pain that migrates to the RLQ is very specific for appendicitis, while epigastric pain that localizes to the right upper quadrant (RUQ) is classic for biliary disease.

Does the pain radiate anywhere?

The pain of biliary colic may radiate to the right infrascapular region; the pain of pancreatitis to the midback. Pain that radiates to the flank or genitals may represent a kidney stone or ruptured AAA.

How did the pain begin (sudden vs. gradual onset)? How long have you had the pain?

Sudden or abrupt onset of abdominal pain often indicates a serious underlying disorder. Fainting or collapsing with such pain is worrisome for conditions such as a ruptured AAA, perforated ulcer or ectopic pregnancy. Inflammatory causes of pain (cholecystitis, appendicitis, diverticulitis) tend to develop over hours to days and generally are less severe at the onset. Pain for >6 hours or <48 hours duration, or pain that is steadily increasing in intensity is more likely to require surgical intervention.

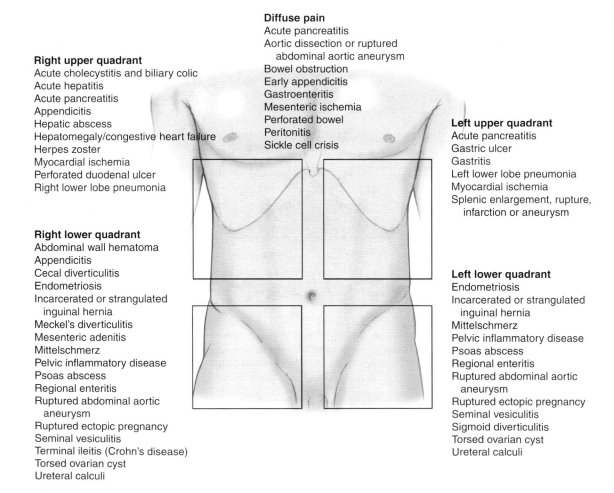

Diffuse pain
Acute pancreatitis
Aortic dissection or ruptured
  abdominal aortic aneurysm
Bowel obstruction
Early appendicitis
Gastroenteritis
Mesenteric ischemia
Perforated bowel
Peritonitis
Sickle cell crisis

Right upper quadrant
Acute cholecystitis and biliary colic
Acute hepatitis
Acute pancreatitis
Appendicitis
Hepatic abscess
Hepatomegaly/congestive heart failure
Herpes zoster
Myocardial ischemia
Perforated duodenal ulcer
Right lower lobe pneumonia

Left upper quadrant
Acute pancreatitis
Gastric ulcer
Gastritis
Left lower lobe pneumonia
Myocardial ischemia
Splenic enlargement, rupture,
  infarction or aneurysm

Right lower quadrant
Abdominal wall hematoma
Appendicitis
Cecal diverticulitis
Endometriosis
Incarcerated or strangulated
  inguinal hernia
Meckel's diverticulitis
Mesenteric adenitis
Mittelschmerz
Pelvic inflammatory disease
Psoas abscess
Regional enteritis
Ruptured abdominal aortic
  aneurysm
Ruptured ectopic pregnancy
Seminal vesiculitis
Terminal ileitis (Crohn's disease)
Torsed ovarian cyst
Ureteral calculi

Left lower quadrant
Endometriosis
Incarcerated or strangulated
  inguinal hernia
Mittelschmerz
Pelvic inflammatory disease
Psoas abscess
Regional enteritis
Ruptured abdominal aortic
  aneurysm
Ruptured ectopic pregnancy
Seminal vesiculitis
Sigmoid diverticulitis
Torsed ovarian cyst
Ureteral calculi

Figure 9.1
Differential diagnosis of acute abdominal pain by location. Adapted from Wagner DK. *Curr Topic* 1978;1(3).

What were you doing when the pain began?

Severe pain that awakens a patient from sleep is concerning and may represent perforation or ischemia. This history of abdominal pain following trauma raises the possibility of an intra-abdominal injury to the solid organs or bowel.

What does the pain feel like?

The significance of the patient's characterization of pain (visceral, somatic, referred) is described in detail earlier in this chapter. Classic descriptions of pain include the burning or gnawing pain of peptic ulcer disease, the sharp pain of biliary colic, the penetrating pain of pancreatitis, the tearing pain of an aortic dissection, and the crampy intermittent pain of intestinal obstruction.

On a scale of 0–10, how severe is the pain?

Unfortunately, the patient's quantification of pain severity is often inconsistent and generally unreliable in determining the specific cause of pain. Studies have shown that elderly patients tend to have a higher pain threshold than younger patients. In general, nonsurgical causes of pain tend to be less painful than surgical etiologies. Although acute nephrolithiasis (kidney stone) may present with severe, incapacitating pain, the majority of patients will spontaneously pass their stone without surgical intervention. The finding of severe pain "out of proportion" to physical examination is worrisome for mesenteric ischemia.

Does anything make the pain better or worse?

Parietal peritoneal pain is aggravated by movement, such as hitting bumps on the car ride to the hospital or with walking. This finding necessitates the exclusion of appendicitis. The pain of peptic ulcer disease typically improves with eating, whereas biliary colic worsens with meals. Pain accentuated by reclining and relieved by sitting upright should raise suspicion for a retroperitoneal process such as pancreatitis. Abdominal pain relieved by vomiting suggests a gastric or proximal bowel problem, whereas relief of pain after a bowel movement suggests a colonic process.

Have you had the pain before?

Some patients with abdominal pain have had prior similar episodes. It has been reported that prior pain events occur in up to 71% of patients with cholecystitis and in 18% of patients with appendicitis.

Associated symptoms

Gastrointestinal

Ask about nausea, vomiting, anorexia, constipation, diarrhea or bleeding. Nausea and vomiting may result from irritation of intra-abdominal organs or obstruction of an involuntary muscular tube (i.e., intestine, bile duct, ureter). Consequently, nausea and vomiting are common to many abdominal processes, including appendicitis. However, vomiting may also be slight or absent from many serious surgical conditions (ectopic pregnancy, intussusception). The temporal relationship of abdominal pain and vomiting is another key historical finding. Classically, patients with appendicitis or other surgical causes of abdominal pain develop pain prior to vomiting. The reverse is often true in medical conditions, where vomiting may precede pain. Any child presenting with bilious vomiting raises concern for an acute bowel obstruction.

Contrary to popular belief, anorexia is not a requisite finding for the diagnosis of appendicitis, as it is absent in 10–30% of cases. Constipation and diarrhea occur with equal frequency (15% of cases) in appendicitis. Diarrhea may accompany a partial small bowel obstruction (SBO) despite the common misconception that any bowel movement excludes this condition. Bloody diarrhea is suggestive of inflammatory bowel disease or infectious enterocolitis. A bloody or "currant jelly" (blood and mucus) stool may indicate intussusception, although this is generally a late finding. Failure to pass flatus or feces could be associated with an intestinal obstruction.

Genitourinary

Ask about dysuria, frequency, urgency and hematuria. Though dysuria and urinary frequency are classic symptoms of a urinary tract infection (UTI), they can also occur as the result of bladder irritation by an inflamed appendix or pelvic organ. Gross hematuria may indicate bladder irritation (infection, tumor) or nephrolithiasis.

Gynecologic

Ask about pregnancy, menses, contraception, fertility, sexual activity, sexually transmitted infections (STIs), vaginal discharge or bleeding and dypareunia. Previous gynecologic history including surgeries, previous pregnancies and infections are also important to identify. A patient may mistake abnormal vaginal bleeding for their menses. Painful menses in a patient without a history of dysmenorrhea should raise concern for a serious gynecologic condition. Ectopic pregnancy should be considered in <u>all</u> female patients between the ages of 9 and 50 years with abdominal pain.

Pregnancy not only alters the diagnostic possibilities of a patient with acute abdominal pain but can also change the clinical findings. Advanced pregnancies make the diagnosis of appendicitis more difficult – not only does the location of the appendix change with the progression of the pregnancy, but these patients tend to have fewer clinical findings than non-pregnant patients.

Cardiopulmonary

Ask about cough, dyspnea and chest pain. Pneumonia, pulmonary embolism (PE) and acute MI may present with abdominal pain as the chief complaint. Abdominal pain may be the result of other extra-abdominal causes (Table 9.1).

Table 9.1 Important extra-abdominal causes of abdominal pain

Systemic causes	Pneumonia
Diabetic ketoacidosis	Pulmonary embolism
Alcoholic ketoacidosis	Herniated thoracic disk
Uremia	
Sickle cell disease	**Genitourinary**
Porphyria	Testicular torsion
Systemic lupus	Renal colic
erythematosus	
Vasculitis	**Infectious**
Glaucoma	Strep pharyngitis (more
Hyperthyroidism	often in children)
	Rocky Mountain spotted
Toxic	fever
Methanol poisoning	Mononucleosis
Heavy metal toxicity	
Scorpion bite	**Abdominal wall**
Black widow spider bite	Muscle spasm
	Muscle hematoma
Thoracic	Herpes zoster
Myocardial infarction	
Unstable angina	

Adapted from Purcell TB. Nonsurgical and extraperitoneal causes of abdominal pain. *Emerg Med Clin North Am* 1989;7:721–740.

Past medical

Previous abdominal surgery is an important risk factor for bowel obstruction due to adhesions. Patients with a history of cardiovascular disease, hypertension or atrial fibrillation are at risk for mesenteric ischemia and AAA. Ongoing medical illnesses such as diabetes, heart disease, or chronic obstructive pulmonary disease (COPD) may complicate the evaluation and stabilization of patients with abdominal pain. Certain medications (non-steroidal anti-inflammatory drugs (NSAIDs), corticosteroids, antibiotics, immunosuppressants) may lead to abdominal pain or make its evaluation more challenging. Alcohol consumption places patients at risk for pancreatitis, hepatitis or cirrhosis.

Physical examination

The primary goal of the physical examination is to localize the organ system responsible for disease. It is important not only to examine the abdomen but other body areas as well that may provide clues to the etiology of the pain, especially the pelvic (women), genitourinary (men), back, and rectal areas.

General appearance

The general appearance of a patient is an important clinical observation. As a general rule, patients with pallor or distress are generally more acutely ill. Patients whose disease process has progressed to peritonitis tend to lie still to avoid exacerbating their pain. Patients with ureteral colic or mesenteric ischemia may writhe in pain because they cannot find a position of comfort. Nonspecific abdominal pain, gastroenteritis and ureteral colic are usually less aggravated by movement.

Vital signs

The absence of a fever, often used as a marker to identify infection, can be deceiving in patients with abdominal pain. Diseases such as appendicitis and cholecystitis may present with temperatures <100.2°F (37.8°C). Elderly or immunocompromised patients may not mount a fever despite serious underlying illness. The majority of elderly patients with acute appendicitis or cholecystitis are afebrile in spite of higher rates of perforation and sepsis.

The presence of fever should alert the physician to the possibility of infection as the cause of pain. An acute onset of a high fever and chills make appendicitis less likely than pneumonia or pyelonephritis in the appropriate clinical setting.

Other vital signs may be helpful in assessing the degree to which a patient is affected by his or her illness. Hypotension may be a result of dehydration, sepsis or internal hemorrhage, and is a worrisome finding in an elderly patient. Tachycardia may signify occult blood loss, sepsis, volume contraction or pain. However, medications such as beta-blockers may blunt the patient's ability to mount such a response. An increased respiratory rate may result from severe pain, acidosis or an extra-abdominal cause such as PE, pneumonia or MI.

Abdomen

Inspection

Inspection may reveal distention, masses, bruising, scars from prior surgeries or cutaneous signs of portal hypertension. Cullen's sign (a bluish umbilicus) and Grey Turner's sign (discoloration of the flank) are signs of internal hemorrhage, although infrequently seen in the acute setting.

Auscultation

Auscultation is performed prior to palpation because the latter may induce peristalsis artificially. Contrary to conventional teaching, absent or diminished bowel sounds provide little useful clinical information. In one investigation, approximately half the patients with confirmed peritonitis had normal or increased bowel sounds.

High-pitched or tinkling sounds can be associated with SBO, especially in the presence of abdominal distention. Low-pitched and less frequent bowel sounds are classically associated with a large bowel obstruction. The auscultation of bruits might indicate the presence of a AAA in an elderly patient. In the pregnant patient, assess for fetal heart tones, which can be heard in 90% of patients by 12 weeks gestation.

Percussion

Percussion is useful for determining the size of organs and for distinguishing between distention caused by air or fluid. Tympany may be due to excessive gas in the bowel or peritoneal cavity; shifting dullness or a fluid wave suggests ascites.

Palpation

For palpation of the abdomen to be effective, it is important to first calm the patient and gain his or her cooperation. Having the patient flex the legs at the knee and hip may relax abdominal musculature, making palpation more effective. Be gentle. A rough or painful examination is not only distressing to the patient but may mislead the examining physician. Palpation should be performed systematically, beginning as far as possible from the patient's perceived location of pain. It is important to observe the patient's facial expressions for signs of pain during palpation. In older patients, careful palpation of the abdomen may also reveal a pulsatile mass suggestive of a AAA.

It is rare for a serious abdominal condition to present without abdominal tenderness. By localizing tenderness to a specific abdominal region, the clinician often can narrow the possible diagnoses to the organs within that anatomic region. Complicating matters, however, is the fact that some patients with inflamed intra-abdominal organs do not have localizable tenderness. For example, only two-thirds of patients with appendicitis have RLQ tenderness on examination.

In addition to localizing tenderness, the patient should be assessed for signs of peritoneal irritation, the hallmark of surgical disease.

Guarding

Guarding is the reflex spasm of the abdominal wall musculature in response to palpation or underlying peritoneal irritation (Figure 9.2).

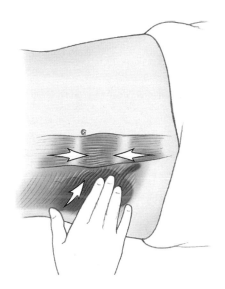

Figure 9.2
Guarding.

Voluntary guarding can occur as a response to the physician's cold hands, fear, anxiety or being ticklish. Involuntary guarding, which has greater clinical significance, is more likely to occur with surgical illness and is not relieved by physician encouragement.

Rebound tenderness

Rebound tenderness is elicited by slow, gentle, deep palpation of an area of tenderness followed by abrupt withdrawal of the examiner's hand (Figure 9.3). Though rebound tenderness has classically been a hallmark of surgical disease, several recent studies have questioned its sensitivity and specificity as well as its lack of prospective utility for surgical conditions. As a result, some physicians have condemned the procedure as a cruel and uninformative holdover from the past.

Alternatives to classic rebound testing include the *cough test*, where the examiner has the patient cough and looks for evidence of post-tussive abdominal pain, such as grimacing, flinching or grabbing the belly, and the *heel drop sign*, where the patient experiences pain on dropping the heels to the ground after standing on his or her toes. In children, this may be tested by having them jump up and down.

Special signs or techniques

A positive *Murphy's sign* is elicited when a patient abruptly ends deep inspiration during palpation of the RUQ. Murphy's sign is very sensitive for acute cholecystitis and biliary colic. The *psoas sign* (Figure 9.4) is performed by having the patient flex the thigh against resistance. The *obturator sign* (Figure 9.5) is performed by having the patient internally and externally rotate their flexed hip. Pain elicited by either the psoas or obturator maneuvers can indicate irritation of the respective muscles by an inflammatory process such as acute appendicitis, a ruptured appendix or pelvic inflammatory disease (PID).

A positive *Rovsing's sign* is pain in the RLQ precipitated by palpation of the left lower quadrant (LLQ). This is also suggestive of appendicitis. *Carnett's sign* is increased tenderness to palpation when the abdominal muscles are contracted, as when the patient lifts his or her head or legs off the bed, and may be useful to distinguish abdominal wall from visceral pain.

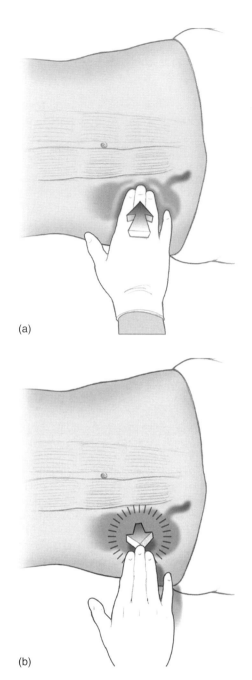

(a)

(b)

Figure 9.3
Rebound (a) hand down (b) hand up.

Pelvic

A pelvic examination is mandatory in any woman of childbearing age with abdominal pain. The pelvic examination may help differentiate a gynecologic cause of pain from other causes. Cervical appearance, cervical motion tenderness (CMT), adnexal tenderness or masses, uterine

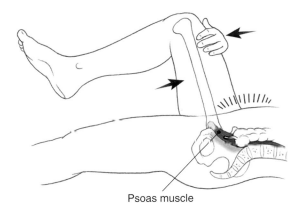

Figure 9.4
Psoas sign.

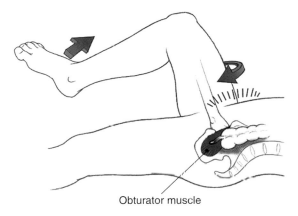

Figure 9.5
Obturator sign.

size, and the presence or absence of discharge, pus or blood should be noted. While women with appendicitis or PID may have CMT or adnexal tenderness, the presence of pus at the cervical os suggests PID. A woman with severe PID may also experience RUQ tenderness due to perihepatic inflammation (Fitz–Hugh–Curtis syndrome).

Genital

Just as every woman of childbearing age needs a pelvic examination, every male with abdominal pain should have a genital examination. The groin should be inspected and palpated for hernias which may be the cause of an acute bowel obstruction. The external genitalia and scrotum should also carefully be evaluated for any tenderness, masses, or abnormalities.

Rectal

Recent literature has questioned the utility of the rectal examination in the diagnosis of appendicitis, as it is neither sensitive nor specific for the disease. However, the rectal examination still remains a necessary component of the evaluation of patients with abdominal pain. The diagnosis of prostate or perirectal disease, stool impactions, rectal foreign bodies and gastrointestinal (GI) bleeding all depend on the digital rectal examination. Occult blood in the right clinical setting should raise suspicion for intestinal ischemia.

Back

Gently percussing the costovertebral angles (CVA) of the back with a fist will elicit pain in patients with pyelonephritis or obstructive uropathy.

Head-to-toe

Abdominal pain may be elicited by extra-abdominal causes, such as pharyngitis, pneumonia and MI. These conditions can be missed without a comprehensive physical examination.

Differential diagnosis

Table 9.2 lists conditions causing abdominal pain by diagnosis.

Table 9.2 Differential diagnosis of abdominal pain

Diagnosis	Symptoms	Signs	Work-up
Appendicitis	Classically vague periumbilical or epigastric pain that migrates to the RLQ Anorexia, nausea, vomiting Diarrhea Low grade fever	Abdominal tenderness Fever (mean temperature 38°C) Voluntary or involuntary guarding Rebound tenderness Rovsing, psoas, or obturator signs CMT	Clinical diagnosis Abdominal CT Ultrasound (preferred in children and pregnant patients)

(continued)

Table 9.2 Differential diagnosis of abdominal pain (*cont*)

Diagnosis	Symptoms	Signs	Work-up
Biliary colic, cholecystitis, cholangitis	Acute crampy, colicky RUQ or epigastric pain May radiate to the subscapular area Nausea, vomiting Fever/chills may be present with cholecystitis and cholangitis	RUQ tenderness Murphy's sign Fever with cholecystitis, cholangitis	Ultrasound (preferred ED study) Radionuclide scan Liver function tests Amylase, lipase
Bowel obstruction	Crampy diffuse abdominal pain Nausea, vomiting No flatus or stool passage Bloating History of previous surgery or bowel obstruction	Abdominal distention Abdominal tenderness Fever Abnormal bowel sounds Peritoneal signs may indicate strangulation	Abdominal plain films Abdominal CT
Diverticulitis	LLQ abdominal pain Nausea, vomiting Change in stool pattern (frequency or consistency) Constipation Diarrhea Rectal bleeding	LLQ tenderness, guarding, rebound Fever Heme-positive stools If perforation, potential for tachycardia, high fever, sepsis	Clinical diagnosis Abdominal CT Ultrasound Barium contrast enema
Ectopic pregnancy	Abdominal or pelvic pain Vaginal bleeding Amenorrhea Nausea, vomiting Dizziness May complain of shoulder pain (referred)	Abdominal or pelvic tenderness Adnexal tenderness Adnexal mass	Urine or serum pregnancy test Quantitative β-hCG Endovaginal ultrasound Culdocentesis Rh type Hematocrit
Gastroenteritis	Intermittent, crampy abdominal pain Poorly localized Diarrhea Nausea, vomiting	Nonspecific abdominal examination Absence of peritoneal signs Fever	Testing usually not necessary for uncomplicated gastroenteritis
Intussusception	Episodic colicky abdominal pain Nausea, vomiting Bloody stool Diarrhea Poor feeding Episodes of crying and drawing legs up	Palpable abdominal mass Abdominal tenderness Occult blood in stool Currant jelly (mucoid, bloody) stool Dehydration and lethargy between episodes	Abdominal series Barium or air contrast enema – gold standard, sometimes therapeutic Ultrasound CT
Mesenteric ischemia	Gradual to acute onset Poorly localized, unrelenting abdominal pain Nausea, vomiting, diarrhea	Classically, pain "out of proportion" to examination Physical examination varies depending on the duration of ischemia May develop hypovolemia and sepsis	Serum lactate Plain films: may show *pneumatosis intestinalis*, portal vein gas or thumbprinting Abdominal CT Gadolinium-enhanced MRA Angiography
Ovarian torsion	Abrupt onset Severe unilateral abdominal or pelvic pain Nausea, vomiting	Unilateral abdominal or pelvic tenderness Tender adnexal mass	Transvaginal ultrasound with color doppler Exclude pregnancy

(continued)

Table 9.2 Differential diagnosis of abdominal pain (*cont*)

Diagnosis	Symptoms	Signs	Work-up
Pancreatitis	Severe, dull epigastric or LUQ pain Radiation to back	Abdominal tenderness Vomiting Abdominal distention Volume depletion	Amylase Lipase Abdominal CT (with contrast)
Pelvic inflammatory disease	Lower abdominal pain – dull, constant or poorly localized Vaginal discharge Abnormal vaginal bleeding Urinary symptoms Dyspareunia	Lower abdominal tenderness Adnexal mass or tenderness CMT Mucopurulent endocervical or vaginal discharge Fever	Cultures for GC, chlamydia Pregnancy test Pelvic ultrasound to exclude tubo-ovarian abscess Consider syphilis, HIV testing
Perforated peptic ulcer	Sudden severe abdominal pain May radiate to back with posterior ulcers Nausea, vomiting Older patients may have minimal pain	Diffuse abdominal pain Acute peritonitis Rigid abdomen Volume depletion Hypotension, tachycardia, fever	Abdominal series: free air Abdominal CT
Ruptured or leaking abdominal aortic aneurysm	Severe abdominal pain Flank or back pain Radiation to groin, thigh Syncope	Pulsatile abdominal mass Diffuse abdominal tenderness Abdominal bruit, decreased pulses Hypotension Hematuria	Straight to OR Abdominal plain films ED ultrasound Abdominal CT
Testicular torsion	Sudden onset severe pain May be felt in the lower abdomen, scrotum or inguinal area Nausea, vomiting Previous episodes resolving spontaneously (41%)	Swollen, tender, firm hemiscrotum High-riding testis with transverse lie Loss of cremasteric reflex	Straight to OR Color doppler imaging Radionuclide technetium scan
Ureteral colic	Abrupt onset of severe pain in the flank Radiates to the groin Nausea, vomiting Writhing in pain	Cannot find a comfortable position CVA percussion tenderness Benign abdominal examination Fever suggests infection Hematuria	Urinalysis may show hematuria Unenhanced CT IVP Ultrasound + KUB
Volvulus	Sudden severe colicky abdominal pain Abdominal distention May have had recurrent episodes Nausea, vomiting Constipation	Diffuse abdominal tenderness Abdominal distention Tympany Palpable mass with cecal volvulus Peritoneal signs, fever, shock with bowel infarction	Abdominal plain films: extremely distended colon Barium enema Sigmoidoscopy

CMT: cervical motion tenderness; CVA: costovertebral angle; CT: computed tomography; ED: emergency department; GC: gonococcus; hCG: human chorionic gonadotropin; HIV: human immunodeficiency virus; IVP: intravenous pyelogram; KUB: kidney, ureter and bladder X-ray; LLQ: left lower quadrant; LUQ: left upper quadrant; MRA: magnetic resonance angiography; OR: operating room; PID: pelvic inflammatory disease; RLQ: right lower quadrant; RUQ: right upper quadrant.

Diagnostic testing

Laboratory studies

Complete blood count

A complete blood count (CBC) is frequently ordered in patients with abdominal pain. Despite the association of an elevated white blood cell (WBC) count with many infectious and inflammatory processes, numerous studies have demonstrated that many patients with surgically-proven appendicitis have initially normal WBC counts. Even serial WBC counts have failed to discriminate between surgical and nonsurgical illness. In the patient with abdominal pain, an elevated WBC does not necessarily imply serious disease, detecting only 53% of patients with severe abdominal pathology in one study. In fact, elevations of the WBC count may lead to additional tests and increased costs without providing additional information. The CBC should never be used to make the sole diagnosis of abdominal pathology, nor should it be used in isolation to exclude reasonable diagnostic possibilities. The bottom line is that decision-making in cases of abdominal pain rest primarily on a carefully taken history and thorough physical examination, not the WBC count.

Urinalysis

The urinalysis is a rapid, cost-effective adjunctive laboratory test that needs to be interpreted with caution in patients with abdominal pain. Findings suggestive of UTI include pyuria, positive leukocyte esterase, positive nitrites and the presence of bacteria. However, up to 30% of patients with appendicitis may present with blood, leukocytes or even bacteria in their urine. A mild degree of pyuria may be present in elderly patients at baseline. Be wary of ascribing abdominal pain to a UTI when the clinical picture does not fit. Red blood cells (RBCs) in the urine are consistent with infection, trauma, tumors and stones. The patient with acute flank pain and hematuria suggests renal colic but also may represent a leaking or ruptured AAA.

Pregnancy test

All female patients of childbearing age with abdominal pain should have a pregnancy test. A positive pregnancy test expands the differential diagnosis (i.e., ectopic pregnancy), influences the choice of medications or adjunctive studies, and may impact disposition. Do not omit pregnancy testing in patients who report sexual abstinence, tubal ligation or contraceptive use.

Amylase/lipase

Though a serum amylase is commonly ordered when looking for pancreatitis, it may be normal in as many as a third of patients with pancreatitis. The serum amylase may also be elevated in other conditions including peptic ulcer or liver disease, SBO, common duct stones, bowel infarction, ectopic pregnancy, ethanol intoxication and diabetic ketoacidosis (DKA). Serum lipase has a higher sensitivity and specificity for pancreatitis than total amylase, and is therefore the most useful test in a patient with suspected pancreatitis.

Other laboratories

Liver function tests may be elevated in patients with biliary or hepatic disease. Serum electrolytes may be abnormal in patients with significant vomiting or diarrhea, symptoms >24 hours duration, diuretic use, or a history of kidney or liver disease. Serum phosphate and serum lactate may be elevated in cases of bowel ischemia.

Electrocardiogram

Electrocardiograms (ECGs) should be considered for all patients with unexplained epigastric or abdominal pain. They are particularly essential in the evaluation of elderly patients with vague, poorly localized abdominal complaints. An acute coronary syndrome (ACS) or inferior MI can present with epigastric pain, diaphoresis and vomiting. Though a normal ECG in the setting of abdominal pain does not exclude an MI, it makes it less likely.

Radiologic studies

Plain films

Abdominal plain films are markedly overutilized, difficult to interpret (even in experienced hands), and rarely provide useful clinical information. Plain films are unlikely to be helpful in patients with nonspecific abdominal pain, suspected appendicitis, and UTIs. In fact, they may cloud the diagnosis leading to delays in management. Plain films of the abdomen should be restricted to patients with suspected bowel obstruction,

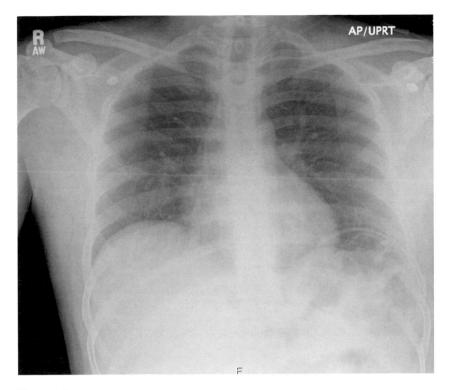

Figure 9.6
Pneumoperitoneum. AP erect chest X-ray reveals free air beneath the left hemidiaphragm consistent with pneumoperitoneum.

perforated viscus or foreign bodies. Even in these presentations, computed tomography (CT) scanning provides much more detailed information. When evaluating plain abdominal radiographs, look for abnormalities such as dilated loops of large or small bowel, air-fluid levels, abnormal calcifications of the abdominal aorta or urinary tract, gallstones, and free air under the diaphragm (Figure 9.6).

Ultrasound

Ultrasound has emerged as an extremely useful diagnostic modality in patients with abdominal pain. Advantages of ultrasound include lack of ionizing radiation, low cost and widespread availability. It is the preferred imaging approach for evaluating patients with RUQ pain. In patients with acute cholecystitis, ultrasound may detect gallstones, gallbladder wall thickening, pericholecystic fluid or a sonographic Murphy's sign.

Ultrasound is also commonly used to make the diagnosis of acute appendicitis, particularly in children, thin adults, women of reproductive age and pregnant patients. The primary sonographic

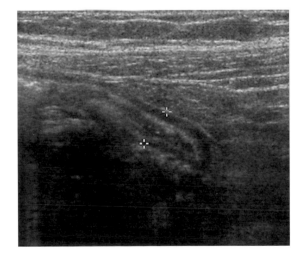

Figure 9.7
Appendicitis on ultrasound. Gray scale longitudinal ultrasound demonstrates enlarged non-compressible appendix (cursors) >7 mm, consistent with acute appendicitis. *Courtesy*: GM Garmel, MD.

criterion of appendicitis is demonstration of a swollen, noncompressible appendix >7 mm in diameter with a target configuration (Figure 9.7).

Additionally, ultrasound is useful in imaging the pelvic organs; the transvaginal approach is preferred and superior to the transabdominal approach for the diagnosis of ectopic pregnancy.

Limited bedside ED ultrasonography can be used for:

1. confirming an intrauterine pregnancy which dramatically lowers the risk of ectopic pregnancy;
2. screening for the presence of a AAA (Figure 9.8);
3. screening for the presence of free intraperitoneal blood in patients with abdominal trauma (see Appendix E).

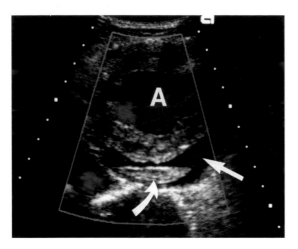

Figure 9.8
Ruptured abdominal aortic aneurysm (AAA) on transverse color Doppler sonogram. Note color flow within aneurysm (A) and retroperitoneal clot and hemorrhage posterior to AAA (arrows). *Courtesy*: R. Brooke Jeffrey, MD.

Ultrasound may be difficult to perform in obese patients and those in severe pain. As ultrasound requires considerable skill, findings are operator-dependent and interpretation errors can occur. A negative ultrasound does not exclude the diagnosis of either appendicitis or ectopic pregnancy.

Abdominal computed tomography

Abdominal CT has fast become the modality of choice in patients with undifferentiated abdominal pain who require imaging, as it allows for a panorama-like visualization of the structures of the peritoneal and retroperitoneal space, uninhibited by the presence of bowel gas or fat. Due to its exceptional accuracy, CT is often the primary imaging modality in patients with suspected appendicitis. CT findings of appendicitis

(Figure 9.9) include a swollen, fluid-filled appendix often with a calcified appendicolith or inflammatory changes in the periappendiceal mesenteric fat. After perforation, a phlegmon or abscess may be visible. CT is also useful for determining the diagnosis (and in many cases, the clinical severity) of conditions such as renal colic, bowel obstruction, bowel perforation, bowel ischemia, diverticulitis, pancreatitis, intra-abdominal abscess and AAA. The major drawbacks of CT are the cost, radiation dose and availability.

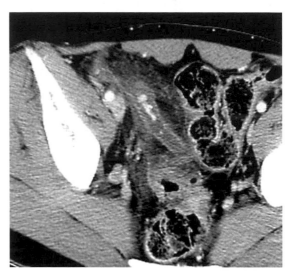

Figure 9.9
Acute appendicitis on contrast enhanced CT. Note enlarged appendix with multiple appendicoliths. Periappendiceal fat stranding is apparent. *Courtesy*: R. Brooke Jeffrey, MD.

General treatment principles

As with all ED patients, treatment begins with the ABCs (Airway, Breathing, Circulation). The main goals of treatment are physiologic stabilization, symptom relief and preparation for surgical intervention when warranted.

Volume repletion

Not all patients with abdominal pain need intravenous (IV) access or IV fluids. However, many patients have some degree of volume contraction resulting from poor intake, vomiting and diarrhea, or third-spacing. Other patients may have volume loss secondary to internal bleeding (e.g., ectopic pregnancy). Crystalloids are the initial fluids of choice in both children and adults. The rate of repletion is determined by the degree of hypovolemia, the cardiovascular status of the patient, and the response of the patient to initial therapy. Under certain circumstances, such as life-threatening hemodynamic collapse, blood products may be the initial resuscitation fluid.

Pain relief

Despite the long held opinion that narcotic analgesia masks peritoneal signs of an acute abdomen, there is no clear evidence supporting this notion. In fact, recent studies have revealed that the administration of moderate doses of analgesia and the ensuing pain relief do not cloud diagnostic findings; instead, this approach actually may aid in the diagnosis of surgical disease. In the acute setting, pain relief is typically achieved with IV titration of opioid analgesics such as morphine sulfate or fentanyl.

When combined with narcotic agents, IV ketorolac provides pain relief for patients with biliary and renal colic. Patients with epigastric discomfort may gain relief from a GI cocktail (varied combinations of an antacid, viscous lidocaine and/or donnatal). Though the GI cocktail may be therapeutic, it is not diagnostic, as even pain from an acute MI may be relieved by this therapy.

Antibiotics

Antibiotics are indicated in patients with abdominal sepsis, suspected perforation, or the presence of peritonitis (local or diffuse). Abdominal infections are often polymicrobial and necessitate coverage for enteric Gram-negatives, Gram-positives, and anaerobic bacteria. The specific regimen must take into account the patient's presentation, comorbid conditions, and local bacterial drug sensitivities and drug-resistance patterns.

Other

The control of emesis can be achieved by a number of agents. Patients in whom surgery is anticipated should be kept from eating or drinking (NPO). A nasogastric (NG) tube may be of benefit in patients with vomiting refractory to antiemetic administration or confirmed bowel obstruction.

Special patients

Elderly

Several factors make the diagnosis and management of abdominal pain in elderly patients challenging. Surgical causes of abdominal pain increase in incidence with advancing age, whereas nonspecific abdominal pain becomes less common. Typically, surgical illness in elderly patients is more rapidly life-threatening than in younger patients. Older patients are at much greater risk for vascular catastrophes such as ruptured AAA, mesenteric ischemia and MI. Elderly patients are more likely to present without the classic or expected historical or physical examination findings associated with a common disease. Because of atypical presentations and comorbidities, patient mortality and rates of misdiagnosis increase exponentially each decade after age 50. This highlights the importance of considering surgical illness (and surgical consultation) in most elderly patients with abdominal pain. About 40% of all patients >65 years of age presenting to the ED with abdominal pain ultimately require surgery.

Pediatric

The diagnosis of abdominal pain in children presents its own unique challenges. Histories must often be obtained from the children and caregivers. Children are not always able to articulate their complaint or describe their symptoms. Consequently, younger children tend to present with late symptoms of disease and have a higher incidence of perforated appendicitis compared to adults. The usual etiologies of abdominal pain in children vary from those in adults (Table 9.3). Gastroenteritis, non specific abdominal pain and appendicitis are more common in children, whereas biliary disease, pancreatitis and vascular disease are relatively rare. Illnesses relatively unique to children include intussusception, volvulus, pyloric stenosis and Hirschsprung's disease. Any child presenting with bilious vomiting should be presumed to have a bowel obstruction.

Immune compromised

In addition to ordinary afflictions such as appendicitis, patients with human immunodeficiency virus (HIV) presenting with abdominal pain may also have:

1. enterocolitis with profuse diarrhea and dehydration;
2. large bowel perforation associated with cytomegalovirus (CMV);
3. bowel obstruction from Kaposi's sarcoma, lymphoma or atypical mycobacteria;
4. biliary tract disease from cryptosporidium or CMV;
5. drug-induced pancreatitis.

Table 9.3 Causes of abdominal pain by age of onset

Birth to 1 year	2–5 years	6–11 years	12–18 years
Constipation	Appendicitis	Appendicitis	Appendicitis
Gastroenteritis	Constipation	Constipation	Constipation
Hirschsprung's disease	Gastroenteritis	Functional pain	Dysmenorrhea
Incarcerated hernia	Henoch–Schönlein	Gastroenteritis	Ectopic pregnancy
Infantile colic	purpura	Henoch–Schönlein purpura	Gastroenteritis
Intussusception	Intussusception	Mesenteric lymphadenitis	Mittelschmerz
UTI	Pharyngitis	Pharyngitis	Ovarian torsion
Volvulus	Sickle cell crisis	Pneumonia	PID
	Trauma	Sickle cell crisis	Testicular torsion
	UTI	Trauma	Threatened abortion
	Volvulus	UTI	

PID: pelvic inflammatory disease; UTI: urinary tract infection.
Adapted from Leung AKC, Sigalet DL. *Acute abdominal pain in children. Am Fam Physician* 2000;67(11).

The use of antibiotics, steroids or other immunosuppressants may mask abdominal examination findings usually associated with infection, so consideration should be given to any abdominal pain complaint, no matter how slight. Steroid use can lead to demargination of leukocytes, making interpretation of the WBC count more difficult. Steroids also promote peptic ulcer disease, leading to an increased incidence of perforated viscus.

Disposition

Surgical consultation

Patients with an acute abdomen or confirmed surgical illness require urgent surgical consultation. Life-threatening diagnoses such as ruptured AAA or ectopic pregnancy require emergent consultation and expedited treatment. The most common causes of abdominal pain requiring surgical consultation are appendicitis, intestinal obstruction, perforated ulcer and acute cholecystitis. These patients should be kept well-hydrated and NPO. Early diagnosis and surgery for appendicitis prevents perforation and the associated acute (abscess formation, sepsis) and late (scar formation with bowel obstruction/infertility) complications.

Serial evaluation

Observation with serial examinations allows the emergency physician an extended evaluation of a patient with an early or atypical presentation of appendicitis or another acute abdominal process.

These patients are kept in the ED or admitted to the hospital for serial abdominal examinations. Serial evaluation, preferably by the same physician, allows a patient's clinical picture to evolve or resolve over a period of time. Studies have shown that observation and repeated examinations of patients with suspected appendicitis improve diagnostic accuracy without increasing rates of perforation.

Discharge

After a thorough work-up in the ED or serial observation, patients without evidence of concerning medical or surgical illness may be discharged. Despite a patient's expectation of a firm diagnosis, it is perfectly acceptable to diagnose the patient with nonspecific or undifferentiated abdominal pain. In fact, the majority of patients are discharged from the ED with this diagnosis. Avoid forcing a diagnosis on the patient such as acute gastroenteritis. True gastroenteritis requires the presence of vomiting and diarrhea.

When discharging a patient with undiagnosed abdominal pain, it is important to arrange for a repeat evaluation within 8–10 hours (either in the ED or with an outpatient clinic) and make it clear to the patient to return to the ED if symptoms worsen. Typically, patients are placed on a clear liquid diet and narcotic analgesics are avoided. For patients returning to the ED with worsening symptoms, the additional opportunity to establish the diagnosis should be welcomed. Typically, these patients are more likely to have appendicitis or bowel obstruction. Patients in whom reliable follow-up cannot be arranged or assured may require admission.

Pearls, pitfalls, and myths

- Do not restrict the diagnosis solely by the location of the pain.
- Consider appendicitis in all patients with abdominal pain and an appendix, especially in patients with the presumed diagnosis of gastroenteritis, PID or UTI.
- Do not use the presence or absence of fever to distinguish between surgical and medical causes of abdominal pain.
- The WBC count is of little clinical value in the patient with possible appendicitis.
- Any woman with childbearing potential and abdominal pain has an ectopic pregnancy until her pregnancy test comes back negative.
- Pain medications reduce pain and suffering without compromising diagnostic accuracy.
- An elderly patient with abdominal pain has a high likelihood of surgical disease.
- Obtain an ECG in elderly patients and those with cardiac risk factors presenting with abdominal pain.
- A patient with appendicitis by history and physical examination does not need a CT scan to confirm the diagnosis; they need an operation.
- The use of abdominal ultrasound or CT may help evaluate patients over the age of 50 with unexplained abdominal or flank pain for the presence of AAA.

References

1. American College of Emergency Physicians (ACEP). Clinical policy. Critical issues for the initial evaluation and management of patients presenting with a chief complaint of nontraumatic acute abdominal pain. *Ann Emerg Med* 2000;36(4).
2. Coluciello SA, Lukens TW, Morgan DL. Assessing abdominal pain in adults: a rational, cost-effective evidence based approach. *Emerg Med Prac* 1995;1(1).
3. DeGennaro BA, Jacobsen SJ. Abdominal pain. In: Harwood-Nuss A (ed.). *The Clinical Practice of Emergency Medicine*, 3rd ed., Philadephia: Lippincott Williams & Wilkins, 2001.
4. Gallagher EJ. Acute abdominal pain. In: Tintinalli JE (ed.). *Emergency Medicine: A Comprehensive Study Guide*, 5th ed., McGraw Hill, 2000.
5. Graff LG, Robinson D. Abdominal pain and emergency department evaluation. *Emerg Med Clin North Am* 2001;19(1).
6. Kamin RA, Nowicki TA, Courtney DS, Powers RD. Pearls and pitfalls in the emergency department evaluation of abdominal pain. *Emerg Med Clin North Am* 2003;21(1).
7. King KE, Wightmen JM. Abdominal pain. In: Marx JA (ed.). *Rosen's Emergency Medicine: Concepts and Clinical Practice*, 5th ed., St. Louis: Mosby, 2002.
8. Leung AKC, Sigalet DL. Acute abdominal pain in children. *Am Fam Physician* 2000;67(11).
9. Marincek B. Nontraumatic abdominal emergencies: acute abdominal pain: diagnostic strategies. *Eur Radiol* 2002;12(19):2136–2150.
13. Newton E, Mandavia S. Surgical complications of selected gastrointestinal emergencies. *Emerg Med Clinic North Am* 2003;21(4).
10. Nicholson V. Abdominal pain. In: Hamilton GC (ed.). *Presenting Signs and Symptoms in the Emergency Department: Evaluation and Treatment*. Baltimore: Williams and Wilkins, 1993.
11. Silen W. *Cope's Early Diagnosis of the Acute Abdomen*, 20th ed., New York: Oxford University Press, 2000.
12. Thomas SH, Silen W. Effect of diagnostic efficiency of analgesia for undifferentiated abdominal pain. *Br J Surg* 2003;90:5–9.

10 Abnormal behavior

Tim Meyers, MD and Gus M. Garmel, MD

Scope of the problem

Patients manifesting abnormal behavior are common in emergency departments (EDs). They represent one of the most challenging classes of patients the emergency physician must treat. The causes of abnormal behavior are exceedingly diverse and require physicians to maintain a high level of vigilance to determine whether an underlying medical disorder exists. In 1998, it was estimated that nearly 4% of the approximately 100.4 million ED visits in the US were for behavioral problems. Many of these patients present "for medical clearance" prior to an intended psychiatric hospitalization. It is important that these patients be treated with the same sensitivity as every patient in the ED. "Medical clearance" should include a comprehensive medical evaluation to identify any potential underlying medical problem that may be responsible for the changes in behavior.

Pathophysiology

The physiology of behavior represents a complex interplay of human physiology and the environment in which it exists. Historically, changes in behavior have been classified as being of functional (psychiatric) or organic (medical) etiology. These classifications are dated, as neuropathophysiologic mechanisms of psychiatric disease have advanced over the past decades. Examples include aberrations in neurotransmitter transduction in depression (serotonin), schizophrenia (dopamine) and Alzheimer's disease (acetylcholine). Pharmacologic therapy directed at modulation of these neurotransmitters has greatly advanced the treatment and prognosis of patients suffering with these illnesses.

History

Prior to obtaining the history, the safety of the patient and staff should be ensured. Patients who are altered or violent may be unable or unwilling to give an adequate history. It is important to seek additional sources of information from paramedics, police, family members or witnesses.

Is this an acute or chronic condition?

The temporal nature of these behavioral changes is a good place to start when obtaining the history. Sudden behavioral changes in a previously healthy person are more likely to herald an underlying medical disorder. In contrast, dementia is characterized by progressively worsening cognitive function.

If acute, what were the events leading up to the change in behavior?

Is there an antecedent history of trauma, ingestion, medication noncompliance, or new medication(s) that might explain the patient's symptoms? Has the patient had a recent social stressor such as difficulty with work, family or a relationship that serves as the precipitant.

Does the patient have a history of psychiatric illness?

Patients with a history of psychiatric illness are more likely to have an underlying functional disorder as the cause of their abnormal behavior. Ask the patient if he or she has a history of depression, mania, schizophrenia or anxiety. Does the patient have a psychiatrist or psychotherapist? If so, it is important to attempt to contact that individual for additional history and consultation about disposition once underlying medical illnesses have been excluded. Many patients suffer from undiagnosed depression. The mnemonic SIG-E-CAPS is helpful when evaluating patients for possible depression (Table 10.1).

Table 10.1 SIG-E-CAPS mnemonic for depression screening

S	sleep disturbances
I	interest in hobbies decreases
G	guilt (feelings of worthlessness)
E	energy decreases
C	concentration decreases
A	appetite (usually less, may be variable)
P	psychomotor movements
S	suicidal ideations or thoughts

What medication does the patient take? Is there a suspected ingestion?

Medications are commonly implicated as the etiology of acute behavioral changes. When taking a history regarding medication usage, the following information should be considered:

1. What are the prescribed and over-the-counter medications taken by the patient?
2. Is there a new medication that could be causing an adverse reaction (e.g., mefloquine for malaria prophylaxis causes psychosis) or altering behavior through a drug–drug interaction?
3. Is there a possibility of an accidental or intentional overdose?
4. Is the patient sharing or taking someone else's medications?

Many medications are well known for causing alterations in mental status (Table 10.2). The patient should be questioned about any recent dosage adjustments. Even when patients have been on regularly scheduled doses, worsening renal or hepatic insufficiency may cause medications to become supratherapeutic (e.g., digoxin toxicity in the dehydrated elderly patient with worsening renal function) and precipitate alterations in behavior.

Table 10.2 Drugs that cause behavior changes

Anxiolytics	Lorazepam
Antibiotics	Isoniazid, rifampin, metronidazole
Anticonvulsants	Phenytoin, phenobarbital, valproate
Antidepressants	Selective serotonin reuptake inhibitors, monoamine oxidase inhibitors
Cardiovascular drugs	Digoxin, beta-blockers, methyldopa
Others	Antihistamines, cimetidine, corticosteroids, disulfiram, mefloquine, chemotherapy agents

Is the patient suicidal? Is there a history of suicide attempts or gestures? Is the patient homicidal? Can the patient care for him/herself?

These questions are essential in identifying patients who require involuntary psychiatric admission for evaluation and treatment. Immediate steps should be taken to keep these patients from harming themselves or others. Inquire about "red flags" for suicidality. These include guns or weapons at home, pills or access to them, previous suicide attempts or recent stresses (job, finances, relationships, health). In addition, the physician has a "duty to warn" parties who may be endangered as the result of a homicidal ideation. When trying to assess whether or not a patient is "gravely disabled," determine if the patient is able to shower or bathe, feed adequately, ambulate safely, manage finances, and make reasonable judgments. The conditions under which a person can be placed on an emergency psychiatric hold are a matter of state law and will be discussed later in this chapter.

Is there a history of substance or physical abuse?

Abnormal behavior is often the result of acute recreational drug or alcohol ingestion, or a withdrawal syndrome. Research reports that drugs and alcohol account for 21–60% of cases of abnormal behavior seen in EDs. There is a higher incidence of substance abuse in patients who suffer from psychiatric illness; similarly, patients with a history of substance abuse are more likely to have an underlying psychiatric condition. For patients who are depressed, substance abuse is an independent risk factor for suicide. It is important to ask patients, especially those with abnormal behavior, whether or not they are victims of physical, emotional, or sexual abuse.

Associated symptoms

- *Head, eye, ear, nose and throat (HEENT)*: headache, diplopia, vision loss, pain.
- *Chest*: pain, cough, shortness of breath.
- *Gastrointestinal (GI)*: pain, nausea, vomiting, diarrhea, incontinence, constipation.
- *Genitourinary (GU)*: pregnancy, bleeding, pain, discharge, incontinence, dysuria.
- *Skin*: rash, lesions.
- *Neurologic*: weakness, numbness, difficulty walking, vertigo, tinnitus.
- *Psychiatric*: mood, hallucinations (visual or auditory), anxiety, depression, suicidal, homicidal.

Physical examination

The physical examination represents a key aspect in the identification of underlying medical pathology in patients with behavioral changes. In addition, it may provide clues to specific underlying psychiatric diagnoses. Physicians and psychiatrists infrequently perform complete physical examinations in patients with abnormal behavior. The medicolegal literature has documented cases of fatal medical disorders inappropriately diagnosed as psychiatric illness. It is important that emergency physicians are meticulous in their data gathering from history and physical examination to avoid missing medical illnesses responsible for abnormal behavior.

General appearance

The general appearance of the patient is a key feature of the physical examination. Is the patient alert? Is the patient violent or are there signs of impending violence, such as increased motor activity, pressured speech, threatening posture and gestures? Is the patient clean, well groomed and appropriately attired?

Vital signs

These should be obtained as soon as safety allows. Any vital sign abnormality warrants a thorough evaluation. Many patients with underlying psychiatric illness who are evaluated in the ED do not have a complete set of vital signs documented. In particular, the temperature is frequently not obtained. An incomplete set of vital signs is a common pitfall. Alterations in vital signs may be the only clue to an underlying medical disorder, such as bacterial meningitis, sepsis, pneumonia or other infection, or a toxidrome.

Head

The head should be inspected for any evidence of trauma, including signs of a basilar skull fracture (Battle's sign or raccoon's eyes), soft tissue swelling or lacerations. Palpate the scalp for occult hematomas. Closely examine the head for the presence of surgical scars or shunt hardware.

Eyes

The ocular examination warrants close attention as it may be the only abnormality detected on physical examination in a patient with an underlying medical problem. Pinpoint pupils (miosis) can be caused by narcotics, cholinergic toxicity, brainstem lesions or clonidine use. Dilated pupils (mydriasis) are associated with sympathomimetics, anticholinergics, withdrawal states and post-anoxic injury. If papilledema is present, immediate computed tomography (CT) of the head should be performed, as this may signify increased intracranial pressure. Asymmetry of the pupils (anisocoria) may indicate a space-occupying central lesion, although this may be a normal finding. Attention should also be directed to the extraocular movements (EOMs). Alterations in EOMs can be seen with Wernicke's encephalopathy or brainstem lesions. The presence of nystagmus is another important feature associated with drug intoxication, but may be present in brainstem and posterior fossa lesions.

Neck

Assess for evidence of trauma, surgical scars, masses, nuchal rigidity, bruits, or thyromegaly.

Cardiopulmonary

Careful inspection and auscultation for evidence of pneumonia, murmurs, extra heart sounds, trauma or surgical scars is very important.

Abdomen

Distension or pain with palpation may suggest possible underlying surgical pathology. Hepatomegaly and ascites in the setting of abnormal behavior may suggest hepatic encephalopathy. A rectal examination should be performed to assess for signs of trauma, foreign body, drugs or melena/hematochezia.

Genitourinary

In women, a careful pelvic examination should be performed to look for evidence of foreign body, rape, trauma or infection. In older men, particularly those with diabetes, Fournier's gangrene of the scrotum and perineum or prostatitis may cause abnormal behavior due to infection.

Skin

Assess skin turgor for signs of dehydration and malnutrition. Inspect for the presence of petechiae, purpura or ecchymosis. Is there evidence of intravenous (IV) drug usage (track marks, "skin popping," abscesses or scars from previous I&Ds), burns, or excoriations. Are there lesions suspicious for Kaposi's sarcoma that might signify underlying acquired immune deficiency syndrome (AIDS) encephalopathy?

Neurologic

The neurologic examination is essential in differentiating medical from psychiatric illness. A retrospective review of patients admitted to psychiatric hospitals demonstrated the neurologic examination to be the most frequently undocumented portion of the physical examination. The examination should be performed in a systematic fashion, with assessment of orientation, memory, cranial nerves, motor, sensory, reflexes and cerebellar function included and documented.

Psychiatric

Is the patient suicidal or homicidal? Determine the patient's orientation (day, date, time and location), mood (emotional state), affect (flat vs. elevated), thought content (delusions), cognitive function (mini-mental status examination), speech quality (rapid, clear) and presence of hallucinations (auditory vs. visual) (Table 10.3).

Another helpful mnemonic in distinguishing functional from organic disorders is OMI-HAT (Orientation, Memory, Intellect, Hallucinations, Affect, Thinking). An organic etiology is more often associated with alterations in the OMI, while functional disorders are more associated with abnormalities in HAT.

The confusion assessment method (CAM) may be the most useful tool for diagnosing delirium. Delirium is an acute disturbance of consciousness with associated impaired cognition not accounted for by pre-existing dementia. CAM identifies the criteria necessary for diagnosis; other criteria that are not necessary for diagnosis (although common in delirium) include abnormal psychomotor activity, sleep–wake cycle disturbances, hallucinations, delusions and tremor. CAM can detect delirium even in the presence of dementia. The diagnosis of delirium requires both features 1 and 2 to be present with either feature 3 or 4 (Table 10.4).

Table 10.3 Mini-mental status examination

Orientation

What is the: (year) (season) (date) (day) (month)?	5 points
Where are we: (state) (county) (town) (hospital) (floor)?	5 points

Registration

Name three objects, ask patient to repeat	3 points

Attention and calculation

Serial 7 subtraction or spell *world* backwards	5 points

Recall

Ask the patient to rename the three objects stated earlier	3 points

Language

Name a pencil and watch	2 points
Repeat the following: "No ifs, ands or buts."	1 point
Follow a three-stage command: "Take this paper from my hand, fold it in half, and drop it on the floor."	3 points
Read and follow the printed command: "Close your eyes."	1 point
Write a sentence	1 point
Copy a design	1 point

Source: Folstein MF, Folstein SE, McHugh PR. Mini-mental state: a practical method for grading the cognitive state of patients for clinicians. *J Psych Res* 1975;12:189–198.

A score of ≤23 may indicate the presence of dementia or an underlying cognitive problem.

Table 10.4 Confusion assessment method

Feature 1	Acute onset and fluctuating course
Feature 2	Inattention
Feature 3	Disorganized thinking
Feature 4	Altered level of consciousness

Source: Inouye SK, van Dyck CH, Alessi CA, Balkin S, Siegal AP, Horwitz RI. Clarifying confusion: the confusion assessment method. *Ann Int Med* 1990;113:941–948.

Differential diagnosis

The differential diagnosis of abnormal behavior is broad, and includes medical and traumatic illness, effects of medications or intoxicants, and psychiatric disorders. Alterations in behavior can run the gamut from minor changes in speech to florid psychosis. Historically, several features

Table 10.5 Organic vs. functional etiology for abnormal behavior

Organic	Functional
Age <12 or >40 years	Age 12–40 years
Sudden onset (hours to days)	Gradual onset (weeks to months)
Fluctuating course	Continuous course
Disorientation	Scattered thoughts
Decreased consciousness	Awake and alert
Visual hallucinations	Auditory hallucinations
No psychiatric history	Previous psychiatric history
Emotionally labile	Flat affect
Abnormal vital signs/ physical examination	Normal vital signs/ physical examination

Table 10.6 Differential diagnosis of delirium

Cause	Etiology
Infectious	Sepsis, encephalitis, meningitis, neurosyphilis, CNS abscess
Withdrawal	Alcohol, barbiturates, sedatives
Acute metabolic	Acidosis, electrolyte abnormality, hepatic or renal failure, hypoglycemia
Trauma	Head trauma, burns
CNS disease	Hemorrhage, CVA, vasculitis, seizure, tumor
Hypoxia	COPD, respiratory failure, hypotension
Deficiencies	B_{12}, niacin, thiamine
Environmental	Hypo- or hyperthermia
Acute vascular	Hypertensive emergency, subarachnoid hemorrhage
Toxins/drugs	Medications, recreational drugs, alcohols, pesticides, industrial poisons (carbon monoxide, cyanide, solvents)
Heavy metals	Lead, mercury

COPD: chronic obstructive pulmonary disease; CNS: central nervous system; CVA: cerebrovascular accident.

help differentiate organic from functional disease (Table 10.5).

There are many organic causes of behavioral changes. Frequently, these are manifestations of an underlying medical problem. The mnemonic "I WATCH DEATH" is one of several proposed for the differential diagnosis of delirium, and serves as a good reminder when evaluating a patient in the ED with acute behavioral changes (Table 10.6).

Diagnostic testing

As with all patients seen in the ED, diagnostic testing should be guided by a careful history and physical examination. Patients with a prior history of psychiatric illness, normal vital signs and a normal physical examination may not require diagnostic tests in the ED. In a recent survey of emergency physicians, most felt that "routine" laboratory testing was not a necessary part of the medical screening examination of psychiatric patients. However, nearly one-third of those respondents reported that "routine" testing is required by their local psychiatric treatment facilities.

Few studies have examined the yield of routine laboratory testing as part of the medical screening examination of the psychiatric patient. At a large county ED, Henneman prospectively studied the utility of a standardized medical evaluation of 100 alert patients 16–65 years of age, presenting with first time psychiatric symptoms without obvious signs of intoxication or suicidality. This evaluation included a complete H&P, complete blood count (CBC), creatine phosphokinase (CPK), electrolyte and renal panel, prothrombin time, calcium, drug and alcohol screening, head CT and lumbar puncture if febrile. They reported that 63 patients had an underlying medical condition, with H&P being positive in 33 patients, CBC in 5, electrolyte and renal panel in 10, CPK in 6, drug and alcohol screen in 28, head CT in 8 and lumbar puncture in 8. The authors noted that all infections were detected by fever or lumbar puncture. This literature sharply contrasts the majority of literature that reports a yield for routine screening as low as 0.05%. Most emergency physicians agree that mandatory testing is costly and time-consuming, and clinically insignificant abnormalities may subject an otherwise medically stable patient to unnecessary additional testing and delays in transfer. However, selected or directed diagnostic testing is always appropriate.

Specific diagnostic testing

In patients with normal behavior, self-reporting of drug or alcohol use has been shown to be 92% sensitive and 91% specific for identifying a positive drug screen. Drug screens and alcohol levels are frequently ordered on emergency patients in the evaluation of abnormal behavior. These tests can assist with the diagnosis in obtunded patients. In addition, the absolute value of the blood alcohol level can be used to estimate the rate at which an intoxicated patient should sober (30–60 mg/dl/hour). Many newer recreational drugs that cause abnormal behavior, such as ecstasy, gamma hydroxybutyrate (GHB), and ketamine are not detected by routine urine drug screens.

Some literature states that hypoglycemia is responsible for up to 10% of abnormal behavior seen in ED patients. Based upon these numbers and the rapidity in which treatment should be rendered, immediate bedside testing of blood sugar is important for all patients who present with acute alterations in behavior.

Screening electrocardiograms (ECGs) are generally not necessary in the evaluation of abnormal behavior unless the patient has abnormal vital signs, symptoms or exam findings suggestive of acute coronary syndrome, or significant risk factors for a cardiac event (age >50 years, cocaine or stimulant use/abuse, or strong family history). If there is a suspicion that the patient has ingested a tricyclic antidepressant, beta-blocker, calcium channel blocker, antiarrhythmic or other medication known to affect cardiac conduction, an ECG should be obtained and reviewed.

Chest radiography is indicated in patients with cough, tachypnea, fever or hypoxia. A low threshold for obtaining a chest X-ray in an elderly patient is essential, as pneumonia may present with abnormal behavior as its sole finding. CT scanning of the brain is reserved for patients with a headache, focal neurologic deficits, or those at risk for subdural hematomas (elderly, anticoagulant use, recent falls, trauma, or dialysis).

Lumbar puncture should be performed in patients suspected of having a subarachnoid hemorrhage (despite a negative head CT) or central nervous system (CNS) infection. As a rule, anyone with fever, nuchal rigidity and altered mental status should have a lumbar puncture (LP). Patients who are immunocompromised may not mount a fever even in the presence of fulminant meningitis; therefore, they should have an LP whether or not fever is present. Most clinicians advocate obtaining a CT scan prior to lumbar puncture in anyone who exhibits focal neurologic findings in order to assess for masses or radiologic signs of increased intracranial pressure.

General treatment principles
Ensure safety

The primary treatment principle of any patient presenting with abnormal behavior is ensuring the safety of the staff and the patient. The patient must be prevented from harming him/herself or others. As a general rule, safety measures should be instituted as needed in a rapid, collaborative, rehearsed and stepwise fashion proceeding from the least to the most restrictive.

The setting for obtaining the history is important, especially with a potentially violent patient. The interview should be conducted in an environment of privacy but not isolation. Security personnel should be stationed outside the room in which the interview is being conducted. While in the room, the examiner should always remain between the patient and the door. Ideally, the room should have two points of exit so that both the physician and the patient have access to an exit should they feel threatened. During the H&P, the physician should act as an advocate for the patient, not an adversary. Decompress the situation by allowing the patient to feel in control, while setting limits to what is appropriate behavior. Interviewing the patient in a seated position has been shown to be effective in decompressing violent patients. Avoid prolonged eye contact and talk in a calm manner without being condescending. If at any time an examiner feels unsafe, he or she should leave!

Rule out conditions that require immediate action

Once the safety of the patient and staff has been established, the next step is to determine whether the altered behavior is a symptom or sign of an underlying medical problem. Blood glucose, oxygenation status, fever and hemodynamic compromise should be rapidly addressed.

Determine the need for emergency pyschiatric admission

Every state has conditions and laws set forth to provide for the involuntary admission of a mentally ill patient. The purpose of these laws allows for a patient to be held for a set period of time (usually 72 hours) for further psychiatric evaluation and treatment if they are deemed dangerous to themselves, to others, or gravely disabled. Some states also have laws specific to alcohol or drug intoxication that make it possible to hold a patient for evaluation and treatment.

Implement physical or chemical restraint when necessary

Many patients who are agitated can be "talked down" using a calm and soothing voice. Inform the patient that you are his or her advocate and want to help. Speak clearly while remaining non-judgmental. Ask the patient why he is upset and what could be done about it. For some patients, it may be appropriate to bargain using food or drink to gain control of the situation. The patient can be offered medication, either oral or parenteral, to calm him down. If these verbal interventions fail, proceed to a higher level of intervention called a "show of force." A minimum of five trained staff are needed, one to control each extremity and one to control the head. An additional person serves as the leader. To begin, the security personnel gather around the leader to promote an image of confidence. The leader tells the patient to calm down or he will be restrained. The patient is then given a few seconds to back down. Many patients will respond to this demonstration of force. If a patient remains agitated or combative, it is then necessary to apply physical restraints. At the signal of the leader, the team controls the patient's extremities and head. Caution should be exercised at all times, as violent patients are prone to kick, swing, bite, spit and scratch while being restrained. The patient is taken down in a backward motion and then rolled over. The leader informs the patient why restraints are necessary. Restraints are then applied and the patient is properly positioned in either a prone or recumbent orientation. Avoid placing patients in the supine position as this is uncomfortable and increases the risk of aspiration.

Physical restraints are usually only a bridge to chemical restraint. The goal of chemical restraint is rapid tranquilization. Two classes of drugs are used in the ED for chemical restraint: antipsychotics and anxiolytics. It is important to be familiar with the use of these medications in the emergency setting. Cooperative patients should be offered oral medications as first-line agents. Traditionally, antipsychotics (known as neuroleptics) are the preferred first-line agent for controlling the agitated or violent patient. Haloperidol (Haldol) is the most common antipsychotic used in the ED for rapid chemical control of the agitated patient. The recommended adult dose is 5–10 mg IV, which is not approved by the Food and Drug Administration (FDA) but is generally accepted as safe, or intramuscular (IM), repeated every 15–30 minutes until sedation is achieved. Haloperidol is a "low-potency" antipsychotic. It is associated with increased risk of extrapyramidal symptoms (EPS) that include dystonia (acute torticollis, oculogyric crisis and opisthotonos), akathisia, pseudoparkinsonism and tardive dyskinesia in the case of chronic use. The incidence of EPS is low and occurs $<1\%$ of the time. EPS typically responds to anticholinergic medications, such as diphenhydramine 25–50 mg PO/IM/IV and benztropine 1–2 mg PO/IM/IV. "High-potency" antipsychotics, such as chlorpromazine, are associated with lower rates of EPS but have a higher incidence of prolonged sedation, cardiovascular toxicity, and orthostatic hypotension, making them poorly suited for controlling the acutely agitated patient. Risperidone and olanzapine are newer "atypical" antipsychotics that are available in an oral formulation.

The FDA recently approved the atypical antipsychotic ziprasidone for IM injection to rapidly control agitated behavior and psychotic symptoms in patients with acute exacerbations of schizophrenia. To date, no studies in the ED setting have compared haloperidol and ziprasidone. Ziprasidone has been shown to have a greater capacity to prolong the QT interval compared to haloperidol.

Droperidol, formerly a favorite medication of many emergency physicians, has received a "black box" warning by the FDA due to its potential to precipitate torsades de pointes in patients with underlying QT prolongation. One study estimates the incidence to be 4/1100. It is important to note that many of the antipsychotics can precipitate torsades. Antipsychotics should not be used in pregnant or lactating females, phencyclidine overdose or anticholinergic-induced psychosis.

Anxiolytics may be used as single-line agents (especially when drug or alcohol intoxication or withdrawal is suspected) or as an adjunct to antipsychotics for control of the violent patient. Benzodiazepines are the anxiolytics of choice in this situation – especially those with rapid onset and short half-lives. Lorazepam is one mainstay and can be given at a dose of 1–2 mg PO/IM/IV every 30 min. Numerous studies have shown that anxiolytics decrease the dosage requirements of antipsychotic agents when they are used in conjunction. Patients require lower doses of medication and the incidence of EPS is lower. "HAC" is a commonly used ED mnemonic for Haldol (5 mg), Ativan (2 mg) and Cogentin (1 mg). This combination of medication can be given as a single IM injection. Care should be exercised when using multiple agents in elderly patients, as oversedation is a concern. Midazolam is another short-acting benzodiazepine with very rapid onset of action, and has been given safely at a dose of 5 mg IM.

Frequent rechecks

The medical and psychiatric evaluation or transfer of a patient often takes time to complete. It is important that patients with abnormal behavior are frequently rechecked for over- or undersedation, abnormal vital signs, seizures, emesis or respiratory compromise. Patients who are older or those with abnormal vital signs should be monitored while their disposition is being established. Patients who are agitated may need additional medication for sedation. Patients who are physically restrained should be frequently rechecked for extremity trauma, aspiration, respiratory compromise, pressure sores and skin injury.

Special patients

Elderly

Elderly patients who manifest behavioral changes represent a special population. Alterations in behavior have been reported to be more common precursors of physical illness than fever, pain or tachypnea. Urinary tract infections are often implicated as a cause of abnormal behavior in the elderly; thus, a low threshold should exist for obtaining a urinalysis. If the ED evaluation of an elderly patient is unrevealing, yet a concern for an underlying medical problem remains, the patient should be admitted to a medical floor for further observation and evaluation.

Pediatric

In a national review by Sills, it is estimated that there are over 400,000 pediatric mental health visits annually, accounting for 1.6% of all ED visits by individuals under 18. Unspecified neurotic state was diagnosed in 13.1% of patients, depressive disorder in 12.9%, anxiety state in 11.4% and psychosis in 10.8% of patients. Nearly 14% of the patients were seen for suicide attempts. The World Health Organization estimates that by the year 2020, childhood psychiatric disorders will become one of the top five causes of morbidity, mortality and disability among children. Over the past few decades an increasing number of children have been prescribed psychoactive medications.

There is a higher incidence of ingestions and psychiatric illnesses in pediatric patients with abnormal behavior than adults. When a child with a psychiatric illness presents to the ED, there is often a breakdown of the family's support system. It is important to attempt to uncover what is not working smoothly in the home situation. Furthermore, school, work, or social stressors may be even more challenging without a supportive home environment.

Suicide is currently the fourth leading cause of death in children 10–14 years of age and the third leading cause in children 15–19 years old. A retrospective study by Porter demonstrated that adolescents with somatic complaints were infrequently screened for depression in the ED. ED visits provide an opportunity to intervene in children at risk for major depression or suicide.

Pediatric and adolescent patients requiring admission for psychiatric evaluation and treatment typically go to specialized facilities that deal only with pediatric patients. There is a nationwide shortage of pediatric psychiatric beds, which often results in pediatric patients experiencing extended stays in the ED.

Immune compromised

Patients who are immunocompromised may not demonstrate abnormal vital signs even with serious medical illness. This is frequently demonstrated in patients with AIDS. In patients with a history of HIV, it is important to determine the history of any AIDS-defining illness. The patient and any medical records should be queried for recent lymphocyte counts. A low threshold for diagnostic testing should be maintained. Patients with HIV are susceptible to CNS infections such as toxoplasmosis, cytomegalovirus (CMV), herpes encephalitis, cryptococcal and bacterial meningitis or CNS lymphoma with minimal focal neurologic findings. For this reason, any immunocompromised person with abnormal behavior, even if afebrile, should have a CT scan of the brain as part of the medical work-up before a lumbar puncture.

Disposition

Admission

Patients with underlying medical problems require admission to the hospital for further evaluation and treatment. Patients with progressive dementia may no longer be safe in their current living situation and might benefit from a social services evaluation or admission. Patients in whom underlying medical pathology cannot be safely eliminated should be admitted to a medical bed for further testing. Patients who are suicidal, homicidal or gravely disabled should be placed on an emergency psychiatric hold, and be admitted to a psychiatric facility for further evaluation and treatment.

Depressed patients who do not actively endorse suicidal ideation can be difficult to disposition. One mnemonic and scoring system for the assessment of suicide risk is SAD PERSONS (Table 10.7). Scores of ≤6 are associated with low risks of suicide, while scores >6 represent a higher risk of suicide and warrant hospitalization. Caution is warranted in any patient with the possibility of suicidal behavior, and liberal use of consulting psychiatric services is recommended.

Table 10.7 SAD PERSONS: Assessment for suicide risk

Sex: Male	1 point
Age: <19, >45 years	1 point
Depressed	2 points
Previous suicide attempt	1 point
Ethanol or any substance	1 point
Rational thinking absent	2 points
Separated or divorced	1 point
Organized suicide plan	2 points
No social support	1 point
Stated future attempt	2 points

Consultation

Maintain an on-call list of psychiatric care providers at your hospital who are available to evaluate and treat patients with psychiatric emergencies. Attempts should be made at contacting the patient's primary psychiatrist, psychologist or therapist to assist with the disposition. When contacting a psychiatric care provider, be certain

to relay the events leading up to the ED visit, all treatment rendered in the ED, and the status of the "medical clearance."

Transfer

Depending on the hospital, patients requiring involuntary or voluntary psychiatric admission may have to be transferred to a psychiatric care facility after the medical screening examination has been completed. It is important that physician-to-physician communication occurs prior to transfer, and for the staff to confirm bed availability. Furthermore, it is never appropriate to allow a family member or taxi service to transfer a patient for involuntary psychiatric admission. Caution should be used for transfer arrangements for voluntary psychiatric admissions as well.

Observation/discharge

Most patients with abnormal behavior will not be released unless they are observed for an extended period in the ED. Patients who are discharged should have emergency medical and psychiatric causes of their abnormal behavior excluded. Family members or a responsible adult (preferably with transportation) should be involved in the discharge process. Patients suffering from mild drug ingestions or alcohol intoxication are frequently discharged from EDs after observation. In addition, patients with a stable psychiatric condition may be discharged if they are not suicidal (danger to self), homicidal (danger to others), or gravely disabled. In this situation, speaking directly with the patient's primary mental health provider is always preferred. Patients who are discharged should have intact support networks, a safe place to stay, and reliable follow-up, preferably arranged prior to discharge. Next day appointments or contact from the patient's psychiatrist or therapist is most desirable.

Pearls, pitfalls, and myths

- Limited history from limited sources
- Incomplete review of systems
- Incomplete review of medications without considering drug–drug interactions or adverse effects
- Failure to document vital signs
- Failure to address abnormal vital signs

- Limited or incomplete physical examination, including neurologic
- Unreasonable assumption of psychiatric illness without considering medical or traumatic etiologies or ingestion and intoxication.

References

1. Armitage DT, Townsend MG. Emergency medicine, psychiatry and the law. *Emerg Med Clinic North Am* 1993;11(4):869–887.
2. Folstein MF, Folstein SE, McHugh PR. Mini-mental state: a practical method for grading the cognitive state of patients for clinicians. *J Psych Res* 1975;12:189–198.
3. Reeves RR, Nixon FE. Assessment for medical clearance. *Ann Emerg Med* 1995;25(6):852–853.
4. Reeves RR, Pendarvis EJ, Kimble R. Unrecognized medical emergencies admitted to psychiatric units. *Am J Emerg Med* 2000;18(4):390–393.
5. Stuart P, Garmel GM. Psychiatric disorders in the emergency department. *Hosp Phys* 2000;6(4):1–11.
7. Tintinalli JE, Peacock FW, Wright MA. Emergency evaluation of psychiatric patients. *Ann Emerg Med* 1994;23:859–862.
6. Tueth MJ. Diagnosing psychiatric emergencies in the elderly. *Am J Emerg Med* 1994;12(3):364–369.
8. Williams ER, Shepard SM. Medical clearance of psychiatric patients. *Emerg Med Clinic North Am* 2000;18(2):185–198.

11   Allergic reactions and anaphylactic syndromes

Steven Go, MD

Scope of the problem

In the emergency department (ED), it is not uncommon to compare the pain of minor procedures to a "bee sting." However, the estimated prevalence of acute anaphylactic reactions to insect stings is as high as 0.8% of the US population, resulting in about 40 deaths annually. In the broader scheme, anaphylaxis from any cause has been estimated to occur at rates as high as 1 in every 3000 patients, with 500 deaths per year in the US. Despite the predominantly subtle presentations, lethal allergic reactions do occur. Failure to rapidly diagnose and treat these conditions will likely result in untoward outcomes. Therefore, it is imperative that emergency physicians have a solid understanding of allergic reactions and anaphylaxis. It is important to remember that the symptoms of allergic reactions occur on a spectrum – from mild cases of pruritis to cardiovascular collapse.

Pathophysiology

The term *"anaphylaxis"* comes from the Greek words for "against" and "protection." The mechanism begins when the body produces immunoglobulin E (IgE) during initial exposure to an antigen. On subsequent exposure, IgE binds to mast cells, causing release of vasoactive products. These products, histamine being chief among them, lead to smooth muscle spasm, bronchospasm, mucosal edema, angioedema, and increased capillary permeability. Such reactions are generally immediate; however, it has been suggested that mast cells or basophils can also release new mediators in a delayed fashion, which results in a second phase of symptoms.

Anaphylactoid reactions are syndromes that present as anaphylaxis, but not through an IgE-mediated mechanism. In addition, they often do not require a prior exposure to the antigen. From a practical perspective, however, anaphylaxis and anaphylactoid reactions are often clinically indistinguishable, and will therefore be addressed together as *anaphylactic syndromes*.

Inciting causes of anaphylactic syndromes are legion, including but not limited to insect bites and stings, food exposure, medications (especially by parenteral administration), latex exposure, exercise (with or without concurrent food exposure), seminal fluid, and idiopathic factors.

History

Although history is important in confirming both the diagnosis and etiology of acute allergic syndromes, it is vital to remember that the length of the history must be proportional to the stability of the patient.

Do you have trouble breathing or talking?

As always, airway management must take top priority. In allergic syndromes, airways can be compromised by angioedema, and the sometimes brief window of opportunity for securing the airway may close rapidly. If impending airway collapse is not quickly recognized by the emergency physician, a bad outcome is almost certain to follow. An affirmative nod to this question requires immediate transfer to a monitored area of the ED, where airway emergencies can be adroitly handled.

When did the symptoms start and how long have they been going on?

The symptoms of anaphylaxis typically start within seconds to minutes of exposure to the offending antigen; however, they may start as late as 24 hours after exposure. In general, the sooner symptoms appear after exposure, the more severe the clinical course. The possibility of a biphasic response, where severe symptoms recur up to 8 hours after the initial symptoms resolve (in about 20% of treated patients) has been described in the literature. Persistent anaphylactic reactions consist of continual symptoms for 5–32 hours despite medical therapy.

Do you have any known allergies? Any new exposures? Has this happened before?

Identification of the inciting antigen is not always possible, but should be attempted in order exposure to that antigen (e.g., new ~~ume~~, topical medication). Previous ~~known~~ allergies may provide a clue ~~y~~ of the current attack or point to ~~reactivities~~ that may exist (i.e., peni-~~cephalosporins~~). Frequent previous ~~identify~~ carcinoid syndrome, hereditary angioedema, or factitious anaphylaxis.

What were the surrounding events when the symptoms occurred?

If the symptoms occur in conjunction with the introduction of emotional stress, a vasovagal reaction may be suspected. If the symptoms begin during or shortly after a meal, a potential food antigen is possible. Since restaurants do not generally disclose the precise ingredients in their dishes, many patients may not realize they have consumed foods that they know cause them problems. Anaphylaxis can occur in conjunction with vigorous exercise, especially in conditioned athletes in adverse climates.

Has anyone in your family had symptoms like this before?

If affirmative, hereditary angioedema should be suspected. Many antigens and exposures cause difficulty for an entire family.

Associated symptoms

Anaphylactic syndromes can present in various ways (Table 11.1). Increased vascular permeability can appear as urticaria, angioedema, and is sometimes preceded by a feeling of flushing and warmth. Laryngeal edema can quickly lead to airway compromise and may present with stridor, hoarseness, a feeling of airway obstruction, and dysphagia. Nasal congestion can further hamper respirations. Bronchospasm presents with dyspnea, wheezing, and "tightness" in the chest. Hypotension can present with syncope or dizziness, which are sometimes harbingers of vascular collapse. Other associated symptoms include gastrointestinal (GI) symptoms such as nausea, vomiting, abdominal pain, and diarrhea, which may sometimes be bloody. Signs and symptoms of shock may be present in severe cases. Uterine muscle contractions can cause pelvic cramping, and in pregnancy, miscarriage. In anaphylaxis, any of these symptoms can be present, either together or in isolation. Skin findings are present in up to 90% of cases. However, the absence of skin signs in no way rules out the presence of an anaphylactic syndrome.

Past medical

Patients with a history of cardiac or pulmonary disease are at greater risk of death. Patients taking β-blockers who develop anaphylaxis are

Table 11.1 Symptoms and signs of anaphylactic syndromes

Presentation	Symptoms	Signs
Airway edema	Sensation of throat tightness, dysphagia, dysphonia	Respiratory distress, stridor, muffled voice or hoarseness, coughing, sneezing, nasal congestion
Angioedema	Swelling without pruritis	Edema: especially of face, eyelids, lips, tongue, uvula, eyes, hands, and feet
Bronchospasm	Dyspnea, chest tightness	Wheezing, coughing, retractions, tachypnea
Distributive shock	Dizziness, syncope, near-syncope, anxiety, weakness, confusion	Hypotension, tachycardia
Gastroenteritis .	Nausea, vomiting, diarrhea, bloating, abdominal cramping	Diffuse abdominal pain without peritoneal signs. May have normal examination
Increased secretions	Rhinorrhea, bronchorrhea, increased lacrimation	Nasal congestion, increased tracheal and bronchial secretions. Drooling, tearing, conjunctival erythema
Urticaria	Pruritis or tingling, rash or swelling, flushing	Raised erythematous welts of various sizes on the skin surface. Usually pruritic

often refractory to therapy and are at extremely high risk.

Physical examination

General appearance

The general appearance of the patient is of crucial importance. Patients experiencing allergic reactions who appear sick are probably ill or about to be very ill. Any difficulty speaking, respiratory distress, or agitation should provoke immediate treatment. An expressed fear of impending doom is often prescient.

Vital signs

Temperature is usually normal. Cardiovascular involvement is suggested by hypotension, tachycardia, and dysrhythmias. Pulse oximetry is typically normal until airway compromise is nearly complete; therefore, a normal reading does not rule out airway involvement.

Integument

Inspection may reveal urticaria (Figure 11.1), angioedema, erythema, flushing, and pruritis. Diaphoresis and/or cyanosis indicates the presence of shock.

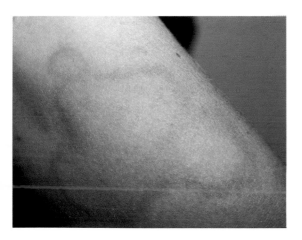

Figure 11.1
Urticaria. *Courtesy*: Steven Shpall, MD.

Head and neck

Inspection may reveal swelling of the eyelids, lips (Figure 11.2), tongue, and oral mucosa. Lip or facial cyanosis indicates severe respiratory

compromise. The presence of drooling, the inability to manage secretions, and the size and appearance of the uvula and tongue should all be noted. The posterior oropharynx should be inspected for patency. A hoarse or muffled voice signals potential airway compromise, as does dysphagia. Stridor should be identified. Eye itching, conjunctival injection, and tearing can occur. Nasal congestion, rhinorrhea, and sneezing may also be present. Observing the patient's Mallampati classification (Figure 2.8) may be useful in helping determine what type of airway stabilization method is appropriate if acute airway compromise occurs, but its role in the management of anaphylaxis has not been clearly delineated in the literature.

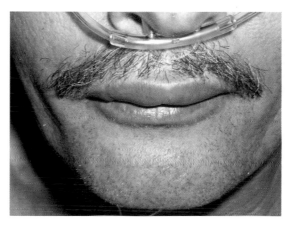

Figure 11.2
Angioedema involving the upper lip. *Courtesy*: Leland Robinson, MD and Steven Go, MD.

Lungs

Wheezing indicates bronchospasm if enough air flow is present to wheeze. A quiet chest is an even more dangerous sign because it indicates severe compromise of the patient's ventilatory status. Increased respiratory effort is also dangerous.

Heart

Tachycardia is most common, but other dysrhythmias may be present.

Abdomen

Crampy abdominal pain as a result of edema, smooth muscle contraction or vascular engorgement can be present. However, true peritoneal signs should not be present. Tenesmus can also occur.

Extremities

Patients with anaphylaxis commonly have a rapid, weak, thready pulse. Cyanosis of the nail beds occurs with severe respiratory compromise.

Neurologic

Altered mental status, agitation, lightheadedness, or unconsciousness are signs of a severe reaction. Seizures are uncommon, but may occur. Otherwise, the neurologic examination should be normal.

Differential diagnosis

There are numerous entities that can mimic anaphylaxis. It can be very difficult to differentiate them in the acute phase. Therefore, clinical syndromes that appear to be anaphylaxis should be treated as anaphylaxis until proven otherwise (Table 11.2).

Diagnostic testing

Diagnostic testing is of little utility in the emergent diagnosis and management of anaphylactic syndromes in the ED.

Laboratory studies

Serum histamine and tyramine levels have been mentioned in the literature to possibly confirm the diagnosis of anaphylaxis. However, histamine has an extremely short half-life; therefore, a meaningful level is difficult to measure. More importantly, these tests are more appropriate to confirm the diagnosis after the patient has been stabilized. They should play no role in determining whether to suspect anaphylaxis or to treat it.

Electrocardiogram and radiologic studies

Electrocardiogram (ECG) and radiologic studies are generally nonspecific. Confirmational skin testing is beyond the scope of emergency medicine.

General treatment principles

The guiding treatment principle is to rapidly determine that the patient needs treatment. Anaphylaxis often occurs without warning, and a delay in appropriate therapy may prove fatal. Therefore, a high level of suspicion must be maintained. In addition, for obvious reasons, there are few prospective controlled trials for the treatment of anaphylactic shock. Therefore, it should be remembered that the treatment recommendations in the literature are largely based on anecdotal clinical experience.

Although the following treatment strategies should occur simultaneously, it is helpful to conceptualize them in a few basic categories.

Antigen removal

If the inciting antigen is still present (e.g., the stinger of a bee, article of clothing), it should be removed promptly.

Epinephrine administration

Epinephrine administration is the cornerstone of treatment. It should be given when anaphylaxis is suspected. The usual dose of epinephrine is 0.3–0.5 mg of 1:1000 solution given subcutaneously (SC) or intramuscularly (IM). The IM route has been touted as being the more efficacious. Some experts have even recommended intravenous (IV) administration, but given the potential hazards of this route (e.g., dysrhythmias, myocardial infarction, cerebral vascular events, organ ischemia) and the lack of conclusive advantages, it is probably prudent to avoid the IV route except in cases of cardiopulmonary arrest. Epinephrine should be used with care in those with known cardiac disease or pregnancy; however, as always, the benefits of the treatment must be weighed against its risks. Epinephrine should be used with caution in patients on β-blockers (see Special patients).

Airway control

The most common mistake in airway management is the failure to recognize the need for early airway control. For any patient with an allergic reaction, the status of the airway must be determined, documented, and monitored closely. An oral airway is preferable to a surgical airway, if possible. If early laryngeal edema is present, early elective airway control is preferable to expectant management. By the time extreme respiratory distress develops, achieving an airway may be impossible. Rapid sequence intubation (RSI) should be used with great caution in these patients, as unseen lower airway edema may

Table 11.2 Differential diagnosis of anaphylaxis-like syndromes

Diagnosis	Symptoms	Signs	Workup
Carcinoid syndrome	Recurrent episodes of flushing of the face and neck, palpitations, facial swelling, GI symptoms (especially diarrhea, which can be debilitating). Dyspnea may also occur	Hypotension, no urticaria. Facial edema, malar telangiectasia, flushing, wheezing. May hear murmur if cardiac involvement	Increased serum and urine levels of serotonin metabolite, 5-HIAA
Chinese restaurant syndrome (MSG symptom complex)	Proximity to eating MSG-containing foods. Dyspnea, flushing, sweating, tightness in the chest, burning sensation at the back of the neck into arms and chest, headache, nausea, palpitations, oral numbness and burning	Wheezing, flushing, hypotension, and dysrhythmias can occur. True anaphylaxis may occur	History. No definitive test. Symptoms typically resolve in 2 or 3 hours
Factitious anaphylaxis	Anxiety present	No objective signs of anaphylaxis	History and examination. Diagnosis of exclusion. Munchausen's anaphylaxis is true anaphylaxis that the patient causes surreptitiously
Hereditary angioedema	Swelling of lips, tongue, and upper airway with possible respiratory compromise. Sometimes abdominal pain or non-pruritic swelling of extremities. Often develops after trauma (e.g., dental procedure). Lack of antigen exposure. Family history of these events and/or history of recurrent episodes in the absence of antigen	Angioedema is usually seen in the lips, face, and oral mucosa. Absence of urticaria or pruritis	Decreased C1-esterase inhibitor levels. Decreased serum C4. Fiberoptic laryngoscopy may reveal upper airway edema
Pheochromo-cytoma	Headache, sweating, palpitations, tremor, nausea, weakness, constipation, abdominal pain, weight loss	Hypertension, fever, weight loss, pallor, tremor, neurofibromas, café au lait spots, tachydysrhythmias	Elevated levels of urine catecholamines. Hyper-glycemia, hypercalcemia, erythrocytosis
Scombroid poisoning	Exposure to fish of the Scombridae family or related fish (tuna, mackerel, mahi-mahi, sardines, anchovies). Rapid onset of facial flushing, peppery taste, dizziness, palpitations, nausea, headache, diarrhea, abdominal pain	Diaphoresis, facial rash, urticaria, edema, abdominal tenderness. Respiratory distress, tongue swelling, blurred vision, and vaso-dilatory shock may occur	Elevated level of urine histamine. FDA analysis of tainted fish. Typical resolution of symptoms in within 8–10 hours
Serum sickness	Fever, malaise, headache, arthralgias, GI symptoms, associated with urticaria occur 7–10 days after exposure to antigens	Fever, rash (may be scarlati-niform, urticarial, morbilliform, or polymorphous) lymph-adenopathy, arthritis, arthralgias. Rarely cardio-pulmonary involvement	Elevated sedimentation rate. Possible elevated creatinine. CBC with eosinophilia. Depressed complement levels
Systemic mastocytosis	Not associated with a particular antigen exposure	Presents as anaphylaxis	No available test to differ-entiate from anaphylaxis
Vasovagal reactions	Occurs during stress (e.g., injection, dental procedures) No pruritis. Absence of respiratory obstruction or skin symptoms	Slow, strong, steady pulse. Blood pressure normal or elevated. Skin cool. Pallor without cyanosis	Monitoring and ED observation. Symptoms relieved by recumbency
MCSLC	See specific disorder	See specific disorder	See specific disorder

CBC: complete blood count; ED: emergency department; FDA: Food and Drug Administration; GI: gastrointestinal; 5-HIAA: 5-hydroxyindoleacetic acid; MCSLC: miscellaneous causes of sudden loss of consciousness (i.e., seizure, cardiac dysrhythmias, pulmonary embolism, foreign-body aspiration); MSG: monosodium glutamate.

preclude an oral endotracheal airway. In such cases, giving paralytics would be unwise. If *immediately available*, fiberoptic intubation may be a safer option. In any event, equipment and personnel necessary for the establishment of an emergent surgical rescue airway should ideally be close at hand when managing the airway.

Ventilatory support

Any component of bronchospasm should be treated with bronchodilators, supplemental oxygen, and corticosteroids. Arterial blood gases may be useful in determining the level of ventilatory compromise, although the decision to intubate for ventilatory compromise remains largely a clinical one.

Circulatory support

Fluid resuscitation with normal saline or colloid should be given for hypotension and other signs of shock. Large quantities may be required to maintain a satisfactory blood pressure. Central venous pressure monitoring may be helpful in guiding therapy. For refractory cases, vasopressors such as norepinephrine may be required. The patient should be kept recumbent until blood pressure stabilizes.

Secondary medications

Antihistamines can be useful in treating cutaneous manifestations of allergic reactions, but there is debate regarding their efficacy in acute anaphylaxis. Therefore, they should be viewed as adjunctive treatments to epinephrine and fluids in this circumstance. It has been shown that in acute allergic urticaria, the addition of H_2-blockers to H_1-antagonists results in improved outcomes (resolution of urticaria, with or without angioedema) in patients compared with treatment with H_1-blockade alone.

Corticosteroids likely have no benefit in the acute phase of anaphylaxis, given their delayed onset of action. However, they may reduce the possibility of a biphasic reaction. Therefore, they should probably be given early to all patients, unless contraindications exist.

Aminophylline has traditionally been thought to be useful in treating bronchospasm, stimulating respiratory drive, augmenting cardiac contractions, and promoting diaphragmatic contractility. However, the utility of this medication in the emergency treatment of acute bronchospasm has been questioned in the literature, and its use remains controversial.

Norepinephrine and glucagon may be useful in refractory hypotension. Glucagon may be particularly useful in hypotensive patients taking β-blockers.

Special patients
Taking β-blockers

β-blockers are proallergenic, and also amplify the production of anaphylactic mediators which potentiate the severity of allergic reactions. β-blockers may also blunt the usually favorable response to epinephrine treatment. Glucagon may be useful in treating hypotension in anaphylaxis patients who are taking β-blockers. In addition, these patients may develop severe hypertension upon epinephrine administration, secondary to unopposed α-adrenergic effects. Dysrhythmias may also occur. Adverse reactions may also occur during epinephrine therapy in patients who are using tricyclic antidepressants or monoamine oxidase inhibitors. Epinephrine should be used at reduced dosages in these cases, and phentolamine (to treat hypertension) and lidocaine (to treat dysrhythmias) should be readily available.

Resistant bronchospasm

Resistant bronchospasm may occur in patients who are taking β-blockers. Sometimes higher than usual dosages or frequency of bronchodilators (β-agonists and anticholinergics) are necessary for these patients. Inhaled epinephrine may be useful when SC epinephrine fails to relieve bronchospasm. Other therapies mentioned in the literature include IV magnesium, vitamin C, naloxone, atrial natriuretic factor, and glucagon; however, evidence of benefit for these medications is inconclusive.

Disposition

Much like treatment, disposition recommendations in the literature are generally based on clinical experience.

Patients with mild allergic reactions limited to peripheral cutaneous findings (not involving the airway) without evidence of anaphylaxis may be treated symptomatically and discharged with careful follow-up instructions, including avoidance of the inciting antigen.

Patients with more severe reactions (e.g., mucosal swelling, wheezing), but without evidence of shock should be treated aggressively, and observed for at least 8 hours. If the patient makes a prompt recovery without complications and remains asymptomatic, he may be safely discharged with cautionary discharge instructions, corticosteroids to prevent a late-phase reaction, and close follow-up. In the absence of contraindications, patients should also be given a prescription for an epinephrine injector and instructions on how to use it. However, the subset of these patients with significant pre-existing comorbidities (e.g., advanced age, cardiopulmonary disease) should probably be admitted for observation. In addition, some experts suggest admitting any patient who requires multiple doses of epinephrine, regardless of response to therapy.

All other patients with anaphylactic syndromes should be admitted for observation.

For all discharged patients, the prevention of future allergic reactions should be stressed. The patient should be urged to remove inciting antigens from their environment. This may require a physician's note to an employer to request that the patient be allowed to avoid a workplace antigen. In certain cases, where desensitization for unavoidable antigens may be necessary, referral to an allergist is appropriate. Finally, the inciting antigen (if known) should be well-documented in the patient's medical record, especially if the antigen is a medication or latex.

Pearls, pitfalls, and myths

Pitfalls

- Failure to recognize the subtle early presentation of anaphylaxis.

Table 11.3 Anaphylactic syndrome drug dosages

Drug	Adult dose	Pediatric dose
Parenteral adrenergic agents		
Epinephrine	0.3–0.5 mg 1 : 1000 solution IM or SC q 15 minutes 0.1 mg 1 : 10,000 solution slow IV push	0.01 mg/kg (minimum 0.1 ml) 1 : 1000 solution SC q 15 minutes 1 mcg/kg (minimum 0.1 ml) 1 : 10,000 solution slow IV push
Epinephrine (intravenous) infusion	1–10 mcg/minute titrate to effect	0.1–1.0 mcg/kg/minute titrate to effect
Inhaled β-agonists		
Albuterol	0.5 ml 0.5% solution in 2.5 ml NS nebulized q 15 minutes	0.03–0.05 ml/kg 0.5% solution in 2.5 ml NS via nebulizer q 15 minutes
H₁-receptor blockers		
Diphenhydramine (Benadryl)	25–50 mg IV/IM q 4–6 hours 50 mg PO q 4–6 hours	1–2 mg/kg IV/IM q 4–6 hours 2 mg/kg PO q 4–6 hours
H₂-receptor blockers		
Ranitidine (Zantac)	50 mg IV over 5 minutes 150 mg PO bid	0.5 mg/kg IV over 5 minutes 0.25–2 mg/kg/dose PO q 12 hours (maximum of 150 mg q 12 hours)
Cimetidine (Tagamet)	300 mg PO/IV/IM q 6 hours	Not recommended for children
Corticosteroids		
Methylprednisolone (Solu-Medrol)	40–250 mg IV/IM q 6 hours	1–2 mg/kg IV/IM q 6 hours
Prednisone	20–60 mg PO qd	1 mg/kg PO qd
Antidote, refractory hypotension		
Glucagon	1 mg IV q 6 minutes until hypotension resolves, followed by 5–15 mcg/minute infusion	Dosing not definitively established

BID: two times a day; IM: intramuscular; IV: intravenous; NS: normal saline; PO: per os; QD: four times a day; SC: subcutaneous.

- Failure to recognize the need for acute and definitive airway management.
- Failure to administer epinephrine early in the patient's treatment.
- Failure to recognize the contraindications for RSI in anaphylaxis patients.
- Failure to anticipate difficulties in the treatment of patients taking β-blockers.
- Failure to observe patients for an adequate length of time.
- Failure to admit high-risk patients.
- Failure to anticipate the possibility of a biphasic allergic reaction.
- Failure to appropriately administer and prescribe corticosteroids.
- Failure to counsel the patient to avoid antigen triggers.
- Failure to prescribe an epinephrine injector for susceptible patients and to properly instruct them regarding its use.

Myths

- Patients with anaphylaxis always look sick on initial presentation.
- Airway compromise always follows a linear time course.
- Antihistamine agents are first-line treatments for anaphylaxis.
- Once patients get better, they never relapse.
- If the patient does not react immediately after exposure to an antigen, they cannot have a significant anaphylactic reaction.

References

1. Bochner BS, Lichtenstein LM. Anaphylaxis. *New Eng J Med* 1991;324:1785–1790.
2. Brown AFT. Therapeutic controversies in the management of acute anaphylaxis. *J Accid Emerg Med* 1997;15:89–95.
3. Freeman TM. Anaphylaxis diagnosis and treatment. *Primary Care* 1998;25:809–817.
4. Gordon BR. Prevention and management of office allergy emergencies. *Otolaryn Clin North Am* 1994;25:119–134.
5. Heilborn H, et al. Comparison of subcutaneous injection and high-dose inhalation of epinephrine. Implications for self-treatment to prevent anaphylaxis. *J Allergy Clin Immunol* 1986;78:1174–1179.
6. Jacobs RL, Rake Jr GW, Fournier DC, et al. Potentiated anaphylaxis in patients with drug-induced beta-adrenergic blockade. *J Allergy Clin Immunol* 1992;92:277–296.
7. Joint Task Force on Practice Parameters. The diagnosis and management of anaphylaxis. *J Allergy Clin Immunol* 1998;101:S465–S528.
8. Land GM. Anaphylactoid and anaphylactic reactions: hazards of beta-blockers. *Drug Safety* 1995;12:299–304.
9. Lip GYH, Metcalfe MJ. Adrenaline in allergic emergencies. *Br Med J* 1992;304:1443.
10. Lin RY, et al. Improved outcomes in patients with acute allergic syndromes who are treated with combined H1 and H2 antagonists. *Ann Emerg Med* 2000;36:462–468.
11. Metcalf DD. Acute anaphylaxis and urticaria in children and adults. In: Schocket AL (ed.). *Clinical Management of Urticaria and Anaphylaxis*. New York: Marcel Dekker, 1992. pp. 70–96.
12. Portier P, Richet C. D l'action anaphylactique de certains venins. *C R Soc Biol* (Paris) 1902;54:170–172.
13. Roberts-Thomson P, Heddle R, Kupa A. Adrenaline and anaphylaxis. *Med J Aust* 1985;142:708.
14. Sampson HA. Fatal food-induced anaphylaxis. *Allergy* 1988;53:125–130.
15. Sim, TC. Anaphylaxis: how to manage and prevent this medical emergency. *Postgrad Med* 1992;92:277–296.
16. Smith GB, Taylor BI. Adrenaline in allergic emergencies. *Br Med J* 1992:304:1635.
17. Soto-Aguilar MC, deShazo RD, Waring NP. Anaphylaxis: why it happens and what to do about it. *Postgrad Med* 1987;82:154–170.
18. Sullivan TJ. Cardiac disorders in penicillin-induced anaphylaxis. Association with intravenous epinephrine therapy. *JAMA* 1982;248:2161–2162.
19. Terr AI. Anaphylaxis. *Clin Rev Allergy* 1985;3:3–23.
20. Valentine MD, Sheffer AL. The anaphylactic syndromes. *Med Clin North Am* 1969;53:249–257.
21. Winberry SL, Lieberman P. Anaphylaxis. *Immunol Allergy Clin North Am* 1995;15:447–477.

12 Altered mental status

Barry Simon, MD **and Flavia Nobay,** MD

Scope of the problem

The patient with altered mental status (AMS) represents a great challenge for emergency physicians: potential life threat, rapid decision-making and astute detective work. The etiology might be chronic or acute, life-threatening or benign, reversible or irreversible. One of nearly a dozen different organ systems might be implicated or perhaps harmed by the event. The knowledgeable, diligent emergency physician will be able to narrow the differential to a manageable number of diagnoses within minutes and correctly treat the majority of patients.

Terminology

AMS is an alteration of a patient's level of cognitive (knowledge-related) ability, appearance, emotional mood, and speech and thought patterns.

Level of consciousness relates to one's level of awareness and responsiveness to his or her surroundings.

Lethargy is generally referred to when one is suffering from a mild to moderate depression in level of consciousness. It implies an abnormal state of drowsiness or sleepiness in which it may be difficult to arouse the patient.

Stupor is a more profound depression of one's level of consciousness. One might say that stupor is an extreme form of lethargy requiring a greater stimulus to produce a lesser degree of arousal.

Coma is an abnormal state of deep unconsciousness from which a patient cannot be awakened.

Organic illness refers to impairment of normal anatomic and/or physiological activity resulting in impaired mental functioning. *Functional illness* generally refers to a physical disorder with no known or detectable organic basis to explain the symptoms.

Delirium is an acute confusional state with an organic etiology. The key to this definition is that there is an alteration in both the level and the content of consciousness. Unrecognized delirium can result in significant morbidity and mortality. If treated, it is reversible in the majority of cases.

Dementia is an insidious deterioration of higher cortical function with an organic etiology. In distinct contrast to delirium, affected patients will have a normal level of consciousness. Although acute insults and deterioration in mental status may be reversible, underlying dementia is rarely completely corrected.

Acute psychosis is the functional disease that needs to be distinguished from delirium and dementia. Loss of the ability to distinguish reality from fantasy is the hallmark of psychosis. It can be very difficult to distinguish an acutely psychotic patient from one who is delirious.

Abulic state (akinetic mutism) is the inability to respond or act. For example, responsiveness may be so depressed in a patient with frontal lobe dysfunction that it may take the patient several minutes to answer a question.

Locked-in syndrome from destruction of pontine motor tracts may leave the patient unable to respond, except for the ability to move the eyes in upward gaze.

Psychogenic unresponsiveness is a form of functional, nonphysiologic unresponsiveness.

Delirium vs. dementia vs. acute psychosis

The emergency physician must make a concerted effort to identify patients who are delirious. The distinction can be difficult to make but may be critical to the ultimate well-being of the patient. The etiologies of delirium are extensive, and many of the causes have the potential for serious morbidity or mortality. Distinguishing features between these three conditions are identified in Table 12.1.

Anatomic essentials

Arousal requires a healthy functioning reticular activating system (RAS) and cerebral cortex. The midbrain portion of the reticular system is the key and may be viewed as a driving center for the higher structures; loss of the midbrain reticular formation (MRF) produces a state in which the

Table 12.1 Delirium vs. dementia vs. acute psychosis

	Delirium	Dementia	Acute psychosis
Definition	Acute confusional state	Insidious deterioration in higher cortical functions	Loss of the ability to distinguish reality from imaginary
Organic vs. functional	Organic disease	Organic disease	Functional disease
Onset/course	Hours to days Fluctuating course	Months Progressive course	Hours to days Stable course
Level of consciousness	Altered	Normal	Normal
Hallucinations	Visual – common	None	Auditory – common
Orientation	Altered	Altered	Normal
Vital signs	Widely variable and fluctuating	Normal	Variable
Miscellaneous	Extreme agitation is common Reversible in >80%	Consider medications, thyroid disease and infections as a cause for exacerbations	Fixed delusions First attack common in patients <40 years old

cortex appears to be waiting for the command to function. This ascending midbrain reticular activating system extends upward into the hypothalamus to the thalamus. It is stimulated by every major somatic and sensory pathway, directly or indirectly. Awareness and arousal also depend on the proper functioning of the cerebral cortex. Unconsciousness will result if there is severe disruption of anatomic or physiologic functioning of either the MRF or both cerebral hemispheres. These critical structures may be compromised by structural, chemical or infectious etiologies. Unilateral insults to the cerebral cortex will not result in unconsciousness unless the brainstem is also affected.

History

What is/was the timing and course of events since the onset of change in mental status or level of consciousness?

A critical distinction between dementia and delirium is the time course. Therefore, this is a key question for the patient and family member(s). Dementia is generally insidious in onset compared with delirium, which is acute and dramatic. With respect to acute psychosis vs. delirium, the distinction is less clear. However, patients suffering from a state of delirium will often have a waxing and waning course compared with the continuous nature of functional disease.

What methods can the physician use to help overcome the inability to obtain a detailed history from the patient?

As with most medical problems, the quality of the history will often dictate the success and timeliness of the emergency department (ED) evaluation. One of the major inherent difficulties in the evaluation of patients with AMS is the inability to get a meaningful and reliable history from the patient. All other sources for recent and past medical history must be tapped: paramedics, relatives, friends, medic alert tag, wallet, personal physician, hospital records, pill bottles, etc. Social services support may be critical in the search for information about these patients. In addition to recent history, the importance of obtaining past medical history (including suicidal ideation/suicide attempts), current medications and social history (substance abuse) cannot be overemphasized.

Physical examination
Vital signs

A thorough physical examination along with rapid bedside tests may be more enlightening than with many other problems that present to the ED. The five vital signs may offer a number of important clues. The respiratory rate and pattern may suggest an intracranial pathology or an acid–base disorder. The heart rate, rhythm, and electrocardiogram (ECG) findings can offer a number of clues about toxins (digoxin, tricyclic antidepressants (TCAs), beta blockers), metabolic derangements (high or low calcium or potassium) or closed head injury with deep inverted T waves. An elevated temperature can lead one to an infectious etiology or, if pathologically high ($\geq$106 °F), may suggest heat stroke or an intracranial process. Elevated blood pressure, a widened pulse pressure (systolic minus diastolic pressure) and slow heart rate (Cushing reflex) may be consistent with elevated intracranial pressure. Pulse oximetry may direct the practitioner to focus on causes of hypoxia and whether or not low oxygenation relates to the patient's overall presentation.

Head, ears, eyes, nose and throat

There are a number of components of the general physical examination that are particularly helpful. *Breath odor* can quickly clue one to the presence of diabetic ketoacidosis (DKA), liver failure (fetor hepaticus) or a number of toxins, such as alcohol, insecticides (onion odor), paint or glue, gasoline, cyanide (bitter almonds) and arsenic (garlic). The head needs to be examined for signs of acute or recent trauma (hemotympanum, cephalohematoma, cerebral spinal fluid (CSF) leak, Battle's sign, raccoon eyes) and for past surgery (shunt, cranial defect).

Eyes

The pupillary exam is an essential part of the physical examination, as it can provide information about structural and metabolic abnormalities. One must look for pupillary size and the presence of asymmetry. Examining the direct and consensual response to light will determine the integrity of the afferent function of the optic nerve. A unilateral dilated pupil in an altered patient is secondary to herniation until proven otherwise (Figure 12.1). The mass causing the pathology is usually on the same side as the dilated pupil, as demonstrated in the figure. In the awake, alert patient, the only life-threatening cause for a unilateral dilated pupil is compression of cranial nerve III by a mass such as a posterior communicating aneurysm. There are a number of other causes for pupillary dilation that are not serious (traumatic mydriasis, intentional or accidental topical medications, Adie's pupil, anisocoria). Bilateral pupillary constriction (pinpoint pupils) may represent an opiate overdose or pontine lesion.

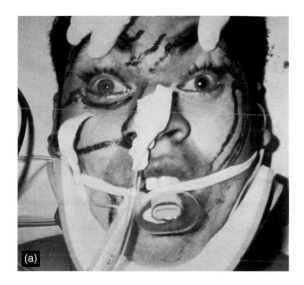

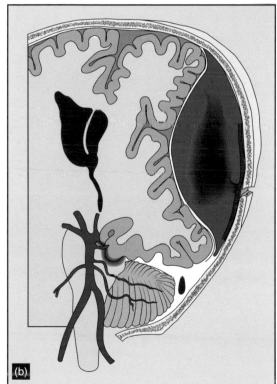

Figure 12.1
(a) Photograph of patient with transtentorial herniation from blunt head trauma. The right pupil is constricted normally; the patient's left pupil is fixed and dilated. (b) Illustration of an epidural hematoma with acute mass effect and compression of the ipsilateral cerebral peduncle resulting in uncal herniation. Reproduced from D. Mandavia et al, *Color Atlas of Emergency Trauma*, Cambridge, Cambridge University Press, 2003.

The *fundoscopic examination* is a critical, often underutilized component of the eye examination. Flame hemorrhages are characteristic of hypertensive bleeds. Increased intracranial pressure will produce changes associated with papilledema (Figure 12.2), in which the disc margins of the optic nerve are not sharp. Early, more subtle findings of increased intracranial pressure include absent venous pulsations, although this is not specific. Eventually, the findings will include blurred disc margins and engorged vessels. Fundoscopic changes associated with diabetes (neovascularization, hemorrhages, exudates) or with methanol ingestion (optic disc hyperemia

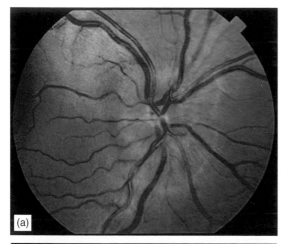
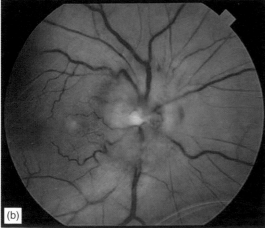

Figure 12.2
(a) Early papilledema with disc elevation, blurring of the margins, hyperemia, and venous engorgement in the right eye. (b) Acute papilledema with increased elevation and hemorrhages on the disc surface in the right eye. Reproduced with permission from Tasman W et al. Wills Eye Hospital Atlas of Clinical Ophthalmology, 2 ed., Lippincott Williams & Wilkins, 2001.

and retinal edema) may provide clues to the cause of the patient's altered level of consciousness.

Eye movements are generally more helpful than commonly thought. Assuming the brainstem is intact, most comatose patients exhibit slowly roving eye movements. In contrast, malingering or hysterical patients feigning coma have spontaneous eye movements that tend to be rapid and rigid. It is important to note that if both eyes cross midline, the brainstem is intact. When the eyes are fixed in one direction, commonly they will "look" toward the side of a hemorrhage or away from a destructive lesion.

Eyelid tone may help to differentiate organic disease from hysteria. Hysterical patients may offer some resistance to the examiner's attempt to open the eyes. They tend to close the lids quickly. "Fluttering" eyelids are commonly seen in patients who are feigning unresponsiveness. Patients with organic coma offer no resistance to lid opening, and then close the lids slowly and incompletely. Unilateral ptosis may be seen in patients with a third cranial nerve palsy or when there is disruption of the sympathetic chain in association with a *Horner's syndrome*.

The *oculocephalic reflex (doll's eyes)* (Figure 12.3) depends upon the medial longitudinal fasciculus (MLF), which receives constant input about the patient's head position from the semicircular canals. Without cortical input, the eyes are typically directed straight ahead and remain fixed in the orbit as the head is turned. The oculocephalic reflex is elicited by rotating the head briskly from side to side. If the brainstem is intact, the eyes deviate opposite to the direction of the rotation of the head (head rotated right, eyes deviate left). Confusion often arises because the patient's eyes continue to look straight ahead. In other words, they remain focused in the same direction, possibly giving one the impression that they did not move. The examiner needs to remember that in order for the eyes to remain fixed in a given direction when the head is turned, the eyes had to move. Cervical spine injury must be excluded before performing this maneuver.

Oculovestibular testing (cold calorics) (Figure 12.4) is another underutilized ED maneuver which can yield important clinical information about the integrity of the brain and the brainstem. The test is performed by positioning the patient supine with the head elevated 30° in order to isolate the input of the horizontal semicircular canals. 10–20 cc of ice-cold water or saline are injected into the auditory canal. Cooling of the mastoid bone causes alteration in endolymphatic flow

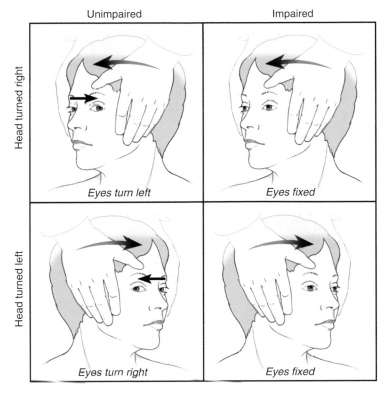

Figure 12.3
Oculocephalic reflex (Doll's eyes).

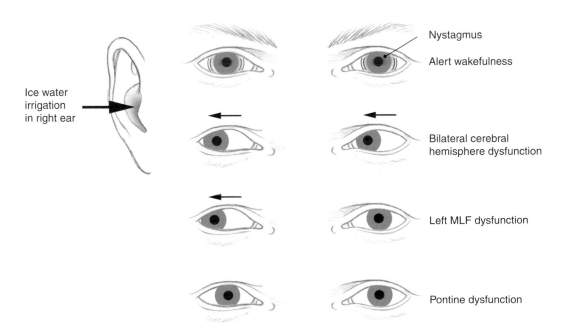

Figure 12.4
Oculovestibular testing (cold calorics). MLF: medial longitudinal fasciculus.

within the canals. Information is then transmitted to vestibular nuclei and pontine gaze centers, triggering the eye movements.

If the practitioner always uses cold water and remembers three points described in Table 12.2 and Figure 12.4, the examination can be extremely helpful.

Table 12.2 Cold calorics

Response	Interpretation
Both eyes deviate, nystagmus (slow phase toward stimulus, fast back to midline)	Patient is not comatose
Both eyes tonically deviate toward cold water	Coma, but intact brainstem
No eye movement or movement only of eye ipsilateral to the stimulus	Brainstem damage Internuclear ophthalmoplegia (brain-stem structural lesion)

Neck

The neck must be examined for the presence of nuchal rigidity (meningismus) that often occurs when the meninges become inflamed by blood or infection. Thyroid or parathyroid disease may be the cause for an alteration in mental status or level of consciousness. The neck should be examined for an enlarged thyroid or the presence of a surgical scar suggesting previous thyroid or parathyroid surgery.

Pulmonary

Hypoxia and hypercarbia are uncommon causes of an altered level of consciousness. However, findings consistent with severe lung disease and respiratory distress should raise consideration for these entities. One must look for the barrel chest of the patient with emphysema, wheezing and a prolonged expiratory phase in patients with obstructive lung disease, and for evidence of consolidation in those with pneumonia.

Cardiac

The cardiovascular system is rarely the primary source for mental status changes. Yet dysrhythmias,

valvular heart disease and severe heart failure can be implicated. The heart should be examined for the presence of an irregular rhythm and for extra heart sounds including an S3, murmurs and/or rubs.

Abdomen

A thorough abdominal examination should be performed to look for signs of infection, organomegaly, mass or obstruction. Any cause of abdominal infection can lead to an alteration in consciousness, especially in elderly patients. Localized tenderness, absent bowel sounds, rebound tenderness and rigidity are all signs of a serious intra-abdominal infection. Liver failure is a common cause of altered consciousness. An enlarged liver or a small, hard nodular liver may be noted during examination. Late findings of catastrophic abdominal processes such as pancreatitis and ruptured abdominal aortic aneurysm include periumbilical ecchymosis (Cullen's sign) and flank ecchymosis (Grey Turner's sign).

Rectal

Rectal examination may identify a mass suggestive of a malignancy or melena associated with an upper gastrointestinal bleed.

Skin

The skin is an often underappreciated component of the physical examination. Signs of local or systemic disease may be found. Skin temperature and state of hydration offer clues about infection, blood sugar (moist with low glucose and dry with elevated blood glucose) and some toxins (cholinergic and anticholinergic agents). The brow covered with "uremic frost" may suggest renal disease. Spider angiomas, palmar erythema and jaundice may be present in patients with long-term liver disease. Hypothyroid patients will often develop coarse dry hair, thinning of the lateral aspect of the eyebrows and dry, rough, pale skin. Needle tracks, petechiae and other rashes may often be significant clues of underlying disease processes.

Neurologic

The neurologic examination for patients with AMS must be thorough. This part of the examination begins with observation. *Automatisms*

Table 12.3 Progressive brainstem dysfunction – rostral caudal progression with increasing pressure

Level of lesion	Respiratory pattern	Other
Early brainstem compression	Cheyne-Stokes	Small but reactive pupils Plantar reflex becomes extensor
Midbrain and upper pons	Central neurogenic hyperventilation	Dilated nonreactive pupils Will see spontaneous decerebrate posturing
Pons and upper medulla	Quiet respirations – normal rate	Loss of Doll's eyes + Cushing reflex No response to painful stimuli
Medulla	Slow irregular respirations leading to apnea	Widely dilated, fixed pupils, hypotension

(involuntary acts carried out as protective mechanisms) such as yawning, hiccups, sneezing and swallowing may be present with brainstem or frontal lobe pathology. Respiratory patterns (central neurogenic hyperventilation, apneustic, Cheyne-Stokes, ataxic) are suggestive of lesions at various levels of the brainstem (Table 12.3). The key is to recognize an abnormal respiratory pattern, not remembering the exact level of the brainstem that may be implicated. Body posture is also important, and will be discussed in the section on the motor examination.

Mental status assessment

Glasgow Coma Scale (GCS): This is a fifteen point scale developed to assess head-injured patients; however, it is commonly used to communicate the mental status of a patient or compare the mental status of a patient at different periods of time. The lowest score you can receive is three. The score is calculated by assigning the number associated with the patient's best response (Table 12.4).

Table 12.4 Glasgow coma scale

Eye	Verbal	Motor
4 Spontaneous	5 Oriented	6 Obeys
3 Command	4 Confused	5 Localizes
2 Pain	3 Inappropriate	4 Withdraws
1 None	2 Incomprehensible	3 Flexion posture
	1 None	2 Extension posture
		1 None

AVPU: This simplified 4-part scale is used to describe the patient's level of consciousness (Table 12.5).

Table 12.5 AVPU

A	Awake and aware
V	Responds to verbal stimuli
P	Responds to noxious stimuli (Noxious is defined as stimulus that is potentially or actually damaging the body tissue. Typical maneuvers used in the ED include forcefully grinding the knuckles of one's fist into the sternum or squeezing two toes together while a firm object is wedged between them)
U	Unresponsive

Orientation assessment: Person, place and time.
Memory: Test short-term memory by asking the patient to remember three common objects and recall them 3 minutes later.
Specific mental status examinations: Two tests have been developed and studied to assist nonpsychiatrists in the evaluation of mental status. Both tests are easy to perform and are accurate with a high degree of interobserver reliability. The mini-mental status examination (MMSE) is an excellent test, but is geared mostly toward the evaluation of dementia and content of thinking. The best bedside test looking for the presence of delirium is the confusion assessment method (CAM).

The astute physician will perform the CAM while observing the patient's responses during the history and physical examination. The practitioner needs to pay attention to the patient's thinking, communication skills and level of consciousness to complete the assessment. The patient is considered delirious if he or she has an acute onset illness with a fluctuating course, disorganized thinking or altered level of consciousness, and easy distractability. Being easily distracted refers to the patient who interrupts the history and physical examination by striking up a conversation with other patients or health care providers, or by changing the focus to items on the walls, etc. The patient with disorganized thinking will communicate with disconnected sentences or will change topics from moment to moment, making it difficult or impossible to follow the line of thinking.

CAM: To diagnose delirium:

1. Acute onset with a fluctuating course and
2. Easily distracted, inattentive
   And
3. Altered level of consciousness or
4. Disorganized thinking.

A positive test includes numbers 1 AND 2 plus number 3 OR 4.

Cranial nerves (CNs) must be tested as part of a thorough neurologic examination. Portions of this examination were completed during the evaluation of the eye. The other CNs must be tested to complete the examination and help localize any lesions that may be present.

Motor/sensory testing is performed to look at tone, focality, and for signs of herniation. Determining the extent or severity of alteration of consciousness is aided by evaluating motor responses to verbal and painful stimuli. Purposeful movements indicate a functioning brainstem and cerebral cortex. Posturing may be apparent in the presence of a diffuse metabolic or toxic insult or secondary to herniation. *Decorticate posturing* (flexion of arms and hyperextension of legs), *decerebrate posturing* (arms and legs extended and internally rotated), or both may occur as herniation progresses, or both may occur as herniation progresses. Assessment of motor tone may be helpful by suggesting an acute cardiovascular accident (CVA) or cord injury if tone is absent. Focality identified on the motor or sensory examination may help identify the level of a cord lesion or confirm that the insult is in the brain. Tone may be increased by the presence of various toxins or neuroleptic malignant syndrome (NMS). Keep in mind that severe hypothermia, massive overdose of sedatives or hypnotics, hypoglycemia and the postictal state can mimic structural neurological diseases.

Reflexes may be helpful to localize the level of lesion or to place the insult in the central or the peripheral nervous system. Symmetry of responsiveness is the key to assessment of deep tendon reflexes. The plantar (Babinski) reflex becomes abnormal in many patients with upper motor neuron pathology, especially related to the corticospinal tracts. The response is abnormal if the big toe dorsiflexes and the other toes fan outward. This response is also significant if it is present and asymmetric.

Differential diagnosis

During the evaluation of patients with AMS, the process of generating and eliminating diagnostic possibilities evolves. The diagnostic possibilities are so numerous and broad that even experienced practitioners need to be organized and systematic in their approach. *It is imperative to develop a process that works for you and to use it routinely.* Many physicians like to use mnemonics to help them focus the broad differential. One commonly-used mnemonic for the altered patient is AEIOU TIPS (Table 12.6). Start from the head and progress down the body, considering diagnostic possibilities that may be associated with each anatomic part and system as they are encountered. The head-to-toe approach is intuitive, simple to remember and apply, and is nearly 100% inclusive (Table 12.7).

Table 12.6 Mnemonic for ALOC differential diagnosis

AEIOU TIPS
A: Alcohol, other toxins, drugs
E: Endocrine, electrolytes
I: Insulin (diabetes)
O: Oxygen, opiates
U: Uremia (renal, including HTN)
T: Trauma, temperature
I: Infection
P: Psychiatric, porphyria
S: Subarachnoid hemorrhage, space-occupying lesion
ALOC: altered level of consciousness; HTN: hypertension.

Table 12.7 Differential diagnosis of altered mental status

Head

1. Supratentorial
   (a) Unilateral hemispheric disease with herniation
      – Abscess
      – Hemorrhage (including traumatic)
      – Infarction
      – Tumor (primary or metastatic)
   (b) Concussion/contusion
   (c) Meningitis/encephalitis
   (d) Seizure (postictal period)/
      nonconvulsive status
   (e) Subarachnoid hemorrhage
   (f) Cerebral vascular accident
   (g) Wernicke's encephalopathy
   (h) Functional (psychiatric)
2. Infratentorial
   (a) Basilar artery occlusion
   (b) Brainstem tumors
   (c) Cerebellar hemorrhage
   (d) Pontine hemorrhage
   (e) Traumatic posterior fossa hemorrhage

Mouth

1. Odors – burns
2. Toxins – medications
3. Toxins – drugs
   (a) Alcohols
   (b) Anticholinergics
   (c) Anticonvulsants
   (d) Barbiturates
   (e) Carbon monoxide
   (f) Cyanide
   (g) Hallucinogens
   (h) Heavy metals
   (i) Opiates
   (j) Phenothiazines
   (k) Salicylates
   (l) Sedative/hypnotics
   (m) Sympathomimetics
   (n) Tricyclic antidepressants

Neck

1. Thyroid disease
   (a) Hyperthyroidism (thyroid bruits, tender goiter, tender neck mass)
   (b) Hypothyroidism (goiter)
   (c) Post-operative endocrinopathies

Chest/heart

1. Hypoxia
2. Hypercarbia
3. Congestive heart failure (CHF)
4. Pulmonary emboli
5. Murmurs
6. Rhythm disturbances

Abdomen

1. Liver – Hepatic encephalopathy
2. Kidney – Renal insufficiency and electrolyte abnormalities
3. Adrenal insufficiency (endocrinopathies)
4. Pancreas (diabetes – hyper- or hypoglycemia)

5. Peritonitis
   (a) Choleycystitis
   (b) Appendicitis
   (c) Spontaneous bacterial peritonitis
   (d) Perforated viscus

Abdomen – vascular

1. Mesenteric ischemia
2. Abdominal aortic aneurysm

Skin

1. Temperature – hypothermia, heat stroke
2. Color – liver failure, renal failure, hypoxia
3. Rash – vasculitis, thrombotic thrombocytopenic purpura (TTP), toxic shock and endocarditis

Others

1. Sepsis
2. Hyperviscosity syndromes

Diagnostic testing

Laboratory and radiographic testing of unstable, critically-ill or confused patients comes in two forms. The first group of helpful tests are those that can be completed in 10 minutes or less. The vast majority of patients presenting with AMS can have a presumptive diagnosis made by the time the history, physical examination, and rapid tests are complete. The following tests yield a tremendous amount of useful information, are inexpensive and can be completed in less than 10 minutes. They are not arranged in any particular order:

1. Glucose (dextrostick or glucometer).
2. Pulse oximetry (hypoxia).
3. Hematocrit (blood loss).
4. Breathalyzer (ethanol).
5. Urinalysis (infection, hyperglycemia, ketosis, dehydration, toxicology).
6. Arterial blood gas (acidosis, hypercarbia, hypoxemia).
7. ECG – monitor (electrolyte abnormalities, toxins, acute cardiac disease).

Other tests to consider:

1. Complete blood count, electrolytes (particularly important is the sodium), blood urea nitrogen (BUN), creatinine (Cr), serum osmolality, calcium and magnesium.
2. Carboxyhemoglobin level.
3. Directed drug screen.
4. Head computerized tomography (CT): done before lumbar puncture (LP) to rule out focal lesions and hemorrhage.

5. LP with CSF analysis.
6. Peritoneal tap.
7. Thyroid function studies.
8. Cervical spine X-rays if trauma cannot be excluded.
9. Chest X-ray.
10. Electroencephalograph (EEG).

General treatment principles

As with all ED patients, treatment begins with the airway, breathing and circulation (ABCs). The main goals of treatment are physiologic stabilization, symptom relief and specific diagnosis-driven treatment plans. The first four recommendations are commonly referred to by the acronym *DON'T* (dextrose, oxygen, naloxone and thiamine).

Dextrose

Dextrose should be administered if glucose testing indicates hypoglycemia. Glucometers are very reliable and rarely miss true hypoglycemia. One ampule of D50 (25 gm of glucose) will raise the serum glucose by about 130 mg/dl (the range is from 30–300 mg/dl). Administer 50 ml of 50% dextrose intravenous (IV) in adults, 4 ml/kg 25% dextrose (0.5–1.0 g/kg) IV in children and 5 ml/kg 10% dextrose (0.5 g/kg) IV in neonates.

Oxygen

Oxygen levels should be checked on all patients with AMS. This can be obtained on most patients by pulse oximetry. Supplemental oxygenation via nasal cannula or face mask is desirable, especially for those patients with oxygen saturations less than 92%.

Naloxone

Naloxone is relatively benign and should be considered in all hypoventilating, altered patients with evidence of opioid ingestion. Naltrexone is a long-acting narcotic antagonist. Its role in the ED is limited because of the risk of sending patients home who may have ingested longer-acting narcotics; these patients may decompensate after discharge. The standard dose of naloxone is 2 mg IV in adults and 0.1 mg/kg IV in children. One can partially reverse the effects of a narcotic ingestion with small aliquots of naloxone in the range of 0.1 to 0.4 mg IV. In contrast, the ingestion of some of the synthetic opioids and combination medications, such as diphenoxylate/atropine, methadone, propoxyphene, and pentazocine may require as much as 10 mg of naloxone to reverse.

Thiamine

Thiamine administration should be considered in all patients with altered consciousness unless the cause is known. Thiamine is a safe, effective and inexpensive treatment for Wernicke's encephalopathy. This thiamine depletion-induced encephalopathy is characterized by the abrupt onset of oculomotor disturbances, ataxia and confusion. If not treated promptly, it may progress to irreversible Korsakoff's psychosis (confabulation, retrograde amnesia, and impaired ability to learn). Although Wernicke's encephalopathy is rare, it is reversible if recognized and treated early. Physicians must remember that alcoholism is not the only cause of thiamine deficiency. Patients are at risk for Wernicke's if they have any cause of malnutrition or vitamin deficiency. Causes include hyperalimentation, anorexia, bulimia, pregnancy and malignancy. Adminster 100 mg IV in adults and 10–25 mg IV in children.

Volume repletion

Many altered patients are dehydrated because of prolonged agitation and excessive stimulation over hours to days. Care must be taken as diseases such as renal failure or water intoxication may produce delirium in volume-overloaded patients.

Temperature control

Fever may be a manifestation of a disease process, and can contribute to ongoing cell damage. Whether fever is secondary to heat stroke, sepsis, aspirin toxicity or drug overdose, it should be treated with appropriate interventions. One may use ibuprofen or acetaminophen, cooling blankets, wet sheets with a fan, or ice packs in the axillae or groin to reduce temperature elevations.

Flumazenil

Flumazenil is a competitive benzodiazepine antagonist. Independently, the drug is benign. Its use is limited in emergency medicine practice because blocking benzodiazepines from their receptor sites can unmask epileptogenic potential. Patients addicted to benzodiazepines may seize from this pharmacologically-induced withdrawal state. Patients who ingested drugs or medications that can cause seizures along with benzodiazepines may seize once the "protective" effect of the benzodiazepines has been removed. Yet flumazenil may serve a diagnostic and therapeutic role in selected cases. Administration of flumazenil may awaken patients who may have ingested benzodiazepines, preventing unnecessary endotracheal intubation. It may also eliminate the need for expensive testing and possible admission. The risk of causing seizures may be ameliorated by titrating the dose of flumazenil; using the smallest dose recommended in increments may decrease the chance of seizure. One should not eliminate flumazenil from the arsenal of critical care medications solely based on the risk of seizures. As with all medications, the risks and benefits must be carefully considered before its administration. The dose of flumazenil is 0.2–1.0 mg IV in adults.

Physostigmine

Physostigmine is a cholinergic drug that can diagnose and treat overdoses of anticholinergic substances and agents with anticholinergic-like properties. The goal of physostigmine administration is to reverse the patient's anticholinergic signs and symptoms. Physostigmine is administered IV in small 0.5 mg aliquots up to a maximum total of 2.0 mg. End points of administration include clear reversal of anticholinergic signs and symptoms, the development of cholinergic symptoms (salivation, lacrimation, defecation, gastric irritation, emesis), or delivery of 2.0 mg of drug. Physostigmine must be used with great caution; many centers do not use this drug at all. When administered to patients who have co-ingested agents that cause myocardial depression (such as tricyclic antidepressants), the result can be cardiac standstill. If used, the dose of physostigmine is 0.5–2.0 mg IV in adults.

Antibiotics

Antibiotics are indicated in patients with a suspected infectious cause for their AMS. When considered, these drugs should be administered early in the ED course, often before a source of infection is clearly identified. Infections implicated include the urinary tract, lungs, skin, genitalia, or meninges. The choice and dose of antibiotic must be directed by the organisms suspected. Blood and urine cultures should be obtained prior to the administration of antibiotics.

However, in suspected meningitis, it is recommended that antibiotics be administered immediately before performing the LP.

Others

The myriad of possible etiologies for AMS preclude a discussion of all the possible treatments. The potential exists to prepare the patient for neurosurgery, to treat significant metabolic abnormalities, begin treating thyroid dysfunction, or to support the patient until drugs are metabolized or the postictal period passes. Specific antidotes and treatment for drug ingestions are discussed in greater detail in Chapter 36.

Special patients
Geriatric

The geriatric population is at special risk for alterations of mentation for a myriad of reasons. Some studies indicated that 40% of all geriatric patients over 70 years have some degree of AMS. Of these, approximately 25% had alterations in their level of consciousness, 25% had delirium and 50% had cognitive impairment. The most common cause of AMS was multifactorial, followed by medication (22–39% of all cases), infection, metabolic disturbance (such as diabetes mellitus), trauma, neoplasm, cardiovascular disease, pain, and dehydration/nutritional abnormalities. Not surprisingly, in addition to the predisposition of being altered for a given physiological alteration, elderly patients had greater morbidity and mortality compared to younger populations. Acute confusional states are more likely to herald an infectious process in the elderly than the classic symptoms of fever, pain and tachycardia seen commonly in younger patients.

Pediatric

In contrast to the elderly, children and infants with AMS usually present with treatable causes that often lead to favorable outcomes. The most common cause of the altered pediatric patient is toxicologic in nature. The critical factors in pediatric patients are early detection and prompt treatment with gut decontamination and antidotes. Other causes of coma in children include infections, trauma, metabolic derangements and child abuse. Complications unique to pediatrics need to be recognized and anticipated. For example, unlike in adults, hypoglycemia and metabolic derangements are commonly seen following beta-blocker ingestions, exposure to alcohols and perfumes. Failure to consider the unique causes of hypoglycemia in children could lead the provider down the wrong treatment algorithm.

Immune compromised

The immunocompromised altered patient can be a medical quagmire. This patient population includes those with malignancies, immunosuppressive therapies, and immunocompromising diseases such as acquired immune deficiency syndrome (AIDS). Not only are these patients at risk for greater complications of any given disease, but they also are at risk for pathology not seen in the usual clinical setting. For instance, toxoplasmosis in the HIV+ patient is a serious condition that may present with subtle findings, making it difficult to diagnose. Other central nervous system (CNS) diseases and organisms that threaten this patient population, commonly causing altered levels of consciousness include cryptococcus, cytomegolovirus, herpes simplex, bacterial infections and CNS malignancies such as lymphoma. It is important to remember that significant chronic illness and IV drug use also predispose individuals to opportunistic infections. History taking must include meticulous attention to medication lists – both prescribed and over the counter, recent changes in diet (increased protein in renal dialysis patients) and environmental exposures, as these are critical in the evaluation of the altered immunocompromised patient.

Disposition

Altered mental status is a medical emergency. Most patients have reversible causes for their altered state and will clear their sensorium – usually from the metabolism of substances such as alcohol, recreational drugs, prescription medications or by recovery from their postictal state. However, physicians must be meticulous because a small but significant number of patients can progress to coma or death unless rapid evaluation and treatment are successful. Despite the risk of significant morbidity and mortality, the majority of young patients have a benign cause for their condition and will eventually be discharged from the ED following an extended period of observation.

Patients who present with an altered sensorium as the result of an intentional ingestion will need acute psychiatric evaluation once they have been medically stabilized and cleared of any toxic side effects, such as dysrhythmias, hypoglycemia, or gastrointestinal (GI) bleeding. These patients will also need to be stabilized with regard to their coexisting medical conditions. Diabetics often present to the ED with hypoglycemia. In most cases, the cause is related to a change in diet, dietary noncompliance, a change in activity or inadvertent medication error. Once infectious causes of their glucose disturbance have been ruled out, these patients may be safely discharged home after treatment and education, preferably with a friend or family member who can offer assistance. Patients with hypoglycemia secondary to long-acting oral agents must be admitted to the hospital for further observation and treatment.

Elderly and immunocompomised patients are far more complex and often require hospitalization regardless of the ultimate cause of their AMS. It is not unusual for this population to experience a persistent decline in their baseline level of functioning with a loss of at least one activity of daily living. Not surprisingly, elderly hospitalized patients have longer hospital stays, higher mortality rates, and increased rates of institutional care after hospitalization. Patients with underlying dementia often suffer significant deterioration in their sensorium despite seemingly minor medical insults. Hospitalization is often required to deal with the social as well as medical concerns in this patient population.

Pearls, pitfalls, and myths

The clinical arena that includes altered states of consciousness is complex and high-risk. There are many pitfalls, but with meticulous evaluation, most can be avoided.

- The first critical branch point is to recognize the importance of distinguishing delirium from dementia and psychosis. Traveling down the wrong path at this juncture can result in harm to the patient.
- Recognize the difficulty obtaining a quality history. Do not lose sight of the importance of that history, and aggressively overcome any obstacles to obtaining it.
- Consider the enormous differential without narrowing the possibilities too early.

- Remember the basics: DON'T, hydration, temperature control, and a thorough physical examination that includes the eyes, the skin, breath odor and mental status examination utilizing the CAM.
- An awake, alert patient with a unilateral dilated pupil has a posterior communicating aneurysm until proven otherwise.
- The intracranial mass is on the same side as the dilated pupil in about 85% of cases.
- The largest organ in the body, the skin, is often overlooked when considering causes for AMS.
- Patients with delirium have a 15% mortality, but the causes are reversible 80% of the time.

References

1. Clinical policy for the initial approach to patients presenting with AMS. *Ann Emerg Med* 1999;33:2.
2. Doyon S, Roberts JR. Reappraisal of the "coma cocktail." *Emerg Med Clin North Am* 1994;12:301.
3. Frame DS, Kercher EE. Acute psychosis: functional vs. organic. *Emerg Med Clin North Am* 1991;9:123–136.
4. Gueye PN, et al. Empiric use of flumazenil in comatose patients: limited applicability of criteria to define low risk. *Ann Emerg Med* 1996;27(6):730–735.
5. Hoffman RS, Goldfrank LR. The poisoned patient with altered consciousness. *J Am Med Assoc* 274(7):562–569.
6. Inouye SK, et al. Clarifying confusion: the confusion assessment method – a new method for detection of delirium. *Ann Int Med* 1990;113:941.
7. Kanich W, Brady WJ, Huff SJ, et al. Altered mental status: evaluation and etiology in the ED. *Am J Emerg Med* 2002;20(7).
8. Lewis LM, et al. Unrecognized delirium in ED geriatric patients. *Am J Emerg Med* 1995;13(2):142–145.
9. Luekoff SE, et al. Identification of factors associated with the diagnosis of delirium in elderly hospitalized patients. *J Am Geriatr Soc* 1988;36:1099.
10. Marx JA (ed.). *Rosen's Emergency Medicine: Concepts and Clinical Practice*, 5th ed., St. Louis: Mosby, 2002.
11. Naughton BJ, et al. Delirium and other cognitive impairment in older adults in an emergency department. *Ann Emerg Med* 1995;25:751.
12. Plum F, Posner J. *Diagnosis of Stupor and Coma*, 4th ed., Philadelphia: FA Davis, 1984.
13. Rudberg M, et al. The natural history of delirium in older hospitalized patients a syndrome of heterogeneity. *Aging* 1997;26.169.
14. Wofford JL, Loehr LR, Schwartz E. Acute cognitive impairment in the elderly ED patients: etiologies and outcomes. *Am J Emerg Med* 1996;14(7):649–653.

13 Chest pain

Jeffrey A. Tabas, MD and Susan B. Promes, MD

Scope of the problem

Acute chest pain is the presenting complaint in roughly 3% of emergency department (ED) patients. The diagnostic possibilities range from the immediately life-threatening (myocardial infarction (MI), unstable angina (USA), aortic dissection (AD), pulmonary embolism (PE), ruptured esophagus) to the self-limiting (chest wall strain), and the common (gastroesophageal reflux disease) to the unusual (herpes zoster). Although the etiology of the chest pain may remain unidentified in a significant proportion of patients, which can be frustrating to both the patient and provider, it is imperative that the clinician recognizes and treats life-threatening causes.

Anatomic essentials

When considering the differential diagnosis of the patient with chest pain, it is helpful to consider the five organ systems in the thorax: cardiac (heart and pericardium), pulmonary (lungs and pleura), gastrointestinal (esophagus and upper abdominal contents), vascular (aorta and great vessels), and musculoskeletal (chest wall). *Visceral pain* from internal structures such as the heart, lungs, esophagus, and aorta may be difficult for the patient to define. Pain may be described as a discomfort or strange sensation, and it is often challenging for the patient to discern an exact location. *Somatic pain*, from chest wall structures, is often more localizable and easier for the patient to characterize. Pain may be sharp or stabbing, brought on by movement or position, and can often be pinpointed. *Referred pain*, from irritation or inflammation of the upper abdominal contents, may be perceived as pain in the chest or upper back. A differential diagnosis based on these structures is given in Table 13.1.

History

A careful and focused history may uncover important clues to the etiology of chest pain. To avoid a common pitfall, ask open-ended questions when possible. "Why did you come to the emergency department today?" may yield more initial information than "How often do you get this chest pain?" Additionally, ask about chest discomfort rather than pain, since a patient may deny pain and admit only to chest pressure. The mnemonic LMNOPQRST (location, medical history, new, other symptoms, provoking/palliative, quality, radiation, severity, timing) may be helpful in obtaining a complete history. Whether or not you use this mnemonic, it is important to obtain a picture of the patient's symptoms which includes the following aspects:

Table 13.1 Differential diagnosis of chest pain

Heart
Myocardial infarction
Cardiac angina
Pericarditis
Myocarditis
Valvular diseases (especially aortic stenosis)

Lungs
Pneumonia/other infections
Pneumothorax
Pulmonary embolism
Chronic obstructive pulmonary disease exacerbation

Esophagus
Esophagitis (e.g., candidal)
Gastroesophageal reflux disease
Spasm (nutcracker esophagus)
Foreign body
Rupture (Boerhaave's)

Aorta
Dissection
Aneurysm
Aortitis

Upper abdomen
Gallbladder disease (cholecystitis or cholelithiasis)
Pancreatitis
Duodenal or peptic ulcer
Hepatic disease

Chest wall
Costochondritis (Tietze's disease)
Contusion
Rib fracture
Muscle strain or tear

Location

The location of pain may help define the abnormality. If a patient can point to a specific spot that is extremely tender to palpation and worsens with position change, this may be consistent with a musculoskeletal etiology. As mentioned previously, visceral pain may be difficult to localize.

Medical history

While classic risk factors for coronary artery disease have not been shown to be predictive in the acute setting, many clinicians extrapolate their importance from studies of long-term atherosclerotic disease. These include hypertension, smoking, diabetes, increased cholesterol, obesity, and family history of premature heart disease. Cocaine use is a risk factor for both cardiac ischemia and aortic dissection. A history of rheumatic fever or a murmur can suggest valvular disease. Patients with a history of cerebral or peripheral vascular disease or coronary artery disease (CAD) are at risk for acute coronary syndrome (ACS). Patients with a history of hypertension or Marfan's disease are at risk for aortic dissection. Patients with vomiting or a recent esophageal procedure may be at risk for esophageal perforation. A heavy smoking history suggests underlying chronic obstructive pulmonary disease (COPD). Risk factors for PE include recent surgery, family history, cancer, and estrogen use or pregnancy. Patients with PE have no identifiable risk factor in 20% of cases.

New

It is important to discover whether the patient has had similar episodes of chest pain in the past, if they have been of similar severity, and what medical diagnosis and treatment, if any, they received. A history of multiple similar episodes of pain associated with previous COPD exacerbations is an important clue that this may be another similar exacerbation.

Other (associated) symptoms

Nausea, vomiting, shortness of breath, syncope, near-syncope, and palpitations may increase the clinician's suspicion for serious illness, such as cardiac ischemia or dysrhythmia. Shortness of breath, productive cough, and fever may suggest a respiratory infection. Any neurologic deficit in the setting of pain should immediately suggest aortic dissection.

Provoking/Palliative

Pain that is worse with a deep breath is termed pleuritic. Pleuritic pain is associated with pulmonary etiologies such as pneumonia, pulmonary embolus, or COPD exacerbation. Pain that is worse lying flat and improves sitting up suggests pericarditis. Chest discomfort due to angina may be associated with exertion and often improves with rest or nitroglycerin (NTG). Burning pain that is associated with meals may suggest a gastrointestinal (GI) etiology.

Quality

Chest discomfort may be described in numerous ways, such as sharp, burning, stabbing, pinching, squeezing, heaviness, or pressure. It is important to begin with open-ended questions, such as "tell me about this discomfort in your chest," rather than "how long have you had this chest pain?" If a patient cannot provide a description of the character, you can use prompts such as "is it sharp, burning, stabbing, heavy, squeezing or pinching?" Pressure, heavy or squeezing pain is often consistent with cardiac ischemia. Sharp or stabbing pain suggests a non-cardiac cause, although cardiac ischemia can present in a multitude of ways. A patient's demonstration of pain by a clenched fist against his or her chest is termed *Levine's sign*. One small study showed a high correlation with this description and acute cardiac ischemia.

Radiation

Radiation of pain to the neck, jaw, shoulder, or arm is often consistent with cardiac ischemia. Pain that radiates to the back may be associated with aortic dissection.

Severity

"On a scale of 0 to 10, how severe is the pain?" Severe chest pain should always raise concern for a life-threatening emergency. A 0–10 scale may be used to rate the pain. A rating of 1 is almost undetectable, while a rating of 10 is the worst pain ever experienced. Severity of pain is not predictive of disease, but should be followed over time to document the effect of interventions. The goal of the practitioner is to relieve pain as rapidly as possible, especially in a patient with a high suspicion of acute cardiac ischemia.

Timing (duration and onset)

"How long have you had this discomfort? Is it constant, waxing/waning, or intermittent?" Pain lasting seconds or more than 24 hours is less likely to be cardiac in origin. However, use caution when questioning about symptom duration. Discomfort that has been intermittent for several days and recently became severe differs from pain that has remained constant for the last 72 hours. Be certain to ask questions about today's episode of pain, distinguishing it from previous episodes. "Do you get this pain with exertion?" would receive a different response depending on whether you are referring to prior anginal type pain or today's nonexertional chest pain due to acute MI (AMI). Sudden or abrupt onset of chest pain may indicate a serious underlying disorder, such as MI, PE, or aortic dissection.

Physical examination

The physical examination in patients with chest pain may be unrevealing. However, a thorough examination is essential to identify important diagnostic clues if present.

General appearance

The general appearance of a patient is an important clinical observation. Patients who appear markedly uncomfortable or present with pallor, diaphoresis, or respiratory distress should be considered acutely ill. Evaluation and treatment should proceed in parallel rather than sequentially.

Vital signs

Vital signs are vital, and should be verified. Hypotension suggests shock or impending shock, and may be due to decreased cardiac output, intravascular volume depletion, or sepsis. Note any difference in blood pressure between arms, or between arms and legs. This may suggest aortic dissection. Tachycardia may suggest systemic illness, dysrhythmia, or pain. In addition to reviewing the recorded vital signs, observe the patient's respiratory pattern and rate. Abnormal respirations may be a clue to a pneumothorax, congestive heart failure (CHF), PE, COPD exacerbation, or other pulmonary abnormalities. Fever or hypothermia may suggest an infectious process. Think of pulse oximetry as the "fifth vital sign," and measure it in all patients with chest pain. A low measurement may suggest a pulmonary disorder or poor perfusion from a cardiac or vascular event, especially if it is decreased from the patient's baseline.

Pulsus paradoxus is a loss of the pulse during inspiration. It represents the fall in systolic pressure from expiration to inspiration that can be felt or auscultated. As the cuff is slowly deflated, note that pressure at which any pulse is first detected, and then the pressure at which every beat is detected. Normally, the fall in systolic arterial pressure is less than 10 mmHg during inspiration. Presence of a "pulsus" classically suggests cardiac tamponade, although it may also be present in pulmonary conditions such as emphysema or asthma.

Skin

Note the degree of perfusion, pallor, or diaphoresis. Visual examination of the chest may identify the cause for the pain, such as contusion or ecchymosis suggesting traumatic injury, or vesicular rash suggesting herpes zoster.

Pulmonary

Inspection of the chest and surrounding structures may reveal increased respiratory effort or accessory muscle use. Auscultation may reveal normal, abnormal, or diminished breath sounds. Bilaterally decreased breath sounds with poor air movement suggest severe reactive airway disease or emphysema. Unilaterally decreased breath sounds suggest consolidation, pneumothorax, or pleural effusion. If there are decreased breath sounds unilaterally, the position of the trachea should be examined for signs of tracheal deviation suggestive of tension pneumothorax. Check for "E to A" changes (egophony) throughout the lungs. Their presence indicates consolidation. Increased inspiratory to expiratory (I:E) ratio should be noted (normal is 2:1). A prolongation of the expiratory phase suggests significant obstructive airway disease. Adventitial sounds such as wheezes suggest reactive airway disease. Rales or crackles may be consistent with atelectasis, infiltrate, or edema. The location and extent of these should be documented (e.g., one-third of the way up bilaterally, or right lower lung field). "Velcro-like" rales are consistent with chronic interstitial fibrosis. Percussion may be useful for localizing dullness, suggesting infiltrate, mass, or fluid, or hyperresonance, suggestive of pneumothorax. Palpation of the chest wall may be helpful to identify crepitus, or to localize tenderness when a musculoskeletal source is suspected.

Cardiac

Inspection of the chest may reveal previous surgical scars, implanted devices such as pacemakers or cardioverter defibrillators (ICDs), and hyperdynamic states. Palpation should assess for location and quality of the left ventricular systolic impulse. Normal location of this impulse is in the fifth intercostal space at the mid-clavicular line. Placing the fingers of the right hand at the left sternal border in each rib space allows appreciation of a right-sided heave. Auscultation of heart sounds should proceed over all four cardiac listening areas, first with the diaphragm and then with the bell. The regularity of the heart sounds and any murmurs, rubs, or gallops should be noted. The most commonly heard murmurs and methods to distinguish them are listed in Table 13.2.

Carotid arteries

Auscultation of the carotid arteries should be performed using the bell of the stethoscope to assess for bruits (often unilateral) or transmitted murmurs (bilateral). Pressing too firmly on the carotids may create a false bruit. If there is confusion as to the source of the bruit (carotid vs. cardiac), auscultation in the region of the sternal notch will either confirm the presence or absence of a transmitted murmur. Palpation of the carotid pulses should also be performed to confirm normal strength and upstroke.

Jugular venous pressure (JVP)

Findings of right heart failure include jugular venous distension, hepatic congestion and peripheral edema. Patients may have right-sided heart failure from left-sided failure (most common etiology), pulmonary hypertension (COPD, PE), or impaired right-sided filling (pericardial tamponade, tension pneumothorax). The jugular venous pressure (JVP) is noted in the anterior triangle of the neck (Figure 13.1). The patient should rest with the head of the bed at 30° and the chin rotated left of midline by 30°. The pulsation is most often visible just above the clavicle. The jugular pulse is distinguished from the carotid pulse by its double wave and lack of palpability. It can further be confirmed by noting a rise in the

Table 13.2 Most commonly heard cardiac murmurs and methods to distinguish them

Three common systolic murmurs
1. Systolic ejection (flow)
   (a) Heard across the precordium with the diaphragm of the stethescope
2. Aortic stenosis
   (a) Harsh, crescendo/decrescendo, heard with diaphragm
   (b) Radiates to carotids (heard with bell of the stethescope)
3. Mitral regurgitation
   (a) Heard at apex with the bell, radiating to axilla
   (b) Blowing, holosystolic
   (c) Heard best with patient turned slightly into left lateral decubitus position
   (d) Increased with Valsalva maneuver

Two common diastolic murmurs
1. Mitral stenosis
   (a) Low, rumbling
2. Aortic regurgitation
   (a) Blowing, decrescendo or holodiastolic

Other cardiac sounds
1. Idiopathic hypertrophic subaortic stenosis (IHSS)
   (a) Late systolic murmur without radiation
2. Pericardial rub
   (a) Triple phase (mid-systole, mid-diastole, pre-systole), scratchy
3. S3
   (a) Heard best with bell at apex in left lateral decubitus position
   (b) Sounds like Kentucky (Ken = S1, tu = S2, cky = S3)
   (c) Represents heart failure in an adult.
   (d) Normal finding in small children
4. S4
   (a) Heard best with bell at apex
   (b) Sounds like Tennessee (Te = S4, nne = S1, ssee = S2)
   (c) Represents atrial filling of stiff ventricle in an adult
   (d) Always pathologic in a child

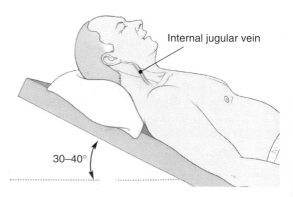

Figure 13.1
Jugular venous pressure assessment.

height of the JVP by lowering the bed or by compressing the liver (hepatojugular reflux).

Extremities

Pulses should be assessed including symmetry between sides and between upper and lower extremities. Changes of peripheral vascular disease, such as decreased pulses, hair loss, or shiny reddened skin may provide evidence of underlying atherosclerotic disease. Bilateral lower extremity edema may represent right heart failure (usually secondary to left heart failure or pulmonary disease), especially in the presence of elevated JVP. Another common cause of bilateral lower extremity edema is venous insufficiency. Liver failure, hypoalbuminemia, and nephrotic syndrome also should be considered as causes of edema. Asymmetric edema should raise concern for deep venous thrombosis (DVT), especially in the presence of cords or venous distension. When asymmetry is present, the size of each leg should be measured and recorded.

Abdomen

Always perform the abdominal exam with the head of the bed flat (so the patient is completely supine), both knees bent (to relax the abdominal musculature), and both arms down by the sides. This allows the most accurate and reproducible exam. The examination of the abdomen should progress sequentially with observation, auscultation, percussion, and palpation. It is particularly important to evaluate for non-thoracic causes of chest pain, such as diseases of the gallbladder (cholecystitis or cholelithiasis). Note the presence of bruits or pulsatile masses suggesting abdominal aortic aneurysm, a potential life-threatening emergency.

Rectal

Rectal examination should be performed to assess for gross blood, melena, or occult blood. The presence of gastrointestinal bleeding may impact imminent therapy (anticoagulant or fibrinolytic therapy), or be the source of significant blood loss leading to cardiac ischemia.

Neurologic

A complaint-directed neurologic examination should be performed. Any new neurologic deficits in the setting of chest pain should be presumed due to aortic dissection and considered an emergency, unless proven otherwise.

Differential diagnosis

Table 13.3 provides an extensive list of possible chest pain causes.

Table 13.3 Differential diagnosis of life-threatening causes of chest pain

Diagnosis	Classic symptoms	Signs	Work-up
Acute myocardial infarction	*High-risk features include:* 1. Advanced age 2. Known CAD 3. Diabetes 4. Pain like prior AMI or worse than usual angina 5. Pain that is pressure-like or squeezing 6. Radiation to neck, left shoulder, or left arm. *Low-risk features include:* 1. Pleuritic, sharp, or stabbing pain 2. Pain reproducible with palpation or movement 3. Younger age 4. Pain lasting for seconds or constant for more than 24 hours. However, 22% of patients with AMI have pain that is sharp or stabbing, 13% have partially pleuritic pain, and 7% have pain completely reproduced by palpation.	Physical examination is most helpful when there are findings of decreased cardiac output: rales, hypotension, an S3, new or worsening mitral regurgitation murmur. Otherwise, it is often unremarkable.	Diagnosed by an elevation of serum cardiac markers and one of the following: 1. Clinical history of ischemic-type chest discomfort *or* 2. Serial changes on ECG *or* 3. Urgent vascularization

(continued)

Table 13.3 Differential diagnosis of life-threatening causes of chest pain (*cont*)

Diagnosis	Classic symptoms	Signs	Work-up
Aortic dissection	Presentation: pain (95%), abrupt onset (85%), severe or worst ever (90%), tearing or ripping (50%), chest (75%) and/or back location (50%), syncope (10%), hypertension history (70%).	Hypertension (50%), hypotension (5%), aortic insufficiency murmur (30%), pulse deficit (15%), neurologic deficit.	CXR may reveal abnormalities (Table 13.5). Helical CT or echocardiogram sensitive and specific.
Aortic stenosis	Classic progression of symptoms over time from chest pain to syncope to CHF.	Harsh, systolic, crescendo–decrescendo murmur radiating to carotids. Weak, delayed pulses, narrow pulse pressure.	ECG may show left ventricular hypertrophy. Diagnosis by echocardiography or cardiac catheterization.
COPD exacerbation	Patients may complain of dyspnea and pleuritic chest pain. Symptoms of respiratory infection may be present.	Vital signs may show tachypnea, tachycardia, and hypoxia. Breath sounds are typically decreased, wheezing is variable depending on the amount of air movement.	Obtain CXR to exclude pneumonia or pneumothorax as exacerbating factor. Diagnosed when symptoms respond to beta-agonist therapy.
Esophageal rupture	Chest pain in the setting of vomiting or recent esophageal procedure. Progressively increasing symptoms with diagnostic delays.	Early physical examination can be remarkably benign. As disease progresses, infectious mediastinitis develops.	Laboratory analysis may be unremarkable. Chest radiography may reveal abnormal air in the mediastinum (pneumomediastinum) or may be normal. Definitive diagnosis by CT scan, gastrograffin esophography (avoid barium given risk of extravasation), or endoscopy.
Pericardial tamponade	Often presents with shortness of breath or weakness rather than chest pain.	Tachycardia is an early presentation. Pulsus paradoxus is present. With progression, distended jugular veins and hypotension develop. The classic presentation of Beck's triad (muffled heart tones, distended neck veins and hypotension) is actually uncommon.	ECG usually reveals low voltage. Electrical alternans (alternating size of the QRS complex) is highly suggestive. Definitive diagnosis by ultrasound demonstrates impaired relaxation of the right atrium and ventricle during diastole.
Pericarditis	Sharp or burning pain, often of several days duration, pleuritic component, worse lying down, better sitting forward, may have prodrome of fever and malaise. Uremia from renal failure is a common predisposing factor.	Scratchy or squeaky pericardial friction rub heard best in left lower sternal border using the diaphragm – usually triphasic, but may have just two components. Varying degree of fever. An increased pulsus paradoxus is concerning for tamponade.	Four stages on ECG: 1. Diffuse ST elevation, PR depression, and peaked T waves most common 2. Normalization 3. Deep, symmetric, diffuse T wave inversion 4. Normalization. Diagnosis is suggested by pericardial effusion on echocardiography, although an effusion may be present in the absence of pericarditis.

(*continued*)

Table 13.3 Differential diagnosis of life-threatening causes of chest pain (*cont*)

Diagnosis	Classic symptoms	Signs	Work-up
Pneumonia	Productive cough, fever, shortness of breath. Symptoms may be less impressive in immunocompromised states (diabetes, HIV, chronic alcoholism).	Fever, tachypnea, hypoxia, and/or findings of consolidation such as rales or E to A changes (egophony).	Leukocytosis on CBC. Chest radiography demonstrates an infiltrate. PA and lateral films are more sensitive and specific than a portable AP film. Consider tuberculosis, pneumocystis in the HIV patient.
Pneumothorax	Often associated with history of trauma. Spontaneous pneumothorax typically occurs in tall, thin individuals, 20–40 years old, male > female. Secondary pneumothorax may occur in smokers, patients with emphysema or asthma, or patients with pneumocystis. Symptoms include pleuritic chest pain and shortness of breath.	Decreased breath sounds, tachypnea, hypoxia may or may not be present. Tracheal deviation may be noted with tension pneumothorax.	Chest radiography reveals pneumothorax. A diagnosis of tension pneumothorax should never be made radiographically, since it should be diagnosed clinically and treated immediately.
Pulmonary embolism	Risk factors include recent pelvic or low abdominal surgery, family or patient history of thromboembolism, cancer, paralysis, LE casting or immobility, CHF, estrogen use or pregnancy, LE extremity or pelvic trauma, age >40 years. Twenty percent of patients with PE have no risk factors.	Respirations >20/minute (70%), rales (51%) tachycardia (30%), leg swelling (28%), loud P2 (23%), temperature >38.5°C (13%), wheeze (5%).	V/Q scan, helical CT, or pulmonary angiography are diagnostic tests of choice. A negative result of a high sensitivity D-dimer test in a low-risk patient may be adequate to exclude disease.
Unstable angina	Angina is discomfort, induced by exercise, relieved by rest or NTG. USA is either: 1. Angina at rest (usually >20 minutes) 2. New onset exertional angina (<2 months) with walking 1–2 blocks or 1 flight of stairs *or* 3. Increased severity within 2 months at above exertion level.	Often absent.	Difficult to diagnose in an emergency setting. Dynamic ECG abnormalities or elevated cardiac markers define a high-risk group. Diagnosis made by noninvasive stress testing or cardiac catheterization.

AMI: acute myocardial infarction; AP: anteroposterior; CAD: coronary artery disease; CBC: complete blood count; CHF: congestive heart failure; COPD: chronic obstructive pulmonary disease; CT: computed tomography; CXR: chest X-ray; ECG: electrocardiogram; HIV: human immunodeficiency virus; LE: lower extremity; NTG: nitroglycerin; PA: posteroanterior; PE: pulmonary embolism; USA: unstable angina; V/Q: ventilation–perfusion.

Diagnostic testing

Laboratory studies

Complete blood count

A complete blood count (CBC) is frequently ordered in patients with chest pain. A low hematocrit may indicate a reason for symptoms of cardiac ischemia, or may be due to bleeding associated with the source of pain (gastric ulcer). Most authorities recommend maintenance of the hematocrit in a patient with cardiac ischemia above 30 mg/dl to maximize O_2 delivery. A high white count may represent demargination due to stress, pain, or a catastrophic event (e.g., sepsis from delayed diagnosis of esophageal rupture). However, this test is rarely illustrative.

Chemistry panel

Chemistry panels generally provide little help in the evaluation of the patient with chest pain. They may suggest acidosis (low bicarbonate), especially in the presence of an anion gap. If intravenous (IV) contrast imaging is to be performed to evaluate the aorta, it is important to obtain a creatinine level prior to the administration of IV dye. Renal insufficiency, suggested by elevated creatinine level, is a relative contraindication to contrast injection, as in computed tomography (CT) or cardiac catheterization. Elevated glucose may reveal previously unsuspected diabetes, a risk factor for coronary artery disease.

Cardiac markers

Serial serum cardiac marker measurements can be used to rule out AMI at an appropriate interval from symptom onset (Table 13.4). However,

Table 13.4 Measurements of serial cardiac markers to rule out AMI

Cardiac marker characteristics	Rise (hours)	Peak (hours)	Return to baseline
Myoglobin	<3	4–9	<24 hours
CK-MB mass	3–8	9–30	1–3 days
CK-MB subforms	1–3	4–6	18–24 hours
cTnT	2–6	10–24	10–15 days
cTnI	2–6	10–24	7–10 days

	Hours post pain onset
Myoglobin	Does not exclude
CK-MB mass	6–10
CK-MB subforms	6–10
cTnT	8–12
cTnI	8–12

Serial marker testing for rapid exclusion of AMI in low-risk patients – ACEP policy
Obtain an initial marker on arrival. Obtain a second marker at least 6 hours from chest pain onset for CK and 8 hours from onset for Troponin. Note that serial marker testing excludes MI but does not exclude USA. ACEP: American College of Emergency Physicians; AMI: acute myocardial infarction; CK-MB: creatine kinase, cTnI: cardiac troponin I; cTnT: cardiac troponin T; MI: myocardial infarction; USA: unstable angina.

serial cardiac markers are only found to be elevated in 10–30% of cases of unstable angina (USA) and therefore cannot be used to exclude this condition.

Liver function tests

Liver function tests may be elevated in patients with biliary or hepatic disease, or due to passive congestion of the liver in heart failure.

Amylase/lipase

When an abdominal source of pain is suspected, or tenderness is elicited in the mid-epigastrium, pancreatitis should be considered. This is especially true in the presence of risk factors (alcohol use, biliary disease, and diabetes).

Urinalysis

Evaluation of the urine is rarely helpful in the chest pain patient, except when glucosuria (possible screen for diabetes) or bilirubinuria (possible screen for biliary duct obstruction or hepatic disease) are present.

Pregnancy test

Consider a pregnancy test in all female patients of childbearing age, especially if they may undergo radiologic imaging.

Urine toxicology screen

Cocaine has been associated with ACS, AMI, and aortic dissection, especially in the first hour after use.

D-dimer

D-dimers are degradation products of circulating cross-linked fibrin. Sensitivity and specificity for thromboembolism vary, depending on the type of test. Newly developed rapid tests appear to be adequately sensitive to exclude PE in low-risk patients. In a patient with suspected PE, D-dimer testing should only be performed when the type of test used is known to be sensitive for thromboembolism.

Arterial blood gas

Arterial blood gas sampling is useful to assess ventilatory status (CO_2 level), serum pH, and to confirm a low pulse oximetry reading. In the assessment of a patient with suspected PE, it has been shown to lack significant predictive value. In one study, 26% of patients with PE had a partial pressure of O_2 (PO_2) greater than 80 mm. A low oxygen saturation, either from pulse oximetry or ABG that lacks an adequate explanation (i.e., pneumonia, heart failure or COPD) should raise suspicion for pulmonary embolism.

Electrocardiogram

An attempt should be made to perform an electrocardiogram (ECG) within 10 minutes of arrival for all patients with unexplained chest pain (recommendation of the American College of Emergency Physicians and the American College of Cardiology). In studies of patients with AMI, ECGs are diagnostic in 30–50%, nonspecific in 40–70%, and normal in up to 10%. Findings of acute ischemia include new or presumed new ST elevation, ST depression, or inverted T waves (Figure 13.2). Known findings on ECG that

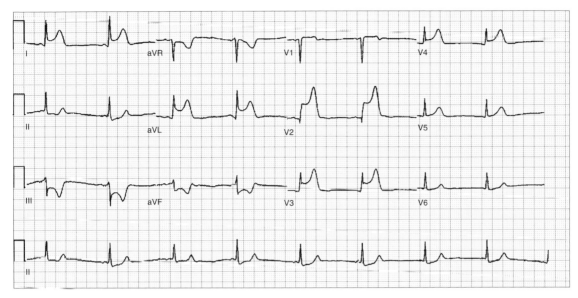

(a)

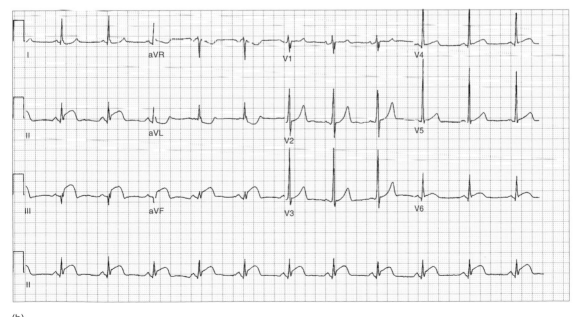

(b)

Figure 13.2
(a) ECG in a patient with anterolateral MI demonstrating ST-segment elevations in leads I, aVL, and V_2–V_4. Note the reciprocal ST-segment depressions in leads II, III, and aVF. (b) ECG in a patient with inferoposterior MI demonstrating ST-segment elevations in leads II, II and aVF, and prominent R waves in leads V_1–V_3. *Courtesy*: Amal Mattu, MD.

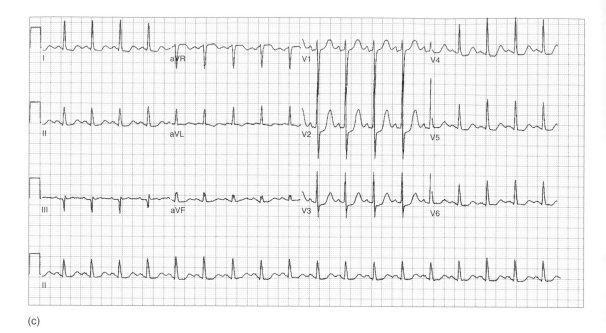

(c)

Figure 13.2 (*cont*)
(c) ECG in a patient with posterior MI demonstrating prominent R waves in leads V_1–V_3 and ST-segment depression in leads V_2–V_3. *Courtesy*: Amal Mattu, MD.

obscure the assessment of ischemia include bundle branch block (especially left bundle branch block) and left ventricular hypertrophy with repolarization abnormality (strain pattern). American Heart Association guidelines recommend posterior and right-sided ECG leads when there are findings of ischemia such as ST elevation, ST depression, or T-wave abnormalities on the traditional 12-lead ECG (Figure 13.3). Patients with ST- or T-wave abnormalities in the inferior leads (II, III, and aVF) or ST depression in the septal leads (V1 and V2) are most likely to have abnormalities on posterior and right-sided ECGs.

The ECG may also reveal evidence of pericarditis (Figure 13.4) or a pericardial effusion.

Radiologic studies

Chest radiography

Chest radiography is most helpful when it points to a definitive diagnosis such as pneumothorax or pneumonia. Although chest radiography is often normal or nonspecific in conditions such as AMI, PE, and aortic dissection, it may also suggest the diagnosis (Figures 13.5 and 13.6). Tables 13.5 and 13.6 describe CXR findings in aortic dissection and PE, respectively.

Helical computed tomography

Helical CT may be extremely helpful in the evaluation of a stable patient with chest pain. It is reasonably sensitive (70 to >90%) and specific (90 to >95%) for PE depending on scanner technology and the expertise of the radiologist. It often provides additional information either suggestive or supportive of a final diagnosis in patients without PE. It is 95–100% sensitive and specific for aortic dissection (Figure 13.5b). In the rare occasion that helical CT is inconclusive for aortic dissection or PE, and the pre-test probability for the diagnosis is high, angiography should be performed.

Echocardiography

This test can prove helpful in the evaluation of chest pain, especially in the unstable patient. Transthoracic echocardiography can evaluate the cardiac chamber sizes, wall motion, systolic function, valvular function, and aortic integrity. Remarkable findings include valvular disease, pericardial effusion with tamponade physiology, regional wall motion abnormalities suggesting ischemic cardiac disease, right heart failure suggesting acute PE, and aortic dissection.

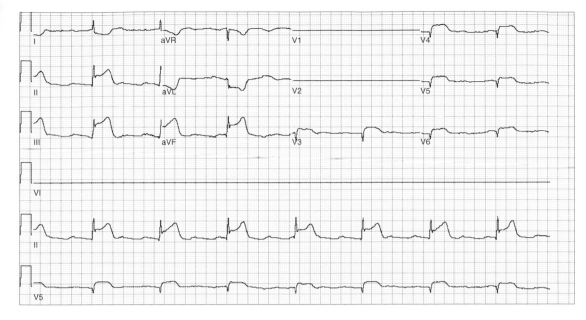

Figure 13.3
Right-sided ECG in a patient with right ventricular infarct demonstrating ST-segment elevation in lead V₄R.
Courtesy: S.V. Gurudevan, MD.

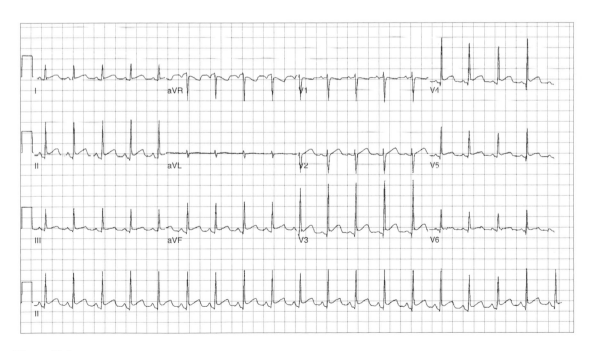

Figure 13.4
ECG in a patient with pericarditis demonstrating PR-segment depression, PR-segment elevation in aVR, and diffuse ST-segment elevations. *Courtesy*: Amal Mattu, MD.

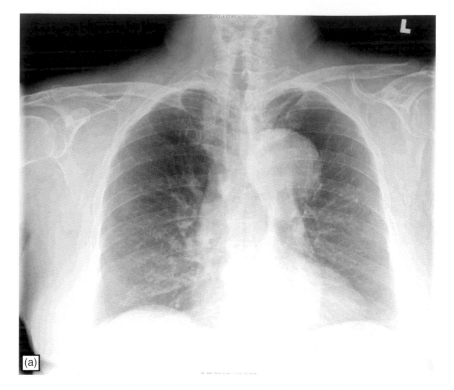

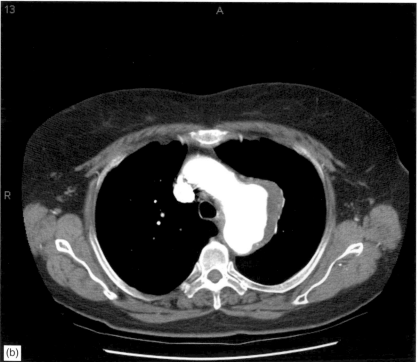

Figure 13.5
(a) Abnormal chest X-ray and (b) chest CT revealing aortic dissection.
Courtesy: Gus Garmel, MD.

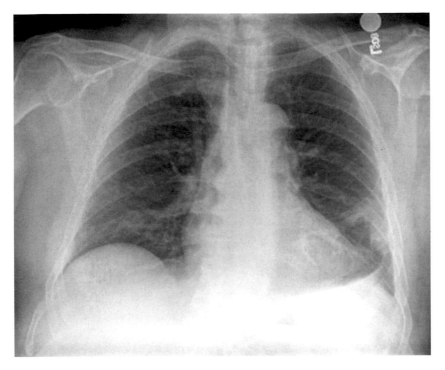

Figure 13.6
Hampton's hump. Reprinted from Journal of Emergency Medicine, 24(3), Tarleton GP, Manthey DE, The elusive Hampton's hump, pages 329–330, 2003, with permission from Elsevier.

Transesophageal echocardiography is more sensitive than transthoracic echocardiography in detecting aortic dissection.

Table 13.5 Chest X-ray findings in aortic dissection

- Normal (10–30%)
- Wide mediastinum or abnormal aorta (70–80%)
- Wide paraspinal shadow
- Pleural effusion
- Tracheal shift
- Aortic calcification displacement
- "Lump" distal to vessels

Table 13.6 Chest X-ray findings in pulmonary embolism

- Classic presentation is normal X-ray in patient with dyspnea and hypoxia
- Atelectasis or parenchymal abnormality (68%)
- Elevated hemidiaphragm
- Pleural effusion
- Hampton's hump is a wedge-shaped pleural-based density (Figure 13.6)
- Westermark's sign is distension of pulmonary vasculature proximal to embolism with loss of vascular markings distally (rare)

General treatment principles

As with all ED patients, treatment begins with the ABCs. The goals of treatment are stabilization, symptom relief, and limitation of morbidity and mortality due to the disease entity.

Patients with chest pain should receive a high triage level, indicating that they have a potentially life-threatening medical problem. They should be placed in a room expeditiously. The initial assessment of the chest pain patient should focus on the patient's stability. If the patient has unstable vital signs or appears ill, an accelerated assessment and treatment plan should be used. The American Heart Association guidelines for assessment of patients with potential ACS recommend performance and interpretation of an ECG within 10 minutes of arrival to the ED.

Initial assessment and interventions

- ABCs
- Patient appearance
- Vital signs including O_2 saturation

- Place IV line, administer O$_2$, and place on cardiac monitor
- ECG within 10 minutes of arrival
- Directed H&P (includes pulmonary and cardiovascular examination).

If immediate life-threatening disease is found or suggested, initiate rapid and directed treatment. Otherwise perform a secondary assessment and treatment.

Secondary assessment and interventions

- ASA 325 mg po (unless patient allergy, appropriate dose already taken, or ischemia excluded)
- Complete H&P
- Provide pain relief
- Consider additional ECGs, radiologic and laboratory evaluation as indicated.

Acute coronary syndrome (ACS)

Aspirin

Aspirin should be given to everyone with suspected ACS who is not allergic. Its efficacy is equivalent to that of costly thrombolytics, and contraindications are infrequent. There is a 23% reduction in 30-day mortality in patients with AMI. In patients with USA, there is a 50% reduction in the rate of progression to AMI.

Dosing: 325 mg oral (or rectal).

Nitrates

Nitrates are recommended in AMI, although a clear benefit on morbidity or mortality has not been proven. Nitrates act to vasodilate the coronary arteries, and reduce both preload and afterload. Hypotension, a frequent and unacceptable adverse effect, should be avoided at all costs; therefore, blood pressure should be monitored before each additional dosage. Sublingual NTG is recommended in patients with suspected ACS, except those with contraindications such as allergy, bradycardia less than 50 beats per minute, tachycardia, or hypotension. The use of agents for erectile dysfunction, sildenafil or vardenafil within 24 hours, or tadalafil within 48 hours, is an absolute contraindication to use of nitrates because of the risk of prolonged and exaggerated vasodilatation. NTG should be used with caution in patients with right ventricular infarct who are often sensitive to preload reduction. IV NTG

is indicated in patients with persistent ischemia, CHF, hypertension, or a large anterior AMI.

Dosing: Treatment should begin with sublingual tablet or spray dosing of 0.4 mg every 5 minutes until pain free. Three doses are commonly recommended but not a limit. Check blood pressure before each additional dose. If symptoms are relieved with sublingual therapy, apply 1–2 inches of nitropaste to the anterior chest wall. Indications for IV therapy include the first 24 to 48 hours for patients with definite USA or AMI who experience ongoing or recurrent ischemic discomfort, hypertension, or signs of congestive heart failure, or for controlled titration of therapy. Start an infusion at 10–20 mcg/minute and titrate by 10–20 mcg/minute every 3 to 5 minutes until symptom relief.

Morphine

Morphine is used as an analgesic for the relief of ischemic chest pain. Any patient with significant discomfort should receive treatment with analgesics, although the benefit of narcotics for pain relief in patients with AMI is inferred rather than clearly supported by literature.

Dosing: Depending on the patient's previous exposure to narcotics, an initial IV dose of 2–4 mg is recommended with titration to effect.

Beta-blockers

Beta-blockers have been shown to decrease morbidity and mortality in patients with AMI and USA. They should be used in all patients except those with contraindications, such as CHF, history of significant COPD or asthma, atrioventricular (AV) node disease, bradycardia, or hypotension.

Dosing: 5 mg of metoprolol is given IV three times at 5 minute intervals. Vital signs should be checked before each dose. If this is tolerated, then 25–50 mg of metoprolol is given orally.

Heparin

The significant benefit shown from heparin use in patients with unstable angina was largely from the pre-aspirin era. A meta-analysis comparing heparin plus aspirin to aspirin alone revealed a 2.4% reduction in death or MI which did not reach statistical significance. Heparin is recommended for all patients with suspected AMI. It is part of the treatment protocol for most thrombolytic regimens, except streptokinase. Low molecular weight heparin has several advantages over IV unfractionated heparin. These include ease of use in the inpatient and outpatient setting, weight-based dosing, lack of need for laboratory monitoring, and lower rates of heparin-induced thombocytopenia. Bleeding rates and efficacy are equivalent, and when nursing and laboratory costs are included, overall cost of therapy is equivalent. Precautions include extremes of weight (<45 or >100 kg) and renal insufficiency.

Dosing: IV unfractionated heparin is given as an 80 unit/kg IV bolus and an 18 unit/kg/hour infusion. A nomogram should be used for dose adjustment. If given with alteplase, reteplase, or tenecteplase the dosing is reduced to 60 unit/kg IV bolus and 12 units/kg/hour infusion. For low molecular weight heparin, Enoxaparin is given 1 mg/kg SQ BID or Dalteparin 120 IU/kg SQ BID.

Thrombolysis

Thrombolysis is indicated in patients with AMI with ST-segment elevation (1 mm in 2 or more contiguous leads) or presumed new left bundle branch block and symptoms <12 hours (Table 13.7). Relative mortality is reduced by 21%, with

Table 13.7 Thrombolysis indications and contraindications

Indications for thrombolysis
- ST elevation (≥0.1 mm in ≥2 contiguous leads) or *new* left bundle branch block (not known to be old) *and*
- Symptoms <12 hours which are continuing

Contraindications to thrombolysis
- Active internal bleeding (not including menses)
- Suspected aortic dissection
- Uncontrollable hypertension (>180/110)
- History of hemorrhagic CVA
- History of non-hemorrhagic CVA within 1 year

Relative contraindications
- Presenting blood pressure >180/110
- History of chronic severe hypertension
- Active peptic ulcer
- Pregnancy
- Internal bleeding within 4 weeks
- Noncompressible vascular puncture(s)
- Trauma/surgery or CPR within 2–4 weeks
- Current use of anticoagulants in therapeutic doses (INR ≥ 2–3) or known bleeding diathesis
- History of prior CVA or known intracerebral pathology not mentioned in contraindications

CVA: cerebrovascular accident;
CPR: cardiopulmonary resuscitation.

the greatest reduction occurring in patients with bundle branch block. There is no evidence of benefit in patients with proven AMI lacking ECG criteria; in fact, outcomes may be worse. Every hour of delay to thrombolytics increases death by 1.6 per 1000 patients treated. Complications, however, are not benign. These include intracranial hemorrhage in 0.5–1.0% of treated patients. Blood transfusions are required in 5–15%. The GUSTO trial of 40,000 patients provides the main support for the use of alteplase (t-PA) over streptokinase. Thirty-day mortality of alteplase plus heparin was 6.3%, while that for streptokinase was 7.3%. Tenecteplase (also called TNKase) is a modified form of alteplase which can be delivered by weight-based single bolus dosing. Comparison with front-loaded alteplase in the ASSENT-2 trial showed equivalent mortality and complication outcomes.

Dosing: Streptokinase: 1.5 million units IV over 60 minutes.

Alteplase: 15 mg IV bolus, then 0.75 mg/kg (50 mg maximum) over 30 minutes, then 0.5 mg/kg (35 mg maximum) over the next 60 minutes. Concurrent heparin infusion.

Tenecteplase: Single IV bolus over 5 seconds based on body weight: ≤60 kg = 30 mg, 60–69 kg = 35 mg, 70–79 kg = 40 mg, 80–89 kg = 45 mg, ≥90 kg = 50 mg.

Glycoprotein IIB/IIIA inhibitors

Glycoprotein IIB/IIIA (GP IIB/IIIA) inhibitors block platelet aggregation by inhibiting binding of fibrinogen at the GP IIB/IIIA platelet receptor. They have been shown to be of significant benefit when given to patients receiving percutaneous coronary intervention (PCI). It remains controversial whether patients with USA and non-ST-segment elevation MI (NSTEMI) benefit from IIB/IIIA receptor antagonism. Recommended indications for their use include elevated cardiac markers, continuing ischemia, or transient ST changes >0.5 mV despite aspirin and heparin therapy.

Percutaneous coronary intervention

Percutaneous coronary intervention (PCI) is an alternative to thrombolysis if performed within 90 minutes of presentation. Operator experience has been shown to have a significant impact on outcome. High volume centers have recently been shown to produce significantly better results compared to the administration of thrombolytics, while low volume centers have been shown to produce outcomes inferior to that of thrombolysis. Indications for PCI include: an alternative to thrombolysis in patients if performed within 90 minutes of presentation, persisting or recurring pain despite aggressive noninvasive therapy, presence of cardiogenic shock >36 hours after AMI, and when thrombolysis is contraindicated.

Angiotensin-converting enzyme inhibitors

Angiotensin-converting enzyme (ACE) inhibitors are recommended in all patients with AMI (especially with CHF and systolic blood pressure greater than 100 mmHg) based on the ISIS-4 and GISSI-3 trials. Treatment should begin within the first 24 hours but not necessarily in the ED.

Dosing: Begin at the lowest starting dosage for the chosen ACE inhibitor.

Clopidogrel

Clopidogrel is an adenosine diphosphate receptor antagonist that acts to inhibit platelet aggregation. It is indicated instead of aspirin when a patient is aspirin-allergic. The recent clopidogrel in unstable angina to prevent recurrent events (CURE) trial showed that clopidogrel in addition to aspirin improved outcomes when given to high-risk patients; that is, those with dynamic ECG changes or elevated cardiac markers. Outcomes were worse when clopidogrel was given to patients who underwent coronary artery bypass grafting.

Dosing: 300 mg oral load, then 75 mg/day.

Aortic dissection

The goal of aortic dissection (AD) treatment in the ED is to decrease shearing stress on the aorta by decreasing cardiac inotropy and lowering blood pressure. Any patient with a high suspicion for dissection should be started immediately on a beta-blocker, achieving a desired heart rate of 50–60 beats per minute. Options include metoprolol or labetalol, which has the additional benefit of some alpha-blockade, or esmolol, which has the benefit of an ultra-short acting effect (seconds to minutes). If beta-blockers are contraindicated, calcium channel blockers with negative inotropic effects, such as diltiazem, should be given. For additional control of SBP, nitroprusside is often recommended.

Management depends on the location of involvement. Dissection which involves any portion of the ascending aorta (Type A) requires emergent surgical repair. If involvement is limited to portions of the aorta distal to the right brachiocephalic takeoff (Type B), attempts at medical management are warranted.

Pulmonary embolism

Initial treatment of PE is with heparin. If IV unfractionated heparin is used, weight-based dosing and treatment algorithms improve the rate of therapeutic heparinization. Patients with sub-therapeutic heparinization in the first 24 hours experience up to 15 times the rate of recurrent thromboembolism compared with patients who reach therapeutic anticoagulation. Low molecular weight heparins (enoxaparin and tinzaparin) are approved for patients with PE who have documented DVTs. Clinical trials in PE, although limited, show equivalence between heparins in complications and efficacy. Coumadin should be started in the first 24 hours. Coumadin is contraindicated in pregnancy. Weight-based dosing for IV unfractionated heparin is 80 units/kg bolus, followed by an 18 units/kg/hour infusion. The goal is a partial thromboplastin time (PTT) of 46–70 seconds. For low molecular weight heparins, dosing of enoxaparin is 1 mg/kg SQ BID and dosing of tinzaparin is 175 anti-Xa IU/kg SQ daily.

Indications for *vena caval filters* include: recurrent thromboembolism despite adequate anticoagulation, active bleeding or high risk for bleeding, or history of heparin-induced thrombotic thrombocytopenia. Indications for *thrombolysis* include hemodynamic instabililty due to PE or massive iliofemoral venous thrombosis (phlegmasia cerulea dolens). Indications for *thrombectomy* include chronic thromboembolic pulmonary hypertension or massive PE in patients with contraindication to thrombolysis.

Disposition
Admission vs. discharge

Admission rates are high for patients with chest pain, since it is difficult to exclude life-threatening disease without an extended period of observation. Admission rates vary in studies from 30% to 70%. Any patient with chest pain who has concerning findings, such as abnormal vital signs, an abnormal ECG, or elevated cardiac enzymes requires admission. In addition, any patient with a potentially life-threatening cause for symptoms who is awaiting definitive testing to exclude disease should be admitted (or transferred to a hospital where the study is available) if testing cannot be performed in a reasonable time period given the clinical situation. In a patient with possible ACS, repeat evaluation with serial examinations, repeat ECGs, and cardiac marker testing is required. In addition, a noninvasive evaluation such as exercise treadmill testing is needed to exclude USA. If it is possible to obtain these in the setting of a *chest pain observation unit*, it may not be necessary to admit these patients. In a patient with suspected aortic dissection, a normal CT scan of the chest is reassuring for safe discharge if other concerning etiologies have been excluded. In the patient with suspected PE, negative CT pulmonary angiography or low-probability ventilation/perfusion scanning excludes disease in the low-risk patient. Moderate- or high-suspicion patients must receive further testing. Any patient who is discharged with chest pain should have close follow-up arranged, with clear instructions to return for concerning symptoms such as recurrent or increasing pain, shortness of breath, lightheadedness, neurologic symptoms, or other concerns.

Pearls, pitfalls, and myths

- Given the range of potentially life-threatening conditions associated with the complaint of chest pain, the history, physical examination, diagnostic testing, and treatment of such patients should proceed in parallel.
- Consider other diagnostic possibilities in addition to cardiac ischemia in patients with chest pain.
- Do not exclude diseases such as PE or ACS simply on the basis of lack of risk factors.
- Recognize the limitation of emergency testing (laboratories, ECG, CXR) to exclude the presence of life-threatening diseases such as ACS, PE, and AD.

- Do not ignore high-risk findings, even in a patient with many low-risk findings.
- Beware of using a single negative cardiac marker to exclude AMI.
- Negative cardiac markers do not exclude USA.

References

1. Braunwald E, Antman EM, et al. ACC/AHA Guideline update for the management of patients with unstable angina and non-ST-segment elevation myocardial infarction – 2002: Summary article: a report of the American College of Cardiology/American Heart Association Task Force on Practice Guidelines (Committee on the management of patients with unstable angina). *Circulation* 2002;106(14):1893–1900.
2. Edhouse J, Brady WJ, et al. ABC of clinical electrocardiography: acute myocardial infarction – Part II. *Br Med J* 2002;324(7343):963–966.
3. Green GB, Hill PM. Approach to chest pain and possible myocardial ischemia In: Tintinalli JE, Kelen GD, et al. (eds). *Emergency Medicine: A Comprehensive Study Guide*. New York: McGraw-Hill Health Professions Division, 2000. pp. 341–351.
4. Hagan PG, Nienaber CA, et al. The International Registry of Acute Aortic Dissection (IRAD): new insights into an old disease. *J Am Med Assoc* 2000;283(7):897–903.
5. Kline JA, Johns KL, et al. New diagnostic tests for pulmonary embolism. *Ann Emerg Med* 2000;35(2):168–180.
6. Morris F, Brady WJ. ABC of clinical electrocardiography: acute myocardial infarction – Part I. *Br Med J* 2002;324(7341):831–834.
7. Panju AA, Hemmelgarn BR, et al. Is this patient having a myocardial infarction? *J Am Med Assoc* 1998;280(14):1256–1263.

14 Constipation

Victoria Brazil, MBBS

Scope of the problem

Constipation may be defined as either stool frequency of less than three per week or, more generally, as difficulty in passing stool. In either case it should be recognized that constipation is a symptom, not a medical diagnosis.

It has been estimated that the prevalence of constipation in the adult population of industrialized nations is as high as 20%. There are approximately 2.5 million physician visits per year in the US for this symptom, and at least 20% of the population habitually use over-the-counter laxative preparations.

Constipation is a surprisingly frequent chief presenting complaint in the emergency department (ED) despite the medical community's attitude of it being a "minor" problem. It is particularly common in the elderly and those with multiple medical problems, complicating both their assessment and treatment for other conditions.

It is important to recognize constipation as a preventable adverse outcome of an ED visit, and to consider selecting discharge medications with this in mind.

Anatomic essentials

Normal bowel function has two components – colonic transit and defecation.

Colonic transit is maintained by smooth muscle function via bowel wall myenteric plexuses regulating motility and submucosal plexuses regulating absorption, with overall control by the parasympathetic nervous system. Transit time is also affected by bowel contents, specifically fiber and water.

Defecation is a complex series of events in which rectal distension triggers a series of reflexes to relax sphincters and pelvic floor muscles. This is coordinated with an increase in intra-abdominal pressure to facilitate expulsion of rectal contents. In infants, this is entirely a reflex act. Voluntary control of the external anal sphincter is physiologically possible from the second year of life, after which children generally become "toilet trained." Neurologic disease including spinal cord injury may obliterate voluntary control of this reflex in adults.

History

It is important to establish what exactly the patient means when he/she complains of constipation.

How often do you have bowel movements? When did you last have a bowel movement?

The answers to these questions will help establish the nature and significance of a patient's complaints. There is a wide variation in frequency of bowel movements; adults generally have between three bowel movements per day to one every 3 days.

What is the consistency of the stool? Do you ever have difficulty or pain passing stool?

Many patients with normal stool frequency present with a change in consistency of their stool, or with pain on defecation. These symptoms are equally as important as stool frequency in suggesting abnormal bowel function. A history of gradually diminishing or changing stool caliber may indicate an obstruction or mass, such as colon cancer.

How long have you had problems with constipation?

This information helps ascertain the acuity of the problem. Long-term problems which have slowly worsened may focus the management on *therapy* to relieve symptoms, while a new problem or sudden change prompts a more rigorous focus on *diagnostic* evaluation. Acute constipation may represent intestinal obstruction, tumor, stricture, or volvulus.

Other symptoms

Although sometimes constipation may be a sole presenting complaint, it is frequently part of a symptom complex. It is preferable to ask about associated symptoms as an open question initially, but specific enquiry should be made with regard to the following sentinel-associated symptoms:

Abdominal pain

It is important to recognize that constipation is a *symptom*, and should not be attributed as a cause of abdominal pain without a thorough search for more sinister etiologies, such as obstruction caused by colon cancer. This is particularly important in elderly patients.

Rectal bleeding or dark stools

Hemorrhoids and minor anal trauma causing bright bleeding are common in those with constipation. However, attributing bleeding to these causes should be done only after endoscopic or other evaluation has excluded malignancy, inflammatory bowel disease or diverticulitis. Risk of malignancy increases with increasing age.

Weight loss

This may occur in conjunction with constipation due to malignancy or hypothyroidism.

Diarrhea, flatulence, foul-smelling feces

Inconsistent bowel habits require investigation for tumors or malabsorption, or may suggest constipation with overflow diarrhea. Inability to pass flatus should raise a concern for bowel obstruction. Diarrhea alternating with constipation suggests an obstructing colonic lesion or irritable bowel syndrome. Flatulence and bloating may represent a malabsorption syndrome.

Vomiting

Vomiting rarely accompanies a benign cause of constipation and may suggest bowel obstruction.

Past medical

Specific inquiry should be made regarding diabetes, renal failure, neurologic disorders, spinal cord lesions, thyroid disease, and depression, as constipation is common in these conditions.

Medications

Patients should be asked what medications they take regularly, both prescribed and over-the-counter. Specific questions regarding herbal medications and treatments should be asked. This is to ascertain medications *causing* constipation (Table 14.1), and what *treatment* has been attempted. Medications responsible for constipation are best discontinued or modified.

Table 14.1 Medications commonly associated with constipation

- Analgesics
  - Morphine, codeine, tramadol, vicodin, other opiates
  - NSAIDs
- Medications with anticholinergic properties
  - Tricyclic antidepressants
  - Antihistamines
  - Phenothiazines (e.g., antipsychotics)
  - Antispasmodics (e.g., hyoscyamine, baclofen, atropine)
  - Antiparkinsonian agents
- Antacids (aluminium-containing)
- Laxative abuse
- Cardiac medications – diuretics, calcium channel blockers, ACE inhibitors, lipid-lowering agents
- Others – iron, phenytoin, barium, bismuth

ACE: angiotensin converting enzyme;
NSAID: non-steroidal anti-inflammatory drug.

Dietary habits

Inadequate dietary intake of fiber and water is responsible for constipation in the majority of patients who present with this complaint.

Other lifestyle factors

Immobility due to illness or injury or a sedentary lifestyle make constipation more likely. Irregular routines such as traveling or shiftwork also affect bowel function. Neurovegetative features such as sleep disturbance or anhedonia may suggest depression, which has been associated with constipation.

Physical examination
General appearance and vital signs

Those individuals with uncomplicated constipation should look well. Abnormal vital signs or a patient in significant pain or discomfort suggests that the constipation represents a more serious problem, such as bowel obstruction, perforation of colonic diverticulum, or ischemic bowel. Signs of sepsis in a patient with constipation are always concerning.

Abdomen

Careful and thorough abdominal examination should be performed. There may be mild distension and tympany. In thin patients, stool may even be palpable on abdominal exam. However, significant distension, masses, abnormal bowel sounds or signs of localized peritoneal inflammation should prompt an urgent search for significant pathology. Any abdominal wall scars should be noted.

Rectal

Examination of the anus and rectum may reveal rectal blood, tumors, strictures, or fissures. Significant discomfort on examination is suggestive of anal trauma from hard feces. Impacted feces may be felt on digital examination. This finding may indicate mechanical obstruction requiring manual disimpaction, possibly under some form of sedation. Anal fissures are a common cause of constipation in young children.

Head-to-toe

The ED examination should be thorough but focused. Patients should routinely be examined for signs of hypothyroidism, such as dry, cool skin, fine or brittle hair, recent weight gain, lethargy, and hoarse voice. A neurologic examination should also be performed (Table 14.2). Examination of other systems should be made according to historical information and as suggested by abdominal findings.

Table 14.2 Clinical features suggestive of neurologic disease as the etiology of constipation

- Paraplegia – previous trauma, tumor, surgery, stroke, or congenital cause
- Acute spinal pathology – abnormal tone, power, reflexes or sensation in lower limbs, particularly if bilateral and symmetrical
- Autonomic dysfunction – lability of heart rate or blood pressure, orthostatic hypotension, urinary retention, or incontinence
- Parkinson's disease – fine tremor, shuffling gait
- Demyelination, polyneuropathies – focal neurologic deficits in any of spinal, peripheral or upper motor neuron distributions

Differential diagnosis

Most common

- Inadequate fiber and fluid in the diet

- Lifestyle factors – immobility, medications (Table 14.1)
- Pregnancy
- Painful perianal region – hemorrhoids, abscesses, fissures, herpes infection
- Irritable bowel disease
- General debility
- Chronic laxative abuse

In this group, the etiology is frequently multifactorial.

Less common

- Metabolic – hypothyroidism, hypokalemia, hypercalcemia, renal failure
- Intrinsic bowel lesions – tumors, strictures
- Inflammatory bowel disease
- Diverticulitis
- Volvulus, hernias, adhesions, pelvic or abdominal masses
- Neurogenic disorders
  - Autonomic dysfunction, including diabetes
  - Spinal cord lesions
  - Multiple sclerosis
  - Amyotrophic lateral sclerosis
  - Parkinson's disease
    Cerebral palsy

Uncommon

- Scleroderma
- Lead poisoning

Pediatric considerations

- Imperforate anus, colonic or rectal atresia
- Meconium ileus
- Hirschsprung's disease
- Cystic fibrosis
- Intussusception

Diagnostic testing

History and examination should allow the emergency physician to determine the urgency with which diagnostic testing should be undertaken in the patient presenting with constipation. In those previously investigated having an exacerbation of a chronic problem, diagnostic testing may not be necessary.

Laboratory studies

These tests should be ordered as directed by history and examination. *Hypokalemia* and *hypercalcemia* may cause constipation. Tests of *thyroid* and *renal function* may be helpful in a patient not previously evaluated, as thyroid disease, renal disease, and dehydration may cause or contribute to constipation. *Iron deficiency anemia* may be present in a patient with colon carcinoma, so a complete blood count (CBC) should be considered.

Radiologic studies

Erect and supine abdominal radiographs may assist in evaluating possible bowel obstruction, particularly in patients with prior abdominal surgery, vomiting, significant abdominal distension, abdominal pain or an acute/subacute history of constipation. Erect chest films may be useful to look for free air under the diaphragm associated with bowel perforation. Visualization of "fecal loading" on plain abdominal radiographs rarely changes management and should not be used as a diagnostic test in the absence of other indications.

Abdominal computed tomography (CT) is a low yield test in the ED for evaluation of constipation alone, but may be extremely useful if the evaluation is part of a work-up for abdominal pain or malignancy.

Outpatient studies

Patients referred to their primary care physician from the ED may ask what investigations might be performed as an outpatient. These may include colonoscopy, endoscopy, intestinal transit studies, or anorectal manometry.

General treatment principles

Assess whether the constipation is part of a symptom complex (e.g., with abdominal pain) representing a life-threatening emergency?

As always, identify and treat any immediate life threats first. This might occur in patients with a perforated colon carcinoma, ischemic bowel, or ruptured appendix.

Red flags for serious conditions include abnormal vital signs, a "sick" patient, rebound or guarding on abdominal examination, and co-morbidities such as advanced age, chronic steroid treatment, or previous abdominal operations.

Action includes evaluation of the airway, breathing, and circulation (ABCs), resuscitation as appropriate, and a thorough investigation, usually in consultation with a surgeon.

Decide whether this presentation represents an acute crisis or complication in a patient for whom constipation is a long-term problem?

An acute crisis may occur in patients who develop bowel obstruction or become completely impacted, or in those who have developed new medical problems or have changed medications. These patients require a focus on *diagnostics* in the ED.

Specific therapy

Treatments need to be tailored to the individual patient. Attention to dietary and lifestyle factors may be sufficient for mild cases of constipation and will likely improve the success rate of other treatments. More than 700 laxative preparations are available over-the-counter. Review of the medical literature reveals little difference in effectiveness between laxatives. Common regimens for the treatment of constipation are provided in Table 14.3.

Table 14.3 Common regimens for the treatment of constipation

Mild constipation
- Senna and docusate (Senakot-S): 2 tablets PO qd for 3–4 days until relief *or*
- Psyllium (metamucil): up to 30 grams PO per day in 2–3 divided doses *or*
- Magnesium hydroxide (milk of magnesia): 30–60 ml regular strength liquid PO

Moderate constipation
as above plus
- Lactulose: 15–30 ml (syrup) or 10–20 grams (powder for oral solution) PO qd *and/or*
- Glycerin: One adult or infant suppository PR as needed *or*
- Sodium phosphate (Fleet enema): 1 adult or pediatric enema PR (Caution if renal failure or insufficiency) *or*
- Magnesium citrate: 150–300 ml PO divided qd-BID (Caution if renal failure or insufficiency)

Severe constipation
as above plus
- polyethylene glycol with electrolytes (GoLytely): 2–4 L over PO 4 hours *and/or*
- Soap suds enema in the ED

BID: two times a day; ED: emergency department; PO: per os; PR: per rectum; QD: every day.

Therapeutic manual disimpaction may be required, and patients may require sedation for the procedure. Laxative preparations will be required after the procedure to establish normal bowel habit.

Disposition

Assess whether anything in the systems review suggests a more extensive investigation is needed. If so, where should this be performed?

Inpatient evaluation may be required for patients who have severe symptoms such as pain, and for those with new diagnoses of severe hypothyroidism, significant anemia, or neurologic deficit on clinical examination. Referral to an inpatient specialist should occur after reversible causes have been treated in the ED.

Oupatient referral to a gastroenterologist should be made for patients with:

1. chronic constipation associated with weight loss, anemia, or change in stool caliber;
2. refractory constipation, and;
3. constipation requiring chronic laxative use.

Is it appropriate for the patient with uncomplicated constipation to receive symptomatic relief with laxatives or enemas at home?

This requires that bowel obstruction has been excluded, and that other social and medical considerations have been taken into account. These include the patient's level of self-care, ability to administer treatment, other co-morbidities, ability to follow-up with a primary care physician, and the ability to return to the ED if the problem worsens.

Discharge instructions should include discussion of diet (including fluid intake) and behavior modification such as exercise and "normalizing" daily routines.

Special patients
Elderly

Constipation in the elderly is more common, more difficult to treat, and more frequently represents serious pathology. Elderly patients are less likely to be able to manage treatment at home, and more likely to develop complications from constipation or from treatment. However, the general principles and approach are unchanged.

Pediatric

Bowel habits vary more commonly in children, so the problem of constipation is more difficult to define. The etiology is less commonly organic in nature and more frequently functional or behavioral. This should not preclude a thorough evaluation and investigation for organic causes. Presentations of organic etiologies may be non-specific including poor feeding, irritability, or even dyspnea. Referral to a pediatrician or family practitioner is essential for appropriate ongoing care. Neonates are a special group, and the diagnoses of imperforate anus, meconium ileus and Hirschsprung's disease must be considered.

Neurologic disease

Patients with neuromuscular disorders or spinal cord lesions generally have recurrent problems with constipation. Spinal patients can often train defecation reflexes to come under "voluntary" control (e.g., stroking their inner thigh). The condition of *autonomic dysreflexia* presents as high and labile blood pressure and diaphoresis in patients due to overwhelming autonomic nervous system stimulation. When this critical condition occurs, patients usually appear unwell. Fecal impaction with rectal distension is a recognized precipitant and needs to be treated urgently.

Pearls, pitfalls, and myths

- Do not attribute abdominal pain to constipation without careful consideration – they are both symptoms, not diagnoses.
- Simple fecal loading does not cause signs of peritonitis on abdominal examination, or abnormal vital signs.
- Feces evident on plain radiographs is normal – imaging is not a diagnostic modality for constipation. Imaging should be used to exclude alternative pathologies.
- Most constipation is caused by lifestyle, dietary factors and medications that are amenable to modification.
- Although thorough evaluation of constipation is warranted in all age groups, most patients can be investigated as outpatients in the absence of complicating features on history or physical examination.
- Consider constipation as a potential adverse outcome of all ED visits. Carefully consider all discharge medications, and advise patients accordingly.

References

1. Borum ML. Constipation: evaluation and management. *Prim Care* 2001;28(3): 577–590, vi.
2. Bulloch B, Tenenbein M. Constipation: Diagnosis and management in the pediatric emergency department. *Pediatr Emerg Care* 2002;18(4):254–258.
3. Cullen N. Constipation. In: Marx JA (ed.). *Rosen's Emergency Medicine: Concepts and Clinical Practice*, 5th ed., St Louis: Mosby, 2002.
4. Lamparelli MJ, Kumar D. Investigation and management of constipation. *Clin Med* 2002;2(5):415–420.
5. Sadosty AT, Browne BJ. Vomiting, diarrhoea and constipation. In: Tintanelli JE (ed.). *Emergency Medicine: A Comprehensive Study Guide*, 5th ed., McGraw Hill, 2000.
6. Zenni EA. Constipation. In: Harwood-Nuss A (ed.). *The Clinical Practice of Emergency Medicine*, 3rd ed., Philadelphia: Lippincott Williams and Wilkins, 2001.

15   Crying and irritability

Lee W. Shockley, MD

Scope of the problem

Small children cry and cry and cry. In part, this is due to the limited repertoire of communication skills they possess. They cry because crying is remarkably effective; there is no other infant behavior that elicits an adult's attention and response more reliably than the cry. At 2 weeks of age, the average crying time of a normal infant is 2 hours per day. By age 6 weeks, that increases to nearly 3 hours per day. Fortunately, it decreases to about 1 hour per day by 12 weeks of age.

Inconsolable crying is a very challenging presentation for several reasons: the child (usually under 2 years of age) may have nonspecific symptoms (or no symptoms at all except for the crying), and the associated diseases can range from benign to life-threatening. Inconsolable crying is also very challenging for parents. The primary focus of the emergency practitioner should be to search for and rule out serious causes of crying and irritability. Benign etiologies, although more common, should be established only after first considering the serious etiologies.

Pathophysiology

Crying is one of the only ways by which an infant communicates discomfort or distress. In that sense, it is a nonspecific form of communication. However, the infant's cry is probably more than a distress signal. Studies of the acoustic qualities of infant cries indicate that the cry probably contains "encoded" messages about the state of early neurologic development. These characteristics are the result of various muscular factors of the vocal anatomy combined with autonomic influences and central nervous system control. It is well recognized that infants with neurologic immaturity have abnormal cries; the cries of infants who are small for gestational age (SGA) correlate with the ability to modulate their state and quality of alertness. Infants suffering from meningitis, birth asphyxia, or hyperbilirubinemia classically are described as having high-pitched cries delivered in short bursts. The distinctive *cri-du-chat* ("cry of the cat") is associated with trisomy 18.

There is no single acoustic characteristic that differentiates a normal infant's cry from that of an abnormal infant. Several characteristic cries that may be associated with neurologic impairment have been described:

- Very high or low pitch;
- Extreme changes in pitch, little or no change in pitch, or rapidly fluctuating sounds;
- Extreme variation in length of individual cry bursts;
- Very short to very long latency to cry (very high or low threshold to cry after a stimulus);
- Flat, atonal, or stark cry with no harmonic quality, fullness, or overtones;
- Non-harmonic sounds that interrupt the cry.

Parents are unlikely to bring an infant to an emergency department (ED) for a cry they believe is normal. Parents tend to bring their child in for evaluation of the crying when:

1. they cannot identify the source,
2. they cannot console the infant,
3. the crying is longer than usual.

The words that the parents use to describe the crying may be very helpful in determining its etiology.

History

Physicians must rely on the parents and care providers to give a history. It is important to ascertain the onset, frequency, and duration of crying. Parents often report a distinctive cry for various situations; the infant may have one cry that communicates hunger and another that communicates fatigue. Abnormal characteristics of an infant's cry often elicit a parental response of concern, prompting a visit to the pediatrician or the ED. The complaint of an abnormal cry may be the only clue to a serious condition. However, a careful history can provide clues for the cause of abnormal crying in approximately 20% of cases.

The child's medical history (including birth history, pregnancy complications, hospitalizations, illnesses, surgeries, and allergies) should be reviewed. The clinician should ask about recent medication use, illnesses, and immunizations. Excessive persistent crying is a well-documented side effect of the diphtheria, pertussis, and tetanus (DPT) vaccine and is probably related to a painful local reaction at the site of the vaccination. Furthermore, parents may be able to provide valuable clues by exploring feeding habits (including changes in the diet), bowel habits, urination, fever, sick contacts, level of activity, and ability to be consoled.

Physical examination

The primary goal of the physical examination is to identify painful conditions which might lead to excessive crying. A careful physical examination can find the cause for abnormal crying in an additional 40% of infants (on top of the 20% diagnosed by the history alone). Although it is important to conduct a thorough physical examination, there are several high-yield examinations to perform (Table 15.1)

Table 15.1 High-yield examinations in the crying or irritable child (in descending order)

Otoscopy
Rectal examination
Fluorescein staining of the cornea
Inspection of skin underneath clothing and diapers
Palpation of bones
Oral examination
Auscultation of the heart
Laryngoscopic examination of the hypopharynx
Eversion of the eyelid
Palpation of the anterior fontanelle
Retinal examination
Neurologic examination

General appearance

The general appearance of the infant should be noted with particular attention to observations of the cry and consolability with the parents. Will the child take a bottle? Does feeding calm the child? What is the child's tone and posture? How are the parents reacting to the child? Is the child interactive with the examiner?

Vital signs

Special attention should be paid to the vital signs. In particular, what is the heart rate and the respiratory rate when crying and when calm? A rectal temperature should be used to assess the child's core temperature. Hypothermia as well as hyperthermia may be signs of sepsis. Pulse oximetry should be performed to assess for hypoxia. The child's weight should be measured and compared to previous weights to assess hydration and nutritional status. It is also important for calculating medication and fluid doses, and in assessing the child's growth curve at subsequent visits.

Skin

Undress the child completely to examine for rashes, bruising, insect or spider bites, open diaper pins in children wearing cloth diapers, and other signs of trauma. The state of hydration and perfusion should also be assessed.

Head, eyes, ears, nose, and throat

Examine the head for any signs of trauma and anterior fontanelle fullness. The ears should be examined for otitis externa, otitis media, and foreign bodies. Examine the eyes for symmetric pupillary activity or retinal hemorrhages. Evert the upper eyelids to identify foreign bodies or lashes under the lid. Apply fluorescein to the corneas and examine them for corneal abrasions under ultraviolet light. Examine the nose and throat for foreign bodies and infection. Examine the mouth, tongue, and hypopharynx for new tooth eruptions, trauma, infections, aphthous ulcers, lesions, vesicles, foreign bodies, and scald burns on the buccal mucosa or tongue from milk heated in a microwave oven. A tongue depressor or laryngoscope (used as a tongue depressor) may be necessary to visualize the hypopharynx.

Neck

Examine the neck for masses, lymphadenopathy, tenderness, and rigidity (which may be absent even in an infant with bacterial meningitis).

Chest

Assess for tachypnea and retractions, and auscultate for abnormal breath sounds.

Abdomen

The abdomen should be evaluated for bowel activity, distention, tone, tenderness, and masses. A mass in the left upper quadrant is suggestive of constipation; a vertical sausage-shaped mass is the classic (although rare) finding in intussusception. An olive-sized mass in the epigastrium in an infant with post-prandial vomiting is described in pyloric stenosis. Cellulitis or abnormal discharge around the umbilicus or umbilical stump should be identified.

Genitourinary

Examine for hernias (Figure 15.1) and masses. In boys, examine the genitalia for testicular torsion, paraphimosis, and strangulation of the penis or testes from a hair or thread tourniquet. In girls, examine for evidence of trauma.

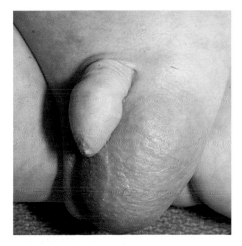

Figure 15.1
Left inguinal hernia with erythema of the overlying hemiscrotum. Reprinted from Atlas of Pediatric Physical Diagnosis, 4th ed., Eds Zitelli BJ, Davis HW. Copyright 2002, with permission from Elsevier.

Rectal

Perform a visual examination of the perineum looking for blood or fissures. Using the tip of the examiner's small finger, perform a gentle digital rectal examination. Although "currant jelly" stool is a classically described finding in intussusception, it is often a late finding indicating bowel necrosis. An earlier finding is occult blood in the stool on guaiac testing.

Musculoskeletal

Inspect and palpate the extremities. Specifically, examine for focal tenderness along bones and hairs or thread tourniquets wrapped around the digits (Figure 15.2). Test the range of motion of the joints, especially the hips, for tenderness and limitation of motion suggestive of septic arthritis.

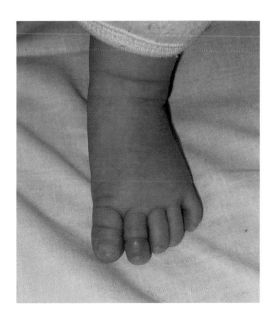

Figure 15.2
Hair tourniquet of 2nd toe.
Courtesy: S.V. Mahadevan, MD.

Neurologic

The neurologic examination should include an assessment of the infant's overall level of activity, responsiveness, and ability to be consoled. The examination should assess movement of all of the extremities and muscle tone.

Differential diagnosis

Causes of inconsolable crying are legion. They may be classified as follows.

Head and neck

Head

- Encephalitis
- Headache
- Head trauma (skull fracture, intracranial hemorrhage, shaken baby syndrome)
- Meningitis

Eye

- Corneal abrasion
- Foreign bodies
- Glaucoma

Ear

- Foreign bodies
- Otitis media or externa
- Mastoiditis

Mouth or throat

- Aphthous ulcers, herpangina
- Burns
- Foreign bodies
- Oral thrush
- Teething
- Stomatitis

Chest

Cardiac

- Anomalous left coronary artery
- Coarctation of the aorta
- Congestive heart failure
- Dysrhythmia

Respiratory

- Hypoxia
- Pneumonia/pneumonitis
- Rib fractures
- Upper respiratory tract infection

Abdomen

- Anal fissure
- Appendicitis
- Celiac disease
- Constipation
- Gastric distention
- Gastroenteritis
- Gastroesophageal reflux
- Incarcerated hernia
- Intussusception
- Milk intolerance or cow's milk allergy
- Peritonitis
- Volvulus

Genitourinary

- Balanitis
- Hair tourniquet syndrome
- Meatal ulceration
- Testicular or ovarian torsion
- Urinary tract infection
- Urethral foreign body

Extremities

- Arthritis
- Bites
- Burns (immersion, cigarette, etc.)
- Contusions
- Fractures
- Hair tourniquet syndrome
- Insect or spider bites
- Open diaper pin
- Osteomyelitis

Metabolic or toxic

- Aspirin overdose
- Drug reactions
- Electrolyte abnormalities
- Hypoglycemia
- Inborn errors of metabolism
- Metabolic acidosis
- Neonatal drug withdrawal
- Phenylketonuria
- Pre- or perinatal cocaine exposure
- Sepsis
- Sickle cell crisis
- Vitamin A toxicity

Miscellaneous

- Autism
- Caffey disease (infantile cortical hyperostosis)
- Colic
- Dermatitis, skin infections
- Discomfort (cold, heat, itching, hunger)
- Emotional or physical neglect
- Idiopathic
- Immunization reactions
- Maternal depression
- Night terrors
- Overstimulation
- Parental expectations or responses
- Persistent night awakening
- Temperment

A study of 56 infants ages 4 days to 24 months, presenting to the ED of the Children's Hospital of Denver over a 1-year period with acute, unexplained, excessive crying, revealed numerous etiologies (Table 15.2).

Approximately half of the patients seen in the ED at the Children's Hospital were referred from community pediatricians, the remaining half were "walk-in" patients. Sixty-one percent of the infants in this study had a condition that was considered serious as determined by a panel of

Table 15.2 Diagnoses in children with excessive crying

Diagnosis	Frequency (%)
Idiopathic	10/56 (18)
Otitis media	10/56 (18)
Colic	6/56 (11)
Corneal abrasion	3/56 (5)
Constipation	3/56 (5)
Viral illness with anorexia and dehydration	2/56 (4)
Supraventricular tachycardia	2/56 (4)
Urinary tract infection	1/56 (2)
Mild prodrome of gastroenteritis	1/56 (2)
Herpangina	1/56 (2)
Herpes stomatitis	1/56 (2)
Foreign body in the eye	1/56 (2)
Foreign body in the oropharynx	1/56 (2)
Tibial fracture	1/56 (2)
Clavicle fracture	1/56 (2)
Brown recluse spider bite	1/56 (2)
Hair tourniquet syndrome	1/56 (2)
Intussusception	1/56 (2)
Gastroesophageal reflux with esophagitis	1/56 (2)
Subdural hematoma	1/56 (2)
Encephalitis	1/56 (2)
Pseudotumor cerebri	1/56 (2)
Vaccine reaction	1/56 (2)
Inadvertent pseudoephedrine overdose	1/56 (2)
Night terrors	1/56 (2)
Overstimulation	1/56 (2)
Glutaricaciduria, type 1	1/56 (2)

three pediatricians not participating in the study. A serious condition determination was made if two or three of the panel members felt the infant had a condition that required prompt treatment or had the potential for harm if the condition was not recognized and treated.

Special attention should be paid to the diagnosis of infant colic (paroxysmal fussiness, infantile colic, evening colic, 3-month colic). Infant colic is a syndrome characterized by:

- sudden attacks, usually in the evening;
- loud, almost continuous cry lasting several hours;
- the infant's face is flushed, occasionally with circumoral pallor;
- abdomen is distended and tense;

- legs drawn up, feet are often cold (legs may extend periodically during forceful cries);
- fingers are clenched;
- relief with the passage of flatus or feces;
- not quelled for long by feeding;
- terminates from apparent exhaustion.

The etiology of infant colic is not well understood. The condition affects up to 20% of newborns. Infant colic is most common at 1 month of life and most often resolves by 3 months.

Diagnostic testing

In general, focused diagnostic studies should be ordered based on suspicions raised from the history and physical examination or when the history and physical examination do not reveal or suggest the etiology of the crying.

Radiologic studies

Chest X-ray

A chest X-ray is indicated to diagnose pneumonia or aspirated foreign bodies. Radiolucent foreign bodies may be suspected on the basis of air trapping. This finding is most pronounced in an expiratory film. In the crying infant, it may be extremely difficult to coordinate the timing of the film exposure with expiration; in these circumstances, bilateral decubitus films can be ordered. The dependent lung is compressed by the child's own weight, simulating expiration.

Skeletal X-rays

Focal areas of tenderness, bruising, or deformity should prompt the ordering of skeletal X-rays. In addition, the "skeletal survey" is useful to look for signs of previous trauma. Several patterns of skeletal injuries are highly correlated with non-accidental trauma (NAT) (Table 15.3).

Table 15.3 Skeletal injuries associated with non-accidental trauma

Spiral fracture of a long bone (Figure 15.3)
Metaphyseal chip fracture
Multiple fractures at different stages of healing
Fractures at unusual sites, such as ribs, lateral clavicle, sternum, or scapula

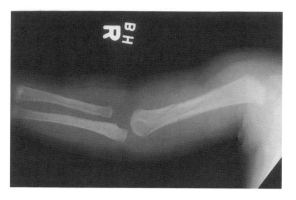

Figure 15.3
Spiral fracture. A spiral fracture courses from the distal portion to the upper third of the diaphysis. There is moderate soft-tissue swelling. Reprinted from Atlas of Pediatric Physical Diagnosis, 4th ed., Eds Zitelli BJ, Davis HW. Copyright 2002, with permission from Elsevier.

Head computed tomography

In the infant with an abnormal neurologic examination (especially lateralizing findings), retinal hemorrhages, signs of head trauma, or suspicion for NAT, head computed tomography (CT) is indicated. This study provides information about brain injuries (contusions and hematomas) as well as most skull fractures. It may also be helpful in diagnosing hydrocephalus or other congenital abnormalities. An inconsolable crying infant may have to be sedated and closely monitored in order to obtain this study. It is important, however, that indicated studies be obtained regardless of the need for sedation and monitoring, and the increase in work that such diagnostic tests cause.

Barium enema

A barium or air-contrast enema is indicated when concerns for intussusception must be answered. These tests are not only diagnostic but often therapeutic, reducing the intussusception. Consultation with a pediatric surgeon and radiologist are warranted prior to the study in the case that emergent surgical intervention is necessary (i.e., for bowel perforation). Abdominal ultrasonography has a role in the diagnosis of intussusception, depending on the skill of the radiologist.

Esophagram

An esophagram may be necessary to diagnose esophageal abnormalities, such as tracheo-esophageal (TE) fistula, webs, reflux, but is rarely necessary from the ED.

Electrocardiogram

An electrocardiogram (ECG) is indicated to evaluate the infant with an abnormally fast or slow heart rate or an irregular pulse. An echocardiogram can also provide information about structural and flow abnormalities of the heart.

Laboratory studies

Complete blood count and blood culture

A complete blood count (CBC) and blood culture are included in the workup of a suspected septic infant (toxic-appearing or febrile without an obvious source of infection). For a more detailed discussion, see Chapter 23.

Glucose

A bedside dextrostick can rapidly identify hypo- or hyperglycemia. Hypoglycemia in the infant is often associated with sepsis, errors of metabolism, and certain toxic ingestions. Hyperglycemia may be the first indication of diabetes.

Electrolytes

Serum electrolytes may be indicated in the evaluation of a crying infant to look for hyper- or hyponatremia, hyper- or hypokalemia, metabolic acidosis, and hypocalcemia.

Urinalysis and culture

A urinalysis and culture are indicated in crying infants. Urinary tract infections are common in infants, particularly girls younger than 12 months, boys younger than 6 months, and uncircumcised boys younger than 12 months. They may present with nonspecific symptoms such as inconsolable crying.

Lumbar puncture

A lumbar puncture with cell count and differential, Gram stain, glucose and protein determination, and culture should be performed if meningitis is suspected as the cause of inconsolable crying.

Toxicologic screening

Toxicologic screening may be indicated in infants where acute or chronic exposures are considered. Be aware, however, that many toxins are not routinely screened for. Toxicologic screening may also be negative in cases of drug withdrawal.

Liver enzymes

Liver transaminases and bilirubin may be used as a screening test for liver injuries associated with blunt abdominal trauma. If the clinical suspicion of abdominal trauma is high or the liver enzymes are elevated, the clinician should proceed to CT scanning of the abdomen.

Amino and organic acid studies

Amino and organic acid studies may be ordered in cases in which an inborn error of metabolism is suspected. These studies are rarely indicated in the ED, however.

General treatment principles

There is no single medication that can be recommended for the crying infant because of the large variety and spectrum of etiologies responsible.

Several treatments have been advocated for infant colic, including:

- use of a pacifier;
- motion, such as rocking the infant, a bounce chair, a car ride, or a car seat on top of a dryer;
- softly massaging the infant's back or abdomen;
- playing relaxing music;
- simethicone drops;
- changing the infant's diet, feeding schedule, or techniques.

Unfortunately, none of these is guaranteed.

Special patients

Infants who were premature or are immunocompromised are at special risk for infectious etiologies as the cause of inconsolable crying.

Risk factors for NAT include:

- Unwanted children: accidental pregnancies, illegitimate births, the opposite sex from what the parents desired, being born during periods of crisis or a former relationship.
- Difficult to rear: poor feeders, fussy behavior, abnormal sleep patterns, excessive crying, retardation, hyperactivity, behavior disorders, handicaps, or chronic disease.
- Poor maternal–child bonding: premature infants, infants separated from their mothers because of illness, stepchildren, or foster children.

- A parent who is an abuser of alcohol or other drugs.
- Intergenerational patterns of abuse.
- A parent with poor impulse control or very rigid and unrealistic expectations of children.

Be suspicious for NAT in:

- inconsistent or discrepant histories;
- injuries that are inconsistent with the child's age and development;
- alleged self-inflicted injuries;
- unexplained injuries;
- accusatory histories;
- delays in seeking medical care;
- past histories of abuse (or abused siblings);
- presentations for apparently unrelated complaints;
- unusual bruising;
- unusual burns;
- skeletal injuries in different stages of healing, multiple fractures, metaphyseal injuries, and an exaggerated periosteal reaction;
- intracranial injuries;
- retinal hemorrhages;
- intra-abdominal injuries;
- renal injuries;
- bruising and laceration of the upper lip, frenulum, and floor of the mouth;
- psychiatric complaints;
- developmental delay.

Disposition

The disposition of the infant with persistent crying and irritability will likely be dictated by the ultimate diagnosis. The conditions that are serious should prompt consultation and hospitalization. Most of the etiologies are benign and can be followed as an outpatient. If an etiology cannot be established after a thorough evaluation, the family is reliable and will return should the infant's condition change, and adequate follow-up arrangements can be made, the infant can be discharged. If the decision to discharge the patient is contemplated, it should be done only after a period of observation in the ED (perhaps 2–4 hours). If there are concerns about parental reliability or safety, the child is best admitted to the hospital.

Pearls, pitfalls, and myths

- Ask about medication use, including over-the-counter medications and medications used by a breast-feeding mother. This should include topical medications that a breast-feeding mother may apply to her nipples.

- Listen to the parents' descriptions of the cry and document their words. It can occasionally be helpful in making the diagnosis.
- Undress the infant completely and perform a comprehensive physical examination.
- Always consider the possibility of NAT.
- The diagnosis of excessive crying should be made using a process of elimination, after ruling out the more dangerous causes.
- Paradoxical inconsolability (an increase in crying associated with efforts at consolation, such as lifting or rocking) can be associated with meningitis, peritonitis, fractures, arthritis, or abuse.
- All infants who are not admitted need good follow-up care arranged prior to leaving the ED. Included in the instructions should be a list of things which should prompt a return to the ED for reevaluation.
- Children with infant colic often show decelerated growth. Failure to thrive should make one suspicious about the diagnosis of infant colic.
- Sedatives (chloral hydrate, phenobarbital, alcohol, antihistamines) should not be used for the treatment of inconsolable crying.
- All 50 states have laws for the mandatory reporting of *suspected* NAT in children.

References

1. Behrman RE, Kliegman RM, Jenson HB (eds). In: *Nelson Textbook of Pediatrics*, 16th ed., Philadelphia, PA: WB Saunders Co, 2000. pp. 167.
2. Brazelton TB. Crying in infancy. *Pediatrics* 1962;29:579–588.
3. Charney EB, Ditmar MF. Growth, development and behavior. In: Polin RA, Ditmar MF (eds). *Pediatric Secrets*, Philadelphia: Hanley & Belfus, 1989. pp. 137–150.
4. Ditmar MF. Crying. In: Schwartz MW (ed.). *The Five Minute Pediatric Consult*, 2nd ed., Philadelphia: Lippincott Williams & Wilkins, 2000. pp. 24–25.
5. Forsyth BW. Colic and the effect of changing formulas: a double-blind, multiple-crossover study. *J Pediatr* 1989;115(4): 521–526.
6. Garrison MM, Christakis DA. A systematic review of treatments for infant colic. *Pediatrics* 2000;106(1 pt 2):184–190.
7. Henretig FM. Crying and colic in early infancy. In: Fleisher GR, Ludwig S (eds). *Textbook of Pediatric Emergency Medicine*, Baltimore: Williams & Wilkins, 1993. pp. 144–146.
8. Jakobsson I, Lindberg T. Cow's milk as a cause of infantile colic in breast-fed infants. *Lancet* 1978;2(8087):437–439.
9. Lester BM, Zeskind PS. A biobehavioral perspective on crying in early infancy. In: Fitzgerald H, Lester B, Yogman M (eds). *Theory and Research in Behavioral Pediatrics*, Vol. 1. New York: Plenum Publishing, 1982.
10. Lucassen PL, Assendelft WJ, Gubbels JW, et al. Infantile colic: crying time reduction with a whey hydrolysate: a double-blind, randomized, placebo-controlled trial. *Pediatrics* 2000;106(6):1349–1354.
11. McKenzie S. Troublesome crying in infants: effect of advice to reduce stimulation. *Arch Dis Child* 1991;66(12):1416–1420.
12. Poole SR. The infant with acute, unexplained, excessive crying. *Pediatrics* 1991;88:450–455.

16 Diabetes-related emergencies

Christopher R.H. Newton, MD

Scope of the problem

Diabetes mellitus affects an estimated 11 million people in the US and over 100 million worldwide. Approximately 90% of these patients have type 2 or non-insulin-dependent diabetes. The remainder are classified as type 1 or insulin-dependent diabetics.

Diabetes is characterized by chronic hyperglycemia that often requires lifelong treatment. Untreated, chronic hyperglycemia eventually leads to both micro- and macrovascular complications affecting virtually every organ system. As a result, diabetics frequently present to the emergency department (ED) with complications such as severe infections, myocardial infarction (MI), stroke, renal disease, and lower extremity ischemia and skin ulcerations.

This chapter focuses on the diagnosis and management of acute metabolic derangements frequently encountered in diabetic patients. These consist of diabetic ketoacidosis (DKA), hyperglycemic hyperosmolar state (HHS), and hypoglycemia.

Diabetic ketoacidosis

DKA is a potentially life-threatening medical emergency. It occurs predominantly in type 1 diabetics and accounts for the initial presentation of glucose-related problems in about 25% of diabetics. Despite advances in treatment, the mortality rate for this condition remains 2–4%.

DKA is a syndrome characterized by hyperglycemia, ketonemia, and metabolic acidosis caused by either relative or absolute insulin deficiency. The treatment consists of fluid and electrolyte replacement, together with continuous low-dose insulin infusion.

Precipitating causes for DKA include infection, MI, trauma, pregnancy, or stress. In many cases, there isn't an intercurrent disease process, and noncompliance with insulin therapy is recognized as a significant precipitant of DKA. Errors of insulin dosage may occasionally be a contributing factor.

Pathophysiology

The primary abnormality in DKA is an absolute or relative insulin deficiency. This leads to a rise in the counter-regulatory hormones (catecholamines, glucagon, growth hormone, and cortisol). Changes in these hormone levels produce three major effects:

1. Hyperglycemia resulting from decreased glucose utilization and increased hepatic gluconeogenesis;
2. Increased lipolysis leading to ketone body formation;
3. Increased metabolism of protein and reduction in protein synthesis.

Hyperglycemia causes a profound osmotic diuresis resulting in progressive dehydration. Ketonemia and acidosis may lead to nausea and vomiting, which exacerbates fluid and electrolyte losses.

History

Have you had increased thirst or urinary frequency?

Typically, patients describe the gradual onset of polyuria (increased urinary frequency) and polydipsia (increased thirst) with fatigue and progressive weight loss.

Have you had nausea, vomiting, or abdominal pain?

A combination of increased ketones and prostaglandin release is thought to contribute to nausea and vomiting. This can lead to a misdiagnosis of gastroenteritis in early DKA. Abdominal pain is frequently reported in DKA and has many causes, including gastric distension and ileus.

Have you been following your usual insulin schedule recently? Have you missed insulin doses or changed your diet?

This has been increasingly recognized as a precipitant of DKA, particularly in adolescents who often find it more difficult to comply with insulin regimens and eat regular scheduled meals.

Have you had a fever, painful urination, cough, or shortness of breath? Have you had any chest pain or dark stool?

Infection, acute MI, and gastrointestinal (GI) bleeding are all common precipitants of DKA. Systemic inquiry should be directed at uncovering these precipitants.

Physical examination

The vital signs are often abnormal in DKA. Tachycardia is most frequently observed. As fluid deficits increase, orthostatic hypotension is common. An elevated temperature is rarely caused by DKA itself and suggests the presence of infection. Hypothermia can also be associated with infection, and has an increased mortality rate in the setting of DKA.

As the metabolic abnormalities progress, the patient becomes acidemic, leading to direct stimulation of the respiratory center in an attempt to compensate. This leads to an increased rate and depth of respiration, referred to as *Kussmaul respirations*. Systemic ketosis is often associated with an unusual fruity odor that may be detected by some clinicians on the breath of patients. Progressive dehydration may also lead to changes in mental status or coma. A careful abdominal examination is particularly important in patients presenting with abdominal pain.

Evidence of infection should always be sought on examination of diabetics, with particular attention to the feet, genitourinary (GU) and rectal areas of elderly diabetics.

Diagnostic testing

Once intravenous (IV) access is established, a bedside capillary blood glucose test should be performed. This is usually accurate to around 500 mg/dl. If the bedside capillary glucose is above 300–400 mg/dl, fluid resuscitation should be initiated prior to obtaining formal laboratory results.

The laboratory investigations needed include serum electrolytes, blood urea nitrogen, creatinine, glucose, calcium, magnesium, phosphate, and a complete blood count. Serum ketones should also be ordered, as the urine dipstick for ketones can be falsely negative. A blood gas should be obtained to document the pH. Recent literature has shown a significant correlation between venous and arterial blood gases; therefore, a venous sample is now often used for diagnostic purposes.

The serum potassium level is extremely important. Patients are usually severely potassium depleted, yet may have high serum levels on the first sampling. This is caused by acidosis that enhances potassium release from cells in exchange for hydrogen ions in an attempt to normalize the pH. Pseudohyponatremia is common and is caused by hyperglycemia. The sodium level can be corrected by adding 1.6 meq of sodium for every 100 mg of glucose above 100 mg/dl.

Patients with abdominal pain should also have amylase, lipase, and liver function tests ordered.

A septic work-up, including blood and urine cultures and a chest X-ray should be considered, especially in febrile patients, but depends on the patient's presentation.

An electrocardiogram (ECG) is essential to look for evidence of hyperkalemia and to search for a possible precipitant of DKA, such as myocardial ischemia.

Guidelines published by the American Diabetic Association outline a triad of biochemical requirements for the diagnosis of DKA:

1. Glucose >250 mg/dl;
2. Arterial pH <7.35, venous pH <7.30, or bicarbonate <15 meq/l;
3. Ketonemia or ketonuria.

General treatment principles

Many EDs now have clinical guidelines and pathways available for the management of DKA. Treatment is usually initiated after obtaining a history suggestive of DKA and a confirmatory high bedside glucose.

1. Fluid replacement

Vigorous fluid resuscitation is mandatory and should be initiated prior to laboratory results being available. Fluid restores intravascular volume and improves perfusion to vital organs. It also begins to lower the serum glucose. The initial fluid of choice is normal saline. Generally, in adults, the first 2 liters should be given over the first 2 hours. An additional 2 liters should then be given over the next 4 hours. After that, fluid can be titrated to the patient's clinical improvement and perceived hydration state. A number of studies suggest that hypotonic solution should be used after the initial resuscitation. A 5% dextrose-containing fluid should be used when the glucose level falls below 300 mg/dl.

Excessive fluid replacement has been previously cited as a cause of important complications, such as cerebral edema and adult respiratory distress syndrome. However, it is more common that patients are under-resuscitated then fluid overloaded. It is now recognized that fluid resuscitation probably has little or no role in the development of these complications.

2. Insulin therapy

Insulin therapy is usually initiated once the serum electrolytes become available to ensure that the patient is not hypokalemic. This is due to the fact that insulin drives potassium intracellularly and can cause life-threatening dysrhythmias or respiratory paralysis in hypokalemic patients. Insulin therapy is administered by an initial 0.1 units/kg IV bolus followed by a continuous infusion of short-acting insulin, usually at a rate of 0.1 units/kg/ hour (maximum usually 10 units/hour initially). The IV tubing should be flushed prior to starting the infusion because insulin adheres to its walls, which can make the initial dosing erratic. A bedside capillary glucose should be monitored hourly when an insulin infusion is used.

The insulin infusion should be continued until the serum ketones are cleared and the patient's anion gap (sodium minus chloride and bicarbonate) has normalized (<12–14). Resolution of hyperglycemia usually occurs prior to this, so dextrose must be provided to ensure normoglycemia.

3. Potassium replacement

Patients with DKA usually have profound depletion of total body potassium caused by insulin deficiency, acidosis, osmotic diuresis, and vomiting. However, the initial potassium is usually normal or even high secondary to acidosis that drives hydrogen intracellularly and potassium extracellularly. Once fluid and insulin replacement are initiated, potassium is forced intracellularly and the serum level can drop dramatically. The decision to replace potassium is made after the serum electrolytes become available because of the potentially life-threatening consequences of giving potassium to a patient with hyperkalemia. Peaked T-waves, prolonged PR intervals, and widened QRS complexes on the ECG provide early evidence of hyperkalemia prior to the serum electrolytes becoming available. For this reason, a stat ECG is included in the initial evaluation. A stat potassium may be run off arterial blood from an ABG.

Potassium replacement should be initiated in all patients unless the serum level is greater than 5.5 meq/liter or the patient is anuric. Potassium is usually given as potassium chloride at an IV rate not faster than 5–15 meq/hour. Patients with an initial potassium less than 3.5 meq/liter need more aggressive replacement <u>prior</u> to initiation of the insulin infusion. The goal is to maintain potassium in the normal range of 4–5 meq/liter while avoiding life-threatening hypo- or hyperkalemia.

Bicarbonate replacement is controversial and is not routinely recommended for the emergency management of patients in DKA. Despite a number of clinical trials assessing the efficacy of bicarbonate, none has shown improvement in clinical outcomes. Bicarbonate can be considered for patients with an initial pH of less than 7.0.

The replacement of phosphate remains controversial and it is not routinely done in the ED. Despite theoretical benefits, there appears to be no clinical benefit from the routine administration of phosphate in patients with DKA.

Serum glucose and electrolytes should be checked at 0, 2, and 4 hours from presentation and then every 4 hours during insulin infusion and potassium replacement. Capillary glucose should be checked at 0, 1, and 2 hours after presentation and then every 1–2 hours while on the insulin drip.

Many hospitals now use DKA flow sheets that keep track of vital signs and laboratory results, which makes both patient management and documentation more efficient and reliable.

Special patients

Pediatric patients in DKA have a higher rate of developing cerebral edema. The exact reasons for this are unknown. A recently published study showed that children with DKA who have low partial pressures of arterial carbon dioxide and high serum urea nitrogen concentrations at presentation, and who are treated with bicarbonate are at increased risk for cerebral edema. Children should have fluid replaced judiciously and be admitted to a specialist knowledgable in the management of pediatric DKA.

Pregnancy predisposes individuals to both diabetes (gestational) and DKA. Pregnant patients in DKA have higher rates of complications for mother and baby. Maternal acidosis decreases fetal blood flow, and may cause fetal demise. As with children, pregnant patients in DKA should be cared for by specialists comfortable with the care of diabetes in pregnancy.

Patients with congestive heart failure can be particularly difficult to manage. They require fluid resuscitation, yet can easily become fluid overloaded because of poor cardiac function. Although usually unnecessary, monitoring of central venous pressure or pulmonary artery wedge pressure should be considered for patients with a history of prior congestive heart failure.

Patients with renal failure and DKA require careful fluid and potassium replacement. Management often requires input from a nephrologist or critical care specialist.

Disposition

The vast majority of patients with DKA require admission to a setting where frequent monitoring of vital signs and serial blood draws can occur. Patients with altered mental status, hypotension, or severe acidosis should be admitted to the intensive care unit. Many hospitals have policies that dictate admission criteria for DKA patients on insulin drips.

Complications

Cerebral edema and adult respiratory distress syndrome (ARDS) are rare but life-threatening complications of DKA. Cerebral edema occurs primarily in pediatric patients. It manifests as progressive deterioration in mental status 6–10 hours after the initiation of therapy. There are no warning signs or clinical predictors. Patients who develop cerebral edema should be aggressively treated with mannitol and dexamethasone in collaboration with an intensivist.

Dyspnea, hypoxemia, and diffuse pulmonary edema on chest X-ray are the classic findings of ARDS. Patients often require ventilatory support. As with cerebral edema, mortality is high.

Iatrogenic complications include pulmonary edema from over-aggressive fluid resuscitation, hypoglycemia from inadequate glucose monitoring and failure to add glucose to the fluids when the serum glucose falls below 300 mg/dl, and hypokalemia. Strict nursing adherence to DKA management guidelines minimizes the risk of these complications.

Hyperglycemic hyperosmolar state

HHS or hyperosmolar hyperglycemic non-ketotic syndrome (HNKS) is characterized by hyperglycemia, hyperosmolarity, and dehydration. Ketosis and acidosis are usually minimal or absent. HHS is most frequently observed in poorly-controlled or undiagnosed type 2 diabetics. Altered level of consciousness is a common finding and may progress to coma, leading to the former name hyperosmolar nonketotic coma (HNKC). However, this term is confusing as the majority of these patients are not actually comatose. Mortality in HHS is much greater than in DKA, usually between 15% and 30%. This higher rate is likely related to both the underlying disease precipitants and the elderly population that it affects.

Pathophysiology

Insulin resistance leads to inadequate tissue utilization of glucose, resulting in hyperglycemia. Hepatic gluconeogenesis and glycogenolysis further elevate the serum glucose level. As the serum glucose increases, it creates an osmotic gradient that draws water out of the intracellular space and into the intravascular compartment. When the serum glucose level exceeds the kidneys' capacity to reabsorb it, glucose spills into the urine, creating glucosuria and an osmotic diuresis.

Patients may be able to keep up with the volume losses; however, many elderly patients in nursing homes do not have access to fluids or are unable to keep up with the excessive fluid losses. Therefore, they become progressively dehydrated. These fluid losses often exceed 20% of total body weight.

The absence of ketoacidosis in patients with HHS has a number of potential causes, including lower levels of counterregulatory hormones, higher levels of insulin, and inhibition of lipolysis by the hyperosmolar state.

History

HHS is usually seen in elderly patients with a variety of nonspecific complaints, including weakness and fatigue. If able to answer questions, patients may complain of polyuria and polydipsia for days or weeks prior to seeking medical attention.

Inquiries about symptoms consistent with precipitants of HHS, such as infection, MI, stroke, or GI bleeding should be made.

Physical examination

Altered mental status and abnormal vital signs are the most frequently encountered findings in

HHS. It is important to remember that elderly patients often have a degree of baseline cognitive impairment, making it essential to obtain a detailed history from the family or caregiver about any change from that baseline. The degree of lethargy and coma exhibited correlates well with their serum osmolality.

Patients in HHS usually exhibit evidence of volume depletion, such as poor skin turgor, dry mucus membranes, and orthostatic hypotension. Evidence of cellulitis or melena should be sought during the physical examination.

Diagnostic testing

The initial diagnostic work-up for HHS is similar to that for DKA, with the addition of sending a serum osmolality. An ECG should be performed as early as possible. Precipitants of HHS should be considered when ordering other studies. Blood cultures, cardiac enzymes, chest X-ray, head computed tomography (CT), and lumbar puncture should be guided by the clinical presentation. Arterial blood gases are usually unnecessary unless there is a pulmonary component to the acid–base abnormality.

HHS is defined by a serum glucose greater than 400 mg/dl and a calculated plasma osmolality greater than 315 mOsm/liter in the absence of ketosis. In practice, the serum glucose level is usually greater than 600 mg/dl and the osmolality is greater than 350 mOsm/liter, with marked electrolyte abnormalities. Acidosis and ketones can be seen occasionally and are usually explained by the precipitant of the HHS.

General treatment principles

1. Fluid replacement

The initial resuscitation is aimed at restoring adequate tissue perfusion and decreasing serum glucose. The average fluid deficit in HHS is 8–12 liters, often double the deficit encountered in DKA. Half of this fluid deficit should be replaced IV over the first 12 hours, with the remainder over the next 24 hours. The actual rate of fluid administration is highly variable and depends on the estimated fluid deficit, the patient's weight, and the degree of renal and cardiac impairment. Isotonic saline (0.9% NS) is the most appropriate crystalloid for initial volume restoration. This can then be substituted for half-normal saline (0.45% NS) when vital signs have normalized and there is adequate urine output.

2. Potassium replacement

All patients with HHS have deficits in total body potassium. An IV infusion of potassium at 10 meq/hour should be initiated in all patients who are making urine and are not hyperkalemic. Higher rates of potassium replacement may be necessary if the patient is hypokalemic initially. Potassium levels should be monitored every hour until consistently in the normal range.

3. Insulin infusion

After adequate fluid replacement and determination of the serum potassium, regular insulin may be given as a continuous IV infusion at 0.1 units/kg/hour. The insulin infusion should be discontinued when the blood glucose is less than 250 mg/dl. At this point, 5% dextrose should be added to the maintenance fluid to prevent hypoglycemia.

Special patients

HHS most commonly occurs in the elderly, who may have underlying cardiac or renal disease. As discussed in the DKA section, this makes therapy much more complicated and results in higher morbidity and mortality.

Disposition

Most patients with HHS require admission to an intensive care unit for frequent evaluation, monitoring of vital signs, and serial blood tests.

Hypoglycemia

Although there is no universal definition, hypoglycemia is best defined as a low serum glucose (usually less than 50 mg/dl) with symptoms that resolve upon administration of glucose or carbohydrate. The glucose level at which patients become symptomatic is highly variable, as many patients report symptoms with normal serum glucose levels, while others remain asymptomatic at serum levels less than 50 mg/dl.

Hypoglycemia is most commonly encountered in type 1 diabetics who have missed meals, increased their exercise, or increased their dose of insulin. It occurs more frequently in young diabetics as a result of an increased emphasis on tight glycemic control. It is also encountered in diabetics taking oral hypoglycemic agents both during the course of normal therapy and as a result of an intentional overdose. Sepsis, alcohol intoxication, starvation, and liver disease also may result in hypoglycemia. Adolescents and the elderly are at increased risks of hypoglycemia.

Hypoglycemia should be considered in any patient presenting to the ED with altered mental status or focal neurologic deficits. Rapid diagnosis is essential, as a delay in the restoration of carbohydrate substrate can lead to permanent neurologic deficits, even death.

Pathophysiology

Glucose homeostasis involves the intake of food as well as the complex interactions between insulin, glucagon, and other counter-regulatory hormones.

Following a meal, insulin is the major regulatory hormone enhancing glucose utilization for fuel and storage, while also inhibiting glucose production.

In the fasting state, low insulin levels promote mobilization of stored fuel. Hepatic glycogen is broken down first and is depleted in 24–48 hours in a person with normal nutritional status. With prolonged fasting, gluconeogenesis becomes the primary source of glucose, with possible breakdown of adipose tissue and protein.

Alcohol inhibits hepatic gluconeogenesis and causes problems when malnourished alcoholics use up already depleted glycogen stores. Sepsis also inhibits gluconeogenesis, which in turn can lead to hypoglycemia.

The brain requires a continuous supply of glucose for normal function. When glucose levels fall, patients develop neurologic symptoms directly from a lack of glucose at the brain, and likely develop adrenergic symptoms from increased levels of counter-regulatory hormones.

History and physical examination

Hypoglycemia is a great mimic and has a variety of clinical presentations that can fool even the most experienced physician.

Adrenergic symptoms are most prominent when there is an abrupt fall in the blood glucose. These consist of anxiety, nervousness, irritability, nausea, vomiting, palpitations, tremors, diaphoresis, and sweating. They are often referred to as the "classic warning symptoms" of hypoglycemia. Diabetics are usually able to recognize these symptoms, and respond by ingesting glucose. For this reason, they are not commonly encountered in

the ED. Adrenergic symptoms are less prominent or may be absent in some patients, especially those on beta-blockers. For these patients, symptoms related to decreased cerebral glucose predominate. They range from lethargy and confusion to combativeness and agitation. Hypoglycemia can also cause seizures, focal neurologic deficits, and coma.

Diagnostic testing

The diagnosis of hypoglycemia can be made at the patient's bedside with a capillary glucose level, which can be confirmed with laboratory serum glucose testing. As discussed previously, rapid diagnosis is imperative so that treatment can be instituted in a timely fashion. Early diagnosis can also minimize costly work-ups for patients with altered mental status or focal neurologic deficits.

Further evaluation depends on the patient's clinical improvement and possible precipitants. The response to IV dextrose is usually rapid. However, hypoglycemia and altered mental status can be an initial presentation of sepsis. Therefore, if the clinical picture fits, the patient should undergo further work-up including blood cultures, lumbar puncture, antibiotics, and admission.

General treatment principles

Once the diagnosis of hypoglycemia is made or suspected, treatment should be initiated immediately. In adults, this consists of 1 g/kg of 50% dextrose IV (initially 1–2 ampules of D50W). In children less than 8 years old, 1 ml/kg of 25% dextrose is administered; 10% dextrose is used in neonates. These doses can be repeated if the patient remains unresponsive. An infusion of either D5W or D10W can then be started to maintain the glucose above 100 mg/dl.

In patients without IV access, 1 mg glucagon can be given intramuscularly or subcutaneously. It usually takes 5–20 minutes before clinical effects are seen.

If the patient is awake and alert, they can be given a drink containing sugar, such as orange juice, and then a meal of complex carbohydrates.

IV thiamine should be administered to alcoholic patients prior to dextrose due to the theoretical risk of precipitating Wernicke's encephalopathy. IV corticosteroids should be considered for hypoglycemia resistant to dextrose therapy.

Special patients

All patients on oral hypoglycemic agents (i.e., sulfonylureas) should be admitted for observation because these drugs have long biological half-lives and a propensity for causing prolonged and severe hypoglycemia.

Homeless and alcoholic patients may require a more prolonged period of observation. They may also benefit from seeing a social worker who can help them with referrals to appropriate outpatient care, and psychological or possibly financial support.

Geriatric patients being discharged may benefit from having pre-filled insulin syringes or a home nurse to assist them with their medications. Social services are integral to their care.

Disposition

Patients with diabetes who are not on oral hypoglycemic medications can be discharged home following a short period of observation if they have an appropriate response to treatment and are able to eat without difficulty. They should be instructed to follow-up with their primary care physician, including a phone call that day or the next. Advice should be given regarding consumption of regular meals, including small snacks, and the warning symptoms of hypoglycemia. If they are on insulin, the dose can be cut until they follow-up with their physician who manages their diabetes.

Pearls, pitfalls, and myths

- A search for precipitants of DKA, HHS, or hypoglycemia, such as MI, stroke, infection, and GI bleeding should always be performed. It is particularly important to examine the urine, feet, and perineal area of elderly diabetics for a source of infection.
- The two main ketoacids produced in DKA are acetoacetate and beta-hydroxybutyrate. The nitroprusside test for urine ketones detects acetoacetate but not beta-hydroxybutyrate. Beta-hydroxybutyrate often predominates in early DKA; hence, false-negative results can occur if serum ketones are not measured in addition to urine testing for ketones.
- Excessive fluid replacement has been previously cited as a cause of complications in the management of DKA. However,

patients are more commonly under-resuscitated.
- Always remember to replace potassium in DKA and HHS when the initial potassium is in the normal or high–normal range *unless* the initial potassium level is greater than 5.5 meq/liter or the patient is anuric.
- In patients with DKA, an insulin drip must be continued until the anion gap is normal. This will usually require adding dextrose to the IV fluids when the glucose level falls below 300 mg/dl.
- Check a bedside capillary glucose; if it is low, give glucose to patients presenting with seizures, new neurological deficits, or coma.
- The capillary glucose should be rechecked regularly on patients presenting with hypoglycemia.
- All patients on long-acting oral hypoglycemic agents presenting with hypoglycemia should be admitted for observation.

References

1. Glaser N. Risk factors for cerebral edema in children with diabetic ketoacidosis. The Pediatric Emergency Medicine Collaborative Research Committee of the American Academy of Pediatrics. *New Engl J Med* 2001;344(4):264–269.
2. Goldman L, Ausiello D. *Cecil Textbook of Medicine*, 22nd ed., W.B. Saunders, 2003.
3. Harwood-Nuss AL. *The Clinical Practice of Emergency Medicine*, 3rd ed., Philadelphia, PA: Lippincott Williams and Wilkins, 2001.
4. Herbel G. Hypoglycemia. Pathophysiology and treatment. *Endocrinol Metab Clin North Am* 2000;29(4):725–743.
5. Magee MF. Management of decompensated diabetes. Diabetic ketoacidosis and hyperglycemic hyperosmolar syndrome. *Crit Care Clin* 2001;17(1):75–106.
6. Marx JA. *Rosen's Emergency Medicine: Concepts and Clinical Practice*, 5th ed., St. Louis: Mosby, 2002.
7. Rakel RE, Bope ET. *Conn's Current Therapy 2005*, W.B. Saunders, 2004.
8. Tintinalli JE. *Emergency Medicine: A Comprehensive Study Guide*, 6th ed., New York, NY: McGraw Hill, 2003.
9. Williams RH (ed.). *Williams Textbook of Endocrinology*, 10th ed., W.B. Saunders, 2002.

17 Diarrhea

Rawle A. Seupaul, MD

Scope of the problem

There are estimated to be over 100 million cases of acute diarrhea in adults in the US each year. Diarrhea accounts for approximately 5% of emergency department (ED) visits. This complaint is even more common in children <3 years of age. Worldwide, diarrheal illnesses affect 3 to 5 billion people a year, accounting for over 5 to 10 million deaths in developing countries. Etiologies range from benign conditions such as viral gastroenteritis to life-threatening invasive diarrheal illnesses. The most common causes of acute diarrhea are infectious agents.

Pathophysiology

Diarrhea is defined as the rapid passage of excessively fluid stool, passing stool that takes form of the container rather than remaining in its natural form, or frequency of stool greater than three times a day. The gastrointestinal (GI) tract resorbs over 9 liters of fluid a day (the majority by the small intestine), leaving approximately 100 ml/day excreted in stool. Alteration in this process may lead to diarrhea. This can occur from an increase in the volume load presented to the GI tract, diminished ability to resorb fluids by the bowel, inflammatory processes, or an increase in gut motility.

Osmotic diarrhea occurs when unabsorbable or poorly absorbable molecules such as lactulose and laxatives challenge the small intestine.

Inflammatory diarrhea occurs with inflammation of bowel mucosa, which limits its ability to resorb fluid. This can occur with numerous agents, for example *Shigella* and *Giardia*. Toxigenic agents (*Vibrio cholerae* and *Escherichia coli*) result in secretory diarrhea by increasing the amount of fluid secreted into the bowel beyond the amount absorbed. Diarrhea caused by increased gut motility can be seen in patients with irritable bowel syndrome or gut-altering surgery.

It is important that physicians attempt to distinguish between gastroenteritis and dysentery. *Gastroenteritis* refers to patients who have both diarrhea and vomiting, while *dysentery* refers to diarrhea containing blood and purulence.

History

The exact etiology of diarrheal illnesses is rarely determined in the ED. However, a thorough yet focused history is critical in identifying important pathogens and noninfectious etiologies (Table 17.1). Ensure privacy and empathy, as many patients are uncomfortable discussing diarrhea.

How would you describe the diarrhea?

Loose, watery, or bloody stools may suggest an invasive process or GI bleeding. Abnormal rectal discharge, greasy or foul-smelling stools may suggest malabsorption or giardiasis.

Table 17.1 Historical information relevant to diarrhea

Character of stools	Temporal characteristics	Exogenous factors	Associated symptoms	Past history
Amount	Acute	Diet	Fever	GI disease
Consistency	Chronic	Medications	Nausea	HIV/AIDS
Color	Recurrent	Travel	Vomiting	Endocrine
Odor	Frequency	Exposure to	Abdominal pain	Diabetes
Mucus	Duration	others with	Oral intake	Adrenal
Blood		same symptoms		insufficiency
Pus		Sexual habits		Uremia

Adapted from Bitterman R in Rosen P. *Emergency Medicine: Concepts and Clinical Practice*, 5th ed., St. Louis, MO.: Mosby, 2002
AIDS: acquired immunodeficiency syndrome; GI: gastrointestinal; HIV: human immunodeficiency virus.

How many episodes of diarrhea?

The greater the number of daily stools may confer a greater risk of dehydration or electrolyte abnormality.

How long have you had symptoms?

Distinguishing acute versus chronic diarrheal diseases lends insight into etiology as well as possible co-morbid conditions. Acute disease is usually <3–4 weeks, whereas chronic disease occurs beyond this time frame. Patients with advanced human immunodeficiency virus/ acquired immune deficiency syndrome (HIV/ AIDS), pancreatitis, inflammatory bowel disease, or complex gastric or bowel surgery may suffer from chronic diarrhea requiring long-term therapy. Acute illness, the more common presentation, usually requires only a short course of symptomatic treatment. Acute illnesses are more commonly viral or food-borne diseases which are self-limiting.

What do you think caused your symptoms?

Most patients attribute their acute illness to something they ate or being around someone with the same illness. This is helpful if a history of ingesting fried rice, seafood, or egg-based products is obtained. Food poisoning should be considered when the patient's symptoms begin 1 to 6 hours after eating a high-risk meal. It is important to take a complete history and perform a thorough physical examination, however, before accepting the patient's conclusions.

Have you traveled recently?

Travel to foreign countries where water purification and food handling is not well-regulated may suggest bacterial or parasitic causes of diarrhea. The most notable of these disorders is *Montezuma's revenge* (traveler's diarrhea) caused by enterotoxigenic *E. coli*. Patients who give a history of camping and drinking water from lakes or streams may be suffering from giardiasis.

Have you started any new medications?

Many classes of drugs can cause acute diarrheal illnesses including laxatives, cholinergic drugs, antacids, and alcohol. Antibiotics are by far the most common cause of drug-induced diarrheal illness. Disruption of the native colonic bacterial flora can lead to overgrowth of other species, as occurs with *Clostridium difficile* colitis.

Associated symptoms

Most patients with diarrhea complain of nonspecific abdominal cramps, nausea, and vomiting. Significant potassium loss may occur causing weakness or muscle cramps. Patients with fever or bloody diarrhea may have a more serious invasive disease caused by *E. coli*, *Shigella*, *Salmonella*, *Yersinia*, or *Campylobacter*. In children and the elderly, severe dehydration, sepsis, and death can occur without adequate therapy. Weight loss suggests prolonged disease, malabsorption, or carcinoma. Flatulence may suggest malabsorptive diseases or parasitic infection.

Past medical

Patients with certain co-morbid illnesses may have chronic diarrhea requiring long-term care. These include but are not limited to AIDS, known irritable bowel or malabsorption syndromes, renal disease, certain malignancies and chemotherapy, and certain endocrine disorders.

Social

Sexual habits or HIV risk factors may be a critical clue in facilitating the diagnosis of a diarrheal illness in an immunocompromised host. Work history may also be helpful. For example, food handlers, day-care workers and health-care workers may require work restriction to prevent the spread of diarrheal illnesses.

Physical examination

The physical examination assists emergency physicians in the diagnosis as well as helps them gauge the patient's clinical status. The most important initial clinical assessment in a patient complaining of diarrhea is *volume status*. As with any chief complaint, consideration of all organ systems is important to avoid missed diagnoses.

General appearance

The general clinical impression of whether a patient is sick or not is a critical piece of clinical information. In patients who appear toxic with high fever, tachycardia, and/or hypotension, suspect invasive disease causing bacteremia and sepsis. Patients with more benign diseases generally appear mildly uncomfortable or relatively well.

Vital signs

The presence of tachycardia or hypotension suggests dehydration. In the presence of fever, an invasive etiology should be considered, although this finding is neither sensitive nor specific.

Head, eyes, ears, nose, throat and neck

Dry mucous membranes, sunken fontanelle in children, poor skin turgor, sunken eyes, or poor capillary refill suggest severe volume depletion. Also inspect the thyroid gland for a mass, which may suggest hyperthyroidism.

Abdomen

Most patients have generalized mild abdominal tenderness and increased bowel sounds. Patients with inflammatory bowel disease will often have mild focal findings. In general, peritoneal signs are not present.

Neurologic

Alteration in mental status may be related to volume loss or electrolyte abnormalities. It may be associated with specific infectious agents such as *Salmonella typhi*, *Shigella*, and *Campylobacter*.

Skin and extremities

Poor skin turgor and/or poor capillary refill suggest dehydration.

Rectal

Rectal examination should be performed gently on the majority of patients complaining of diarrhea. Extraintestinal manifestations of inflammatory bowel disease may be suggested if perianal fissures or fistulae are found. Grossly bloody stool, pus, or mucus support inflammatory, invasive, or ischemic processes. In elderly patients and those

with Hirschprung's disease, fecal impaction can result in diarrhea or liquid stool passing around the impaction ("overflow diarrhea").

Differential diagnosis

Tables 17.2 and 17.3 summarize pertinent differential diagnoses for patients with diarrhea, divided by infectious and non-infectious causes.

Table 17.2 Infectious causes of diarrhea

Toxin producers
- *Ciguatera* fish toxin
- *Bacillus cereus*
- *Staphylococcus aureus*
- *Clostridium perfringens*
- *Vibrio cholerae*
- Enterotoxigenic *Escherichia coli*
- *Klebsiella pneumoniae*
- *Aeromonas* species
- Enteropathogenic/adherent *Escherichia coli*
- *Giardia* organisms
- *Cryptosporidium*
- *Helminthes*
- *Clostridium difficile*
- Hemorrhagic *Escherichia coli*

Invasive organisms
- Rotavirus
- Norwalk agent
- *Salmonella*
- *Campylobacter*
- *Aeromonas* species
- *Vibrio parahaemolyticus*
- *Yersinia*
- *Shigella* species
- Enteroinvasive *Escherichia coli*
- *Entamoeba histolytica*

Parasites
- *Giardia lamblia*
- *Isospora belli*
- *Entamoeba histolytica*
- *Cryptosporidium*

Table 17.3 Non-infectious causes of diarrhea

- Lactose intolerance
- Reaction to medications
- Inflammatory bowel disease
- Irritable bowel disease
- Bowel-altering surgery
- Mesenteric ischemia
- Bowel obstruction
- Cancer
- Hyperthyroidism
- Laxative abuse

Diagnostic testing

Diagnostic testing is rarely necessary for patients presenting to the ED with diarrhea. Testing should be driven by clues obtained in the history and physical examination. Patients with chronic diarrhea can usually be managed in an outpatient setting. Patients who appear toxic or have bloody diarrhea, however, may warrant diagnostic testing.

Laboratory studies

Complete blood count

A complete blood count (CBC) should be obtained in patients with significant blood loss or systemic toxicity. Nonspecific findings may include a leukocytosis with a leftward shift. Eosinophilia is rarely seen and is most likely associated with *Strongyloides stercoralis.* Anemia may be seen with any agent causing bloody diarrhea, such as *Shigella* or *Salmonella.*

Electrolytes

Electrolytes should be obtained in patients with signs or symptoms of severe dehydration or those suffering from co-morbid illnesses that may lead to electrolyte alteration. Patients on diuretics, those with diabetes and the elderly may be more susceptible to rapidly-developing electrolyte disturbances. Hypokalemia, hyponatremia, and metabolic acidosis may be found secondary to bicarbonate loss.

Fecal leukocytes (Wright's stain)

Normally, stool should not contain leukocytes. The presence of fecal leukocytes suggests a bacterial etiology. As leukocytes are not present in stool, this test is highly sensitive and specific.

Stool cultures

Cultures may be helpful in patients with a history and physical examination consistent with invasive diarrhea, when public health concerns exist (food handlers, day-care workers, health-care workers) or when stool Gram's stain is positive for fecal leukocytes. Stool cultures may be the most useful in children, toxic patients, immunocompromised patients, patients with bloody diarrhea, or those with diarrhea for more than 3 days.

Stool ova and parasites

This study should be obtained if the patient has traveled to an endemic area or has chronic diarrhea. Immunocompromised patients with prolonged diarrheal illnesses who have failed standard antibiotic therapy should also have these stool studies performed.

Giardia-*specific antigen*

Giardia-specific antigen (GSA) is the most common diagnostic method for visualizing *Giardia* cysts. This test may be useful in disease outbreaks and for diarrhea occurring at day-care settings.

Clostridium difficile *toxin*

This stool test should be ordered if *C. difficile* colitis is suspected in patients with a diarrheal illness preceded by antibiotic use.

Escherichia coli *O157 : H7 toxin*

This stool study should be ordered in afebrile patients having bloody or nonbloody diarrhea who are at risk for exposure to this toxin (contaminated beef or water, or exposure to someone with known disease). The laboratory should be informed that this disease process is suspected, since a special media is needed (MacConkey sorbitol agar).

Pregnancy test

While not essential to the diagnosis of acute diarrheal illnesses, this test should generally be obtained in women of childbearing age with any abdominal complaint (cramping, burning, pain). Pregnancy should be considered when recommending medications to treat or relieve symptoms.

Blood cultures

Blood cultures may be appropriate in patients who demonstrate signs or symptoms of systemic toxicity or sepsis.

Radiologic studies

Radiographic studies are rarely indicated unless another process is suspected (e.g., small or large bowel obstruction with overflow diarrhea, or toxic megacolon).

General treatment principles

Rehydration and electrolyte repletion

Initial treatment consists of restoring hydration status. Mild dehydration can be treated with oral fluids. Oral solutions should contain some glucose, which stimulates resorption of water by the small intestine. Milk products should be avoided since some patients develop a temporary deficiency of lactase. Moderate to severe dehydration should be treated with intravenous (IV) fluids. One to two liters of normal saline or D5 normal saline will usually suffice. In patients with electrolyte abnormalities, the most common being hypokalemia and hypochloremia, IV fluids can be administered in the ED to correct these imbalances.

Antimotility agents

Some experts warn that antimotility agents such as loperamide and diphenoxylate should be used cautiously in individuals with infectious diarrhea. They argue that these agents may precipitate toxic megacolon or delay the excretion of pathogens leading to prolongation of symptoms. However, there is little evidence to support this claim. Caution should be taken in recommending diphenoxylate in children, particularly those 2 years of age and younger (Table 17.4).

Table 17.4 Various agents that can be used in the management of diarrheal illness

Agent	Adult dosage	Pediatric dosage	Indication
Ciprofloxacin	500 mg PO BID for 3–5 days.	Not recommended.	Empiric first-line therapy for presumed bacterial etiologies
Trimethoprim–sulfamethoxazole	1 DS tablet PO BID for 3–5 days.	>2 months: 0.5 ml susp/kg PO BID for 10 days; Max 20 ml susp/dose.	Empiric second-line therapy for presumed bacterial etiologies.
Metronidazole	250–500 mg PO TID for 10 days.	30–50 mg/kg/day PO divided TID for 10 days; not to exceed adult dose.	Giardia, protozoa, anaerobic organisms, *Clostridium difficile* colitis.
Vancomycin	500 mg PO QID for 10–14 days.	40–50 mg/kg/day PO divided QID for 10–14 days; not to exceed 2 g/day.	Second-line therapy for *Clostridium difficile* colitis.
Cefixime	400 mg/day PO QD for 7–10 days.	8 mg/kg/day PO QD for 7–10 days.	Gram-negative bacteria.
Ceftriaxone	1–2 g IV/IM q 24 hours.	50 mg/kg/day IV/IM divided QD/BID for 7–10 days; not to exceed 2 g/day.	Gram-negative and Gram-positive bacteria.
Furazolidone	100 mg PO QID for 7–10 days.	5 mg/kg/day PO divided QID for 7–10 days.	Parasitic disease.
Iodoquinol	650 mg PO TID for 20 days.	30–40 mg/kg/day PO divided TID for 20 days; not to exceed adult dose.	Parasitic disease.
Loperamide	4 mg once, followed by 2 mg after each loose stool; do not exceed 16 mg/day.	*Initial doses*: 2–6 years: 1 mg PO TID; 6–8 years: 2 mg PO BID; 8–12 years: 2 mg PO TID. Maintenance: 0.1 mg/kg PO after each loose stool, not to exceed initial dose.	Antimotility.
Diphenoxylate HCl–atropine sulfate	2 tablets PO QID until the diarrhea is controlled.	<2 years: not recommended; 2–5 years: 2 mg of diphenoxylate PO TID; 5–8 years: 2 mg of diphenoxylate PO QID; 8–12 years: 2 mg of diphenoxylate five times/day.	Antimotility.
Bismuth subsalicylate	525 mg PO QID; not to exceed 4.2 g/day.	<12 years: not established. >12 years: administer as in adults.	Cytoprotective for gastrointestinal mucosa.

BID: two times a day; DS: double strength; IM: intramuscular; IV: intravenous; PO: per os; QD: every day; QID: four times a day; susp: suspension; TID: three times a day.

Antibiotics

The use of antibiotics for acute diarrheal illnesses should be scrutinized since the offending agent is viral in 50–70% of cases. Of the empiric therapies available, the fluoroquinolones offer the best proven advantage. Resistance to this class of antibiotics is low, and they do not interfere with the endogenous colonic flora. Also, unlike other antibiotics, quinolones do not appear to prolong the carrier state associated with *Salmonella* infections. In general, antibiotics decrease the length of disease by about 1 day and may be indicated in individuals with fever, fecal leukocytes, bloody diarrhea, symptoms for more than 3 days, or travelers.

Other agents

Other symptomatic treatments include anti-motility agents and bismuth subsalicylate (Table 17.4).

Dietary restriction

There are several agents that should be avoided until the patient's diarrhea subsides. These include raw fruits, caffeine (increases motility), milk or lactose-containing products, and sorbitol (increases the osmotic load).

Special patients

While most diarrheal illnesses are self-limited and otherwise benign, special care needs to be taken with certain patients. Individuals who are immunocompromised, elderly, have multiple co-morbidites, and children may have less reserve to withstand even minor fluid, electrolyte, hematologic, or hemodynamic abnormalities. In these individuals, treatment should be dictated by their underlying condition.

Pediatric

The major concern in children is hydration status. This can be assessed historically by determining changes in urine output, oral intake, and the number of wet diapers. The majority of diarrheal illnesses in children are of viral origin, with rotavirus accounting for up to 50% of cases. Fortunately, the duration of illness is usually short and self-limited.

Elderly

The elderly may succumb to any of the aforementioned etiologies of diarrheal disease but, like children, may become ill faster. They may require more aggressive therapy, diagnostic testing, and possibly hospital admission.

Immune compromised

Those with immune-compromising illness such as HIV/AIDS may present with unusual infections caused by *Isospora belli*, *Cryptosporidium parvum*, *Mycobacterium avium-intracellulare*, and cytomegalovirus. They may also require more diagnostic studies including stool ova and parasites and stool cultures. Those with CD4 counts less than 200 will tend to suffer from severe volume loss, weight loss, and intractable illness despite appropriate therapy.

Travelers

Travelers with diarrheal illness are usually infected with *E. coli*, *Rotavirus*, *Salmonella*, or *Campylobacter*. Fortunately, this disease process is self-limited and usually resolves in a few days requiring only a short course of antibiotics and/or symptomatic therapy.

Disposition

Most patients with diarrhea can be safely discharged from the ED with symptomatic therapy. They should be instructed to drink clear fluids containing some sugar and a eat simple diet (e.g., bananas, rice, applesauce, and toast, known as the BRAT diet). Patients should be instructed to use strict hand-washing, limit unnecessary contacts (e.g., school, food handlers, day care) to prevent spread, and follow up with their primary care physician as needed. Patients who have persistently abnormal vital signs, continued nausea, vomiting, or copious stool output should be considered for admission for hydration, observation, and other therapies such as antibiotics.

All patients should be instructed to follow up with their primary care physician or asked to return to the ED if their symptoms worsen. Public health officials should be notified when *E. coli* O157:H7 toxin is diagnosed or strongly suspected. Other infectious agents may require reporting to public health officials as well.

Pearls, pitfalls, and myths

Pearls

1. Diarrhea is a common presenting complaint to the ED requiring thorough understanding of its pathophysiology and treatment.
2. Focus the history to include recent travel, medications, co-morbid disease(s), and associated symptoms.
3. Disease severity should be assessed based on the vital signs and physical examination.
4. Grossly bloody diarrhea is almost always from invasive bacteria and not viral pathogens.
5. The hallmark of treatment in any diarrheal illness begins with rehydration.
6. Laboratory and radiographic studies are rarely warranted for patients with diarrhea unless dictated by physical findings (hypotension, tachycardia, severe dehydration, mental status changes).
7. All diarrheal illnesses are not infectious.

Pitfalls

1. Not performing a thorough history and physical examination.
2. Not addressing abnormal vital signs (tachycardia, fever, hypotension, tachypnea).

Myths

1. The use of antidiarrheal agents should not be pursued for symptomatic relief because they may precipitate toxic megacolon.
2. Antibiotics prolong *Salmonella* carrier state.

References

1. Braunwald E. *Harrison's Principles of Internal Medicine*, 15th ed., New York: McGraw-Hill Medical Publishing Division, 2001.
2. Hamilton GC. *Emergency Medicine: an Approach to Clinical Problem-Solving*, 2nd ed., Philadelphia, PA.: Saunders, 2003.
3. Harwood-Nuss A and Wolfson AB. *The Clinical Practice of Emergency Medicine*, 3rd ed., Philadelphia, London: Lippincott Williams & Wilkins, 2001.
4. Hogan DE. The emergency department approach to diarrhea. *Emerg Med Clin N Am* 1996;14(4):673–694.
5. Marx J. *Emergency Medicine : Concepts and Clinical Practice*, 5th ed., St. Louis, Mo.: Mosby, 2002.
6. Reisdorff E, Pflung V. Infectious diarrhea: beyond supportive care. *Emerg Med Rep* 1996;17(14):141–150.
7. Rosen P. *5 minute Emergency Medicine Consult*, Philadelphia: Lippincott Williams & Wilkins, 1999.
8. Tintinalli JE, et al. *Emergency Medicine : a Comprehensive Study Guide*, 5th ed., New York: McGraw-Hill Health Professions Division, 2000.

18 Dizziness and vertigo

Andrew K. Chang, MD

Scope of the problem

Dizziness, a common complaint in patients presenting to the emergency department (ED), is a disorder of spatial orientation. It is the most common complaint in patients over the age of 75 years. Approximately 7% of ED patients present with dizziness, and dizzy patients account for 1.5% of admitted patients.

Evaluating the dizzy patient can be challenging, since it is a nonspecific symptom and is difficult to objectively measure. Although most cases are usually benign, emergency physicians need to be wary about life-threatening causes of dizziness, such as cardiac dysrhythmias and cerebrovascular events. In some cases, however, the patient can be cured at the bedside.

Pathophysiology

Two studies performed approximately 30 years apart have confirmed that there are four general subtypes of dizziness: vertigo, near-syncope, disequilibrium, and psychophysiologic dizziness. It is important to realize, however, that a person may describe more than one subtype, but rarely will describe elements of all four.

Pertinent anatomy that contributes to dizziness includes the vestibular, visual, proprioceptive, cardiac, and central nervous systems (CNS).

Vertigo

Vertigo is defined as an illusion of motion. The CNS coordinates and integrates sensory input from the visual, vestibular, and proprioceptive systems. Vertigo occurs when there is a mismatch of information from two or more of these systems. Vertigo is divided into central and peripheral causes (Table 18.1). *Central vertigo* indicates involvement of the cerebellum or the vestibular nuclei within the pons and medulla. *Peripheral vertigo* indicates involvement of either the eighth cranial nerve (CN) or the vestibular apparatus of the inner ear, and is usually benign. Benign positional vertigo (BPV), the most common cause of vertigo, results from the inappropriate presence of calcium particles (otoliths) in the semicircular

Table 18.1 Differentiating between peripheral and central causes of vertigo

	Peripheral	Central
Onset	Sudden	Gradual
Intensity	Severe	Mild
Duration	Seconds	Continuous
Nystagmus	Fatigable	Non-fatigable
Direction of nystagmus	Unidirectional	Multidirectional
Associated neurologic findings	None	Usually present
Hearing loss or tinnitus	May be present	None
Associated nausea or vomiting	Frequent, severe	Infrequent, mild

canals. Movement of the head causes these otoliths to inappropriately trigger receptors in the semicircular canal, causing the sensation of vertigo. In Ménière's disease, there is an increase in the volume of endolymph associated with distension of the endolymphatic system (endolymphatic hydrops), causing vertigo, fluctuating sensorineural hearing loss, and tinnitus. Ruptures of the membranous labyrinth are thought to cause the sudden episodic attacks of Ménière's disease.

Near-syncope

Near-syncope is the sensation of feeling faint. Like vertigo, it is a common experience. Unlike vertigo, there is no illusion of motion. Near-syncope is due to the global reduction of blood flow to the brain. Since people rise from the supine and sitting positions multiple times a day, a complicated neural reflex has evolved; the CNS puts out a stimulus causing vasoconstriction to combat gravitational pooling of blood in the lower extremities while preserving blood flow to the brain. There are many things that can interfere with this reflex, such as orthostatic hypotension, cardiac disease, vasovagal syndrome, hyperventilation, and environmental factors. When this neural reflex fails, pallor, nausea, rubbery legs, diaphoresis, and constriction of the visual fields occur. These warning signs are the brain's way of signaling the person to lie down, making it easier to perfuse the brain. If the person is unable to lie down, he may progress from near-syncope to syncope. If this still does not cause him to lie horizontally, the body will make antigravity postures that may be misinterpreted as a seizure. This unfortunate chain of events can lead to unnecessary work-ups.

Disequilibrium

The third category of dizziness is disequilibrium. Disequilibrium occurs because of disruption between the sensory inputs and motor outputs, which often results in an unsteady gait. This is usually a disease of the elderly, as there is an age-related decline in the ability of the CNS to process sensory inputs as well as control postural reflexes. Disequilibrium is often exacerbated by unfamiliar surroundings, uneven ground, or poor lighting. The most common cause of disequilibrium is cervical spondylosis, which leads to spinal cord myelopathy. Patients have poor proprioception in the legs, which leads to a stiff-legged gait. These patients usually demonstrate a positive Romberg test, in which disequilibrium with the eyes closed and feet together suggests impaired proprioception. Other causes of disequilibrium are listed in Table 18.2.

Table 18.2 Causes of disequilibrium

- Cervical spondylosis
- Parkinson's disease
- Cerebellar disease
- Hydrocephalus
- Multi-infarct syndrome
- Peripheral neuropathy
- Bilateral vestibulopathy

Psychophysiologic dizziness

The fourth category of dizziness is psychophysiologic dizziness. The mechanism is poorly understood but is felt to result from impaired central integration of sensory signals. Patients experience feelings of dissociation, as though one has left one's own body. These patients are often in a hypervigilant state and constantly monitor themselves for any signs of impending dizziness. Their exaggeration of reactions to normal changes often induces great psychologic stress, including hyperventilation. In reality, their symptoms are actually quite mild, and anxiety is felt to be the *sine qua non* of psychophysiologic dizziness. Indeed, dizziness is the most common somatic symptom associated with panic disorder.

History

The medical history provided by the patient or witnesses is the most important source of information in the evaluation of the dizziness. Two office-based studies found that the etiology of dizziness could be made using history alone in approximately 70% of patients.

What do you mean, dizzy?

In emergency medicine, time frames are often constrained and history is usually obtained in the form of closed-ended questions. However, the dizzy patient is best approached using open-ended questions. It is counterproductive to suggest definitions for patients, such as asking them whether the room spins or whether they feel lightheaded. Patients who present with dizziness are often very suggestible and tend to answer affirmatively to suggestive questions. In addition, their symptoms can persist or recur. Their history thus becomes distorted and can cause confusion for future emergency physicians or consultants.

Patients with vertigo will offer that the "room is spinning." However, other descriptions such as rocking, tilting, somersaulting, or descending in an elevator may also be used to describe vertigo.

Patients with near-syncope generally respond that they feel like they are "going to faint."

Patients with disequilibrium typically respond that they feel like they are "going to fall" or that they feel "unsteady on their feet."

Patients with psychophysiologic dizziness commonly share that they feel as if they have "left their own body," or that they are "floating or swimming." Some patients describe a spinning sensation inside their head. Unlike vertigo, this type of spinning is not associated with an illusion of motion of the environment, and the patient does not have nystagmus on examination. In some cases, patients may be unable to describe their dizziness using words other than "dizzy."

Have you had any (recent or past) history of head trauma?

Since BPV is generally a disease of the elderly, the emergency physician should ask younger patients about a history of head trauma, even if it occurred years ago (head trauma can dislodge the otoliths from the utricular macule, allowing them to enter the semicircular canal).

Do you have any new neurologic symptoms?

Diplopia, dysarthria, dysphagia, gait abnormality, or other focal neurologic complaints are concerning for a central cause of vertigo and dizziness.

Have you recently had a viral illness?

The patient should be asked about current or recent viral illnesses, which are often associated with labyrinthitis and vestibular neuritis.

How long do your symptoms of vertigo last?

In general, episodes of vertigo vary depending on the disease process. For BPV, episodes last for seconds; for a transient ischemic attack (TIA) or vertebrobasilar insufficiency, episodes last for minutes; for Ménière's disease and migraines, episodes last for hours; and for vestibular neuritis and labyrinthitis, episodes last for days.

The duration of symptoms is helpful in differentiating BPV from labyrinthitis and vestibular neuritis. The patient with BPV has episodes of vertigo that last only seconds at a time and are caused by head movements. However, the patient may describe that he has been having continuous vertigo when in fact he is experiencing many attacks during the day. For this reason, it is important for the emergency physician to elicit how long each *individual* episode of vertigo lasts. Labyrinthitis and vestibular neuritis, on the other hand, tend to be continuous and last for several days. These may or may not be worsened with head movement. Therefore, during history taking, if a patient states that the room is spinning and his head is still (and has not been manipulated or moved), the diagnosis is probably not BPV.

Is your hearing affected?

The key to the diagnosis of Ménière's disease is fluctuating hearing levels in patients with episodic vertigo. Hearing is also affected in labyrinthitis, which distinguishes it from vestibular neuritis.

Cerumen impaction, otitis media, and cerebellopontine angle tumors may also result in hearing loss. Tinnitus (the perception of sound in the absence of an acoustic stimulus) occurs with Ménière's disease, acoustic neuromas, and medication toxicity.

Do you have a headache?

Vertigo associated with migraine is thought to be due to vasospasm or to an inherited metabolic defect. Vertebrobasilar insufficiency is usually caused by atherosclerosis of the subclavian, vertebral, and basilar arteries. Vertigo and headache may represent infarction of the lateral brainstem or cerebellum.

Do you have chest pain, shortness of breath, or palpitations?

Cardiac dysrhythmias produce spontaneous episodes of dizziness that can occur in any position and can be associated with other cardiac symptoms, such as palpitations and chest pain. Intermittent dysrhythmias may not be identified on a single electrocardiogram, so patients with episodic near-syncope of unknown cause should undergo monitoring to search for sinus pauses, sinus bradycardia, atrial fibrillation, and sustained supraventricular and ventricular tachycardias.

What makes your dizziness worse? Standing from a sitting or reclining position? Exertion? Walking or standing compared with sitting or lying down?

Orthostatic hypotension is usually due to acute blood loss, dehydration, over-diuresis, or anti-hypertensive medications. Gravitational pooling of blood in the legs occurs when the patient stands.

Symptoms that are exacerbated with head turning, lying down, or rolling over in bed are more suggestive of vertigo.

In vasovagal or neurally-mediated near-syncope, the blood pressure is not necessarily reduced immediately upon standing, as it is in orthostatic hypotension.

Disequilibrium is typically worse while walking or standing, but patients are relatively asymptomatic while sitting or lying down.

Do your attacks occur with certain foods?

In susceptible patients, panic attacks can be precipitated by a large number of substances, including caffeine and lactate. One hypothesis is that panic attacks result from loss of central control of the locus ceruleus, leading to the episodic release of catecholamines. These patients often have symptoms of agoraphobia as well.

Additional important historical questions that should be asked include how the dizziness began, previous episodes of dizziness, how frequently the attacks occur, what the provoking and palliating factors are, and associated symptoms.

Past medical

A detailed medical history is important to obtain since there are many factors that cause or exacerbate dizziness. Drug and alcohol abuse, previous psychiatric history, certain medical diseases, such as diabetes and heart disease, as well as certain neurologic diseases, such as seizures and migraine are important to elicit from the patient.

Do you have a history of anxiety or panic attacks?

Hyperventilation, which commonly occurs in anxious patients, lowers the carbon dioxide concentration in the blood. This leads to vasoconstriction of cerebral blood vessels which may contribute to near-syncope. However, it is important to be aware that the panic attack may actually be intermittent episodes of supraventricular tachycardia, which can also cause anxiety and palpitations.

What medications do you take?

A medication history is important, as many medications are vestibulotoxic. Common examples include aspirin and aminoglycosides. However, vertigo itself is rarely caused by medications, since both sides are usually affected equally.

Physical examination

General appearance

The general appearance of the dizzy patient varies widely, from the healthy young adult to the frail elderly patient. Patients who are dizzy and vomiting generally appear extremely uncomfortable, and may even be ashen and diaphoretic.

Vital signs

Blood pressure

Hypertension in a dizzy patient should raise concern for vertebrobasilar insufficiency, cerebellar infarction, or hemorrhage as a possible cause. Hypotension can lead to decreased cerebral perfusion and may be associated with near-syncope. Orthostatic vital signs can be checked but are notoriously unreliable in elderly patients. Differences in blood pressures between arms can indicate subclavian steal syndrome (which may result in vertebrobasilar insufficiency) or aortic dissection.

Heart rate

Both tachycardia and bradycardia can impair cardiac output and lead to near-syncope via cerebral hypoperfusion.

Respiratory rate

As mentioned earlier, hyperventilation can contribute to hypoperfusion of the brain through vasoconstriction of cerebral blood vessels.

Temperature

Fever alone may produce a sensation of dizziness and also may accompany CNS or other infections.

Head, eyes, ears, nose, and throat

Eyes

The emergency physician should ask the patient to look to the right and left to check for the presence of nystagmus. Avoid having the patient fixate on an object, such as a pen or finger, since visual fixation can inhibit nystagmus. The physician should note the nature of the nystagmus (horizontal, rotary or torsional, horizontal-rotary, vertical, or vertical-rotary), its direction (based on the direction of the fast component), and its duration. With vestibular disease, the fast component usually beats toward the side of the lesion. In peripheral vertigo, spontaneous nystagmus usually continues in one direction even when the direction of the gaze changes. In contrast, central causes (such as cerebellar or brainstem infarction, or hemorrhage) result in nystagmus that changes direction with change in the gaze direction. The nystagmus of peripheral vertigo is typically fatigable (extinguishes with repeated testing), while the nystagmus of central vertigo is not. There are exceptions to this rule, such as BPV caused by cupulolithiasis, which results in non-fatigable nystagmus. In addition, the presence of nystagmus at extreme end-gaze is seen in up to 60% of normal people.

Ears

- External auditory canal: this should be inspected for vesicles (Ramsay Hunt syndrome), cerumen, and cholesteatoma.
- Tympanic membrane: this should be visualized for signs of otitis media. A perforated or scarred tympanic membrane may indicate a perilymphatic fistula. This can be confirmed with pneumatic otoscopy.
- Hearing should also be tested. The emergency physician can use either the ticking of a watch or the rubbing of fingers near the patient's ears. Unilateral hearing loss is suggestive of labyrinthitis, cerumen impaction, Ménière's disease, or acoustic neuroma, although the latter usually presents with gradual hearing loss.

Cardiovascular

The heart should be auscultated for the presence of dysrhythmias and murmurs. The presence of murmurs may indicate aortic stenosis or hypertrophic obstructive cardiomyopathy, both which may decrease cardiac output. In addition, the carotid arteries should be auscultated for the presence of bruits, which may indicate carotid stenosis as a contributing cause of cerebral hypoperfusion.

Neurologic

All patients with dizziness need a comprehensive neurologic examination, with special attention to the CNs, cerebellar examination, and gait testing.

Cranial nerves

CN abnormalities strongly suggest a central process:

- CN I dysfunction is suggested by uni- or bilateral decrease in or loss of smell.
- CN II dysfunction is suggested by loss in visual acuity and abnormalities on funduscopic examination (papilledema, optic atrophy).
- CN III, IV, VI dysfunction is suggested by dysconjugate gaze with formal EOM testing.
- CN V dysfunction is suggested by weak or absent contraction of the temporal and masseter muscles or decrease in or loss of facial sensation. Loss of the corneal reflex also suggests CN V dysfunction.
- CN VII dysfunction is suggested by facial droop or weakness of one side of the face.

- CN VIII dysfunction is suggested by decreased hearing.
- CN IX, X dysfunction is suggested by hoarseness or a nasal quality to the patient's voice, a history of swallowing difficulty, and asymmetric movements of the soft palate and pharynx when the patient is asked to say "aah."
- CN XI dysfunction is suggested by atrophy or weakness of the trapezius and plastysma muscles.
- CN XII dysfunction is suggested by dysarthria and deviation of the protruded tongue towards the involved side.

Cerebellar

Cerebellar function can be evaluated using rapid alternative movements or point-to-point testing. The slow, irregular, and clumsy movements that occur with rapid alternating movements are called *dysdiadochokinesis* and indicate cerebellar disease. Cerebellar disease also results in movements that are clumsy, unsteady, and inappropriately varying in their speed, force, and direction.

The Romberg test is a functional test of position sense (Figure 18.1). The patient stands with his feet together and is then told to close his eyes. In ataxia due to loss of position sense, vision

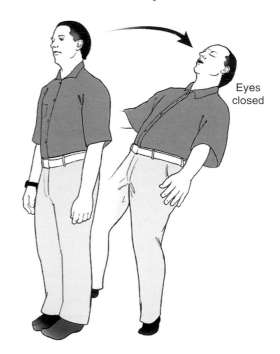

Eyes closed

Figure 18.1
Positive Romberg test.

compensates for the sensory loss. When the eyes are closed, the patient loses balance resulting in a positive Romberg sign. With cerebellar ataxia, the patient has difficulty standing with his or her feet together regardless of whether the eyes are open or closed.

Gait testing

Whenever possible, gait should be tested. Ataxia (a gait that lacks coordination with reeling and instability) may be due to cerebellar disease, loss of position sense, or intoxication. Tandem walking may bring out an ataxia not previously obvious. The broad-based ataxic gait of cerebellar disorders is readily distinguished from the milder gait disorders seen with vestibular or sensory loss.

Rectal

A rectal examination may be useful to suggest anemia from gastrointestinal bleeding, and should be considered in the dizzy patient with a history consistent with near-syncope.

Clinical tests

Orthostatic vital signs

Orthostatic hypotension is generally defined as a fall in systolic blood pressure of at least 15–20 mmHg within 2 minutes of standing upright. Orthostatic vital signs may help suggest hypovolemia, but are very nonspecific, especially in the elderly, and should not be considered pathognomonic.

Hallpike test

For patients with a history consistent with vertigo, a Hallpike test (also known as the Dix–Hallpike, Nylan–Barany, or Barany test) should be performed at the bedside. This is performed as follows: the patient sits upright in the gurney with the head turned 45° to one side. The patient is then guided down to the supine position with the head overhanging the edge of the gurney. The eyes are viewed for evidence of torsional nystagmus and the patient is questioned regarding reproduction of symptoms. By turning the head 45° to one side, the posterior semicircular canal becomes aligned in the direction of

movement when the head is laid down. This serves as the most provocative way to move the otoliths and reproduce symptoms. The patient is then returned to the sitting position and the eyes are viewed again (Figure 18.2). With BPV, the direction of nystagmus will be opposite in the head-hanging and sitting positions. In the head-hanging position, the eyes beat upward (toward the forehead) and toward the affected ear in the fast phase. The nystagmus fatigues with repeated positioning, and there is usually a brief latency from the time the head-hanging position is achieved to the onset of nystagmus. The test is then repeated with the head turned in the opposite direction. This test does not need to be done rapidly, as it is a "positional" as opposed to a "positioning" test. Although it is theoretically possible to have bilateral BPV, generally only one side tests positive in patients with BPV. This positive side serves as the starting point for the Epley maneuver, described in the treatment section.

Head-thrust test

This test should be performed if unilateral peripheral vestibular loss is suspected, as in vestibular neuritis or labyrinthitis. The patient's head is quickly rotated about 15° to the side while the patient fixates on the examiner's nose. With unilateral peripheral vestibular loss, the eyes cannot maintain focus, and a saccade (quick rotation of the eyes from one fixation point to another) will occur bringing the eyes back to the examiner's nose.

Hennebert's test

This tests for the presence of a perilymphatic fistula. If the patient develops reproduction of symptoms (vertigo, nausea, and nystagmus) on pneumatic otoscopy, the diagnosis may be perilymphatic fistula. Ménière's disease and otosyphilis can cause false positive tests.

Hyperventilation

A 2-minute hyperventilation challenge is occasionally used when psychophysiologic dizziness is thought to be the cause of dizziness. However, the utility of this test remains unclear, and symptom reproduction cannot be considered diagnostic.

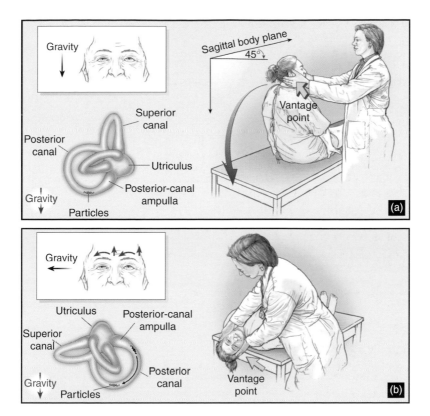

Figure 18.2
The Dix–Hallpike Test of a Patient with Benign Paroxysmal Positional Vertigo Affecting the Right Ear. In Panel A, the examiner stands at the patient's right side and rotates the patient's head 45 degrees to the right to align the right posterior semicircular canal with the sagittal plane of the body. In Panel B, the examiner moves the patient, whose eyes are open, from the seated to the supine right-ear-down position and then extends the patient's neck slightly so that the chin is pointed slightly upward. The latency, duration, and direction of nystagmus, if present, and the latency and duration of vertigo, if present, should be noted. The red arrows in the inset depict the direction of nystagmus in patients with typical benign paroxysmal positional vertigo. The presumed location in the labyrinth of the free-floating debris thought to cause the disorder is also shown. Reprinted from Furman JM, Cass SP, Benign Paroxysmal Positional Vertigo, *N Engl J Med* 1999; 341(21):1590–1596. Copyright 1999 Massachusetts Medical Society. All rights reserved.

Differential diagnosis

Table 18.3 Features of conditions causing peripheral vertigo

	Symptoms	Signs
Benign positional vertigo	Vertigo for seconds at a time	Positive Hallpike test
Cerebellar pontine angle tumors (acoustic neuroma, meningioma, dermoid)	Vertigo, deafness	Ataxia, ipsilateral facial weakness, loss of corneal reflex, cerebellar signs
Cholesteatoma	Facial twitching, various degrees of hearing loss	May have positive insufflation test
Labyrinthitis	Continuous vertigo for hours to days; decreased hearing	Positive head-thrust test, decreased hearing
Ménière's disease	Episodic vertigo, fluctuating hearing loss, ear fullness, roaring tinnitus	Low-frequency hearing loss (unilateral in most cases) *(continued)*

Table 18.3 Features of conditions causing peripheral vertigo (*cont*)

	Symptoms	Signs
Otitis media or tympanic membrane rupture	Vertigo	Bulging or ruptured tympanic membrane
Ototoxic drugs	Vertigo uncommon since both inner ears affected; hearing loss	Ataxia, oscillopsia
Perilymphatic fistula	"Popping" sound, hearing loss, tinnitus	Positive insufflation test
Vestibular neuritis	Continuous vertigo for hours to days	Positive head-thrust test

Table 18.4 Features of conditions causing central vertigo

	Symptoms	Signs
Basilar artery migraine	Vertigo, tinnitus, headache, visual aura	Decreased hearing, diplopia, dysarthria, ataxia, bilateral paresis, bilateral paresthesias, decreased level of consciousness
Cerebellar infarction or hemorrhage	Mild vertigo	Truncal or limb ataxia, abnormal Romberg test
Multiple sclerosis	Discrete episode of vertigo lasting several hours to weeks, usually non-recurrent	Ataxia, optic neuritis
Temporal lobe seizures	Vertigo as part of an aura	Amnesia during seizure, other associated aura symptoms present
Vertebrobasilar insufficiency	Vertigo lasting for minutes, may be provoked by position	May include diplopia, dysphagia, dysarthria, and bilateral loss of vision
Wallenberg syndrome (lateral medullary infarction)	Vertigo, nausea or vomiting, dysphagia and dysphonia	Ipsilateral Horner's syndrome, facial numbness, loss of corneal reflex, paralysis or paresis of the soft palate, pharynx, and larynx

Diagnostic testing

Diagnostic testing should be based on the emergency physician's history and physical examination. For example, patients who have a classic history for BPV, a positive Hallpike test, and a normal neurologic examination do not necessarily need laboratory tests or imaging studies.

Any patient with a focal neurologic examination should receive computed tomography (CT) of the brain and if possible, magnetic resonance imaging (MRI) of the brain.

Laboratory tests

Laboratory testing is rarely helpful in the evaluation of the dizzy patient. A hemoglobin and hematocrit may be helpful to detect anemia, and a glucose level may be useful to exclude hypo- or hyperglycemia, especially in the diabetic patient. In addition, electrolytes, renal function tests, and a toxicology screen may be helpful in certain cases.

Electrocardiogram

An electrocardiogram is appropriate if the emergency physician suspects a cardiac cause for a patient's dizziness, especially if the history is suggestive of near-syncope. The emergency physician should look for evidence of dysrhythmia or ischemia.

Radiologic studies

Any patient with concern for central vertigo or who has focal neurologic deficits on examination should receive an advanced imaging test.

Cranial computed tomography

This study is commonly available but has limited utility when evaluating the posterior fossa. A negative CT in a patient with focal neurologic deficits demands further testing or subspecialty consultation (Figure 18.3).

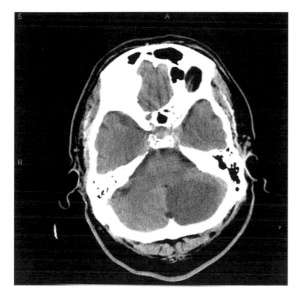

Figure 18.3
Left cerebellar infarct. Non-enhanced head CT revealing left cerebellar hemisphere infarct. *Courtesy*: G. Garmel, MD.

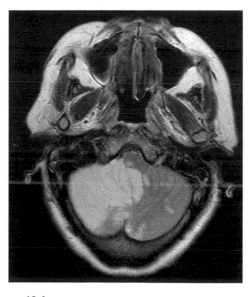

Figure 18.4
Right cerebellar infarct. T2-weighted MRI of the brain revealing high signal intensity consistent with a large right cerebellar infarct. *Courtesy*: Mahesh Jayaraman, MD.

Cranial magnetic resonance imaging

This is more likely to detect subtle brainstem or inferior cerebellar infarction (Figure 18.4).

General treatment principles

Symptomatic care is usually all that is needed for the dizzy patient. If a patient is nauseated or actively vomiting, an intravenous (IV) line should be established and antiemetic medication given along with IV hydration. Fluids should also be given if the physician suspects hypovolemia or dehydration as a contributing cause. If a cardiac cause is being considered, oxygen should be applied and an electrocardiogram obtained.

Peripheral vertigo

After supportive care has been initiated, the emergency physician should determine whether or not the patient has BPV, the most common cause of vertigo. This is based on characteristic historical features and a positive Hallpike test.

The Epley (canalith repositioning) maneuver

Patients with BPV should have the modified Epley maneuver (Figure 18.5) performed as follows: the patient's head is turned 45° to the side causing symptoms (as determined by the Hallpike test). The patient is guided to the supine position with the head hanging over the edge of the gurney. The head is then rotated 90° in the opposite direction with the face upwards, maintaining a dependent position. The patient is then asked to roll onto his side while holding the head in this position. The head is then rotated so that it is facing obliquely downward, with the nose 45° below horizontal. The patient is then raised to a sitting position while maintaining head rotation. Finally, the head is rotated to a central position and moved forward 45°. Each position is held until resolution of nystagmus occurs or for at least 30 seconds. It is not clear if the Epley maneuver should be repeated multiple times. Epley himself has performed the maneuver up to 5 times (personal communication). Other experts perform the maneuver only once since they feel that the particles will continually reintroduce themselves into the canals if the procedure is repeated. The Epley maneuver takes approximately 2–3 minutes to perform and is done at the bedside. Patients are expected to have their symptoms reproduced

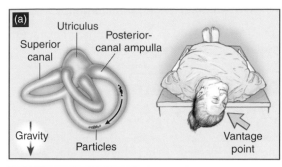

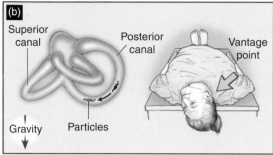

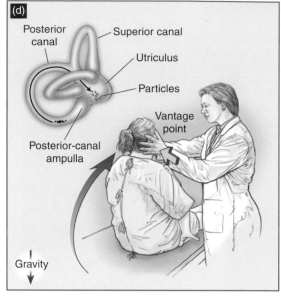

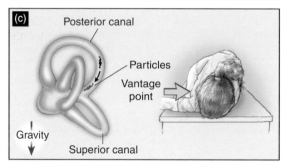

Figure 18.5

Bedside Maneuver for the Treatment of a Patient with Benign Paroxysmal Positional Vertigo Affecting the Right Ear. The presumed position of the debris within the labyrinth during the maneuver is shown in each panel. The maneuver is a three-step procedure. First, a Dix–Hallpike test is performed with the patient's head rotated 45 degrees toward the right ear and the neck slightly extended with the chin pointed slightly upward. This position results in the patient's head hanging to the right (Panel A). Once the vertigo and nystagmus provoked by the Dix–Hallpike test cease, the patient's head is rotated about the rostral-caudal body axis until the left ear is down (Panel B). Then the head and body are further rotated until the head is face down (Panel C). The vertex of the head is kept tilted downward throughout the rotation. The maneuver usually provokes brief vertigo. The patient should be kept in the final, face-down position for about 10 to 15 seconds. With the head kept turned toward the left shoulder, the patient is brought into the seated position (Panel D). Once the patient is upright, the head is tilted so that the chin is pointed slightly downward. Reprinted from Furman JM, Cass SP, Benign Paroxysmal Positional Vertigo, *N Engl J Med* 1999; 341(21):1590–1596. Copyright 1999 Massachusetts Medical Society. All rights reserved.

during each part of the maneuver, which indicates that the maneuver is moving the otoliths within the semicircular canal. Aside from the expected reproduction of symptoms and possible vomiting, no adverse events from performing the Epley maneuver have been reported. After the maneuver, patients are generally advised to stay in an upright position. Once the otoliths enter the utricle where they belong, they need time to reattach

to the utricular macule. The time required for this process is not clear, but it is generally recommended that at least 8 hours are needed before the patient can assume a supine position.

Vestibular suppressants

The use of vestibular suppressants is based on the *sensory conflict theory*. This states that when there is a mismatch of information from any of the three main sensory inputs (vestibular, visual, and proprioceptive), nausea and emesis result in the acute phase, but habituation occurs over time. This mismatch of information is compared to learned prior stimuli. This process is thought to be mediated by three or four neurotransmitters: gamma amino butyric acid (GABA), acetylcholine, histamine and serotonin. Benzodiazepines work by preventing the mismatched information from being compared to prior learned stimuli. However, many experts avoid using benzodiazepines since they prevent the process of vestibular rehabilitation. Anticholinergics work by decreasing the signal-size conflict, and are thought to be the most useful agents. However, atropine is rarely used due to its serious side effects, and scopolamine has an onset of several hours, limiting its use in the ED. Antihistaminics and antiserotonergics block the emesis response. These medications, which include promethazine and meclizine, also have anticholinergic side effects. Intravenous promethazine (Phenergan) is felt by many to be the best medication for the acutely symptomatic patient experiencing vertigo.

Central vertigo

The treatment of central vertigo depends on the cause. Antiplatelet agents should be started in consultation with a neurologist.

Near-syncope

For near-syncope due to orthostatic hypotension, removal of offending medications or correction of volume depletion will often be therapeutic. In patients with autonomic insufficiency, increased salt intake can increase blood volume, and elastic stockings can prevent pooling of blood in the lower extremities. For vasovagal near-syncope, reassurance is usually all that is needed. Patients can also increase their fluid intake and avoid conditions that predispose them to hypotension and dehydration. Near-syncope associated with impaired cardiac output can be a serious warning sign. Cardiac dysrhythmia management depends on the actual rhythm, and many patients can be helped with the insertion of a pacemaker even if the diseased heart cannot be treated. Hyperventilation-induced near-syncope should be treated by educating and reassuring the patient that this is a benign disorder. If associated with panic disorder, pharmacologic treatment (i.e.,

tricyclic antidepressants or selective serotonin reuptake inhibitors) may be considered after discussion with the patient's primary care physician.

Disequilibrium

For disequilibrium, gait and balance training may be beneficial for those patients without cerebellar lesions. Indeed, a cane or walker often helps most patients. Patients with alcoholic cerebellar degeneration may show improvement following their discontinuation of alcohol consumption. Parkinson's disease may be improved with L-DOPA. Hydrocephalus-induced disequilibrium can be reversed with shunt placement.

Psychophysiologic dizziness

For psychophysiologic dizziness, supportive psychotherapy in addition to medications may be helpful. Medications include benzodiazepines, tricyclic antidepressants, and selective serotonin reuptake inhibitors. These medications should be started only after consultation with the patient's primary care physician or specialist.

Special patients
Pediatric

Children rarely complain of dizziness. When they do, they present with similar vestibular and non-vestibular problems as adults. Otitis media and its complications (suppurative labyrinthitis or mastoiditis) can lead to vestibular complaints. Acute cerebellar ataxia can follow a viral infection, and usually occurs in children under the age of 6 years. Infection or volume depletion may be important clues to the diagnosis. Disequilibrium in a young person suggests neurologic disease. Also, near-syncope in a young athlete who is exercising may indicate serious cardiac disease, such as hypertrophic obstructive cardiomyopathy or aortic stenosis.

Elderly

Dizziness becomes more common in the elderly, which can result in falls causing hip fractures and intracerebral hemorrhage. Elderly patients are more likely to present with central causes of vertigo, such as ischemic cerebrovascular disease, and are more likely to be debilitated by symptoms of peripheral vertigo.

Disposition

Admission of patients with dizziness or vertigo should be based on the underlying etiology or associated symptoms. Patients with peripheral vertigo may be discharged home, unless they present with intractable vomiting or vertigo that cannot be controlled in the ED. Patients with an abnormal neurologic examination or those with increased suspicion for a serious neurologic cause should have a formal neurologic consultation or be admitted for observation. Similarly, patients in whom cardiac dysrhythmias are a likely cause should be admitted for observation and cardiac monitoring.

Pearls, pitfalls, and myths

- A detailed neurologic examination is important in differentiating central from peripheral vertigo. Since the cerebellovestibular nuclei are tightly packed with other tracts in the brainstem, any lesion that affects these nuclei will likely affect others as well.
- The Hallpike test should be performed in patients who present with vertigo, but not rapidly. Gently guide the patient into the head-hanging position.
- It is important to differentiate BPV from other causes of peripheral vertigo, such as vestibular neuritis, labyrinthitis, and psychophysiologic dizziness, since the Epley maneuver only works for BPV.
- A chief complaint of dizziness should not result in the knee-jerk reflex to prescribe meclizine. Although meclizine is effective in many cases of vertigo, it may worsen symptoms in other subcategories of dizziness.

References

1. Baloh RW. Vestibular neuritis. *New Engl J Med* 2003;348:1027–1032.
2. Chang AK, Schoeman G, Hill MA. A randomized clinical trial to assess the efficacy of the Epley maneuver in the treatment of acute benign positional vertigo. *Acad Emerg Med* 2004;11:918–924.
3. Drachman DA, Hart CW. An approach to the dizzy patient. *Neurology* 1972;22:323–334.
4. Epley JM. The canalith repositioning procedure: for treatment of benign paroxysmal positional vertigo. *Otolaryngol Head Neck Surg* 1992;107:399–404.
5. Furman JM, Cass SP. Benign paroxysmal positional vertigo. *New Engl J Med* 1999;341:1590–1596.
6. Goldman B. Vertigo and dizziness. In: Tintinalli JE (ed.). *Emergency Medicine: A Comprehensive Study Guide*, 5th ed., New York, NY: McGraw-Hill, 2001. pp. 1452–1463.
7. Kroenke K, Lucas CA, Rosenberg ML, et al. Causes of persistent dizziness. A prospective study of 100 patients in ambulatory care. *Ann Intern Med* 1992;117:898–904.
8. Olshaker JS. Vertigo. In: Rosen P, Barkin R (eds). *Emergency Medicine: Concepts and Clinical Practice*, 5th ed., St. Louis, MO: Mosby, 2002. pp. 123–131.
9. Pigott DC, Rosko CJ. The dizzy patient: an evidence-based diagnosis and treatment strategy. *Emerg Med Pract* 2001;3(3).
10. Raynor EM, Herr RD. Vertigo and labyrinthine disorders. In: Harwood-Nuss AL (ed.). *The Clinical Practice of Emergency Medicine*, 3rd ed., Philadelphia, PA: Lippincott-Raven Publishers, 2001. pp. 120–125.

19   Ear pain, nosebleed and throat pain (ENT)

EAR PAIN

Gregory H. Gilbert, MD and S.V. Mahadevan, MD

Scope of the problem

Ear pain (otalgia) is a common emergency department (ED) complaint. It prompts over 30 million physician visits per year. By the third year of life, 80% of the population will have complained of otalgia at least once. Though many conditions may cause ear pain, otitis media (OM) is by far the most common diagnosis, especially in the pediatric population. The potential for serious causes of otalgia, such as malignant otitis externa (OE) and mastoiditis, underscore the need for early and accurate diagnosis and treatment.

Anatomic essentials

The anatomic ear may be divided into three distinct sections: external, middle and inner (Figure 19.1). The *external ear*, consisting of the auricle (pinna) and the external auditory canal (EAC),

originates at the pinna and ends at the tympanic membrane (TM). The *middle ear* is an air-containing cavity in the petrous temporal bone that houses three auditory ossicles: the malleus, incus and stapes. Though the middle ear is separated from the outer ear by the TM, it connects anteriorly with the nasopharynx via the eustachian tube, and posteriorly with the mastoid air cells. The *inner ear* includes the cochlea, which contains the auditory receptors, and vestibular labyrinth, which contains the balance receptors. Sensory innervation of the ear is derived from branches of cranial nerves (CNs) V, VII, IX and X as well as I, II and III.

Primary otalgia (Table 19.1) is ear pain that results from structures directly within or adjacent to the anatomic ear. OM and OE are the most common causes of primary otalgia.

The development of OM is thought to be associated with dysfunction of the eustachian tube. The eustachian tube protects the middle ear from

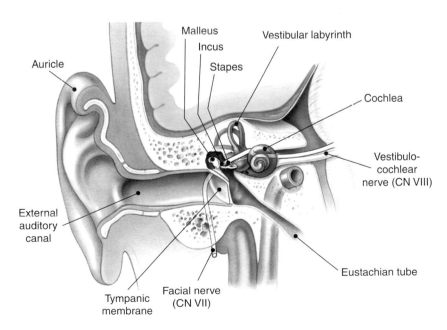

Figure 19.1
Ear anatomy.

nasopharyngeal secretions, allows drainage of middle ear secretions, and helps equilibrate air pressure in the middle ear. Eustachian tube dysfunction may trap fluid, secretions and bacteria within the middle ear and result in an infection.

Mechanical obstruction of the eustachian tube may result due to localized inflammation from an upper respiratory infection (URI), allergies or hypertrophied adenoids. Functional obstruction secondary to eustachian tube collapse may occur in young children due to anatomic differences, such as a shorter length and less cartilaginous support.

OE results from inflammation or infection of the EAC. Prolonged exposure to moisture (i.e., swimming) or local trauma (i.e., cotton swabs or hearing aids) can disrupt the protective outer layer of the EAC, allowing bacterial penetration and ensuing infection. Malignant OE, an invasive necrotizing form, may occur in diabetics or immunocompromised patients and result in severe neurologic sequelae or death.

Not all ear pain originates from the anatomic ear. Otalgia referred from sources outside the anatomic ear (Table 19.1) occurs as a result of shared sensory innervation by the anatomic ear and other head and neck structures. *Referred otalgia* may arise from pathology in the parotid glands, teeth, muscles of mastication, mandible, nasopharynx, paranasal sinuses, thyroid gland, cervical spine, upper gastrointestinal tract or upper respiratory tract (Figure 19.2). Dental disorders are the

Table 19.1 Causes of otalgia (*adapted from* Tintinalli)

Primary	Referred
• Infection	• Dental
– Otitis media	– Temporomandibular joint disease
– Otitis externa	– Caries or tooth abscess
– Mastoiditis	– Malocclusion
– Bullous myringitis	– Poorly-fitting dentures
• Foreign body	– Bruxism
• Cerumen impaction	– Trauma
• Cholesteatoma	• Retro and oropharyngeal
• Neoplasms	– Tonsillitis
• Aerotitis	– Pharyngitis
• Neuralgias	– Abscess
– Herpetic geniculate	– Neoplasm
– Tic douloureux	• Sinusitis
	• Throat and neck
	– Foreign body
	– Thyroid disease
	– Cervical strain
	– Neoplasm

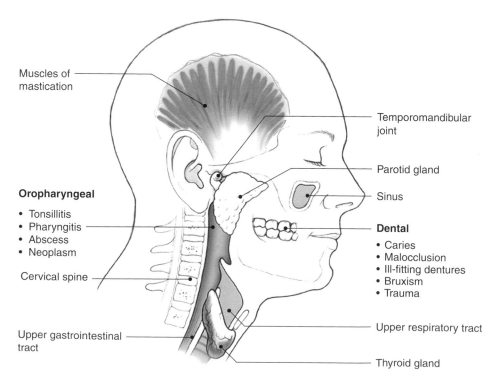

Figure 19.2
Sources of referred otalgia.

most common cause of referred otalgia, especially if the ear examination is normal. Elderly patients are most likely to present with a referred cause of otalgia.

History

Obtaining an accurate history from young patients may be challenging, as a parent or guardian may be describing the patient's symptomatology.

How did the pain begin and how long have you had it?

Most patients present with acute ear pain within 24 hours of its onset. The ear pain may be moderate to severe, leading to difficulty sleeping and prompting an ED visit in the middle of the night. In one study, patients who delayed seeking initial care for OM were more likely to present with complications. Long-standing undiagnosed ear pain may represent an undiagnosed head and neck carcinoma.

Describe the pain?

Constant, sharp, stabbing pain with associated pressure or throbbing is typical of acute OM (AOM). The discomfort from OE may vary from itching to severe pain. Intermittent or variable pain is usually referred and may arise from the temporomandibular joint (TMJ) or teeth. A sudden decrease in pain associated with discharge from the ear is typical of TM rupture. Pediatric patients may pull at their ears rather than complain of ear pain.

What makes the pain better or worse?

Pain exacerbated by eating or chewing may be referred from the TMJ or teeth. AOM is typically worsened with recumbent position. The discomfort from OE is often aggravated by manipulation of the tragus or ear.

How is your hearing?

Patients may describe hearing loss, muffled hearing, popping or crunching sounds. Hearing loss or changes may accompany OM, OE, foreign bodies (FBs) and cerumen impaction.

Any ear discharge?

Otorrhea (discharge from the ear) may occur with a ruptured TM, OE or FB. The discharge may be serosanguinous or purulent. Pain typically precedes otorrhea in OM, whereas in OE it accompanies the drainage. Chronic ear pain and drainage may represent mastoiditis or a cholesteatoma.

Any recent travel or trauma?

Diving or recent air travel could lead to TM perforation from barotrauma. A history of swimming often accompanies OE. A direct blow to the side of the head or noise trauma can also cause TM perforation. The use of a Q-tip to clean the ear canal can result in damage to the external auditory meatus or TM. A whiplash injury or arthritis of the cervical spine can lead to referred otalgia.

Associated symptoms

General

Ask about fussiness, lethargy, fever and URI. While adults and older children can articulate ear pain, infants and toddlers may cry, fuss or refuse food. Very few patients with OM will have a fever greater than 40°C. In these patients, consideration should be given to other etiologies of ear pain, such as OE, trauma, FBs, mastoiditis, meningitis or an abscess. In one prospective study, nearly all patients with OM had ear pain, decreased hearing and URI symptoms, but only 9% of these patients had fever.

Head and neck

Ask about headache, sinus problems, dizziness, bruxism, difficulty swallowing and changes in speech. As otalgia may be referred, a complete review of head and neck symptoms is imperative. Headache may occur with sinusitis, mastoiditis and malignant OE. Headache can also accompany complications of these conditions, such as meningitis, brain abscess and cavernous sinus thrombosis. The presence of dizziness or tinnitus suggests inner ear involvement. Patients who grind their teeth in the middle of the night (bruxism) are more likely to have TMJ syndrome or a dental problem. Difficulty swallowing and speaking can hint that the pain is referred from a retropharyngeal or peritonsillar abscess, or possibly a laryngeal mass.

Past medical

Patients with cervicofacial pain syndromes like myalgias, neuralgias or arthritis may have otalgia.

Children diagnosed with AOM by 1 year of age are more likely to have recurrences, with 33% of patients getting five or more episodes by the age of 6 years. Previous surgery such as myringotomy or tympanostomy tube placement usually indicates either a history of OM with a serious complication or frequent recurrences unresponsive to antibiotic therapy. Patients with allergies also are at increased risk for both sinusitis and AOM; the same is true with craniofacial abnormalities seen in Down's syndrome or cleft palate. A history of sinus problems can suggest a source of the otalgia. Immunocompromised patients and diabetics are at significant risk for developing malignant OE.

Medications

Patients taking medications containing acetaminophen or non-steroidal anti-inflammatory drugs (NSAIDs) for their ear pain may not exhibit a fever. Symptomatic patients with OM who are currently taking antibiotics may require a second-line agent due to penicillin-resistant *Streptococcus pneumoniae*.

Social

A positive correlation exists between smoking and OM. Studies reveal a 2- to 4-fold increase in OM when exposed to second-hand smoke. Smoking also increases the risk of getting sinusitis and cancer of the larynx, both which may cause referred otalgia. Children who attend group day care are at a 2.5-fold increased risk for OM, while breastfed infants have 13% fewer ear infections. Like viruses and the common cold, ear infections are seasonal and tend to occur more frequently in the winter and early spring.

Physical examination

While the history helps establish the problem, a careful physical examination may identify the diagnosis.

General appearance

The importance of assessing the general appearance of a pediatric patient cannot be overemphasized. A toxic-appearing child with altered mental status or lethargy merits consideration of sepsis and meningitis, even if the examination reveals OM.

Vital signs

A fever can occur with AOM, but it is seldom greater than 40°C. Tachycardia is commonly due to fever and dehydration. For every degree (in Celsius) of temperature elevation, expect an increase in the pulse of about 10 beats/minute.

Head, eyes, ears, nose and throat

A complete head, eye, ear, nose and throat (HEENT) examination is essential to proper assessment of the patient with otalgia. Possible serious etiologies identified on examination include mastoiditis, ruptured TM with dislocation of the ossicles, retropharyngeal abscess, meningitis, and malignant OE.

Head and face

The sinuses should be examined to assess for the possibility of sinusitis. The temporal artery should be palpated, as temporal arteritis is a treatable cause of referred otalgia. Periauricular lymphadenopathy may occur with scalp or neck infections. The submandibular, submaxillary and parotid glands should also be inspected and palpated. An infection, tumor or salivary stone affecting the parotid gland, which lies just anterior to the ear, could lead to otalgia.

Ears

External ear

The external ear and periauricular areas should be examined for signs of inflammation. The presence of postauricular erythema, swelling and tenderness with protrusion of the auricle and loss of the postauricular crease suggests acute mastoiditis (Figure 19.3). In patients with malignant OE, the auricle may appear abnormal and grossly deformed.

Ear canal

Begin by selecting the correct speculum size for use with the otoscope. Pain on insertion of the speculum into the canal suggests OE (Figure 19.4). If the canal is occluded with cerumen, debris or discharge, careful removal with an ear curet may

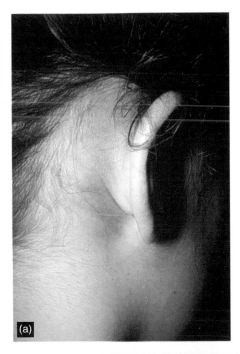

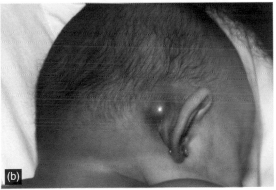

Figure 19.3
(a) Mastoiditis. *Courtesy:* Lawrence Stack, MD. (b) Severe mastoiditis. *Courtesy:* Robert Jackler, MD.

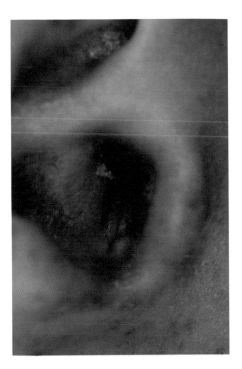

Figure 19.4
External otitis media. Note inflamed and erythematous external auditory canal. *Courtesy:* Lawrence Stack, MD.

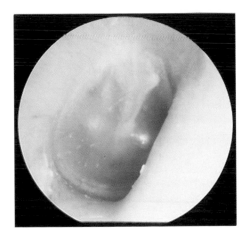

Figure 19.5
A normal tympanic membrane. The drum is thin and translucent, and the ossicles are readily visualized. It is neutrally positioned with no evidence of bulging or retraction. Reprinted from Atlas of Pediatric Physical Diagnosis, 4th ed., Eds Zitelli BJ, Davis HW. Copyright 2002, with permission from Elsevier.

improve visibility. The EAC should be examined for signs of inflammation or the presence of a FB. The presence of erythema or edema of the canal, with ear pain reproduced by pulling on the auricle or tragus, signifies OE.

Tympanic membrane

Pulling the auricle posteriorly and superiorly straightens the external auditory canal and facilitates visualization of the TM. The light reflex, color, translucency and bony landmarks of the TM should be noted. Comparison with the other ear may be helpful. The normal TM is shiny and translucent (Figure 19.5). Erythema may be present with OM, but also crying or fever. A retracted

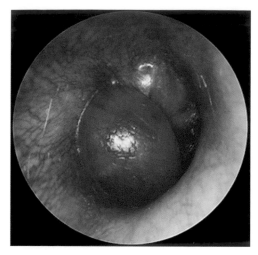

Figure 19.6
Acute otitis media with bullous myringitis. Otoscopy reveals an erythematous bullous lesion, obscuring much of the tympanic membrane. This phenomenon, called bullous myringitis, is caused by the usual pathogens of otitis media in childhood. The bullous lesion commonly ruptures spontaneously, providing immediate relief of pain. Reprinted from Atlas of Pediatric Physical Diagnosis, 4th ed., Eds Zitelli BJ, Davis HW. Copyright 2002, with permission from Elsevier.

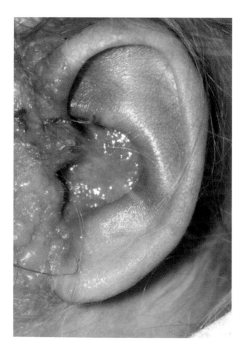

Figure 19.7
Herpes zoster oticus. *Courtesy*: Lawrence Stack, MD.

TM with prominence of the malleus may be found with OM with effusion. The development of bullae indicates bullous myringitis (Figure 19.6); vesicles suggest Ramsay-Hunt syndrome (herpes zoster oticus) (Figure 19.7). The presence of a tympanostomy tube may lead to decreased TM mobility, altered landmarks, opacity and dullness, even in the absence of infection. A defect in the TM suggests perforation (Figure 19.8), while a white mass behind the TM may be a cholesteatoma.

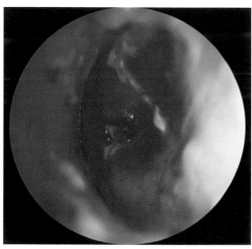

Figure 19.8
Acute otitis media with perforation. In this child, increased middle ear pressure with acute otitis resulted in perforation of the tympanic membrane. The drum is thickened, and the perforation is seen at the 3 o'clock position. Reprinted from Atlas of Pediatric Physical Diagnosis 4th ed., Eds Zitelli BJ, Davis HW. Copyright 2002, with permission from Elsevier.

Pneumatic otoscopy

Following visualization of the TM with the otoscope, air can be insufflated into the canal using a pneumatic bulb. The normal TM should be slightly mobile with insufflation. The lack of TM mobility highly suggests a middle ear effusion, though mobility may also be reduced from middle ear adhesions, TM perforation or eustachian tube dysfunction. An immobile, bulging, erythematous eardrum which has lost its bony landmarks is very predictive of AOM (Figure 19.9).

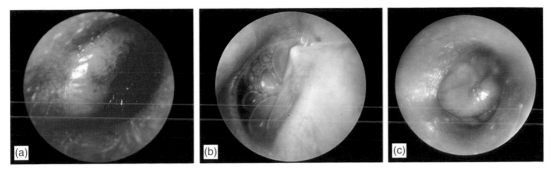

Figure 19.9
Acute otitis media. (a) An erythematous, opaque, bulging tympanic membrane with a reduced light reflex and partially obscuration of the landmarks. (b) The finding of both air and fluid-formed bubbles separated by gray-yellow menisci, combined with fever and otalgia, is consistent with acute infection (even though the drum is not injected). (c) The tympanic membrane is injected at the periphery and a yellow purulent effusion bulges outward from the inferior aspect. Reprinted from Atlas of Pediatric Physical Diagnosis, 4th ed., Eds Zitelli BJ, Davis HW. Copyright 2002, with permission from Elsevier.

If the ear canal is too large to provide a good pneumatic seal, the patient is likely old enough to perform a modified Frenzel maneuver. In this procedure, the patient pinches the nose, gently blows without opening the mouth (cheeks puffing out is okay) and then swallows. Using this technique, the normal TM should move outward initially and then inward with swallowing.

Hearing

Hearing can be evaluated in a cooperative patient, but rarely in the young pediatric patient. Hearing can be measured grossly or using the Weber and Rinne tests. The *Weber test* is performed by placing the base of vibrating tuning fork on the middle of the forehead, equidistant from the ears. Hearing the tone louder in one ear suggests either conductive hearing loss in that ear or sensorineural hearing loss in the opposite ear. Plugging your ear with a finger (to simulate conductive hearing loss) and performing the test will demonstrate this finding. The *Rinne test* is performed by alternating placement of a vibrating tuning fork directly on the patient's mastoid process (bone conduction) and in front of the patient's ear (air conduction). Hearing the tone louder in front of the ear is a positive Rinne test, indicating normal hearing or sensorineural hearing loss. Hearing the tone louder with the tuning fork against the mastoid is a negative Rinne test and indicates conductive hearing loss in that ear.

Mouth and throat

Since dental pain is the most common cause of referred otalgia, the teeth should be carefully examined for dental caries, abscess, impacted molars or poorly-fitting dentures. Dental malocclusion resulting from TMJ dysfunction can cause referred ear pain from masticator muscle spasm. The TMJ should be assessed for clicking, popping and tenderness consistent with TMJ syndrome. Assess the oropharynx for the possibility of pharyngitis, peritonsillar abscess, retropharyngeal abscess, or mass.

Neck

The neck should be evaluated for meningeal signs which must not be missed. Also assess the neck for musculoskeletal disorders, lymph node and thyroid enlargement, or other masses or tenderness. Flexion of the neck may increase otalgia due to degenerative joint disease.

Cranial nerves

Cranial nerve VII dysfunction and resulting facial paralysis may occur in patients with Ramsay-Hunt syndrome, mastoiditis or malignant OE.

Differential diagnosis

Table 19.2 Differential diagnosis of ear pain

Diagnosis	Symptoms	Signs	Special work-up
Acute otitis media (Figure 19.9)	Ear pain; hearing loss; recent URI; pain worse at night; drainage from ear; children may have fever, fussiness, poor appetite, pulling at the affected ear.	Temperature usually <40°C; TM findings: erythema, loss of light reflex, retraction or bulging, impaired mobility with pneumatic otoscopy; absence of pain with manipulation of pinna; drainage if TM ruptured.	
Bullous myringitis (Figure 19.6)	Acute onset of ear pain, usually following a URI (like AOM); hearing loss; serosanguinous ear drainage.	Serous or hemorrhagic blisters (bullae) on the TM; abnormal hearing.	
Cholesteatoma	Progressively worsening hearing loss; malodorous ear drainage and pain.	A cyst of desquamated epithelium or keratin that appears as a whitish area of the TM or polyp protruding through a TM defect.	CT or MRI may reveal local bone erosion.
Dental caries	Throbbing pain, sometimes localized; exacerbated by hot or cold foods, or lying supine.	Poor dentition; pain with percussion of the affected tooth.	
Foreign body	*Children*: ear pain; itching; discharge; foul odor. *Adults*: Usually provide history of FB; may feel motion or buzzing with insect.	Most FBs should be visible; reexamination after removal is important to exclude TM injury, or a retained or additional FB.	
Herpes zoster oticus (Ramsay-Hunt syndrome) (Figure 19.7)	Pain (may be out of proportion to physical findings); rash; facial paralysis; hearing loss and vertigo.	Herpetiform vesicular eruption; vesicles may be seen on the pinna, EAC, TM, oral cavity, face and neck as far down as the shoulder; peripheral CN VII nerve palsy.	
Malignant otitis externa	Fever; severe pain; swelling of the pinna; purulent drainage; headache; facial paralysis; history of diabetes or immunocompromise.	Classic finding is granulation tissue on the floor of the EAC at the bone–cartilage junction; tenderness of bony structures around the ear; cranial nerve involvement is a serious sign.	ESR elevated; CT, MRI, Gallium scintigraphy.
Mastoiditis (Figure 19.3)	Deep severe ear pain; headache; fever, chills, malaise; ear drainage; postauricular ear pain and swelling.	Postauricular erythema, swelling and tenderness; protrusion of the auricle and loss of the postauricular crease; cranial nerve palsies.	Radiographs may be negative; CT or MRI is more useful.
Otitis externa (Figure 19.4)	Varies from itching to severe pain; serous to purulent discharge from the ear canal; systemic symptoms usually absent.	Crusting and drainage in and around the EAC; erythema and edema of the EAC; manipulation of the auricle worsens the pain; the ear canal may be swollen shut leading to conductive hearing loss.	

(*continued*)

Table 19.2 Differential diagnosis of ear pain (*cont*)

Diagnosis	Symptoms	Signs	Special work-up
Pharyngitis, peritonsillar or retropharyngeal abscess	Sore throat; fever; absence of URI symptoms; headache; dysphonia; dysphagia; odynophagia; drooling.	Fever; enlarged inflamed tonsils; exudates; trismus; displacement of the infected tonsil and deviation of the uvula with peritonsillar abscess; oropharyngeal fullness or tenderness with "rocking" the trachea with retropharyngeal abscess.	A lateral neck radiograph or CT will demonstrate the retropharyngeal abscess.
Sinusitis	Headache; facial pain; nasal congestion; purulent nasal drainage; persistent URI symptoms; maxillary toothache; pain exacerbated and relieved with changes in position.	Tenderness with palpation of maxillary or frontal sinuses; mucosal erythema and edema; purulent nasal drainage; transillumination may reveal sinus opacification.	Plain film accuracy best for maxillary sinusitis; diminished for other sinuses; CT is more sensitive and specific.
Temporomandibular joint	Intermittent pain, worsens during the day; typically unilateral; pain associated with chewing or bruxism (teeth grinding).	Clicking and tenderness at the joint; trismus with palpable masseter and internal pterygoid muscle spasm.	Radiographs are generally not helpful.

AOM: acute otitis media; CN: cranial nerve; CT: computed tomography; EAC: external auditory canal; ESR: erythrocyte sedimentation rate; FB: foreign body; MRI: magnetic resonance imaging; TM: tympanic membrane; URI: upper respiratory infection.

Diagnostic testing

Diagnostic testing is generally not indicated in the evaluation of otalgia. In patients with suspected malignant OE, cultures of the purulent discharge may aid pathogen identification and guide antibiotic therapy. Computerized tomography (CT) and/or magnetic resonance imaging (MRI) are indicated to delineate the extent of infection. Patients without an obvious source for otalgia on physical examination may require a CT scan of the head, face or neck to determine the etiology. Thyroid function tests or an erythrocyte sedimentation rate (ESR) may be helpful if thyroiditis or temporal arteritis is suspected. Panorex or dental X-rays may be helpful if suspicion exists for a mandibular or dental etiology.

General treatment principles
Pain relief

While ibuprofen or acetaminophen may be adequate for some patients, others may require a short course of narcotic analgesia. A topical anesthetic like auralgan (antipyrine/benzocaine) may be beneficial in patients with primary otalgia and an intact TM. Viscous lidocaine or benadryl elixir can be gargled to anesthetize the throat and possibly localize referred otalgia to the oropharynx.

Otitis media
Antibiotics

Antibiotics are commonly used to treat AOM. Since the advent of antibiotic therapy for AOM, the rate of complications and deaths from AOM has dropped dramatically. The first-line antimicrobial agent for AOM is typically amoxicillin, given it has few side effects and reasonable efficacy. The use of higher dose amoxicillin (90 mg/kg/day) is more effective against drug-resistant pneumococcus; this therapy should be considered in children who have received antibiotics in the past 3 months, are less than 2 years of age, or are in day care. In penicillin-allergic patients, consider the use of sulfa-containing agents (trimethoprim–sulfamethoxisole, erythromycin–sulfisoxazole) or the macrolides (azithromycin or clarithromycin). Failure to improve after 72 hours of antibiotic therapy is considered a treatment failure. For

Table 19.3 Antibiotic choices for acute otitis media

First line	Dosage
Amoxicillin	Pediatrics: <3 months: 10–15 mg/kg PO BID for 10 days; Max: 30 mg/kg/day 3 months–2 years: 45 mg/kg PO BID for 10 days >2 years: 20–25 mg/kg PO BID for 10 days (Alt: 45 mg/kg PO BID for 5 days; Max: 875 mg/dose) Adults: 500–875 mg PO BID for 10 days
Trimethoprim–sulfamethoxisole	Pediatrics: >2 months: 0.5 ml susp/kg PO BID for 10 days; Max: 20 ml susp/dose Adults: 1 tablet PO BID for 7–14 days
Erythromycin–sulfisoxazole	Pediatrics: >2 months: 10–12 mg/kg (erythromycin component) PO QID for 7–14 days; Max: 2 g/day
Azithromycin	Pediatrics: ≥6 months: 10 mg/kg PO day 1 then 5 mg/kg/day PO QD days 2–5; Max: 500 mg/day Adults: 500 mg PO day 1, 250 mg PO QD days 2–5 (Alt: 500 mg PO QD for 3 days)
Clarithromycin	Pediatrics: 7.5 mg/kg PO BID for 10 days; Max: 1 g/day Adults: 500 mg PO BID for 7–14 days
Second line	**Dosage**
Amoxicillin–clavulanate	Dose based on amoxicillin component Pediatrics: <3 months: 15 mg/kg PO BID for 10 days; Max: 30 mg/kg/day 3 months–2 years: 40–45 mg/kg PO BID for 10 days; Max: 875 mg/dose >2 years: 20–25 mg/kg PO BID for 10 days; Max: 1800 mg/day Adults: 875 mg PO BID for 10 days
Cefuroxime axetil	Pediatrics: 10–15 mg/kg PO BID for 10 days; Max: 1 g/day Adults: 250–500 mg PO BID for 7–10 days
Ceftriaxone	Pediatrics: 50 mg/kg IM × 1 dose; Max: 1 g/dose

alt: alternative; BID: twice a day; IM: intramuscular; Max: maximum; PO: per os; QD: daily; susp: suspension.

patients who fail to respond to initial amoxicillin therapy, the Centers for Disease Control and Prevention recommend amoxicillin/clavulanate, cefuroxime axetil or intramuscular ceftriaxone (Table 19.3).

The need for antibiotic therapy in uncomplicated AOM is controversial. The over-prescription of antibiotics for AOM and emergence of bacterial resistance to commonly-used antibiotics has heightened the urgency to reduce unnecessary antibiotic use. Recent data suggest a lack of benefit to antibiotic treatment in children with uncomplicated OM (the absence of fever and vomiting). The practice of holding antibiotic therapy and watchful waiting is common in Europe and gaining acceptance in the US. Reliable patients with adequate access to follow-up care are given a safety-net antibiotic prescription (SNAP) to be filled only if their symptoms do not resolve during the first 48 hours. During this period of observation, patients are managed with oral analgesics and topical otic anesthetic drops.

Other therapy

The use of antihistamines, decongestants or steroids provides no obvious benefit for patients with AOM.

Otitis media with tympanic membrane perforation

OM with perforation of the TM is treated similarly to AOM. Since the purulent discharge associated with perforation may result in an associated OE, patients are also commonly treated with a topical eardrops containing a steroid–antibiotic suspension, such as corticosporin-HC otic or corticosporin ophthalmic drops. Patients should avoid swimming and diving until the perforation has healed.

Table 19.4 Otic drops for treatment of otitis externa

Name	Components	Dosage
VoSol	Acetic acid and propylene glycol	5 gtts of 2% solution otic TID/QID for 7–10 days
VoSol HC	Acetic acid and hydrocortisone	3–5 gtts of 2% solution otic TID/QID for 7–10 days
Domeboro	Acetic acid and aluminum acetate	3–5 gtts of 2% solution otic every 2–4 hours for 7–10 days
Floxin	Ofloxacin	Age ≥ 1 year to 12 years: 5 gtts of 0.3% solution otic BID for 10–14 days Age >12 years: 10 gtts of 0.3% solution otic BID for 10–14 days
Cipro HC	Ciprofloxacin and hydrocortisone	Age ≥ 1 year; 3 gtts of 0.2% solution otic BID for 7 days
Cortisporin*	Neomycin, hydrocortisone and polymixin	3–4 gtts otic TID/QID for 7–10 days
Colymycin S	Neomycin	3–5 gtts otic TID/QID for 7–10 days
Otobiotic	Polymixin and hydrocortisone	3–5 gtts otic TID/QID for 7–10 days

BID: twice a day; * gtts = drops; HC: hydrocortisone; QID: four times a day; TID: three times a day.

During bathing, the placement of a petroleum jelly-impregnated cotton ball in the outer ear may prevent the entry of water into the EAC.

Otitis externa

The treatment of OE begins with cleansing the external canal through gentle irrigation and suctioning. Though irrigation may be performed with tap water, saline or Burrow's solution, acetic acid has the added benefit of having antifungal and antibacterial properties. Cleansing is followed by treatment with topical antibiotic–steroid otic drops (Table 19.4). In cases where the canal is occluded by edema, the careful placement of a cotton wick facilitates the delivery of medicine throughout the entire ear canal. Consider systemic antibiotics if cellulitis or systemic signs are present.

Foreign bodies

Approaches used for FB removal from the ear include irrigation, suction, direct instrumentation and cyanoacrylate (superglue). The preferred approach reflects the type of FB, available equipment and the physician's proficiency. Warm water irrigation is a simple, noninvasive approach for patients with an intact TM. Avoid irrigation if the suspected FB is made of organic material, as expansion of the object following contact with water may complicate its removal. For insects within the canal, mineral oil or viscous lidocaine is usually applied

to immobilize and kill the insect. Lidocaine has the added benefit of anesthetizing the canal and TM, making extraction less painful. Following the removal of any FB, prophylactic antibiotics may be necessary to prevent OE. If removal of the FB cannot be achieved in the ED, ear, nose and throat (ENT) referral within 24 hours is necessary.

Special patients
Immune compromised

Diabetics and immunocompromised patients are at increased risk for malignant OE, a severe necrotizing infection that originates in the ear canal. As the infection spreads to adjacent structures, it may become destructive and life-threatening. The causative agent is usually *Pseudomonas aeruginosa*. Systemic antipseudomonal antibiotics are usually administered for 4–8 weeks, and surgical debridement may be required.

Disposition
Discharge

The vast majority of patients with otalgia are discharged home with an excellent prognosis. Patients who require subspecialty consultation include those suffering from malignant OE or mastoiditis, and those with worrisome complaints or findings such as severe pain, neurologic deficits, bloody discharge, hearing loss and vertigo.

Most cases of AOM should improve within 48–72 hours. If symptoms persist, patients should be reevaluated for complications or possible treatment failure. Patients with an uncomplicated AOM should be reexamined in 2–3 weeks to ensure resolution of their middle ear effusion. Follow-up with ENT should be arranged for patients with frequent ear infections, craniofacial abnormalities or multiple treatment failures. Patients with otalgia from an undetermined source need follow-up and further evaluation, as an occult tumor may be responsible.

Pearls, pitfalls, and myths

- The most common cause of otalgia is OM.
- Pain typically precedes otorrhea in OM; it accompanies the drainage in OE.
- Few patients with OM have very high temperatures.
- An immobile, bulging red eardrum that has lost its bony landmarks is consistent with AOM.
- The presence of ear pain reproduced by pulling on the tragus or auricle is likely caused by OE.
- Not all discharge from an ear canal is due to OE.
- Not all pain originates from the anatomic ear.
- Dental pain is the most common cause of referred otalgia.
- Not all patients with OM need immediate antibiotics.
- Placement of a wick may aid the treatment of a patient with canal occlusion from OE.
- OE in an immunocompromised host, especially with erythema and/or fever, should be considered malignant OE until proven otherwise.

References

1. Cummings CW, et al. (ed.). *Otolaryngology: Head and Neck Surgery*, 3rd ed., Mosby, 1998.
2. Hamilton GC (ed.). *Emergency Medicine: An Approach to Clinical Problem-Solving*, 2nd ed., Philadelphia: WB Saunders, 2001.
3. Harwood-Nuss A (ed.). *The Clinical Practice of Emergency Medicine*, 3rd ed., Philadelphia: Lippincott Williams & Wilkins, 2001.
4. Kuttila S, et al. *Secondary Otalgia in an Adult Population*, Vol. 127(4). 2001. pp. 401–405.
5. Marx JA (ed.). *Rosen's Emergency Medicine: Concepts and Clinical Practice*, 5th ed., St. Louis: Mosby, 2002.
6. McCracken GH. Diagnosis and management of acute otitis media in the urgent care setting. *Ann Emerg Med* 2002;39(4):413–421.
7. Olsen KD. The many causes of otalgia. Infection, trauma, cancer. *Postgrad Med* 1986;80(6):50–52, 55–56, 61–63.
8. Rakel RE (ed.). *Textbook of Family Practice*, 6th ed., WB Saunders Company, 2002.
9. Roberts JR, Hedges JR (eds). *Clinical Procedures in Emergency Medicine*, 3rd ed., WB Saunders Company, 1998.
10. Sander R. *Otitis externa: a practical guide to treatment and prevention. Am Fam Physician* 2001;63(5):927–936, 941–942.
11. Siegel RM, et al. Treatment of otitis media with observation and a safety-net antibiotic prescription. *Pediatrics* 2003;112:527–531.
12. Tintinalli JE (ed.). *Emergency Medicine: A Comprehensive Study Guide*, 5th ed., McGraw Hill, 2000.
13. Weber SM, Grundfast KM. Modern management of otitis media. *Pediatr Clin North Am* 2003;50(2):399–411.

NOSEBLEED

Gregory H. Gilbert, MD

Scope of the problem

Nosebleeds (epistaxis) are frequently encountered in the emergency department (ED). There is typically a bimodal distribution, with patients commonly 2–10 or 50–80 years of age. Although a relatively small percentage (6–10%) of patients actually seek medical attention, epistaxis affects one out of every seven persons in their lifetime, or 5–15% of the population per year. Though death does occur, it is rare. Surprisingly, one study showed that only a third of emergency personnel in one ED were familiar with basic first aid for epistaxis.

Anatomic essentials

Management of epistaxis requires a basic understanding of the nasal blood supply (Figure 19.10). The nasal circulation is derived from branches of the internal and external carotid arteries. The vascular nature of the nose is essential for its incredible heating and humidification requirements. To further facilitate this function, the vasculature runs just under the mucosa (not the squamous layer), leaving vessels more exposed and at risk for damage. These vessels spread out within this mucosal layer to form an anastomotic meshwork, artificially divided into anterior and posterior segments.

Anterior epistaxis originates from the anterior network of vessels, located in the fleshy part of the nose called Little's area or Kiesselbach's plexus. This collection of vessels is supplied by the anterior ethmoidal, greater palatine, septal branch of the superior labial, and sphenopalatine arteries. Ninety percent of nosebleeds originate from this part of the nose. Examining the nasal septum typically reveals the source in anterior nosebleeds.

Posterior epistaxis occurs in 10% of nosebleeds. Posterior hemorrhage may not be directly visualized, and can be difficult to treat since it occurs in a noncompressible part of the nose. A network of vessels called Woodruff's plexus supplied by the sphenopalatine, posterior ethmoidal and nasopalatine arteries is the most common site of posterior venous bleeds. In the event of an arterial bleed, it is most likely from the sphenopalatine artery. Table 19.5 provides a summary of information about anterior and posterior epistaxis.

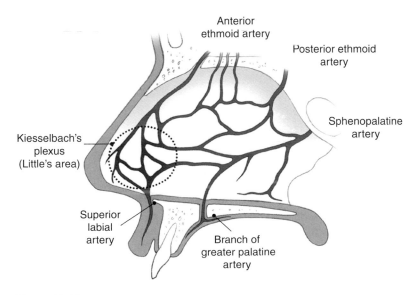

Figure 19.10
Blood supply of the nasal septum.

Table 19.5 Summary of historical and examination distinctions between anterior and posterior epistaxis

	Anterior	Posterior
History	• Presence of an inciting event • Recent use of agents that promote vasoconstriction of the nasal mucosa • Insertion of a foreign body • Recent cold, flu or allergies • Pediatric age group • Unilateral	• Blood flowing down back of throat • Started in both nares • Seen more frequently in the elderly population • Tends to be more severe • Patient unable to control • History of angiofibroma in young males • Squamous cell carcinoma in Asians
Physical examination	• Site of bleeding directly visualized • Bleeding from one nostril • Foreign body identified	• Cannot identify anterior site of bleeding • Bleeding from both nares • Blood continues to trickle down throat despite adequate anterior pack

History

Management of the airway, breathing and circulation (ABCs) and hemorrhage control take precedence over obtaining a complete history. The following information should be obtained once the ABCs are secured and the bleeding is controlled.

How did this begin?

Attempt to determine what precipitated the epistaxis. Was it traumatic or spontaneous? The most common causes of epistaxis include epistaxis digitorum (nose picking), foreign bodies (FBs), and dry air and upper respiratory infection (URI) during the winter months. Think of nasal FBs in children, institutionalized elderly and patients with developmental delay. Consult ear, nose and throat (ENT) early if there has been recent nasal surgery. Traumatic epistaxis may be associated with other serious facial injuries.

Which side did it begin on?

Bleeding from one naris suggests an anterior nosebleed, while bleeding from both sides usually represents a posterior source. However, blood from a brisk anterior nosebleed can reflux into the unaffected side via the posterior choanae, simulating posterior epistaxis.

How severe has it been?

Details regarding the amount of bleeding can be helpful to determine the amount of blood loss that has occurred. This is frequently embellished. Much more accurate predictors of blood loss are the patient's vital signs, symptoms, and physical signs.

How did you attempt to stop the bleeding?

Direct pressure, Afrin or pledgets are common things patients try before coming to the ED. Epistaxis that persists despite these efforts is generally more difficult to treat.

Have you ever had this before?

Nosebleeds that recur should raise concern for intranasal pathology, such as a deviated septum and primary or secondary tumors. This warrants ENT referral and should trigger questions about easy bruising or bleeding, which may suggest coagulopathy. Intranasal pathology predisposes the patient to nosebleeds because of friable vessels and/or engorgement. This is also seen in patients with hypertension, congestive heart failure (CHF), pregnancy or frequent sneezing. Ask the patient about recent ED visits for bleeding and how the bleeding was treated.

Have you been coughing up or vomiting blood?

Massive epistaxis may be initially confused with hemoptysis or hematemesis. In cases of epistaxis without blood clearly dripping from the nose, identification of bleeding from the posterior nasopharynx confirms the diagnosis.

Past medical

It is important to ask about underlying medical conditions such as bleeding disorders or blood dyscrasias (hemophilia, von Willebrand's disease, Osler–Weber–Rendu disease or thrombocytopenia). Ask about easy bruising or bleeding, human immunodeficiency virus (HIV), liver or kidney disease and cancer, as these patients may have drug use, thrombocytopenia, platelet disorders or splenomegaly predisposing them to bleeding.

Past surgical

Has the patient had prior nasal surgery?

Medications

It is important to ask about medications that could make bleeding more likely or treatment more difficult. These include platelet inhibitors like aspirin, dipyridamole and non-steroidal anti-inflammatory drugs (NSAIDs), or anticoagulants like warfarin and heparin. The social history should include questions about alcohol abuse or cocaine insufflation, as both may contribute to or exacerbate bleeding.

Physical examination

A quick look at the patient should make it obvious whether the patient is stable or ill. A focused physical examination should look at the following items.

General appearance and skin

A pale, diaphoretic appearance is an ominous sign. The patient has either lost a large amount of blood, or does not like the sight of it. In either case, placing the patient supine on a gurney will prevent serious injury should the patient lose consciousness. Ecchymosis, petechiae and spider angiomas suggest underlying bleeding disorders. Delayed capillary refill suggests significant blood loss.

Vital signs

It is important to check the blood pressure and pulse rate. Abnormalities suggesting significant blood loss include hypotension, tachycardia or symptomatic blood pressure changes from supine to standing, and should prompt establishment of intravenous (IV) access and administration of fluid. Blood should be drawn for laboratory studies in this situation. Although hypertension has never been shown to cause epistaxis, it can worsen bleeding when present.

Head, eyes, ears, nose and throat

A complete head, eye, ear, nose and throat (HEENT) examination should be performed in all patients with epistaxis. Signs of basilar skull fracture (raccoon eyes, Battle's sign, hemotympanum or cerebrospinal fluid (CSF) rhinorrhea) can complicate therapy, as devices introduced through the nares (i.e., intranasal balloon device) are at risk for perforating the cribriform plate and entering the cranium. Assess for tenderness and stability of the maxilla and other facial bones to help identify Le Fort or orbital wall fractures.

Nose

The key to successful examination of the nose is preparation. Prior to the nasal examination, assemble the proper items for examination, stabilization and treatment (Table 19.6).

First, have the patient blow his nose to clear the nasopharynx, even if the bleeding has stopped. A thorough nasal examination should then be performed. A nasal speculum assists with this task (Figure 19.11). Attempt to locate the source of bleeding. Ninety percent of nosebleeds have a visible source, and careful examination of the nasal septum will reveal a friable vessel. If trauma was the cause, it is important to examine the nasal

Table 19.6 Suggested equipment for the evaluation and treatment of epistaxis

Examination	Stabilization	Treatment
Protective eyewear	Bayonet forceps	Silver nitrate sticks
Two gowns	Pledgets	Electrocautery
Nasal speculum	4% topical cocaine *or*	Gelfoam
ENT headlamp or mirror	1% lidocaine with	Bacitracin
Yankauer and Frazier-tip suction	epinephrine *and*	1/2″ × 6″ petroleum gauze
Emesis basin	4% topical lidocaine	16 fr. Foley or intranasal balloon
Balloon	Afrin spray	Rhino rocket or Merocel sponge
Kleenex or gauze		

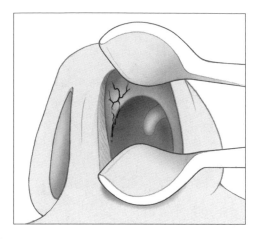

Figure 19.11
Use of a nasal speculum to examine the nose.

septum to exclude septal hematoma, and the facial bones to exclude fracture. An untreated septal hematoma can lead to an abscess or avascular necrosis of the septum. If the bleeding source is not visible on nasal examination, it may be from the posterior circulation. Other findings consistent with posterior epistaxis include bleeding from both nares and hemorrhage into the posterior pharynx. Controlling bleeding in these patients may be extremely difficult. Consider confounding factors like coagulopathy if bleeding persists despite direct pressure, cautery and nasal packing. Consultation with ENT and/or hematology may be necessary in these patients. Nasal examination should look for nasal pathology, such as FBs, perforated or deviated septum, nasal masses or engorged vessels.

Differential diagnosis

Table 19.7 provides several etiologies of epistaxis.

Table 19.7 Etiologies of epistaxis

Traumatic or mechanical
- Epistaxis digitorum (nose picking)
- Congenital or acquired nasal defects
- Direct blow (with or without fracture)
- FB (demented, psychiatric, intentional, children)
- Desiccation (low humidity household, winter, supplemental oxygen)
- Infections/inflammation (allergic or atrophic rhinitis, URI, diphtheria, sinusitis, nasopharyngitis, nasopharyngeal mucormycosis, chlamydial rhinitis neonatorum)
- Local irritants (cocaine abuse, chemical/environmental irritants, OTC nasal sprays)
- Iatrogenic (nasal surgery, NG tube, nasopharyngeal airway, septal perforation, cautery)
- Barotrauma (abrupt changes in pressure – diving or rapid altitude gain)
- Venous congestion (CHF, mitral stenosis, sneezing, coughing, nose blowing, Valsalva, pregnancy)

Tumors (benign or malignant)
- Primary (nasal polyps, juvenile angiofibroma, squamous cell, paranasal sinus tumors, metastatic)
- Secondary (thrombocytopenia due to leukemia, lymphoma or chemotherapy)

Predisposing factors
- Systemic toxins (rodenticide, plant poisoning, glycosides, coumarin, heavy metals)
- Medications (salicylates, NSAIDs, warfarin, heparin, dipyridamole, ticlopidine, thrombolytics)
- Congenital (hemophilia A and B, von Willebrand's disease, inherited platelet disorders)
- Hereditary hemorrhagic telangiectasia (Osler–Weber–Rendu syndrome)

Disease-mediated
- Hypertension and atherosclerotic cardiovascular disease
- Blood dyscrasias (ITP, polycythemia vera, granulocytosis)
- Thrombocytopenia (drug-induced, chemotherapy, ITP, malignancy)
- Vitamin deficiency (scurvy, folic acid, vitamin K)
- Hepatic disease (alcoholism, hepatitis)
- Renal disease (chronic nephritis, uremia, diabetes mellitus)
- Disseminated intravascular coagulation, hypoprothrombinemia, hypofibrinogenemia

Other
- Idiopathic (habitual, familial)
- Migraine headache
- Internal carotid artery aneurysm
- Blood transfusion reactions
- Endometriosis

CHF: congestive heart failure; FB: foreign body; ITP: idiopathic thrombocytopenic purpura; NG: nasogastric; NSAIDs: non-steroidal anti-inflammatory drugs; OTC: over-the-counter.

Diagnostic testing

Laboratory studies

Laboratory studies are not necessary in most cases of epistaxis.

Complete blood count

If there has been a significant amount of blood loss, easy bruising, recurrent epistaxis, history of platelet disorder, cancer or recent chemotherapy, a CBC should be checked. If the blood loss was significant enough to order a CBC, then a *type and screen* should also be ordered.

Partial thromboplastin, Partial thromboplastin time, International Normalized Ratio

These tests are helpful in anticoagulated patients. They may also be helpful in patients with liver disease.

Bleeding time

This test determines if the patient is able to clot normally. An abnormal bleeding time can occur even if the International Normalized Ratio (INR) is normal and could help explain difficulties controlling epistaxis.

Radiologic studies

In the patient with significant facial trauma, computerized tomography (CT) of the facial bones is best to assess the types of fractures present.

General treatment principles

As stated earlier, the ABCs are the first priority. If the bleeding is so severe that the airway and breathing are compromised, intubation should occur along with placement of an epistaxis balloon. While the majority of nosebleeds are stable, patients with significant blood loss need to be placed on a gurney. An attempt to expel all clots from the nose should be performed first, because fibrinolysis of the existing clot can lead to continued bleeding. This will also enable the clinician to see the amount of blood and from which nostril the bleeding is occurring.

Direct pressure

Direct pressure is the first step in controlling epistaxis. With the patient seated, assuming he can tolerate it, tilt the head slightly forward in the sniffing position. The fleshy part of the nose is squeezed between the thumb and a flexed index finger (Figure 19.12). It should look like the patient's nose is in a fist. Have the patient hold pressure for 10–15 minutes. During this time, gather the supplies mentioned previously (Table 19.6) and gown the patient. Dress in appropriate attire, adhering to universal precautions. This includes a gown, eyewear, possibly a facemask or shield, and gloves. A headlamp will help with visualization, and a basin should be placed below the patient's chin. Set up a suction device with a Yankauer or Frazier tip.

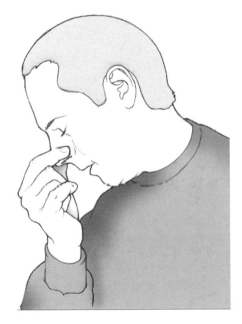

Figure 19.12
Direct pressure.

If bleeding persists after withdrawing direct pressure, the use of pledgets or sprays may arrest the bleeding. The pledget should first be soaked in a lidocaine with epinephrine solution or cocaine and then inserted into the nasal passage (Table 19.8). Be sure to reapply direct pressure. The use of vasoconstrictive agents without an anesthetic is inadequate, as interventions to halt the bleeding will irritate the exquisitely sensitive nasal mucosa. Though phenylephrine spray may also be used, pledgets allow the nasal mucosa to

Table 19.8 Vasoconstrictive and anesthetic agents used for epistaxis

- Afrin or neosynephrine mixed with 4% lidocaine (lidocaine's toxic dose is 4 mg/kg)
- Epinephrine 0.25 ml of 1 : 1000 concentration mixed with 20 ml of 4% lidocaine
- Cocaine (4%) (do not exceed 2–3 mg/kg in adults)

Note: 4% is equal to 40 mg/ml.

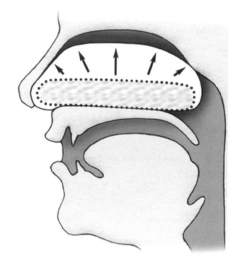

Figure 19.13
Merocel (nasal) tampons.

absorb more agent than spraying alone. Heavy bleeding that persists after three attempts with direct pressure and pledget insertion requires nasal packing. However, if bleeding has slowed to an ooze or stopped, proceed with inspection of the nasal cavity. The effects of these agents are temporary, so bleeding is likely to recur. Using the nasal speculum, headlamp and suction device, evacuate clots and attempt to identify a bleeding source.

Cautery

Silver nitrate sticks can be used for cautery if there is no active bleeding. They are applied to the vessel or friable mucosa for up to 20 seconds. Cauterize in a rolling motion peripherally to centrally and superior to inferior to avoid rendering the stick ineffective with blood. Beware of causing septal perforation with prolonged or overzealous use. Septal necrosis and perforation can also occur with multiple applications to both sides of the septum, so use great care. Cautery has little value in trauma patients, nor should it be attempted if the cause of epistaxis is thought to be cancerous. Persistent bleeding can be treated with Gelfoam or a similar thrombogenic substance. Thermal or electrocautery is extremely difficult and fraught with iatrogenic injury; these modalities are best left to the ENT specialist.

Packing

Anterior

Packing is the next step. Traditionally this was done with Vaseline gauze and forceps. The packing was placed along the floor of the nasal cavity, front to back, back to front, until the entire cavity was filled. This is a difficult, time-consuming process, but when done correctly provides excellent hemostasis. More commonly used devices include nasal tampons (Figure 19.13) or intranasal balloons. Tampons are typically lubricated with

antibacterial ointment prior to insertion. Upon contact with fluid, the tampon expands. One technique uses phenylephrine spray to induce tampon expansion by spraying it on either side. Intranasal balloon catheters should be inserted with water-based lubricants. Petroleum products can cause degradation of the balloon and possible rupture. There are two types of balloons: anterior and anterior/posterior. Tamponade should begin with the anterior balloon since placement of the anterior/posterior balloon usually requires hospital admission. Following packing, the oropharynx is visualized and inspected for further bleeding. Its presence implies either inadequate anterior packing or a posterior source.

Posterior

If these methods fail and bleeding persists, the source of bleeding is likely posterior. Traditionally a posterior pack was performed with silk sutures attached to rolled gauze. This was drawn up through the mouth into the posterior pharynx. Then bilateral anterior packs were placed. Quicker, more comfortable methods have been developed. Treatment can be done with either a 12–16 French Foley catheter with a 30-ml balloon (the distal tip should be cut off for patient comfort) or the anterior/posterior nasal balloon (Figure 19.14). Both are inserted through the naris into the posterior nasal cavity. The balloon is filled with saline and checked prior to insertion for integrity. Following placement, it is pulled into the posterior choana. Care should be taken not to overfill the balloon,

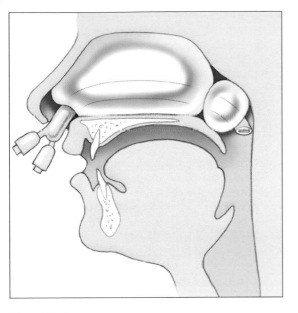

Figure 19.14
Anterior/posterior nasal balloon.

as pressure necrosis or septal damage may occur. This should stop bleeding from the posterior pharynx. Once this has occurred, the anterior balloon may be filled with fluid or an anterior pack placed using one of the above-mentioned methods. Posterior packs may induce suppression of the respiratory drive and hypoxia. Due to the considerable morbidity and mortality associated with posterior packs, ENT consultation and admission are recommended. Patients receiving any nasal packing are at significant risk for sinusitis and possibly toxic shock syndrome. For this reason, antibiotics should be prescribed for all posterior packs and significant anterior packs. (Table 19.9). Furthermore, appropriate analgesia should be considered for posterior packs, as these are often very painful for patients.

Special patients
Elderly

Geriatric patients tend to have multiple medical problems; careful review of the patient's medical history and medications may reveal the cause of the epistaxis. Liver or renal disease, CHF, hypertension, cancer, other coagulopathies, or the use of warfarin or aspirin may play a role in the patient's epistaxis and make it difficult to control.

Pediatric

Most pediatric patients require only direct pressure to control the bleeding. If packing is required, ENT consultation is recommended, as pediatric patients tend to be uncooperative and may need sedation in the operating room. It is especially important to consider the possibility of nasal FB as the cause of bleeding in this population.

Immune compromised

Universal precautions are extremely important in this situation since the clinician is dealing with blood. Patients with HIV may have thrombocytopenia, platelet disorders, splenomegaly or drug use predisposing them to bleeding.

Disposition
Ear, nose and throat consultation

Five to ten percent of ED cases of epistaxis require ENT consultation or admission, particularly if the clinician is unable to control the bleeding. Patients with a posterior packing often need to be admitted to ENT due to increased morbidity and mortality. Pediatric patients who are uncooperative also require ENT consultation.

Table 19.9 Prophylactic antibiotic options for epistaxis with packing

Antibiotic 5-day course	Adult dose	Pediatric dose
First-line		
Cephalexin	250–500 mg PO QID	25–50 mg/kg PO QID; max: 4 g/day
Augmentin	500–875 mg PO BID	15–20 mg/kg PO BID; max: 1.8 g/day
Penicillin-allergy		
Clindamycin	150–450 mg PO QID	3–10 mg/kg PO TID; max: 1.8 g/day
Bactrim DS	1 tablet PO BID	>2 months: 0.5 ml susp/kg PO BID (max 20 ml susp)

BID: twice a day; DS: double strength; max: maximum; PO: per os; QID: four times a day; susp: suspension; TID: three times a day.

Discharge

The majority of patients presenting with epistaxis will be discharged. All patients presenting to the ED with epistaxis need ENT referral for evaluation of possible intranasal pathology. Patients with high risk (posterior or significant anterior) nasal packing need to be placed on antibiotics to prevent sinusitis and reduce the risk of toxic shock syndrome. They require follow-up with ENT in 48–72 hours for removal of the packing and further evaluation of the nasal mucosa. If bleeding recurs prior to the ENT evaluation, the patient should attempt direct pressure two or three times for 10–15 minutes. Patients with bleeding around nasal packing should return to the ED. In dry, cold months, patients without packing may benefit from saline spray, humidifiers and petroleum jelly applied intranasally once or twice a day. Patients should be instructed to avoid blowing or picking their nose, straining or participating in strenuous activities. They should sneeze with their mouths open. Patients should avoid aspirin and NSAIDs for 3–4 days.

Educating patients about prevention and management of recurrences reduces morbidity, mortality and prevents unnecessary future visits.

Pearls, pitfalls, and myths

- Direct pressure should be firmly held over the fleshy part of the nose, not the bridge, for at least 10–15 minutes.
- Ice on the bridge of a nose or in the mouth may help slow bleeding.
- Assuming the patient can tolerate sitting, the head should be above the heart and in the sniffing position, *not* tipped back, which allows blood to run down the back of the throat.
- Preparation is key to the successful treatment of epistaxis.
- Consider FB in young children presenting with epistaxis.

- Do not waste time doing an anterior pack if a posterior source is suspected.
- Record the amount of fluid used to fill both the anterior and posterior intranasal balloons.
- Consider admitting all patients with posterior packing. They may become hypoxic and hypercarbic due to hypoventilation and thus have increased mortality. They also can get bradycardic or develop dysrhythmias or coronary ischemia.
- Improper packing can lead to pressure necrosis of the columella or nasal ala.
- Patients who start bleeding around anterior packing need to be reevaluated, repacked, or have ENT consultation.
- Patients with high risk nasal packing should be started on antibiotics, due to an increased risk for sinusitis and toxic shock syndrome.

References

1. Hamilton GC (ed.). *Emergency Medicine: An Approach to Clinical Problem-Solving*, 2nd ed., Philadelphia: WB Saunders, 2001.
2. Harwood-Nuss A (ed.). *The Clinical Practice of Emergency Medicine*, 3rd ed., Philadelphia: Lippincott Williams & Wilkins, 2001.
3. Marx JA (ed.). *Rosen's Emergency Medicine: Concepts and Clinical Practice*, 5th ed., St. Louis: Mosby, 2002.
4. McGarry GW, Moulton C. The first aid management of epistaxis by accident and emergency department staff. *Arch Emerg Med* 1993;10(4):298–300.
5. Tintinalli JE (ed.). *Emergency Medicine: A Comprehensive Study Guide*, 5th ed., McGraw Hill, 2000.
6. Wild DC, Spraggs PD. Treatment of epistaxis in accident and emergency departments in the UK. *J Laryngol Otol* 2002;116(8):597–600.

THROAT PAIN

Michelle Huston, MD

Scope of the problem

Throat pain is the third most common complaint seen by all healthcare providers. Pharyngitis is by far the most common cause of throat pain. The etiologies, work-up and treatment of tonsillitis and pharyngitis are identical, so it is common to refer to both as pharyngitis. Viruses are the most common cause of pharyngitis, accounting for 40% of cases. Group A beta-hemolytic streptococcus (GABHS) accounts for up to 40% of pediatric cases, but less than 15% of adult cases of pharyngitis.

Although most patients presenting with sore throat have a mild, self-limiting illness, throat pain may be the hallmark of life-threatening illness. Recognizing and treating both common and serious causes of sore throat is an essential skill for emergency providers.

Anatomic essentials

The throat or pharynx is divided into three areas extending from the base of the skull to the inlet of the esophagus (Figures 19.15a and b): the nasopharynx (soft palate and posterior nasal cavity), oropharynx (posterior to the mouth down to the upper edge of the epiglottis) and hypopharynx (between the epiglottis and the cricoid cartilage). Sore throat may be caused by a disorder affecting any of these areas, as well as processes affecting the ears, tongue, esophagus and upper thorax. Throat pain is commonly associated with ear pain because cranial nerves IX and X provide sensory innervation to the pharynx and larynx as well as the ear.

Deep space infections of the lower face and neck may cause sore throat. A polymicrobial cellulitis of the submandibular spaces of the head and neck causes Ludwig's angina. There are seven spaces in the neck which may also become infected: the peritonsillar, parapharyngeal, retropharyngeal, prevertebral, pretracheal, carotid, and danger (lying between the prevertebral and retropharyngeal spaces). The supraglottic structures become infected in epiglottitis.

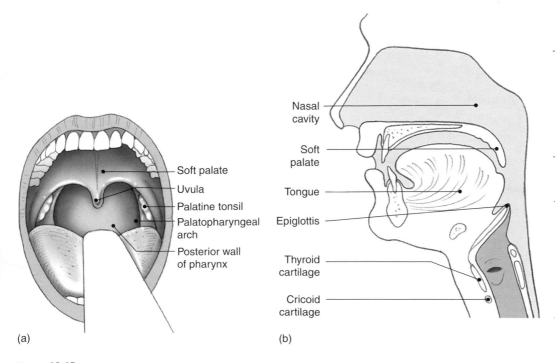

Figure 19.15
(a) Anatomy of the pharynx and (b) sagittal anatomy.

History

Life-threatening illnesses should be ruled out in all cases of sore throat. These include deep space infections, epiglottitis, foreign bodies (FBs), laryngeal trauma and burns. All of these entities may cause sudden airway obstruction with asphyxia. Additionally, deep space infections may lead to carotid artery and jugular vein thrombosis and hemorrhage, mediastinitis, pericarditis, empyema and sepsis.

Where is the pain located?

Lateralization of symptoms is suggestive of peritonsillitis, a cellulitis or abscess of the peritonsillar space. Patients with retained FBs are often able to describe the exact location of the pain.

How long has the pain been present?

If the pain has been present less than 72 hours, it is unlikely that a deep space infection is present. A sore throat of greater than 2 weeks duration in a patient over the age of 40 years should be considered cancer until proven otherwise.

How did the symptoms begin?

Sudden onset of pain during eating suggests a FB. The presence of a FB can be easily missed in children and those with mental illness or swallowing dysfunction if these patients and their companions are not carefully questioned. Similarly, trauma is not always mentioned without the examiner specifically asking.

Have you had the pain before?

Many patients with GABHS pharyngitis have experienced their symptoms with previous episodes.

Describe the character of the pain (quality and severity)

Throat pain ranges from a sensation of scratchiness to severe pain. The gradual onset of a scratchy sensation evolving into pain is consistent with a viral infection.

Any close contacts with similar symptoms?

A positive answer to this question supports either a viral or bacterial source of infection.

Are there any measures that make the discomfort worse or better?

Pain with swallowing (odynophagia), especially hot or acidic fluids, is seen with many causes of throat pain, including pharyngitis and cancer.

Associated symptoms

Potential airway obstruction

Ask about swallowing function, drooling, voice change, trouble breathing and apprehension. Dysphagia (difficulty swallowing) and the inability to swallow must be distinguished from odynophagia, which is present in almost all patients with sore throat. Drooling may represent the inability to swallow. Voice changes may range from mild hoarseness to a muffled voice to complete aphonia. A muffled or "hot potato" voice is often heard with deep space neck infections, epiglottitis, FB and trauma, as well as severe pharyngitis. Dyspnea, tachypnea, "noisy breathing" and apprehension are often reported by patients with impending airway obstruction.

Trismus

Limitation of mouth opening is caused by inflammation of the muscles of mastication. Conditions that may cause trismus include some of the deep space infections of the neck and Ludwig's angina.

Fever

Fever is associated with both viral and bacterial pharyngitis, epiglottitis and deep space infections. Patients with bacterial infections, including those with epiglottitis, typically have high fevers.

Upper respiratory infection

Examples of upper respiratory infection (URI) are rhinorrhea, nasal congestion, cough and coryza. The combination of these symptoms and sore throat is most commonly associated with viral infections.

Ear pain (otalgia)

Pain radiating to the ears is common with pharyngitis and other causes of throat pain, but does not point to a specific etiology of sore throat.

Tooth pain (odontalgia)

Dental pathology and procedures may precede the development of a parapharyngeal abscess, Ludwig's angina or Vincent's angina.

Headache

Headache may be associated with GABHS pharyngitis. Although rare, the deep neck infections and GABHS pharyngitis may spread and cause mastoiditis, cavernous sinus thrombosis or meningitis, which are all serious etiologies of headache.

Neck pain

Posterior or lateral neck pain in the presence of sore throat should raise suspicion for deep space abscess and/or meningeal spread of infection. Anterior neck pain should raise suspicion for epiglottitis or laryngeal injury.

Abdominal pain

Abdominal pain may be associated with GABHS pharyngitis, particularly in children.

Rash

Scarlet fever, which is caused by GABHS, is diagnosed by the presence of a distinctive, diffuse sand-papery red rash. Gonococcal or meningococcal pharyngitis may lead to disseminated rashes.

Vaginal or penile discharge

Ask about a history of sexually transmitted illnesses (STIs) and orogenital sex in sexually active patients with sore throat. These patients are at risk for gonococcal and/or *Chlamydia trachomatis* pharyngitis.

Past medical

Pay special attention to systemic disorders (the immunocompromised host is at risk for opportunistic infections), medications, history of allergic reactions, tobacco and alcohol use (increased risk of cancer), and vaccination history. Ask about a prior history of "strep throat" diagnosed by laboratory measures, and any history of rheumatic fever or rheumatic heart disease. GABHS infection does tend to recur in these patients. Surgical history, particularly previous head or neck surgery, recent intubation, gastric tube placement or recent dental procedure may predispose to retropharyngeal abscess or laryngeal

trauma. Be aware that many patients have already started antibiotics which may mask the clinical picture. Diptheria is now most commonly seen in adults who lack immunization and previous exposure to the bacteria. *H. influenzae* is a rare cause of epiglottitis since the initiation of vaccination programs in 1990.

Physical examination

Diagnosing the cause of sore throat depends on an accurate physical assessment of the oropharynx and, in some cases, the nasopharynx and hypopharynx. The physical examination should focus on the anatomic location of any lesions and potential complications, especially airway obstruction and systemic disease.

General appearance

Assess for "toxicity", a general impression of how ill the patient appears. A patient who prefers to be sitting up or standing with the neck extended and the nose pointed toward the ceiling ("sniffing position") may be self-stenting their airway to avoid complete obstruction. General inspection during history taking may reveal voice alteration and difficulty swallowing with drooling. Other signs of toxicity which require immediate attention include stridor, cyanosis, dyspnea and tachypnea. *Stridor* is a loud, harsh respiratory sound that results from obstruction of the trachea or larynx. Stridor is usually heard during inspiration; in severe cases of obstruction, it may also be heard during expiration.

Vital signs

Fever and tachycardia are nonspecific signs, but demonstrate a systemic impact of the illness.

Oropharynx

Inspection

In cases of suspected epiglottitis (Figure 19.16) or retropharyngeal abscess, a complete examination of the oropharynx should be done cautiously or deferred until reaching the operating room (OR) due to the risk of precipitating airway occlusion. Be cautious in the examination of any patient assuming the sniffing position, in respiratory distress or with drooling. Inability to fully open the mouth may indicate trismus and limit the examination.

If the patient appears stable, examine the oral mucosa, hard and soft palates, oropharynx, tonsillar pillars and tonsils by holding the tongue down

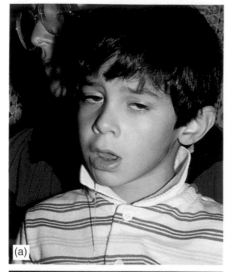

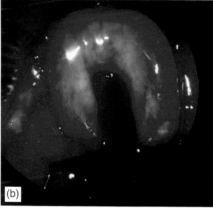

Figure 19.16
Epiglottitis. (a) This 5-year-old, who had been symptomatic for several hours, holds his neck extended with head held forward, is mouth-breathing and drooling, and shows signs of tiring (b) In the operating room, the epiglottis can be visualized and appears intensely red and swollen. It may retain its omega shape. Reprinted from Atlas of Pediatric Physical Diagnosis, 4th ed., Eds Zitelli BJ, Davis HW. Copyright 2002, with permission from Elsevier.

with a wooden blade. Look for erythema, exudates, pseudomembranes, swelling, petechiae (Figure 19.17), lesions (such as vesicles and ulcerations) and masses. A good light source is necessary. Local anesthetic sprays (e.g., Cetacaine) and having the patient assist by holding their own tongue down with a piece of gauze may allow a better examination in the patient with an overactive gag reflex. Having the patient say "ahhh" will also improve your view of the pharynx and tonsils by elevating the uvula and soft palate. Note the size, position and symmetry of the tonsils, looking especially at the degree of airway patency. Abnormal contours

and bulges in the oropharyngeal wall may indicate a deep tissue infection. The oropharyngeal examination in a patient with peritonsillitis typically demonstrates unilateral soft palate swelling anterior and superior to the affected swollen tonsil, with loss of the line between the anterior tonsillar pillar and tonsil (Figure 19.18). The uvula is typically deviated to the opposite side. Unilateral bulging of the posterior pharyngeal wall may be seen with a retropharyngeal abscess. Bulging of the lateral wall of the oropharynx may be seen with a parapharyngeal abscess.

Palpation

Palpation of swelling seen on the soft palate or pharyngeal walls is not recommended due to the potential for disrupting an abscess.

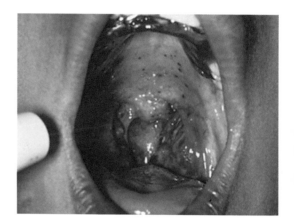

Figure 19.17
Palatal petechiae in a patient with group A beta-hemolytic streptococcal infection. Reprinted from Atlas of Pediatric Physical Diagnosis, 4th ed., Eds Zitelli BJ, Davis HW. Copyright 2002, with permission from Elsevier.

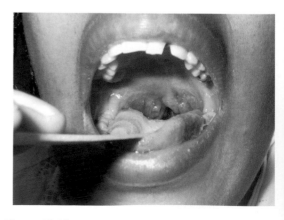

Figure 19.18
Right-sided peritonsillitis. *Courtesy*: S.V. Mahadeven, MD.

Additional head, eyes, ears, nose and neck

Palpate the neck for evidence of enlarged or tender lymph nodes and for evidence of tumor or abscess. Gently palpate the hyoid bone, laryngeal and tracheal cartilages, and the thyroid. To examine the nasopharynx, use a headlight and nasal speculum. Inspect, palpate and percuss the sinuses for evidence or sinusitis or masses. Inspect, palpate, and percuss the teeth and gums of any patient complaining of tooth pain. Prominent papillae on the tongue (strawberry tongue) may be seen with streptococcus infection. Examine the ears for otitis media (OM), as it may manifest as throat pain, and pharyngitis may lead to OM.

Skin

Inspect the skin carefully for rashes or ulcers. Children with GABHS pharyngitis may develop a fine, diffuse papular erythroderma ("sandpaper rash") on the trunk which is worse in the groin and axillae. This scarlatiniform rash in the presence of pharyngitis is virtually diagnostic of GABHS infection with associated scarlet fever.

Lungs and heart

An examination of the lungs and heart should be done in all patients with sore throat, listening for murmurs or asymmetric and irregular breath sounds.

Abdomen

Palpate for tenderness and organomegaly. Splenomegaly and hepatomegaly may be seen with Epstein–Barr virus (EBV) infection. Abdominal tenderness with pharyngitis raises the concern for splenic rupture in this setting.

Special signs/techniques

Unilateral enlargement of the pharynx or tonsil is associated with peritonsillitis, and less commonly neoplasms, vascular lesions and abscesses. *Exudates* are usually white or yellow spots on the tonsils (Figure 19.19). *Pseudomembranes* are usually gray-blue and tightly adherent to the posterior pharyngeal mucosa. When removed, a bleeding surface may be revealed.

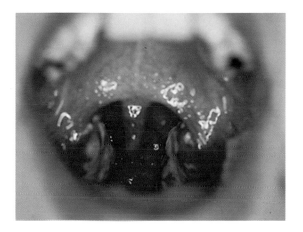

Figure 19.19
Exudative tonsillitis. Reprinted from Atlas of Pediatric Physical Diagnosis, 4th ed., Eds Zitelli BJ, Davis HW. Copyright 2002, with permission from Elsevier.

Differential diagnosis

Table 19.10 provides a comprehensive list of causes of throat pain.

Table 19.10 Differential diagnosis of throat pain

Diagnosis	Symptoms	Signs	Work-up
Agranulocytosis	Sore throat; fever, malaise, nausea, vomiting; bleeding tendency.	Rough-edged ulcers with gray-black membranes on gums, palate and possibly perianal area.	CBC with differential showing low granulocytes; confirmatory bone marrow biopsy.
Associated with flu-like illness (adenovirus, common cold and influenza)	Occur in epidemics; "scratchy" sore throat; absent or low-grade fever, cough, rhinorrhea, sneezing, myalgia and headache.	Mild or absent erythema and edema of pharynx with normal tonsils; adenovirus may mimic GABHS; unilateral conjunctivitis, viral enanthemas and stomatitis associated with adenovirus.	Clinical diagnosis; point-of-care testing available for influenza.

(*continued*)

Table 19.10 Differential diagnosis of throat pain (*cont*)

Diagnosis	Symptoms	Signs	Work-up
Associated with infectious mononucleosus-like illness (EBV, CMV and primary infection with HIV type 1)	Mainly affects 15- to 30-year age group; immuno-compromised children at higher risk; often close contacts with same; risk factors seen with HIV; fluctuating fevers, malaise, anorexia, headache, myalgias and sore throat lasting weeks.	EBV can lead to severely swollen tonsils with exudates and (rarely) airway obstruction; cervical adenopathy in 90% cases; painless splenomegaly and hepatomegaly in 50% EBV cases.	Heterophil antibody test for EBV ("monospot"); other adjunctive tests for EBV include peripheral blood smear, CBC and EBV antigen tests. HIV PCR testing.
Associated with stomatitis (coxsackie and herpes infections)	Affects mainly toddler and school age children; HSV-2 pharyngitis mainly affects young adults; fever precedes oral lesions.	Vesicles and/or ulcers on posterior pharynx with herpangina; on pharynx, lips, tongue and buccal mucosa with HSV gingivostomatitis, and throughout oral cavity and on hands, feet, buttocks with HFM disease. Pharyngeal exudates and tender adenopathy with HSV-2 pharyngitis.	Clinical diagnosis for herpangina and HFM disease (coxsackie viruses) and gingivostomatitis (HSV-1); viral throat culture and cytopathologic scrapings of lesions for HSV-2 pharyngitis.
Bacterial pharyngitis	Fever; odynophagia and dysphagia; associated headache, abdominal pain, nausea and vomiting (especially children with GABHS); dysuria, genital discharge, rash and arthralgias may be reported with disseminated gonorrhea.	Fever typically greater than 38.3°C; exudates, tonsillar swelling, palatal petechiae; tender cervical adenopathy (severe with diptheria); pseudomembrane with diptheria and *A. hemolyticum*. Stridor, myocarditis and neuropathy may be seen with diptheria; scarlatiniform rash may be seen with GABHS.	Controversy surrounding the work-up for GABHS: RAT and throat culture (if RAT negative) versus clinical diagnosis. Laboratory needs notification when diptheria, *A. hemolyticum*, gonorrhea or *C. trachomatis* suspected. Genital cultures or urine probes for suspected gonorrhea or *C. trachomatis*.
Bacterial tracheitis	Similar to epiglottitis except longer viral prodrome; often initially mistaken for croup.	High fever and toxic-appearance; similar to epiglottitis.	Lateral neck radiograph useful for excluding epiglottitis; laryngoscopy is gold standard.
Burns (chemical and thermal)	Hot or caustic liquid exposure by ingestion or inhalation; symptoms may take up to 5 hours to develop; some combination of throat pain, dysphagia, odynophagia, chest, back or abdominal pain, vomiting, hematemesis and respiratory complaints present; injury from hot liquids may cause epiglottitis.	Findings variable; possible mucosal and tongue erythema, swelling and ulceration; may have signs of upper airway obstruction (stridor, drooling, muffled voice); absence of oropharyngeal lesions does not exclude tracheal, esophageal or gastric injury.	Neck and chest radiographs may demonstrate positive findings; laryngoscopy useful.
Candidal pharyngitis	*Risk factors*: immunocompromise, pregnancy, infancy, decreased salivary flow, dentures; burning sore throat, dysphagia, odynophagia.	Pharyngeal erythema and edema; white plaques when scraped off reveal superficial erythematous ulcer.	Clinical diagnosis; yeast seen on KOH preparation of throat swabs.

(*continued*)

Table 19.10 Differential diagnosis of throat pain (*cont*)

Diagnosis	Symptoms	Signs	Work-up
Cancer (laryngeal, tongue, tonsil and soft palate)	Heavy tobacco with or without alcohol. Persistent (>2 weeks) throat pain, hoarseness, dysphagia, cough and/or dyspnea; may have sensation of "lump in throat".	Normal pharyngeal examination; *tongue cancer*: raised white lesion or ulcer usually on posterolateral border of tongue; *tonsil* and *soft palate cancer*: superficial ulcer which may contain impacted food debris.	Urgent referral to ENT for biopsy.
Croup (parainfluenza virus, influenza virus and RSV)	Affects infants and toddlers peaks in spring and fall; barking cough worse at night; often 2–3 days common cold prodrome.	Inspiratory stridor; hoarseness; expiratory rhonchi; no dysphagia or drooling.	Clinical diagnosis; lateral neck radiograph; not necessary, but may see "steeple sign".
Epiglottitis	Most common in African Americans, males and smokers. Classically rapid onset severe sore throat, odynophagia and dysphagia; may have 1–2 day prodrome of cold symptoms; atypical presentations increasingly reported.	Classically toxic-appearing with high fever, stridor, tongue protrusion, muffled voice and assuming the "sniffing" or "tripod" position; may be more subtle with absence of fever (up to 50%) and pain out of proportion to examination; often coexisting pharyngitis. Tenderness to palpation of anterior neck over hyoid and with moving larynx or upper trachea is a reliable finding.	Lateral neck radiograph shows "thumbprint" sign; gold standard is laryngoscopy; blood cultures positive in 80–90% bacterial cases.
Foreign body	Peanuts and popcorn in children; dentures, meat and bones in adults. Choking episode, dyspnea, throat pain, dysphagia, chest pain, vomiting and unexplained cough; pain may persist after FB dislodged.	May cause high-pitched inspiratory stridor, barking cough, focal wheezing, dysphonia and drooling; FB may be seen lodged near tonsil on oropharyngeal examination.	Plain radiographs only helpful if FB radiopaque; fiberoptic scope examination frequently reveals FB or abrasion in lingual or palatine tonsils or pyriform sinus.
Laryngeal trauma	Rare, but many cases unrecognized; occurs after motor vehicle crashes, assaults and sports injuries; may be asymptomatic initially; earliest symptom may be subtle voice change; *Other:* throat pain, dysphagia dyspnea, cough, hemoptysis.	May see swelling, bruising, seatbelt mark, laryngeal/tracheal tenderness and crepitus; signs often absent.	Plain neck and chest radiographs may show air in soft tissues; CT will demonstrate fractures and dislocations; indirect laryngoscopy also useful.
Laryngitis	Mild sore throat; hoarseness predominant; viral URI symptoms.	Hoarseness; otherwise normal oropharyngeal examination.	Clinical diagnosis.
Lingual tonsillitis	Rare, but seen in patients without palatine tonsils; may be acute or chronic; may cause sleep apnea; throat pain (above hyoid bone) worse with tongue motion; sensation of throat swelling; dysphagia.	May have muffled voice; Normal-appearing pharynx; Cervical adenopathy.	Indirect laryngoscopy.

(continued)

Table 19.10 Differential diagnosis of throat pain (*cont*)

Diagnosis	Symptoms	Signs	Work-up
Ludwig's angina	Usually preceded by dental procedure or infection; ≥48 hours of symptoms: progressive throat pain, odynophagia, dysphagia, anterior neck pain and swelling, alteration in voice, drooling and halitosis.	Usually toxic-appearing with high fever and dehydration; lymphadenopathy; stridor if severe; bilateral submandibular swelling ("bull neck") with marked tenderness (may have "woodiness" or crepitus on palpation; elevation of floor of mouth with tongue protrusion.	Lateral neck radiograph shows swelling of submandibular tissues; CT scan of the face and neck with IV contrast for confirmation and surgical planning.
Parapharyngeal abscess	Rare; spread from dental infection (30%); ≥48 hours of symptoms: fever, lateral neck pain and swelling.	Usually toxic-appearing with fever and dehydration; lymphadenopathy; examination may be limited by trismus; stridor when supine if severe; lateral neck swelling and mass below angle of mandible.	Lateral neck radiograph of limited use; CT of neck and mediastinum with IV contrast for confirmation and surgical planning.
Peritonsillitis (peritonsillar abscess)	Most common deep space infection; adolescents and young adults; increased risk in diabetes, immunocompromise; preceded by pharyngitis, ≥48 hours of symptoms often despite antibiotics; fever, progressive throat pain, odynophagia, dysphagia, alteration in voice, drooling and halitosis.	Toxic-appearing with high fever and dehydration; lymphadenopathy; trismus may limit examination in severe cases; stridor in supine position if severe; unilateral swelling anterior and superior to tonsil with loss of line between anterior tonsillar pillar. Tonsil and uvula deviation to contralateral side.	Clinical diagnosis confirmed by needle aspiration; aspirated pus sent for gram stain and culture; if diagnosis suspected and needle aspiration negative CT with IV contrast or US.
Retropharyngeal abscess	≥48 hours of symptoms; fever, drooling, poor feeding and irritability in infants; neck pain, dysphagia in older children and adults.	Classically toxic-appearing with fever and dehydration; lymphadenopathy; stridor in supine position if severe; unilateral bulging of lateral or posterior wall of or opharynx; meningismus and torticollis may be present.	Lateral neck radiograph is a screening measure; CT of neck and mediastinum with IV contrast for confirmation and surgical planning.
Vincent's angina (ANUG)	Poor dental hygiene; abrupt onset severe throat pain, odynophagia and foul taste; fever, malaise.	Gray exudates over gums and tonsils; gingival ulcers; submandibular adenopathy	Clinical diagnosis.
Uvulitis	Throat pain and/or FB sensation.	Uvula red and swollen.	Clinical diagnosis. RAT and throat culture may reveal GABHS as etiology.

ANUG: acute necrotizing ulcerative gingivitis; C. trachomatis: *Chlamydia trachomatis*; CBC: complete blood count; CMV: cytomegalovirus; CT: computed tomography; EBV: Epstein–Barr virus; ENT: ear, nose, throat; FB: foreign body; GABHS: group A beta-hemolytic streptococcus; HFM: hand-foot-mouth; HSV: herpes simplex virus; IV: intravenous; RAT: rapid antigen test; RSV: respiratory syncytial virus; URI: upper respiratory infection; US: ultrasound.

Diagnostic testing

Laboratory studies

White blood cell count

Ordering a white blood cell (WBC) count is of little value in most cases of sore throat. It may be useful if infectious mononucleosus (atypical lymphocytosis), serious bacterial infection, leukemia or an immunocompromised state are concerns.

Blood cultures

Blood cultures should be obtained in patients with deep space infections (except most cases of peritonsillitis), immunocompromised states, sepsis and epiglottitis (once the patient's airway is secure).

Rapid diagnostic tests for group A beta-hemolytic streptococcus

Rapid antigen tests (RATs) and throat cultures aid in the diagnosis of GABHS pharyngitis. The tonsils and posterior pharyngeal wall should be swabbed vigorously to obtain an accurate specimen for both RATs and throat cultures. RATs are generally considered to have good positive predictive values, but insufficient sensitivities to rule out GABHS infection (most being 79–95% sensitive). Specificities range from 31% to 100%, with most being 90–98% specific depending upon which commercial test is used. Results for RATs usually return in 10–30 minutes. Both RATs and cultures identify the Group A antigen, not active infection. Since 15–20% of the population are chronic carriers of GABHS, treating all positive RATs or cultures with antibiotics inevitably results in overtreatment.

Throat cultures

All negative RATs should be confirmed with culture; otherwise, a significant number of cases of GABHS pharyngitis will be missed. Culture for GABHS is 90–95% sensitive and 94–100% specific. About one-third of patients with infectious mononucleosus and diptheria have positive GABHS cultures, which may lead to misdiagnoses. The true gold standard for determining GABHS infection is with acute and convalescent antistreptolysin-O (ASO) titers. However ASO titers are not practical in an outpatient setting and are rarely done.

Table 19.11 lists situations in which obtaining throat cultures are indicated.

Table 19.11 Situations in which throat cultures should be obtained

- Evidence of epiglottitis, peritonsillitis or retropharyngeal abscess (once airway secured).
- Presence of a pharyngeal membrane: culture for *A. hemolyticum* and *Corynebacterium diptheriae* (laboratory should be notified).
- History of or suspected immunocompromised state (including status-post splenectomy).
- History of possible gonorrhea (laboratory should be notified).
- History of prolonged and/or severe pharyngitis: consider obtaining cultures for *Yersinia*, *A. hemolyticum*, *C. diptheriae* and a monospot test.
- Pediatric patients (controversial).

Heterophil antibody test (monospot test)

The monospot test, used to detect EBV infectious mononucleosus, may not be positive until 1–2 weeks of illness. The test's sensitivity declines as the patient's age decreases, with a 95% sensitivity in adults but only a 30% sensitivity in those less than 20 months of age. This test is almost always negative in persons of Japanese ancestry for unknown reasons. False positives may occur with some systemic illnesses, such as leukemia.

Electrocardiogram

An electrocardiogram (ECG) would be useful in the patient with throat discomfort, a negative pharyngeal examination, and a history compatible with acute coronary syndrome (ACS).

Radiologic studies

Plain films

A soft tissue lateral view of the neck is useful in the work-up of croup, epiglottitis, lingual tonsillitis, retropharyngeal abscess, Ludwig's angina, laryngeal trauma and suspected FBs. However, plain radiographs may be normal despite the presence of these illnesses. Any patient who appears unstable should not leave the emergency department (ED) for radiographs.

The "steeple sign" (narrowing of the airway) due to glottic and subglottic edema is a reliable finding of croup, although an X-ray is not commonly needed. A soft tissue lateral radiograph of the neck is abnormal in 90% cases of epiglottitis. Positive findings include an enlarged, misshapen epiglottis ("thumbprint" sign) and swelling of the retropharyngeal soft tissues (Figure 19.20).

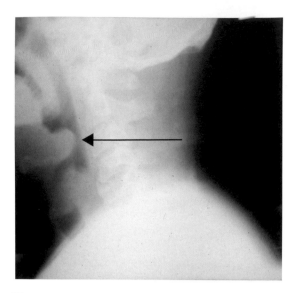

Figure 19.20
Epiglottitis. Lateral view of the cervical soft tissues demonstrating marked swelling of the epiglottis *(thumbprint sign)* with obliteration of the vallecula. *Courtesy*: Edward Damrose, MD.

Plain films are useful for excluding epiglottitis in cases of bacterial tracheitis and croup.

Abnormal retropharyngeal soft tissue swelling may be also seen with retropharyngeal abscess (Figure 19.21). Nonspecific soft tissue swelling may be seen in a patient with a parapharyngeal abscess. Patients with Ludwig's angina may have swelling of the submandibular soft tissues, airway narrowing and gas collections on plain film. Air in the soft tissues may also be seen on plain film in patients with laryngeal trauma or burns. If a FB is radiopaque, it may be seen.

Ultrasound

Ultrasound (US) is useful in the evaluation of deep space infections when the goal is to distinguish between cellulitis and abscess. US has the advantage over computerized tomography (CT) in critically ill patients, who should not be transported from the ED.

Computerized tomography

CT with intravenous (IV) contrast is useful in the evaluation of throat pain with a suspected neck mass or laryngeal trauma. CT may also help distinguish abscess from cellulitis, and assist in surgical planning for deep space infections. CT will demonstrate fractures of the hyoid, cricoid and thyroid cartilages, and dislocation of the cricoarytenoid joints. The patient's airway must be stable prior to transport to CT.

Laryngoscopy

Patients with drooling, inability to swallow, FB sensation, dysphonia and/or laryngeal neck pain require complete visualization of the pharynx if history, physical and diagnostic imaging do not identify the etiology of the illness. Laryngoscopy is used to definitively diagnose epiglottitis, bacterial tracheitis, lingual tonsillitis, FB, injury from laryngeal trauma, and chemical and thermal burns. Visualization of a swollen epiglottis ("cherry red") is seen in epiglottitis. Erythematous,

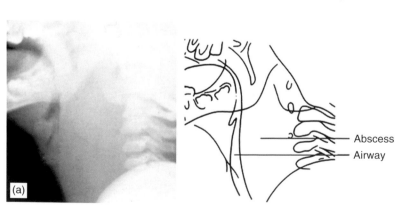

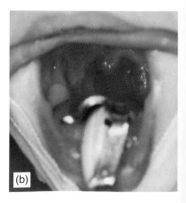

Figure 19.21
Retropharyngeal abscess. (a) A lateral neck radiograph and associated line diagram reveal prominent prevertebral soft tissue swelling that displaces the trachea forward. (b) Pharyngeal examination in the operating room revealed an intensely erythematous, unilateral swelling of the posterior pharyngeal wall. Reprinted from Atlas of Pediatric Physical Diagnosis, 4th ed., Eds Zitelli BJ, Davis HW. Copyright 2002, with permission from Elsevier.

swollen lingual tonsils covered with exudates are seen with lingual tonsillitis. A FB or abrasion in the lingual or palatine tonsils or pyriform sinus may be seen. Laryngoscopy may show mucosal tears, cartilaginous fractures or dislocations in patients with trauma. Edema, burned tissue, erythema and ulcerations may be seen on laryngoscopy in a patient with a chemical or thermal burn.

General treatment principles

Most management decisions relevant to the patient with sore throat concern antibiotic use and palliative measures. More serious considerations involve airway management and emergency anesthesiology or ENT consultation for procedures.

Airway management

Patients with illnesses associated with upper airway involvement (e.g., epiglottitis, deep space infections, trauma, burns and FBs) should be handled carefully to avoid precipitating sudden complete airway obstruction. Allow patients to maintain the position in which they are most comfortable. Pediatric IV lines should not be established in the ED unless the child is already in extremis. Never leave these patients alone! Difficult airway equipment should be ready for use at the bedside. Definitive airway management is usually best accomplished by an otolaryngologist and anesthesiologist in the OR with the neck prepped for a tracheostomy.

Volume repletion

Patients who are not tolerating sufficient oral hydration should be given IV crystalloid fluids.

Pain relief

Anesthetic lozenges, throat sprays and salt water gargles may help mild to moderate discomfort. Viscous lidocaine or Xylocaine may be used for acute temporary relief, but should not be used frequently or chronically because they may mask an underlying disorder and cause toxicity. These agents also decrease the gag reflex and may lead to aspiration. Gargling with benadryl elixir is another option, although the pain relief is brief. Patients with mild to moderate pain may do well with acetaminophen or ibuprofen alone. Elixirs (even in adults) may be better tolerated than tablets. Patients with severe pain may require oral or IV narcotics. Other palliative measures include air humidification and voice rest.

Antibiotics

Antibiotics are indicated in patients with suspected bacterial infections. Despite patients' misconceptions, antibiotics will not help most sore throats. The disadvantages of overtreating with antibiotics include increased bacterial drug resistance, decreased immune response, disruption of natural microbial ecology, antibiotic-associated side effects and patients' expectations for antibiotics with repeated episodes of sore throat. GABHS pharyngitis resolves spontaneously in 3–5 days without antibiotics. However, untreated GABHS infection may result in significant sequelae, including rheumatic fever, peritonsillitis, and glomerulonephritis. A recent resurgence in invasive streptococcal infections (e.g., scarlet fever and streptococcal toxic shock syndrome) has also influenced the aggressive treatment of pharyngitis. Early antibiotic treatment has been shown to shorten the course and severity of illness and decrease transmission of GABHS.

Controversy exists concerning the selection of patients with pharyngitis for laboratory testing and antibiotic treatment. One popular strategy is based on the adult scoring system for GABHS. The presence of two or more risk factors (Table 19.12) indicates a 56% probability of disease; thus, empiric oral antibiotic therapy is indicated.

Table 19.12 Adult scoring system for GABHS

Risk factors
• Pharyngeal exudates
• Tender anterior cervical adenopathy
• Fever >38°C
• Absence of cough and coryza

GABHS: Group A beta-hemolytic streptococcus.
Modified from: Centor RM, Witherspoon JM, Dalton HP, Brody CE, Link K. The diagnosis of strep throat in the emergency room. *Med Decis Making* 1001;1:000 016.

The general consensus is that patients with a history of rheumatic fever or a family member with a history of rheumatic fever (or documented GABHS infection), evidence of scarlet fever and/or partially treated pharyngitis should also be empirically treated with antibiotics. Many experts recommend empiric treatment for GABHS pharyngitis in the midst of a GABHS, rheumatic fever or glomerulonephritis outbreak. Some believe that those who will be unavailable for follow-up (transient and noncompliant patients) should be empirically treated for GABHS pharyngitis, since cultures take 24–48 hours to return. Patients with less than two risk factors should undergo RAT and throat culture if RAT negative, and only be treated if either result is positive. Despite the fact that many providers empirically prescribe antibiotics for the above-mentioned situations, the American Academy of Pediatrics (AAP), the American Heart Association (AHA) and the Infectious Disease Society of America (IDSA) all recommend doing at least one laboratory test before the decision to administer antibiotics is made. The best strategy for an individual clinician depends upon the prevalence of streptococcal disease in the population, the ease of follow-up, and the availability and accuracy of the specific RAT used.

Antibiotic therapy for GABHS pharyngitis should be initiated within 9 days of symptom onset to prevent acute rheumatic fever. The treatment of choice for GABHS infection remains penicillin. A one-time dose of parenteral benzathine penicillin should be given to patients who cannot tolerate per os (PO) or in whom poor compliance is suspected.

Erythromycin is the main alternative to penicillin, although several alternative regimens exist. Antibiotic treatment is also indicated for lingual tonsillitis, gonococcal and chlamydial pharyngitis, diphtheria (which also requires treatment with antitoxin), *A. hemolyticum* pharyngitis, Vincent's angina, epiglottitis and deep space infections. Candidal pharyngitis should be treated with oral fluconazole or itraconazole. Patients with evidence of herpes pharyngitis should be treated with acyclovir or famcyclovir.

Steroids

Steroids may be useful with severe bilateral tonsillar swelling in infectious mononucleosis and some cases of lingual tonsillitis. Research has demonstrated that steroids slightly reduce time to resolution of pain in severe cases of pharyngitis, although this is not common practice. Steroid use for epiglottitis, Ludwig's angina and caustic ingestion is controversial. A single dose of steroids is useful in the treatment of croup.

Racemic epinephrine

Racemic epinephrine is useful in reducing airway edema in moderate and severe croup. It has reportedly been used for epiglottitis and lingual tonsillitis. Evidence-based studies are needed prior to recommending it for use in these circumstances.

Needle aspiration and incision and drainage

Until recently, incision and drainage or immediate tonsillectomy was the recommended treatment for peritonsillitis caused by an abscess. Currently, needle aspiration is recommended by either a trained physician or otolaryngologist. It has been shown to be equally effective, safer and less painful compared to incision and drainage. The technique has been well described. Patients with severe trismus or those who cannot cooperate (young children) are best served by having this procedure or a tonsillectomy done in the OR by an otolaryngologist. Surgical drainage for Ludwig's angina is reserved for patients with crepitance and abscess, and may be done to eradicate dental infections as well. Most cases of retropharyngeal abscess require surgical drainage.

Special patients
Elderly

The incidence of infectious pharyngitis declines with age. Persistent sore throat without obvious physical findings in an elderly patient should prompt a search for neoplasm, particularly if there is a history of tobacco use.

Pediatric

Children with GABHS pharyngitis should receive antibiotics for 24 hours prior to returning to school. Gonococcal pharyngitis may be seen in sexually abused children and sexually active adolescents.

Immune compromised

Any immunocompromised patient with pharyngitis who is going to be discharged needs to be followed closely as an outpatient. Asplenic patients are at risk for developing streptococcal sepsis and should be admitted. Leukopenic patients should only be discharged if they have an adequate granulocyte count. Candidal infection is the most common type of pharyngitis in patients with acquired immunodeficiency syndrome (AIDS). A patient with a candidal infection without an obvious underlying risk factor should be evaluated for potential neoplasm or an immunocompromised state.

Infectious mononucleosus

Patients should be informed that infectious mononucleosus may persist for weeks to months. Steroids may help reduce severe tonsillar edema. Any patient with infectious mononucleosus and abdominal pain should undergo immediate US or CT to detect splenic rupture, which typically occurs after 4–6 weeks of illness. If given amoxicillin or ampicillin, 90% of patients with EBV infection will develop a diffuse macular rash, often mistaken for an allergic reaction. All patients with infectious mononucleosus should be seen by their primary care physician within 1 week of their diagnosis for follow-up.

Post-tonsillectomy

About 10% of patients will present with bleeding 5–10 days after tonsillectomy. The majority of these patients are in the pediatric age group and have minor bleeding from the tonsillar veins that can be controlled with direct pressure. About 1% of patients presenting with post-tonsillectomy bleeding (usually males in the age 15–24-year age group) have major bleeding which requires emergent airway control and massive transfusion. ENT should be consulted emergently in these patients.

Disposition

Emergent ear, nose and throat consultation and admission

The following are admission criteria for patients with throat pain:

1. Evidence of or at risk for airway compromise (includes all suspected cases of epiglottitis, retropharyngeal abscess, Ludwig's angina and diptheria).*
2. Cannot maintain hydration or swallow.
3. Require IV antibiotics.
4. Patients whose pain is intolerable despite maximal oral analgesia.
5. Controversy still exists concerning whether the patient with a peritonsillar abscess should be treated in the ED and discharged or hospitalized. This depends not only upon the appearance of the patient but the preference of the ENT consultant.
6. Evidence of disseminated spread of infection.
7. Evidence of deep neck space infection, including necrotizing fasciitis.*
8. Evidence of or significant risk for sepsis (often in immunocompromised patients).*
9. Post-tonsillectomy patients with any bleeding other than the most minor.*

Any patient with a chronic sore throat or evidence of carcinoma of the oropharynx should be referred to ENT to be seen within 5–7 days for further work-up of a potential neoplasm.

Observation/serial evaluation

Patients with peritonsillitis may benefit from observation over a several hour period, during which time they receive IV hydration, antibiotics and a PO challenge. All of these patients must have close follow-up within 24 hours with an otolaryngologist to check for abscess formation.

Discharge

Most patients with sore throat can be safely discharged. If an antibiotic treatment is planned pending culture results, it is important to establish a detailed plan for follow-up.

Pearls, pitfalls, and myths

- Recognize the signs of impending complete airway obstruction: sniffing position, apprehension, tachypnea, drooling, voice alteration and stridor. Patients with these signs should be allowed to assume the position in which they are most comfortable.
- ENT and anesthesia should be consulted emergently and the OR prepared for patients who appear to have impending or actual airway obstruction.
- Always be prepared for complete airway obstruction and other catastrophic complications (sepsis, carotid artery hemorrhage) in any patient with a deep space infection or epiglottitis.
- Despite epiglottitis becoming relatively uncommon in the pediatric population, it is often overlooked, resulting in fatal consequences. Consider this diagnosis in those with rapid onset of sore throat, throat pain out of proportion to examination, respiratory symptoms accompanying the

---

*These patients are usually admitted to the ICU or go directly to the OR.

sore throat or the sensation of a "lump" in the throat.

- Do not fail to recognize an abscess or impending abscess in the potential spaces of the head and neck.
- Plain radiographs of the neck may be useful for detecting retropharyngeal abscess and epiglottitis. Advanced imaging in a stable patient with a secure airway is useful for further diagnosis, distinguishing abscess from cellulitis, and surgical planning.
- Antibiotics should be tailored to the specific disease process suspected. Understand the common rationale and criteria for testing and empiric antibiotic prescribing for pharyngitis.
- Needle aspiration of a suspected peritonsillar abscess should only be attempted by trained physicians because of potential significant complications (puncture of major vessels of the neck).
- A patient with a chronic sore throat (especially one who has an alcohol or tobacco history) needs prompt referral to ENT for work-up of a potential cancer.

References

1. Bradley CP. Taking another look at the acute sore throat. *Br J Gen Pract* 2000;50:780–781.
2. Centor RM, Witherspoon JM, Dalton HP, Brody CE, Link K. The diagnosis of strep throat in the emergency room. *Med Decis Making* 1981;1:239–246.
3. Fernandez-Franckelton M, Turbiak TW. Bacteria. In: Marx JA (ed.). *Rosen's Emergency Medicine: Concepts and Clinical Practice*, 5th ed., St. Louis, MO: Mosby, 2002:1785–1788.
4. Garlington JC, Nemiroff PM. Emergency aspects of head and neck neoplasms. In: Harwood-Nuss A (ed.). *The Clinical Practice of Emergency Medicine*, 3rd ed., Philadelphia, PA: Lippincott Williams & Wilkins, 2001:124–127.
5. Greenough G. Sore throat. In: Davis MA, Votey SR, Greenough PG (eds). *Signs and Symptoms in Emergency Medicine*, 1st ed., St. Louis, MO: Mosby, 1999:400–411.
6. Hackeling TA, Triana RJ. Disorders of the neck and upper airway. In: Tintinalli JE, Kelen GD, Stapczynski JS (eds). *Emergency Medicine: A Comprehensive Study Guide*. 5th ed., New York, NY: McGraw-Hill, 2000:1556–1565.
7. Jerrard D. Infectious mononucleosis. In: Harwood-Nuss A (ed.). *The Clinical Practice of Emergency Medicine*, 3rd ed., Philadelphia, PA: Lippincott Williams & Wilkins, 2001:814–816.
8. Joyce SM. Acute sore throat. In: Hamilton GC (ed.). *Emergency Medicine: An Approach to Clinical Problem-Solving*, 1st ed., Philadelphia, PA: WB Saunders, 1991:547–560.
9. Melio FR. Upper respiratory tract infections. In: Marx JA (ed.) *Rosen's Emergency Medicine: Concepts and Clinical Practice*, 5th ed., St. Louis, MO: Mosby, 2002:969–990.
10. Perkins A. An approach to diagnosing the acute sore throat. *Am Fam Physician* 1997;55:131–138.
11. Pichichero M. Cost-effective management of sore throat. *Arch Pediatr Adolesc Med* 1999;153:672–673.
12. Pichichero M. Sore throat after sore throat after sore throat. *Postgrad Med* 1997;101:205–225.
13. Picken CA. Acute infections of the adult pharynx. In: Harwood-Nuss A (ed.). *The Clinical Practice of Emergency Medicine*, 3rd ed., Philadelphia, PA: Lippincott Williams & Wilkins, 2001:80–85.
14. Quayle KS, Fuchs S, Jaffe DM. Otitis and pharyngitis in children. In: Tintinalli JE, Kelen GD, Stapczynski JS (eds). *Emergency Medicine: A Comprehensive Study Guide*. 5th ed., New York, NY: McGraw-Hill, 2000:791–794.
15. Renicks M. Sore throat. In: Hamilton, GC (ed.) *Presenting Signs and Symptoms in the Emergency Department: Evaluation and Treatment*, 1st ed., Baltimore, MD: Williams & Wilkins, 1993:438–446.
16. Sonnad SS, Van Harrison R, Standiford CJ, Bernstein SJ. Issues in the development, dissemination, and effect of an evidence-based guideline for managing sore throat in adults. *J Qual Improv* 1999;25:630–640.
17. Stewart CE. Not just a sore throat. *Emerg Med Serv* 2000;29:56–66.
18. Wright MS. Acute pharyngitis in the pediatric patient. In: Harwood-Nuss A (ed.). *The Clinical Practice of Emergency Medicine*, 3rd ed., Philadelphia, PA: Lippincott Williams & Wilkins, 2001: 1108–1109.

20 Extremity trauma

Dan Garza, MD and Gregory W. Hendey, MD

Scope of the problem

Trauma to an extremity is a common reason for a patient to present to the emergency department (ED). According to the Centers for Disease Control and Prevention, there were nearly 15 million visits to the ED in the year 2000 for injuries involving the extremity. The most common sites of injury were the wrist and hand, followed by the ankle and shoulder. It is important to perform a thorough but efficient history and physical examination in order to accurately diagnose and provide initial treatment for these injuries. When improperly treated, extremity injuries may lead to long-term pain and disability for the patient.

Anatomic essentials

Each extremity can be viewed as a group of individual bones held together by a musculo-ligamentous apparatus. Careful attention must be paid to the vascular and nerve supply to each extremity; injury to these structures may be overlooked when fractures are present. Each extremity is encased in soft tissue that is often subdivided into fascial compartments. The clinician should

Table 20.1 Bones, ligaments, arteries and nerves of the upper extremity

	Bones	Ligaments	Arteries	Nerves
Shoulder (Figure 20.1)	Scapula Humerus Clavicle	Acromioclavicular Coracoclavicular Coracoacromlal Coracohumeral Capsular ligaments Transverse ligaments of humerus	Axillary Anterior circumflex humeral Posterior circumflex humeral	Axillary Musculocutaneous
Elbow (Figure 20.2)	Humerus Radius Ulna	Annular Ulnar collateral Radial collateral	Brachial Inferior ulnar collateral Superior ulnar collateral Radial collateral	Median Radial Ulnar
Wrist (Figure 20.3)	Radius Carpals	Ulnar collateral Radial collateral Palmar radiocarpal Dorsal radiocarpal	Radial Ulnar	Median Radial Ulnar
Hand (Figures 20.3 and 20.4)	Carpals • Scaphoid • Lunate • Triquetral • Pisiform • Trapezium • Trapezoid • Capitate • Hamate Metacarpals	Intercarpal ligaments Palmar carpometacarpal Dorsal carpometacarpal Palmar and collateral metacarpophalangeal ligaments Deep transverse metacarpal Superficial transverse metacarpal	Deep palmar arch Superficial palmar arch Common palmar digital	Median • Muscular branch • Common palmar digital Ulnar • Superficial branch • Deep branch • Common palmar digital
Digits (Figure 20.4)	Proximal phalanges Intermediate phalanges (except thumb) Distal phalanges	Palmar and collateral ligaments of proximal interphalangeal joints and distal interphalangeal joints	Palmar digital	Palmar digital

become familiar with the normal anatomy and pathology of an extremity in this context: bones and ligaments, muscles and tendons, nerves and vessels, and soft tissue (compartments). The examination is complete only when all of these structures in the relevant area have been assessed (Tables 20.1 and 20.2).

Sensory and motor innervation of the extremities can be rapidly assessed. When evaluating sensorimotor function due to an extremity

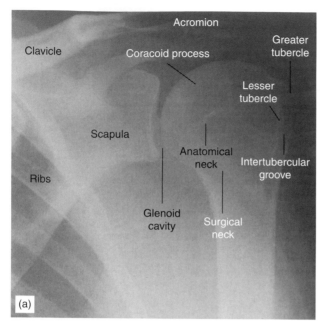

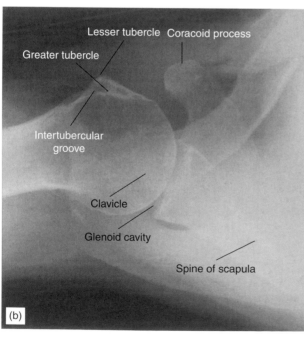

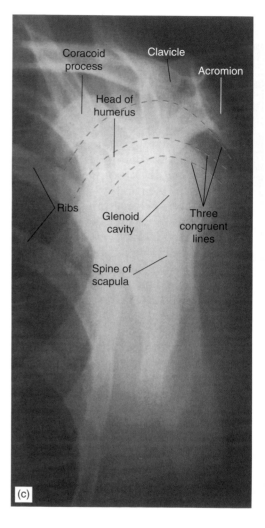

Figure 20.1
(a) Anteroposterior, (b) axillary, and (c) lateral radiographic projections of the shoulder. Reproduced from Butler et al, *Applied Radiological Anatomy*, Cambridge, Cambridge University Press, 1997.

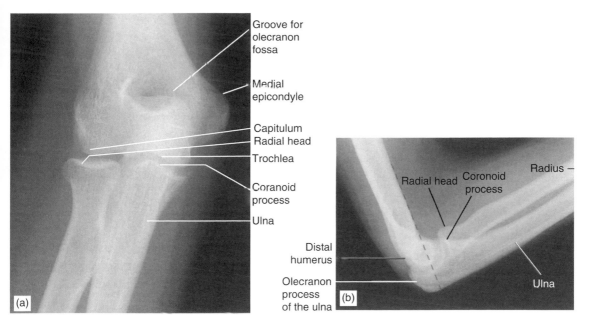

Figure 20.2
(a) Anteroposterior and (b) lateral radiographs of the elbow. Reproduced from Butler et al, *Applied Radiological Anatomy*, Cambridge, Cambridge University Press, 1997.

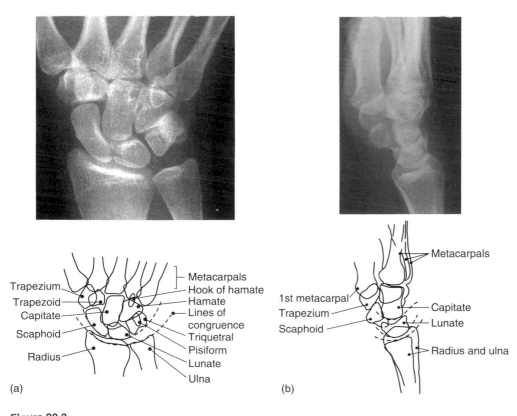

Figure 20.3
(a) Anteroposterior and (b) lateral radiographs of the wrist. Reproduced from Butler et al, *Applied Radiological Anatomy*, Cambridge, Cambridge University Press, 1997.

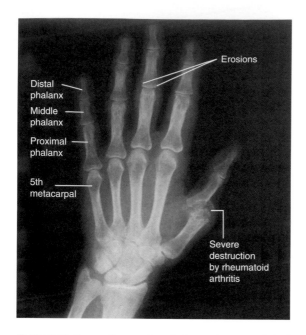

Distal
phalanx

Middle
phalanx

Proximal
phalanx

5th
metacarpal

Erosions

Severe
destruction
by rheumatoid
arthritis

Figure 20.4
Radiograph of the hand. Reproduced from Butler et al,
Applied Radiological Anatomy, Cambridge, Cambridge
University Press, 1997.

Table 20.2 Bones, ligaments, arteries and nerves of the lower extremity

	Bones	Ligaments	Arteries	Nerves
Hip (Figure 20.5)	Pelvis Femur	Iliofemoral Pubofemoral Ischiofemoral Round	Femoral Profunda femoris Medial femoral circumflex Lateral femoral circumflex Inferior gluteal	Femoral Obturator Sciatic
Knee (Figure 20.6)	Femur Tibia Fibula	Anterior cruciate Posterior cruciate Medial collateral Lateral collateral Anterior and posterior ligaments of head of fibula	Popliteal Anterior tibial Descending genicular Medial and lateral superior genicular Medial and lateral inferior genicular Descending branch of lateral femoral circumflex Anterior tibial recurrent Circumflex fibular	Tibial Common peroneal Medial and lateral sural cutaneous Saphenous
Ankle (Figure 20.7)	Tibia Fibula Talus	Lateral • Anterior tibiofibular • Anterior talofibular • Posterior talofibular • Calcaneofibular Medial • Deltoid (talar, calcaneal, navicular)	Anterior tibial Posterior tibial	Superficial peroneal Deep peroneal Saphenous Tibial Sural
Foot (Figure 20.8)	Calcaneus Talus Navicular Cuboid Cuneiforms • Medial • Intermediate • Lateral Metatarsals Phalanges	Bifurcate • Calcaneocuboid • Calcaneonavicular Interosseus talocalcaneal Plantar calcaneonavicular Plantar calcaneocuboid Long plantar	Medial plantar Lateral plantar Plantar arch Dorsalis pedis Arcuate Medial and lateral tarsal Dorsal metatarsal Plantar metatarsal Common plantar digital Proper plantar digital Dorsal digital	Medial plantar Lateral plantar Deep peroneal Common plantar digital Proper plantar digital Dorsal digital

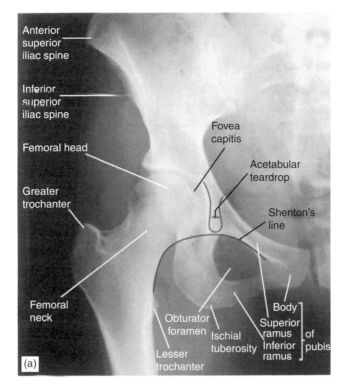

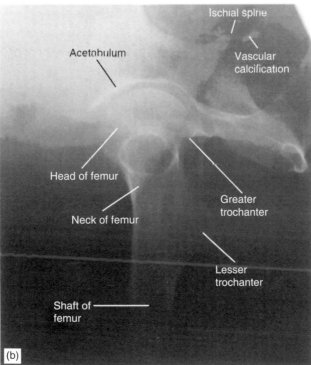

Figure 20.5
(a) Anteroposterior and (b) lateral radiographs of the hip.
Reproduced from Butler et al, *Applied Radiological Anatomy*,
Cambridge, Cambridge University Press, 1997.

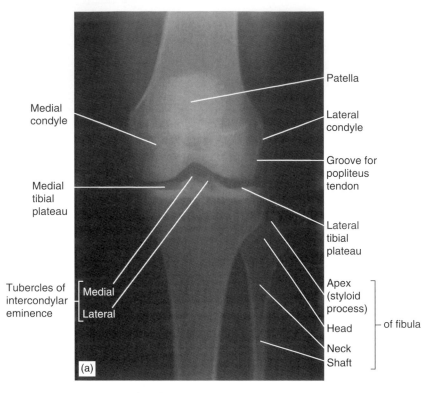

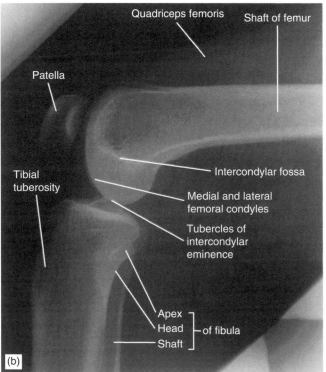

Figure 20.6
(a) Anteroposterior and (b) lateral radiographs of the knee. Reproduced from Butler et al, *Applied Radiological Anatomy*, Cambridge, Cambridge University Press, 1997.

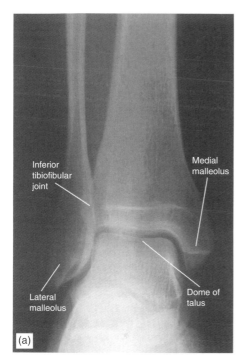
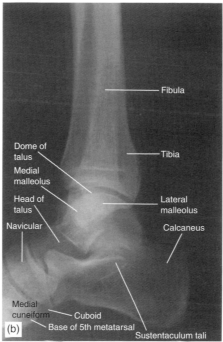

Figure 20.7
(a) Anteroposterior and (b) lateral radiographs of the ankle. Reproduced from Butler et al, *Applied Radiological Anatomy*, Cambridge, Cambridge University Press, 1997.

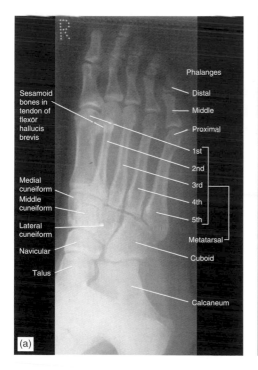
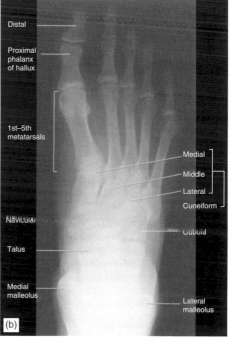

Figure 20.8
(a) Anteroposterior and (b) lateral radiographs of the ankle. Reproduced from Butler et al, *Applied Radiological Anatomy*, Cambridge, Cambridge University Press, 1997.

Table 20.3 Peripheral nerves: sensory and motor function

Nerve	Sensory	Motor
Axillary (C5,6)	Lateral aspect of deltoid	Shoulder abduction
Median (C6–8)	Lateral palmar aspect of hand (including lateral palmar half of ring finger)	Abduction of thumb
Radial (C6–8)	Lateral dorsum of hand	Thumb/wrist extension
Ulnar (C8,T1)	Medial palmar aspect of hand (including medial palmar half of ring finger)	Finger abduction
Femoral (L2–4)	Anterior aspect of thigh	Knee extension
Saphenous (L2–4)	Medial aspect of leg and foot	
Sciatic (L4–S3)	Posterior aspect of thigh	Knee flexion
Tibial (L4–S3)	Sole of foot	Plantar flexion (posterior compartment)
Common peroneal (L4–S2)	Posterior aspect of lower leg	
Superficial peroneal (L4–S2)	Lateral aspect of lower leg Dorsum of foot	Foot eversion (lateral compartment)
Deep peroneal (L4–S2)	First toe web space	Dorsiflexion (anterior compartment)

Table 20.4 Compartments of the leg

Compartment	Contents
Anterior	Muscles • Tibialis anterior • Extensor digitorum longus • Extensor hallucis longus • Peroneus tertius Anterior tibial artery Deep peroneal nerve
Lateral	Muscles • Peroneus brevis • Peroneus longus Superficial peroneal nerve
Deep posterior	Muscles • Tibialis posterior • Flexor digitorum longus • Flexor hallucis longus Posterior tibial artery Peroneal artery Posterior tibial nerve
Superficial posterior	Muscles • Gastrocnemius • Plantaris • Soleus Sural nerve

injury, the examiner should focus on peripheral nerves rather than nerve root and dermatomal distribution, as is the case with vertebral injury (Table 20.3).

Each extremity is divided into compartments by longitudinal fascia. Best seen on cross section, these compartments are named according to their anatomic position. For example, the compartments of the leg and the structures they contain are shown in Table 20.4 and Figure 20.9.

History

How did the injury occur?

The nature, magnitude, and direction of forces applied to the extremity help determine the likely resulting injury. Crush injury may predispose to compartment syndrome or rhabdomyolysis. A shearing force onto gravel or dirt raises suspicion for foreign bodies that must be removed to avoid the risk of wound infection or osteomyelitis. Falls from a height, significant collisions, or loading of a patient's entire weight on a single joint increases the likelihood of fracture. Trauma that involves force imparted across the transverse axis of a bone raises the possibility of a transverse fracture, whereas a force along the long axis will more likely lead to compression or impaction fractures. Table 20.5 summarizes classic injuries resulting from common mechanisms.

When did the injury occur?

Depending on the nature of the injury, the time elapsed since its onset may be important. As the amount of time between injury and wound care for a laceration or open fracture increases, the risk of infection also increases. Depending on location, lacerations may need to undergo delayed closure if >6–12 hours have passed. In the case of vascular injury, blood flow must be returned within 6 hours for a meaningful chance of limb salvage.

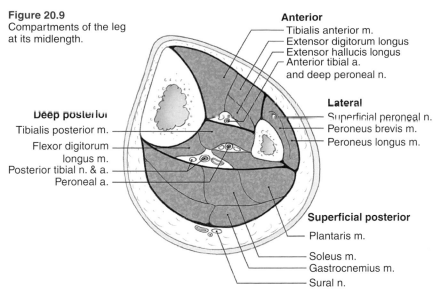

Figure 20.9
Compartments of the leg at its midlength.

Anterior
— Tibialis anterior m.
— Extensor digitorum longus
— Extensor hallucis longus
— Anterior tibial a. and deep peroneal n.

Lateral
— Superficial peroneal n.
— Peroneus brevis m.
— Peroneus longus m.

Deep posterior
Tibialis posterior m. —
Flexor digitorum longus m. —
Posterior tibial n. & a. —
Peroneal a. —

Superficial posterior
— Plantaris m.
— Soleus m.
— Gastrocnemius m.
— Sural n.

Table 20.5 Common injuries with associated mechanisms

Mechanism	Possible injury
Fall onto shoulder	Acromioclavicular joint separation Shoulder dislocation Humerus fracture
Seizure Electrical injury	Posterior shoulder dislocation
FOOSH	Radial head fracture Colles fracture Scaphoid fracture
Pulling child's arm	Radial head subluxation (Nursemaid's elbow)
Striking knee against dashboard in high-speed collision	Posterior hip dislocation Femur fracture
Landing on feet after fall from height	Calcaneus fracture Tibial plateau fracture Vertebral compression fracture
Ankle inversion	Malleolus fracture Fracture of base of fifth metatarsal
Rotary ankle force	Malleolus fracture Maisonneuve injury
Inversion, medial or lateral stress to midfoot	Midfoot dislocation (Lisfranc injury)

Modified from Tintinalli JE (ed.). *Emergency Medicine: A Comprehensive Study Guide*, 5th ed., McGraw-Hill, 2000. FOOSH: fall on outstretched hand.

Is the patient right- or left-handed? What is the patient's occupation?

It is appropriate to assess the relative importance of an affected upper extremity to a patient's quality of life. Although all patients should receive optimal care, an injury to the dominant hand of a professional illustrator may be treated more aggressively by a consultant.

What is the patient's tetanus status?

Although rare, the potentially fatal consequences of tetanus can be easily avoided with appropriate prophylaxis (Table C.4, Appendix C). This may be overlooked in complicated fractures or lacerations requiring time-consuming repair. The most likely individuals to have inadequate prior immunization are those older than 60 and immigrants. If a patient's tetanus status is unknown or uncertain, he or she should receive the complete series.

When was the patient's last meal?

The patient's injury may require reduction under conscious sedation or general anesthesia; assessing the risk of aspiration requires knowledge of the time since the patient's last meal. Acceptable limits may vary according to institution and injury.

Associated symptoms

Is the extremity weak, cold, or numb?

These symptoms might indicate a nerve or vessel injury in the affected extremity. The clinician must perform a thorough neurovascular examination distal to the injury. An obvious bony deformity or joint dislocation should be reduced promptly in an attempt to restore any neurovascular deficit.

Past medical

Of particular concern is the patient with a coagulopathy, in whom hemodynamic status and serial hematocrits may need to be followed closely. Those taking warfarin require coagulation studies. Hemophiliacs should have the appropriate factor replacement transfused. Other considerations include allergies to analgesics or anesthetics and a history of prior surgeries or surgical hardware in the affected extremity.

Physical examination

The physical examination should begin with adequate exposure. Patients will often present with various bandages or splints applied, which must be carefully removed. While the tendency to "just order an X-ray" may seem efficient, the few minutes required to carefully examine the injury may save unnecessary radiographs or reveal unexpected findings that demand immediate attention. In addition, jewelry and clothing that may form a tourniquet due to swelling should be removed immediately. Analgesia should not be withheld pending a definitive diagnosis. In fact, the use of parenteral, regional, or local anesthesia may assist the examiner by making it easier for the patient to comply with the physical examination. It is recommended to perform a sensory examination before blocking any sensory input with a local or regional nerve block.

Vital sign abnormalities (tachycardia, hypertension) tend to be a response to pain. The failure of tachycardia to resolve with adequate analgesia should raise suspicion for blood loss.

The general approach to the assessment of extremity injuries includes evaluation of the following:

Bones and ligaments

Bony deformities are often obvious, but more subtle clues to fractures include crepitus, marked swelling, point tenderness, and ecchymosis. Knowledge of local anatomy should allow the examiner to palpate any structures of concern.

Sprains or ligamentous injuries may be characterized as first-, second-, or third-degree. First-degree sprains are tears of only a few fibers and result in minimal swelling, point tenderness, and normal joint motion and stability. Second-degree sprains are more significant tears of the ligament, although not complete disruptions. Signs include more significant swelling, tenderness, and functional loss, although joint motion and stability remain normal. Third-degree sprains are complete disruptions of the ligament with marked swelling, tenderness, functional loss, and abnormal motion and laxity at the joint.

Muscles and tendons

Rupture of tendons may result from repetitive stress or excessive loading, or from deep lacerations that directly disrupt the tendon. Regardless of cause, functional compromise should be evident on physical examination. In the case of lacerations, the tendon should be directly visualized through its full range of motion. Strains (injuries to muscle fibers) have a similar classification to sprains. First-degree strains are disruptions of a few fibers and are characterized by mild localized pain exacerbated by stretch. Second-degree strains are more significant, although not complete disruptions, with more marked tenderness and ecchymosis. Third-degree strains are complete disruptions with significant tenderness, ecchymosis, and loss of function. Larger muscles, such as the biceps, may display obvious deformities when ruptured.

Nerves and vessels

Care must be taken to assess the neurovascular status distal to an injured extremity. Neurovascular damage may result from direct trauma, disruption due to a severely displaced fracture or dislocation, or from fracture fragments. Injuries to nerves are more common than vascular injury, and range in severity from neuropraxia (secondary to contusion), which results in eventual recovery, to complete disruption or destruction. Complete assessment should include sensory, motor and deep tendon reflex (DTR) examinations. Table 20.6 lists common injuries associated with possible nerve deficits.

Although not as common, vascular injuries are potentially devastating. Complete assessment involves capillary refill time, palpating pulses, and noting color and temperature changes. If pulses are not palpable, a Doppler stethoscope should be

Table 20.6 Extremity injuries and associated nerve deficits

Injury	Possible nerve deficit
Anterior shoulder dislocation/fracture	Axillary nerve Musculocutaneous nerve
Humeral shaft fracture	Radial nerve
Fracture of distal third of radius	Radial nerve
Supracondylar fracture of humerus	Median nerve Radial nerve Ulnar nerve
Posterior elbow dislocation	Median nerve Ulnar nerve
Wrist fracture/dislocations	Median nerve
Posterior hip dislocation	Sciatic nerve
Anterior hip dislocation	Femoral nerve
Knee fracture/dislocations	Peroneal nerve Tibial nerve
Proximal fibula fracture	Peroneal nerve

used to confirm flow. Table 20.7 lists common injuries associated with possible vascular deficits.

Soft tissue (compartments)

Bound by stiff fascial walls, limb compartments are susceptible to dangerously high pressures when there is an increase in volume. When trauma results in muscle swelling or extravasation of blood, there is little room within the compartment to expand. As intra-compartmental pressures rise, blood flow to the nerves and muscles decreases

Table 20.7 Extremity injuries and associated vascular deficits

Injury	Possible vascular deficit
Anterior shoulder dislocation/fracture	Axillary artery
Supracondylar fracture of humerus	Brachial artery
Posterior elbow dislocation	Brachial artery
Knee dislocations	Popliteal artery

and, if unrelieved, muscle necrosis occurs. This process represents *compartment syndrome* and is classically characterized by the five "Ps:"

- *Pain*
- *Pallor*
- *Paralysis*
- Pulselessness
- Paresthesias

Unfortunately, by the time all of these signs and symptoms are present, permanent damage has usually occurred. The key is to maintain a high index of clinical suspicion. Certain fractures are more commonly associated with compartment syndromes; tibial fracture with anterior tibial artery involvement or supracondylar fracture of the humerus with brachial artery involvement are two examples. The earliest manifestation is pain in the affected extremity followed by paresthesias. Pain can often be exacerbated by passive extension of the fingers or passive flexion of the toes.

Regional

Shoulder

Examination of the shoulder begins with inspection and palpation of the clavicle and acromioclavicular joint. Deformity, swelling, or tenderness of the clavicle may represent a fracture. Superior displacement or prominence of the lateral clavicle is seen with complete (Grade 3) acromioclavicular separations (Figure 20.10), whereas incomplete separations (Grades 1 and 2) often present only with point tenderness at the joint. Tenderness, swelling, or bruising over the proximal humerus may represent a fracture.

Anterior shoulder dislocations (Figure 20.11), which are far more common than posterior dislocations, present with the patient holding the arm fully adducted. There is a loss of the normal rounded contour of the lateral aspect of the shoulder. A simple method to rule out a shoulder dislocation requires the examiner to gently internally and externally rotate the shoulder, followed by asking the patient to place the hand of the injured extremity across his chest and on the opposite shoulder. Free rotation of the humeral head is painful and difficult in the presence of a shoulder dislocation, and the ability to perform these maneuvers virtually rules out a dislocation. The musculocutaneous branch of the axillary nerve may be injured in anterior dislocations, resulting in weakness in shoulder abduction and

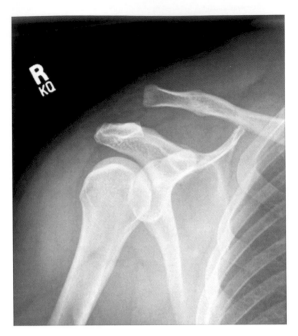

Figure 20.10
Complete (Grade 3) acromioclavicular separation. AP radiograph of the right shoulder showing diastasis of the AC joint, with superior displacement of the distal clavicle and widening of the coraco-clavicular distance. *Courtesy*: S.V. Mahadevan, MD.

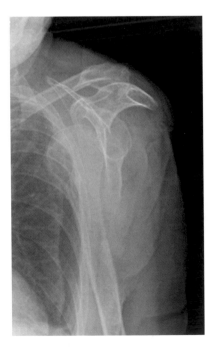

Figure 20.11
Anterior shoulder dislocation. Trans-scapular Y-view of the left shoulder showing the humeral head lying anterior and inferior to the glenoid. *Courtesy*: S.V. Mahadevan, MD.

diminished sensation over the lateral aspect of the shoulder.

Rotator cuff tears are disruptions of the muscles that permit shoulder abduction and rotation: subscapularis, infraspinatus, supraspinatus, and teres minor. Consequently, patients present with weak and painful active abduction and external rotation, as well as tenderness over the greater tuberosity (the insertion site of supraspinatus). Passive range of motion may be pain-free. In the *drop arm test*, the patient abducts the shoulder to 90° and then is asked to slowly lower the arm. In the presence of a rotator cuff tear, the patient is unable to lower the arm slowly and smoothly.

Examination of the scapula requires palpation along its entire surface. As significant force is required to fracture the scapula, the mechanism is usually a direct blow or fall from height. Fractures of the scapula may be associated with pneumothorax, rib fractures, and vertebral compression fractures. As abduction beyond 90° involves scapular rotation, this motion should produce pain in a scapular fracture.

Elbow

Deformity at the elbow may represent a fracture or dislocation, and radiographs are needed to differentiate the two. Important clues include tenting of the posterior aspect of the elbow by the olecranon in a posterior dislocation, isolated tenderness of the proximal radius in a radial head fracture, or point tenderness and swelling of the olecranon in olecranon fractures. Any effusion identified either clinically or radiographically in the setting of trauma is concerning for fracture (Figure 20.12).

Supracondylar fractures (Figure 20.13) occur most commonly in children who have fallen on an outstretched hand. Displacement of the distal humeral fracture fragment posteriorly may cause injury to the brachial artery or median, radial, and ulnar nerves. It is therefore important to document distal neurovascular findings in patients with a supracondylar fracture. Patients with supracondylar fractures are at risk of compartment syndrome of the forearm, leading to muscle necrosis and contractures of flexor muscles (Volkmann's ischemic contractures). Orthopedic consultation for appropriate disposition is mandatory, with hospitalization, reduction, and surgery if the fracture is significantly displaced.

Nursemaid's elbow is a subluxation of the radial head that results from longitudinal traction applied along the radius. This usually occurs when a child's arm is pulled to prevent him from

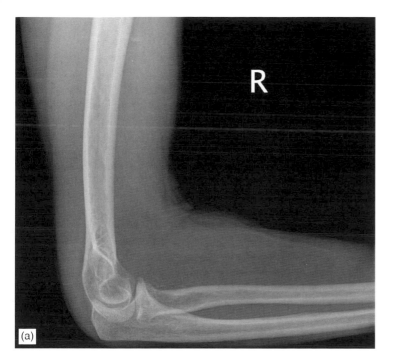
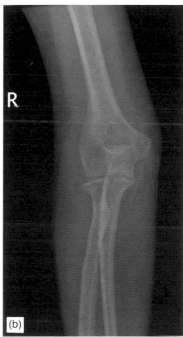

Figure 20.12
Radial head fracture. Lateral (a) and AP (b) X-rays of the right elbow showing a posterior fat pad sign indicative of a joint effusion, and a fracture of the radial head. *Courtesy*: S.V. Mahadevan, MD.

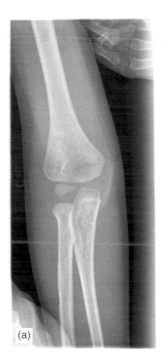
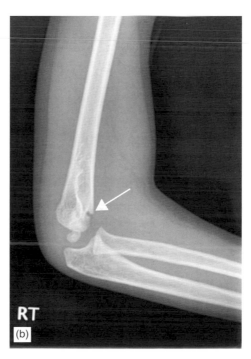

Figure 20.13
Supracondylar fracture. AP (a) and lateral (b) radiographs of the right elbow of a child demonstrating a supracondylar fracture. *Courtesy*: S.V. Mahadevan, MD.

falling or to redirect his path. The child is usually <5 years old and presents with the arm held in passive pronation and dangling to the side. Patients typically refuse to use the affected limb (i.e., refusal to reach for any offered objects, such as keys). Nursemaid's elbow is a clinical diagnosis; routine radiographs are not indicated unless a fracture is suspected.

Wrist

Examination of the distal radius and ulna may reveal characteristic deformities on inspection. Dorsal angulation of the radius after a fall on an outstretched hand is the typical presentation of a Colle's fracture (Figure 20.14), whereas volar angulation represents a Smith's fracture. Minimally displaced fractures of either the radius or ulna may present with minimal swelling and point tenderness. A thorough examination of all bony landmarks is essential.

Vascular integrity of the radial and ulnar arteries can be assessed by the *Allen test*. The examiner applies pressure to both arteries and asks the patient to lift his hand in the air and repeatedly pump his fist. The examiner then releases the radial artery and determines the time required for the blanched hand to return to its normal color. The process is repeated for the ulnar artery. Significant differences in refill time between the two arteries or between the affected and unaffected hand suggest vascular injury, and requires consultation.

Examination of the carpal bones requires careful palpation of each bone, as fractures may not be immediately apparent on radiographs. This is typical of scaphoid fractures (Figure 20.15), the most common carpal fracture. As missed scaphoid fractures significantly increase the likelihood of avascular necrosis, the physical examination is more important than radiographs. Two sensitive signs for a scaphoid fracture include tenderness in the anatomic snuffbox and pain with axial loading of the thumb. Clinical suspicion based on either of these findings and a history of falling on an outstretched hand (FOOSH) mandates appropriate splinting and follow-up in 10–14 days for repeat films.

Triquetral fractures are the second most common carpal fracture, often as a result of a FOOSH mechanism. These may often only be visualized on a lateral radiograph (Figure 20.16). Patients

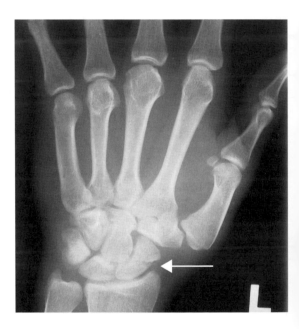

Figure 20.15
Scaphoid fracture. AP X-ray of the left hand showing a fracture through the waist of the scaphoid. *Courtesy*: S.V. Mahadevan, MD.

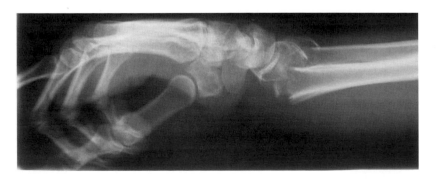

Figure 20.14
Colles fracture. Lateral radiograph showing a fracture of the distal radius, with dorsal displacement of the distal fragment. *Courtesy*: S.V. Mahadevan, MD.

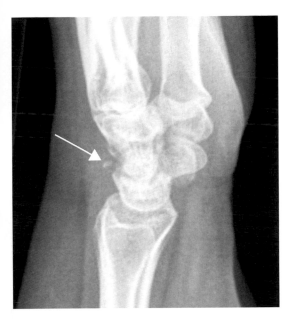

Figure 20.16
Triquetral fracture. Lateral X-ray of the wrist revealing avulsion fracture of the triquetral carpal bone. *Courtesy*: S.V. Mahadevan, MD.

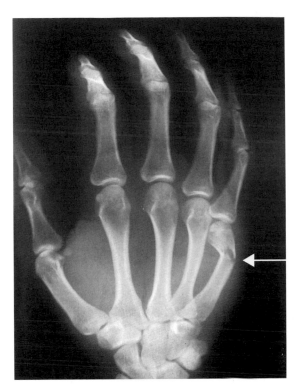

Figure 20.17
Boxer's fracture. AP radiograph showing an angulated fracture through the neck of the fifth metacarpal. *Courtesy*: S.V. Mahadevan, MD.

present with tenderness just distal to the ulnar styloid. Lunate fractures, although less common, are potentially devastating because, like the scaphoid, they carry a significant risk of avascular necrosis (Kienbock's disease). Patients generally complain of centrally located wrist pain after a fall. On examination, tenderness is just distal to Lister's tubercle. As with scaphoid fractures, clinical suspicion alone mandates splinting and orthopedic follow-up.

Ligamentous disruption can also occur between carpal bones, the most common of which causes scapholunate dissociation. Particular attention should be paid for tenderness at the joint, which is immediately ulnar to the anatomic snuffbox. *Watson's test* for scapholunate instability is considered positive if pain or subluxation is elicited when the patient moves the wrist from ulnar to radial deviation while the examiner applies pressure at the scaphoid tubercle.

Hand

Bony deformities are often obvious in fractures and dislocations of the hand. It is important that not only angulation and displacement be noted, but also rotational deformities. All three factors must be addressed in an adequate reduction. Palpation of each metacarpal and phalanx may

reveal point tenderness suspicious for a fracture (Figure 20.17).

Any injury to the hand should prompt an examination of the sensorimotor function of the median, radial, and ulnar nerves (Table 20.3). The sensory examination of the hand is best assessed by two-point discrimination. The patient should be able to distinguish between two discrete blunt points at a minimum distance of 5 mm at the fingertips and 10 mm at the base of the palm. This examination can be performed with a paper clip whose ends have been separated to 5 mm.

Tendon injuries may be apparent upon initial inspection. Flexor tendon injuries may result in the finger held in relative extension compared to other digits, whereas extensor tendon injuries result in relative flexion (Figure 20.18). Deficits or pain on active range of motion indicate injury to the tendon being assessed. Care must be taken to assess the function of flexor digitorum superficialis (FDS) and flexor digitorum profundus (FDP) tendons separately. To test FDP function, have the patient flex the distal interphalangeal (DIP) joint. When assessing the FDS, the examiner must isolate the digit by holding all other fingers in extension. Otherwise, adjacent FDS tendons may assist in flexion of the proximal interphalangeal (PIP) joint and mimic normal function.

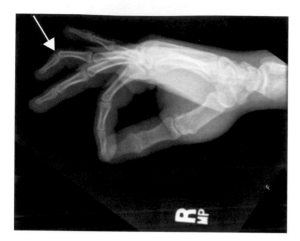

Figure 20.18
Mallet finger. Lateral radiograph of the right hand with a fixed flexion deformity of the distal interphalangeal joint. *Courtesy*: S.V. Mahadevan, MD.

Hip

The position in which the affected leg is held upon presentation can be a significant clue to the underlying pathology. Anterior dislocations and femoral neck fractures (Figure 20.19) present with the leg abducted, externally rotated, and, in fractures, shortened. Posterior dislocations present with the leg shortened, adducted, and internally rotated. Palpation may reveal tenderness at the site of fracture or may reveal a dislocated femoral head. It is important to assess range of motion and stability with respect to flexion/extension, abduction/adduction, and internal/external rotation.

Knee

Asymmetry of the knees, particularly loss of the peripatellar groove, can indicate a joint effusion resulting from meniscal or ligamentous disruption. Palpation for joint effusion includes:

1. Testing for a fluid wave by tapping the lateral aspect of the knee while simultaneously compressing the medial and superior aspects.

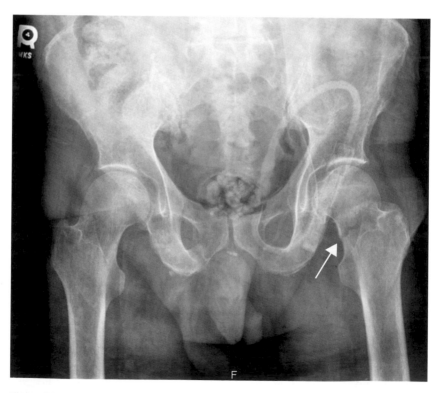

Figure 20.19
Left femoral neck fracture. AP X-ray of the pelvis demonstrating a trans-cervical fracture of the left femoral neck. *Courtesy*: S.V. Mahadevan, MD.

2. Ballottement of a patella "floating" in an effusion by pressing against the femoral condyle and eliciting a tapping sensation.

Additional landmarks important for palpation are the patella and fibular head (tenderness indicates suspicion for fracture), and the joint line (tenderness is suspicious for meniscal/collateral ligament injury). While an effusion may distort the anatomy of the affected knee, the position of the patella should be compared with that of the unaffected knee to rule out patellar dislocation, which almost always occurs laterally, or patellar fracture (Figure 20.20).

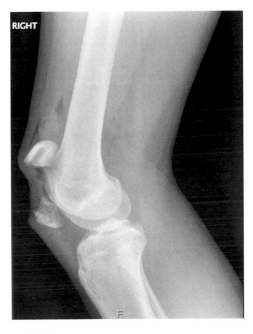

Figure 20.20
Patella fracture. Lateral X-ray of the knee with a transverse fracture of the patella, and significant retraction of the fracture fragments. *Courtesy*: S.V. Mahadevan, MD.

The anterior cruciate ligament (ACL) is commonly injured when the foot is planted and a lateral force or torsion is applied to the knee. It can be readily assessed by two maneuvers. The *Lachman test* (Figure 20.21) is performed with the patient supine and the knee flexed 20–30°. The examiner grasps the distal fibula with one hand and the proximal tibia with the other hand. The lower leg is given a brisk forward tug in an attempt to identify a discrete endpoint. A positive test (indicative of injury) occurs when no endpoint is appreciated or there is increased anterior translation of

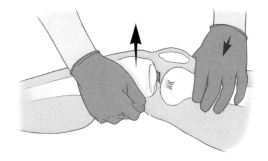

Figure 20.21
Positive Lachman test.

the tibia relative to the unaffected side. The *anterior drawer test* (Figure 20.22) is performed with the patient supine and the knee flexed to 90°. Both hands are placed around the proximal tibia with the thumbs approximated at the anterior tibial plateaus. The examiner quickly pulls anteriorly, without rotation, and feels for a discrete endpoint. The test is positive if no discrete endpoint is reached, especially compared to the unaffected side.

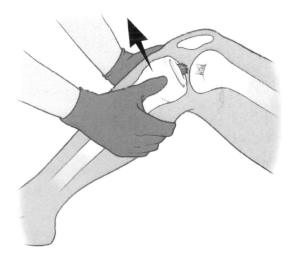

Figure 20.22
Positive anterior drawer test.

Posterior cruciate ligament (PCL) stability is commonly assessed by the *posterior drawer test*. This test is performed with the patient supine and the knee flexed to 90°. There are two different ways it may be performed. The first is the opposite of the anterior drawer test. Absence of a discrete endpoint with posterior force applied to the tibia is considered positive. The second approach is positive if anterior force applied to the tibia corrects a posterior subluxation or "sag" of the affected knee.

Integrity of the menisci is assessed by the McMurray test and the Apley compression test. The *McMurray test* is performed with the patient supine and the examiner grasping the medial aspect of the affected knee with one hand and the patient's heel with the other hand. A valgus force is generated and the tibia internally rotated as the knee is moved from a fully flexed position to full extension. The test is repeated while externally rotating the tibia. Any "popping" or pain along the joint line is considered a positive test. The *Apley compression test* (Figure 20.23) is performed with the patient prone and the knee flexed to 90°. A downward force is generated along the long axis of the tibia while simultaneously externally rotating it. If pain is increased, the test is positive.

Injuries to the collateral ligaments are assessed by stress tests. The *valgus stress test* is performed with the patient supine and the knee in 20° of flexion. With one hand on the lateral aspect of the knee and the other on the foot, the examiner gently abducts and externally rotates the lower leg. Increased laxity compared to the unaffected side is considered a positive test for medial collateral ligament (MCL) injury. In the *varus stress test*, the examiner adducts and internally rotates the lower leg to assess the stability of the lateral collateral ligament (LCL).

Regardless of the maneuver attempted to diagnose ligamentous injury, pain and effusion may make adequate examination of the knee impossible. Analgesia prior to examination is important. If an adequate examination cannot be performed, the patient should be treated conservatively with a knee immobilizer and/or crutches. Expeditious follow-up for re-examination (once the swelling has decreased) should be arranged.

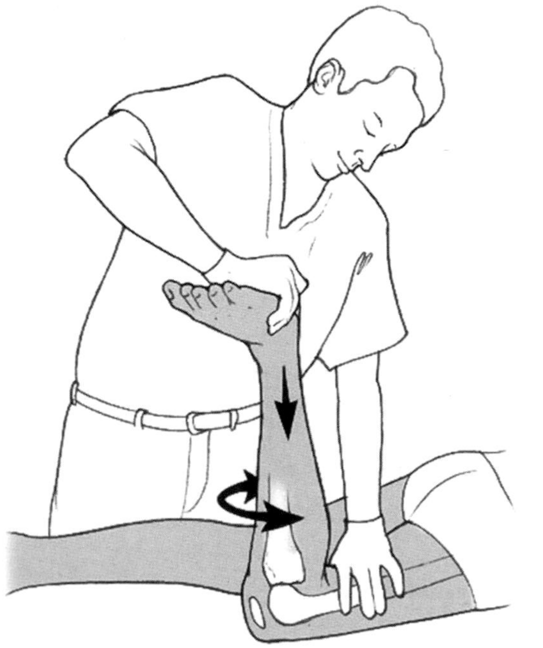

Ankle

Both ankle sprains and fractures may present with marked swelling and point tenderness. The major ligaments of the ankle are assessed by placing stress on them in an attempt to elicit instability. These maneuvers are frequently limited by soft tissue swelling and pain. Therefore, adequate analgesia and immediate application of rest, ice, compression, and elevation (RICE) assists in the ankle examination. If the examination is questionable or inadequate, and orthopedic consultation is not indicated, then conservative treatment and follow-up for repeat assessment (once swelling and pain has subsided) is appropriate.

The *anterior drawer test* (Figure 20.24) assesses the stability of the anterior talofibular ligament. The examiner exerts a downward force on the tibia while simultaneously attempting to "lift up" the foot while grasping behind the heel. A significant difference from the unaffected side (>2 mm) or dimpling of the anterior skin (suction sign) is considered positive.

Figure 20.23
Apley compression test.

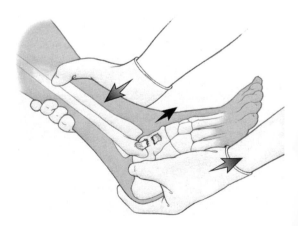

Figure 20.24
Positive anterior drawer test.

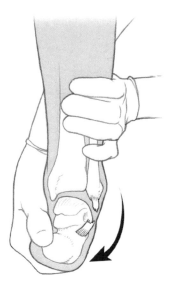

Figure 20.25
Positive talar tilt test.

The *talar tilt test* (Figure 20.25) may also be used to assess the integrity of the anterior talofibular ligament. The examiner plantar flexes and inverts the patient's ankle; an increase in laxity compared with the unaffected side is considered a positive test.

Any tenderness over the medial aspect of the ankle warrants an examination of the proximal fibular head to assess for a possible Maisonneuve fracture. A result of external rotation of the ankle, the Maisonneuve fracture is a spiral fracture of the fibular head found in association with fractures of the medial malleolus or deltoid ligament injury (Figure 20.26).

Integrity of the Achilles tendon is assessed by the *Thompson test*. The examiner squeezes the calf with the patient prone. If the foot does not plantar flex, the test is positive for Achilles tendon disruption.

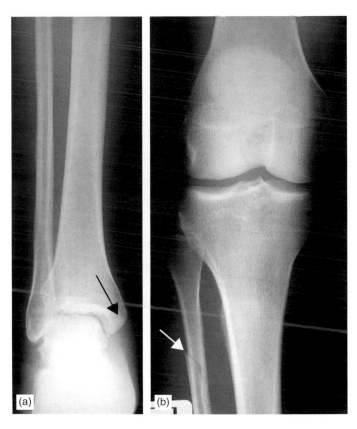

(a) (b)

Figure 20.26
Maissoneuve fracture. (a) AP radiograph of the ankle showing a small avulsion fracture of the medial malleolus, with widening of the mortise joint and (b) a spiral fracture of the proximal fibula. *Courtesy*: Kathryn Stevens, MD.

Foot

Care must be taken to assess the foot separately from the ankle. While the deformity of dislocated metatarsophalangeal or interphalangeal joints may be obvious, fractures may present with only minimal swelling and point tenderness. Stress fractures occur most commonly in the second and third metatarsals and often cannot be seen on initial radiographs. Injury to the base of the fifth metatarsal may be seen with inversion injuries of the ankle (Figure 20.27). Injuries to the calcaneus are associated with a fall onto the feet or with a severe twisting mechanism, and result in heel pain and soft tissue swelling. In falls which produce axial loading, a careful search for coincident lower extremity injuries and compression fractures of the thoracolumbar spine should occur. The Lisfranc injury (Figure 20.28) is a tarsometatarsal dislocation that occurs when there is a direct axial load on a foot that is plantar flexed. Radiographs are often negative, although a fracture of the base of the second metatarsal is pathognomonic. Any examination revealing tenderness at the tarsometatarsal joint or base of the second metatarsal should prompt the clinician to consider a Lisfranc injury.

Diagnostic testing

Radiographs

Radiographs are important in evaluating extremity trauma. By revealing the nature of a fracture or dislocation, they assist in decisions regarding the need for reduction or operative repair, the length of time required for immobilization, or potential complications during rehabilitation. However, indiscriminate use of radiographs for extremity pain leads to higher health care costs, unnecessary radiation exposure, and increased length of stay in the ED. Therefore, the challenge to the emergency physician is to order radiographs *when appropriate*. Research on judicious film utilization in patients with extremity injuries continues to evolve. The Ottawa ankle, foot, and knee rules (Table 20.8) represent guidelines

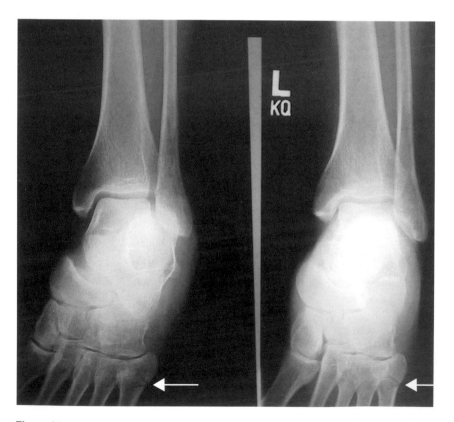

Figure 20.27
5th metatarsal fracture. AP views of the left ankle showing a fracture of the base of the fifth metatarsal. *Courtesy*: S.V. Mahadevan, MD.

derived from high-quality evidence in large studies.

Once the decision is made to order radiographs, the clinician should follow several important principles. First, it is important to formulate a presumptive diagnosis based on history and examination. Some injuries, such as a scaphoid fracture or posterior shoulder dislocation, may require special visualization techniques not included in a normal series. Also, injuries such as a scaphoid fracture, non-displaced radial head fracture, and metatarsal stress fracture may not be apparent on initial films. If these injuries are suspected, patients should be treated as though they have such an injury despite negative radiographs, and appropriate follow-up for repeat

imaging should be arranged. The use of weight-bearing films to diagnose a Lisfranc injury or acromioclavicular (AC) separation is often not feasible in a busy ED; conservative treatment and follow-up radiographs are appropriate for these patients.

The clinician should also ensure that the radiographs taken are adequate to visualize structures of concern. At least two views, taken perpendicular to one another, are necessary for most bones and joints. Sometimes a third (oblique) view may be necessary. A fracture of a long bone is often associated with a nearby dislocation or additional fracture along the shaft; therefore, films should include the joints above and below the injury. Finally, if any reduction has been attempted,

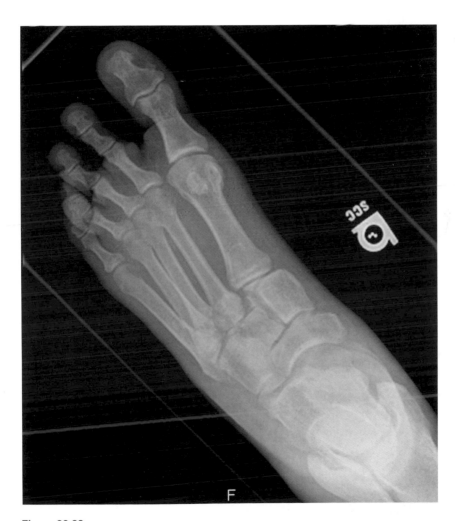

Figure 20.28
Lisfranc fracture-dislocation. DP oblique radiograph of the left foot showing fractures through the bases of the second and third metatarsals, and lateral dislocation of the metatarsals. *Courtesy*: Kathryn Stevens, MD.

Table 20.8 Ottawa rules for extremity radiographs

Ottawa ankle rules
Order ankle radiographs only if the patient has ankle pain and either of the following:
1. Inability to bear weight for four steps, both immediately and in the ED
2. Bone tenderness at the posterior edge or distal 6 cm of either medial or lateral malleolus

Ottawa foot rules
Order foot radiographs only if the patient has foot pain and either of the following:
1. Inability to bear weight for four steps, both immediately and in the ED
2. Bone tenderness at the navicular or base of the fifth metatarsal

Ottawa knee rules
Order knee radiographs only if the patient has knee pain and any of the following:
1. Age 55 years or older
2. Isolated tenderness of the patella
3. Tenderness over the head of the fibula
4. Inability to flex to 90°
5. Inability to bear weight for four steps, both immediately and in the ED

post-reduction films should be ordered after the extremity is splinted to assess adequacy of reduction and identify small fractures which might have been initially obscured.

Description of fractures

Once a fracture is visualized on the radiograph, it is essential that the emergency physician communicate to a consultant the location and nature of the injury. An accurate verbal description will enable the consultant to make an informed decision regarding disposition and indications for operative repair. The terms below are commonly used by orthopedists in fracture description and therefore facilitate communication.

Exposure

Perhaps the most important description, and therefore the first that should be mentioned, is whether the fracture is open or closed. An *open fracture* is exposed to the environment and often requires parenteral antibiotics as well as operative repair. The bone may be obviously protruding through the skin or there may be only a small laceration overlying the fracture. It is therefore important to clean and thoroughly examine the extremity for skin integrity. A *closed fracture* is present when the skin overlying a fracture is intact.

Location

Description of fracture location can involve both general anatomic terms and landmarks specific to a particular bone. Fractures of long bones can be described as being either *midshaft* or in the *proximal* or *distal thirds*. Describing the length of the fracture from either the proximal or distal end provides additional information.

Specific anatomic descriptions exist for a variety of fractures; often this nomenclature is used because these fractures may require operative repair or because of specific associated complications. Examples include *intertrochanteric* and *femoral neck* fractures of the femur, and *supracondylar* fractures of the humerus.

Orientation

Figure 20.29 illustrates nomenclature based on the direction of the fracture line. A *transverse* fracture runs perpendicular to the long axis of the bone. *Oblique* fractures run at an angle to the long axis of the bone, usually between 45 and 60°. A *spiral* fracture results from torsion on the bone. A *comminuted* fracture consists of more than two fracture fragments, often in a "shattered" pattern. A *segmental* fracture consists of a single free-floating fracture fragment between two fracture lines.

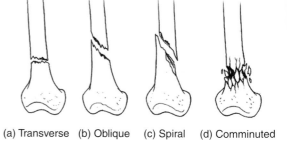

(a) Transverse (b) Oblique (c) Spiral (d) Comminuted

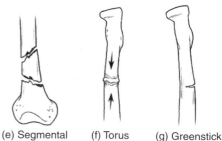

(e) Segmental (f) Torus (g) Greenstick

Figure 20.29
Fracture orientation.

Two fracture patterns found in pediatric populations deserve special mention. A *torus* fracture is demonstrated by "buckling" of the bone cortex, whereas a *greenstick* fracture is an incomplete fracture with disruption of only one cortical aspect on the radiograph.

Displacement

Displacement refers to the amount of offset of a fracture fragment as expressed in millimeters or percent. It is may be modified by the anatomic direction in which the distal fragment is displaced. In the Figure 20.30a the tibia fracture is fifty percent laterally displaced.

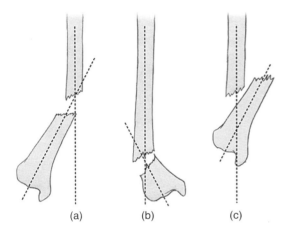

Figure 20.30
Fracture displacement and angulation.

Separation/shortening

Separation refers to the distance by which two fragments have been pulled apart. Shortening refers to the distance by which the bone's length has been reduced. Shortening occurs as a result of impaction of one fragment into another, or as a result of complete displacement allowing one fragment to "slide over" the other. It is measured in millimeters or centimeters.

Angulation

Angulation describes the relationship between the long axes of the respective fracture fragments. The direction of angulation is determined by the apex formed by these two axes; Figure 20.30b demonstrates a fracture with 30 degrees of lateral angulation. Figure 20.30c demonstrates a fracture with 30 degrees of medial angulation, 100 percent

displacement, and shortening of an undetermined length.

Joint involvement

The clinician must pay particular attention to fractures located near any joint. A fracture that enters the joint is termed *intra-articular* and deserves special attention by the consultant. In addition, fractures near a joint may be associated with a dislocation. Such fracture–dislocations often require operative repair; therefore, joint alignment should always be assessed prior to communicating with a consultant.

General treatment principles

As with any patient presenting to the ED, initial assessment of extremity trauma begins with the Airway, Breathing, and Circulation (ABCs). In isolated extremity trauma, circulation deficits, as indicated by diminished or absent pulses, may be the most worrisome initial finding. If an obvious deformity is present, immediate reduction with appropriate analgesia should be performed in an attempt to restore circulation. Once a patient can answer questions reliably and clinical suspicion for other injuries "masked" by the pain of the extremity injury is sufficiently low, treatment can be focused on the affected limb.

Analgesia should be administered as soon as possible to patients who are hemodynamically stable. Options include local anesthesia, regional nerve blocks, and parenteral analgesia. In cases requiring extremely painful maneuvers such as reduction, conscious sedation should be used. Oral analgesia should never be given until the need for immediate operative repair or conscious sedation is ruled out.

Fractures and dislocations can undergo reduction by the emergency physician, depending upon individual proficiency. Most emergency physicians are comfortable reducing the majority of dislocations, but any reduction with which the clinician is not familiar or that is unsuccessful requires orthopedic consultation. *Fractures or dislocations with signs of neurovascular compromise should undergo emergent reduction in the ED*, even before radiographs are obtained.

The majority of extremity injuries require immobilization, especially following reduction. Appropriate immobilization reduces pain by decreasing movement, inflammation, and the chance of bleeding. Casts are rarely applied in the ED, as patients generally present after an acute injury, and continued swelling confined by a hard cast may lead to compartment syndrome. Therefore, the preferred method of immobilization in the ED is non-circumferential splinting. Individual injuries require specific splinting techniques; a summary of common injuries and appropriate immobilization is listed in Table 20.9.

Several general principles apply to patients with extremity trauma. RICE (rest, ice, compression, elevation) remain effective in reducing swelling and discomfort for the patient, and should be started in the ED. Ice should never be applied to exposed skin; a towel placed underneath the ice pack prevents skin damage. The extremity should be elevated (above the level of the heart, if possible), and the use of gentle compression with an elastic bandage augments venous and lymphatic drainage.

Special patients

Pediatric

Children present with a different set of injuries following extremity trauma owing to their developing bones being more pliable. Unique fractures such as torus, buckle, and greenstick have already been discussed. Of particular concern are fractures involving the growth plate, as they may result in lifelong morbidity. Injuries to the growth plate are classified according to the involvement of metaphysis, epiphyseal plate, and epiphysis.

The Salter-Harris classification consists of five different types of growth plate fractures based on the location of the injury (Figure 20.31). In general, the higher the number, the worse the prognosis. *Salter Type I* fractures are through the epiphyseal plate. *Salter Type II* fractures are the most common and involve a fracture of the metaphysis with extension through the epiphyseal plate (Figure 20.32). *Salter Type III* fractures extend from epiphysis into the epiphyseal plate. *Salter Type IV* fractures involve a fracture through the metaphysis, epiphysis, and epiphyseal plate. *Salter Type V* fractures are crush injuries to the epiphyseal plate and are most common in the knee and ankle.

Any tenderness at a joint in pediatric patients should be treated conservatively, as they are more likely to suffer growth plate fractures than ligament sprains. Even in the setting of negative radiographs, the clinician should maintain a low threshold to treat with immobilization and obtain

Table 20.9 Extremity injuries and recommended immobilization

Injury	Immobilization
Shoulder dislocation	Sling and swathe
Rotator cuff tear	Sling and swathe
Acromioclavicular joint sprain	Sling
Clavicle fracture	Sling
Elbow dislocation	Long arm posterior splint
Supracondylar fracture	Long arm posterior splint
Radial head fracture	Sugar tong splint
Olecranon fracture	Long arm posterior splint
Subluxation of radial head	No post-reduction immobilization required
Midshaft ulnar fracture	Long arm posterior splint
Radial and ulnar fracture	Long arm posterior splint
Wrist fracture	Long arm posterior or sugar tong splint
Navicular fracture	Short arm thumb spica splint
Thumb metacarpal fracture	Short arm thumb spica splint
Metacarpal fracture	Ulnar gutter or radial gutter splint
Metacarpophalangeal joint dislocation	Short arm posterior splint
Ulnar collateral ligament tear	Short arm thumb spica splint
Phalangeal tuft fracture	Aluminum splint
Proximal phalanx fracture	Short arm posterior splint
Middle phalanx fracture	Aluminum splint or dynamic splinting
Interphalangeal joint injury	Aluminum splint

Adapted from Hamilton GC (ed.). *Emergency Medicine: An Approach to Clinical Problem-Solving*, 1st ed., Philadelphia: W.B. Saunders, 1991.

appropriate orthopedic follow-up for a presumed Salter-Harris fracture. In fact, given the presence of multiple ossification centers (six alone in the elbow), the clinician may actually "over-read" a

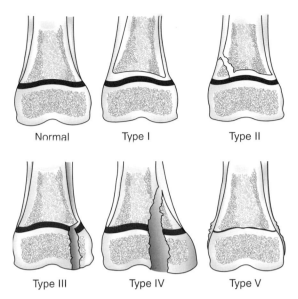

Normal   Type I   Type II

Type III   Type IV   Type V

Figure 20.31
Salter-Harris classification. Reproduced from
D. Mandavia et al, *Color Atlas of Emergency Trauma*,
Cambridge, Cambridge University Press, 2003.

fracture where there is not one present. If the
emergency physician is unfamiliar with pediatric
radiographs or a radiologist is not available, one
option may be to obtain plain films of the unaffected joint for comparison.

Elderly

Elderly patients are likely to have osteoporosis
and sustain fractures with even minimal trauma.
Falls are a source of considerable morbidity. The
threshold for ordering radiographs should be low.
Elderly patients may have substantial difficulties
wearing splints and using crutches. Social support
considerations and temporary care arrangements
may become necessary. Beware of occult hip fractures in the elderly patient with negative radiographs but significant pain on weightbearing.

Disposition

Although it is impractical to provide an exhaustive list of injuries requiring consultation for possible admission, in general, the following injuries
meet such requirements:

1. Open fractures
2. Open joint injuries
3. Vascular injuries
4. Hip fractures and dislocations
5. Compartment syndrome

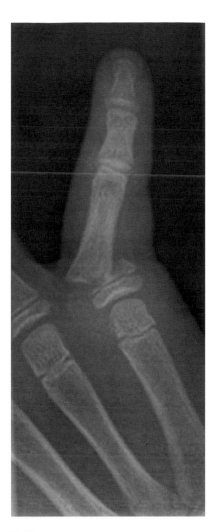

Figure 20.32
Salter-Harris 2 fracture. AP radiograph of the 5th digit
demonstrating a type II Salter-Harris fracture through the
base of the 5th proximal phalanx. *Courtesy:* Kathryn
Stevens, MD.

6. Dislocations or displaced fractures that
   cannot be reduced in the ED.

Any injury with which the clinician is not familiar
or comfortable mandates at least a phone consultation to secure adequate guidance and follow-up.
Depending on the nature of the injury, the patient
may require immobilization, non-weightbearing
status, or weightbearing as tolerated. Follow-up
may be with the primary care physician, orthopedic specialist, or hand surgeon.

As discussed earlier, RICE is the mainstay of
treatment for extremity injuries and should be
continued at home. Although rest is essential,
assistive devices such as crutches should be used

to ensure that a patient does not become bed-bound. Resumption of activities of daily living as early as appropriate is an important consideration.

Pain reduction to a tolerable level, not pain elimination, is a realistic goal while in the ED. Outpatient analgesic/narcotic combinations are often effective in maintaining adequate analgesia. Patients should be instructed to return for signs of neurovascular compromise, infection, pleuritic chest pain suggesting embolus, severe pain not controlled by appropriate analgesia, or a splint that feels too tight.

Pitfalls

- Failure to warn patients that some hairline or non-displaced fractures may not become apparent on radiographs until 7–10 days later.
- Failure to repeat radiographs when the affected area is inadequately visualized.
- Missed open fracture because the extremity is not inspected or cleaned adequately to reveal an overlying laceration.
- Missed foreign bodies due to inadequate irrigation and exploration.
- Missed tendon injury due to inadequate visualization and examination through the entire range of motion.
- Failure to document a complete neurovascular examination prior to administering local or regional anesthesia.
- Missed injuries due to focusing on obvious trauma without performing a complete physical examination.
- Failure to update tetanus immunization status in open fractures, or in extremity injuries in which skin integrity is compromised.

References

1. *Closed Injuries of the Upper Extremity* from Hamilton GC (ed.). *Emergency Medicine: An Approach to Clinical Problem-Solving*, 1st ed., Philadelphia: W.B. Saunders, 1991.
2. Harwood-Nuss A (ed.). *The Clinical Practice of Emergency Medicine*, 3rd ed., Philadelphia: Lippincott Williams & Wilkins, 2001 (Chapters are Approach to musculoskeletal injuries, Shoulder injuries, Elbow injuries, Hand, Wrist and elbow injuries, Hip injuries, Knee injuries, Injuries of the ankle and foot).
3. Hill S, Wasserman E. Wrist injuries: emergency imaging and management. *Emerg Med Prac* 2001:3(11).
4. Hill S, Wasserman E. Ankle injuries in the ED: how to provide rapid and cost-effective assessment and treatment. *Emerg Med Prac* 2002:4(5).
5. Marx JA (ed.). *Rosen's Emergency Medicine: Concepts and Clinical Practice*, 5th ed., St. Louis: Mosby, 2002 (Chapters are Wrist and forearm, Humerus and elbow, Shoulder, Injuries of the proximal femur, Knee and lower leg, Ankle and foot).
6. Roberts J, Hedges J (eds). *Clinical Procedures in Emergency Medicine*, 3rd ed., Philadelphia: W.B. Saunders, 1998 (Chapters are Management of common dislocations, Splinting techniques, Compartment syndrome evaluation).
7. Solomon DH, Simel DL, Bates DW, et al. The rational clinical examination. Does this patient have a torn meniscus or ligament of the knee? Value of the physical examination. *J Am Med Assoc* 2001;286(13): 1610–1620.
8. Tintinalli JE (ed.). *Emergency Medicine: A Comprehensive Study Guide*, 5th ed., McGraw Hill, 2000 (Chapters are Injuries to the bones, joints, and soft tissues, Musculoskeletal disorders in children).

21 Eye pain, redness and visual loss

Janet G. Alteveer, MD

Scope of the problem

Eye complaints are very frequent in the emergency department (ED), although the actual number of visits per year is not known. Patients may complain of redness, swelling, pain, foreign body sensation, flashing lights, floating spots, visual field defects, blurred and/or decreased vision. The diagnoses may be common and benign, such as allergic conjunctivitis, or uncommon and vision-threatening, such as acute angle closure glaucoma (AACG), corneal ulcers, or central retinal artery occlusion (CRAO). Careful attention to the history and physical examination helps delineate the problem and define the treatment.

Anatomic essentials

The bony structure of the orbit is formed by a confluence of the frontal, maxillary, and zygomatic bones. The walls of the orbit are referred to by their anatomic location: superior, inferior, medial, and lateral. The inferior orbital wall or plate is quite thin and often fractured following a direct blow to the globe or orbit. The eyelids, the lacrimal gland (tucked away under the upper lid), and the canalicular system that drains tears into the nasal cavity make up the adnexal structures of the eye (Figure 21.1).

The globe (Figure 21.2) is divided into two sections: the anterior and the posterior segment. The anterior segment includes the cornea, limbal conjunctiva, iris, anterior chamber, and the lens. The conjunctiva is a thin, transparent mucus membrane that covers the sclera (bulbar conjunctiva) and the inner surface of the eyelids (palpebral conjunctiva). The sclera is a tough layer of collagen and elastic fiber that surrounds the entire globe with the exception of the cornea. The sclera gives the eye its white appearance. The cornea is made up of a dense layer of collagen 500–600 μm thick. It consists of 5 layers including Bowman's and Decemet's membranes. The cornea is the anterior-most aspect of the eye. It is transparent and allows light to be transmitted and focused through the pupil. The iris is a diaphragm anterior to the lens and is responsible for eye color. It has two layers: the stromal and the pigmented layers. The iris has two sets of muscles: the constrictor and the dilator muscles, that are innervated by separate nerves. The pupil

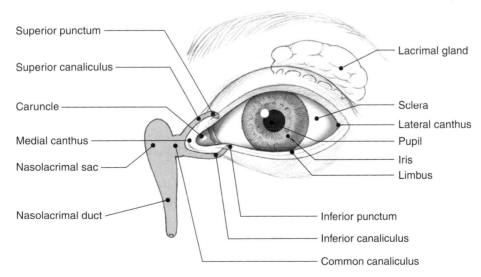

Figure 21.1
Anterior view of the eye and adnexal structures. Lacrimal gland is situated superotemporally. The superior and inferior puncta drain into the canalicular system, which eventually empties into the nasal cavity.

is the circular aperture in the iris that controls the amount of light entering the eye based upon the tone of the iris dilator and constrictor muscles. The trabecular meshwork, located anterior to the iris insertion in a circumferential pattern around the globe, filters and removes the aqueous humor; malfunction can result in elevated intraocular pressure (IOP). The *ciliary body*, located posterior to the iris in an inner-tube configuration circumferentially around the globe, has two main functions:

1. Production of aqueous humor, a transparent protein-free liquid contained in the anterior and posterior chambers that provides oxygen and nutrients to the avascular cornea and lens.
2. Control of accommodation by changing the shape of the crystalline lens. The lens sits behind the iris and is responsible for focusing light upon the retina. When the ciliary body contracts, the lens thickens, increasing the eye's ability to focus up close. When looking at a distant object, the ciliary body relaxes and the lens becomes thinner, adjusting the eye's focus for distance vision.

The lens thickens and becomes less compressible with age, and is the site of cataract formation. The lens also establishes the anterior boundary of the posterior chamber.

The posterior segment of the globe contains the vitreous humor, choroid, retina, and optic nerve. The vitreous humor is a clear hydrogel that fills the vitreous cavity. It is 98–99% water on a collagen framework. The choroid is the vascular structure between the sclera and the retina's pigmented epithelium. It is responsible for cooling the retina, which has a high metabolic rate and the highest blood flow per gram of tissue in the human body. The retina contains 10 layers and is a complex interplay of neuronal elements, supporting tissue, photoactive cells, and blood vessels. When the rods and cones absorb light energy, an electrical potential is created. This is then amplified and conducted through the optic nerve to the occipital cortex. The nerve fiber layer of the retina enters the optic disk of the optic nerve, makes a 90° turn posteriorly, and exits the globe. The optic disk (optic nerve head) is also referred to as the blind spot. The optic nerve is a bundle of myelinated nerve fibers that exits the globe through the superior orbital fissure.

The eye is under the influence of both the sympathetic and parasympathetic nervous systems. The sympathetic fibers exit the spinal cord with the T11–T12 outflow. These fibers then travel up the neck in the sympathetic plexus to the nasociliary and long ciliary nerves. These nerves innervate the dilator muscle of the iris. Increased sympathetic tone results in pupillary dilation. Horner's syndrome, an interruption of these sympathetic fibers, often by an apical lung tumor, results in pupillary constriction (miosis). The parasympathetic fibers travel to the eye via the oculomotor nerve and the ciliary ganglion.

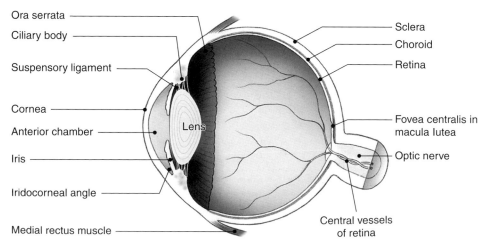

Figure 21.2
The globe in cross section. The iris diaphragm outlines the margins of the pupil. The anterior surface of the lens abuts the posterior surface of the iris. Zonular suspensory fibers are seen emanating from the ciliary body, adjacent to the iris root.

These fibers innervate the constrictor muscle of the iris. Increased parasympathetic tone causes pupillary constriction. Compression or injury of the oculomotor nerve results in pupillary dilation.

Table 21.1 Glossary of terms

Conjunctivitis	Inflammation of the conjunctiva
Keratitis	Inflammation of the cornea
Anterior uveitis	Inflammation of the iris and ciliary body (also called iritis)
Scleritis	Inflammation of the sclera
Episcleritis	Inflammation of the subconjunctival tissue and blood vessels
Blepharitis	Inflammation of the eyelids
Oculus dexter	Right eye
Oculus sinister	Left eye
Ocular uterque	Both eyes

History

Is your eye red?

Injection of the conjunctiva is a finding shared by many infectious, inflammatory, and allergic conditions. Eye redness alone does not distinguish vision-threatening from benign eye conditions.

Does your eye hurt? How would you describe the pain?

A sharp pain, accompanied by the sensation that something is in the eye, is characteristic of corneal foreign bodies, corneal abrasions, infections, or ulcers. Pain made worse by light or accommodation is typical of acute anterior uveitis. Deeper pain often accompanies inflammation of the sclera or anterior uvea. A deep boring pain made worse by movement of the eyeball is often present in optic neuritis, while severe pain accompanied by a headache on the same side is common in acute angle closure glaucoma (AACG). The absence of pain is significant – acute conjunctivitis is almost never painful.

Is your eye sensitive to light?

Photophobia and increased pain on exposure to bright light suggests anterior uveitis. It is caused by spasm of the ciliary muscle that may accompany corneal abrasions, blunt trauma to the eye, infections, or inflammatory processes. Certain corneal abrasions or keratitis may cause light sensitivity, as the incident light irritates the eye due to refraction.

How is your vision?

Benign conditions such as bacterial, viral, or allergic conjunctivitis generally do not affect visual acuity. Mild to moderate vision loss may accompany anterior uveitis, scleritis, herpes simplex virus (HSV), or herpes zoster virus (HZV) infections of the eye. Severe deficits in vision may occur with optic neuritis, AACG, central retinal artery occlusion (CRAO), central retinal vein occlusion (CRVO), central corneal abrasions, or ulcers. A halo around lights is characteristic of acute glaucoma, while loss of color vision is common in optic neuritis.

Have you noticed a discharge and what is it like?

A purulent discharge is pathognomonic of acute bacterial conjunctivitis. Patients often wake up with their lids and lashes crusted together, and may need to apply warm water to remove the crust and open their eyes. The discharge of gonococcal (GC) conjunctivitis is so profuse that it is described as welling up as soon as it is wiped away. By contrast, adenoviral infections produce a copious watery discharge. These patients often describe a clear puddle on their pillow. Chlamydia infection and certain types of allergic conjunctivitis produce a mucoid discharge. Neither scleritis, anterior uveitis, glaucoma, nor optic neuritis result in discharge. It is important to differentiate tearing in response to pain or light from discharge.

Is there any itching?

The presence of itching is a hallmark for an allergic process.

How long has your eye been bothering you?

Patients with a corneal foreign body or abrasion are usually able to tell you the moment their problem began. Acute angle closure glaucoma often occurs at night, or after emerging from a darkened location – dilation of the pupil in response to decreased light often precipitates the crisis. Bacterial conjunctivitis often occurs overnight.

A more indolent onset is typical of inflammatory processes, such as scleritis, uveitis, or optic neuritis.

Is it one eye or both eyes?

Corneal foreign body, abrasion, acute glaucoma, central retinal artery or vein occlusion, optic neuritis, periorbital and orbital cellulitis (respectively, POC and OC) generally develop in one eye. Conjunctivitis, both bacterial and viral, may start in one eye and rapidly spread to the other. Inflammatory conditions such as thyroid-related ophthalmopathy, scleritis, and allergic conjunctivitis are generally bilateral.

Have you had a recent exposure to someone with a red eye?

Adenoviral infections often present in epidemic form, often in schools, dormitories, military barracks, and swim clubs. HSV, gonorrhea, and chlamydia infections are transmitted via direct contact.

Do you wear contact lenses?

Contact lens wearers are at increased risk of corneal infections and ulcers (infectious keratitis or epidemic keratoconjunctivitis, EKC). A "simple" corneal abrasion in a contact lens wearer can progress overnight to a vision-threatening ulcer if the appropriate history is not obtained. Contact lens users are also at risk for rare parasitic infections.

Did you rub your eye?

Rubbing the eye may result in a mechanical corneal abrasion.

Were you hit in the eye?

Traumatic anterior uveitis may develop several days after a blow to the eye. These patients will complain of pain, tearing, and photophobia, but may forget to tell you about the trauma. Eye trauma accompanied by visual impairment is an ophthalmologic emergency.

What kind of work do you do?

Machinists, drill workers, those who do any type of metal-on-metal work are at risk for metallic foreign bodies. Welders, boaters, and skiers, particularly those who do not use proper eyewear, are at risk for ultraviolet (UV) burns to the cornea.

Are you using any eye drops?

Allergic conjunctivitis may develop from the use of certain eye preparations, particularly those containing neomycin. Patients who are on long-term topical steroid drops are at risk for glaucoma or cataracts.

Have you ever had this before?

Thirty percent of patients with HSV infection will have a recurrent episode. Allergic phenomena and some inflammatory conditions (such as scleritis or optic neuritis) can remit and recur.

Do you use eye make-up?

Contamination of mascara and liquid eyeliners may result from or occur due to bacterial or viral conjunctivitis. This is especially true with shared products. Patients with these conditions should be counseled to discard these products.

Have you had recent eye surgery?

Recent eye surgery has been associated with acute keratitis as well as endophthalmitis (a severe vision-threatening infection of the globe).

Do you have any chronic medical conditions?

Immunosuppression is associated with fungal infections. Rheumatoid arthritis and systemic lupus erythematosus (SLE) are associated with scleritis. There is an association between multiple sclerosis (MS) and optic neuritis.

Physical examination

The physical examination of the eye and surrounding structures is critical to narrowing the differential diagnosis. It needs to be conducted in a systematic fashion.

Vital signs

A complete set of vital signs is essential. Note whether the patient is febrile, tachycardic, or hypertensive. Patients with glaucoma may be dehydrated from the nausea and vomiting that often accompanies this condition. Fever may be a clue to an infectious process. Hypertension and visual loss may point to a vascular etiology.

Visual acuity

This is the vital sign of the eye and *must be recorded* on every patient with an eye complaint. It may be obtained using the following sequence.

Snellen eye chart

This standard chart, using progressively smaller letters, is found on a wall in every ED and many primary care offices. It should be used for all patients who are able to stand and follow simple instructions. Patients who regularly wear glasses (other than for reading) should wear them for the examination. This should be noted in the chart. Cover one eye and have the patient begin identifying the largest letters. Repeat with the other eye and then both eyes together. For non-readers a "tumbling E" chart may be used. Patients indicate with their hands which way the E is facing. A chart with pictures is often used for children and serves the same purpose. Note the smallest row in which the patient is able to correctly identify more than half the letters/symbols. Record the visual acuity as the number of this row under 20 (i.e., 20/30 OD, 20/40 OS, 20/30 OU).

Near chart

For those too sick to stand, a "near card" held 14 inches from the face may be used, following the same procedure as with the Snellen chart.

Pinhole testing or ophthalmoscope

If the patient wears corrective lenses and does not have them with him/her, or to ascertain if the visual deficit can be corrected mechanically, utilize pinhole testing or a handheld ophthalmoscope. Ask the patient to read the eye chart while looking through the pinhole or have the patient look at a near chart through a handheld ophthalmoscope. Ask the patient to "dial" the ophthalmoscope until they can see the letters and record the setting (i.e., 20/40 using lens −10). If either method corrects the visual deficit, the problem is optical and not pathologic.

Gross visual acuity testing

In patients with vision less than 20/400, gross visual acuity may be quantified in terms of the patient's ability to count fingers, detect hand motion (waving), or perceive light.

Orbit and adnexal structures

Inspect the orbits and the tissue around the eyes for redness, swelling, lesions (i.e., vesicular eruption from an HZV infection), and asymmetry. Proptosis (protruding eye) suggests that an orbital infection, inflammation, or tumor is forcing the eye forward (Figure 21.3). This condition is best assessed looking from above the head downward toward the eyes. Keratoconus differs from proptosis in that the cornea is cone-shaped while the globe does not protrude. Examine the eyelashes carefully for crusting, lashes pointing in the wrong direction, or lice.

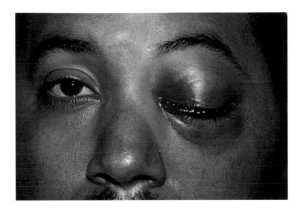

Figure 21.3
Orbital cellulitis. Presenting with massive swelling, chemosis, erythema, and poor ocular motility.
Reproduced with permission from Tasman W et al, Wills Eye Hospital Atlas of Clinical Ophthalmology, 2nd ed., Lippincott Williams & Wilkins, 2001.

Ocular motility

It is particularly important to evaluate the motility of the globe in cases of eye trauma, suspected infection, and double vision. While standing directly in front of the patient, have them hold their head still and follow your finger with their eyes. Study the movement of one eye at a time as you move your finger first up and down, and then from side to side. The extraocular muscles (EOMs) responsible for eye movements are innervated by cranial nerves III, IV, and VI (Figure 21.4, Table 21.2).

Entrapment of the inferior rectus muscle within a fracture of the inferior orbital plate may result from a direct blow to the eye. Orbital infection, tumor, inflammation, compression, or ischemia of the individual nerves anywhere from the eye to the brainstem, or by aneurysms of the circle of Willis, may result in diplopia. Monocular diplopia is usually the result of problems of the cornea, iris, lens, or retina of that particular eye, and is almost always pathologic.

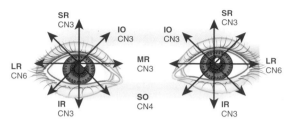

Figure 21.4
Depiction of extraocular muscle innervation by cranial nerves III, IV, VI, and the direction of eye movements that result with contraction of the different extraocular muscles. CN: cranial nerve; SR: superior rectus; MR: medial rectus; LR: lateral rectus; IR: inferior rectus; SO: superior oblique; IO: inferior oblique. *Source*: Figure 18.1, page 199, ISBN 0 521 00980 4, *Principles and Practice of Emergency Neurology*, Eds Shah SM, Kelly KM.

Table 21.2 Ocular motility

Nerve	Muscle	Lesion
Oculomotor (cranial nerve III)	Superior rectus Inferior rectus Medial rectus Superior oblique	*At rest*: eye deviated down and out *With activity*: unable to look up or adduct
Trigeminal (cranial nerve IV)	Inferior oblique	*At rest*: eye externally rotated (extorted) Patients tilt their head to compensate
Abducens (cranial nerve VI)	Lateral rectus	*At rest*: eye slightly adducted *With activity*: unable to abduct

Pupillary

Note the size, shape, and symmetry of the pupils and their reaction to direct light. An asymmetric or teardrop-shaped pupil following trauma may indicate injury to the iris or a ruptured globe. Topical medications can affect the size of the pupil. Sympathomimetic (tropicamide) and anticholinergic drops (homatropine or scopolamine), also known as *mydriatics*, will dilate the pupil. Beta blockers (timolol) and cholinergic preparations (pilocarpine), both called *miotics*, result in pupillary constriction.

The swinging flashlight test

The swinging flashlight test is used to test for "paradoxical" pupillary dilation in response to light. Abnormal results are referred to as a relative afferent pupillary defect (RAPD) or a Marcus–Gunn pupil involving the affected eye (Figure 21.5). This test is performed in a darkened room by shining a bright light in the patient's eye for 1–2 seconds followed by swinging the light to

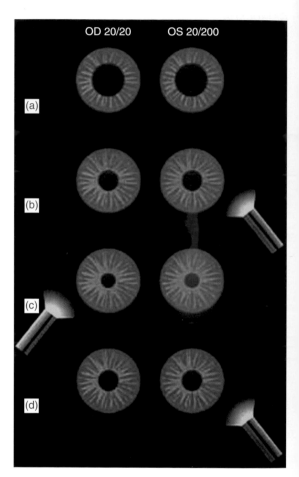

Figure 21.5
Relative afferent pupillary defect (RAPD). Vision in the right eye is 20/20, but vision in the left eye is 20/200 because of optic neuropathy. (a) The pupils in dim light are equal. (b) Light directed into the left eye results in a partial and sluggish contraction in each eye. (c) Light directed into the right eye results in a brisk and normal reaction in each eye. (d) The light quickly redirected into the left eye results in a dilatation of both pupils. It is possible to detect RAPD even in the presence of a dilated, dysfunctional pupil, as in a traumatic mydriasis or cranial nerve III palsy, by observing the other pupil. Reproduced with permission from Tasman W et al, Wills Eye Hospital Atlas of Clinical Ophthalmology, 2nd ed., Lippincott Williams & Wilkins, 2001.

stimulate the other eye, and then repeating the process in each eye. A normal physiologic response is constriction of the pupil with direct light stimulation. Pupillary dilation in response to direct light stimulation indicates an afferent (sensory) visual lesion, most commonly an optic neuropathy. Failure of pupil to constrict with either direct or consensual light stimulation indicates an efferent pupillary defect.

Anisocoria

Lesions that result in anisocoria (unequal pupils) include:

1. *Adie's tonic pupil*: A dilated pupil that responds poorly to direct light but will constrict with accommodation. The lesion is in the cranial nerve III ciliary ganglion, usually the result of a viral infection or local inflammation.
2. *Argyll–Robertson pupil*: A small irregular pupil that reacts poorly to light. It develops over months to years and is associated with central nervous system (CNS) syphilis.
3. *Horner's syndrome*: A miotic pupil that reacts to light. There is often accompanying ptosis of the lid of the affected side as well as anhydrosis of the ipsilateral face. It is the result of sympathetic denervation from apical lung tumors, trauma to the spinal cord, brainstem lesions, or syringomyelia.
4. *Essential anisocoria*: A small percentage of the population has unequal pupils of idiopathic etiology.
5. *Factitious dilated pupil*: Occasionally a patient will self-medicate with anticholinergic drops (scopolamine or homatropine). They will present with a fixed and dilated pupil. The administration of two drops of 1% pilocarpine can be diagnostic, as a "normal" pupil will constrict over 45 minutes, while a "medicated" pupil will remain dilated.

Visual fields

Visual field testing will detect disorders affecting the retina, optic nerve, optic chiasm, and visual cortex. Patients with visual complaints (irrespective of their visual acuity) should always be screened for visual field defects. Confrontational visual fields are measured for one eye at a time and can detect segmental retinal detachments (often a horizontal defect) or intracranial pathology (usually a vertical defect obeying the midline). Care must be taken to ensure that the non-examined eye of the patient is completely covered. The visual field examination may detect a central scotoma, common in optic neuritis, a localized defect due to a retinal detachment, or bitemporal hemianopsia indicative of a lesion affecting the optic chiasm, such as a pituitary tumor (Figure 21.6).

Anterior segment

General inspection and slit lamp examination will detect abnormalities of the anterior segment, including the conjunctiva, sclera, cornea, iris, lens, and anterior chamber. The conjunctiva and the sclera should be examined for discharge, injection, chemosis (swelling), or foreign bodies. When discharge is present, its amount, quality, and color should be noted. The pattern of erythema (generalized vs. focal) should also be noted. Acute conjunctivitis usually results in diffuse erythema, while cases of anterior uveitis present with redness largely around the cornea (perilimbic erythema). The white sclera may become very thin in scleritis, resulting in a bluish hue to the eye.

Topical anesthetics

Patients with eye pain, infection, inflammation, or foreign body often require the application of a topical anesthetic to facilitate the examination. Instill a few drops of a preparation such as 0.5% proparacaine in the inferior palpebral sulcus. Prompt relief of symptoms following application of a topical anesthetic is almost diagnostic of a corneal abrasion. Never dispense a topical anesthetic for outpatient use; extended application has been associated with persistent corneal defects, infections, ulcers, and increased risk of additional trauma.

Eyelid eversion

After instillation of a topical anesthetic, the eyelids should be everted to look for adherent foreign bodies. With the patient looking down, apply a cotton-tipped applicator to the mid-portion of the upper lid. Gently grab the upper lashes and pull the eyelid over the applicator. When the patient then looks up, this action reverses the eversion.

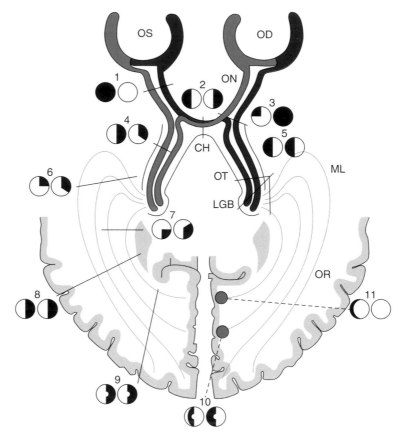

Figure 21.6
Schematic illustration of the **visual pathway** and **visual field defects** produced by lesions in various areas of the pathway. ON, optic nerve; CH, chiasm; OT, optic tract; LGB, lateral geniculate body; ML, Meyer's loop; OR, optic radiations. (1) Compromise of the left optic nerve results in a central scotoma in the left eye, with a normal right visual field. (2) A lesion of the optic chiasm may cause a bitemporal hemianopia. (3) A lesion at the junction of the right optic nerve and the chiasm results in a central scotoma in the right eye and a superior visual field defect that respects the vertical meridian in the left eye. This effect results from compromise of the inferior nasal crossing fibers from the left eye, which extend into the prechiasmal portion of the right optic nerve (i.e., Wilbrand's knee). The resulting visual field defect is known as a junctional scotoma, which is localized at the junction of the optic nerve and chiasm. (4) Complete interruption of the optic tract produces a homonymous hemianopic field defect. Subtotal lesions produce highly incongruous homonymous hemianopias. (5) Complete interruption of the optic tract, lateral geniculate body, and optic radiations results in a total contralateral homonymous hemianopia. (6) Fibers originating in the ipsilateral inferior temporal retina and the contralateral inferior nasal retina sweep anteriorly and laterally around the temporal horn (i.e., Meyer's loop) before transversing posteriorly. As a result, lesions of the temporal lobe characteristically produce superior, often incongruous homonymous quadrantanopias. (7) Parietal lobe lesions may interrupt visual pathway fibers from the superior retinas pursuing a more direct posterior course. This results in an inferior homonymous quadrantanopia. (8) Complete interruption of the optic radiations results in contralateral total homonymous hemianopia. (9) Posterior occipital lobe lesions result in homonymous hemianopic defects, which may spare the macula. Subtotal occipital lesions produce exquisitely congruous visual field defects because the fibers are more highly segregated in the occipital area. (10) Lesions affecting the posterior portion of the occipital lobe may spare the more anteriorly placed unpaired crossing peripheral nasal retinal fibers, resulting in a preserved temporal crescent in an otherwise congruous homonymous hemianopia. (11) Focal lesions involving the anterior-most portion of the occipital lobe may affect the receptive area for the unpaired crossing fibers from the contralateral nasal retina, resulting in a unilateral peripheral temporal visual field defect. Reproduced with permission from Tasman W et al, Wills Eye Hospital Atlas of Clinical Ophthalmology, 2nd ed., Lippincott Williams & Wilkins, 2001.

The slit lamp examination

The ideal method of examining the cornea, the iris, and the anterior chamber is the slit lamp microscope because it allows magnification of these structures. Normally, the anterior chamber is optically clear. However, careful inspection under magnification may reveal proteinaceous debris (flare), red blood cells (hyphema), or purulent exudate (hypopyon). Flare resembles a motion projector beam in a dark smoky room. The presence of cells and flare in the anterior chamber is commonly associated with anterior uveitis (also known as iritis or iridocyclitis).

The oblique flashlight test

This test estimates the depth of the anterior chamber of the eye, and may demonstrate a narrow or closed angle in AACG (Figures 21.7 and 21.8).

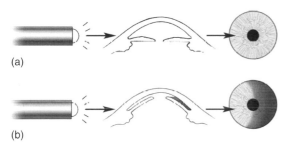

(a)

(b)

Figure 21.7
Oblique flashlight test: (a) normal and (b) shallow anterior chamber.

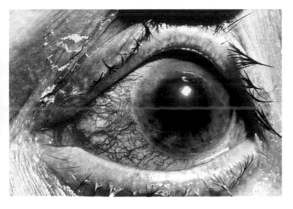

Figure 21.8
Acute angle closure glaucoma. Typical external appearance of acute angle closure caused by pupillary block, with diffuse hyperemia of the conjunctiva, mid-dilated pupil, and steamy cornea. The intraocular pressure is 64 mmHg. Reproduced with permission from Tasman W et al, Wills Eye Hospital Atlas of Clinical Ophthalmology, 2nd ed., Lippincott Williams & Wilkins, 2001.

A penlight is held to the side of the patient's head, with the beam parallel to the iris and shining across the anterior chamber. If the entire iris is illuminated, the "angle" is open. If there is a shadow projected on the nasal part of the iris, the "angle" is narrow or closed. If the cornea of the affected eye is too hazy to perform this test effectively, perform it on the other eye. While AACG usually occurs in only one eye, both eyes will have "narrow" or "closed" angles.

Fluorescein staining

The cornea should be examined for clarity, surface irregularities, and foreign bodies. Fluorescein dye is used to identify epithelial defects of the cornea. After the application of a topical anesthetic, a fluorescein-coated strip is lightly applied to the lower conjunctival sulcus, and the patient is asked to blink a few times. The damaged corneal epithelium picks up the dye and fluoresces brightly when the cornea is examined with a cobalt blue light (Figure 21.9). The slit lamp provides superior

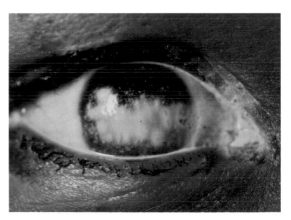

Figure 21.9
Corneal abrasion. A large traumatic corneal abrasion stains brightly with the cobalt blue light after topical fluorescein instillation. *Courtesy:* Lawrence Stack, MD.

visualization of any epithelial defects. Fluorescein staining will identify scratches from a foreign body, corneal ulcers (Figure 21.10), as well as the "grape-like clusters" of herpetic infections (dendrites) (Figure 21.11). Removal of contact lenses prior to the application of fluorescein will prevent permanent staining.

Posterior segment (fundoscopy)

Fundoscopy is rarely useful in the evaluation of the red eye; however, it may identify the cause of visual loss or eliminate possible etiologies. The fundoscopic examination may be facilitated by dilation of the pupils with topical mydriatics (e.g., tropicamide) or cycloplegics (e.g., cyclopentolate). Prior to inducing pupillary dilation, patients should have a complete pupillary examination and be screened for contraindications to dilation of the pupil, such as suspicion of globe rupture, history of angle closure glaucoma, or narrow anterior angles.

Fundoscopy may reveal abnormalities of the retina, optic nerve, or vitreous cavity. A diminished red reflex may result from corneal edema, cataract formation, vitreous hemorrhage, or a large retinal detachment. A classic (late) finding in Central Retinal Artery Occlusion (CRAO) is a pale retina with a "cherry red spot" indicating the spared blood supply to the fovea (Figure 21.12). Venous congestion and hemorrhage may be evident in Central Retinal Vein Occlusion (CRVO), with the retina being described as having a "blood and thunder" appearance (Figure 21.13). Some patients with optic neuritis may present with edema of the optic disk. The fundoscopic evidence of a retinal detachment may explain a patient's sudden visual loss (Figure 21.14). Any patient with acute vision loss thought to be due to posterior segment disease should be referred immediately to an ophthalmologist for a further evaluation.

Intraocular pressure

A portable Tonopen (electronic tonometer), Schiotz pressure tonometer, or applanation tonometer (part of the slit lamp microscope) can be used by non-ophthalmologists to measure

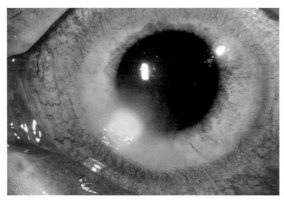

Figure 21.10
Corneal ulcer. Infected corneal ulcers are characterized by corneal infiltrates associated with overlying epithelial defects and an anterior chamber reaction. This ulcer caused by Staphylococcus aureus extends toward the center of the cornea and is associated with surrounding corneal edema. Reproduced with permission from Tasman W et al, Wills Eye Hospital Atlas of Clinical Ophthalmology, 2nd ed., Lippincott Williams & Wilkins, 2001.

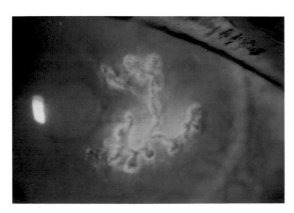

Figure 21.11
Herpetic simplex dendrites. The hallmark of herpes simplex keratitis is the dendrite, a branching, epithelial ulceration with swollen, raised edges and terminal bulbs. Reproduced with permission from Tasman W et al, Wills Eye Hospital Atlas of Clinical Ophthalmology, 2nd ed., Lippincott Williams & Wilkins, 2001.

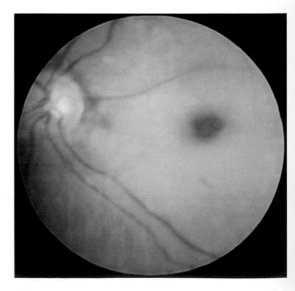

Figure 21.12
Central retinal artery occlusion. An acute central retinal artery obstruction with superficial retinal whitening and a cherry red spot in the fovea. Reproduced with permission from Tasman W et al, Wills Eye Hospital Atlas of Clinical Ophthalmology, 2nd ed., Lippincott Williams & Wilkins, 2001.

IOP. These techniques require topical anesthesia prior to direct application of the device over the surface of the cornea. Measurement of IOP is therefore contraindicated in cases of globe rupture or infections. Normal IOP's range between 12 and 21 mmHg. People who have pressures between 21 and 30 mmHg with normal optic disks have ocular hypertension. While any value over 30 mmHg is abnormal, a measurement of greater than 50 mmHg suggests acute glaucoma.

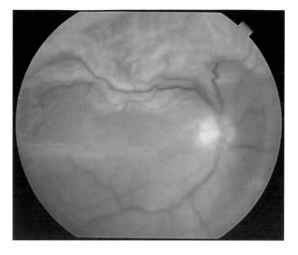

Figure 21.14
Retinal detachment. Corrugated, opaque appearance of the detached retina in a patient with rhegmatogenous retinal detachment. Reproduced with permission from Tasman W et al, Wills Eye Hospital Atlas of Clinical Ophthalmology, 2nd ed., Lippincott Williams & Wilkins, 2001.

General physical

The general physical examination is used to assess the overall health of the patient and is important to search for clues to the nature of the eye problem. Joint deformities may indicate a connective tissue disease, while signs of malnourishment may indicate chronic or acute immunosuppression. The skin should be examined for lesions that may indicate systemic infection or autoimmune disorders.

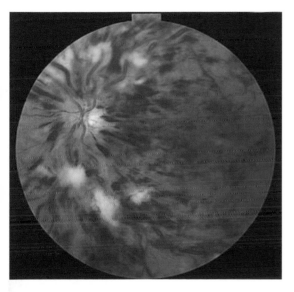

Figure 21.13
Central retinal vein occlusion. Fundus examination shows dilated and tortuous retinal veins, a swollen optic disc and retinal hemorrhages. Reproduced with permission from Tasman W et al, Wills Eye Hospital Atlas of Clinical Ophthalmology, 2nd ed., Lippincott Williams & Wilkins, 2001.

Differential diagnosis

Tables 21.3 and 21.4 describe causes of the red eye and etiologies of visual change or vision loss, respectively.

Table 21.3 The red eye

Diagnosis	Symptoms	Signs	Workup
Acute angle closure glaucoma	Severe unilateral eye pain, decreased vision, halos around lights. May have nausea/vomiting, headache, abdominal pain or constitutional symptoms.	Red eye; hazy ("steamy") cornea; mid-dilated, minimally reactive pupil. Elevated IOP (>50 mmHg).	Evaluate other eye for shallow anterior chamber. Measure IOP using tonometry (Tonopen, Schiotz, or applanation). Consult an ophthalmologist immediately.

(continued)

Table 21.3 The red eye (*cont*)

Diagnosis	Symptoms	Signs	Workup
Acute anterior uveitis (iritis, iridocyclitis)	Pain, tearing, photophobia, and mildly decreased vision (may have history of trauma several days before).	Marked perilimbal conjunctival injection (ciliary flush); "cells" (WBCs) and "flare" (protein) may be visible in the anterior chamber on slit lamp examination.	None if unilateral, first occurrence. Refer to an ophthalmologist for a further workup.
Allergic conjunctivitis	Itching, burning, redness, and tearing.	Inflamed and watery eye, may have chronic changes on the lids and/or conjunctivae.	None.
Bacterial conjunctivitis (non-gonococcal)	Redness and mucopurulent discharge from one eye, then the other; foreign body sensation; normal or decreased vision.	Diffuse conjunctival injection, purulent discharge, pre-auricular node formation.	Culture and sensitivity of discharge (for severe or refractory cases).
Blepharitis	Eye irritation, foreign body sensation, crusting, and swelling of the lids.	Chronic scaling, edema, or erythema of lid margins. May have abnormal apposition of lids.	None.
Chalazion	Typically painless slowly-growing erythematous nodule of the eyelid.	Lump usually located on the conjunctival portion of eyelid; often an incidental finding.	None.
Chlamydial conjunctivitis	Redness and mucoid discharge, foreign body sensation.	Looks like viral conjunctivitis; follicular conjunctival changes.	Chlamydia culture. Refer to an ophthalmologist immediately.
Corneal abrasions	Sudden-onset of excrutiating pain, tearing, photophobia; decrease in vision, foreign body sensation.	Conjunctival injection, blepharospasm, light sensitivity, and corneal defect on fluorescein staining.	Evert the lids to search for retained foreign body. Topical anesthetics provide immediate pain relief.
Corneal ulcers	Pain, decreased vision, foreign body sensation, photophobia.	Focal white corneal infiltrate. Raised borders and crater with slit lamp exam. Intense staining with fluorescein if there is an epithelial defect.	Corneal scrapings for smear and culture. Refer to an ophthalmologist immediately.
Dacrocystitis	Pain, redness, swelling over the lacrimal sac; may have tearing, discharge, and fever; may be recurrent. Associated with nasolacrimal duct obstruction.	Erythematous, tender swelling over nasal aspect of lower eyelid; a purulent discharge may be expressed with gentle compression.	Culture and sensitivity of discharge. Refer to ophthalmologist.
Episcleritis	Acute localized redness and mild pain in one or both eyes.	Localized engorgement of episcleral blood vessels; may be a small nodule.	Topical phenylephrine 2.5%, may reduce the redness and differentiate it from scleritis.
Gonococcal conjunctivitis	Redness, acute onset, and profuse purulent discharge.	"Angry eye": bloody conjunctival injection and red swollen lids; "waterfall of pus": the discharge is so copious, it reaccumulates after wiping.	GC culture and Gram's stain. Refer to an ophthalmologist immediately.
Herpes simplex keratitis	Irritation, tearing, decreased vision, and photophobia; may have history of previous episodes.	Decreased visual acuity; decreased corneal sensation in 80% (test blink reflex with cotton applicator). Characteristic dendrites on fluorescein staining.	Refer to an ophthalmologist immediately.

(continued)

Table 21.3 The red eye (cont)

Diagnosis	Symptoms	Signs	Workup
Herpes zoster ophthalmicus	Eye pain, redness, and decreased vision. May have prodrome of HA, fever and malaise.	Pseudodendrites on fluorescein staining. Vesicular lesions on the tip of the nose (Hutchinson's sign) suggest ocular involvement.	Refer to an ophthalmologist immediately.
Hordeolum	Localized pain and swelling of one eyelid.	Localized swelling of eyelid, sometimes with "pointing" inside lid or on lid margin.	None.
Orbital cellulitis	Similar to POC; may have headache, blurred vision or diplopia.	Similar to POC, but testing EOMs may produce pain. May also have proptosis, restricted ocular motility and decreased vision.	CT scan to evaluate the extent of orbital involvement and to prepare for possible surgical debridement. Refer to an ophthalmologist immediately.
Periorbital cellulitis	Swelling, redness, and pain around one eye.	Unilateral swelling, redness, and tenderness around the eye, including the lids. Often with fever.	CT scan to rule out spread to the orbit and to evaluate the sinuses.
Scleritis	Severe boring eye pain, redness, and decreased vision.	Inflammation of scleral, episcleral and conjunctival blood vessels. If severe, the bluish hue can be seen.	Evaluate for underlying connective tissue disease. Refer to an ophthalmologist immediately.
Superficial keratitis (UV keratitis, Welder's flash)	Pain, redness, tearing, and photophobia; may have history of UV light exposure.	Conjunctival injection. Fluorescein staining may show pinpoint corneal epithelial defects.	None.
Viral conjunctivitis	Redness, burning and watery discharge; often profuse; normal vision. May have had a recent URI or contact with someone with a red eye.	Diffuse conjunctival injection; red, edematous eyelids; watery discharge; pre-auricular node.	Contact precautions for 2 weeks, consider DFA for adenovirus.

CT: computed tomography; DFA: direct fluorescent antibody; EOMs: extraocular muscles; GC: gonococcus; HA: headache; IOP: intraocular pressure; POC: periorbital cellulitis; URI: upper respiratory tract infection; UV: ultraviolet; WBC: white blood cell.

Table 21.4 Visual change or vision loss

Diagnosis	Symptoms	Signs	Workup
Central retinal artery occlusion	Sudden painless vision loss.	Severe vision loss. Afferent pupillary defect. Pale edematous retina with cherry red spot (late).	Refer to an ophthalmologist immediately. Obtain ESR in elderly patients to evaluate for giant cell arteritis.
Amaurosis fugax	Transient sudden, painless, monocular vision loss. Vision often returns prior to ED visit.	Hollenhorst plaque (embolus composed of cholesterol) variably present in the retinal circulation. Exam may be normal.	Search for the source of the embolus: ECG, echocardiogram and carotid doppler. Obtain ESR in elderly patients to evaluate for giant cell arteritis.

(continued)

Table 21.4 Visual change or vision loss (*cont*)

Diagnosis	Symptoms	Signs	Workup
Binocular diplopia	Present when both eyes are open. May occur when looking in only one direction. Resolves with closing either eye.	May have abnormalities on EOM examination. May have signs of external eye trauma.	Evaluate for diabetes, thyroid disease, and neuromuscular disorders (myasthenia gravis, botulism). CT scan of the oribit and brain (especially in cases of trauma). MRI for suspicion of brainstem lesion. MRA for suspicion of circle of Willis aneurysm.
Central retinal vein occlusion	Abrupt or gradual decrease in vision.	Mild to very severe vision loss. Retinal hemorrhages, dilated veins in four quadrants with optic disc edema.	Evaluate for hypertension, DM, ASCVD, and hyperlipidemia, glaucoma.
Functional vision loss	Varies from blurry vision to complete vision loss, monocular or binocular.	Normal examination: normal pupillary light reflex, normal optokinetic testing.	Psychiatric consult. Consider ophthalmology consult.
Monocular diplopia	Double vision in one eye.	May see cataract or dislocated lens.	Evaluate for refractive error involving the patient's contact lenses or bifocal glasses. Inquire about trauma, eye surgery, flashing lights or floating spots (retinal detachment, posterior vitreous detachment).
Optic neuritis	Progressive visual loss – over hours to days. Periorbital pain, worse with movement of eye. Alterations in color vision. Age <50.	Decreased visual acuity. Normal disk although 1/3 may have disc edema. Afferent pupillary defect.	MRI within 2 weeks for possible MS. Tests for Lyme, syphilis, toxoplasmosis. Refer to an ophthalmologist immediately.
Retinal detachment	Sudden onset of light flashes or floaters; a "curtain" or "shade" descending over a field of vision. Visual loss or a visual field defect.	Pigmented cells in the vitreous, vitreous detachment, retinal detachment, or retinal break. An afferent pupillary defect may be present.	Refer to an ophthalmologist immediately.
Temporal arteritis	Sudden painless visual loss. May have unilateral headache, pain with chewing (jaw claudication), proximal muscle and joint aches (polymyalgia rheumatica), weight loss, anorexia, or fever. Rare under 65 years of age.	Afferent pupillary defect; devastating visual loss; pale, swollen optic disc. May have tenderness over the temporal artery.	ESR (usually >100) must be >50. Temporal artery biopsy. Refer to an ophthalmologist immediately.
Vitreous hemorrhage	Sudden painless visual loss. Visual "floaters" or "cobwebs."	Decreased or absent red reflex, pigmented cells in the vitreous.	Evaluate for DM, trauma, leukemias, thrombocytopenia. Refer to an ophthalmologist immediately. Evaluate for retinal break or detachment.

ASCVD: arteriosclerotic cardiovascular disease; CT: computed tomography; ECG: electrocardiogram; ED: emergency department; EOM: extraocular muscle; DM: diabetes mellitus; ESR: erythrocyte sedimentation rate; MRA: magnetic resonance angiography; MRI: magnetic resonance imaging; MS: multiple sclerosis.

Diagnostic testing

Laboratory studies

Very few laboratory tests are used in evaluating the red eye (Table 21.3) or acute visual loss (Table 21.4).

The red eye

1. A *Gram's stain* may be useful for GC conjunctivitis, but is rarely helpful in other cases of conjunctivitis.

2. A *corneal culture* and *scraping* is useful in the evaluation of a corneal ulcer, but bacterial sensitivities often do not correlate with the clinical response.
3. *Blood cultures* may be useful in defining the infectious agent in orbital cellulitis.
4. Specific blood tests for collagen vascular disorders or autoimmune diseases may be useful in the evaluation of scleritis.

Vision loss

1. *Erythrocyte sedimentation rate (ESR)*: This test should only be ordered if the clinical suspicion of temporal (giant cell) arteritis is high. Ask the patient about the nature and location of headache; presence of scalp tingling, jaw claudication, temporal artery tenderness and throbbing; unexplained weight loss in the presence of visual acuity loss or field defect. In this scenario, a erythrocyte sedimentation rate greater than 50 in an older individual in the clinical setting of headache and/or visual change is highly suggestive of temporal arteritis.
2. *Electrolytes, blood urea nitrogen (BUN), creatinine*: A patient with AACG may have electrolyte abnormalities or dehydration from nausea and vomiting.
3. *Glucose, lipid profile*: Diabetes and hyperlipidemias are associated with CRAO.

Radiologic studies

Computed tomography (CT) of the brain, orbits, and sinuses may be useful in delineating infectious, inflammatory, and malignant processes. CT will differentiate between a POC (superficial) and OC (deep). It will also define any co-existing conditions, such as sinusitis, abscess, or tumor.

Magnetic resonance imaging (MRI) is often used to evaluate for optic neuritis, primarily to look for demyelinating lesions of Multiple Sclerosis (MS). As many as 40% of individuals determined to have MS initially present with symptoms of retrobulbar or optic neuritis. In this setting, the MRI does not have to be done emergently. MRI is contraindicated in patients with metallic intraocular or intraorbital foreign bodies because of the risk of further injury from movement of these objects.

General treatment principles

Treatment of eye disorders is predicated on the specific diagnosis.

The red eye

Common disorders not requiring specialty care.

Allergic conjunctivitis

Treatment depends on the etiology. For example, in individuals sensitive to cat dander, avoidance of the allergen may be all that is required. Topical over-the-counter vasoactive drops, oral antihistamines, or both may help in the short run. Mast cell stabilizer ophthalmic drops are effective, but usually take 2 weeks to exert any effect.

Bacterial conjunctivitis

While generally considered benign and self-limited, the course of bacterial conjunctivitis can be shortened by the use of broad-spectrum topical antibiotics. Inexpensive drops such as sulfacetamide or gentamicin are perfectly acceptable. The decision of which agent to use is based on cost, availability, local resistance patterns, and local practice. Neomycin preparations should be avoided because of the high incidence of allergic conjunctivitis.

Blepharitis

Treatment includes a daily regimen of lid hygiene, including warm compresses, lid massage, and cleaning of the lids with diluted (1:10) baby shampoo.

Chalazion

Warm compresses for 15 minutes 4 times daily. The use of antimicrobial ointments is controversial; they are not recommended in ophthalmology texts, but are commonly used in practice. Steroid injection and elective excision should be left to the ophthalmologist.

Corneal abrasions

Corneal abrasions are commonly treated with a short-course of topical broad spectrum antibiotic ointment and short-acting topical cycloplegics (cycopentolate). Topical non-steroidal anti-inflammatory drug (NSAID) preparations significantly reduce the pain associated with corneal abrasions. Oral narcotic pain medications may also be prescribed for patient comfort. Corneal abrasions associated with contact lens use should not be patched due to an increased risk of *Pseudomonas* infections. These corneal abrasions should be treated with broad-spectrum topical antibiotics with good anti-pseudomonal coverage (gentamicin, polymixin/bacitracin, or tobramycin). Tetanus status should be investigated and updated as needed. Under no circumstances should the patient be prescribed outpatient topical anesthetics.

Episcleritis

Topical or oral NSAIDs are often effective for episcleritis.

Hordeolum (stye)

Warm compresses as for chalazion. Topical antibiotics should be prescribed if the inflammation extends beyond the immediate area of the stye. Surgical drainage with an 18-G needle or No. 11 blade may speed resolution if the hordeolum is already pointing, but runs the danger of scarring if done incorrectly (i.e., on the external lid surface). Only if the stye is pointing directly into the lid margin and affecting vision should it be drained, and only by someone with experience.

Superficial keratitis

Broad-spectrum topical antibiotics, cycloplegics (if associated anterior uveitis is present) and oral pain medication usually control the symptoms and generally prevent complications.

Viral conjunctivitis

There is no specific treatment for viral conjunctivitis. Adults who are capable of good hygiene may return to work if they have a negative direct fluorescent antibody (DFA) test to the viruses which cause EKC. In the presence of a positive DFA for EKC, the patient should remain off work for 2 weeks to control the spread of this debilitating disease. Children who cannot wash their hands meticulously need to be kept home from school.

The following conditions threaten vision and require immediate consultation.

Acute angle closure glaucoma

If untreated, acute angle closure glaucoma will result in blindness. The initial treatment targets lowering the IOP. Accepted components of acute medical therapy include topical beta blockers (timolol 0.5%), low-dose parasympathomimetics (pilocarpine 0.2%), topical steroids (prednisolone 1%), topical alpha-2-agonists (apraclonidine 0.5%), and oral or IV acetazolamide. Acetazolamide should be avoided or given with caution in patients with significant pulmonary disease because of the combined effects of metabolic and respiratory acidosis. IV mannitol is effective in lowering IOP, but is relatively contraindicated in patients with congestive heart failure (CHF) or renal failure because of the significant osmotic load. Immediate consultation with an ophthalmologist is necessary. Reduction of the IOP may take hours, and repeated installation of medications to achieve lowering of IOP is mandatory, under close management by an ophthalmologist.

Anterior uveitis

Topical steroids are the mainstay of therapy. As steroids (Prednisolone) themselves are associated with complications (cataract formation, glaucoma, and pupillary abnormalities), they should only be prescribed after consultation with an ophthalmologist. Intermediate-acting cycloplegics, such as homatropine or scopolamine, are used to alleviate ciliary spasm, which is responsible for much of the pain associated with anterior uveitis.

Corneal ulcers

Immediate referral to an ophthalmologist is necessary. Never attempt to treat a suspected corneal ulcer without ophthalmologic consultation. The medicolegal ramifications of undertreated disease are profound.

Gonococcal conjunctivitis

These patients often require parenteral antibiotics (Ceftriaxone), ocular saline lavages, and daily ophthalmologic evaluations.

Herpes zoster keratitis

Oral antivirals and topical antibiotics (to prevent a secondary bacterial infection) are used to treat the skin lesions of HZV ophthalmicus. Topical antivirals have not been shown to be effective.

Topical steroids are used if anterior uveitis or deep stromal keratitis is present, although only following direct consultation with an ophthalmologist. As 50% of division I trigeminal nerve HZV infections involve the cornea and have the potential for scarring, these cases should be referred to an ophthalmologist.

Herpetic simplex keratitis

For disease limited to the epithelium, either topical (trifluridine, vidarabine, idoxuridine) or oral antivirals (acyclovir, famcyclovir, and valacyclovir) are effective in the vast majority of cases. When corneal ulcers are present, both an oral and a topical agent are used. Steroid preparations should be used only in consultation with an ophthalmologist. Oral acyclovir at prophylactic doses has been shown to prevent recurrences of HSV eye disease.

Suspected globe rupture/perforation

Shield the eye immediately and discontinue the examination. This condition is a surgical emergency that threatens the entire globe. Care should be rapidly transferred to an ophthalmologist.

Visual change or vision loss

Most of these conditions require immediate or urgent ophthalmologic consultation.

Central retinal artery occlusion

Few interventions have much effect on the generally poor outcome from CRAO. While awaiting the arrival of the ophthalmologist, some low-risk (and potentially beneficial) actions may be taken. Ocular massage (5 seconds on 5 seconds off) for 15–30 minutes may manually dislodge the clot. Rebreathing carbon dioxide (CO_2) by breathing into a paper bag may result in vasodilation of the central retinal artery. Acetazolamide IV has also been advocated as it may lower IOP. Paracentesis of the anterior chamber is no longer recommended as a therapeutic intervention by an emergency practitioner.

Central retinal vein occlusion

No specific medical therapy is effective for CRVO. Surgery and thrombolytic therapy are still considered experimental. Some patients may be candidates for laser surgery. An ophthalmologist should be involved in the care of patients with CRVO.

Optic neuritis

IV methylprednisolone 250 mg 4 times daily for 3 days improves the short-term visual outcome, and may slow the progression of MS over the subsequent 2 years. Oral prednisone is contraindicated because of adverse visual outcomes. Always consult with an ophthalmologist or neurologist.

Retinal detachment

Suspected retinal detachments should be urgently referred to an ophthalmologist. No specific sight-saving therapy can be instituted in the ED. Identification of the problem and urgent consultation are the major services that the emergency physician can offer the patient.

Temporal (giant cell) arteritis

The suspicion of temporal arteritis and the presence of visual symptoms warrants the administration of oral or parenteral steroids prior to the establishment of a definitive diagnosis by temporal artery biopsy. This condition warrants immediate ophthalmologic referral.

Special patients
Pediatric

1. *Neonatal conjunctivitis*: Caused by GC and HSV acquired during passage through the birth canal; can be vision- and life-threatening. Requires a full septic workup, admission, IV antibiotics and antivirals. Chlamydia infection, acquired in the same manner, is more benign and can be treated as an outpatient.
2. *Periorbital* or *orbital cellulitis*: Since the advent of the *Haemophilus influenzae* type B (HIB) vaccine, POC or OC have become much less common. As *H. Influenza* has an aggressive nature largely due to hematogenous spread, a full septic workup and IV antibiotics are recommended for suspected cases of POC or OC. In the post-HIB era, POC or OC has largely become associated with sinusitis or contiguous spread from trauma or skin infections. In patients over the age of 12 months, and in the absence of orbital or intracranial involvement, POC may be

treated as an outpatient if the parents are compliant and reliable follow-up can be arranged. OC still requires urgent referral and admission.

3. *Kawasaki disease*: A multisystem disease occuring primarily in children under 8 years. Bilateral conjunctival injection that spares the perilimbic area is one component of the disease. The incidence of coronary artery aneurysms, a cause of significant morbidity, can be significantly reduced by the administration of IV gamma globulin and high-dose aspirin.

4. *Acute dacrocystitis (AD)*: Neonates, infants, and small children with AD require admission for IV antibiotics covering *Staphylococcus* and *Streptococcus* bacterial species. These patients also require ear, nose, and throat (ENT) or ophthalmologic consultation for nasolacrimal duct probing. Cases associated with facial fractures may require stenting of the duct. Adults with AD may be discharged on oral antibiotics and warm compresses with next day follow-up.

5. *Congenital nasolacrimal duct obstruction* and *chronic dacrocystitis*: Chronic duct obstruction usually resolves by 1 year of age and is managed by instructing the parents to "milk"

the sac and duct, which may improve drainage. Chronic dacrocystitis requires topical antibiotics and subsequent referral to an ophthalmologist.

6. *Suspected shaken baby syndrome (child abuse)*: Ophthalmology consultation should be obtained to look for retinal hemorrhages, which are pathognomonic for shaken baby syndrome in the appropriate setting.

Immune compromised

Patients with diabetes, hematologic malignancies, those on immunosuppressive drugs, and generally debilitated individuals are susceptible to mucormycosis, an aggressive fungal infection. This infection begins in the sinuses and spreads contiguously to the orbits. Mucormycosis presents as a unilateral swelling of the eye, accompanied by proptosis and decreased vision. Treatment is surgical debridement and IV antifungal agents. Immediate ophthalmologic referral is essential (Table 21.5).

Disposition

See Table 21.5.

Table 21.5 Ophthalmologic referral of disposition

Disease	Emergent ophthalmology consult	Urgent ophthalmology consult	"Next day" ophthalmology consult	Admission
Acute angle closure glaucoma	Yes			Yes
Anterior uveitis			Yes	No
Corneal abrasion		Yes (in contact lens wearer)	Yes	No
Corneal ulcer	Yes			If compliance issues
CRAO	Yes			Yes
CRVO		Yes		Yes
GC conjunctivitis	Yes			Often, depends on compliance
Globe rupture/perforation	Yes			Yes
HSV keratitis	Yes			Not usually
HZV keratitis	Yes			Not usually

(*continued*)

Table 21.5 Ophthalmologic referral of disposition (*cont*)

Disease	Emergent ophthalmology consult	Urgent ophthalmology consult	"Next day" ophthalmology consult	Admission
Neonatal conjunctivitis	Yes if <1 month of age			Yes, if GC or HSV
Optic neuritis		Yes (<24 hours)		IV steroids if <72 hours onset
Orbital cellulitis	Yes			Yes
Periorbital cellulitis			Yes	If <12 months, toxic compliance issues
Retinal detachment	Yes			No
Scleritis		Yes	Yes	No
Temporal arteritis (with visual changes)		Yes		Yes (IV steroids)

CRAO: central retinal artery occlusion; CRVO: central retinal vein occlusion; GC: gonococcus; HSV: herpes simplex virus; HZV: herpes zoster virus.

Pearls, pitfalls, and myths

Pearls

- Pay attention to the history, it will often point you in the right direction.
- Remember to ask about chronic conditions, sexual contacts, job-related exposures, and trauma.
- Do not forget the vital sign of the eye, the visual acuity.
- Age-related vision loss: <50 years, optic neuritis; >65 years, temporal arteritis.

Pitfalls

- Do not patch corneal abrasions associated with contact lens use.
- Do not confuse a herpetic dendrite with a corneal abrasion.
- Remember to measure IOP in an older patient with sudden onset of unilateral eye pain and redness; it may be due to acute angle closure glaucoma.
- Remember to look under the lids for a foreign body in patients with corneal abrasions.
- Be wary of iris prolapse in the setting of ocular trauma, which may have the appearance of a corneal foreign body.
- The use of any steroid preparation in the eye should be done with extreme caution and only following direct consultation with an ophthalmologist.
- Patients with corneal abrasions or injuries should **never** be prescribed (or go home with) topical anesthetic preparations.

Myths

- All patients with red eyes and tearing need topical antibiotics. Viral conjunctivitis requires only attention to hygiene, and allergic conjunctivitis may respond to antihistamines, vasoactive drops, or mast cell stabilizers. Only patients with a purulent discharge should be treated with a short course of broad-spectrum topical antibiotics.
- Patching corneal abrasions are a necessary part of treatment. This common practice is controversial as several studies have demonstrated no improvement in relief of pain with patching abrasions less than 10 mm in size. Patching the eye is specifically contraindicated in contact lens wearers.

References

1. Alteveer JG, McCans KM. The red eye, the swollen eye, and acute vision loss: handling

non-traumatic eye disorders in the ED. *Emerg Med Pract* 2002;4(6).

2. Alward WLM. Medical management of glaucoma. *New Engl J Med* 1998;339(18):1298–1307.

3. Barone SR, Aiuto LT. Periorbital and orbital cellulitis in the *Haemophilus influenzae* vaccine era. *J Pediatr Ophthalmol Strab* 1997;34(5):293–296.

4. Cuculino GP, DiMarco CJ. Common ophthalmologic emergencies: a systematic approach to evaluation and management. *Emerg Med Rep* 2002;23(13).

5. Harwood-Nuss A (ed.). *The Clinical Practice of Emergency Medicine*, 3rd ed., Philadelphia: Lippincott Williams and Wilkins, 2001.

6. Laskowitz D, Liu GT, Galetta SL. Acute visual loss and other disorders of the eyes. *Neurol Clin* 1998;16(2):323–353.

7. Leibowitz HM. The red eye. *New Engl J Med* 2000;343(5):345–351.

8. Mahadevan SV, Savitsky E. Emergency management of traumatic eye injuries. *Trauma Rep* 2001;2(4).

9. Marx JA (ed.). *Rosen's Emergency Medicine: Concepts and Clinical Practice*, 5th ed., St. Louis: Mosby, 2002.

10. Morgan A, Hemphill RR. Acute visual change. *Emerg Med Clin North Am* 1998;16(4):825–843, vii.

11. Schein OD. Contact lens abrasions and the nonophthalmologist. *Am J Emerg Med* 1993;11(6):606–608.

12. Shah SM, Kelly KM (eds). *Principles and Practice of Emergency Neurology: Handbook for Emergency Physicians*, 1st ed., Cambridge University Press, 2003.

13. Shovlin JP. Orbital infections and inflammations. *Curr Opin Ophthalmol* 1998;9(5):41–48.

14. Tintinalli JE (ed.). *Emergency Medicine: A Comprehensive Study Guide*, 5th ed., McGraw Hill, 2000.

15. Wald ER. Conjunctivitis in infants and children. *Pediatr Infect Dis J* 1997;16(suppl. 2):S17–S20.

Eye pain, redness and visual loss

22 Fever in adults

Tamas R. Peredy, MD and Gus M. Garmel, MD

Scope of the problem

Accounting for 5–10% of all adult emergency department (ED) visits, fever is ubiquitous to the human experience. It is popularly felt to be either harmful in and of itself or a sign of an underlying serious disease. Most often young, previously healthy adults suffer self-limited illnesses that are well-tolerated and respond to symptomatic therapy. Morbidity and mortality from infectious causes of fever rise sharply with age. As opposed to children whose temperature elevations are overwhelmingly likely to be due to infection, adults have a broader differential of both infectious and noninfectious etiologies. Responses to elevated body temperature readings in the ED must first be taken in the context of the stability of the patient and then regarding the presumptive cause. Fever may not always be a component of initial concern but may be identified on measurement of the initial vital signs. Patients may also present with a history of feeling "feverish" that has resolved spontaneously or with home therapy. Disease entities that are being considered in febrile patients cannot be ruled out simply by the momentary absence of fever.

Pathophysiology

It is important to distinguish whether a high temperature is from a fever (defined as a deliberate hypothalamus-controlled reflex elevation of body temperature) or hyperpyrexia (an uncontrolled heat accumulation overwhelming compensatory mechanisms). This distinction is typically not difficult but has important immediate diagnostic and therapeutic implications. Antipyretics are ineffective in hyperpyrexia, while rapid cooling of a patient with a febrile response may intensify the body's efforts to reach the new set point temperature.

In order to define fever, an understanding of "normal" temperatures and the circadian cycle is necessary. A healthy, unclothed adult can maintain euthermia within 1°F (0.5°C) in dry ambient air between 55°F and 140°F (13–60°C). Sample populations exhibit ranges of baseline temperatures between 97.6°F and 99.4°F (36.4–37.4°C) +/− 0.7°F (0.4°C). Women experience well-known menstrual cycle-related temperature changes. Healthy elderly persons do not have lower core temperatures as is popularly believed.

Temperatures vary throughout the day by as much as 3.6°F (2°C) from a trough mean oral temperature of 97.6°F (36.4°C) from 4–6 a.m. to a peak mean of 99.4°F (37.4°C) between 4 and 10 p.m. The lower limit of an abnormally elevated oral temperature may thus be considered 100°F (37.8°C). Taking into account thermometer precision, fever is conservatively defined as a temperature of at least 100.4–101°F (38–38.5°C). It is generally believed that the fever response has a physiologic upper limit between 105.8°F and 107.6°F rectally (41–42°C). Infectious causes rarely lead to hyperpyrexia and collapse of compensatory thermoregulatory mechanisms in the normal host.

Systemic fever response

Normally, body temperature is controlled within a narrow range that predictably varies over the course of a day. Compensatory mechanisms ensure thermal homeostasis through autonomic nervous control by inducing changes in smooth muscle tone, shunting blood flow to and away from peripheral vascular beds, and provoking heat-seeking or heat-avoidance behaviors. Exogenous substances such as bacterial cell wall components (lipopolysaccharides), bacterial breakdown products, endotoxins, drugs, immune complexes, and activated complement factors induce polymorphonuclear cells to release a group of endogenous pyrogenic cytokines. These cellular mediators, known as interleukins (IL)-1 and IL-6, tumor necrosis factor (TNF), and interferon G induce the production of prostaglandin E2 (PGE2) by endothelial cells. In a vascular area near the preoptic nucleus of the anterior hypothalamus, PGE2 diffuses the short distance to the neurons of the thermoregulatory center. Upon stimulation, efferent discharge increases peripheral heat-generating processes until a new temperature set point is established. The thermoregulatory center is also influenced directly by toxic or hormonal mediators, or by direct central nervous system (CNS) insult. Cyclooxygenase

(COX) inhibitors that suppress fever by blocking synthesis of PGE2 include aspirin, acetaminophen, non-steroidal anti-inflammatory drugs (NSAIDs), and COX-2 selective inhibitors.

Clinically, chills (or less frequently rigors) subside within minutes of reaching the newly-established febrile set point. During the fever peak, adults may experience a mild delirium that is more prominent in the elderly. Myalgias and arthralgias represent increased muscle tone and circulating inflammatory mediators. The hypermetabolic state causes an acceleration in pulse (increased 10 beats/min/°F) and respiratory rate. Defervescence brings about predominantly heat-dissipating processes, including sweating, facial flushing, and the sense of being uncomfortably warm. Experimental models confirm that fever-inducing agents introduced directly into the bloodstream can generate clinical signs within minutes (Table 22.1).

The orchestrated febrile response enhances host defense mechanisms by increasing neutrophilic migration and T-cell proliferation (cellular immunity). Tissue levels of antiviral interferon and TNF are also increased (humoral immunity). Antibacterial substances such as cytotoxic-free radicals are generated by polymorphonuclear cells (PMNs) in greater quantity. Iron, a bacterial growth substrate, is sequestered. Metabolism is shifted away from glucose toward increased protein and fatty acid breakdown.

This transiently more protective state comes at a cost to the host. For each degree Fahrenheit of temperature rise, the basal metabolic rate is increased 7%. Increased caloric demands are compounded by increased utilization of less efficient protein and fat fuels. Tissue oxygen demands are also elevated despite a temperature-induced shifting of the oxygen-hemoglobin dissociation curve to the right. Tachycardia occurs from a combination of direct catecholamine stimulation and relative dehydration, as circulation shifts to the periphery. The most vulnerable organ to heat injury is the CNS. Subtle damage is first detected as a mild delirium, especially in the elderly. Convulsions, solely as a result of fever, are rarely seen in adults.

Hyperpyrexia

Hyperpyrexia represents a critical imbalance of heat-producing and heat-dissipating processes, and should be considered at temperatures above 105°F (40.5°C). Spiraling temperature elevations can occur from excess heat generation, impaired heat loss, or a direct CNS insult. The mechanism of heat rise in hyperpyrexia is independent of pyrogenic cytokine production and does not involve resetting of the thermoregulatory set point. Antipyretics are ineffective. Clinically, high temperatures are not seen until compensatory mechanisms have failed. It is important to act quickly to correct the heat imbalance before irreversible neurological injury, rhabdomyolysis, cardiac dysrhythmias, and circulatory collapse occur (Table 22.2).

Table 22.1 Common causes of fever

Infectious	Noninfectious
Viruses	Allergic reactions
Bacteria	CNS injury
Fungi	Inflammatory conditions
Parasites	Medications
	Neoplasm
	Hyperthyroidism
	Thromboembolic disease

Table 22.2 Causes of hyperpyrexia

Excess heat	Impaired heat loss	CNS dysfunction
Exertional heat stroke	Classic heat stroke	CNS trauma
Delirium tremens	Phenothiazines	Tumor
Stimulant abuse	Anticholinergics	Encephalitis
Salicylism	Spinal cord injury	Stroke
Thyroid storm	Bundling	
Pheochromocytoma		
Status epilepticus		
Neuroleptic malignant syndrome		
Malignant hyperthermia (anesthetic)		
Muscle tetany		
Serotonin syndrome		
CNS: central nervous system.		

Local fever response

Inflammatory stimuli activate a cascade of cellular and cytokine changes that assume control of local homeostatic mechanisms at the site of the affected body part. These changes manifest in a characteristic but site-specific fashion. If local control is not soon achieved, a systemic febrile response may result. This spillover is more likely in areas with a high concentration of immunologically-active cells or that are richly vascular.

Classically described changes of the local inflammatory response have been appreciated for centuries. These include *rubor* (erythema from vasodilatation), *dolor* (activation of pain fibers), *calor* (local temperature increase), and *tumor* (swelling or edema). Drainage of purulent material may also signify infection.

History

Patients presenting with fever represent a potential exposure risk to the health care team. Policies of universal precautions including glove, gown, and face-shield use must be strictly adhered to, in order to prevent direct blood-borne pathogen-laden fluid contact. Indirect contact via stethoscope, thermometer, bed railing, or aerosolized droplet may transmit disease. Additional measures such as patient isolation or the use of a negative pressure room are necessary for highly contagious diseases (e.g., active tuberculosis, SARS, Ebola).

The amount of history-gathering prior to the initiation of treatment must be tailored to the severity of illness and the potential for life-threatening processes (Tables 22.3 and 22.4).

How long have you been sick? What was your temperature, and how did you take it? Have you appreciated a daily fever pattern?

General characteristics of the fever pattern, magnitude, and duration may be of some clinical value. Continuous fevers are seen in lobar Gram-negative pneumonias, rickettsial disease, typhoid fever, and CNS disorders. Intermittent relapsing fevers are characteristic of endocarditis, osteomyelitis, and deep tissue abscesses. The amplitude or maximum temperature reading is an insensitive sign for distinguishing a viral from bacterial source. Patients with high fevers tend to appear more ill and have a higher overall incidence of serious bacterial illness. Purulent complications of common viral upper respiratory tract illness, such as sinusitis, otitis or pneumonia often manifest following a prodrome of 3–10 days. Fevers greater than 2 week's duration should prompt an appropriate work-up, focused on uncovering inflammatory, immunologic, endocrinologic, toxic, or iatrogenic causes. Response to antipyretics provides little value.

What medications, including antibiotics, do you take? Have you recently stopped any medication? Do you take steroids?

Most patients who are able to recall their medication describe their daily routine. Patients typically omit mention of medications taken intermittently, inhalers, eye drops, oral contraceptives, non-prescription supplements, and even insulin.

Table 22.3 Immediate life-threats associated with fever

Associated signs	Concerns
Airway compromise	Epiglottitis, pharyngeal abscess
Respiratory distress	Pneumonia, empyema
Circulatory collapse	Septic shock
Altered mental status	Meningitis, encephalitis, brain abscess
Peritonitis	Perforated bowel, cholangitis, abscess, spontaneous bacterial peritonitis, appendicitis

Table 22.4 Organization framework for history of present illness (HPI)

Fever descriptors
Duration, magnitude, pattern

Contagion risks
Known sick contacts
Exposure to nosocomial infections (time spent in nursing home or hospital)
Travel
Occupation (restaurant, farm, industry, day care)
Dietary (raw seafood, home canning)
Social habits (sex, alcohol, tobacco, IV drug use)

Host factors
Relevant medical conditions (diabetes, sickle cell, HIV, systemic lupus erythematosus)
Immunization status
Medical hardware (indwelling catheter, pacemaker, shunts)
Medications (including antipyretics)

Unless directly asked, patients may not volunteer that they have taken samples of someone else's medication (e.g., leftover antibiotics for a fever). All patients should be encouraged to carry an updated list of medications and allergies for their own protection.

Have you been exposed to individuals at home, school, or work with similar symptoms? Do you have any special risks for infection?

It is crucial to ascertain any special circumstances or contagion risks. These include sick household contacts, extended exposure at a hospital, nursing home or day care facility, recent foreign travel, dietary and occupational risks, new or symptomatic prior sexual partners, and intravenous (IV) drug habits. Although most patients can recall a colleague or friend being ill, patterns of similar symptoms in several close contacts may be helpful. High-risk dietary habits include the practice of eating raw or undercooked meats or fish, home canning, and "direct from source" food use (milk, honey, chickens).

Do you have any chronic medical conditions that may make you susceptible to infection?

A multitude of comorbidities predispose patients to infection. This may be through the inability of the immune system to access the affected part, as in the case of peripheral vascular disease. Defenses are attenuated in individuals with diabetes, or deliberately suppressed in organ transplant recipients. Patients who are asplenic have increased risk for infection and sepsis. Conditions requiring the use of glucocorticoids further diminish already vulnerable host defenses.

Do you have any indwelling or implanted medical devices?

Implanted medical devices have great potential for hematogenous contamination in the setting of transient bacteremia. Nonnative heart valves and indwelling vascular and urinary catheters are at greatest risk. Implantable cardioverter-defibrillators (ICDs), pacemakers, breast and penile implants, artificial joints and medication pumps are vulnerable immediately following surgical placement, but diminish their seeding potential after several months.

Are your immunizations or booster shots current?

Immunization status is important and should include questions regarding childhood vaccine series, subsequent titers, hepatitis B series, pneumovax, tetanus boosters, and influenza prophylaxis. Newer vaccines are being developed that will alter our current approaches to certain diseases. Other vaccines represent protection from biological weapon threats.

Associated symptoms

Acquisition of a detailed history often points to focal examination findings and identification of the source of fever (Table 22.5). Conceptually, fever is a systemic sign that forces clinicians to consider causes anywhere from head to toe, including the skin and external sources, like drugs or drug–drug interactions. It therefore makes sense to organize the approach to the history by physiological systems as opposed to anatomical location. Each organ system will have characteristic but non-pathogen specific signs and symptoms.

Table 22.5 Associated localizing symptoms by organ system

Respiratory	Dyspnea, cough, phlegm or sputum, pleuritic pain
Gastrointestinal	Nausea, vomiting, cramping, diarrhea, anal pain/itching, blood
Skin/soft tissue	Pain, rash, red streaks, induration, drainage
Musculoskeletal	Pain on movement or palpation, swelling, inability to bear weight
Genitourinary	Dysuria, discharge, dyspareunia, pelvic pain
Head and neck CNS	Nasal drainage, tooth, throat or ear pain, difficulty swallowing, confusion, neck stiffness, vomiting, headache, back pain

Past medical

An extensive list of comorbidities exists that impede normal defense mechanisms and put patients at special risk. These include chronic cardiopulmonary disease, cancer, chronic renal failure, human immunodeficiency virus (HIV), diabetes mellitus (DM), hemoglobinopathies, and transplanted organs. Recent surgery, childbirth or exacerbation of chronic conditions may critically lower host defenses. Prior infections recently treated with antibiotics are a risk factor for the development of drug-resistant organisms, including methicillin-resistant *Staphylococcus aureus* (MRSA), drug-resistant *Streptococcus pneumoniae* (DRSP), vancomycin-resistant enterococci (VRE), and fluoroquinolone-resistant enterics. The loss of protective non-pathogenic flora may result in vaginitis or colitis.

Physical examination

A thorough history will often allow the clinician to concentrate on target areas of the physical examination. Local inflammatory-mediated changes provide clues to the presumptive source of fever. If no such associated localizing findings are identified, treatment is based largely upon host factors. Young, previously healthy adults with physical examination findings consistent with benign viral illnesses such as nasal discharge, head congestion, cough, diffuse myalgias and arthralgias, or non-bloody loose stools can be safely discharged with symptomatic therapy only. In contrast, the elderly or immune compromised hosts with few historical or physical examination findings require careful consideration for further work-up and possible empiric antibiotic treatment.

General appearance

The term "toxic-appearing" applies to those who "look ill from across the room." Behavioral clues such as responsiveness to voice, posture, hygiene, and energy level provide insight into the severity of illness. The inability to sit up in a stretcher or ambulate to the bathroom without assistance is a gross marker of functional impairment.

Temperature

Factors influencing temperature measurement include environmental conditions, testing technique, anatomical site, and site-specific confounders. The distinction of core versus shell temperature is most important in extreme states of hyper- and hypothermia. Invasive methods to determine temperature are usually not necessary, but include pulmonary artery catheters, and esophageal or urinary bladder probes. Peripheral temperatures are typically obtained from the tympanic membrane, mouth, or rectum. Measurements on the forehead, either by palpation or via thermosensitive strips, as well as axillary temperature measurement have proved less reliable.

The accuracy of an appropriately calibrated infrared tympanic thermometer is expected to be within 0.2°F (0.1°C) between 98°F and 102°F (37–39°C). Outside this narrow range, accuracy diminishes. Temperatures less than 95°F (35°C) or greater than 104°F (40°C) should prompt the clinician to take additional measurements by alternate methods. Tympanic thermometers have gained popularity because they are noninvasive and calibrate quickly, and do not rely on direct contact with the tympanic membrane. Errors occur through improper positioning, anatomical abnormalities, cerumen, or local inflammatory processes such as otitis media or externa. Many authors do not favor the use of the tympanic thermometer as a sensitive screen for fever in the ED, especially in the elderly.

Rectal, oral, and tympanic temperatures correlate poorly with one another. On average, rectal temperatures are 0.8°F (0.4°C) higher than oral and 1.6°F (0.8°C) higher than tympanic readings. Rectal temperatures are maximal at a depth of 2.5 inches (6.4 cm). Fecal impaction and shock states may falsely reduce temperatures, while elevated fecal bacterial counts and proctitis may erroneously increase readings. Sublingual or oral temperature measurements require cooperative patients able to breathe with their mouths closed. Mastication, smoking, recently ingested foods, and respiratory distress may affect readings.

Since temperatures can vary during the ED, it may be prudent to repeat temperature measurements. A high degree of clinical suspicion in the setting of a normal temperature should prompt at least one or more rechecks during a patient's stay, and consideration of measurement at other anatomical sites. Patients at the extremes of age or with significant comorbidity may have a serious infection in the absence of fever.

Vital signs

Review of the remaining vital signs (Chapter 1) may provide clues to the source of fever. For example, an increased respiratory rate with lower than expected oxygen saturation suggests pneumonia or other respiratory causes of fever.

Central nervous system

Despite its protective barriers, devastating CNS infections can occur as a result of direct (e.g., otitis media, sinusitis) or hematogenous spread of pathogens. Fever may impair cognitive function, particularly in the elderly, and result in agitation or decreased responsiveness. This makes discerning a primary CNS infection from a systemic problem very difficult. An effort should be made to detect signs of meningeal irritation or increased intracranial pressure (ICP). *Meningismus*, defined as pain due to irritation of the meninges that surround the brain and spinal cord, is often a late finding, non-specific, and unreliable below 18 months of age. Maneuvers which demonstrate meningismus include difficulty with or resistance to neck or hip flexion. Increased ICP, if progressing slowly, may manifest subtly as mental status or personality changes, bulging fontanelle, papilledema, or less often focal neurologic abnormalities. The absence of signs of increased ICP or abnormal neurological findings does not exclude the presence of a serious CNS infection. Fever and an abnormal sensorium or neurological examination should raise immediate concern for meningoencephalitis and prompt consideration of empiric antimicrobial or antiviral therapy. In the setting of a clinically suspected CNS infection, broad-spectrum antibiotics that cross the blood-brain barrier may be given prior to lumbar puncture (LP), and may be lifesaving. Despite controversy, IV dexamethasone has been recommended prior to antibiotics in cases of acute bacterial meningitis.

Upper respiratory tract

The upper respiratory tract is the most commonly infected site in humans. Colonized by diverse flora, a delicate balance exists at this strategic opening to the respiratory and digestive systems. Droplet transmission of potential pathogens upon inhalation initially seeds the nasal mucosa.

A detailed examination should include the eyes and surrounding structures, the nares, the oropharynx including teeth, gums, tonsils, and mucosal surfaces. Tender anterior cervical adenopathy may provide clues to a current or recent facial or oral infection. The paranasal sinuses should be gently percussed. The ear canal, tympanic membrane, mastoid bone, and posterior cervical lymph nodes should also be evaluated. It is important to remember that skin abscesses can manifest anywhere on the body and may be hidden behind an ear, beneath the hair, or in the perianal or rectal area. Neck stiffness may be a manifestation of severe pharyngitis or soft tissue neck abscess, or a component of diffuse myalgias. Palpation of the salivary and

thyroid glands and auscultation of the upper airway are part of the complete examination.

Lower respiratory tract

Acute bronchitis and pneumonia are common infections resulting from translocation of upper respiratory flora or infrequently from aspiration of gastric contents. Other insults such as smoking render this area extremely vulnerable to pathogenic seeding. An overall global assessment of the respiratory status of a patient includes his or her work of breathing (WOB), respiratory rate, pulse oximetry, and breath sounds. Normal values on pulse oximetry accompanied by tachypnea, abnormal breath sounds, or increased WOB provide little reassurance. Asymmetric or rhoncherous breath sounds suggest air space disease, air sac collapse, or an effusion. A complete lung examination includes auscultation anteriorly, posteriorly, and in the axillae, with intentional cough, phonation, and forced exhalation to elicit sounds not otherwise heard. Sputum, if produced, may be collected in a sterile container for gram stain and culture, but is rarely helpful.

Cardiovascular

A pleural or pericardial rub may point to inflammatory processes. Any new murmur, especially in the setting of IV drug use, should prompt immediate concern for endocarditis, as fever may be the only symptom. Evidence of impaired cardiac function such as congestive heart failure may indicate myocarditis. Rheumatic heart disease or known cardiac valve abnormalities should also be considered.

Gastrointestinal

Analogous to the skin, the gut represents an important protective barrier against pathogens. Any weakening from systemic or local bowel disease can allow translocation of intraluminal disease-causing agents. One of the first concerns is whether peritonitis is present. Reflexively- or persistently-increased abdominal wall muscle tone, worsening pain with movement of the abdomen, and the loss of bowel sounds in the appropriate setting should prompt surgical consultation. Evaluation of the abdomen by quadrant can help narrow the large list of abdominal causes of fever, taking into account significant anatomical overlap. Special consideration should be made to examine liver size, texture and tenderness, gallbladder prominence and tenderness with and without inspiration, pain isolated to the right lower quadrant or unilateral flank. A rectal examination is invaluable in identifying a perirectal abscess or prostatitis. The perineum should be visually inspected for soft tissue abnormalities.

Genitourinary

Urinary tract infections (UTIs) proceed in an ascending manner from the introitus cephalad. Initially, local irritation or burning at the urethral opening can progress to classic signs of cystitis including dysuria, urgency, and frequency. Flank pain may represent stretch or irritation of the kidney's fibrous capsule due to pyelonephritis. Upper tract signs are not reliably present to distinguish cystitis from pyelonephritis. A thorough inspection of the foreskin, glans, penile skin, and scrotal structures in males, as well as inguinal lymph nodes, is important. In females, a speculum and bimanual examination are important given the high prevalence of pathogens transmitted by sexual intercourse.

Soft tissue and musculoskeletal

Diffuse transient myalgias and arthralgias are common to many pathogens. However, isolated pain localized to the soft tissue or one joint should be thoroughly investigated. Areas of special concern include the perineum, feet, and areas of continuous external pressure. All debilitated patients need to be log-rolled on both sides using at least two providers to examine these areas, especially the sacrum. When examining cutaneous wounds, the presence of drainage, spreading erythematous margins, crepitus, and functional impairment need to be considered. Recent shaving, body piercing, and tattoos can be a nidus of infection or inflammation. Skin abscesses (carbuncle, furuncle) from "skin popping" are most common in the forearms of IV drug users, but abscesses can occur anywhere, including in axillae, lactating breast, and groin.

Skin

Characteristic skin lesions often accompany febrile adults. It is important to be familiar with proper dermatological terminology so that rash categorization algorithms may be appropriately utilized. A wide variety of infectious and non-infectious processes manifest as a limited number of skin lesions (Table 22.6). Petechiae are worrisome vasculitic lesions seen in meningococcemia, most often on the lower legs.

Table 22.6 Infections presenting with fever and rash

Maculopapular
Central
Rubeola, rubella, roseola, erythema infectiosum
Lyme disease
Drug reactions
Peripheral
Erythema multiforme
Secondary syphilis

Petechiae
Meningococcemia, rocky mountain spotted fever (RMSF), viral hemorrhagic fevers, thrombotic thrombocytopenic purpura (TTP)

Diffuse erythema
Scarlet fever, toxic shock syndrome (TSS)
Scalded skin syndrome
Ehrlichiosis

Vesicles/pustules
Varicella, *Herpes zoster*
Gonococcemia
Impetigo

Nodules
Erythema nodosum, fungus

Differential diagnosis

The differential diagnosis of the febrile adult is protean and includes a large number of infectious and noninfectious causes. Diagnostically, it is important to focus on:

1. what illness or injury may have occurred causing host vulnerability and allowing the infection to take hold;
2. what site-specific pathogens are usually responsible for disease, and exist in the local community;
3. what special exposure risks may have occurred from professional or personal habits.

The most difficult diagnoses are in patients with systemic illness without an obvious cause or portal of entry. This may prompt a broad search for suspected causes. From an emergency provider's perspective, it is easier to organize this search by organ system (Table 22.7). Local Departments of Health require physician reporting of infectious diseases of public health concern.

Table 22.7 Differential diagnosis of infectious causes of fever

Diagnosis	Symptoms and signs	Etiologic agents	Work-up considerations
Systemic			
AIDS	Altered mental status, dyspnea, diarrhea, vesicular rash	HIV	Western blot, ELISA, CBC, CD4, viral load, chest X-ray, ABG, acid-fast sputum, brain CT with contrast precedes LP, fecal leukocytes
Malaria	Malaise, myalgias, headache, chest pain, diarrhea, anemia, hepatosplenomegaly	Plasmodia species	Travel history, CBC, thick and thin blood smears
Rabies	Malaise, paresthesias, agitation, coma	Rabies virus	PCR saliva
Sepsis	Altered mental status, ↓BP, respiratory distress, tachycardia	Gram-positive, Gram-negative, rarely anaerobes, fungus	CBC, blood cultures, urine cultures
Tetanus	Muscle rigidity, lockjaw, sardonic smile, opisthotonus	*Clostridium tetani*	Electrolytes, control of airway, muscle spasms
Toxic shock syndrome	BP↓, erythroderma, desquamation, sore throat, diarrhea, myalgias	*Staph. aureus* (toxin-mediated) Groups A, B, C, G *Strep. pyogenes*	Removal FB, CBC, blood cultures
Head and neck			
Brain abscess	Altered mental status, headache	Streptococci, bacteroides, Enterobacteriaceae, *Staph. aureus*, *Toxoplasma gondii* (HIV+)	Brain CT
Epidural abscess	Fever, back pain, signs of spinal cord involvement	*Staph. aureus*, *Pseudomonas*, TB	Spine CT, myelogram, MRI, LP
Meningitis/ encephalitis	Meningismus, headache, altered mental status, nausea, vomiting, seizure	Depends on age of patient, chronicity, and immunocompetence: viral, *Strep. pneumoniae* (especially post-neurosurgical or CSF leak), *N. meningitidis, Listeria monocytogenes* (unlikely if young and immunocompetent), Gram-negative bacilli (*H. influenza* rare), herpes simplex, chemical/drug	Brain CT, LP
Periorbital/ orbital cellulitis	Facial swelling, painful eye movement	*Strep. pneumoniae, H. influenzae, M. catarrhalis, Staph. aureus,* anaerobes, Group A *Streptococcus*, occasional Gram-negative bacilli post-trauma	Facial CT if concerns with orbital cellulitis or abscess
Respiratory			
Lung abscess/ empyema	Toxic, dyspnea, chest pain	*Strep. pneumoniae*, Group A *Streptococcus, Staph. aureus, H. influenzae*, other	Chest X-ray, thoracentesis, drainage by chest tube thoracostomy, interventional radiology, or surgery

(continued)

Table 22.7 Differential diagnosis of infectious causes of fever (*cont*)

Diagnosis	Symptoms and signs	Etiologic agents	Work-up considerations
Pharyngeal abscess	Stridor, sore throat	*Strep. viridans*, Group A *Streptococcus*, Mixed oral flora	Soft tissue neck X-ray, neck CT, I&D
Pneumonia	Cough, sputum, dyspnea, rhonchi, chest pain	Factors include community- or hospital-acquired, tobacco, age, and comorbidities: viruses, mycoplasma, *Strep. pneumoniae*, *H. influenzae*, *M. catarrhalis*, TB, *Legionella* and *Pseudomonas* species	Chest X-ray
Sinusitis/otitis media/pharyngitis/dental	Localized pain	*Strep. pneumoniae*, *H. influenzae*, *M. catarrhalis*, Group A *Streptococcus*	None
URI/bronchitis	Cough	Viruses	None
Cardiac			
Endocarditis	Murmur, microemboli, myalgias, weakness, Osler's nodes, Roth's spots, Janeway lesions, petechiae	Depends on native or prosthetic valve, IV drug abuse: *Strep. viridans*, *S. bovis*, *S. epidermidis*, *Staph. aureus*, other streptococci, enterococci, and enterobacteriaceae species	Blood count, TEE, infectious disease consultation recommended
Gastrointestinal			
Colitis (toxic, ulcerative, Crohn's)	Abdominal pain, diarrhea	Enterobacteriaceae, anaerobes	*C. difficile* toxin
Diverticulitis/abscess	Abdominal/pelvic pain, peritonitis	Enterobacteriaceae, enterococci, bacteroides species, anaerobes	CT scan, surgical consult
Gastroenteritis	N/V/D	Viral, enteric bacteria, including *Shigella*, *Salmonella*, *E. coli* 0157:H7, *Campylobacter*, *C. difficile*, *E. histolytica*, parasites	Fecal leukocytes, stool tests, *C. difficile* toxin
Hepatitis	N/V/D, jaundice	Hepatitis A, B, C, D	Hepatitis screen, LFTs
Spontaneous bacterial peritonitis	Abdominal pain	Enterobacteriaceae, *Strep. pneumoniae*, enterococci, anaerobes	Paracentesis and Gram stain/culture
Genitourinary			
Epididymitis/orchitis	Testicular pain	Mumps, treponema, other viruses	Urine dip, scrotal US to rule out testicular torsion
Herpes simplex	Burning pain, itching	HSV 1, 2	Tzanck, DFA
Pelvic inflammatory disease/tubo-ovarian abscess	Purulent vaginal discharge, cervical motion tenderness, abdominal pain, shuffling gait	*N. gonorrhoeae*, *C. trachomatis*, bacteroides, Enterobacteriaceae, Streptococci, *Trichomonas vaginalis*	UA, DNA probe, cervical/rectal/throat swab, CBC, joint aspirate, pelvic US
Perirectal abscess	Pain, purulent drainage	Enterobacteriaceae, occasional *P. aeruginosa*, bacteroides species, enterococci	I&D

(continued)

Table 22.7 Differential diagnosis of infectious causes of fever (*cont*)

Diagnosis	Symptoms and signs	Etiologic agents	Work-up considerations
Prostatitis	Dysuria, abdominal pain	Etiology depends on age, chronicity, and sexual practices: *N. gonorrhoeae*, *C. trachomatis*, Enterobacteriaceae (coliforms), other (including unknown)	Urine dip
Pyelonephritis/abscess	Dysuria, flank pain	Enterobacteriaceae (*E. coli*), enterococci, occasional *P. aeruginosa*	Urine dip, UA, urine culture, renal CT
1° Syphilis, chancroid, lymphogranuloma venereum (LGV)	Chancre (painful versus nonpainful), lymphadenopathy	*Treponema pallidum*, *Hemophilus ducreyi*, *Chlamydia trachomatis*	RPR, VDRL, FTA-ABS, DNA probe
Skin/soft tissue			
Cellulitis/fasciitis	Pain, swelling, redness, possible drainage, occasional crepitus	Group A *Streptococcus*, other *Streptococcus* species, *Staph. aureus*, anaerobes, *Clostridium* species (fasciitis is often polymicrobial)	CBC, I&D, fasciotomy
Folliculitis/skin abscess	Pain, swelling, redness, possible drainage	*Staph. aureus*, *S. epidermidis*, candida, anaerobes, *P. aeruginosa* (hot tub)	I&D, US if concern for FB
Osteomyelitis	Pain	*Staph. aureus*, *P. aeruginosa*, may be polymicrobial (especially if chronic). *Salmonella* common in sickle cell anemia. *S. epidermidis* possible post-operative	I&D
Septic arthritis	Pain with range of motion	*Staph. aureus*, *N. gonorrhoeae*, Streptococci, anaerobes	Aspiration via arthrocentesis

ABG: arterial blood gas; CBC: complete blood count; CP: chest pain; DFA: direct fluorescent antibody; ELISA; enzyme-linked immunosorbent assay; FB: foreign body; HSV: herpes simplex virus; I&D: incision and drainage; LFT: liver function tests; LP: lumbar puncture; N/V/D: nausea/vomiting/diarrhea; TB: tuberculosis; TEE: transesophageal echocardiography; UA: urinalysis; URI: upper respiratory infection; US: ultrasound.

Strep: *Streptococcus*; Staph: *Staphylococcus*; H. influenzae: *Haemophilus influenzae*; E. histolytica: *Entameba histolytica*; C. difficile: *Clostridium difficile*; P. aeruginosa: *Pseudomonas aeruginosa*; N. gonorrhoeae: *Neisseria gonorrhoeae*; S. epidermidis: *Staphylococcal epidermidis*; N. meningitidis: *Neisseria meningitidis*; M. Catarrhalis: *Moraxella catarrhalis*; C. trachomatis: *Chlamydia trachomatis*.

Infections can be divided into viral, bacterial, fungal, and parasitic. Viral infections are the most common pathogens and include a variety of upper respiratory, gastrointestinal, blood-borne, CNS, skin, and genital pathogens. A variety of hemorrhagic and mosquito-borne viral illnesses are common outside the US, but do occur (West Nile Virus, Rabies). Bacterial illness is typically divided into Gram-positive skin and respiratory organisms and Gram-negative gastric and urinary pathogens. The disruption or translocation of ordinary flora is often the cause of disease.

Encapsulated organisms pose a special threat to asplenic patients (e.g., sickle cell disease). Prompt initiation of antibiotics has greatly reduced mortality, but has also resulted in the evolution of drug-resistant organisms. The practice of treating unknown or noninfectious illnesses with antibacterial agents in healthy adults is not justified.

Most EDs have instituted policies of universal precautions, isolation and environmental controls to prevent the spread of drug-resistant organisms. Fungi can cause devastating disease in immunosuppressed hosts, but rarely have significant impact upon healthy individuals. In the US, parasitic infections are generally limited to adverse social conditions or special occupational and recreational exposures, and have special vectors of transmission. As with all infectious diseases, a careful exposure history including recent travel is important.

Noninfectious causes of fever

Medication/drug fever

Often a diagnosis of exclusion, drug fever is not often made based on a single ED visit. Fevers may develop from the administration of irritating substances that cause phlebitis, sterile abscesses, or aseptic meningitis. Other drugs may have intrinsic properties that interfere directly in the thermoregulatory process. A classic febrile response to the treatment of pathogens such as syphilis is the *Jarisch–Herxheimer* reaction. Febrile reactions to inhalational anesthetics and agents that induce red cell hemolysis can occur in those with genetic predisposition. The widely held belief that drug fever patients appear well, have a relative bradycardia and eosinophilia, and routinely manifest cutaneous signs have not held true. The most common drugs associated with drug fever are cardiovascular agents such as α-methyl dopa, quinidine, procainamide, antineoplastic agents, antibiotics, antiepileptics, and rarely cimetidine. Drug combinations that increase synaptic serotonin induce autonomic hyperactivity, including fever. Exposure to neuroleptics may induce a progressive state of fever and rigidity, although this is rare.

Thromboembolic disease

Between one-quarter and one-third of patients with angiographically-proven pulmonary embolus (PE) will have a low-grade (<101°F or 38.5°C) fever. Many conditions that predispose patients to PE, such as malignancy, may be responsible for this temperature elevation. No difference in fever frequency occurs with or without complications such as pulmonary infarction. The presence of thrombophlebitis or deep venous thrombosis in the absence of PE may also produce temperature elevation.

Tumor fever

A variety of solid organ and hematogenous neoplasms cause persistent fever. Fever is common among leukemias and lymphomas due to the proliferation of neoplastic cells capable of endogenous pyrogen release. Liver, CNS, and renal cell cancers also typically produce temperature elevations. Since both the cancer and its treatment cause immune compromise, it is important that infection be ruled out. If a patient is neutropenic and develops a fever, empiric antibiotics should be administered promptly, even in the absence of any source.

Inflammatory/immunological disease

Diseases that induce a chronic inflammatory state that may manifest with fever include Systemic Lupus Erythematosus, Juvenile Rheumatoid Arthritis, and Polyarteritis Nodosa. Although there may be localizing signs, the systemic nature of these diseases can cause diffuse symptoms. A relative immunodeficient state exacerbated by immunosuppressive therapy increases the risk of infection, particularly to Gram-negative bacteria and fungi. A history of inflammatory bowel disease raises concern for an intra-abdominal abscess. Pancreatitis can lead to a cascade of enzymatic auto-digestion and profound inflammatory-mediated third-space fluid losses resulting in shock. Many vasculitides also present with unexplained low-grade fever.

Environmental/occupational

Heat stroke is divided into classic and exertional forms. *Classic heat stroke* typically affects deconditioned or elderly individuals, those with chronic morbidity or a history of drug or alcohol use, and individuals on medication that may exacerbate fluid losses or prevent heat dissipation. *Exertional heat stroke* occurs more commonly in young males involved in endurance training. Despite the fact that exertional heat stroke patients retain the ability to sweat, they have overwhelmed their reparative mechanisms and require aggressive management. Metal and polymer fume fevers are examples of environmental exposures that can masquerade as flu-like illnesses with fever. Welders are particularly at risk. Aerosolized metals induce symptoms that may be delayed by several hours, and may last 1–2 days until exposure is discontinued.

Miscellaneous

A variety of conditions causing a hypermetabolic state may present to the ED with fever. Hyperthyroidism, pheochromocytoma, carcinoid syndrome, as well as anaphylaxis induce increases in the basal metabolic rate and catecholamine secretion. Other diagnoses associated with fever include hyperlipidemia and factitious fever.

Diagnostic testing

Laboratory tests

Prior to any ancillary studies being ordered, the clinician should have a clear idea of what treatable disease process is being ruled in or out. Objective data should be viewed as confirmatory for the history and physical examination. In the majority of febrile ED patients, the source of illness is determined clinically, prior to objective testing. Examples of conditions occurring in healthy hosts that do not require confirmatory diagnostic testing include rhinitis, bronchitis, gastritis, and enteritis.

When laboratory studies are indicated, every effort should be made to obtain adequate sample quantities of appropriate specimens. Failure to collect specimens prior to the initiation of antimicrobial therapy may cloud the future clinical picture. Specimen types collected include blood, urine, sputum, stool, cerebrospinal fluid (CSF), throat, penile, cervical and wound swabs, and pleural or joint aspirates.

Blood tests

Complete blood count

The complete blood count (CBC) is the most commonly ordered laboratory test in the ED. It is neither sensitive nor specific for identification of bacterial versus nonbacterial illness. Cutoff values of white blood cell (WBC) counts greater than $15,000/mm^3$ suggest a higher likelihood of serious illness. Leukocytosis occurs first through demargination of existing mature WBC stores, and then by increased bone marrow production and release of mature and immature forms (left shift). Demargination and leukocytosis as high as $30,000$ WBC/mm^3 occur under many conditions of physiological stress. Emotional upset, glucocorticosteriod use, myeloproliferative disorders, and pregnancy are conditions with baseline leukocytosis. Automated white cell typing accompanies the standard CBC report. Manual differentials that identify immature forms are generally only performed above laboratory-established total cell count cutoffs, unless specifically requested. A lower than normal WBC level may represent transient viral bone marrow suppression or the host's inability to mount a significant immune response. WBC counts greater than $40,000/mm^3$ can occur in severe infections but should prompt consideration for a myelodysplastic disorder or leukemia.

Most admitted patients or those undergoing specialty consultation will have a CBC drawn, as consultants prefer to follow the WBC count as a marker of physiologic response to treatment. In patients who have received chemotherapy, the CBC is important to exclude neutropenia.

Acute phase reactants

C-reactive protein (CRP), serum amyloid A, pro-calcitonin, haptoglobin, and fibrinogen are examples of acute phase reactants. Pyrogenic cytokines stimulate production of this group of proteins during the acute inflammatory process. Considerable literature now reveals these tests add little to the clinical impression except in special circumstances. These serum markers may be useful in following the clinical progression of infections such as epidural abscesses, septic arthritis, and chronic inflammatory conditions (rheumatoid arthritis or temporal arteritis). The erythrocyte sedimentation rate (ESR) in mm/hour is an indirect marker of the level of acute phase proteins in the blood, but suffers the same limitations as the direct markers. Decisions regarding treatment or disposition should not be made based solely on these tests, except in rare circumstances.

Blood cultures

Blood cultures should be drawn prior to antibiotic therapy on patients who have a likelihood of bacteremia. Two sets of blood cultures, two bottles each (one anaerobic and one aerobic), with 15 ml blood in each set should be drawn from two distinct puncture sites. One site should include any indwelling vascular catheter. The positivity rate of blood cultures in the ED is surprisingly low (10%), thus care should be taken to order blood cultures selectively. Blood cultures drawn from afebrile patients are of limited value. Therefore, limit blood culture testing to patients being admitted for systemic infection, patients with impaired defenses who will be placed on empiric antibiotics, and patients who may have uncommon or atypical bacterial growth.

Other blood tests

Liver function tests (LFTs), lipase and hepatitis screens should be considered in febrile patients with right upper quadrant pain or diffuse abdominal pain. Rapid HIV testing is important in patients who possess risk factors for HIV or present with a suspected opportunistic infection. Patients suspected of having an acute presentation of HIV (fever, flu-like symptoms, myalgias, sore throat, adenopathy) should be tested for the p24 Antigen or viral load, as rapid HIV testing may initially be negative. When suspecting malaria, thin and thick smears are important for establishing the diagnosis by direct visualization of intracellular pathogens.

Urine tests

Urine dipstick

The multi-test urine dipstick is an accurate point-of-care screening test for lower UTI in young, healthy adults. Classic symptoms of cystitis such as dysuria, urgency, frequency, and suprapubic pain require no further confirmatory tests. Pyuria and the presence of urea-splitting bacteria render the leukocyte esterase (LE) and nitrite tests positive in over 90% of UTIs. False readings can occur from improper dipstick storage, poor collection, and incorrect interpretation. Vaginitis, menses, and some medications such as Pyridium can confound results. Clean catch specimen collection is only appropriate if clinical suspicion is such that confirmatory urine culture is not needed. Care must be taken to consider other infectious and noninfectious processes that can cause pyuria, such as appendicitis. Interpretation of dipstick results cannot be read instantly upon exposure to the sample, but require colorimetric development over several minutes. Urine odor and turbidity are most often caused by calcium phosphate precipitates, and are not reliable markers of infection. Urine dipstick performance is less reliable in the evaluation of abdominal pain without dysuria (lower pretest probability), early pregnancy, and high-risk hosts.

Urinalysis

A formal urinalysis (UA) consists of dipstick-type interpretation performed by laboratory personnel and additional microscopic examination of cells present in a spun and/or unspun specimen. The microscopic analysis is useful in identifying adequacy of sample quality and visual confirmation of pathogens (e.g., bacteria, trichomonads). Asymptomatic bacteriuria is common in the elderly, especially among institutionalized males, and requires no intervention. Patients who have an ileal conduit for urinary diversion have chronic pyuria even in the absence of infection.

Urine culture

The urine culture represents the gold standard for detecting bacteria in urine. Urine cultures are performed routinely according to predetermined laboratory protocols on abnormal UAs unless otherwise specified. The practice of obtaining urine culture irrespective of host factors, dipstick results, and specificity of lower urinary symptoms is unnecessarily costly. Definitions of true urinary tract infection vary, but are most often considered to be the growth of 10^5 colony-forming units (CFUs) of a single species. Counts below 10^5 CFUs may represent contaminants or chronic colonization. Some authors suggest that, given the link between UTI and fetal demise in early pregnancy, all symptomatic pregnant patients have urine cultures done regardless of UA results. Patients with chronic indwelling suprapubic or bladder catheters are often colonized with bacteria and represent a special diagnostic challenge.

Other urine tests

The qualitative urine pregnancy test may have importance regarding antibiotic treatment choices. A number of antibiotic classes are contraindicated during pregnancy. It is important to check the pregnancy and lactation safety information for every drug given to pregnant or nursing mothers.

Other specimen tests

Stool

Bacterial enteritis is uncommon in the US unlike other parts of the world. Stool specimens are therefore not necessary in the setting of a well-appearing patient with diarrhea. Fever, abdominal cramping, bloody diarrhea, immune compromise, and recent foreign travel make a bacterial cause more likely. Potential exposure to pathogens, such as a history of a recent camping, may prompt further testing. Fecal leukocyte detection (entero-invasive disease) represents the best screening test for a potential bacterial cause of diarrheal illness.

Routine stool cultures can identify common bacterial pathogens including Campylobacter, Salmonella, and Shigella. Special specimen processing is necessary to serotype *Escherichia coli* 0157:H7. Stool ova and parasites can be ordered if *Giardia* or other parasites are suspected. *Clostridium difficile* toxin detection should be checked in patients with possible toxic colonic bacterial overgrowth due to recent antibiotic use.

Cerebrospinal fluid (CSF)

Lumbar puncture is necessary in all patients with suspected CNS infection, especially those with fever, altered sensorium, headache, neurologic changes, meningismus, or localized spinal tenderness. At least 10 ml of CSF should be collected with care not to contaminate the specimen with skin flora. Repeated puncture attempts increase the likelihood of a bloody tap, which may diminish the interpretation accuracy (Table 22.8).

Table 22.8 Lumbar puncture order set

Tube 1	Cell count and differential
Tube 2	Protein, glucose
Tube 3	Gram's stain, bacterial culture, viral culture (herpes, etc.)
Tube 4	India Ink, cryptococcal antigen, bacterial antigen (CIE, ELISA). Repeat cell count and differential

CIE: countercurrent immunoelectrophoresis; ELISA: enzyme-linked immunosorbent assay.

Throat swab and culture

The detection of group A beta-hemolytic *Streptococcus* (GABHS) historically has been important given its well-known link to rheumatic heart disease (RHD). GABHS pharyngitis classically causes fever, throat pain, tonsillar exudates, and tender anterior cervical lymphadenopathy in the absence of upper respiratory infection (URI) symptoms such as cough or coryza. Patients younger than 35 years of age are at greatest risk for the development of RHD from serotypes of GABHS now very uncommon in the US. Young patients with at least intermediate probability for strep pharyngitis in the absence of symptoms suggestive of viral illness should undergo rapid antigen testing (rapid *Strep* screen). A second swab for throat culture is simultaneously collected, as confirmatory throat cultures should be sent if the screen is negative. Positive results of either warrant treatment that can be delayed up to one week without increased risk of RHD. Contrary to popular belief, antibiotics provide little symptomatic relief. Sexually transmitted infections, such as gonorrhea, can manifest as pharyngitis (see below).

Genital swabs

Mucosal surfaces have the potential to become infected through sexual contact. A low threshold to test for disease should be maintained for high-prevalence diseases such as Chlamydia, Trichomonas, Gonorrhea, and Syphilis among sexually-active teenagers and adults. Patients may be infected for long periods of time despite no or few symptoms. Failure to treat sexual partners and medication noncompliance represent the greatest challenges to prevent disease recurrence. Traditional endocervical collection and culture practices are being replaced by methods of rapid urine detection with deoxyribonucleic acid (DNA) probes and amplification techniques. Herpetic vesicular lesions can be treated based upon their classic clinical appearance. Ulcerative areas should be vigorously cultured prior to the initiation of prophylactic antibiotics. Scrapings of fluid or tissue lesions can be sent for special testing, such as culture, direct fluorescent antibody (DFA), or enzyme-linked immunosorbent assay (ELISA).

Joint aspiration

Localized pain, erythema, and swelling of a joint causing painful limited range of movement in the setting of systemic fever should prompt consideration of a septic joint until proven otherwise. Aspiration and analysis of synovial fluid is crucial to the diagnosis, and can help distinguish sterile processes such as aseptic synovitis or crystal arthropathy from an infectious cause. Bedside ultrasound may guide sample collection. Joint aspirates should be tested for cell type and count, the presence of bacteria on Gram's stain, culture, and crystals under polarizing microscopy. Leukocyte counts greater than $50,000/mm^3$ are likely the result of infection, and should prompt immediate antibiotics and orthopedic consultation. Cultures have a high rate of detection of *Staphylococcus* and *Streptococcus*, but are less sensitive for gonorrhea.

Radiological studies

Chest X-ray

The chest X-ray is the gold standard for the identification of pneumonia but may lag symptoms by several days. Two views of the chest are helpful to improve identification of retrocardiac processes. Community-acquired pneumonia (CAP) may be lobar or a diffuse interstitial process ("walking pneumonia"). Focal infiltrates represent consolidation and fluid accumulation within air spaces, resulting in the loss of air–solid interfaces on radiograph. Plain radiographs may not be helpful in distinguishing infection from other causes of consolidation such as atelectasis (air sac collapse). Effusions, particularly unilateral, may represent complications from abscess (empyema) or airway obstruction. Endobronchial processes such as reactive airway disease or bronchitis rarely demonstrate clinically important radiographic findings. Pregnancy testing and proper shielding with lead can reduce inadvertent exposure.

Other plain radiographs

Soft tissue neck X-rays may help in the diagnosis of epiglottitis. The classic thumbprint replaces the normally thin epiglottic shadow. Prevertebral soft space width may be increased due to retropharyngeal abscess. Air in the soft tissues may represent a gas-forming organism. Films of suspected extremities are usually unnecessary unless there is suspicion of foreign body, necrotizing fasciitis, or a long-standing deep infection. Osteomyelitis is the slow destruction of bony architecture that may be apparent after more than 1 week of symptoms.

Ultrasound

Ultrasound (US) can accurately and rapidly identify fluid-filled structures such as deep tissue abscesses (perinephric, subhepatic, tubo-ovarian) without risk of radiation exposure. US is also the modality of choice in identifying biliary tract disease. Gallbladder wall thickening greater than 3 mm, pericholecystic fluid, or ductal dilatation in a patient with pain, tenderness, and fever should prompt an immediate surgical consultation. The increased availability of bedside US to physicians, and their increasing comfort with this technique has resulted in greater use, such as in joint aspiration and abscess drainage.

Computed tomography

Computed tomography (CT) scanning provides definitive anatomic information regarding deep infections, especially in those areas inaccessible by US or obscured by bone or air-filled structures, such as the brain, paranasal sinuses, or deep abdomen. Attenuation differences among tissues are enhanced by the administration of contrast material. Appropriate contrasting methods (PO, IV, rectal) and delays of 2–4 hours are necessary for maximal accuracy (especially in thin patients). All patients must be evaluated for any contraindications to contrast such as prior allergy, pregnancy, or renal insufficiency. Patients should be adequately hydrated, and metformin use should be discontinued briefly.

Other radiological tests

Magnetic resonance imaging (MRI) is rarely necessary for the initial work-up of fever. Spinal cord impingement from a suspected epidural abscess may be one exception. Radionucleotide-tagged bone scintillography may be useful in isolating a recurring fever of unknown etiology.

General treatment principles

The duration of patient interview must be tailored to the severity of illness, which in turn is most often related to the host's ability to fight disease rather than the particular pathogen. Febrile adults presenting with abnormal vital signs, altered sensorium, airway compromise, respiratory or circulatory distress require rapid simultaneous diagnostic testing and resuscitative therapy. Recognition of the severity of illness and transfer to a resuscitation area in the ED with the appropriate personnel is essential. The standard management priorities of the ABCs take precedence over treatment of the fever itself. Immediate interventions include assuring airway patency, providing supplemental oxygen or supporting inadequate ventilatory efforts, and obtaining adequate vascular access for fluid resuscitation.

Further history gathering may be limited by the severity of illness, resulting in the need for alternative sources of pertinent history. These include reports from emergency medical services, accompanying family members, transfer or medical records, or the primary care physician. Families of elderly patients often understand that infection is a frequent cause of death. Care must be taken that any advance directive, if available, be adhered to prior to initiating invasive diagnostic and stabilizing measures.

Antipyretics

The administration of antipyretics for fever has become standard practice to provide patient comfort. It is important to inquire about the time and dose of the most recently administered antipyretic. Acetaminophen is the most common anti-fever drug used in the ED, and can be used concurrently with an NSAID such as ibuprofen. Large studies have demonstrated similar efficacies between acetaminophen and ibuprofen in the treatment of fever, although NSAIDs may result in greater gastrointestinal irritation and reduction in renal blood flow, which may limit their use in some patients. Although extremely dangerous in the overdose setting, acetaminophen has a wide margin of safety in doses up to the current recommendations of 1 g every 4 hours (maximum 4 g/day). Hepatic metabolism may limit its use in liver failure. Ibuprofen is inexpensive and may be given in any combination of 2400 mg/24 hours (e.g., 400 mg every 4 hours or 800 mg every 8 hours). Aspirin for febrile illness should be avoided secondary to its association with Reye's syndrome in children. Selective COX-2 inhibitors have no role in the treatment of fever in the ED.

Intravenous fluids

A low threshold should exist for initiating IV fluid therapy in patients with fever who appear ill or dehydrated. Peripheral vasodilation results in a relative decrease in central circulating volume. Fluid losses from vomiting and diarrhea are exacerbated by increased insensible losses from the skin and respiratory system. IV fluids provide a modest cooling effect, replace volume and thus reduce tachycardia and thirst, improving the overall degree of comfort.

Cooling measures

Patients presenting with temperatures confirmed to be greater than 105°F (40.5°C) are more likely experiencing hyperpyrexia. In addition to standard resuscitative efforts, attempts should also be made to immediately lower body temperature. Excessive fluids should be avoided unless there is a clear history of fluid losses or in the setting of oliguric renal failure. Rapid cooling can be achieved through the use of cool sponge baths augmented by moist evaporative cooling from fans. Ice packs to the groin and axillae are effective. The use of alcohol applied to the skin as a cooling agent is discouraged. Invasive techniques of cool cavity lavage are last resorts, and are associated with serious morbidity.

Antimicrobial therapy

The initiation of antimicrobial therapy should be done only after careful consideration and rapid collection of appropriate laboratory specimens. Delaying antibiotic therapy in order to obtain specimens for suspected sepsis or meningitis (e.g., CSF) is not appropriate. Studies indicate that administration of the first-dose of antibiotics while in the ED improves outcome and decreases hospital length of stay in serious bacterial illnesses.

When the likelihood of an infectious cause of fever is sufficiently great, or when the host is vulnerable to systemic illness, empiric antibiotics may be given prior to the identification of a specific source or organism. In cases of potentially life-threatening infections, broad-spectrum antibiotic combinations that cover Gram-negative, Gram-positive, and anaerobic organisms should be given until a specific organism is identified on culture. In cases of localized infections, the spectrum of coverage should then be narrowed to cover the organism(s) most likely responsible for infection (e.g., Gram-positive organisms for an acute uncomplicated cellulitis) and to reduce antibiotic resistance.

The exact antibiotic choice for infections is beyond the scope of this chapter. Most clinicians consult specialized handbooks or computer programs, which are frequently updated. General principles to consider when selecting an antibiotic are to first confirm any drug allergies with the patient and from past medical records, if available. Patients typically do not distinguish adverse reactions such as nausea from true allergic reactions. The likely pathogens at the infected site should then be considered. Decide whether coverage needs to be broadened based upon host defense deficiencies or special exposures. Consider the local pathogen resistance patterns, often posted on the hospital laboratory web site. Drug–drug interactions need to be considered (e.g., warfarin and ciprofloxacin). The route of administration depends upon the drug selected. Of note, more expensive IV medications do not necessarily offer special benefit over highly bioavailable oral preparations, except in the most severely ill patients or those patients with poor gut function (from passive congestion or hypo-perfusion). Dosage may need adjustment in eld-erly patients and those with liver and kidney dysfunction. All patients should be warned about medication side effects and potential complica-tions of therapy, such as candidiasis or colitis. Many antibiotics render oral contraceptives less effective. Patients should be informed to complete the recommended course of antibiotics regardless of symptom improvement, and to discard any tablets that may remain.

Special patients

Pediatrics

Refer to Chapter 23.

Elderly

Geriatric patients and elderly patients residing at skilled nursing facilities represent groups with an increased risk of serious infection. Greater exposures to pathogens that have antibiotic-resistance and decreased immunological respon-siveness make them more vulnerable to adverse outcome. Of note, up to one-third of elderly patients do not mount a fever with systemic infec-tions. Often the reason for transfer from a skilled facility is nonspecific, such as unexplained falls or persistent tachycardia. The presence of delir-ium superimposed on preexisting cognitive defects reduces the ability to rely on history. Greater reliance is therefore placed on a thor-ough physical examination and screening labora-tories. The most common sources of serious infections include urinary (50–60%), respiratory tract, and soft tissue. Noninfectious sources are also more common in elderly patients. Consider admission for any febrile elderly patient with the exception of those not desiring aggressive or inpatient management. Confinement and fre-quent hospitalizations increase the likelihood of antibiotic-resistant organisms.

Immune compromised

Conditions that diminish a host's ability to fight infection frequently encountered in the ED setting include socially-disadvantaged and substance-dependent patients. Crowded living conditions in shelters predispose patients to communicable diseases through contact (scabies) or droplet infection (tuberculosis). Poor nutrition and expos-ure to hostile weather conditions compound these risks. Alcoholics are especially vulnerable to pneumonia due to increased incidence of vomiting and aspiration. The presence of ascites from alcoholic liver disease should key the clin-ician to consider spontaneous bacterial peritonitis as a cause of fever. IV drug users are at risk for local skin abscesses, cellulitis, endocarditis, and blood-borne viruses such as HIV and hepatitis. Diabetics are at risk for chronic fungal and foot infections secondary to impaired microcircula-tion and diminished wound healing. Sickle cell and splenectomized patients are at particular risk for infection by encapsulated organisms such as *Pneumococcus*. Sickle cell patients presenting in crisis should have infectious precipitants ruled out.

HIV-related infections

HIV-related infections are correlated with the CD4 count. Primary HIV infection manifests as a flu-like illness following a 2–4 week incubation period. Opportunistic infections or AIDS-defining illnesses do not present until the CD4 count has fallen below 400 cells/mm^3 and viral loads begin to rise. Once CD4 counts fall below 100 cells/mm^3, a variety of otherwise rare pathogens should be considered: *Pneumocystis carinii* pneumonia, tuber-culosis, cytomegalovirus (CMV), *Mycobacterium avium* complex, *Herpes simplex*, esophageal can-didiasis, toxoplasmosis, and *Cryptococcus*. The incidence of neoplasms such as Kaposi's sarcoma and lymphoma is also high in this patient popu-lation. An acute HIV infection should be con-sidered in a patient with acute febrile illness and adenopathy, pharyngitis, or risk factors.

Fevers may occur from antibiotics used in prophylaxis or treatment, such as sulfonamides or dapsone. Antiretroviral therapy is associated with drug fever, myositis, pancreatitis, and hepatitis. The work-up for patients with advanced HIV should include blood, urine, and possibly sputum and stool tests. A chest X-ray is indicated in essen-tially all HIV-positive individuals with cough and fever. An LDH level is often elevated in patients with PCP, despite the chest X-ray being normal in up to 40% of patients. CT of the brain prior to LP in patients with AIDS is a prudent precaution, as mass lesions such as toxoplasmosis may be present.

Organ transplant

Likely causes of fever in organ transplant patients correlate with the time since transplantation.

Fevers within 1 month are likely to be related to surgical wounds and occasionally to transmitted donor infections. Few fevers are secondary to opportunistic infections this early. In the 1–6 month post-transplant period, there is an increased incidence of viral infections, such as Epstein–Barr virus (EBV), CMV, hepatitis B and C, HIV, and other opportunistic infections. The increased incidence of rejection and fever caused by anti-lymphocytic antibody treatment is also increased. It is not until months or years after transplantation that the causes of fever largely mimic those in the population at large. Organ recipients remain at a somewhat increased risk of malignancy and opportunistic infection due to their immune-modulating therapy. Antibiotic therapy is complex and should involve consultation with the transplant team.

Returned foreign traveler

The returned traveler represents a particular challenge in the ED. In addition to the typical infections prevalent in the US, additional infectious possibilities not typically seen in the US must be considered. It is important to identify all foreign destinations and special exposures, such as travel to farms or jungles. Many travelers routinely query their doctors for immunization recommendations and antibiotic prophylaxis prior to foreign travel.

The most common travel affliction is traveler's diarrhea. Other significant diseases to consider that may present as fever include cholera, dengue and yellow fever, malaria, schistosomiasis, and trypanosomiasis. The Centers for Disease Control and Prevention (CDC-P) maintains a comprehensive updated travel resource for tourists and physicians (http://www.cdc.gov/travel). Patients may require quarantine until the diagnosis can be made, although this is rare.

Neutropenia

Patients undergoing chemo- or radiation therapy often present to the ED with fever. Dramatic drops in neutrophil counts occur 1–2 weeks following cytotoxic therapy. Despite the near obliteration of cells that produce endogenous pyrogens (agranulocytosis), the ability to mount a fever is remarkably preserved. Neutropenia is defined as a blood neutrophil count of less than 500 cells/mm^3. The incidence of bacteremia climbs sharply as neutrophil counts fall below 100 cells/mm^3. Febrile patients who are likely neutropenic should have blood samples for CBC and culture quickly drawn prior to the administration of broad-spectrum antibiotics such as ceftazidime or imipenem. Vancomycin may be added for patients in whom indwelling catheters are the suspected source of infection. Only the most well-appearing, reliable, compliant neutropenic patients should be considered for discharge, and only after discussion with that patient's primary care physician or hematologist/oncologist.

Institutionalized

Patients who have been exposed to nosocomial pathogens are at great risk for colonization with methicillin-resistant *Staphylococcus aureus* (MRSA) or vancomycin-resistant *Enterococcus* (VRE). Although no more virulent than their susceptible counterparts, infections with these organisms are difficult to eradicate and can produce symptomatic infection. Newer strains of fluoroquinolone-resistant enteric bacteria and vancomycin-resistant *Staphylococcus* pose serious future public health risk. It is important that health care providers exercise strict contact precautions. Limiting the inappropriate use of broad-spectrum antibiotics is likely to slow the spread of drug resistance.

Spinal cord injury

The incidence of fever in spinal cord-injured patients is quite high. Decreased mobility and loss of reflexes distal to the lesion predisposes individuals to UTIs, pneumonia, and infected soft tissue decubiti. Nearly all patients who do not void spontaneously become colonized with bacteria from prolonged urine dwell times and self-catheterization. Loss of function above T6 disrupts thermoregulatory neural circuits, impairing shivering and sweating responses. Patients may suffer from autonomic hyperreflexia with intermittent excessive sweating contributing to thermal instability. Despite being insensate in infected areas, spinal cord-injured patients often appreciate spreading infection as vague malaise.

Post-surgical/postpartum

Patients who have recently undergone surgical procedures or childbirth are at risk for the development of fever. The classic 5 W's mnemonic (wind, water, wound, womb, and wonder drug) remains a helpful reminder for the most common sources of fever. The earliest and most common cause of post-operative fever is atelectasis, often occurring within 1–2 days. Bacterial counts at seeded sites may rise to levels that cause symptoms by post-operative day 3. Cesarean section increases the risk of endometritis compared with vaginal delivery. It is important to look closely at all surgical wounds, including episiotomies, for signs of infection.

Disposition

Fever itself is not considered a reason for hospital admission. Healthy patients with acute viral illnesses who quickly respond to antipyretics, antiemetics, IV hydration, and other medication adjuncts do not require hospitalization. Healthy patients with localized bacterial infections who can tolerate oral therapy can also be safely discharged. Appropriate discharge instructions must be provided and follow-up with outpatient clinicians should be arranged in case localized complications develop or general deterioration limits a patient's ability to care for him- or herself. Specific criteria explaining reasons to return to the ED are vital. Patients with significant cardiopulmonary comorbidity, the elderly, alcoholics, the homeless, and those with compromised immune systems (including diabetes) may require admission for infectious processes that could be managed as an outpatient in healthy people.

The following indications for admission may serve as a helpful guide; however, each case depends upon patient preference, social support, and outpatient provider support. Admission should be considered for any patient with:

1. a non-viral systemic infection;
2. serious deep local or regional infections requiring IV antibiotics;
3. infections that require surgical intervention beyond simple incision and drainage;
4. any infection resulting in alterations of behavior or consciousness.

Individuals with limited physiologic reserve and those incapacitated by fever are likely to require admission, even if the source is unknown.

It is the responsibility of the emergency provider to ensure that time-specific return criteria are clear and understood. Most infections treated with antibiotics should symptomatically improve within 72 hours. Those who are not able to follow through on a reasonable outpatient plan by default should be considered for admission.

It is important to be aware of national guidelines now common in the treatment of many serious infections. Severity rating scales, treatment suggestions, and admission criteria are often provided based on clinical research, consensus guidelines, or both. Infectious disease consultation is rarely necessary acutely, but may provide an option for a difficult case or a challenging disposition. Many hospital pharmacies now have policies in place that limit the use of certain antibiotics.

Pearls, pitfalls, and myths

- Fever is a nonspecific symptom with a broad differential including both benign and serious illness. The diagnostic work-up and treatment depend upon host factors and specific causes.
- General resuscitative principles take precedent over the treatment of fever or the identification of specific causative agents.
- Fever must be quickly distinguished from hyperpyrexia. Improper treatment for one may lead to serious morbidity and mortality.
- Universal precautions are protective for the provider and patient. Care must be taken to leave all potentially infective materials safely disposed in the room with the patient.
- Most often the cause of a fever can be made from the history and physical examination alone.
- Special historical questions regarding personal, sexual, occupational, travel, pets, and dietary habits must be asked.
- Infrared tympanic thermometers are inadequate screening tools for fever. A low threshold should exist to recheck the temperature in the appropriate setting by other means and repeatedly, if necessary.
- The diagnostic framework for determining causes of a systemic physiological abnormality such as fever is best done by organ system rather than by anatomic region.
- Expedient laboratory sample collection should occur prior to antibiotic treatment. Antibiotic treatment should not be delayed if sample collection proves difficult.
- Antibiotics are less effective at preventing infection than treating them. Given our current drug-resistance crisis, every effort should be made to limit antibiotic use to those patients with documented or serious bacterial illness.

References

1. Balentine J. Life-threatening infectious disease emergencies. Foresight 2001;50:1–7.
2. Brillman JC, Quenzer RW. Infectious Disease in Emergency Medicine, 2nd ed., Philadelphia: Lippincott Williams & Wilkins, 1998. ISBN 0-316-10950-9.
3. de Gans J, van de Beek D. Dexamethasone in Adults with Bacterial Meningitis. *New Eng J Med* 2002;347(20):1549–1556.
4. ePocrates Rx Pro with QID, Infectious Disease Application, PDA application Palm OS, Version 6.0 Pro, 2002, ePocrates, Inc. http://www.epocrates.com
5. Gilbert DN, Moellering RC, Eliopoulos GM, Sande MA. Sanford Guide to Antimicrobial Therapy 2004, 34th ed., Hyde Park, VT: Antimicrobial Therapy, Inc., 2004. ISBN 1-930808-14-3.
6. Korvek SJ, Villarin LA. 2005 EMRA Antibiotic Guide, 2004. ISBN 1-929854-09-9, http://www.emra.org
7. Mackowiak PA. Fever, Basic Mechanisms and Management, 2nd ed., Philadelphia: Lippincott Williams & Wilkins, 1997. ISBN 0-397-51715-7.
8. McCraig LF, Burt CW. National Hospital Ambulatory Medical Care Survey: 1999 Emergency Department Summary. CDC's Advance Data 2001;320:1–36.
9. Ryan ET, Wilson ME, Kain KC. Illness after international travel. *New Eng J Med* 2002;347(7):505–516.
10. Saxe SE, Gardner P. The returning traveler with fever. *Inf Dis Clin North Am* 1992;6:427–439.
11. Shah SM, Searls L. The febrile adult: Part I. Asystemic approach to diagnosis and evaluation. *Emerg Med Rep* 1998;19(17):173–182.
12. Shah SM, Searles L. The Febrile Adult: Part II, Differential Diagnosis and Management of Infectious and Non-infectious Syndromes, *Emerg Med Rep* 1998;19(18)183–190.
13. Talan DA. New concepts in antimicrobial therapy for emergency department infections. *Ann Emerg Med* 1999;34:503–516.

23   Fever in children

Lynne McCullough, MD and Eric Savitsky, MD

Scope of the problem

Pediatric fever is one of the more common presenting complaints to the emergency department (ED). The objective of ED evaluation of febrile children is to identify and treat the small subset of children who harbor life-threatening bacterial infections. A febrile infant is at risk for a variety of serious bacterial infections (SBIs), including bacteremia, meningitis, osteomyelitis, suppurative arthritis, skin and soft tissue infection, urinary tract infection, gastroenteritis, and pneumonia. Concurrently, an attempt is made to avoid the indiscriminate use of antibiotics in febrile children. The etiology of a child's fever in the majority of cases is an acute viral infection. Unfortunately, considerable overlap exists in the clinical appearance of a child with *occult bacteremia* (presence of pathogenic bacteria in the blood of a well-appearing febrile child without an identifiable focus of infection) and a child with fever due to a viral illness. As a result, the broad spectrum of advocated management practices for febrile children continues to be the subject of much research and controversy.

Pathophysiology

Fever results from body temperature elevation above normal circadian variation due to an increase in the hypothalamic thermoregulatory set point. A febrile response is thought to result from enhanced metabolic activity and is mediated by the release of pyrogens. These pyrogens (e.g., tumor necrosis factor, interleukin-1, and interferon) are released from host leukocytes, which in turn reset the temperature regulatory center in the hypothalamus. In neonates, fever response pathways are not well-developed; consequently, fever is not a uniformly sensitive marker for acute infections. As a result, hypothermic or normothermic children with altered behavior (e.g., poor feeding and weak cry), especially neonates, warrant careful evaluation for acute infections.

A child's immune system matures with age. A neonate relies primarily on passive transfer of protective maternal immunoglobulins (IgG) to ward off infections. A child's immune system becomes more adept at responding to bacterial and viral pathogens over time. Widespread immunization of children has significantly reduced the morbidity and mortality caused by varicella, *Haemophilus influenza* type B, and the poliovirus infections, to name a few. Young infants are unable to mount sustained immunologic responses to certain vaccines (e.g., pertussis vaccine). This delay in immune response renders young infants susceptible to these illnesses.

Elevated body temperatures are often caused by infections, but also result from excessive physiologic stress (e.g., hyperthyroid state), central nervous system (CNS) lesions, inflammation, malignancy, or exposure to chemicals (e.g., drugs). Fever should be distinguished from hyperthermia. *Hyperthermia* is defined as an elevation in body temperature that is not associated with an elevation of the thermoregulatory set point. Hyperthermia is found in conditions characterized by inadequate heat dissipation from the body (e.g., environmental exposure, neuroleptic malignant syndrome, anticholinergic or sympathomimetic toxidromes).

History

How high was the temperature and how was it recorded?

A temperature of $\geq 38.0°C$ (100.4°F) is generally considered the threshold for defining a fever. A rectal temperature is regarded as the most accurate method of detecting core body temperature. A positive correlation between absolute height of fever and the risk for bacteremia has been established. While an elevated temperature itself is not believed harmful, it does impose metabolic demands on the body and predisposes certain children to complications. A small subset of children between the ages of 6 months and 5 years will be predisposed to developing febrile seizures as their body temperature rises. Children with epilepsy are at increased risk for seizures as a result of febrile illnesses.

How ill do the parents perceive their child to be?

The primary factor dictating the extent of a febrile child's ED evaluation is the overall appearance in an otherwise healthy child. A severely ill-appearing child should undergo an extensive fever evaluation and receive empiric antibiotic therapy. A happy, playful child in no visible distress is an ideal candidate for a less aggressive evaluation. Carefully listening to a calm and experienced parent's assessment of how ill their child appears is important. Parents are often more attune to illness subtleties in their children than are healthcare workers practicing in a hurried ED environment. Difficulties with feeding or anorexia are important clinical indicators of SBI and warrant careful evaluation.

Administration of antipyretics to children presenting to the ED with a fever often results in a rapid improvement in their appearance and behavior. Febrile children tend to be more irritable and ill-appearing, often leading to more extensive ED evaluations. Visual and behavioral clues to illness severity are difficult to ascertain in younger patients. Studies utilizing experienced clinicians have demonstrated that with infants below 2 months of age, clinical appearance alone is an insensitive indicator of illness severity. This fact underlies the more conservative approach to the evaluation of fever advocated in younger patients (e.g., neonates).

How long has the child been sick or had a fever?

In order to correctly establish a febrile child's course of illness, careful attention must be paid to the chronology of symptoms. For example, a child with a febrile illness for several days who appears to be improving is less likely to harbor an SBI than a listless and ill-appearing child who is only several hours into their febrile illness.

What are the child's associated symptoms?

Questions regarding the presence of associated symptoms can help identify the source of a child's fever. For example, a preceding history of dysuria and increased frequency of urination in a child are important clues suggesting the diagnosis of pyelonephritis. Infant teething should not be considered as a source of fever. Other symptom constellations may suggest a viral etiology for the fever, such as rhinorrhea, sneezing and cough for viral upper respiratory infection, and vomiting accompanied by diarrhea for acute viral gastroenteritis.

The child's hydration status should be determined by an evaluation inquiring about urine output and oral intake. The current number of wet diapers and the amount of oral fluids should be considered relative to when the child was previously well.

Was there exposure to ill contacts?

Sick household contacts and day-care classmates can be important reservoirs of disease. Inquiries into the specific type of infections (e.g., tuberculosis) that family members are suffering from often provide valuable clues to the etiology of febrile illnesses.

What is the child's medical history?

Prior illnesses or co-morbid conditions often place children at higher risk for suffering complications from SBI. For example, a child with cyanotic congenital heart disease will be less tolerant of an acute pulmonary infection compared to an otherwise healthy patient with a similar illness. Risk factors for SBI in neonates include issues related to birth history, including maternal fever, prolonged rupture of membranes, premature birth, and low birth weight. Prior pneumonia or urinary tract infection would also suggest the possibility of recurrence as the source of fever. Co-morbid conditions (e.g., congenital heart disease) or immunodeficient states (e.g., organ transplant recipients, cancer patients receiving chemotherapy, sickle cell patients with functional asplenia) are risk factors for SBI at any age. Inquiring about a child's immunization status is very important, as a child with an incomplete immunization record is at risk for a wider variety of illnesses and may benefit from more conservative care.

Has there been any travel history? Has there been any exposure to animals?

Travel outside the US may expose children to a variety of infectious diseases (e.g., malaria, typhoid). Noting the geographic areas a patient has traveled or lived within the US may provide useful information (e.g., Rocky Mountain spotted fever association with the East Coast). Inquiring about exposure to animals as well as tick and insect bites may provide important clues to the etiology of infectious illnesses (e.g., cat-scratch disease).

What medications has the child been given recently?

It is important to determine the last time the child received antibiotics, what type was given and for what condition. In the case of recent and recurrent infection, the antibiotic choice may need to be modified to one that has a broader spectrum of coverage to help ensure susceptibility. If the child has become progressively ill despite current antibiotic therapy, the possibility of an incompletely treated meningitis must be entertained.

The amount, type, frequency, and time of the last dose of antipyretic given prior to ED presentation also provides insight into the impact the medication is having on the fever. This information also provides an opportunity for parental education in cases of inadequate dosing or prolonged dosing intervals that may contribute to the persistence of fever in their child.

Physical examination

General appearance

Observation of a child's behavior while acquiring the history of present illness is a care provider's initial clue to illness severity. Attempts to define clinical features as indicators of SBI have been made (e.g., Yale Observation Scale, which includes an objective assessment of a child's alertness, playfulness, interaction with the environment, color, state of hydration, quality of cry, and ability to be consoled). Unfortunately, these clinical tools have been shown to be neither sensitive nor specific for distinguishing young infants with SBI. An assessment of a patient's mental status, activity, temperament, and interaction with their environment are the initial steps in evaluating febrile children.

The assessment of a child's responsiveness should include observation of the child's interaction with the practitioner, their spontaneous visual or physical exploration of the environment, reaching for and playing with age-appropriate toys, consolability with parents, and an observation of feeding behavior in small infants. Toxic children may cry excessively, be irritable, or be lethargic and difficult to arouse. They may demonstrate a lack of interest in the environment or in feeding, and can be inconsolable by their parents. They may appear mottled or pale with tachypnea and grunting respirations, and may be listless with decreased tone and response to external stimuli.

Vital signs

Begin with a review of triage vital signs (Table 23.1). The temperature should be obtained rectally

Table 23.1 Vital signs in children by age

Age	HR (beats/min)	SBP (mmHg)	RR (breaths/min)	Weight (kg)
Preterm	120–180 (140)	40–60 (50)	55–65	2
Term newborn	90–170 (125)	52–92 (72)	40–60	3
1 month	110–180 (120)	60–104 (82)	30–50	4
6 months	110–180 (130)	65–125 (94)	25–40	7
1 year	80–160 (125)	70–118 (94)	20–40	10
2 years	80–130 (110)	73–117 (95)	20–30	12
4 years	80–120 (105)	65–117 (91)	20–30	16
6 years	75–115 (100)	76–116 (96)	18–24	20
8 years	70–110 (90)	79–119 (99)	18–22	25
10 years	70–110 (80)	82–122 (102)	16–20	30
12 years	60–110 (75)	84–128 (106)	16–20	40
14 years	60–105 (75)	84–136 (110)	16–20	50

HR: heart rate; SBP: systolic blood pressure; RR: respiratory rate. Adapted from Barkin RM (ed.) Pediatric Emergency Medicine: Concepts and Clinical Practice, 2nd ed., St. Louis: Mosby, 1997.

in all children less 90 days of age, in those with tachypnea, and in all children too young to cooperate adequately with an oral temperature. The height of the fever should be noted, as it has prognostic value. Higher fevers are associated with an increased incidence of SBI, although the majority of these patients have viral infections. Elevated heart and respiratory rates may be the direct result of a fever. Tachycardia out of proportion to the degree of fever occurs with dehydration, sepsis, and cardiac conditions. Persistent tachycardia or tachypnea despite defervescence may be an indication of SBI. Blood pressure is an insensitive indicator of illness severity in children. Children have resilient cardiovascular compensatory capacity and often maintain normal blood pressures until advanced stages of illness. Pulse oximetry values of less than 95% on room air suggest compromised respiratory function and warrant further evaluation.

Head

The anterior fontanelle should be assessed for bulging that occurs in the presence of elevated intracranial pressure. A bulging fontanelle in a toxic-appearing infant is suggestive of meningitis. The eyes are evaluated for conjunctival injection and discharge, the nasopharynx and oropharynx for erythema, exanthems, or exudates. Injection of the conjunctiva may be seen with viral illness, conjunctivitis, or Kawasaki's disease (Figure 23.1). A careful evaluation of the oropharynx may yield important clues to the etiology of an infant's high fever and anorexia (e.g., mucosal vesicles suggestive of Coxsackie virus infection, a strawberry tongue associated with Kawasaki's disease (Figure 23.2), or late stage scarlet fever). Exudative tonsillitis in a child less than 2 years of age is most often viral in origin. The definitive diagnosis of acute otitis media is made difficult by cerumen, crying, or fever leading to hyperemia of the tympanic membrane. Acute otitis media is typically associated with a middle ear effusion and a hyperemic tympanic membrane with altered landmarks. Decreased movement of the tympanic membrane with insufflation is widely cited as the most accurate method to assess for middle ear effusion.

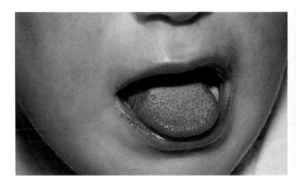

Figure 23.2
Strawberry tongue of Kawasaki's disease. Reprinted from Atlas of Pediatric Physical Diagnosis, 4th ed., Eds Zitelli BJ, Davis HW. Copyright 2002, with permission from Elsevier.

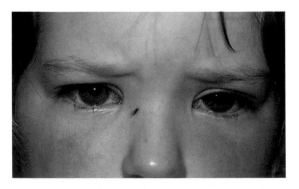

Figure 23.1
Injected conjunctiva of Kawasaki's disease. Reprinted from Atlas of Pediatric Physical Diagnosis, 4th ed., Eds Zitelli BJ, Davis HW. Copyright 2002, with permission from Elsevier.

Neck

The neck is examined for localized masses (i.e., lymphadenopathy and abscesses) and for passive range of motion. In the correct clinical context, nuchal rigidity (resistance to flexion and extension of the neck) suggests meningeal inflammation (i.e., meningitis). This sign is of limited value in young children and infants, as they often fail to develop nuchal rigidity despite having meningitis. In older children, nuchal rigidity may be identified by eliciting pain or spasm with knee extension with the knee and hip flexed at 90° (positive Kernig's sign), and hip flexion that occurs following passive neck flexion (positive Brudzinski's sign), although these signs are not reliable.

Lungs

Pulmonary examination begins with the assessment of work of breathing (i.e., respiratory rate, presence of retractions, or accessory muscle use). Tachypnea is a valuable clue to serious pulmonary infection. Auscultatory findings in pneumonia may demonstrate egophony, crackles, or wheezes. Young children may harbor significant pulmonary infections yet present with minimal auscultatory findings. The finding of diffuse symmetric crackles often signifies acute bronchiolitis. A subset of children with acute bronchiolitis will respond to beta-agonist therapy (e.g., albuterol) with resolution of auscultatory crackles.

Heart

Cardiac evaluation involves assessing heart rate, heart sounds, murmurs, and listening for additional findings (e.g., pericardial friction rub). Many children will have accentuation of innocent heart murmurs (e.g., pulmonary flow murmur and Still's murmur) during febrile illnesses. Any Grade III or higher murmur, diastolic murmur, or friction rub should be deemed pathologic warranting further evaluation. Persistent tachycardias despite defervescence and rehydration may indicate SBI.

Abdomen

The examination of the abdomen is a critical step in the evaluation of febrile children with concurrent gastrointestinal complaints. Hypoactive bowel sounds are an indicator of diminished intestinal motility, and the absence of bowel sounds is a cause for concern. Any focal tenderness, rebound, or guarding is suggestive of a potential surgical abdomen (e.g., appendicitis). Hepatosplenomegaly is associated with a variety of diseases.

A majority of cases of acute appendicitis are misdiagnosed in infants and young children. The accurate diagnosis of appendicitis in young children is confounded because these patients have limited communication skills, are difficult to examine, and typically have benign gastrointestinal illnesses (e.g., viral gastroenteritis) as the etiology of their fevers. Care providers should serially examine the abdomen to ensure the examination is benign in any febrile child with gastrointestinal complaints. In addition, fever and protracted gastrointestinal symptoms (e.g., anorexia and diarrhea) may be the presentation of a perforated appendix with abscess formation.

Extremities

The extremities should be examined for color, capillary refill, and pulse strength. Cool extremities with poor capillary refill and weak pulses are suggestive of diminished peripheral perfusion and sepsis syndrome or shock.

All joints should be examined for the presence of erythema, edema, warmth, or tenderness. Septic arthritis is a noted source of infection in infants.

Skin

The entire body of a febrile child should be inspected for the presence of a rash. The dermatologic manifestations of infectious diseases

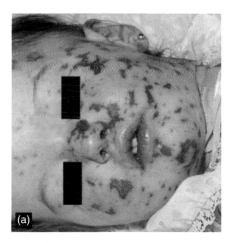

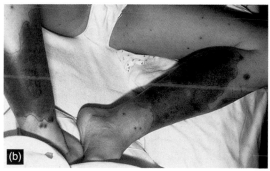

Figure 23.3
Meningococcemia. (a) This youngster manifests the purpuric and petechial rash characteristic of acute meningococcemia; (b) purpura may progress to form areas of frank cutaneous necrosis, especially in patients with DIC. Reprinted from Atlas of Pediatric Physical Diagnosis, 4th ed., Eds Zitelli BJ, Davis HW. Copyright 2002, with permission from Elsevier.

are protean. Nonetheless, familiarity with specific exanthems can provide helpful clues in evaluating febrile patients. The most notable example would be the classic cutaneous manifestations of *Neisseria meningitides* infections (Figure 23.3), including the presence of petechiae and purpura. It is important to distinguish diffuse petechiae from those lesions which occur above the nipple line associated with vigorous coughing or crying, as well as those on the upper extremities following tourniquet placement. Other classic descriptions of rashes include "dewdrop on a rose petal" for the lesions of varicella, and the "slapped-cheek" rash of erythema infectiosum (Figure 23.4).

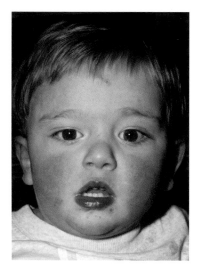

Figure 23.4
Slapped-cheek appearance of erythema infectiosum.
Courtesy: Lawrence Stack, MD.

Lymphatic system

Benign lymph nodes commonly palpated in healthy children are typically 1 cm in size or less, painless, mobile, and devoid of any warmth or induration. Any enlarged, warm, indurated, or fixed nodes warrant further evaluation.

Rectogenital

The circumcision status of a male patient with a fever should be noted, as the presence of foreskin correlates with an increased risk for urinary tract infections. The scrotum and testes should be examined to exclude epididymo-orchitis or testicular torsion as a source of fever. The rectal region should be evaluated to exclude signs of infection (e.g., perirectal abscess). A common finding in infants will be diaper dermatitis. This is differentiated from more serious exanthems by a lack of associated systemic findings, minimal tenderness, and characteristic distribution.

Neurologic

An age-appropriate neurologic examination may provide other clues to the source of the fever. As previously discussed, a diminished level of consciousness, lethargy, or irritability are worrisome for SBI, as well as other serious conditions, such as intussusception (Table 23.2). A reluctance to ambulate or an antalgic gait in an older child with fever may suggest a septic arthritis or osteomyelitis as the source.

Table 23.2 Causes of fever and altered sensorium

- Bacterial sepsis, other than meningitis
- Febrile seizure
- Hypoglycemia, secondary to poor oral intake plus vomiting and diarrhea
- Hyponatremic dehydration
- Intussusception
- Meningitis or encephalitis
- *Shigella* gastroenteritis
- Toxic ingestion
- Unsuspected head trauma, including shaken-baby syndrome with central nervous system bleeding

Adapted from Marx JA (ed.). Rosen's Emergency Medicine: Concepts and Clinical Practice, 5th ed., St. Louis, Mosby, 2002.

Differential diagnosis

Table 23.3 describes the symptoms, signs, and diagnostic tests associated with common diagnoses occuring in febrile children.

Table 23.3 Differential diagnosis of fever in children

Diagnosis	Symptoms	Signs	Diagnostic testing
Acute infectious laryngotracheo-bronchitis (Croup)	Barking cough, hoarse voice.	Stridor, harsh barking cough, occasional coarse crackles, rhonchi.	Clinical diagnosis. Plain radiographs of neck reveal characteristic findings (dilated hypopharynx on lateral view and steeple sign on PA view).
Acute otitis media	Ear pain, crying, hearing loss (typically preceded by an upper respiratory infection).	Bulging tympanic membrane, abnormal tympanic landmarks, middle ear effusion.	Clinical diagnosis. Ear insufflation is used as a screening tool for detecting middle ear effusion.
Acute suppurative adenitis	Painful mass, swelling, redness.	Tenderness, erythema, warmth, firm or fluctuant mass.	Clinical diagnosis. Further diagnostic testing may be indicated (e.g., *Mycobacterium tuberculosis* testing).
Appendicitis	Abdominal pain, anorexia, vomiting, diarrhea.	Abdominal tenderness, rebound, guarding.	Clinical diagnosis. Abdominal ultrasound or CT may assist in equivocal cases.
Bronchiolitis	Cough, rhinorrhea, wheezing, increased respiratory rate.	Tachypnea, crackles, wheezing.	Clinical diagnosis. Chest radiograph will demonstrate characteristic symmetric bilateral perihilar infiltrates. RSV nasal swabs may confirm etiologic agent.
Encephalitis	Altered behavior, headache, seizures.	Altered mental status, focal neurologic deficits, and papilledema.	LP*. The initial analysis is same as for meningitis, additional tests often indicated (e.g., herpes virus testing).
Epiglottitis	Sore throat, voice change, drooling.	Drooling, stridor, dysphonia, tripod posture, toxic-appearing child.	Clinical diagnosis. Plain lateral radiograph often show characteristic "thumbprint" sign. Definitive diagnosis made by direct laryngoscopy.**
Intussusception	Colicky abdominal pain, episodic inconsolability, bilious vomiting follows, 10% have "currant jelly" stool.	Episodes of lethargy or irritability alternating with normal behavior, soft abdomen between episodes, eventually tender or distended-abdomen, 85% mass in right lower quadrant (RLQ) or upper-abdomen, heme-positive stools.	Abdominal X-ray may show dilated loops and no air distal to the obstruction. Ultrasound is operator-dependent, but can have high diagnostic accuracy. Barium or fluoroscopic pneumatic (air) enema diagnostic and therapeutic.
Meningitis	Headache, stiff neck, nausea or vomiting, photophobia, altered behavior.	Photophobia, nuchal rigidity, altered mental status.	LP* Initial analysis includes cell count, Gram's stain, glucose, protein, and bacterial culture.
Occult bacteremia	Fever without a source of symptoms.	Range from well-appearing to lethargic and ill-appearing.	See diagnostic testing.
Orbital or periorbital cellulitis	Redness, pain, swelling around eye.	Pain, erythema, edema of peri-orbital region. Systemic symptoms (e.g., fever) and limited extraocular eye movement define orbital cellulitis.	Clinical diagnosis. Facial CT scan will assist in differentiating peri-orbital from orbital cellulitis in equivocal cases.

(continued)

Table 23.3 Differential diagnosis of fever in children (*cont*)

Diagnosis	Symptoms	Signs	Diagnostic testing
Osteomyelitis	Pain, redness over area, warmth, swelling.	Point tenderness, decreased mobility, swelling, warmth and erythema.	Clinical diagnosis. CBC, ESR, blood cultures, X-rays may be positive if more than 10–20 days of symptoms. CT may show soft tissue changes and swelling at 3 days. MRI is very sensitive after 24–36 hours.
Pharyngitis or tonsillitis	Sore throat, anorexia	Erythema, exudates, ulcerations, vesicles, cervical adenopathy. Displaced uvula and bulge in peritonsillar region are signs of a peritonsillar abscess or cellulitis.	Clinical diagnosis. Organism identification via throat cultures or assay.
Pneumonia	Cough, chest pain, shortness of breath, rapid breathing.	Hypoxia, tachypnea, respiratory distress and adventitial breath sounds.	Chest radiograph typically reveals an infiltrate.
Pyelonephritis	Nonspecific presentation in young children. Flank pain, abdominal pain, and nausea typical in older patients.	Flank tenderness. Physical findings outside of fever may be minimal.	Clinical diagnosis. Urinanalysis is suggestive and urine culture confirmatory of the diagnosis.
Retropharyngeal abscess	Severe throat pain, stiff neck, loss of appetite.	Torticollis, drooling, stridor, bulge in retropharynx.	Plain lateral radiograph of neck. CT imaging is more accurate.
Septic arthritis	Painful joint, can be warm, swollen; if involving the lower extremity, limp.	Exquisite tenderness to range of motion, decreased mobility, erythema, warmth and effusion may be present.	CBC, ESR, glucose, and blood cultures; arthrocentesis. Joint fluid is sent in heparinized tube for Gram's stain, cell count, glucose, and culture.
Viral upper respiratory tract infection	Rhinorrhea, sneezing, sore throat, cough, low-grade headache.	Rhinorrhea, pharyngeal erythema, rhonchi.	Clinical diagnosis.

*Performing an LP without prior neuroimaging in patients with altered mental status and possible CNS infection is controversial.
**Direct laryngoscopy should be performed by skilled endoscopists who are trained in caring for complications of acute airway obstruction.

CBC: complete blood count; CT: computed tomography; ESR: erythrocyte sedimentation rate; LP: lumbar puncture; MRI: magnetic resonance imaging; PA: posteroanterior; RSV: respiratory syncytial virus.

Diagnostic testing

Diagnostic testing of febrile children varies greatly between care providers. There is no uniformly accepted diagnostic approach to febrile children. Febrile child management algorithms incorporate patient age, co-morbidities, general appearance, vital signs, and results of ancillary testing (e.g., white blood cell (WBC) count). Some clinicians rely on prior clinical experience, while others utilize study-based algorithms to dictate their diagnostic evaluations. A list of laboratory studies may be ordered depending on the clinical scenario. A brief summary of significant abnormalities is provided, as well as potential pitfalls in the interpretation of each test.

Laboratory studies

Complete blood count

Leukocytosis with a left shift and bandemia are suggestive, but neither sensitive nor specific for the presence of an SBI. Thrombocytopenia may result from advanced disseminated intravascular coagulation associated with sepsis.

Urinalysis

Healthcare providers should generally obtain a catheterized specimen of urine until children are of school age, or are able to cooperate, to decrease the likelihood of a contaminated specimen. An elevated specific gravity is indicative of the degree of dehydration of the patient. The presence of more than 5 WBCs/high-power field (hpf) as well as a positive nitrite test suggest a bacterial infection. It is important to note that the urine may be normal in some children with urinary tract infections, particularly if obtained late in the day. If clinical suspicion is high, a urine culture should be sent, even if the urinalysis is negative. A Gram's stain positive for the presence of bacteria confirms the diagnosis of a urinary tract infection.

Urine culture

Results are typically not available for 24–48 hours; nonetheless, the urine culture is helpful for the identification of the infecting organism and its sensitivity to commonly prescribed antibiotics.

Blood culture

The delay in obtaining the results of cultures renders them unhelpful in the ED management of the febrile child; nonetheless, blood cultures are invaluable in the evaluation of the febrile child without a source.

Cerebrospinal fluid

Following lumbar puncture (LP), the cerebrospinal fluid (CSF) is routinely sent for glucose, protein, cell count including differential, Gram's stain, and culture. In the case of bacterial infection, a decreased glucose concentration compared with the peripheral blood values and a protein elevated from normal values can be expected. An elevated WBC count in an atraumatic LP needs to be evaluated for a leukocyte predominence, suggestive of a bacterial infection, as compared to a monocytic proliferation which is more indicative of a viral infection of the meninges. Traumatic taps with elevated RBC counts make the interpretation of the numbers and ratios of WBCs to RBCs more problematic. A negative Gram's stain does not conclusively rule out the possibility of bacterial meningitis; if other clinical data suggest a bacterial infection, the patient should be presumed to have bacterial meningitis and treated as such. A CSF culture requires 24–72 hours to be conclusive.

Erythrocyte sedimentation rate/C-reactive protein

The erythrocyte sedimentation rate (ESR) and the C-reactive protein (CRP) level are two non-specific markers of inflammation in the body which tend to be elevated in the presence of SBI. These are typically sent when the somewhat elusive diagnoses of osteomyelitis, septic arthritis, and Kawasaki's disease are being entertained.

Stool studies

The stool of a febrile child with a protracted course of diarrhea or bloody diarrhea can be sent for a number of studies: the number of fecal leukocytes/hpf, bacterial culture, the presence of ova and parasites, and the presence of *Clostridium difficile* toxin in patients who have received an extended course of antibiotics preceeding their diarrhea. A WBC count more than 5/hpf in a stool smear suggests a bacterial etiology of the diarrhea. Bacterial culture results may later define the offending agent.

Radiologic studies

Chest radiographs are indicated in any febrile child who presents with signs of respiratory distress. These include the presence of tachypnea, dyspnea, hypoxia (pulse oximetry on room air below 95%), or abnormal breath sounds. Since young children may harbor significant pulmonary infections with minimal auscultatory findings, a low threshold for radiographic imaging is indicated.

Management algorithms

Baraff et al. (1993) published the most widely publicized study regarding the management of febrile children. They performed a meta-analysis of studies involving the evaluation of febrile children, and developed recommendations for the management of children 0–36 months of age with fever without a source. Fever that has been documented at home by a reliable source should be considered the same as a febrile reading obtained at the doctor's office or in the ED. Fever without a source is defined as an acute febrile illness in which the etiology of the fever is not apparent after a careful history and physical examination. A summary of their recommendations are listed below:

Age below 28 days

A CBC, catheterized urine specimen for UA, urine culture, blood culture and CSF for cell count, glucose, protein, Gram's stain and culture should be obtained on all febrile patients below 28 days of age.

Age 28 days to 3 months

Febrile infants in this age group may be divided into low- and high-risk for invasive bacterial disease. The low-risk criteria include being previously healthy, having no focal bacterial infection on physical examination, and a negative laboratory screening. A negative laboratory screening examination includes a WBC count between 5000 and 15,000/mm^3, a neutrophil band count below 1500/mm^3, UA with less than 10 WBCs/hpf and no bacteria on urine Gram's stain, and CSF with less than 8 WBCs/hpf and no bacteria seen on Gram's stain. Infants meeting these criteria had only a 1.4% chance of a SBI.

Age 3 to 36 months

The major concern in these patients is the presence of occult bacteremia. Although there is no single laboratory test that can immediately exclude this possibility, the height of the WBC count is of some value as a screening test. Obtaining blood cultures is recommended if the WBC count is more than 15,000/mm^3. For febrile patients without a source and a temperature of 39°C or higher, a catheterized urine specimen should be obtained in all male infants up to 6 months of age if circumcized, otherwise until 1 year of age, and in all female patients 24 months or less. A urine culture should also be sent. A stool culture should be sent in the presence of diarrhea with gross blood. Children in this age category having fever of <39°C without a source need no laboratory evaluation, but close outpatient follow-up is warranted.

Age above 36 months

By 36 months of age, a child's immune system has developed such that the likelihood of SBI is less common. The incidence of occult bacteremia increases with higher temperatures and elevated WBC counts. Laboratory studies in febrile children above 36 months of age are dictated by the clinical setting.

The widespread utilization of the *Hemophilus influenzae* type B (HIB) vaccine and recently introduced heptavalent conjugate pneumococcal vaccine (PCV-7) has further challenged traditional diagnostic and therapeutic algorithms. Our approach to febrile children will undoubtedly be modified as the microbiology of occult bacteremia changes in the era of universal vaccination.

General treatment principles
Management of fever

Early and appropriate antipyretic therapy should be instituted in all febrile children to facilitate behavioral observation and relieve the child's discomfort associated with fever. Acetaminophen should be given at a dose of 15 mg/kg either per os (PO) or per rectum (PR) every 4–6 hours. Ibuprofen is also effective and can be given at 10 mg/kg PO every 6–8 hours in combination with acetaminophen.

Aspirin must not be used as an antipyretic in febrile children with viral syndromes (e.g., influenza and varicella), as it has been associated with the development of Reye's syndrome.

Empiric antibiotic therapy

Immediate empiric antibiotic therapy and hospitalization are indicated in any ill-appearing or significantly immunocompromised febrile child. Antibiotics are typically administered immediately following diagnostic evaluation. If a delay in performing diagnostic testing occurs, antibiotics should not be withheld from ill-appearing patients. Initial empiric antibiotic coverage should be targeted at the most likely pathogens. For example, a child with clinical evidence of pneumonia should have antibiotic coverage against typical (e.g., *Streptococcus pneumoniae*) and atypical (e.g., *Mycoplasma pneumoniae*) community-acquired pulmonary pathogens.

In many febrile children, ED evaluation does not reveal a definitive source of infection. These patients are still at risk for occult bacteremia. Initial empiric antibiotic coverage against bacteremia in children is often a third-generation cephalosporin (e.g., ceftriaxone or cefotaxime). The pathogen in a majority of cases of occult bacteremia is *Streptococcus pneumoniae*. Additional antibiotic coverage (e.g., ampicillin) against *Listeria monocytogenes* is recommended in febrile children in the first month of life. This regimen will not provide adequate anaerobic organism coverage, nor will it provide adequate anti-pseudomonal coverage. Additional antibiotic coverage needs to be administered if the aforementioned organisms are likely pathogens.

Additional empiric antibiotic coverage may be indicated (e.g., vancomycin) against cephalosporin-resistant strains of *Streptococcus pneumoniae* in any patient with a life-threatening infection. Finally, any neonate with evidence of a neonatal herpes virus infection should be hospitalized and receive empiric intravenous acyclovir therapy immediately.

All febrile infants below 28 days of age, irrespective of appearance, should have a complete sepsis evaluation and be hospitalized following the administration of parenteral antibiotic therapy. Infants between the ages of 28 days and 3 months meeting low-risk criteria* may be treated with a parenteral dose of ceftriaxone (50 mg/kg), sent home and re-evaluated in 24 hours if logistically feasible. All high-risk infants in this age group warrant empiric antibiotic therapy and careful consideration for hospitalization.

Special patients

Immune compromised

The management of immunodeficient pediatric patients with fever varies greatly depending on the specific immunodeficiency. In general, a lower threshold for diagnostic testing, empiric antibiotic therapy, and inpatient care is important in this patient population. Febrile immune compromised patients (e.g., chemotherapy patients and post-organ transplant) often require initial broad-spectrum antibiotic coverage (e.g., imipenem) while awaiting results of diagnostic testing. Communication with the patient's subspecialty physicians is a crucial part of their ED care. These physicians are excellent sources of additional clinical information that will optimize patient management. In the event these high-risk patients are sent home, careful chart documentation and provision of detailed aftercare instructions are crucial.

---

*Low-risk criteria include being previously healthy, having no focal bacterial infection on physical examination, and a WBC count between 5000 and 15,000/mm^3, a neutrophil band count below 1500/mm^3, UA with less than 10 WBCs/hpf and no bacteria on urine Gram's stain, and CSF with less than 8 WBCs/hpf and no bacteria on Gram's stain.

Patients with indwelling devices

Indwelling devices (e.g., central venous lines) are common sources of infection. A careful inspection of the device's entry site into the skin may reveal signs of infection (i.e., erythema, fluctuance, induration, or tenderness). Patients with indwelling devices represent a management challenge. They are at substantially higher risk of seeding their prosthetic devices or having them serve as a source of infection. A low threshold for obtaining blood cultures in these patients is warranted. Strong consideration for empiric antibiotic therapy and hospitalization should be given to febrile children with indwelling devices with no definitive source of infection.

Disposition

All toxic-appearing febrile children should be hospitalized, irrespective of age. Serial monitoring of vital signs and clinical appearance will influence the selection of an appropriate level of inpatient care (e.g., intensive care unit). As a general rule, any febrile child below 1 month of age (28 days of life), regardless of clinical appearance, is still hospitalized and treated with empiric antibiotic therapy pending culture results from a complete septic workup.

The decision whether to hospitalize patients older than 1 month with a fever is based on a variety of factors. These include presence or absence of systemic symptoms (e.g., respiratory symptoms), co-morbidities, course of illness, access to healthcare, and parental reliability. If a decision is made to discharge such a patient home, a thorough discussion and documentation of aftercare instructions and return precautions are paramount. It is also essential to ensure that the patient has follow-up to assess whether or not the child is improving. Children who remain febrile, or become less interactive with their environment should be reassessed immediately.

Pearls, pitfalls, and myths

- Failing to realize that neonates with SBI may have subtle and nonspecific presentations (e.g., poor feeding).
- The most accurate method for assessing core body temperature in the ED is with a rectal thermometer.
- Always inquire about antipyretic administration prior to ED evaluation.

Antipyretics may temporarily mask a fever and result in omitting an otherwise indicated diagnostic evaluation for a febrile child.

- Do not attribute an infant's fever to teething.
- Normal auscultation of the chest does not exclude the presence of a pneumonia in young febrile children.
- The urinary tract is a common site of bacterial infection in young infants. Failure to obtain a catheterized urine sample will often lead to misleading laboratory results.
- Failing to administer antibiotic coverage (e.g., vancomycin) against cephalosporin-resistant strains of *Streptococcal pneumoniae* in patients with life-threatening infections and organisms likely to be resistant.
- Failing to provide prompt parental antibiotic therapy (e.g., intramuscular route) in ill-appearing febrile children when there is a delay in obtaining intravenous access or completing diagnostic testing.

References

1. Baraff LJ, Bass JW, Fleisher GR, et al. Practice guideline for the management of infants and children 0–36 months of age with fever without a source. *Ann Emerg Med* 1993;22:1198–1210.
2. Baraff LJ. Management of fever without source in infants and children. *Ann Emerg Med* 2000;36:602–614.
3. Barkin RM (ed.). *Pediatric Emergency Medicine: Concepts and Clinical Practice*, 2nd ed., St. Louis: Mosby, 1997.
4. Bonadio WA. Assessing patient clinical appearance in the evaluation of the febrile child. *Am J Emerg Med* 1995;13:321–326.
5. Harwood-Nuss A (ed.). *The Clinical Practice of Emergency Medicine*, 3rd ed., Philadelphia: Lippincott Williams & Wilkins, 2001.
6. Jaskiewicz JA, McCarthy CA, Richardson AC, et al. Febrile infants at low risk for serious bacterial infection. An appraisal of the Rochester criteria and implications for management. *Pediatrics* 1994;94:390–396.
7. Klein JO. Management of the febrile child without a focus of infection in the era of universal pneumococcal immunization. *Pediatr Infect Dis J* 2002;21:584–588.
8. Lee GM, Harper MB. Risk of bacteremia for febrile young children in the post-*Haemophilus influenzae* type B era. *Arch Pediatr Adolesc Med* 1998;152:624–628.
9. Marx JA (ed.). *Rosen's Emergency Medicine: Concepts and Clinical Practice*, 5th ed., St. Louis: Mosby, 2002.
10. Strange GR (ed.). *Pediatric Emergency Medicine: A Comprehensive Study Guide*, 2nd ed., New York: McGraw-Hill, 2002.
11. Tintinalli JE (ed.). *Emergency Medicine: A Comprehensive Study Guide*, 5th ed., McGraw-Hill, 2000.

24 Gastrointestinal bleeding

J. Scott Taylor, MD

Scope of the problem

Bleeding may occur anywhere along the gastro-intestinal (GI) tract. Severity of bleeding may range from asymptomatic rectal bleeding to circulatory collapse from massive blood loss. The serious-ness of the disorder may be difficult to assess ini-tially, presenting a diagnostic and therapeutic challenge for emergency physicians.

GI bleeding (GIB) may occur at any age, most commonly between 40 and 79 years of age. Mor-tality is highest after the age of 60 years. GIB is divided into upper (UGIB) and lower (LGIB). UGIB occurs in 50–150/100,000 adults each year. There are 250,000 hospital admissions each year for UGIB, with costs of almost $1 billion.

Anatomic essentials

The ligament of Treitz crosses the small intestine at the junction of the duodenum and jejunum. Bleeding above the ligament of Treitz is considered UGIB; below this ligament it is considered LGIB. *Hematemesis* is the vomiting of blood. *Coffee-ground emesis* is from GIB in which blood has been in the stomach long enough to have been partially digested by stomach acid. UGIB usually results in the digestion of blood as it transits the small intes-tine. This results in *melena* (dark or black tarry stools), which is often foul-smelling. The passing of maroon or dark red stools is called *hema-tochezia*. This is usually from LGIB; however, this can also occur from brisk UGIB with a fast intes-tinal transit time. Bright red blood per rectum (BRBPR) is often from distal bleeding (descending colon, rectosigmoid, or rectum) or fast transit time.

The distal ileum may have a congenital mal-formation, known as *Meckel's diverticulum*, which may contain gastric tissue and thus result in a local ulceration or GIB.

History

Where are you seeing blood?

Patients can have blood either in their vomitus (hematemesis) or in their stool (hematochezia). Hematemesis occurs in 50% of UGIB. Blood per rectum may be bright red, may appear on toilet paper, or may be mixed with stool. Hematochezia most often signifies LGIB but may be due to brisk UGIB with a rapid transit through the intestinal tract.

Have you had vomit that looked brown or like coffee grounds?

Patients may not recognize that these are symp-toms of UGIB.

Have you had dark black, tarry, or sticky stool (melena)?

Melena occurs in about 70% of patients with UGIB and a third of patients with LGIB. Melena may result from as little as 60 ml of UGIB. Be sensitive to patients who may have visual impairment, diffi-culty with colors, or are elderly and not able to give you information about their stool or vomitus.

How much bleeding have you had?

This is often hard to assess, but ask if the blood in vomitus was merely streaking or frank blood, including the presence of any clots, as this points to larger amounts. Regarding bleeding per rec-tum, patients may see only a small amount on the toilet paper, or may be passing clots. It only takes a small amount of blood to change the color of toilet bowl water (about 5 ml). If possible, try to have the patient quantify their blood loss as a teaspoon or less, between a teaspoon and a cup, or more than a cup of blood.

When did the bleeding start?

Bleeding over days or weeks may appear mild, but can result in large blood loss and critically-ill patients. Heavy bleeding starting just prior to presentation sometimes resolves spontaneously but is more often an ominous sign.

Is the bleeding painful or painless?

Pain is from visceral or somatic nerves. If inflamed, the stomach and intestines can cause visceral pain. The oropharynx and anal verge have somatic pain fibers; bleeding from these areas may result in somatic pain. In cases of UGIB, pain may repre-sent an ulcer or gastritis. In LGIB, pain may be associated with inflammatory bowel disease or infectious diarrhea. Somatic pain may be from anal fissures or external hemorrhoids. Painless bleeding is usually from intestinal sources or internal hemorrhoids, without inflammation.

Did you have vomiting or retching prior to hematemesis?

This suggests a Mallory–Weiss tear of the esophagus.

What other symptoms do you have?

- *Are you dizzy or lightheaded?* Patients with large blood loss may have symptoms of hypovolemia, orthostasis, or shock.
- *Are you having chest pain or shortness of breath?* Blood loss and shock may precipitate cardiac ischemia or cause compensatory increased respiratory drive.
- *Have you had a fever?* This may be seen in patients with inflammatory bowel disease.

Have you ever had gastrointestinal bleeding before?

Bleeding from a previous site recurs in 60% of cases.

What other medical problems do you have?

Previous ulcers or gastritis can point to UGIB. Liver disease with portal hypertension can lead to esophageal varices. Coagulopathies and hemostasis problems (such as hemophilia and thrombocytopenia) can lead to significant bleeding and difficulty in management. Known diverticula can also cause bleeding. Patients with *Helicobacter pylori* infection of the gastric mucosa have a higher incidence of gastritis and risk of UGIB.

What prior surgeries have you had?

Any patient who has had an aortic aneurysm repair is at risk for an aortoenteric fistula. The graft erodes through the aorta into the intestines and can lead to catastrophic blood loss.

Have you ever had an endoscopic procedure?

Documented ulcers, varices, or diverticula can give information about the current bleeding. Previous banding or sclerosing of esophageal varices raises the risk of repeat bleeding due to portal hypertension or hepatic coagulopathy.

What medications do you take?

Aspirin and non-steroidal anti-inflammatory drugs (NSAIDs) can increase the likelihood of bleeding gastric ulcers. Iron ingestion by a child can cause UGIB. Patients on warfarin or outpatient heparin injections can have significant GIB. Steroids increase the likelihood of UGIB. Bismuth and iron can result in black stool that simulates melena. Eating beets can simulate BRBPR.

Do you drink alcohol?

Alcohol use increases the likelihood of gastritis. It also can contribute to coagulopathy and liver disease. Alcoholic cirrhosis can progress to portal hypertension with associated esophageal varices and hemorrhoids.

Physical examination

The primary goal of the physical examination is to assess the severity of the patient's illness and the amount of blood loss. The secondary goal is to establish the location of GIB. Patients with GIB may appear acutely ill with shock or may be asymptomatic except for their bleeding. The physical examination is somewhat limited in utility for localizing bleeding, although the rectal examination is very important.

General appearance

The appearance of cool, clammy, pale skin, decreased level of consciousness, and/or respiratory distress is concerning, as it implies that the patient is acutely ill, in shock, and in need of immediate resuscitation.

Vital signs

Signs of blood loss can be identified in the vital signs. A heart rate greater than 100 beats/minute can be an indicator of blood loss. Abnormal orthostatic vital signs show a trend toward worse outcomes in patients with GIB. Both the pulse and blood pressure are obtained with the patient supine, sitting, and standing. The patient should rest 2 minutes in each position before the recordings are made. Any patient who has symptoms of dizziness or lightheadedness in the sitting position should not be allowed to stand. When the blood pressure drops more than 10 mmHg or the pulse increases more than 20 beats/minute from lying to standing, this suggests volume loss. Orthostatic vital signs can be misleading though, especially in patients taking certain medications (e.g., beta-blockers). Some patients have great reserve and will not drop their blood pressure until dangerously blood-depleted, especially children. Other patients can have postural changes unrelated to blood loss from GIB (e.g., elderly, diabetics with autonomic instability). Patients on antidysrhythmic medication or with pacemakers may also be unable to respond to bleeding with pulse changes. An increase in the respiratory rate can be an indication of blood loss, with increased respiratory drive to compensate for red blood cell loss, or as compensation for metabolic acidosis secondary to poor perfusion.

Head, eyes, ears, nose, and throat

Observe for signs of liver disease such as icteric sclera. Conjunctivae can give a clue to anemia and blood loss if they are pale. Observe the oropharynx for any signs of bleeding from the nose or throat. Posterior epistaxis and oral lacerations can result in swallowed blood, with hematemesis and false positive nasogastric (NG) evaluation. Post-operative tonsillectomy bleeding can result in significant blood loss as the eschar falls off 5–7 days after the procedure. This can cause airway difficulty and requires ear, nose, and throat (ENT) evaluation, even if the bleeding has stopped.

Abdomen

Observe for distension. Auscultate for either increased or decreased bowel sounds, although this finding is nonspecific. Palpation may reveal discomfort in the epigastric region. This can be associated with an ulcer or gastritis. An enlarged or tender liver may be a clue to liver disease. Look for any evidence of peritonitis, as this may point toward an infectious cause. Palpation of an aortic aneurysm should raise the concern for an aortoenteric fistula. Abdominal scars may point to a previous aortic bypass graft with its risk of aortoenteric fistula, or previous surgeries for Crohn's disease. The abdomen may have prominent blue vessels around the umbilicus, known as *caput medusa* (or medusa's head). This dilation of abdominal wall veins occurs in portal hypertension. Ascites suggests liver disease with possible coagulopathy or portal hypertension.

Rectal

The rectal examination is essential in evaluating GIB. Inspection may show anal fissures or hemorrhoids. Digital examination should evaluate for masses or tenderness. The stool is then checked for gross or occult blood. As little as 5 ml of blood in the GI tract will give a positive hemoccult test. Anoscopy may be helpful if the GIB is believed to be from a lower GI source. This allows the anal verge to be visualized to identify a bleeding internal hemorrhoid.

Skin

The skin should be examined for purpura or petechiae, suggesting an underlying coagulopathy. Observe for stigmata of liver failure such as spider angiomata, palmar erythema and jaundice.

Differential diagnosis

Tables 24.1 and 24.2 describe the causes of upper and lower GI bleeding, respectively.

Table 24.1 Differential diagnosis of upper gastrointestinal bleeding

Diagnosis	Symptoms	Signs	Workup
Aortoenteric fistula	Ranges from mild bleeding to severe blood loss. Painless. In patients with history of AAA repair or AAA.	May be in shock from severe bleeding, or have no current bleeding and normal examination.	Urgent vascular surgery evaluation.
Gastritis and esophagitis	Usually hematemesis or coffee-ground emesis. May have epigastric discomfort, melena, hematochezia, or no symptoms.	NG suction positive for blood or coffee-ground material. 10% are false negative.	Early endoscopy within 24 hours.

(continued)

Table 24.1 Differential diagnosis of upper gastrointestinal bleeding (*cont*)

Diagnosis	Symptoms	Signs	Workup
Mallory–Weiss tear	Hematemesis after vomiting. Usually stops spontaneously.	NG suction may be positive. Usually stable.	Early endoscopy within 24 hours.
Ulcer – duodenal	Melena or hematochezia. May have hematemesis, coffee-ground emesis, or abdominal discomfort, but usually not present.	NG suction positive for blood or coffee-ground material. Often negative because bleeding distal to pyloric sphincter.	Early endoscopy within 24 hours.
Ulcer – gastric	Hematemesis or coffee-ground emesis. May have epigastric discomfort, melena or hema-tochezia, or no symptoms.	NG suction positive for blood or coffee-ground material. 10% are false negative.	Early endoscopy within 24 hours.
Varices – esophageal or gastric	Hematemesis may be severe or mild. Usually have melena or hematochezia, but may be delayed due to transit time.	NG suction usually positive and may have clots. May not clear with lavage. May be hemodynamically unstable. Often melena or hematochezia that may be severe.	Early endoscopy within 24 hours. If continued bleeding, more emergent endoscopy necessary. May require Sengstaken–Blakemore tube to stop severe bleeding and stabilize.

AAA: abdominal aortic aneurysm; NG: nasogastric.

Table 24.2 Differential diagnosis of lower gastrointestinal bleeding

Diagnosis	Symptoms	Signs	Workup
Anal fissure	Painful bowel movement with blood on toilet paper.	Seen on external examination and very tender to palpation.	None necessary.
Angiodysplasia	Painless red bleeding from rectum. May have melena.	BRBPR or melena. May be hemodynamically unstable.	Early colonoscopy. If emergent colonoscopy, rapid bowel preparation needed. May need tagged red cell study or angio-graphy to diagnose location. If unstable, consult surgery.
Carcinoma	Weight loss or weight gain. Change in caliber of stool. Often asymptomatic.	May have a palpable abdominal or rectal mass. May be cachectic.	Colonoscopy, biopsy, surgical evaluation.
Diverticulosis	Painless red bleeding from rectum.	BRBPR. May be hemodynamically unstable.	Early colonoscopy. If emergent colonoscopy, rapid bowel preparation needed. May need tagged red cell study or angiography to diagnose location. If unstable, consult surgery.
Hemorrhoid	*External* – painful bleeding on stool and toilet paper. *Internal* – painless red bleeding.	Seen on external examination or anoscopy.	Outpatient surgery evaluation.
Infectious diarrhea	Painful diarrhea with fever and blood or pus in stool.	Heme-positive stool, diarrhea.	Stool cultures, Gram's stain, fecal WBC. Antibiotics indicated.

(*continued*)

Table 24.2 Differential diagnosis of lower gastrointestinal bleeding (*cont*)

Diagnosis	Symptoms	Signs	Workup
Inflammatory bowel disease	Abdominal pain and rectal bleeding. Weight loss. Fever.	BRBPR, melena, or hemo-positive stool. Abdominal tenderness.	CBC, outpatient colonoscopy. May need admission for initial diagnosis.
Ischemic colitis	Severe abdominal pain and rectal bleeding.	Diffuse abdominal pain or peritonitis. May have pain out-of-proportion to examination.	Urgent surgical evaluation. May need angiographic intervention. CT scan for air in intestinal wall.
Meckel's diverticulum	Painless melena or hematochezia. May have abdominal pain.	May have chronic anemia or acute blood loss.	Often requires angiography or tagged red cell scanning. Surgical excision is diagnostic and therapeutic.
Upper GI bleed	May have hematemesis or abdominal pain. Most common cause of massive lower GI bleeding is upper GI bleeding site.	May present in shock.	Immediate GI consultation. CBC, coagulation studies, type and screen vs. crossmatch vs. immediate transfusion depending on clinical condition.

BRBPR: bright red blood per rectum; CBC: complete blood count; CT: computed tomography; GI: gastrointestinal; WBC: white blood cell.

Diagnostic testing

Occult blood

The presence of hemoglobin (Hgb) in the stool is detected using a hemoccult card and specialized developer. Hemoccult testing may detect blood not seen by the naked eye. After developer has been applied to the back of the filter paper (at the stool test site), the presence of a blue color change indicates the presence of Hgb and probable blood. Tests can be positive up to 14 days after a single episode of bleeding. False positive results can occur from consumption of red meat, blood-containing food, iodide, cantaloupe, uncooked broccoli, turnip, radish, or horseradish 3 days prior to the test. False negative results can occur if the blood has not transited the intestinal tract, magnesium-containing antacids have been used, ascorbic acid has been ingested, or the test is performed incorrectly.

Laboratory studies

Complete blood count

An Hgb less than 10 g/dL suggests significant blood loss. Low Hgb may be chronic, and comparison with previous values should be pursued. An Hgb less than 8 g/dL (hematocrit (Hct) less than 25%) usually requires blood transfusion. With fluid therapy, the red blood cell mass becomes diluted and the Hgb decreases. Initial blood counts may be normal if the bleeding has been very recent or is ongoing. Keep this in mind when using initial blood counts to determine therapy or disposition. Serial Hgb measurements are more useful for assessing the degree of blood loss.

The white blood count (WBC) may be elevated in infectious diarrhea or inflammatory bowel processes. Low platelet counts increase the likelihood of bleeding and should be corrected if less than 50,000/ml and bleeding is ongoing.

Blood urea nitrogen and creatinine

Blood urea nitrogen (BUN) greater than 36 mg/dL may suggest GIB in the appropriate clinical setting. It becomes elevated as the protein in blood is digested and absorbed from the GI tract, raising the serum urea level. Be cautious in the diagnostic use of BUN, as it can also be elevated when patients are dehydrated or in the case of renal failure. If the BUN/creatinine ratio is greater than 20, this suggests dehydration, or a "pre-renal" cause of an increased BUN to creatinine ratio.

Type and crossmatch

Whenever the patient's condition allows, it is preferable to provide type-specific blood for transfusion. If the patient is stable, a type and screen may be sent, followed by cross-match should the patient deteriorate.

Prothrombin time

Patients with liver disease, vitamin K deficiency, or taking warfarin may have a coagulopathy that requires correction to stop the bleeding.

Electrocardiogram

Cardiac ischemia may be precipitated by GIB. Any patient over 50 years of age, with a history of heart disease, significant anemia, hypotension, chest pain, shortness of breath, or other evidence of shock should have an electrocardiogram (ECG). The ECG may reveal evidence of ischemia or infarction in the setting of GIB. If ECG changes are seen, early emergent transfusion should be pursued.

Nasogastric tube

A nasogastric (NG) tube should be placed in all patients with UGIB. It is important for determining the location and degree of bleeding. The need for a NG tube is controversial in cases of LGIB. Some apparent LGIB is actually brisk UGIB and is only detected by NG evaluation. If there is any doubt, an NG tube should be placed.

An NG tube may show active bleeding or coffee-ground material. In 10–15% of UGIB patients, bright red blood or clots are found. Gentle *gastric lavage* with saline or sterile water is then done to see if bleeding has stopped; lavage is performed until the blood clears. If bleeding continues, the tube is left in place. If no blood or coffee grounds are found in the NG effluent, the tube can usually be removed. NG suction has a false negative rate of 10%. This can occur with intermittent bleeding, or if the bleeding is duodenal and spasm of the pylorus prevents the reflux of blood into the stomach. If bile is present and no blood is seen, this excludes the possibility of active bleeding above the ligament of Treitz. False positives occur in the case of traumatic tube placement with bleeding from the nasopharynx. The aspirate should be tested for occult blood using either gastroccult or a urine test strip for blood, as both of these tests are pH-independent.

In the case of esophageal varices, an NG tube can be placed carefully. Do not force the tube if resistance is met. No evidence exists that suggests NG tube placement aggravates hemorrhage from varices or Mallory–Weiss tears. Patients who have had gastric bypass surgery or fundoplication usually should not have an NG tube placed. This should first be discussed with the appropriate surgical service.

Anoscopy

Anoscopy can be performed at the bedside to evaluate for the presence of internal hemorrhoids. It is indicated in patients with mild rectal bleeding who do not have an obvious source.

Radiologic studies

Radiographs

Plain films of the abdomen are usually not indicated in most cases of GIB. If there is concern for ruptured viscus associated with vomiting or in suspected cases of gastric or duodenal ulcers, a plain upright chest radiograph is indicated. Free air under the diaphragm may be seen in perforated ulcer, and air in the mediastinum may be due to a ruptured esophagus. If there is concern for cardiac ischemia, a chest radiograph is indicated. A plain abdominal film may show iron tablets in a case of suspected pediatric iron ingestion.

Upper gastrointestinal studies

Barium contrast studies are of limited value in the emergency management of GIB. The use of barium can limit the utility of subsequent endoscopy or angiography.

General treatment principles

The initial treatment approach is the same for upper and lower GI bleeding. Recognition of acutely ill patients is paramount. As with all emergency patients, airway, breathing, and circulation are attended to first. UGIB patients can have airway difficulty if they have severe hematemesis from a bleeding varix or ulcer, and endotracheal intubation may be necessary. Blood loss may result in decreased level of consciousness necessitating intubation if patients are not breathing adequately. If blood loss is severe, patients may be hypotensive and in shock. Supplemental oxygen, a cardiac monitor, and two large-bore intravenous (IV) catheters (18 G or larger) should be placed immediately. If hypotension, tachycardia, or obvious ongoing blood loss is detected, resuscitation should be initiated with a crystalloid bolus, followed by early transfusion with type O blood (unless type-specific blood is available) should the vital signs remain abnormal. An initial bolus of 2 L of crystalloid (adult) or 20 ml/kg (child) should be used.

Upper gastrointestinal bleeding

Esophagogastroduodenoscopy

Esophagogastroduodenoscopy (EGD) is both diagnostic and in many cases therapeutic. In severe bleeding, the airway must be secured before emergency EGD. Endoscopy provides visual evaluation of the esophagus, gastric mucosa, and the proximal duodenum. If performed within 12–24 hours of hemorrhage, EGD identifies lesions in 78–95% of UGIB patients. It allows localization of bleeding, as well as an opportunity for therapeutic intervention. Esophageal varices can either be sclerosed, injected, or banded. Bleeding gastric or duodenal ulcers can be injected and sclerosed if visualized. If complete perforation is detected, surgery can be pursued.

EGD with sclerotherapy has not been found to reduce mortality or rebleeding compared to vasoactive substances or other treatments in the initial treatment of severe UGIB from esophageal varices. It is, however, the diagnostic modality of choice, and repeat sclerotherapy or banding is the long-term treatment of choice for esophageal varices, in addition to treating underlying causes. EGD is not usually performed in the ED, but in the intensive care unit (ICU) or endoscopy suite if the patient is admitted, or the outpatient setting if discharged. UGIB patients rarely need EGD for stabilization. It is difficult to perform endoscopy on extremely critical patients that are bleeding heavily, as large amounts of blood may limit visualization with the endoscope.

Antacids

Antacids should not be used for the treatment of UGIB. They have not been shown to decrease the incidence of bleeding. Antacids also can make urgent or emergent EGD difficult by coating the esophageal or gastric mucosa.

Somatostatin and octreotide

These are vasoactive proteins that cause selective constriction of the splanchnic vascular bed and decrease gastric acid secretion. The use of these medications decreases blood flow to the esophagus, stomach, and duodenum, usually decreasing blood loss from UGIB. Somatostatin is naturally occurring, while octreotide is a synthetic equivalent. These vasoactive substances have shown limited effectiveness in decreasing UGIB, but no difference in mortality or rebleeding compared to endoscopic sclerotherapy. In a recent meta-analysis, use of these agents was associated with a slight decrease in the amount of blood products required. The use of these substances with endoscopic sclerotherapy or banding is a source of ongoing study and discussion.

Vasopressin

Vasopressin is a vasoconstrictor which effects the entire circulatory system, including the splanchnic bed. It is extremely potent and should be used in an exsanguinating patient, when endoscopy is unavailable or not possible. Vasopressin requires cautious use, because end-organ damage may occur.

Histamine blockers and proton pump inhibitors

Histamine (H2) blockers and proton pump inhibitors (PPIs) decrease the acid secretion which contributes to gastric or duodenal ulcer formation. These medications are routinely given to patients with UGIB, not to stop the bleeding, but to initiate ulcer or gastritis treatment. This may reduce further bleeding in the future.

Esophageal tamponade

Direct pressure (tamponade) of bleeding esophageal varices may be performed when vasoactive medications are not effective, and endoscopy is either ineffective or unavailable. Tamponade may temporarily control severe hemorrhage in up to 80% of patients with bleeding esophageal varices. It can be used for 12–24 hours. Tamponade may be accomplished with a specialized gastric tube that incorporates two expanding balloons. One balloon is first expanded in the stomach. A second balloon is then expanded in the esophagus. There is a suction eye at the tip. The Sengstaken–Blakemore tube is the usual multi-lumen tube used for tamponade (Figure 24.1). Some tubes have a modification incorporating suction eyes in the esophagus to decrease the risk of aspiration. A Linton tube has a single stomach balloon which is larger and more effective with gastric varices.

Esophageal tamponade carries significant complications, including esophageal rupture, airway

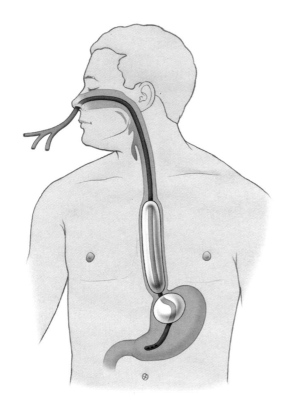

Figure 24.1
Sengstaken–Blakemore tube.

compression from the esophageal tube, and aspiration. Most cases of UGIB can be controlled with endoscopy or medications, but tamponade remains an effective modality for extreme cases.

Surgery

This is the final option for a severe UGIB. Cases where bleeding does not stop or significantly decrease after medication use, endoscopy, or tamponade need surgical intervention. Most UGIB stops after conservative treatment. However, ongoing blood loss, massive blood loss (5 units of red blood cells transfused in 6 hours or 2 units of blood necessary every 4 hours) should prompt surgical intervention. If a patient requires 2 units of blood after crystalloid infusion to maintain blood pressure, surgical consultation should be considered. A surgical team should evaluate patients with other morbidities early in a case of severe UGIB. EGD should be performed in these extreme cases, but usually in the operating room (OR) under general anesthesia to guide surgical treatment or possibly provide direct sclerotherapy.

Due to the risk of aortoenteric fistula, patients with a history of aortic graft placement and current

UGIB should be evaluated emergently by a vascular surgeon.

Lower gastrointestinal bleeding

Colonoscopy

Colonoscopy provides direct visualization of bleeding sources and the opportunity for direct therapeutic intervention. Direct epinephrine injection or electrical coagulation can stop bleeding sources. This is considered the intervention of choice for cases of LGIB. Colonoscopy is difficult on an emergent basis because it is best done after adequate bowel preparation. It is not usually done in the ED. If urgent colonoscopy is anticipated, an emergent bowel preparation can be performed with NG administration of 2 L of polyethylene glycol. This can cause volume loss by osmotic diuresis, so hemodynamic status should be followed closely, usually in the ICU setting.

Sigmoidoscopy

Sigmoidoscopy is performed on an outpatient basis to evaluate the sigmoid colon for diverticulae, polyps or tumors. It is reserved for cases of mild LGIB.

Arteriography

Arteriography can detect 0.5 ml of GIB per minute. Since the advent of endoscopy, it is only used in 1% of UGIB cases. Arteriography is more commonly used in LGIB cases. It can identify the site of bleeding, but rarely diagnoses the cause. If bleeding is detected, vasopressin or epinephrine can be injected locally or embolization can be performed to stop the bleeding. There is a 2% complication rate including dye reaction, arterial dissection, or ischemia related to vasopressin. The use of angiography in the setting of GIB depends on individual institutional practice, availability, and operator expertise. It is usually reserved for significant, persistent, or intermittent LGIB that cannot be localized by endoscopy. It usually is performed outside of the ED setting, after admission to the hospital.

Tagged red blood cell imaging

Technetium (^{99m}Tc) tagged red blood cells can detect LGIB of 0.1 ml/min. An initial scan is done and delayed scans are compared in an attempt to localize bleeding. This scanning is rarely done in the ED setting. Tagged cell scans should be ordered in consultation with either the gastroenterology or surgical service.

Vasopressin

Vasopressin is a vasoconstrictor which effects the entire circulatory system, including the splanchnic bed. It is very potent and should be used only in an exsanguinating LGIB patient. Colonoscopy lacks utility for the initial stabilization of LGIB, so vasopressin may be necessary until surgery or emergent preparation and colonoscopy can be performed. Vasopressin requires cautious use, because end-organ damage may occur.

Surgery

When arteriography is unsuccessful in LGIB, emergent surgery may be necessary. If lower GI hemorrhage is significant and ongoing (5 units of red blood cells transfused in 6 hours or 2 units necessary every 4 hours), surgery may be required. Arteriography provides a guide to the surgical location for hemicolectomy or other intervention.

Indications for transfusion

If a patient has low blood pressure or evidence of volume depletion after an initial crystalloid bolus of 2 L for adults or 20–40 ml/kg in children, transfusion should be started. Patients with severe distress, cardiac ischemia, or massive blood loss should receive blood products as soon as possible. If type-specific blood is not available, then type O blood (Rh-negative in females) should be transfused. Type-specific and then cross-matched blood should be used as soon as possible.

Serial Hgb values should be monitored closely, and if blood losses are ongoing, transfusion should occur. If platelet counts are less than 50,000/ml, platelets should be transfused.

Indications for fresh frozen plasma or vitamin K

Fresh frozen plasma (FFP) should be administered in patients who have GIB and elevated prothrombin times (PT). This occurs in patients with liver disease, vitamin K deficiencies, warfarin therapy, or coagulopathies (e.g., disseminated intravascular coagulation (DIC) or hemophilia). If the PT is elevated and bleeding is ongoing, cross-matched FFP is given. Vitamin K can be given in

the ED; however, its effect is delayed and will not stop acute bleeding.

Special patients

Pediatric

The most common cause of UGIB in children is esophagitis, followed by gastritis, ulcer, varices, and Mallory–Weiss tears. The most common causes of LGIB in decreasing frequency are anal fissures, infectious colitis, inflammatory bowel disease, polyps, and intussusception. Formula intolerance should be considered in infants. Intussusception should be considered in children age 3–12 months with colicky pain and hematochezia. "Currant-jelly" stool is the classic description, but is a late finding. The management of GIB in children is similar to that in adults. More often the cause of bleeding is benign and can be managed on an outpatient basis. The emergency physician should keep in mind that much smaller blood losses may result in hemodynamic instability. Children with large or ongoing blood loss, vital sign abnormalities, or co-morbidities should be admitted.

Elderly

Geriatric patients are often on medications that can make the assessment of hypotension and significant blood loss more difficult. Beta-blockers can obscure the diagnosis of hypovolemia by preventing tachycardia. Geriatric patients are more likely to have vague complaints, and may present with only a change in mental status or weakness. They have a higher morbidity and mortality from GIB; as such, clinicians need to maintain a high level of suspicion. Geriatric patients may have visual difficulties making it difficult to identify blood, hematochezia, or melena. Subsequent problems with cardiac ischemia or respiratory compromise as a result of GIB may occur, as geriatric patients have less hemodynamic and physiologic reserve. Emergency physicians must have a low threshold for admission and further evaluation of these patients.

Immune compromised

Patients with malignancy, human immunodeficiency virus (HIV), and those on immunosuppressants are at a higher risk of infectious complications. Patients treated with steroids have a higher risk of forming ulcers, possibly resulting in GIB. Steroids may also prevent a proper stress response to bleeding and hypovolemia. Supplemental corticosteroids may be necessary for a patient in refractory shock who usually takes steroids.

Disposition

Guidelines for specialty consultation or admission

Any patient who is unstable or has an Hgb less than 10 g/dL should be admitted to the hospital and evaluated by a gastroenterologist. In the case of unstable LGIB, a general surgeon should evaluate the patient if severe bleeding is not controlled with vasoactive medicine or arteriography. Patients with GIB who continue to be unstable, continue to bleed, or have comorbidities should be admitted to the ICU. Ill-appearing patients with inflammatory bowel disease should be admitted for antibiotics and colonoscopy. Patients with LGIB, except from fissures, hemorrhoids, or mild proctitis should be admitted for further evaluation. Patients with UGIB and a history of AAA repair need emergent evaluation by a vascular surgeon. Patients with GIB and comorbidities should also be considered for admission, except in cases that are low-risk for further bleeding and can easily be followed on an outpatient basis.

Guidelines for emergency department observation

A patient with UGIB that has stopped, with a small to moderate amount of bleeding, and an Hgb greater than 10 g/dL may be evaluated in an observation unit for early diagnostic endoscopy. Serial Hgb levels are followed, looking for a drop of 2 g/dL or more, which usually leads to admission. Patients with LGIB are not routinely evaluated in an observation setting, because colonoscopy is usually warranted and is not easily done in a short observation setting.

Guidelines for discharge

Historically, all patients with GIB were admitted. With continuing changes in health care, low-risk patients are often evaluated on an outpatient basis. Stable UGIB patients with a normal Hgb, few or no comorbidities, and a small amount of bleeding that has resolved may be discharged if close follow-up (1–2 days) is available. Patients with LGIB from a benign source (hemorrhoids or fissures) may be discharged with primary care follow-up.

Discharged patients should be given precautions and instructions about any further bleeding, with specific instructions regarding when they should return to the ED or contact their primary care physician. Patients should return if bleeding recurs, or if symptoms of volume depletion (dizziness, lightheadedness, syncope, or near syncope), chest pain, shortness of breath, melena, or hematochezia develop. Patients should also return if they have new symptoms, or any other problems or concerns.

Pearls, pitfalls, and myths

- The most common cause of massive LGIB is an UGIB site with a brisk transit time.
- The Hgb may not initially reflect a large degree of bleeding; serial measurements are necessary.
- NG suction has a 10% false-negative rate.
- Previous aortic aneurysm repair requires early vascular surgery consultation for possible aortoenteric fistula.
- Be very cautious with elderly patients and GIB. Comorbidities make these patients highly susceptible to associated morbidity and mortality.
- GIB is a common cause of altered mental status and generalized weakness in the elderly.

References

1. Bono MJ. Lower gastrointestinal tract bleeding. *Emerg Med Clin North Am* 1996;14:547.
2. Harwood-Nuss A. *The Clinical Practice of Emergency Medicine*, 3rd ed., Philadelphia, PA: Lippincott, Williams, Wilkins, Inc., © 2001. pp. 809–812, 767–771, 1177–1181.
5. Marx JA. *Rosen's Emergency Medicine: Concepts and Clinical Practice*, 5th ed., St. Louis, MO: Mosby, Inc., © 2002. pp. 194–200.
3. McGuirk TD, Coyle WJ. Upper gastrointestinal tract bleeding. *Emerg Med Clin North Am* 1996;14:523.
4. Peter DJ, Dougherty JM. Evaluation of the patient with gastrointestinal bleeding: an evidence based approach. *Emerg Med Clin North Am* 1999;17:239.
6. Talbot-Stern JK. Gastrointestinal bleeding. *Emerg Med Clin North Am* 1996;14:173.
7. Tintinalli JE. Emergency Medicine: A comprehensive study guide, 5th ed., New York, NY: McGraw-Hil, 2000. pp. 520–523.

25 Headache

Gino A. Farina, MD and Kumar Alagappan, MD

Scope of the problem

Headache is a very common complaint, with three out of four Americans experiencing a headache each year. However, only a small percentage of them seek medical care. Headaches account for approximately 2 million emergency department (ED) visits each year in the US. A patient with a headache may have a serious or minor etiology for his or her headache. The differential diagnosis of headache is complex and long. Headache can be divided into primary or secondary disorders (Table 25.1). Primary headaches, such as migraines, cluster, and tension-type headaches account for 90% of headaches in clinical practice. Secondary headaches include tumors, aneurysms, and meningitis, and have an identifiable, distinct pathologic process in which head pain is a presenting symptom. Most patients presenting to the ED have a benign headache requiring symptomatic treatment and referral. A small subset of patients who present with a headache will have a life threatening illness; it is the primary goal of the treating clinician to identify these patients and provide appropriate care.

Table 25.1 Major categories of headaches

Primary
• Migraines
• Tension
• Cluster
Secondary
• Head trauma
• Vascular disorders (stroke, intracranial hematoma, subarachnoid hemorrhage, unruptured vascular malformation, arteritis, venous thrombosis, arterial hypertension)
• Non-vascular intracranial disorder (high or low cerebral spinal fluid pressure, non-infectious inflammatory disease, intracranial neoplasm)
• Substance use or withdrawal
• Infection (meningitis, encephalitis, brain abscess, or acute febrile illness of any type)
• Metabolic disorders (hypoxia, hypercapnia, other metabolic abnormalities)
• Cranial–facial disorders (pathology of cranium, neck, eyes, sinuses, and other cranial–facial structures)
• Neuralgias

Anatomic essentials

The pain from headache can originate from extracranial or intracranial structures. Extracranial structures that can cause pain include skin, blood vessels, muscles, and bone. The brain parenchyma, most of the dura, the arachnoid, and pia mater have no pain fibers and do not produce pain. Intracranial structures with pain fibers include venous sinuses, the dura at the base of the skull, dural arteries, the falx cerebri, and large arteries at the base of the brain.

The fifth cranial nerve (CN) carries pain fibers from structures above the tentorium and supplies most of the facial areas. CNs IX, X, and XI along with upper cervical nerves carry these pain fibers below the tentorium, resulting in pain referred to the neck and back of the head.

History

A detailed history is the most important part of the evaluation of a patient with a headache. A thorough history will identify "danger signs" in patients complaining of headaches (Table 25.2).

Table 25.2 Historical danger signs in patients with headache

• Sudden onset of headache (thunderclap)
• Worst headache of life
• Headache dramatically different from past headaches
• Headache in a patient who is immunocompromised
• New onset of headache after the age of 50
• Headache that begins with exertion

How did the pain begin (sudden vs. gradual onset) and how long has it been present?

These are two crucial questions to ask while obtaining a history. A patient with sudden onset of a severe unprecedented headache, with or without neurologic deficits, should be investigated for ruptured aneurysm or subarachnoid hemorrhage (SAH). Gradual onset of headaches that have persisted for weeks or months suggest tension headaches. New headaches that worsen in intensity over weeks are suspicious for mass effect associated with increased intracranial pressure (ICP). Episodic headaches with symptom-free intervals suggest migraine or cluster headaches. Frontal or occipital headaches that begin 24–48 hours after a lumbar puncture (LP), known as post-dural headaches, may be secondary to a persistent cerebrospinal fluid (CSF) leak.

What time of day is your headache worse?

If a patient complains that they wake up with a headache, one must consider hypertension, cluster, or neoplastic etiologies. However, patients with tension headaches often awaken pain-free and develop their headache as the day progresses.

What were you doing when the pain began?

The activity being performed or the events preceding the onset of headache often provide valuable clues to the etiology. A sudden onset of the "worst headache of my life" at rest or during any activity is highly suggestive of SAH. If the headache begins while in a car with the engine running or the patient is a victim of a fire, carbon monoxide (CO) has to be considered. Headaches and dizziness are the two most common complaints of CO poisoning. A headache that occurs during or immediately after sex may be a coital or post-coital headache. A patient may experience a severe but benign headache after coughing, sneezing, laughing, heavy lifting, stooping, or any Valsalva maneuver. The pain starts within a few seconds of the activity and may last for a few seconds to minutes. The sudden nature and severity of these headaches sometimes simulate an acute SAH. Headache associated with hunger, stress, sleep deprivation, menses, specific types of food ingestion, or oral contraceptive use suggests migraine. Any history of remote or recent trauma prior to the headache also must be ascertained.

What does the pain feel like?

The character of the pain is important, and may be useful in determining an etiology. Severe, intense, sudden onset, or "thunderclap" headaches may be the result of SAH. A pulsatile pain that correlates with the patient's pulse is usually vascular in origin. If the pain is pulsatile but does not correlate with the pulse, it is nonspecific. A dull, constant band-like occipitofrontal headache is characteristic of tension headache.

Where is your pain?

The location of pain may be helpful in narrowing the diagnosis. Unilateral headaches are suggestive of migraines or a mass on the ipsilateral side. Unilateral facial pain is seen with trigeminal neuralgia, sinusitis, and carotid artery dissection. Headaches that progress from unilateral to bilateral may be from increased ICP. Vertex headaches are seen with sphenoid sinusitis and supratentorial lesions. Orbital headaches suggest glaucoma, optic neuritis, cluster headache, and cavernous sinus thrombosis. Occipital headaches suggest cerebellar lesions, muscle spasm, and cervical radiculopathy. However, an acute occipitocervical headache can be associated with intracranial pathology, especially when accompanied by other symptoms.

Does anything make the pain better or worse?

A headache that worsens with coughing, bending, or turning the head may be associated with a mass lesion or sinusitis. Post-dural puncture headaches generally improve or disappear with recumbence and worsen when the patient is upright.

What medications are you taking or have you changed any medications?

Headache is one of the most common side effects of prescribed medications. Medications that commonly cause headaches include nitroglycerine, hydralazine, calcium channel blockers, digitalis, and estrogen. Patients who stop drinking coffee may develop a headache within 24–48 hours of abstinence. The headache resolves following ingestion of caffeine. Alcohol, marijuana, and amphetamines may also induce headaches. A patient who uses cocaine may have a headache due to an intracranial bleed.

Have you had the pain before?

Patients with migraine, cluster and tension headaches often have a history of similar headaches and symptoms. Migraine headaches typically start in childhood, adolescence, or young adulthood, and patients often have a history of previous attacks. A significant change in intensity, location, or character from prior headaches may indicate serious new pathology, such as a SAH. A recent severe headache may represent a *sentinel bleed* from a cerebral aneurysm. Patients with tension headaches may also have a previous history of similar headaches. Periodicity is the main feature of cluster headaches. Suspicion is warranted when an elderly patient complains of a new-onset headache. New headaches in patients over 50 years of age should raise concern for glaucoma, intracranial lesions, and temporal arteritis.

Associated signs and symptoms

Nausea or vomiting

Nausea and vomiting are commonly seen with migraine headaches, in patients with SAH, meningitis, post-LP headaches, or those with increased ICP.

Photophobia

Photophobia can be due to irritation of the meninges from SAH or meningitis, and is a common complaint in migraine headache patients. It can also arise from a pathologic problem with the eyes, such as iritis, uveitis, or acute angle closure glaucoma.

Neck stiffness

Neck stiffness, particularly the inability to flex the neck or resistance to neck flexion, can be a sign of meningeal irritation from SAH or meningitis.

Fever

It is important to ask about fever, as the majority of patients with bacterial meningitis will have a fever on presentation to the ED. Fever is not a specific finding, however, because it can be a secondary cause of a headache.

Other

Unilateral nasal congestion, tearing, and conjunctival injection may be seen with cluster headaches. A patient with temporal arteritis will often complain of polymyalgias. Patients with migraine headaches may develop visual or meningeal findings such as photophobia. Visual field deficits, diplopia, seizures, and syncope are associated with SAH. In a patient who is pregnant, headache may be a sign of preeclampsia.

Past medical and family

A positive family history is present in 70% of patients with migraines. There is no family history with cluster headaches. A family history of SAH is a risk factor for SAH. There is a familial association of cerebral aneurysms with several diseases, including autosomal dominant polycystic disease, coarctation of the aorta, Marfan's syndrome, and Ehlers–Danlos syndrome type IV. A previous history of neurosurgery or malignancy (with potential for metastases) should raise concern for intracranial pathology, including a malfunctioning indwelling shunt.

Physical examination
General appearance

The patient's general appearance is an important clinical observation that helps gauge the degree of distress. It may not help distinguish a life-threatening from benign condition. A patient with a small SAH (sentinel bleed) may be comfortable, particularly if the aneurysm has not yet completely ruptured, as opposed to a patient with a migraine headache who may be in severe discomfort.

Vital signs

Vital signs can be abnormal in patients with a headache. Tachycardia and tachypnea may be secondary to pain. An elevated blood pressure may be seen with SAH. An elevated temperature may indicate an intracranial infection.

Head

Inspection and palpation of the head may reveal evidence of trauma. Tenderness in the area of the sinuses or teeth may be clues to the diagnosis; however, purulent nasal secretions and abnormal sinus transillumination are the best clinical predictors of sinusitis. Always palpate the temporal artery in the elderly patient. Temporal arteritis may present only with a complaint of headache. A tender area of the scalp that exactly reproduces the head pain may indicate neuralgia.

Eyes

A thorough eye examination should be performed in all patients with a headache. The examination should assess the visual acuity, pupil size, extraocular movements, and for evidence of photophobia. Patients with acute angle closure glaucoma may present with a headache. Signs include conjunctival injection, mid-dilated pupil, increased intraocular pressure, and decreased visual acuity. Evaluation of extraocular movements may reveal a CN VI deficit, which may represent a mass lesion or aneurysm. Fundoscopic examination should also be performed to check for spontaneous venous pulsations (SVPs), subtle pulsations of the central retinal vein just where it emerges from the optic disk. The absence of SVPs suggests papilledema, a sign of increased ICP. Subhyaloid or pre-retinal hemorrhages are seen with SAH, whereas retinal hemorrhages and exudates may be secondary to hypertensive encephalopathy. Occasionally a patient may develop a headache because he or she has a refractive error and needs corrective lenses, although the headache is usually not sudden in onset.

Skin

Look for rash associated with meningococcemia (Figure 23.3), Rocky Mountain spotted fever (Figure 30.8), or vasculitis.

Neurologic

A complete neurologic examination on patients with headaches must be performed. This includes assessment of mental status, cranial nerves, motor, sensory, and cerebellar function. The presence of new focal neurologic deficits, seizures, or cognitive impairment mandates imaging studies of the brain. Careful attention to the cranial nerves may reveal abnormal CN III or VI function, which may indicate an intracranial mass lesion, increased ICP, tonsillar herniation, or cerebral aneurysm.

Meningeal signs

Nuchal rigidity

A neck examination should be performed with the patient supine and relaxed, looking for involuntary resistance with passive flexion. Pain or resistance to flexion suggest meningeal inflammation, but may also be due to arthritis or neck injury.

Brudzinki's sign

While passively flexing the neck as described above, watch for flexion of the patient's hips and knees in reaction to this maneuver (Figure 25.1). If present, this also suggests meningeal inflammation. Brudzinki's sign is neither sensitive nor specific for meningitis.

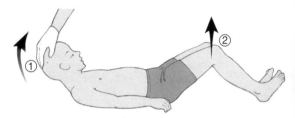

Figure 25.1
Brudzinki's sign.

Kernig's sign

Flex one of the patient's legs at the hip and knee, and then straighten at the knee. Pain or resistance to this suggests meningeal irritation (Figure 25.2). Kernig's sign is neither sensitive nor specific for meningitis.

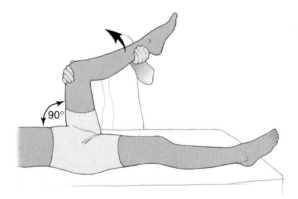

Figure 25.2
Kernig's sign.

Jolt accentuation of headache

This maneuver is performed by asking the patient to turn his or her head horizontally at a frequency of 2–3 rotations per second. Worsening of the baseline headache represents a positive sign. The jolt accentuation sign has a sensitivity of 97% and specificity of 60% for meningitis, but has only been studied in a small sample of patients (Table 25.3).

Differential diagnosis

Tables 25.4. and 25.5 provide a list of primary and secondary causes of headache, with their signs, symptoms, and work-up.

Table 25.3 Physical findings of danger signs in headaches

- Altered mental status
- Meningeal signs, including positive Brudzinki's or Kernig's signs
- Positive "jolt" accentuation sign
- Focal neurologic signs
- Rash suspicious for meningococcemia

Table 25.4 Differential diagnosis of primary headache

Diagnosis	Symptoms	Signs	Work-up
Primary headaches			
Cluster headaches	90% occur in males. No familial predisposition.	Classically unilateral nasal congestion, tearing and conjunctival injection.	No work-up necessary if the diagnosis is clear. CT of the brain may be needed to rule-out CVA or hemorrhage.
Migraine	Often initially unilateral, severe, and associated with an aura. The HA is throbbing and pulsatile in character, and associated nausea, vomiting, photophobia, phonophobia, and scotomas. May be worse lying down.	May vary from mild to severe. In severe cases, patients may be prostrate to stuporous with cold limbs and pale skin. Patients may have conjunctival injection and/or hypesthesia on the affected side. The vein or artery over the temple may be prominent.	No work-up necessary if the diagnosis is clear. CT of the brain may be needed to rule-out CVA or hemorrhage.
Migraine variant	Uncommon. Hemiplegia is a type of aura that may include motor, sensory, or speech disturbances. Lasts >1 hour and <1 week. There is an autosomal inherited form.	As above.	No work-up necessary if the diagnosis is clear. CT of the brain may be needed to rule-out CVA or hemorrhage.
Ophthalmoplegic migraines	Most common in children and adolescents. Transitory paresis of extraocular motor cranial nerves (CNs III, IV, VI). Occurs at the height of the cephalgia but can persist for days to weeks. Paresis is unilateral and pain is periorbital and ipsilateral.	Paresis of extraocular muscles (CNs III, IV, VI).	No work-up necessary if the diagnosis is clear. CT of the brain may be needed to rule-out CVA or hemorrhage. Prognosis for recovery is excellent.
Tension headache	Affects 75% of population. Recurrent pain, most commonly occurs among middle-aged individuals. Little is known about the pathophysiology. Band-like discomfort around head that is non-pulsatile. Usually mild intensity of short duration. Anxiety and depression may coexist with chronic tension HA.	Physical examination is normal.	No work-up necessary if the diagnosis is clear. CT of the brain may be needed to rule-out CVA or hemorrhage.

CT: computed tomography; CVA: cerebrovascular accident; CN: cranial nerve; HA: headache.

Table 25.5 Differential diagnosis of secondary headache

Diagnosis	Symptoms	Signs	Work-up
Secondary headaches			
Acute angle closure glaucoma	Acute onset of a severe HA around the affected eye. May radiate to the forehead, ear, sinuses, or teeth. Patients may see halos around lights, experience blurriness or scotomas, and often complain of nausea and vomiting.	Physical examination reveals a red eye with a fixed, mid-dilated pupil, corneal clouding, and a shallow anterior chamber. The intraocular pressure is >50 mmHg (normal <20 mmHg).	Slit lamp examination and tonometry are mandatory. Urgent ophthalmologic evaluation is required.
Alcohol	Ingestion or withdrawal interferes with cerebral autoregulation and depressed serotonin levels.	May see signs of inebriation.	Supportive treatment.
Bacterial meningitis	HA is severe and worsens rapidly.	Fever with photophobia. Kernig's and Brudzinki's signs may be present. Altered sensorium is not uncommon.	LP with CSF cultures. CT before LP is not required unless there is a concern of a space-occupying lesion. Treatment is with steroids and broad-spectrum antibiotics.
Benign cough headache	Usually bilateral in nature lasting from seconds to minutes following a paroxysm of intense coughing.	Signs depend on the etiology of the cough.	Work-up and treatment should be directed at the etiology of the cough.
Benign exertional headache	More frequent in males >40 years of age. May be precipitated by bending, lifting, sneezing, or defecating. Typically lasts a few seconds but can last for hours. It is bilateral but may be unilateral, severe, and sudden in onset, having a bursting, explosive, or splitting quality.	Physical examination is normal.	History or physical examination do not distinguish this from other more serious pathologies. CT followed by an LP should be performed to rule out a life-threatening condition, particularly SAH. Once the diagnosis of benign exertional HA is confirmed, avoidance of the precipitating factor is recommended.
Brain abscess	HA with fever; may also have vomiting.	Fever, focal neurologic findings and depressed level of consciousness.	CT, antibiotics, and neurosurgical consultation.
Carbon monoxide	Pulsatile and diffuse HA. May be accompanied by nausea and vomiting. Blurred vision occurs with increased HA intensity until a CO level of 30–40% is reached, then obtundation occurs.	Signs are variable. May have findings suggestive of exposure to smoke.	Must have a high index of suspicion, especially when family members living in the same house have similar symptoms. Diagnosis is made by obtaining a CO level from a venous sample. Treatment is 100% oxygen, with some patients requiring hyperbaric oxygen therapy.
Carotid artery dissection	Unilateral HA may be severe and throbbing but may be also be subacute and similar to previous headaches. Acute onset of severe retro-orbital pain in a patient without a history of cluster HAs suggests carotid artery dissection. Patients may also complain of visual disturbances, aphasia and hemiparesis.	Physical findings may include ipsilateral Horner's syndrome and contralateral hemispheric findings (aphasia, neglect, visual disturbances, and hemiparesis).	Diagnosis may be difficult. Initial work-up includes a head CT which may be unremarkable. Future imaging may include duplex carotid artery scanning, magnetic resonance angiography, and carotid angiography.

(continued)

Table 25.5 Differential diagnosis of secondary headache (*cont*)

Diagnosis	Symptoms	Signs	Work-up
Cavernous sinus thrombosis	Limitation of eye movement and facial pain. Fever, nausea, vomiting, and altered level of consciousness often develop. Can be a complication of facial, periorbital, or orbital cellulitis; retrograde spread via the ophthalmic veins leads to cavernous sinus involvement.	Unilateral and then bilateral proptosis with paralysis of CNs III, IV, VI. Meningeal signs, dilation of the episcleral veins, venous engorgement of fundus, and pupillary dilation.	Blood cultures as well as culture of a draining cellulitis if present. CT of the brain warranted. Ophthalmologic and neurosurgical consultation.
Cervicogenic headache	This HA is from conditions related to disorders of the neck. It is a unilateral HA that occurs with movements of the head or neck. HA can occur from a trigger point in the neck, typically unilateral that spreads to the ipsilateral shoulder or arm. Whiplash injury is often associated with these HAs.	Often can elicit a trigger point in the neck or shoulders on careful examination.	Supportive care.
Coital or post-coital headache	Begins as a dull bilateral ache as sexual excitement increases and becomes intense at orgasm. Incidence is unknown because many patients never seek medical attention. Four times more common in males. Risk factors include obesity, hypertension, fatigue, migraine, and peripheral vascular disease.	Physical examination is normal.	Often impossible to distinguish from SAH; therefore, work-up for SAH may be necessary.
Cold stimulus headache	Non-pulsatile. Peaks 25–60 seconds after exposure. Most patients have a history of migraines.	Physical examination is normal.	No work-up required.
Encephalitis	HA severity is variable. May present with fever, confusion, and seizures.	Altered sensorium and focal neurologic findings.	CT and LP with viral cultures.
Epidural hematoma	Classically there is a history of head trauma with LOC, followed by a return to normal mental status. After a period of hours, as the hematoma enlarges, the patient complains of a diffuse HA and may develop hemiplegia and obtundation. This so-called "lucid interval" is neither sensitive nor specific.	Signs may vary from an unremarkable examination to signs of increased ICP (hemiplegia, pupillary dilation, and obtundation) as herniation approaches.	CT and neurosurgical consultation.
Headaches as a side effect of medications	HAs are generally secondary to their vasoactive effects and are typically persistent, generalized, throbbing, and migraine-like in character.	No specific signs.	Generally a diagnosis of exclusion. Stop the offending agent and the headaches should improve.
HIV infections	HA may be from aseptic meningitis, cryptococcus, toxoplasmosis, tuberculous meningitis, or cytomegaloencephalitis.	May be associated with fever and focal neurologic findings.	CT and, if negative, LP with appropriate cultures.

(*continued*)

Table 25.5 Differential diagnosis of secondary headache (*cont*)

Diagnosis	Symptoms	Signs	Work-up
Hypertensive headache	Not a common cause of HA. The rate of rise of the blood pressure is more important than the absolute value. Pain is usually diffuse and occurs in the morning upon awakening. Generally improves as the day progresses.	Diastolic pressures under 130 mmHg are rarely the cause of HA. With hypertensive encephalopathy the blood pressure is around 250/150 mmHg.	Work-up consists of ruling out end-organ damage. In addition, one must consider drug-induced hypertension, eclampsia, and pheochromo-cytoma as alternate etiologies of HA and elevated blood pressure.
Idiopathic intracranial hypertension	Formerly known as *pseudotumor cerebri* or *benign intracranial hypertension*. Relatively common in young obese women of childbearing age. Predisposing factors include use of oral contraceptives, anabolic steroids, tetracyclines, and vitamin A. Visual complaints are common and can become permanent in up to 10%.	Examination may reveal papilledema and visual field defects. No localizing signs on neurologic examination.	Diagnosis is made with neuroimaging and measurement of ICP. An opening spinal pressure >200 mmH$_2$O on LP is associated with an absence of mass lesions or ventricular enlargement on neuroimaging.
Monosodium glutamate (MSG) headache	Chinese restaurant syndrome occurs 20 minutes after ingestion of MSG. HA is throbbing, bifrontal or bitemporal. Often there is pressure or tightness across the face and chest. May also have dizziness, flushing, nausea, and abdominal discomfort.	May see flushing of the skin.	No work-up needed and treatment is symptomatic.
Non-hemorrhagic stroke	HA can be seen with both ischemic and hemorrhagic strokes, and may precede, accompany, or follow the event. Presence of a HA correlates with a large artery thrombotic stroke (less with embolic and least with lacunar strokes). HA is also more common with cortical infarcts compared to deeper lesions.	Cognitive impairment may mask the HA. Neurologic deficits may include slurred speech, cerebellar findings, and hemiparesis.	CT is the study of choice in the initial evaluation of a suspected stroke. Although a CT may not reveal a stroke in the first 24 hours of the event, it is helpful to rule out a hemorrhage and evaluate for the possible use of thrombolytics.
Post-concussive headache	Occurs after mild to moderate head trauma, hours to days after the incident. The syndrome is accompanied by dizziness, fatigue, and insomnia. The HA symptoms resolve spontaneously after several weeks.	Physical examination is normal.	If symptoms or HA persist, CT, MRI and neuropsychiatric testing may be warranted.
Post-dural puncture headache	Usually frontal or occipital headache within 48 hours of an LP. May be associated with nausea, vomiting, dizziness, or tinnitus. The HA results from a persistent CSF leak with subsequent traction on intracranial pain-sensitive structures. Occurs following 10–30% of all LPs.	Symptoms improve or disappear with recumbence.	The diagnosis is usually clear and no work-up is necessary.

(*continued*)

Table 25.5 Differential diagnosis of secondary headache (*cont*)

Diagnosis	Symptoms	Signs	Work-up
Subarachnoid hemorrhage	Sudden onset of the "worst headache" of the patient's life. Loss of consciousness may occur. History of an unusual HA weeks earlier (sentinel bleed) is seen in 1/3 of patients.	Signs include depressed LOC (66%), impaired speech (33%), disorientation (50%), neck stiffness (75%), and seizures (15%). >50% will have ECG changes (prolonged QT, ST elevation or depression, prominent U waves). Close to 70% will have a normal motor examination; around 85% will have a normal CN exam; almost 10% will have abnormal CN III function.	CT of the brain; if, negative, then LP is mandatory. If CT or LP positive then urgent neurosurgical consultation and cerebral angiogram.
Sinus headache	HA is often described as deep, dull, or heavy, made worse by shaking the head or bending forward. Often accompanied by fever and purulent nasal discharge.	Tenderness over sinuses and purulent drainage may be present.	May include a CBC and blood cultures depending on how ill the patient appears. CT of sinuses is the gold standard.
Subdural hematoma	Results from venous bleeding underneath the dura. Symptoms develop more slowly than with epidural bleeds. Many patients present acutely with head trauma and HA. Depending on the extent of bleeding, other symptoms range from mild HA to obtundation. Patients, particularly the elderly, may present several weeks after the initial injury with HAs and personality changes.	Findings may be subtle. If there is continued bleeding, mass effect and signs of increased ICP may develop.	CT and neurosurgical consultation.
Temporal arteritis	Also known as *giant cell arteritis*, this condition results in inflammation of mid- and small-sized arteries. Females are more commonly affected than males, and the age of onset is typically in the early 70s but can occur earlier. HA can be continuous or intermittent, and tends to be worse at night or in the cold. Jaw claudication may also occur secondary to vascular insufficiency. The most serious complication is visual loss if untreated.	Physical examination may reveal tenderness and induration of the scalp arteries.	There is a significant increase in the ESR. Diagnosis is confirmed with arterial biopsy. Treatment is high-dose steroids.
Traumatic subarachnoid hemorrhage	Most common cause of an intracranial hemorrhage following head trauma. May present similarly to non-traumatic SAH. In addition to a HA, may complain of forgetfulness, irritability, poor concentration, fatigue, dizziness, somnolence, insomnia, anxiety, and other global symptoms.	Similar to SAH.	CT and neurosurgical consultation.

(*continued*)

Table 25.5 Differential diagnosis of secondary headache (*cont*)

Diagnosis	Symptoms	Signs	Work-up
Trigeminal neuralgia	Painful, unilateral, brief shock-like pains in the distribution of one or more branches of the trigeminal nerve. Episodes last from seconds to minutes, may occur spontaneously or be invoked by talking, chewing, shaving, or even brushing of teeth.	May see unilateral grimaces during episodes.	Careful neurologic examination with particular attention to the trigeminal nerve distribution. CT or MRI is required to rule out a mass, especially if there is sensory or motor dysfunction.
Tumor headache	HA is the most common symptom occurring in >50% of patients. Most brain tumors are metastases from the lung and breast. These patients tend to be older. Primary brain tumors occur in younger patients. The pain patterns are variable depending on the size and location of the mass. The HA tends to be worse in the morning and may be associated with vomiting.	The neurologic examination depends on the location of the tumor.	Neuroimaging is needed to identify the size and location of the mass. Neurosurgical referral must be made. Steroids should be used for edema.
Vertebral artery dissection	Severe unilateral posterior HA with vertigo, vomiting, ataxia, diplopia, hemiparesis, unilateral facial weakness, and tinnitus.	Hemiparesis, ataxia, and signs of brainstem or cerebellar ischemia.	Same work-up as carotid artery dissection.
Viral meningitis	HA may be severe but more indolent than in bacterial meningitis.	Same as with bacterial meningitis but generally have a normal mental status.	Same as bacterial meningitis. Antibiotics are not required but are often administered pending culture results.

CBC: complete blood count; CN: cranial nerve; CO: carbon monoxide; CSF: cerebrospinal fluid; CT: computed tomography; CVA: cerebrovascular accident; ECG: electrocardiogram; ESR: erythrocyte sedimentation rate; HA: headache; HIV: human immunodeficiency virus; ICP: intracranial pressure; LOC: loss of consciousness; LP: lumbar puncture; MRI: magnetic resonance imaging; SAH: subarachnoid hemorrhage.

Diagnostic testing

Radiologic studies

If the diagnosis of migraine, cluster, tension, or post-dural puncture headache can be made from the history and physical examination, then imaging studies are unnecessary. If the diagnosis is unclear then computed tomography (CT) of the head or magnetic resonance imaging (MRI) of the brain should be performed to delineate lesions that may be responsible for the headache. CT is preferred for the detection of acute intracranial hemorrhage, increased ICP, and hydrocephalus. In a patient with a headache and human immuno-deficiency virus (HIV), CT with contrast may reveal a ring-enhancing lesion suggestive of toxo-plasmosis (Figure 25.3). A CT can also identify approximately 90% of patients with SAH, and is best when performed in the first 24 hours follow-ing headache onset (Figure 25.4).

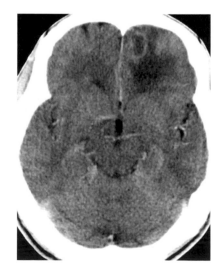

Figure 25.3
Cerebral toxoplasmosis. Head CT post-contrast enhance-ment demonstrates ring-enhancing lesion of left frontal lobe with vasogenic edema. *Courtesy*: Mahesh Jayaraman, MD.

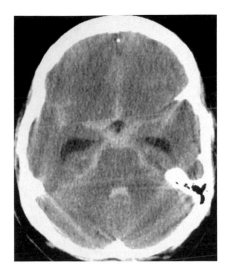

Figure 25.4
Subarachnoid hemorrhage. Non-enhanced CT of the head reveals diffuse subarachnoid hemorrhage, intraventricular hemorrhage and hydrocephalus.
Courtesy: Mahesh Jayaraman, MD.

MRI is generally not required in the initial work-up of a patient with a headache. When available, however, it is preferred in certain clinical situations. MRI has a higher sensitivity than CT for the detection of SAH after 24 hours and non-hemorrhagic strokes in the first 24–48 hours. MRI is also superior to CT at visualizing the posterior fossa, localizing tumors and focal infections, and diagnosing cavernous sinus thrombosis and carotid artery dissection.

Laboratory studies

Laboratory tests may be performed depending on the clinical scenario. For example, if an infection is suspected, blood cultures and a complete blood count (CBC) may be required. However, patients with meningitis may have a normal white blood cell count. The erythrocyte sedimentation rate (ESR) is elevated in patients with temporal arteritis; physicians should consider ordering this test in an elderly patient with a headache. A CO level should be obtained when there is a suspicion of CO poisoning. One should not rely on pulse oximetry or an arterial blood gas (ABG) alone to rule out CO poisoning. The arterial oxygen concentration and hence the calculated oxygen saturation reported on an ABG are usually normal since CO does not affect dissolved oxygen in the serum. Co-oximetry can measure oxygen saturation directly. The measured oxygen saturation will be less than the calculated oxygen saturation by the amount roughly equal to the percent of CO-hemoglobin present. Serum chemistries should be performed when there is concern for electrolyte abnormalities, such as in patients with profuse vomiting, prolonged diarrhea, diabetes mellitus, or seizures.

CSF analysis is required when there is suspicion of intracranial infection, or when SAH is suspected and CT of the head does not demonstrate subarachnoid blood. When SAH is likely, the CSF analysis should include a cell count from the first and last tube collected. This is done to distinguish a traumatic LP from SAH. If the number of red blood cells (RBCs) does not significantly decrease from the first to the last tube (which suggests possible SAH), the patient needs a neurosurgical evaluation and a cerebral angiogram (Figure 25.5). The CSF also needs to be examined for xanthochromia, a yellowish discoloration of the CSF caused by pigment released from the breakdown of RBCs in the CSF (Figure 25.6). This may be done visually, but is more accurately done with a spectrophotometer. Presence of xanthochromia also warrants neurosurgical evaluation and a cerebral angiogram. When performing an LP, an opening pressure should be measured. An opening spinal pressure >200 mmH$_2$O is seen in idiopathic intracranial hypertension or other conditions that may have an increased ICP, such as meningitis.

General treatment principles

All patients presenting with headache to the ED should be evaluated in a timely fashion. All patients deserve symptomatic relief; some will require a work-up. Treatment with analgesics can be initiated while the diagnostic studies are performed. The patient should be placed in a quiet and dark area of the ED so as not to exacerbate the symptoms.

After performing a physical examination, if the patient can tolerate oral intake and is not a surgical candidate, the patient may be given oral analgesics. If oral intake cannot be tolerated, intravenous (IV) access must be obtained for hydration and administration of analgesics, and possibly anti-emetics.

Many of the secondary headaches, such as those resulting from cold stimulus, alcohol, exertion, cough, hypertension, MSG, or side-effects of medications improve with treatment of the primary disorder or avoidance of the precipitating event or medication. Symptomatic treatment with acetaminophen may be beneficial.

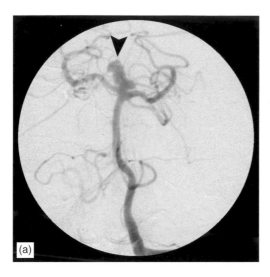 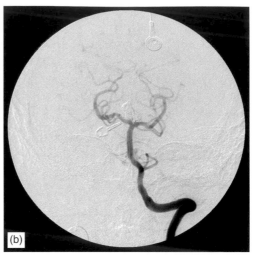

Figure 25.5
Basilar tip aneurysm. (a) Frontal projection from a left vertebral artery angiogram demonstrates a basilar tip aneurysm (BLACK ARROW) with a relatively narrow neck. (b) Frontal projection angiogram following endovascular coil embolization demonstrates no signification residual filling of the aneurysm. *Courtesy*: Mahesh Jayaraman, MD.

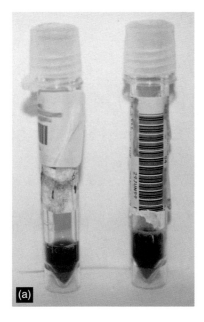 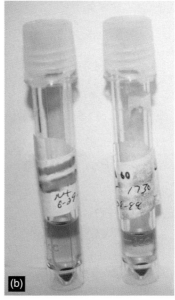

Figure 25.6
CSF tubes demonstrating: (a) bloody CSF representing subarachnoid hemorrhage (SAH); (b) xanthochromia in CSF fluid, note the golden yellow-brown appearance of the translucent CSF. *Courtesy*: Gus M. Garmel, MD.

Migraines

For mild to moderate attacks, acetaminophen, aspirin, or non-steroidal anti-inflammatory drugs (NSAIDs) are recommended. For moderate to severe attacks, if the patient cannot tolerate oral intake, intramuscular or subcutaneous dihydroergotamine or sumatriptan are excellent options. IV prochlorperazine, chlorpromazine, or metoclopramide are also commonly used. Parenteral ketorolac or meperidine may be of value as well. Refractory attacks (status migrainosus) are best treated with parenteral dihydroergotamine and IV steroids (Table 25.6).

Table 25.6 Pharmacologic options for the treatment of acute migraines and related headaches

Drug	Indications	Dose and route	Comments
NSAIDs			All contraindicated if allergy to aspirin or NSAIDs
Ibuprofen	Mild/moderate headache	600–800 mg PO	Gastrointestinal upset
Naproxen sodium	Mild/moderate headache	275–550 mg PO	Gastrointestinal upset
Indomethacin	Mild/moderate headache	25–50 mg PO or 50 mg PR	Gastrointestinal upset
Ketorolac	Moderate/severe headache	30 mg IV or 30–60 mg IM	Gastrointestinal upset; avoid in elderly patients and those with renal insufficiency.
Serotonin agonists			
Dihydroergotamine	Moderate/severe migraine, cluster	1 mg IV or IM may be repeated in 1 hour	Gastrointestinal upset (pretreat with antiemetic). Cannot be used if sumatriptan already taken. Contraindicated with hypertension, coronary artery disease, peripheral vascular disease, and pregnancy.
Sumatriptan	Moderate/severe migraine, cluster	6 mg SQ; may be repeated once in 1 hour if partial response	Chest pain, throat tightness, flushing. Contraindicated with hypertension, coronary artery disease, peripheral vascular disease, and pregnancy. Cannot be used within 24 hours of ergot usage.
Dopamine antagonists			
Prochlorperazine	Moderate/severe migraine	10 mg IV or IM may be repeated in 30–60 minutes	Sedation and dystonic reaction.
Chlorpromazine	Moderate/severe migraine	12.5–25 mg IV	Significant orthostatic hypotension; therefore, saline bolus should be administrated before use of this medication. Sedation and dystonic reaction.
Metoclopramide	Moderate/severe migraine	10 mg IV	Dystonic reaction.
Steroids			
Dexamethasone	Status migrainosus, intractable episodic cluster	10–20 mg IV	Interval medication until other agents take effect. Gastrointestinal bleeding, infection, cataracts, aseptic necrosis, memory disturbances.
Opioids			
Meperidine		50–100 mg IM or IV	Last resort, most of the other regimens provide superior pain relief.
Hydromorphone		1–4 mg SQ or IV	Last resort, most of the other regimens provide superior pain relief.
Morphine sulfate		1–10 mg IM or IV	Last resort, most of the other regimens provide superior pain relief.

IM: intramuscular; IV: intravenous; NSAIDs: non-steroidal anti-inflammatory drugs; PO: per os; PR: per rectum; SQ: subcutaneous.

Cluster headaches

High flow oxygen followed by subcutaneous sumatriptan are preferred. Dihydroergotamine parenterally has also been shown to be effective. Intranasal application of lidocaine to produce anesthesia of the sphenopalantine region has been advocated but not proven to be effective. Steroids have also been used.

Tension and cervicogenic headaches

Treatment is symptomatic with analgesics, ice, relaxation techniques, and trigger point injections.

Subarachnoid hemorrhage

The initial management of SAH includes resuscitation, stabilization, and emergent neurosurgical consultation. The main goals are to prevent recurrent bleeding, prevent further increase in ICP, mitigate the effects of vasospasm, and treat acute medical and neurologic complications. Continued or recurrent bleeding is worsened by uncontrolled elevations in blood pressure. To reduce the likelihood of an ischemic stroke, nimodipine should be started soon after the diagnosis of SAH is made. The recommended dose is 60 mg every 4 hours by mouth or nasogastric tube. Blood pressure must be monitored closely to prevent hypotension. Patients with a Hunt and Hess classification grade III or higher SAH are at risk for respiratory depression, which can lead to hypercapnia and worsening ICP (Table 25.7). These patients may require early endotracheal intubation with precautions to prevent elevation in ICP. Analgesics should be used and NSAIDs, including aspirin, must be avoided because of their antiplatelet effects. Antiemetics may be required. Agents that lower the seizure threshold should be avoided, since these patients are at an increased risk for seizures. Prophylactic anticonvulsant therapy is controversial and should be instituted in consultation with neurosurgery. Most of these patients require monitoring in an intensive care setting.

Epidural hematoma

Patients with an epidural hematoma can deteriorate rapidly; they require emergent neurosurgical evaluation and intervention. Definitive treatment is surgical.

Subdural hematoma

Patients with a subdural hematoma also require emergent neurosurgical evaluation. The neurosurgeon may opt to observe the patient rather than rushing him or her to an operating room, depending on the size, location, and duration of the hematoma.

Giant cell arteritis

Giant cell arteritis must be treated promptly once the diagnosis is suspected due to the risk of permanent visual loss. Steroids are the mainstay of therapy. The recommended initial oral dose of prednisone is 60–120 mg/day. Therapy needs to be continued for months, although symptomatic response may be seen within several days of initiation of steroids. The ESR needs to be closely monitored. A definitive diagnosis requires a temporal artery biopsy, which should be performed within 1 week of starting steroid therapy. A positive result may be seen up to 1 month later.

Idiopathic intracranial hypertension

Treatment involves lowering the ICP as well as symptomatic treatment of the headache. Acetazolamide decreases CSF production and lowers the ICP. Steroids have also been used. Repeated LPs are sometimes used to remove CSF, but such therapy is typically not well-tolerated by patients. In patients with impending visual loss, a ventricular shunt may be indicated.

Tumor headache

Urgent neurosurgical consultation is required once this diagnosis is made. Treatment includes managing increased ICP and seizures. ICP elevation from a brain tumor is initially managed with steroids.

Table 25.7 Hunt and Hess clinical grading scale for subarachnoid hemorrhage

Grade	Condition
0	Unruptured aneurysm
1	Asymptomatic or minimal headache and nuchal rigidity
2	Moderate or severe headache, nuchal rigidity, no neurologic deficit other than cranial nerve palsy
3	Drowsiness, confusion, or mild focal deficit
4	Stupor, moderate or severe hemiparesis
5	Deep coma, decerebrate posturing, moribund appearance

Dexamethasone is a high-potency steroid used to treat edema associated with brain tumors. The starting dose is 10 mg IV followed by 4 mg every 6 hours. Seizures are managed with agents such as phenytoin, valproic acid, or carbamazepine.

Meningitis

The specific treatment of the varied types of meningitis is beyond the scope of this chapter. Empiric treatment with broad-spectrum anti-biotics pending cultures is prudent. IV steroids are now recommended prior to antibiotics for patients with bacterial etiologies.

Acute angle closure glaucoma

Urgent ophthalmologic consultation is required once the diagnosis of acute angle closure glaucoma is made. The initial treatment involves lowering the intraocular pressure with topical beta-blockers (such as timolol maleate) and oral or IV acetazolamide. Miotics (such as pilocarpine) are used to constrict the pupil. Definitive management requires an ophthalmologist.

Trigeminal neuralgia

Carbamazepine, phenytoin, and baclofen are effective in the treatment of trigeminal neuralgia. However, all of these therapies have high failure rates, and surgical management may be required.

Post-dural puncture headache

Once identified by history, the patient should be treated with hydration, bed rest, and analgesics. Oral or IV caffeine can produce symptomatic relief (i.e., 500 mg of caffeine sodium benzoate in 1 liter of normal saline over 1 hour). When conservative methods have failed, an epidural blood patch (placed by an anesthesiologist) can be highly effective.

Carbon monoxide

Treatment is with 100% oxygen. Some patients may require hyperbaric oxygen therapy depending on the CO level and their symptomatology.

Carotid and vertebral artery dissection

Treatment is aimed at stroke prevention from embolization, and includes early anticoagulation followed by antiplatelet therapy.

Cavernous sinus thrombosis

Treatment requires high-dose IV antibiotics that cover staphylococcal, streptococcal, and *Haemophilus influenza* organisms. In addition, neurosurgical consultation as well as ophthalmologic or otolaryngologic consultation, depending on the location of the primary infection, should be obtained in a timely fashion.

Special patients
Elderly

Elderly patients with headache need special consideration. Chronic disease and normal physiologic changes with aging contribute to atypical presentations in the elderly. Elderly patients can present with only a mild headache and have a subacute or chronic subdural hematoma from a minor traumatic event. Up to 20% of patients with a chronic subdural hematoma have no identifiable precipitant or present with symptoms up to 3 months following a known traumatic event. Certain diseases, such as temporal arteritis, present later in life. It is rare for an elderly patient to develop a new migraine headache. A thorough work-up including a low threshold for a CT scan is required for any elderly patient who presents with a headache.

Immune compromised

Immunocompromised patients can suffer from any of the headaches described above, but require special consideration because of their immune status. This group of patients is at risk for opportunistic central nervous system infections, including mycobacteria, spirochetes, viruses (herpes simplex, herpes zoster, cytomegalovirus, and HIV), fungi (*Cryptococcus*), protozoa (toxoplasma), and actinomycetes. These patients are also at risk of central nervous system lymphoma and Kaposi's sarcoma. Noncontrast and contrast CT scan must be performed on any immunocompromised patient with a headache to rule out a space-occupying lesion, especially if an LP is being considered.

Pediatric

Headache is common in children and adolescents; 40% of children will experience a headache by the age of 7 years and 75% will experience a headache by the time they are 15 years old. Migraine is one of the most common causes of headache in childhood, occurring in 1% of children by the age of 7 and 5% of children by 15 years of age.

An acute headache may accompany many infectious processes. Nonspecific viral illnesses represent the most common diagnoses in children presenting with headaches. Care must be taken to exclude serious illnesses, such as meningitis, hypertension, and SAH as the cause. Pediatric patients with meningitis usually present with a history of headache accompanied by other systemic symptoms, such as changes in behavior, lethargy, seizures, and shock. Patients with mildly or severely elevated blood pressure may present with headache, and require rapid assessment to determine the etiology of their elevated blood pressure. Pediatric patients with SAH present similarly to adult patients with severe headache. They usually have neurologic abnormalities or a change in consciousness.

Pregnant

The most common type of headache occurring during pregnancy is a muscle contraction headache. Most patients have a previous history of headaches prior to the pregnancy. Eighty percent of women with classic migraine headaches have remission from attacks during pregnancy; thus, any headache other than a muscle contraction headache requires investigation.

Brain tumors enlarge during pregnancy and shrink temporarily postpartum. Most tumors become symptomatic during the second half of pregnancy. Brain tumors account for 10% of maternal deaths during pregnancy.

Pseudotumor cerebri associated with pregnancy usually occurs in obese women and begins between the third and fifth months of pregnancy. Symptoms usually resolve spontaneously after 1–3 months.

Spontaneous SAH accounts for 10% of maternal deaths. The most common cause of SAH in women younger than 25 years is a berry aneurysm. For women older than 25 years, it is an arteriovenous malformation. Nearly one-third of spontaneous SAHs are the result of bleeding disorders, bacterial endocarditis, metastatic tumors, or sickle cell disease.

Patients with eclampsia present with the sudden onset of focal neurologic deficits in addition to headache, seizure, or altered consciousness. The most common cause of death in patients with eclampsia is cerebral hemorrhage, occurring in 60% of patients who die after becoming eclamptic.

Disposition

Most patients presenting with a headache to the ED can be managed as outpatients. Specific treatment modalities are discussed in Table 25.6. Table 25.8 lists indications for hospitalization of patients with headache.

Table 25.8 Indications for hospitalization of patients with headache

- Central nervous system infections
- Vascular diseases
  - Subarachnoid hemorrhage
  - Cerebral ischemia
  - Severe hypertension
  - Spontaneous dissection of carotid artery
  - Temporal arteritis
- Space-occupying lesions
- Toxic metabolic encephalopathy
- Idiopathic intracranial hypertension not responding to usual measures
- Headache associated with severe medical illness
- Severe intractable headache
- Continuous vomiting, electrolyte abnormalities or inability to maintain oral hydration
- Complex drug interactions
- Social situations preventing appropriate outpatient management

Pearls, pitfalls, and myths

- Consider SAH in any patient who presents with the first or worst headache of their life.
- SAH and meningitis need to be considered in patients presenting with a change in the character, location, or intensity of their headache.
- Always perform a thorough eye examination on patients with a headache. The headache may be due to acute angle closure glaucoma. Identifying this condition may prevent unnecessary testing and delays in treatment.
- The typical patient with idiopathic intracranial hypertension is young, female, overweight, with acne on tetracycline. Fundoscopic examination typically reveals papilledema. A normal head CT and an elevated opening pressure confirm the diagnosis.
- Consider CO poisoning when a patient presents with a headache and nausea, and other family members have similar symptoms.
- Always consider giant cell arteritis in an elderly patient who presents with a headache, especially if it is unilateral.

- CT scanning is not 100% sensitive for the detection of SAH. A negative head CT must be followed by a negative LP to exclude the diagnosis.
- Be wary of assigning the diagnosis of "new-onset migraines" to an elderly patient with their first headache.

References

1. Diamond S, Diamond ML. Emergency treatment of migraine: insights into current options. *Postgrad Med* 1997;101:169.
2. Edlow JA, Caplan LR. Avoiding pitfalls in the diagnosis of subarachnoid hemorrhage. *New Engl J Med* 2002;342:29.
3. Edmeads J. Emergency management of headache. *Headache* 1988;28:675.
4. Gallagher EJ, Birnabaum AJ. Headache. In: Harwood-Nuss A (ed.). *The Clinical Practice of Emergency Medicine*, 3rd ed., Philadelphia: Lippincott Williams & Wilkins, 2001. pp. 969–978.
5. Hunt WE, Hess RM. Surgical risk as related to time intervention in the repair of intracranial aneurysm. *J Neurosurg* 1968;28:14.
6. Kanner RM. Headache and facial pain. In: Portenoy RK, Kanner RM (eds). *Pain Management: Theory and Practice*. Philadelphia: FA Davis, 1996.
7. Kwiatkowski T, Alagappan K. Headache. In: Marx JA, Hockberger RS, Walls RM (eds). *Rosen's Emergency Medicine, Concepts and Clinical Practice*, 5th ed., St. Louis: Mosby, 2002. pp.1456–1467.
8. Newman LC, Lipton RB. Emergency department evaluation of headache. *Neurol Clin* 1998;16:285.
9. Raskin NH. On the origin of head pain. *Headache* 1988;28:254.
10. Saper JR. Headache disorders. *Med Clin North Am* 1999;83:663.
11. Schull M. Headache and facial pain. In: Tintinalli JE, Ruiz E, Krome RL (eds). *Emergency Medicine in a Comprehensive Study Guide, American College of Emergency Physicians*, 5th ed., New York: McGraw Hill Co., 1996, pp. 1422–1430.
12. Uchihara T, Tsukagoshi H. Jolt accentuation of headache: the most sensitive sign of CSF pleocytosis. *Headache* 1991;31:167–171.
13. Welch KMA, et al. Headache in the emergency room. In: Olesen J, Tfelt-Hansen P, Welch KMA (eds). *The Headaches*, 2nd ed., Philadelphia: Lippincott Williams & Wilkins, 2000.

26 Hypertensive urgencies and emergencies

Loretta Jackson-Williams, MD and Robert Galli, MD

Scope of the problem

Hypertension (HTN) affects more than 20% of the adult and 3% of the pediatric populations. It is a disease process that contributes to the development of cardiovascular and renal diseases. It appears to be a polygenic, multifactorial disorder with several genes interacting with environmental factors. It is defined by a systolic blood pressure (SBP) greater than 140, diastolic blood pressure (DBP) greater than 90, or someone requiring antihypertensive medications for control of sustained elevations of blood pressure (BP).

As a disease process, HTN was born out of epidemiological studies that showed chronic BP elevation decreased life expectancy; that treatment of HTN reduces stroke, coronary artery disease (CAD), and heart failure; and that most hypertensive patients require more than one agent to achieve BP control.

HTN is an asymptomatic disease process. The exception is a hypertensive emergency. Hypertensive emergencies and urgencies, also known as hypertensive crises, can cause end-organ dysfunction and require controlled management. These hypertensive crises can be viewed as a continuum of the disease process in some patients.

A *hypertensive emergency*, also known as malignant HTN, is defined as an acute elevation in BP (DBP >130 mmHg in general) with end-organ dysfunction or damage. It requires prompt parenteral treatment with a goal of 25% reduction in mean arterial pressure (MAP) within 30–60 minutes.

A *hypertensive urgency* is defined as moderately severe to severe HTN with DBP 120–140 mmHg without presenting signs or symptoms of malignant HTN or a concomitant emergency medical condition. However, these patients are at risk for imminent end-organ damage. Hypertensive urgencies require controlled lowering of BP over several days, which can generally be accomplished in the outpatient setting.

Pathophysiology

The primary event for initiating any hypertensive crises is an increase of arterial pressure. The triggers for this rapid rise in pressure are unknown. They likely include a combination of cellular, organ, and environmental systems. It is clear that the rate of rise in arterial pressure is more important than the absolute level of pressure. Without prompt control of arterial pressure, fibrinoid necrosis of small arterioles occurs with resultant ischemia and infarction of end organs. This is followed by end-organ dysfunction and damage.

The process of fibrinoid necrosis of small arterioles begins when vessels in the capillary beds dilate to accommodate the sustained elevation in BP. Presumably, the shear force causes damage to the endothelium with resultant vascular wall injury. Response to this injury is the activation of coagulation and cell proliferation mediators. Fibrin is deposited within the damaged vascular walls. The process is continuously repeated and results in progressive narrowing and stiffening of the arterioles.

Flow through the vessels in the capillary beds is autoregulated to ensure that end organs are adequately perfused. This autoregulation occurs within specific ranges of BP in end organs. Beyond these specific ranges, autoregulation of blood flow does not occur, and hypo- or hyperperfusion of end organs results. In patients with sustained elevations in BP, the specific range of autoregulation is shifted higher. Therefore, acutely lowering the BP in hypertensive patients can result in evidence of hypoperfusion of end organs, since autoregulation of blood flow has been disrupted.

Changes in blood flow through end organs have clinical relevance. Stroke, intracerebral hemorrhage, and hypertensive encephalopathy can occur as a result of hyperperfusion of the brain. Angina, myocardial infarction, and acute left ventricular dysfunction with resultant pulmonary edema can occur as a result of hypoperfusion through the coronary arteries. In the kidneys, renal impairment and failure result from hypoperfusion. Aortic dissection may result from hyperperfusion to this structure.

History

The evaluation of a patient with elevated BP in the emergency department (ED) should focus on determining the presence of any end-organ dysfunction or concomitant emergency medical conditions. Primary areas of focus include the neurologic, cardiovascular, pulmonary, and renal systems.

What were the onset and duration of presenting signs and symptoms?

This information will help determine appropriate disposition and referral. Patients with long-standing HTN may not present with evidence of malignant HTN because of autoregulatory mechanisms previously discussed. Hypertensive emergencies typically present with acute onset and rapid progression within minutes to hours.

Neurologic

Does the patient have a severe headache?

In general, headache in hypertensive patients is a nonspecific sign and is not a reliable indicator of elevated BP. Severe headache may represent hypertensive encephalopathy or intracranial hemorrhage.

Does the patient have any speech or gait abnormalities, focal sensory or motor deficits, or mental status changes?

These questions address areas of the neurologic examination related to specific stroke syndromes. Focal deficits secondary to hypertensive encephalopathy may not follow a single anatomic pattern. In addition, autonomic instability manifested by dizziness, syncope, tremor, or abnormal sweating should be assessed.

Ophthalmologic

Does the patient have visual disturbances or loss of vision?

Decreased visual acuity or the presence of visual field defects may indicate the development of retinopathy. In addition, amaurosis fugax or painless monocular blindness identifies a stroke involving the internal carotid artery and the anterior circulation of the brain.

Cardiovascular

Does the patient complain of dyspnea or chest pain?

Acute left heart failure will result in the sensation of breathlessness or dyspnea, especially with exertion. Patients may also develop right heart failure and complain of the development of or worsening peripheral edema. Acute coronary syndromes can be precipitated by severe elevations in BP.

Does the patient complain of abdominal or back pain?

Patients with these complaints should be assessed for an aortic dissection or aneurysmal dilatation.

Obstetric

Is the patient pregnant?

Because of profound changes in circulatory physiology during pregnancy, hypertensive events may occur at lower-than-expected BPs. These patients should be assessed for pre-eclampsia.

Renal

Does the patient complain of hematuria?

HTN can precipitate or exacerbate existing renal insufficiency or failure.

Past medical

In general, historical information should include the age of the patient, known prior diagnosis of HTN, cardiovascular or renal diseases, present or past antihypertensive medications, compliance history with those medications, and known concomitant medical conditions, such as diabetes. The patient should be specifically asked about the use of drugs, such as monoamine oxidase inhibitors, cocaine, amphetamines, and alcohol, and the abrupt discontinuation of antihypertensive drugs, such as clonidine or β-blockers. The sudden withdrawal of clonidine and β-blockers may result in catecholamine excess and rebound HTN.

Physical examination

Most hypertensive patients presenting to the ED are without distinguishing signs on physical examination. As with the history, it is important to look for manifestations of end organ dysfunction. This information will help determine if the patient is having a hypertensive emergency requiring prompt treatment, or a hypertensive urgency requiring specific follow-up.

Areas of the physical examination to address include all of the following:

Vital signs

The BP should be checked more than once while the patient is in the ED with an appropriately-sized cuff. A cuff that is too short will produce an erroneously high reading. Most BP devices depend on occluding the artery of an extremity with an inflatable cuff, and measure BP either by oscillometry or detection of Korotkoff sounds. Oscillometric or automatic devices are subject to greater error than auscultating for Korotkoff sounds by manual pressure measurement. BP measurements (Table 26.1) can be different

Table 26.1 Normal blood pressure ranges for children and adults

| Age (years) | Blood pressure (mmHg) | |
	Systolic	Diastolic
0–2	60–110	40–65
3–6	80–120	55 70
7–10	90–130	60–75
11–15	90–140	60–80
>15	90–139	60–89

between arms. However, differences greater than 20 mmHg for systolic or 10 mmHg diastolic pressures raise concern for a vascular abnormality that should be further investigated. If autonomic instability is suspected, the BP should be checked in three positions – prone, upright sitting, and upright standing. BP measurement from the patient with a gravid uterus should be obtained in the left lateral recumbent position. Otherwise, the BP reading can be erroneously low due to compression of blood return from the inferior vena cava by the gravid uterus. In addition to BP measurements, it is important to note whether the patient is tachypneic or hypoxic.

Fundoscopic

The retinae are examined for vascular changes, hemorrhages and exudates. The optic disc margins are examined for edema (Figure 26.1). Acute hypertensive changes include papilledema, fundal hemorrhages, and vasospasm. Chronic hypertensive changes include arteriovenous nicking, hard exudates, and silver wiring.

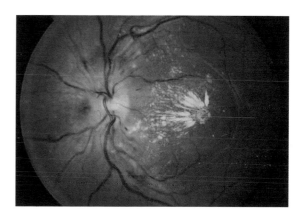

Figure 26.1
Hypertensive retinopathy. The eye has retinal hemorrhages and hard exudates in the form of a hemimacular star. Reproduced with permission from Tasman W et al, Wills Eye Hospital Atlas of Clinical Ophthalmology, 2nd ed., Lippincott Williams & Wilkins, 2001.

Neurologic

The mental status examination should specifically address whether the patient is alert and aware. Alertness requires normal functioning of the reticular activating system. Awareness requires alertness plus normal functioning of the cerebral hemispheres. Mental status changes may indicate hypertensive encephalopathy. Focal abnormalities of speech, cranial nerves, motor or sensory systems, or reflexes may be the result of subarachnoid hemorrhage, stroke, or pre-eclampsia (in a pregnant patient).

Cardiovascular

The focus of this examination is the identification of pulse abnormalities and the presence of murmurs and gallops. Diminished extremity pulses may be found in patients with coarctation of the aorta or aortic dissection. Patients with heart failure may have dusky or pale skin, tachycardia, pulsus alternans, jugular venous distension (JVD), peripheral edema, or hepatojugular reflux (HJR).

Pulmonary

The physical findings of left heart failure include tachypnea and pulmonary rales or crackles. Rhonchi and wheezing may be present secondary to airway edema, referred to as "cardiac asthma."

Abdomen

The abdomen should be examined for a bruit or a palpable pulsatile mass that may indicate the presence of an abdominal aortic aneurysm (AAA).

Differential diagnosis

Table 26.2 describes diagnoses associated with acute hypertension.

Diagnostic testing

The purpose of diagnostic testing of hypertensive patients in the ED is to identify end organ damage and to determine the presence of concomitant diseases or complications. Commonly utilized tests include hematocrit, electrolytes, blood urea nitrogen (BUN), creatinine (Cr), glucose, urinalysis, urine pregnancy test, electrocardiogram (ECG), and computerized tomography (CT) of the brain.

Table 26.2 Diagnoses associated with acute hypertension

Diagnosis	Symptoms	Signs	Workup
Acute coronary syndrome	Chest discomfort or pain, dyspnea, nausea, sweating	Diaphoresis, pallor, restlessness	ECG, cardiac enzymes
Acute pulmonary edema	Dyspnea, orthopnea, DOE, PND	Rales or crackles	CXR, BNP, cardiac enzymes
Acute renal failure	Dizziness, oliguria	Edema, decreased skin turgor	Urinalysis, serum and urine electrolytes (especially potassium), serum Cr, BUN
Aortic dissection	Chest, back, or abdominal pain; dyspnea, weakness	Diminished pulses, new murmur	CXR, chest CT, aortography, echocardiography, possibly MRI
Hypertensive encephalopathy	Severe headache, nausea, vomiting, confusion, seizure, stupor, decreased vision	Obtundation, retinopathy, papilledema, localized neurologic deficits without anatomic pattern	Vital signs, laboratories to rule out other end-organ damage, brain CT
Illicit drug use	Headache, chest pain, dyspnea	Diaphoresis, tachycardia, tachypnea, hyperthermia	Toxicologic studies
Intracerebral hemorrhage	Headache, focal weakness, confusion, vomiting	Aphasia, focal paresis or paralysis, decreased consciousness	Brain CT
Medication withdrawal	Chest pain, nausea	Diaphoresis, piloerection	Ask the patient, review medical record and recent medications
Pheochromocytoma	Anxiety, palpitations, headaches, chest or abdominal pain in paroxysms	Diaphoresis, pallor	24-hour urine catecholamines
Pre-eclampsia/eclampsia	Headache, visual disturbances, seizure	Edema	Urinalysis, coagulation studies, CBC, renal and liver function tests
Subarachnoid hemorrhage	Headache, vomiting, syncope	Stiff neck, decreased consciousness	Brain CT, lumbar puncture if CT negative

BNP: β-natriuretic peptide; BUN: blood urea nitrogen; CBC: complete blood count; Cr: creatinine; CT: computed tomography; CXR: chest X-ray; DOE: dyspnea on exertion; PND: paroxysmal nocturnal dyspnea.

Selected test ordering should be presentation-and patient-specific.

Laboratory studies

Complete blood count

The complete blood count (CBC), which includes the hematocrit, serves as a general measure of a patient's health. Anemia is found in a variety of chronic diseases, including renal insufficiency due to sustained elevations of BP. It is not required for the diagnostic work-up.

Electrolytes

The primary electrolyte of interest is potassium. Abnormal potassium levels could indicate hyperaldosteronism, renovascular disease or advanced renal insufficiency. This information would be helpful to the primary health care provider and allows him or her to determine if further diagnostic tests are needed.

Urinalysis

The renal status of the patient is assessed by the presence of protein, blood, and glucose in the urine. Examination of urine sediment provides important information regarding renal parenchymal disease. Although BUN and Cr are insensitive markers of renal function, they do provide a long-term marker of progressive decline. Glucose determination is also important in determining the potential for diabetes. The selection of antihypertensive therapy would be affected by the presence of diabetes.

Pregnancy test

Women of childbearing age with HTN should have a pregnancy test completed if appropriate. This determines if further studies are needed and the type of referral necessary.

Toxicologic testing

In any hypertensive patient in whom illicit drug use is suspected, toxicologic screening would be appropriate to clarify clinical management.

Electrocardiogram

The ECG identifies patients with left ventricular hypertrophy that occurs with sustained elevations of BP. Specific criteria exist which demonstrate HTN by ECG voltage criteria. The most specific is an R wave in lead aVL > 11 mm.

In addition, patients with prior asymptomatic myocardial infarctions and HTN should be identified because of an increased risk of cardiovascular complications.

Radiologic studies

In patients with focal neurologic signs or symptoms, a brain CT is required. This is not necessary on all patients with elevated BP and headache. Clinical judgment and discretion is required. A chest CT is indicated for patients with suspected aortic dissection. This test can be substituted for aortography or done in conjunction with it. Abdominal CT is recommended if AAA is suspected. In the proper hands, abdominal ultrasound may be satisfactory, and can be performed more quickly and safely at the bedside.

General treatment principles

An asymptomatic, hypertensive patient presenting to the ED does not require emergent treatment. There is no evidence to suggest that the acute reduction of BP in these patients reduces the complications of HTN. There is evidence, however, that stroke, deterioration in renal function, and cardiac ischemia or infarction can occur as a result of rapid, uncontrolled BP reduction.

As a general guideline for treatment of HTN, a diuretic should be started as initial drug therapy, especially in the elderly, when there are no concomitant medical conditions or a hypertensive emergency. As an alternative, β-blockers could be used if there are no contraindications (i.e., bronchospasm, bradycardia, heart block, previous sensitivity to β-blockers). Some patients with concomitant medical conditions have specific treatment recommendations. These include angiotensin-converting enzyme (ACE) inhibitors in diabetics with proteinuria, ACE inhibitors or diuretics in patients with heart failure, diuretics or calcium channel antagonists in patients with isolated systolic HTN, and β-blockers or ACE inhibitors in patients with prior myocardial infarction.

Acute BP reduction is contraindicated for hypertensive urgencies. If a noncompliant patient had been on an antihypertensive regimen, the prior therapy could be resumed. The dose of one medication should be increased in a compliant patient. Newly-diagnosed patients should be started on monotherapy. All of these patients need follow-up within a week to be reevaluated following the initiation of therapy and to make necessary adjustments in therapy.

The goal of therapy in the treatment of hypertensive emergencies is to limit the damage to end organs with controlled reduction in BP. The general target pressure reduction is no more than 25% of the MAP within 2 hours. These patients must be closely monitored, ideally with invasive continuous arterial measurements. Antihypertensives used in the management of hypertensive emergencies are listed in the Tables 26.3 and 26.4.

Table 26.3 Medication recommendations for hypertensive emergencies

Emergency	Drug(s) of choice	Alternative drug(s)
Acute coronary syndrome	Nitroglycerin, β-blockers	Nitroprusside, labetalol
Acute pulmonary edema	Nitroglycerin, nitroprusside	Fenoldopam, ACE inhibitors
Adrenergic crises	Phentolamine; nitroprusside with β-blockers	Labetalol
Aortic dissection	β-blockers followed by nitroprusside	Labetalol, esmolol, trimethaphan
Hypertensive encephalopathy	Nitroprusside, fenoldopam	Labetalol, nicardipine
Intracranial hemorrhage	Labetalol	Nitroprusside, nicardipine
Pre-eclampsia/eclampsia	Hydralazine	Nicardipine, labetalol

ACE: angiotensin-converting enzyme.

Table 26.4 Pharmacologic agents in the treatment of hypertension emergencies

Agent	Dose	Comments
Captopril	Sublingual use 25–50 mg has gained increasing popularity in ED, especially patients with HTN and CHF.	Cautions include symptomatic hypotension following the first dose. Especially useful in HTN crisis associated with CHF or myocardial ischemia. Adverse reactions include ACE inhibitor-induced cough, angioedema.
Esmolol	Loading dose 250–500 mcg/kg/minute infusion for 1 minute, followed by a maintenance infusion of 50 mcg/kg/minute × 4 minutes; repeat loading dose and follow with maintenance infusion using increments of 50 mcg/kg/minute (for 4 minutes). May repeat up to four times as needed. Once desired BP is approached, reduce maintenance infusion from 50 mcg/kg/minute to 25 mcg/kg/minute or less.	Test β-blocker safety and tolerance in patients with history of COPD, asthma, or CHF who are at risk of bronchospasm from β-blockade. When used with nitroprusside for treatment of aortic dissection, its use should precede nitroprusside to prevent reflex tachycardia and increased dP/dT. Contraindications include documented hypersensitivity, uncompensated CHF, bradycardia, cardiogenic shock and AV conduction abnormalities.
Fenoldopam	Continuous infusion (inability to bolus may preclude its use in the ED). Dose 0.1–1.6 mcg/kg/minute (usual dose 0.3 mcg/kg/minute). Also recommended to use 0.1 mcg/kg/minute increased by 0.05–0.1 mcg/kg/minute at 15 minutes intervals.	Primarily used in patients with renal impairment.
Hydralazine	Dose 5–20 mg IV q4–6 hours prn initial dose; increase dose prn. Change to PO as soon as possible.	Used in the treatment of eclampsia.

(continued)

Table 26.4 Pharmacologic agents in the treatment of hypertension emergencies (*cont*)

Agent	Dose	Comments
Labetalol	Initial dose 20 mg IV over 2 minutes; follow with 20–80 mg q10–15 minutes until BP controlled. Maintenance dose 2 mg/minute continuous infusion; titrate up to 5–20 mg/minute; not to exceed a total dose of 300 mg.	Contraindications include coronary or cerebral arteriosclerosis, renal impairment, or documented hypersensitivity.
Nicardipine	Initial infusion 5 mg/hour, titrate 2.5 mg/hour every 5–15 minutes. Maximum 15 mg/hour, maintenance 3 mg/hour.	Contraindications include aortic stenosis, known or previous hypersensitivity to calcium channel blockers. Pheochromocytoma 0.5–2 mg boluses repeated as needed. Pre-eclampsia/eclampsia, initial dose 1 mcg/kg/minute, titrate 0.5 mg/hour (usual dose 0.7 mcg/kg/minute).
Nitroglycerin	Dose 5–10 mcg/minute IV titrating upward to keep SBP > 90 mmHg or to decrease MAP by 25%. Continuous 0.1–1 mcg/kg/minute IV infusion. Doses may reach over 100 mcg/minute pending hemodynamic tolerance.	Side effects include headache, hypotension, tachycardia.
Nitroprusside	Dose 0.3–10 mcg/kg/minute in D5W.	Must protect from light by wrapping in aluminum foil. Contraindications include documented hypersensitivity, idiopathic hypertrophic sub-aortic stenosis (IHSS), atrial fibrillation or flutter. Caution in renal or hepatic insufficiency, as levels may increase and can cause cyanide or thiocyanate toxicity, especially with prolonged use and with doses greater than 4 mcg/kg/minute. Arterial invasive monitoring recommended.

ACE: angiotensin-converting enzyme; BP: blood pressure; CHF: congestive heart failure; COPD: chronic obstructive pulmonary disease; D5W: 5% dextrose in water; ED: emergency department; HTN: hypertension; IV: intravenous; MAP: mean arterial pressure; PO: per os; SBP: systolic blood pressure.

Special patients

Pregnant

HTN in pregnancy contributes significantly to maternal and fetal morbidity and mortality. In pregnancy, HTN is defined as a BP of 140/90 mmHg or greater, or a 20 mmHg rise in the systolic pressure or a 10 mmHg rise in the diastolic pressure from baseline. The threshold for the diagnosis of HTN in pregnancy is therefore lower than in the nonpregnant patient. The hypertensive emergencies of pregnancy include pre-eclampsia and eclampsia. Hydralazine has classically been the antihypertensive drug of choice in hypertensive crises of pregnancy because it preserves uterine blood flow. Calcium channel antagonists and β-blockers are effective, safe alternatives. Magnesium sulfate is effective in reducing the incidence of eclampsia in women with severe pre-eclampsia. Delivery of the infant is the only cure for pre-eclampsia and eclampsia.

Pediatric

HTN in children is uncommon. It is defined as a systolic or diastolic pressure greater than the 95th percentile for age and sex. Generally, children with significant HTN have underlying renal or renovascular causes. These children should be referred to primary care pediatricians or pediatric nephrologists for further diagnostic evaluation.

Disposition

All patients with identified hypertensive emergencies must be admitted to an intensive care or telemetry setting for appropriate monitoring. Patients with identified hypertensive urgencies can be referred for close primary care follow-up, preferably within one week. Patients with elevated BP in the ED and concomitant medical conditions should have the presenting conditions stabilized, with referral to primary care for follow-up within a few weeks for a BP recheck. Patients with elevated BP in the ED without concomitant medical conditions should be referred to primary care for a BP recheck within one month, sooner if possible.

Occasionally, patients present to the ED with a primary complaint of elevated BP that has been noted on a screening examination. If no prior history of HTN exists, the above guidelines for referral should be followed. If a patient was treated in the past for HTN, appropriate drug therapy could be reinstated with primary care referral within a month.

Pearls, pitfalls, and myths

- Not all patients who present with elevated BP require emergent treatment. Evidence of acute end-organ damage defines a hypertensive emergency and the need for prompt, controlled therapy. Treat the patient, not the number.
- Patients with evolving ischemic strokes frequently have elevated BP. A rapid reduction of BP may cause extension of neurologic damage due to decreased cerebral blood flow. Therefore, expedient lowering of the BP should be avoided. In addition, oral and sublingual medications that cannot be titrated should not be used.
- Patients with asymptomatic HTN can be managed as outpatients in a primary care setting.
- Patients presenting with HTN and heart failure should be treated for fluid overload first, with precautions for cardiac ischemia or other cardiac events.
- Pregnant patients are considered hypertensive at lower absolute BP measurements than nonpregnant patients. Pre-eclampsia and eclampsia are two serious conditions specific to pregnant or post-partum patients.

References

1. Braunwald E, Fauci A, Kasper D, Hauser S, Longo D, Jameson JL (ed.). *Harrison's Principles of Internal Medicine*, 15th ed., Washington, DC: McGraw-Hill, 2001.
2. Burt V, Welton P, Roccella E, Brown C, Cutler J, Higgins M, Horan M, Labarthe D. Prevalence of hypertension in the US adult population; results from the Third National Health and Nutrition Examination Survey, 1988–1991. *Hypertension* 1995;25:305.
3. Flack J, Peters R, Mehra V, Nasser S. Hypertension in special populations. *Cardiology Clinics* 2002;20:303.
4. Furberg C, Wright J, Davis B, et al. Major outcomes in high-risk hypertensive patients randomized to angiotensin-converting enzyme inhibitor or calcium channel blocker vs diuretic the Antihypertensive and Lipid-Lowering treatment to prevent Heart Attack Trial (ALLHAT). *J Am Med Assoc* 2003;288:2981.
5. Hamilton G (ed.). *Emergency Medicine: An Approach to Clinical Problem-Solving*, 2nd ed., Philadelphia: W.B. Saunders Company, 2003.
6. Harwood-Nuss A (senior editor). *The Clinical Practice of Emergency Medicine*, 4th ed., Lippincott Williams & Wilkins, 2001.
7. Laragh J, Brenner B (eds). *Hypertension Pathophysiology, Diagnosis, and Management*, 2nd ed., New York: Raven Press, 1995.
8. Marx J (ed.). *Rosen's Emergency Medicine: Concepts and Clinical Practice*, 5th ed., St Louis: Mosby, 2002.
9. Oparil S, Weber M (eds). *Hypertension: A Companion to Brenner and Rector's The Kidney*. Philadelphia: W.B. Saunders Company, 2000.
10. Sixth Report of the Joint National Committee on Prevention, Detection, Evaluation and Treatment of High Blood Pressure. *Arch Int Med* 1997;157:2413.
11. Tintinalli J (editor-in-chief). *Emergency Medicine: A Comprehensive Study Guide*, 5th ed., New York: McGraw-Hill, 2000.
12. Weber M (ed.). *Hypertension Medicine*. Totowa, New Jersey: Humana Press, 2001.

27 Joint pain

Douglas W. Lowery, MD and Melissa J. Lamberson, MD

Scope of the problem

Non traumatic joint pain is a common presenting complaint for patients in the emergency department, and emergency medicine practitioners should be knowledgeable in the evaluation of the "red hot joint." While rarely life-threatening, joint pain is important because it may be the harbinger of more serious systemic diseases and infections. Furthermore, even mild diseases of many joints, especially the hands and weight-bearing joints, can result in significant short- and long-term disability. Accurate evaluation and treatment may reduce the severity and duration of disability.

Anatomic essentials

In order to determine the cause of joint pain, one must understand the underlying anatomy of the joint (Figure 27.1). The sources of joint pain may be classified into two major anatomic categories: articular structures (joint capsule and its contents) and periarticular structures (structures superficial to the joint capsule).

A joint is the union of the ends of two or more bones. On each bony surface lies a cushion, the articular cartilage, a compressible matrix of collagen fibers and proteoglycans which serves to prevent bone-on-bone contact. Adherent along the margins of the articular cartilage is a synovial membrane, which creates the synovial cavity. The synovial membrane also secretes high-viscosity synovial fluid, which fills the synovial cavity in order to lubricate the joints and facilitate mobility. A fibrous joint capsule encloses the synovial membrane, thus creating the unit known as the joint space.

The joint is strengthened and supported by ligaments, which are bands of fibrous tissues connecting bones or cartilages. Additional support is provided by tendons, which are cords of fibrous tissue continuous with muscle fibers attaching muscle to bone or cartilage. More than 150 sacs of synovial fluid, known as bursae, are situated throughout the body around joints where friction occurs. Examples include the olecranon bursa beneath the skin superficial to the olecranon process, and the subacromial bursa between the acromion and supraspinatus muscle.

A variety of maladies may lead to joint pain, and the pathophysiology behind this is frequently the result of disruption of the normal articular or periarticular anatomy and physiology. Mechanical trauma may lead to imbalance of the anabolic and

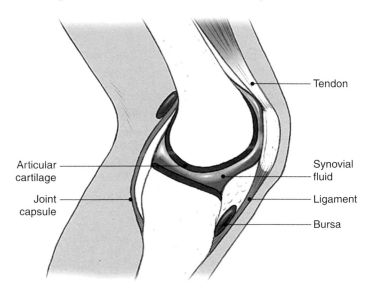

Articular cartilage

Joint capsule

Tendon

Synovial fluid

Ligament

Bursa

Figure 27.1
Joint anatomy.

catabolic processes maintaining normal joint homeostasis. Inflammatory reactions may be triggered by various stimuli, including bacteria, crystals, trauma, or systemic inflammatory conditions. Inflammation of either the articular or periarticular structures is associated with the movement of polymorphonuclear cells (PMNs) into the synovial cavities, and a subsequent decrease in the viscosity of the synovial fluid. Lysosomal enzymes released from these PMNs attack the joint structures, invoking a severe inflammatory response. Unlike cartilage, synovium is rich in pain receptors, so that even minor inflammation leads to severe pain and disability.

History

The most important historical information to obtain in a patient with joint pain is that which enables determination of whether the pain involves the entire joint capsule (articular) or the structures surrounding the joint capsule (periarticular). If the pain is articular, the number and distribution of the joints guide the differential diagnosis (Table 27.1).

Table 27.1 Causes of joint pain

Articular		Periarticular
Monoarticular	**Polyarticular**	
Gout	Acute rheumatic	Bursitis
Hemarthrosis	fever	Cellulitis
Osteoarthritis	Drug-induced	Tendinitis
Pseudogout	arthritis	
Septic arthritis	Gonococcal	
Trauma	arthritis	
	Immune complex	
	Lyme disease	
	Reiter's syndrome	
	Rheumatoid arthritis	
	Seronegative	
	spondyloarthropathies	
	Systemic lupus	
	erythematosus	
	Viral arthritis	

Where is the pain located?

Articular pain is often described as a generalized sensation of joint pain because the inflammatory process affects all parts of the joint. Periarticular pain, in contrast, is more readily localized to a specific site of inflammation.

When did the pain begin?

Acute pain may be secondary to an injury, infection or inflammatory process, or may be due to an acute exacerbation of a chronic condition. Patients with chronic arthritic conditions will often provide a history of recurrent acute episodes.

What makes the pain worse?

As synovial tissue is rich in stretch receptors, articular pain is often exacerbated by both active and passive motion of the joint. It may even occur at rest, as is often seen in arthritic conditions (e.g., inflammatory or septic arthritis). Periarticular pain is usually exacerbated with active or passive movement involving the affected muscles or tendons. It is commonly seen with overuse conditions in which repetitive motion results in inflammation of the involved tissues (e.g., shoulder bursitis/tendinitis in a baseball player).

How many joints are involved?

Periarticular disease, such as bursitis, tendinitis, and cellulitis, typically involves a single joint. Articular disease may be monoarticular or polyarticular. Examples of monoarticular arthritides include septic and gouty arthritis. Polyarticular arthritis may be acute (e.g., viral arthritis, Lyme disease, or gonoccocemia) or chronic (e.g., systemic lupus erythematosus (SLE), psoriatic arthritis, or dermatomyositis); it may also be symmetric (rheumatoid arthritis (RA), drug-induced arthritis) or asymmetric (rubella, gonococcal arthritis, acute rheumatic fever).

Which joints are involved?

Certain arthritic conditions are often recognized by joint pain in distinctive locations. Osteoarthritis commonly affects the proximal interphalangeal (PIP) and distal interphalangeal (DIP) joints of the hand. Rheumatoid arthritis commonly affects the metacarpophalangeal (MCP) and PIP joints of the hand. Gout commonly affects the great toe metatarsophalangeal (MTP) joint (known as *podagra*), the ankle, and the knee. However, a patient may present with joint pain that may actually be referred from a bony metastatic lesion in the setting of an underlying malignancy.

Associated symptoms

Eliciting other specific information will assist in making the right diagnosis in a patient with joint pain. A low-grade fever is not unusual with inflammatory conditions of the joint. However, the presence of a high fever and chills must alert one to the possibility of septic arthritis. Constitutional symptoms are also commonly seen not only in infection but also in RA. Skin lesions should increase suspicion for a systemic or autoimmune disease (e.g., track marks of intravenous drug abuse (IVDA) in endocarditis, malar rash of SLE). Purulent urethritis suggests gonococcal disease. The combination of conjunctivitis and urethritis suggests Reiter's syndrome. Uric acid nephrolithiasis may be associated with gouty arthritis.

Past medical

Obtaining information about the medical history may yield additional clues to the etiology of joint pain. One must inquire about autoimmune disease, gout, other known arthritic conditions, hemophilia, and even malignancy. The medication history may prove useful. Thiazide diuretics increase uric acid levels and may precipitate gout. Isoniazid, procainamide, and hydralazine therapy may lead to a lupus-like syndrome with arthritis. Chronic arthritides have a familial predisposition, so inquiring about family history may be helpful. Social history is often a clue to making a definitive diagnosis. Inquire about overuse activities, sports, injection drug use, and sexual history. Just as important is a vocational history. Certain joint conditions are characteristically associated with particular occupations due to distinct injuries or repetitive stress (e.g., anterior cruciate ligament (ACL) tear in a football player or prepatellar bursitis in a housemaid). Tick bites may lead to Lyme disease in endemic areas.

Physical examination

Once a thorough history has been elicited, an appropriate physical examination is important in enabling practitioners to develop a differential diagnosis. The basic principles of physical examination of the musculoskeletal system are inspection, palpation, and range of motion.

General appearance

Patients with acute inflammatory or infectious joint conditions will present with varying degrees of pain and distress. However, an acutely ill or toxic-appearing patient with joint pain likely has a significant infection or an underlying systemic condition that may or may not have been previously diagnosed.

Vital signs

In the presence of a high fever, look for signs of joint infection. Other suggestive signs include tachycardia or possibly hypotension if there is a systemic infection. Inflammatory conditions more commonly present with a low-grade or normal temperature, and possibly mild tachycardia or tachypnea due to pain.

Musculoskeletal

Inspection

Redness of the overlying skin is often associated with periarticular processes (e.g., cellulitis of the skin or bursitis/tendinitis from overuse or injury), and should alert providers to the possibility of infection of the underlying joint. This warrants immediate orthopedic evaluation.

Swelling within the joint (an effusion), may be secondary to blood from an injury, purulence from infection, or excessive amounts of synovial fluid from synovitis. Such fluid is usually palpable. However, fluid may also be periarticular, originating from similar causes involving the tissues surrounding the joint (e.g., prepatellar bursitis).

Wounds may be superficial, indicating a minor injury, or may be contiguous with the joint space necessitating urgent orthopedic intervention to prevent or treat a potential infection. Other lesions may be pustular, indicating a potential systemic infection such as gonococcemia (Figure 27.2).

Muscle atrophy is evidence of disuse due to pain in the involved joint.

Deformities frequently enable immediate diagnosis if they are fractures or dislocations, or are characteristic of specific conditions, such as tophaceous lesions of gouty arthritis or Heberden's nodes of osteoarthritis.

In chronic arthritic conditions, the distribution of joint involvement may suggest a specific diagnosis. For example, in osteoarthritis, there is a predilection for the first carpometacarpal joint, the first MTP joint, the DIP joints, and the knees, hips, cervical and lumbosacral spine. In contrast, RA affects the wrists, MP joints, PIP joints, and feet. Symmetry of deformities on both sides of the body is typical of rheumatoid arthritis.

Palpation

Warmth suggests inflammation, and should be compared to the surrounding tissues or the opposite joint. It may be due to arthritis, infection, or acute trauma.

Tenderness often reveals the underlying pathology if localized to a specific anatomic structure. Generalized tenderness may imply involvement of the entire joint.

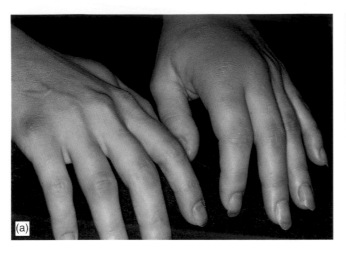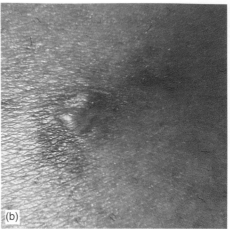

Figure 27.2
Disseminated gonococcal infection (a) Erythema and swelling of the joints of the left hand; a single vesicle is present on the right hand; (b) More advanced lesion with a hemorrhagic and necrotic base; the central hemorrhagic area is the embolic focus of the gonococcus. Permission granted from Habif, TP; Reprinted from Clinical Dermatology, 4th ed., Habif TP, page 333, Copyright 2004, with permission from Elsevier.

Table 27.2 Clues to specific arthritic diseases

	Findings	Diseases
Skin Figure 27.2b	Pustules (Figure 27.2b)	Gonococcemia
	Malar rash	SLE, dermatomyositis
	Rash on elbows/knees	Psoriasis
	ECM (Figure 27.3)	Lyme disease
	Hyperkeratotic lesions	Reiter's syndrome
	Tophi	Gout
	Track marks	Injection drug use
	Erythema marginatum	Rheumatic fever
	Subcutaneous nodules	Rheumatoid arthritis
Eyes	Iritis, uveitis	Seronegative spondyloarthropathy
	Conjunctivitis	Reiter's syndrome
	Scleral icterus	Hepatitis
Mouth	Ulcerations	Reiter's syndrome
Cardiac	Friction rub	Rheumatoid arthritis, SLE
	Murmurs	Endocarditis, rheumatoid arthritis
Pulmonary	Pleuritis	SLE, rheumatoid arthritis
Gastrointestinal	Enlarged, tender liver	Hepatitis
Genitourinary	Purulent urethral discharge	Reiter's syndrome, gonococcemia

ECM: erythema chronicum migrans; SLE: systemic lupus erythematosus.

Swelling, particularly a joint effusion, may be palpable if not easily visualized as described above.

Range of motion

Range of motion varies from person to person, but no musculoskeletal examination is complete without taking a joint through its full range of motion. Decreased range of motion may be present secondary to pain from inflammation, infection, or injury, even if no abnormalities are noted on inspection or palpation. It may also be seen with increasing age. Increased range of

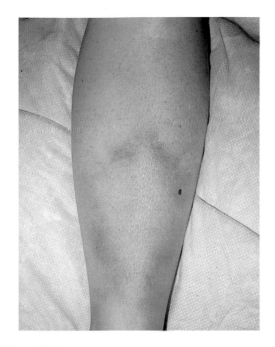

Figure 27.3
Erythema chronicum migrans of Lyme disease. Broad oval area of erythema that has slowly migrated from the central bite puncture. Permission granted from Habif, TP; Reprinted from Clinical Dermatology, 4th ed., Habif TP, page 519, Copyright 2004, with permission from Elsevier.

motion may occur with joints that are unstable (e.g., ligamentous injury) or associated with hyperelastic connective tissue (e.g., Ehlers-Danlos syndrome). Look for symmetry of range of motion.

The presence of pain with range motion is not a specific finding, as it may be found with numerous pathologies involving the joint. It is usually more helpful if it can be localized to a specific structure. Involvement of periarticular structures commonly results in pain only with active range of motion. Another maneuver to perform in assessing range of motion is pain with axial loading or weight-bearing, which is more likely to be seen with arthritic conditions or an injury to the joint.

Head-to-toe

In addition to a focused examination of the joint, a more thorough examination involving the remainder of the organ systems is required in the presence of other patient complaints, signs or symptoms. A detailed examination will help identify any evidence of underlying systemic disease which may not have initially been suspected based on the chief complaint of joint pain (e.g., skin tightening in scleroderma or heart murmur of endocarditis) (Table 27.2).

Differential diagnosis

Table 27.3 describes causes of joint pain.

Table 27.3 Differential diagnosis of joint pain

Diagnosis	Symptoms	Signs	Work-up
Acute rheumatic fever	Polyarticular (symmetric or asymmetric) arthritis, usually affecting the large joints. May accompany carditis, valvulitis, rash, or chorea after Group A β-hemolytic streptococcal infection of the pharynx	Patients may demonstrate *erythema marginatum*, a pinkish, non-pruritic rash with central clearing on the trunk and proximal limbs. Sub-cutaneous nodules are firm, non-tender overlying bony prominences. In addition to symmetric polyarthritis, patients may have evidence of cardiac disease, including pericarditis, CHF, or valvular abnormalities. The major neurologic manifestation is chorea with sparing of sensory function	ESR, CRP, ASO titer, and pharyngeal cultures. The synovial fluid is inflammatory with a negative culture. ECG may show evidence of carditis or pericarditis, and echocardiography may demonstrate valvular dysfunction
Drug-induced arthritis	Polyarticular, symmetric arthritis, associated with lupus-like systemic symptoms. History of procainamide, hydralazine, or isoniazid treatment	Mild to moderate arthritis and synovitis with effusions, symmetrically distributed. Other systemic signs of the lupus-like syndrome may be present	Synovial fluid shows non-inflammatory picture, although in severe cases the cell counts may suggest inflammatory picture

(continued)

Table 27.3 Differential diagnosis of joint pain (*cont*)

Diagnosis	Symptoms	Signs	Work-up
Gonococcal arthritis	Polyarticular (symmetric or asymmetric) arthritis, affecting one to several joints – typically the knee, ankle, or wrist. Associated with rash, fever, chills, and rarely urethritis or cervicitis	Fever often present. The rash (70%) is characterized by hemorrhagic, necrotic pustules starting on the distal extremities. Acute inflammation in the joints of the knee, ankle, and wrist or the tendon sheaths of the hands or wrists is common	WBC count and ESR may be elevated. Blood cultures are positive for *N. gonorrhoeae* less than 50% of the time, but should be sent. Cultures for *N. gonorrhoeae* should be obtained from pharynx, rectum, cervix, and urethra. Synovial fluid analysis shows inflammatory fluid, and Gram's stain for the organism is more often positive than cultures
Gout	Monoarticular symptoms, with >75% occurring in the MTP joint of the great toe. Pain severe at onset. Systemic symptoms uncommon	Affected joints are erythematous, warm, and exquisitely sensitive to touch or movement. Fever uncommon	Serum uric acid may be normal in acute attacks. Synovial fluid analysis demonstrates negatively-birefringent, needle-shaped crystals and high WBC counts. Septic arthritis must be ruled out by Gram's stain and culture, as the presence of gout crystals does not rule out septic arthritis
Lyme disease	Polyarticular (symmetric or asymmetric) arthritis is a late manifestation of this disease, caused by spirochete *Borrelia burgdorferi* from the deer tick, *Ixodes dammini*. Tick bite leads to rash, fever, malaise, myalgias, and arthralgias. Occasionally, the patient may have neurologic (Bell's palsy or other mononeuritis) or cardiac (syncope) symptoms	Arthritis of the large joints occurs in more than half of patients. Large joint effusions are common. The rash of *erythema chronicum migrans* appears at the site of the tick bite, and may spread to the thigh, axilla, and groin	Lyme serologies may not be positive for 6 weeks following initial exposure, but are often positive by the time arthritis develops. Synovial fluid demonstrates inflammatory changes
Osteoarthritis	Monoarticular arthritis acutely flared up in a joint with longstanding chronic disease. The patient usually has no systemic symptoms. The hands, knees, and first MTP joints are most commonly affected	Patients are usually more than 50 years old, and have crepitus and swelling in the affected joints. *Bouchard's nodes* (PIP) and *Heberden's nodes* (DIP) are osteophytic spurs often present in the hands	WBC count is often normal, although ESR may be slightly elevated. Radiography demonstrates formation of osteophytes and joint space narrowing. Synovial fluid analysis typically shows a non-inflammatory picture (WBC counts <2000 cells/mm^3)
Pseudogout	Monoarticular arthritis usually occurring in the knee, wrist, ankle, and elbow. Sometimes more than one joint is involved. Typically less acute and less severe than gout	Affected joints are erythematous, warm, and exquisitely sensitive to touch or movement. Systemic systems are less common than with gout	WBC count often elevated, as is ESR. Radiographs may show calcifications (*chondrocalcinosis*) in joints, tendon insertions, ligaments, and bursae. Synovial fluid shows rhomboidal, weak positively-birefringent crystals of calcium pyrophosphate. Septic arthritis must be ruled out by Gram's stain and culture

(continued)

Table 27.3 Differential diagnosis of joint pain (*cont*)

Diagnosis	Symptoms	Signs	Work-up
Rheumatoid arthritis	Polyarticular, usually symmetric, arthritis with acute flare-ups occurring in the context of chronic disease. The hands (MCP and PIP joints), wrists, elbows, and feet (MTP joints) most often affected. Patients often complain of fatigue, malaise, and joint pain lasting months	Joints are warm, tender, and swollen. Long-term changes of rheumatoid arthritis include severe deformities (swan neck and boutonniere deformities in the hand), muscle atrophy, and Baker's cysts in the knees. Subcutaneous nodules may be present	CBC may show mild anemia. ESR is often elevated. RF, an antibody against IgG, is positive in 85% of patients but is nonspecific. X-rays demonstrate soft tissue swelling and joint space narrowing. Synovial fluid is typically inflammatory
Septic arthritis	Monoarticular joint pain, warmth, and swelling. More than two-thirds of cases involve the knee, hip, or shoulder. Joint symptoms associated with fever (80%), chills (20%), and malaise	Affected joints are erythematous	WBC count often, though not always, elevated. ESR often elevated. Blood cultures may grow etiologic agents (50%). Synovial fluid analysis shows markedly elevated WBC count with predominance (>75%) of PMNs. Gram's stain may demonstrate organisms (50–70%), although synovial fluid culture is the gold standard. X-rays not helpful unless underlying etiology being considered
Seronegative spondylo-arthropathies	Polyarticular, symmetric arthritis, often associated with other symptoms (psoriatic rash, low back pain from sacroiliitis, urethritis/uveitis) and family history of similar illnesses (ankylosing spondylitis, psoriatic arthritis, arthropathy of IBD, Reiter's syndrome and other reactive arthritides). Onset is subacute, and may occur over several months. Morning stiffness may be a component	In addition to the polyarticular, symmetric arthritis, a variety of clinical signs related to the underlying condition (such as psoriatic rash or uveitis) may be present	Negative RF, although CBC may show mild anemia with elevated WBC. ESR is often elevated. Eighty percent of patients have the HLA-B27 marker. Radiographs may demonstrate sacroiliitis and "bamboo spine" in ankylosing spondylitis. Synovial fluid typically inflammatory
Trauma/hemarthrosis	Monoarticular joint pain and swelling, with history of trauma, or in the case of coagulopathy, no history of trauma. Systemic symptoms are absent, although a personal or family history of bleeding diatheses may be present	Pain and swelling in the affected single joint. Signs of inflammation minimal acutely. Systemic signs, such as fever, typically absent	PT, PTT, bleeding time, and platelet count may demonstrate evidence of coagulopathy if hemarthrosis is atraumatic. Radiographs may demonstrate a fracture if traumatic etiology. Synovial fluid is bloody, with fewer than 10,000 WBCs/mm³. Presence of marrow elements in trauma possible
Viral arthritis (immune complex disease)	Polyarticular (symmetric or asymmetric) concomitantly or following viral syndrome, typically rubella, hepatitis B, parvovirus, mumps, or adenovirus. Typically, the PIP, knee, ankle, and MCP joints	Fever may be present, and signs of hepatitis or other specific viral illness may be noted. The arthritis is typically severe	Elevated WBC count may be noted. Liver function tests may be abnormal in hepatitis, and should be followed with serologies for specific viral etiologies. The synovial fluid is typically non-inflammatory, with cell counts

(*continued*)

Table 27.3 Differential diagnosis of joint pain (*cont*)

Diagnosis	Symptoms	Signs	Work-up
Viral arthritis (*cont*)	most affected. Other symptoms dependent on the temporal relationship of arthritis to the primary viral infection. Fever with swollen lymph nodes may be only other symptoms		<2000 cells/mm^3, although it may develop inflammatory characteristics as disease progresses. Rubella cultures may be performed on the synovial fluid

ASO: antistreptolysin O titer; CBC: complete blood count; CHF: congestive heart failure; CRP: C-reactive protein; DIP: distal interphalangeal; ECG: electrocardiogram; ESR: erythrocyte sedimentation rate; IBD: inflammatory bowel disease; IgG: immunoglobulin G; MCP: metacarpophalangeal; MTP: metatarsophalangeal; *N. gonorrhoeae*: *Neisseria gonorrhoeae*; PIP: proximal interphalangeal; PMNs: polymorphonuclear cells; PT: prothrombin time; PTT: partial thromboplastin time; RF: rheumatoid factor; WBC: white blood cell.

Diagnostic testing

Laboratory studies

Laboratory testing, with the exception of synovial fluid analysis, is rarely useful in evaluating the patient with joint pain. Practitioners generally order a complete blood count (CBC) seeking an elevated white blood cell (WBC) count to confirm an infectious disease or a decreased hemoglobin and hematocrit to suggest systemic rheumatic disease. Another test is the erythrocyte sedimentation rate (ESR); elevations are seen in the context of systemic rheumatic diseases. However, these two commonly ordered tests do not demonstrate adequate sensitivity or specificity to assist in the differential diagnosis. Since septic arthritis is normally the result of hematogenous spread of bacteria to joints, blood cultures may have some utility if this is being considered. If gonococcus (GC) is suspected as a pathogen in septic arthritis (particularly in younger patients), then cultures for GC should be taken from the pharynx, urethra, rectum, cervix, and any skin pustules. In acute gout, serum uric acid levels are often normal.

If the practitioner has suspicion for a systemic rheumatic disease, as would be the case for patients with polyarthritis of more than 6 weeks duration or with an inflammatory synovial fluid, the following laboratory tests should be obtained to aid with diagnosis: CBC, differential, ESR, antinuclear antibody (ANA), rheumatoid factor (RF), creatinine, urinalysis, and antistreptolysin O (ASO) titer.

If the practitioner has suspicion for a viral infectious etiology, such as in polyarthritis of less than 6 weeks duration, the following laboratory tests should be obtained to aid with diagnosis: CBC, differential, liver function tests (to assess for the presence of hepatitis), hepatitis B and C serologies (if indicated by elevations of the liver function tests), and parvovirus serology.

Additional serologies, such as Lyme titers, may be sent if indicated by the clinical picture. In atraumatic hemarthrosis, consideration should be given to a workup for hemophilia with protime, partial thromboplastin time, platelet count, and bleeding time.

Synovial fluid analysis

The most useful diagnostic test for patients with acute joint pain is often synovial fluid analysis. Aspiration and examination of synovial fluid is indicated for patients with joint effusion and/or signs of inflammation. Arthrocentesis is a procedure that involves the puncture and aspiration of synovial fluid from a joint space. Careful aseptic technique must be ensured, and the procedure is contraindicated if there is suspicion or evidence of infection overlying the arthrocentesis landmarks. Typically, synovial fluid analysis includes cell count and differential, Gram's stain and culture, and crystal analysis. Glucose analysis and viscosity may be obtained as well, but are less diagnostic. Synovial fluid should be collected in ethylenediamine tetraacetic acid (EDTA) tubes (lavender top) for cell count and differential, heparin tubes (green top) for crystal analysis, and standard tubes (red top) for chemistries, serologies, and viscosity. Cultures should be plated as soon as possible after aspiration, especially if GC is suspected as a pathogen. A positive Gram's stain is diagnostic for septic arthritis, but a negative Gram's stain does not rule out septic arthritis. Crystal analysis is performed using polarizing

Table 27.4 Analysis of synovial fluid

	Normal	**Non-inflammatory**	**Inflammatory**	**Septic**	**Traumatic**
Color	Colorless	Yellow	Yellow	Yellow	Red
Appearance	Clear	Clear	Cloudy	Cloudy	Cloudy
WBC/ml	<200	<2000	<50,000	>50,000	<10,000
% PMNo	<25	<25	>75	>75	<25
Crystals	None	None	May be present	None	None
Culture	Negative	Negative	Negative	Positive	Negative, though bone marrow elements may be present with fracture
Typical conditions		Osteoarthritis, trauma, viral infection, drug-induced	Crystal-induced arthritides, Lyme disease, acute rheumatic fever, RA, JRA, SLE, spondyloarthropathies, viral infection, sarcoidosis	Bacterial, including GC arthritis	Fracture, ligament injury, hemophilia

GC: gonococcus; JRA: juvenile rheumatoid arthritis; PMNs: polymorphonuclear cells; RA: rheumatoid arthritis; SLE: systemic lupus erythematosus; WBC: white blood cell.

microscopy, with monosodium urate crystals in gout appearing as 2–10 micron, needle-shaped crystals which are negatively birefringent. In contrast, calcium pyrophosphate crystals in pseudo-gout appear as polymorphic (often rhomboid) positively birefringent crystals. High white cell counts are suggestive, but not diagnostic, of infectious etiologies. A low white cell count does not rule out a septic etiology. One must therefore use caution in interpreting these results, as overlap exists between these categories. Synovial fluid cell count may be estimated on a wet mount preparation: two or fewer WBCs per high-power field (hpf) is suggestive of a non-inflammatory effusion, while more than 20 WBC/hpf indicates severe inflammation or infection (Table 27.4).

Electrocardiography

Electrocardiography (ECG) is indicated in patients with clinical symptoms suggestive of cardiac involvement, including chest pain, palpitations, or shortness of breath. Acute rheumatic fever may cause carditis, which leads to prolongation of the P-R interval, and pericarditis, which leads to diffuse S-T segment changes and shortening of the P-R interval. Both of these diagnoses are part of the Jones criteria for the diagnosis of

Table 27.5 Jones criteria for the diagnosis of acute rheumatic fever

Major criteria	**Minor criteria**
Carditis	Clinical findings
Chorea	Arthralgia
Erythema marginatum	Fever
Polyarthritis	Laboratory findings
Subcutaneous nodules	Elevated CRP or ESR
	ECG findings
	Prolonged P-R interval

CRP: C-reactive protein; ECG: electrocardiogram; ESR: erythrocyte sedimentation rate.

acute rheumatic fever (Table 27.5). This requires the presence of either two major criteria, or one major and two minor criteria, in the presence of supporting evidence of prior Group A streptococcal infection. Supporting evidence of prior Group A streptococcal infection includes recent scarlet fever, positive rapid streptococcal test or bacterial throat culture, or increasing or elevated streptococcal antibody titer.

Radiologic studies

Radiographs of painful joints provide the most information in patients with chronic arthritides and late septic arthritis. In the acute setting, X-rays should be reserved for patients with a history of significant trauma or bony point tenderness. In the patient with acute arthritis, the most likely finding is soft tissue swelling, so radiographs cannot be used to rule in or rule out acute septic arthritis. Images should be reviewed for evidence of fracture, neoplasm, osteomyelitis, avascular necrosis (including Legg–Calvé–Perthes disease), slipped capital femoral epiphysis (SCFE) or other bone disease. In case of cellulitis, careful examination of the soft tissues should be performed to rule out foreign body. As early as one week after the onset of septic arthritis, radiographs may show loss of joint space, subchondral bone destruction, and periosteal new bone formation.

General treatment principles

As with all emergency patients, treatment begins with the airway, breathing, and circulation (ABCs). The main goals of treatment are physiologic stabilization, symptom relief, proper utilization of diagnostic tests, and appropriate referral.

Pain relief

Given the severity of pain associated with acute synovitis of any etiology, rapid and effective pain relief is crucial in the treatment of joint pain. Patients may require parenteral opioid analgesics, such as morphine or meperidine, to manage their pain. Adding antiemetics to this regimen decreases the nausea and vomiting that often accompany the administration of these agents. Non-steroidal anti-inflammatory drugs (NSAIDs), such as parenteral ketorolac or oral ibuprofen, may also be effective in reducing the pain of acute synovitis. In osteoarthritis and RA, acetaminophen has been repeatedly demonstrated to improve pain at recommended dosages. Salicylates have been effective in relieving pain from acute rheumatic fever and RA.

In crystal arthropathies, acute synovitis is often treated with a combination of NSAIDs (indomethacin has been a favorite for gout) and colchicine, a microtubule inhibitor that reduces inflammation in the synovium. Colchicine is not as effective for pseudogout as for gout, but may still prove a useful adjunct. Caution is needed in elderly patients, or those with renal or hepatic disease. In resistant cases, a prednisone taper or intramuscular adrenocorticotrophic hormone (ACTH) may prove useful. ACTH may also be used in patients who cannot receive NSAIDs. Uric acid lowering agents, such as allopurinol, have no role in the acute management of gouty arthritis.

Immobilization

Simple splinting of the affected joints often significantly reduces the pain of synovitis, since the synovial receptors are exquisitely sensitive to stretch. However, once the pain has been controlled pharmacologically, patients should be encouraged to remove splints and begin range of motion exercises to avoid loss of function and muscle atrophy that occurs with prolonged splinting.

Antibiotics

Outcomes after septic arthritis, the most serious cause of acute joint pain, are improved with rapid diagnosis and rapid administration of intravenous antibiotics. Specific antibiotic selection should be made with regard to the likely microbial pathogens. It should always include vigorous coverage for Staphylococcus species, given their frequency of occurrence. Ceftriaxone works well against *Neisseria gonorrhoeae*. For early Lyme disease, patients should be treated with 20–30 days of oral doxycycline, amoxicillin, or cefuroxime. Erythromycin is clinically less effective. More severe disease requires intravenous penicillin or ceftriaxone at high doses for several weeks. Acute rheumatic fever is best treated with benzathine penicillin G intramuscularly, or oral penicillin V for 10 days.

Drainage

Patients with septic or gonococcal arthritis require drainage of the affected joints. In the case of bacterial arthritis, this may best be accomplished in the operating room by open incision and drainage, especially if a large joint, such as the knee or hip is involved. For smaller joints or in the case of gonococcal arthritis, repeated daily aspirations with a large bore needle or arthroscope may be recommended. This therapeutic decision should be made in concert with the orthopedic consultant managing the patient. If the patient has osteomyelitis, a joint prosthesis, or is resistant to conservative therapy, open incision and drainage in the operating room should be performed.

Special patients

Pediatric

Septic arthritis in the pediatric population is the result of hematogenous spread from another site, or the result of direct invasion from an area of osteomyelitis prior to growth plate closure. Thus, the clinician must maintain a high degree of suspicion for this diagnosis in febrile children with any joint complaints, even in the presence of a remote source of fever. The diagnosis of septic arthritis in infants is particulary challenging, as infants often present only with irritability and possibly fever. Only the most astute clinicians and parents are likely to notice a decrease in mobility of an extremity in this age group. *Staphylococcus aureus* remains an important etiologic agent across all age ranges. Neonates are at increased risk for *Escherichia coli* and Group B Streptococcus. In toddlers, *S. aureus*, *Kingella kingae*, and *Haemophilus influenzae* are the etiologic agents, although vaccination has reduced the incidence of *H. influenzae* by more than 95%. Pneumococcus and *S. aureus* are the most likely organisms throughout the remainder of the pediatric age group, with *N. gonorrhoeae* becoming more common during adolescence. In children, additional consideration must also be given to conditions like SCFE, osteomyelitis, or Legg–Calvé–Perthes disease (avascular necrosis of the femoral head) that often present with a painful joint.

Elderly

Older adults differ in several ways from the population as a whole with respect to joint pain. First, geriatric patients have a higher incidence of chronic arthritides, which in themselves may flare causing acute joint pain. It is also difficult to interpret acute illness in the setting of chronic joint changes. Additionally, older patients have a higher incidence of septic arthritis. Despite the severity of this condition, they frequently lack the classic symptoms and signs, making the diagnosis more difficult.

Immune compromised

Injection drug users, with or without human immunodeficiency virus (HIV) infection, comprise an increasing proportion of patients presenting with septic arthritis. Typically, septic arthritis in the injection drug user afflicts joints of the axial skeleton more often than the peripheral skeleton.

The most common organisms are *Pseudomonas aeruginosa*, *S. aureus*, *Enterobacter*, and *Serratia marcescens*. Oncology and transplant patients have a higher rate of septic arthritis as well as iatrogenic (drug-associated) gouty arthritis. In these groups, great attention must be given to complaints of joint pain, as the clinical signs of acute inflammation are often mild or absent despite the presence of significant infection. In addition to considering a broader spectrum of bacterial pathogens in these patients, synovial fluid cultures should include evaluation for fungi and mycobacteria. Finally, patients with chronic arthritis, especially RA and crystal arthritis, may be taking immunosuppressive medications, which increases their risk for septic arthritis.

Disposition

Patients in whom septic arthritis is suspected, ruled in, or cannot be excluded require orthopedic consultation and admission for intravenous antibiotics pending culture results. Assuming a non-infectious etiology for joint pain can be established, patients can be discharged if their pain is adequately controlled. If this is not possible, admission for parenteral analgesics may be necessary. Visiting home nursing, assisted living, or skilled nursing care may be required if an episode of acute arthritis leaves a patient unable to perform activities of daily living or increases their risk for falls.

Pearls, pitfalls, and myths

- In patients with monoarticular arthritis, septic arthritis should be presumed until proven otherwise, especially if these patients have systemic signs of toxicity.
- The number of joints involved and their distribution are significant clues to the differential diagnosis.
- Patients with a single painful joint require a detailed physical examination to rule out evidence of systemic disease.
- Never perform arthrocentesis through an area of cellulitis or infection.
- Use caution when interpreting the white cell count of synovial fluid analysis, as overlap exists between etiologies.
- Do not underestimate or undertreat pain caused by synovitis.

References

1. American College of Rheumatology Ad Hoc Committee on Clinical Guidelines. Guidelines for the initial evaluation of the adult patient with acute musculoskeletal symptoms. *Arthritis Rheum* 1996;39:1–8.
2. Brower AC. Septic arthritis. *Radiol Clin North Am* 1996; 34(2):293–309.
3. Braun J, van der Heijde D. Novel approaches in the treatment of ankylosing spondylitis and other spondyloarthritides. *Expert Opin Invest Drug* 2003; 12(7):1097–1109.
4. Chard J, Dieppe P. Update: treatment of osteoarthritis. *Arthritis Rheum* 2002; 47(6):686–690.
5. Davis MA (ed.). *Signs and Symptoms In Emergency Medicine*. St. Louis: Mosby, 1999. Chapter 20 "Joint Pain" and Chapter 21 "Limping Child/Child Won't Walk."
6. Dajani AS, Ayoub E, Bierman FZ, et al. Guidelines for the diagnosis of rheumatic fever: Jones criteria, updated 1992. *Circulation* 1993; 87:302–307.
7. Goldenberg DL. Septic arthritis. *Lancet* 1998; 351(9097):197–202.
8. Greenspan A, Tehranzadeh J. Imaging of infectious arthritis. *Radiol Clin North Am* 2001; 39(2):267–276.
9. Khan MA. Update on spondyloarthropathies. *Ann Intern Med* 2002; 136(12):896–907.
10. Klippel JH (ed.). *Primer on the Rheumatic Diseases*, 12th ed., Atlanta: Arthritis Foundation, 2001.
11. Marx JA (ed.). Chapter 110: Arthritis. *Rosen's Emergency Medicine: Concepts and Clinical Practice*, 5th ed., St. Louis: Mosby, 2002.
12. Massarotti EM. Lyme arthritis. *Med Clin North Am* 2002; 86(2):297–309.
13. Mohan AK, Cote TR, Siegel JN, Braun MM. Infectious complications of biologic treatments of rheumatoid arthritis. *Curr Opin Rheumatol* 2003; 15(3):179–184.
14. Rott KT, Agudelo CA. Gout. *J Am Med Assoc* 2003; 289(21):2857–2860.
15. Schumacher Jr HR. Aspiration and injection therapies for joints. *Arthritis Rheum* 2003; 49(3):413–420.
16. Scott DL. The diagnosis and prognosis of early arthritis: rationale for new prognostic criteria. *Arthritis Rheum* 2002; 46(2):286–290.
17. Song J, Letts M, Monson R. Differentiation of psoas muscle abscess from septic arthritis of the hip in children. *Clin Orthop Relat Res* 2001; (391):258–265.
18. Tallia AF, Cardone DA. Diagnostic and therapeutic injection of the shoulder region. *Am Fam Physician* 2003; 67(6):1271–1278.
19. Tintinalli JE (ed.). Chapter 278: Acute disorders of the joint and bursae. *Emergency Medicine: A Comprehensive Study Guide*, 5th ed., McGraw Hill, 2000.
20. Williamson L, Bowness P, Mowat A, Ostman-Smith I. Lesson of the week: difficulties in diagnosing acute rheumatic fever-arthritis may be short lived and carditis silent. *Br Med J* 2000; 320(7231):362–365.

28   Low back pain

Mel Herbert, MD, MBBS, BMEDSCI **and Mary Lanctot-Herbert**, MSN, FNP-C

Scope of the problem

Back pain affects up to 80% of the general population at some time during their lives. It is one of the most expensive outpatient diseases in medicine and is generally a recurrent problem. Most patients have no serious underlying disease and are termed "uncomplicated." A few patients will have very serious disease necessitating emergent intervention. The process of identifying those with serious disease from the vast majority of patients with uncomplicated back pain can be difficult.

Anatomic essentials

Acute low back pain refers to pain felt in the lumbosacral spine and paraspinal areas. The pain may originate from lumbosacral structures such as bones (lumbar vertebrae, sacrum and coccyx), intervertebral discs, joints (facet, sacroiliac), soft tissues (muscles, tendons, ligaments), vascular structures, and nervous tissue (spinal cord, nerve roots). Low back pain may also be referred from pelvic, retroperitoneal, and abdominal structures due to shared innervation.

The spinal cord is housed in the spinal column, a series of interconnected bones held in place by complex ligamentous and muscular structures. The spinal cord is surrounded by the dura mater and a series of potential spaces. These spaces are important to clinicians because infection and tumor can seed there. The adult spinal cord ends at approximately the L1–L2 junction. The nerve roots at the end of the spinal cord are known as the *cauda equina* (horse's tail). Pressure on the cauda equina can result in bladder and bowel incontinence and saddle anesthesia (decreased sensation over the buttocks, perineum, and proximal medial thighs).

Between each vertebral body lie the shock-absorbing interverterbral discs composed of the nucleus pulposus and surrounding annulus fibrosus. Lateral herniation of the lumbar discs can produce classic sciatica (lateralizing leg pain). Very rarely, central herniation of a disc at or above L1 can produce a cord compression syndrome.

The spinal nerves exit the spinal column between the vertebral bodies. Compression of these spinal nerves can lead to radicular pain, motor and/or sensory loss. Understanding the lumbar dermatomes and myotomes is important for following the progression or resolution of neurologic symptoms, as well as effective medical documentation (Table 28.1).

Table 28.1 Selected dermatomes and myotomes

Site of herniation	Nerve root	Dermatome	Myotome	Reflex
L5–S1	S1	Posterior calf Lateral foot	Plantar flexors	Achilles
L4–5	L5	Anterior calf Medial foot First web space ± great toe	Dorsiflexors	None
L3–4	L4	Medial calf and foot ± great toe	Quadriceps	Patellar
Cauda equina (massive central anterior prolapse)	Multiple	• Saddle anesthesia* • Any or all of the above, usually bilaterally	• Multiple, including any or all of the above • Bladder/bowel dysfunction	• Any or all of the above • Anal wink • Cremasteric

* Saddle area is that part of the buttocks that sits on a traditional bicycle.

History

The overlying concern in the assessment of patients with low back pain is to rule out serious causes (Figure 28.1). Identifying patients with "red flags" on history or physical examination should raise the clinician's suspicion and guide the diagnostic evaluation (Tables 28.2 and 28.3).

How long have you had the pain?

"Acute" low back pain refers to pain lasting less than 2–4 weeks, while "chronic" low back pain has typically lasted more than 12 weeks. Ask the patient about previous episodes and whether or not these episodes were similar.

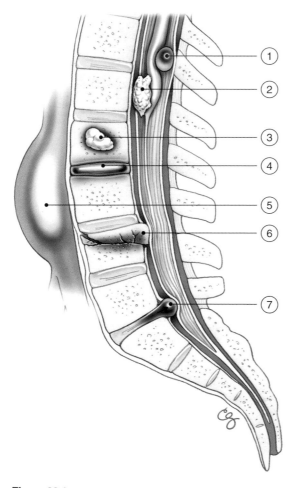

Figure 28.1
Serious causes of low back pain. 1. Epidural abscess; 2. Cancer: spinal cord metastasis; 3. Cancer: primary or metastatic vertebral; 4. Discitis; 5. Abdominal aortic aneurysm; 6. Lumbar vertebra fracture; 7. Cauda equina syndrome.

Table 28.2 Red flags from history

History	Concern
Age <18	Discitis, spinal infection, tumor, spondylolysis, spondylolisthesis
Age >50	Malignancy, fracture, AAA
Trauma, chronic steroid use	Fracture
History of cancer	Metastases
Fevers, chills, night sweats, weight loss	Infection, malignancy
Injection drug use, immunocompromised	Infection
Night pain	Malignancy, infection, ankylosing spondylitis
Unrelenting pain	Malignancy, infection

AAA: abdominal aortic aneurysm.
Reproduced from Della-Giustina, 2000.

Table 28.3 Red flags from physical examination

Physical	Concern
Fever	Infection, malignancy
Anal sphincter laxity, saddle anesthesia	Cauda equina syndrome
Motor weakness	Cauda equina syndrome, spinal cord compression, herniated disc
Abnormal reflexes	Cauda equina syndrome, spinal cord compression, herniated disc
Positive SLR	Herniated disc
Positive CSLR	Herniated disc
Percussion bone tenderness	Fracture, infection
Positive Babinski sign	Upper motor neuron disease (spinal cord compression)
Incontinence, saddle anesthesia	Cauda equina syndrome
Bilateral neurologic deficits	Cauda equina syndrome, spinal cord compression
Unilateral neurologic deficit	Herniated disc

SLR: straight leg raise; CSLR: crossed straight leg raise.
Reproduced from Della-Giustina, 2000.

Where is the pain? Does it radiate?

Pain localized to the paralumbar musculature without dermatomal radiation most likely represents muscular or ligamentous strain. Radiation of pain in a dermatomal distribution implies nerve root compression. Pain radiating to both legs can be seen with cauda equina syndrome. Pain radiating to the groin may be seen with abdominal aortic aneurysm (AAA) or renal calculi. Pain radiating to the abdomen should raise suspicion for a possible visceral cause or sacroiliac disease.

How would you describe the pain?

Deep somatic pain from structures such as the muscles, tendons, and ligaments is often described as a deep, dull ache. Sciatica is often described as a sharp or burning pain radiating down the posterior or lateral aspect of the leg. The pain associated with a ruptured AAA is often acute, severe and constant.

How did the pain begin (sudden versus chronic)? Did you sustain trauma?

The sudden onset of pain suggests disc prolapse, crush fracture, or ruptured AAA, while the gradual onset of pain over years suggests degenerative disease. Pain onset over days to weeks is not reliable in distinguishing the cause. Major trauma, such as motor vehicle collisions or falls from height, as well as minor trauma, such as strenuous lifting in a potentially osteoporotic patient, should raise concern for vertebral fractures.

What makes the pain better or worse?

Mechanical (uncomplicated) back pain improves with rest and is exacerbated by movement and standing. Radicular pain (nerve root compression) is worse with coughing, sneezing, or changing positions. Constant pain not generally altered by rest or position is worrisome for a serious cause, such as cancer or a spinal infection. Similarly, unrelenting pain despite adequate analgesia raises concern for serious disease.

Pain that is worse at night is worrisome for malignancy, infection, or ankylosing spondylitis. Morning stiffness and pain that improves with exercise suggests an inflammatory arthritis, while pain worsening over the course of the day suggests osteoarthritis. Lower extremity pain exacerbated by walking and relieved by sitting (neurogenic claudication) may be due to spinal stenosis.

Have you had any weakness, numbness, or loss of control of your bowel or bladder?

The presence of numbness or weakness suggests nerve root compression or spinal cord involvement. Bladder dysfunction or fecal incontinence in association with low back pain is a very serious symptom, suggesting cauda equina syndrome or higher spinal cord compression. Ask the patient about symptoms of urinary retention, increased frequency, or overflow incontinence.

Do you have a history of cancer or injection drug use?

The most powerful predictor of cancer as a cause of back pain is a prior or current history of cancer (especially breast, lung, and prostate cancers). Metastatic tumors of the vertebrae are 25 times more common than primary tumors, such as multiple myeloma. Metastases to the spinal column and cord may also result in epidural cord compression.

Injection drug use places patients at very high risk of spinal infections, such as osteomyelitis, discitis, or epidural abscess. Other patients at increased risk include those with diabetes, chronic renal failure, alcoholism, or recent spinal surgery. Some authorities recommend that these patients be promptly and aggressively evaluated for spinal infections. Failure to rapidly diagnose an expanding epidural abscess can result in permanent neurologic deficit.

Associated symptoms

The presence of fevers, chills, night sweats, or unexplained weight loss in patients with back pain suggests malignancy or infection. Urinary tract, pulmonary or gastrointestinal (GI) symptoms may identify a referred cause for low back pain.

Past medical

A previous history of back surgery or back problems should be elicited. A history of an aneurysm or aortic graft repair raises concern for a leaking AAA. A previous history of or risk factors for osteoporosis (female, age over 50, steroid use) may predispose the patient to fractures. The dates of the last menstrual period and the possibility of pregnancy should be ascertained, as a normal or ectopic pregnancy can cause low back pain.

Details regarding the patient's profession, pending litigation, or workman's compensation status are important if the injury occurred on the job. A family history of inflammatory arthritis such as ankylosing spondylitis could suggest a potential etiology.

The use of medications, such as corticosteroids, is a risk factor for spinal infections and fractures due to osteoporosis. Over-anticoagulation or thrombocytopenia may place the patient at risk for an epidural hematoma, especially following trauma, lumbar puncture (LP), epidural anesthesia, or spinal surgery. Spontaneous retroperitoneal hemorrhage in patients on warfarin or with bleeding disorders may present with low back pain.

Physical examination

The physical examination of the patient with back pain is focused and intended to select patients with possible serious etiologies.

General appearance

Cachectic patients are at risk for spinal infections from being immunocompromised and vertebral fractures from osteoporosis. Consider whether the underlying cause of cachexia is from injection drug use, human immunodeficiency virus (HIV), or an underlying cancer that has metastasized to the spine.

Vital signs

Fever suggests an infectious cause of back pain, with the rectal temperature being most sensitive. Many patients with spinal infections do not have a fever. Patients with AAA, sepsis, or ruptured ectopic pregnancy may present with hypotension. This finding may be transient and lead to syncope as a presenting complaint.

Abdomen

Gently palpate the abdomen for a pulsatile mass that may be present in 50% of patients with an AAA. Also note any abdominal tenderness or findings that suggest a visceral etiology (e.g., appendicitis or ectopic pregnancy) with pain referred to the back or flank. For low back pain referred to the groin or buttocks, the hips should be assessed for pain and range of motion (ROM).

Back

Examination of the back includes inspection, palpation, and assessment of active ROM. The patient should be assessed for abnormal posture, spinal contour, or pelvic tilt. Such abnormalities may be structural or in response to pain or weakness. The skin overlying the back should be examined for bruising, swelling, or other lesions such as herpes zoster, which can cause lateralized back pain.

The lumbar paravertebral muscles should be palpated for tenderness or spasm. Palpate each spinal vertebral process and sacroiliac joint to identify areas of localized tenderness. Midline bony percussion tenderness is unusual in patients with uncomplicated back pain, and suggests a focal lesion such as a fracture, cancer, or infection. Pain on percussion of the costovertebral angles suggests the presence of kidney pathology such as pyelonephritis.

Active ROM is assessed and described by having the patient flex, extend and bend laterally to each side. Normal ROM is 90° flexion, 15° extension, and 45° lateral flexion.

Rectal

This part of the examination should generally be done with a chaperone. Examine for perianal and saddle sensation by asking the patient "Does the skin in this region feel normal or numb?" Check the rectal tone by having the patient voluntarily contract their anal sphincter after inserting your gloved and lubricated finger. Saddle anesthesia and abnormal sphincter tone suggest a serious cause of back pain, such as cauda equina syndrome.

Neurologic

The legs should be evaluated for sensory changes in a dermatomal distribution by comparing one side to the other (Figure 28.2). In the same way, motor deficits should be sought in a systematic manner, generally starting at the toes and moving to the hips. Each side should be compared against the other. Evidence of major motor weakness is suggested by abnormalities of knee extension (quadriceps weakness), ankle plantar flexion and eversion, and dorsiflexion (footdrop). Documentation is best done with descriptive words rather than any of the variety of scoring systems. For example: "Left great toe dorsiflexion with mild weakness compared to right side," is probably better than: "2+/3 or 4/5 or +++ left great toe." Muscle atrophy can be detected by comparing the circumference of the thighs or calves.

Check for abnormalities of the ankle reflex (tests predominantly the S1 nerve root), and the knee reflex (tests predominantly the L4 nerve root). As reflexes may diminish with age, it is critical to identify asymmetry. The presence of clonus, hyperreflexia, or upgoing toes in response to plantar stimulation indicates an upper motor neuron lesion, such as spinal cord compression.

Gait is an extremely important part of the examination. Check for difficulty with heel walking (ankle and toe dorsiflexors innervated by the L5 and some L4 nerve roots) or toe walking (calf muscles, mostly the S1 nerve root). Inability to walk despite adequate analgesia may suggest serious pathology. This also may assist with disposition, as a patient who cannot walk should not be discharged from the emergency department (ED), unless this situation is chronic and unchanged.

Clinical tests for radiculopathy

The straight leg raise (SLR) test is the standard method of eliciting clinically significant nerve

Nerve root	L4	L5	S1
Pain	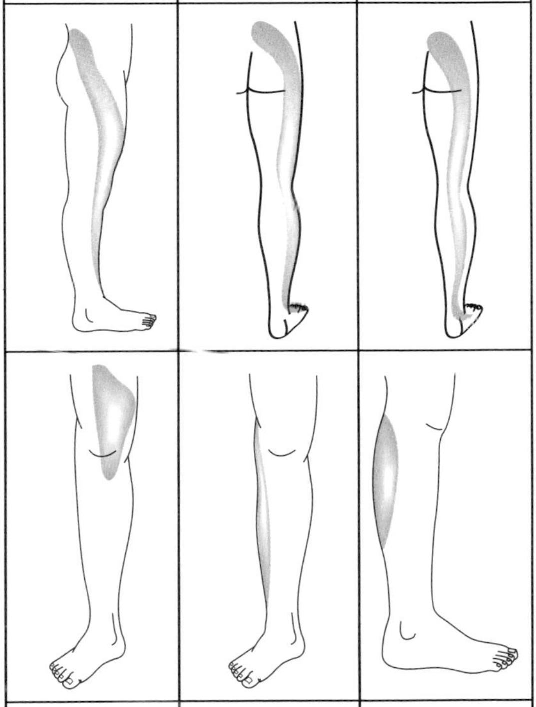		
Numbness			
Motor weakness	Extension of quadriceps	Dorsiflexion of great toe and foot	Plantar flexion of great toe and foot
Screening examination	Squat and rise	Heel walking	Walking on toes
Reflexes	Knee jerk diminished	None reliable	Ankle jerk diminished

Figure 28.2
Testing for lumbar nerve root compromise. Reprinted from Bigos S, Bowyer O, Braen G, et al. Acute Low Back Problems in Adults. Clinical Practice Guideline No. 14. AHCPR Publication No. 95-0642. Rockville, MD: Agency for Health Care Policy and Research, Public Health Service, U.S. Department of Health and Human Services. December 1994.

root compression (Figure 28.3). The SLR test detects tension on the L5 and/or S1 nerve root. The SLR test reproduces posterior or posterolateral leg pain by stretching nerve roots irritated by disc herniation. Pain felt below the knee at less than 70° of straight leg elevation, aggravated by dorsiflexion of the ankle and relieved by ankle plantar flexion or external limb rotation is highly suggestive of tension on the L5 or S1 nerve root from disc herniation. The reproduction of back pain with SLR testing does not indicate significant nerve root tension.

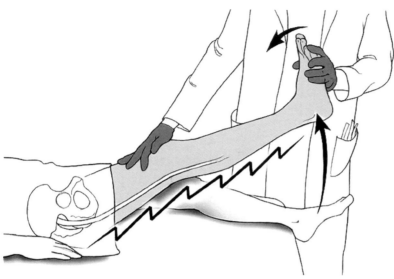

Figure 28.3
Straight leg raise (SLR) test.

SLR instructions include: (1) Have the patient lie as straight as possible on a table in the supine position. With one hand placed above the knee of the leg being examined, exert enough firm pressure to keep the knee fully extended. Ask the patient to relax. (2) With the other hand cupped under the heel, slowly raise the straight limb. Tell the patient, "If this bothers you, let me know, and I will stop." (3) Monitor for any movement of the pelvis before complaints are elicited. True sciatic tension should elicit complaints before the hamstrings are stretched enough to move the pelvis. (4) Estimate the degree of leg elevation that elicits complaint from the patient. Then determine the most distal area of discomfort: back, hip, thigh, knee, or below the knee. (5) While holding the leg at the limit of straight leg raising, dorsiflex the ankle. Note whether this aggravates the pain. Internal rotation of the limb can also increase the tension on the sciatic nerve roots.

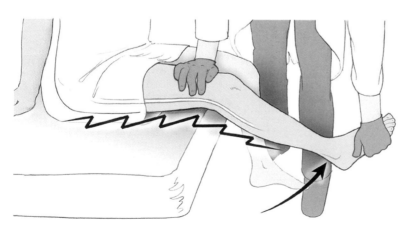

Figure 28.4
Sitting knee extension test (SKET).

SKET instructions include: With the patient sitting on a table, both hip and knees flexed at 90°, slowly extend the knee as if evaluating the patella or bottom of the foot. This maneuver stretches nerve roots as much as a moderate degree of supine SLR.

The crossed straight leg raise (CSLR) test is positive if an SLR test of an opposite (asymptomatic) limb elicits sciatic pain in the symptomatic limb. A positive CSLR is a stronger indication of nerve root compression due to disc herniation than pain elicited from SLR testing in the ipsilateral leg. The reverse straight leg raise (RSLR) test or femoral tension sign detects tension in the L2–L4 nerve roots. With the patient prone, pain elicited in the anterior thigh with extension of the hip or flexion of the knee confirms a positive RSLR test.

The sitting knee extension test (SKET) also tests sciatic nerve root tension (Figure 28.4). The patient with significant nerve root irritation tends to complain or lean backward to reduce tension on the nerve.

Skin

Search for signs of peripheral vascular disease (skin or hair loss over the toes or distal lower extremities, ulcers, absent or weak distal pulses, or the presence of vascular grafts). These findings suggest searching for AAA. The skin should also be screened for lesions suspicious for malignancy, infection, or needle marks.

Cancer screening

As a general screen for cancer, examine the prostate in men, noting if it is hard or irregular. In women, examine the breast for lumps or skin findings that may be associated with cancer. Breast cancer affects women of *all* ages. Examine for lymphadenopathy as a sign of HIV disease, lymphoma, leukemia, or metastatic cancer.

Differential diagnosis

The differential diagnosis of low back pain (LBP) is broad, but the classic mistake is to label LBP as benign (i.e., muscular strain) when a serious cause is present (Tables 28.4 and 28.5). Renal colic is the most common incorrect diagnosis given to patients ultimately found to have AAA.

Table 28.4 Differential diagnosis of low back pain

Mechanical spine etiologies	Non-mechanical etiologies	
	Spinal disorders	**Visceral disorders**
Lumbar strain or sprain[a]	Neoplasia	Pelvic organs
Degenerative disease	Metastatic carcinoma	Prostatitis
Discs (spondylosis)	Multiple myeloma	Endometriosis
Facet joints[b]	Lymphoma and leukemia	Pelvic inflammatory disease
Diffuse idiopathic skeletal hyperostosis[c]	Primary spinal cord or vertebral tumor	Renal disease
Spondylolysis[b,c]	Retroperitoneal tumors	Nephrolithiasis
Spondylolisthesis[d]	Infection	Pyelonephritis
Intervertebral disc herniation	Osteomyelitis	Perinephric abscess
Spinal stenosis	Septic discitis	Vascular disease
Fracture	Paraspinal or epidural abscess	Abdominal aortic aneurysm
Traumatic	Herpes zoster (shingles)	Aortoiliac disease
Osteoporotic	Inflammatory arthritis	GI disease
Congenital disease	Ankylosing spondylitis	Pancreatitis
Severe kyphosis	Reiter's syndrome	Cholecystitis
Severe scoliosis	Psoriatic spondylitis	Perforated bowel
Transitional vertebrae	Inflammatory bowel disease	
Internal disc disruption (discogenic pain)[b]	Paget's disease	
	Scheuermann's disease (osteochondrosis)	

[a] Lumbar strain or sprain can be considered due to nonspecific (idiopathic) musculoligamentous etiology;
[b] The relationship between symptoms and objective findings for these conditions is not clearly established;
[c] Spondylolysis is a defect in the pars interarticularis without vertebral slippage;
[d] Spondylolisthesis is anterior displacement of one vertebra, typically L5, over the one beneath it.
Adapted from Atlas and Deyo.

Table 28.5 Important causes of back pain

Disease	History	Examination	Comments
Abdominal aortic aneurysm	Elderly. Patients with vascular disease (e.g., diabetic, smoker). Pain can also be in the flank or groin.	Feel for an abdominal pulsatile mass. Check for symmetric peripheral pulses.	Best diagnosed with CT or US. Hematuria common – often mistaken for renal colic.
Cancer	Consider in age >50. Continuous pain not relieved with rest. History of cancer (even remote). Recent unexplained weight loss. Night sweats.	Look for spinal tenderness Look for signs of tumors elsewhere (perform breast or prostate examination, feel for enlarged lymph nodes).	This becomes a true emergency when there is spinal cord compression. X-rays may miss the diagnosis. The best test is MRI or CT.
Epidural abscess, osteomyelitis or discitis	Recent skin or urinary infection IV drug users. Immunosuppression. Patients with recent GU manipulation. May occur in patients with prosthetic cardiac valves.	Look for fever (absent 20% of the time). Examine for bony tenderness.	Difficult to diagnose this serious disease. If suspected, the best test is an MRI. Plain radiographs of the spine may not identify this diagnosis.
Fracture	Elderly. Osteoporosis. Trauma (can be minimal in elderly patients). Corticosteroid use. Cancer.	Spinal tenderness over bones.	Plain films are generally adequate for screening in any patient with a question of a fracture. Additional CT scanning may be needed to evaluate the extent of the injury (encroachment into the spinal canal).
Inflammatory arthritis (i.e., ankylosing spondylitis)	Young adult males (<40 years) with pain and stiffness in the morning, not relieved when supine. Improvement with exercise. Family history.	Pain and stiffness throughout back and chest. May have decreased ROM depending on degree of advanced disease.	X-ray may be helpful. MRI better to look for inflammation of the sacroiliac joint. Serum HLA-B27 antigen.
Spinal cord compression or cauda equina syndrome	Urinary retention or dribbling (overflow incontinence). Fecal incontinence. Bilateral leg weakness.	Check the anal wink (diminished or absent). Check anal tone (reduced). Check saddle sensation (reduced). Post-void residual <100 ml makes diagnosis unlikely.	Anything that compresses the spinal cord can produce this syndrome. MRI is the gold standard diagnostic test. CT gives useful bony information.
Spinal stenosis	Elderly patient with long history of low back pain. Pseudo-claudication (LBP, leg weakness, leg pain and paresthesias that occur while standing or walking and are relieved by sitting).	Signs of peripheral vascular disease or hip osteoarthritis absent. Absence of pain when seated. Thigh pain with sustained lumbar extension (30 seconds).	Narrowing of the spinal canal. Diagnosed by CT or MRI.

AAA: abdominal aortic aneurysm; CT: computed tomography; GU: genitourinary; IV: intravenous; LBP: low back pain; MRI: magnetic resonance imaging; ROM: range of motion.

Diagnostic tests

The goal of diagnostic testing is to confirm or exclude serious pathology. Test ordering should be targeted and based on the results of a focused history and physical examination. The overriding concept is to aggressively image patients who have historical or physical exam "red flags," while arranging follow-up for all other patients.

Post-void residual

A post-void residual should be checked in any patient with urinary retention or incontinence. This can be accomplished through urinary catheterization or non-invasive ultrasound. A residual volume greater than 100 ml is reason for concern.

Laboratory studies

The routine use of the complete blood count (CBC) and erythrocyte sedimentation rate (ESR) as screening tools is without merit. Numerous studies note that these tests lack both sensitivity and specificity when applied to the back pain population. The ESR may be elevated in patients with malignancy, inflammatory conditions, or infection.

A urinalysis can screen for pyuria or hematuria. A urine pregnancy test can exclude pregnancy prior to radiography or as a potential etiology of low back pain (i.e., ectopic pregnancy).

Radiologic studies

Though plain lumbosacral spine radiographs may be a useful screening tool for vertebral fractures (Figure 28.5) and spondylolisthesis (may occur in athletes involved in hyperextension sports like golf or gymnastics), it is important to recognize their limitations. Lumbosacral plain films cannot diagnose herniated intervertebral discs or spinal stenosis, and are frequently negative in patients with cancer and spinal infections. Routine use of lumbar spine films to diagnose serious causes of low back pain is a wasteful exercise. In fact, radiation exposure and incorrect imaging sensitivity may preclude more advanced appropriate imaging studies, and therefore may be potentially harmful. In one study, plain lumbosacral radiographs revealed unexpected findings in only 0.04% of patients under the age of 50. A complete lumbosacral plain film series yields nearly 2000 times the gonadal radiation as a single chest X-ray (CXR).

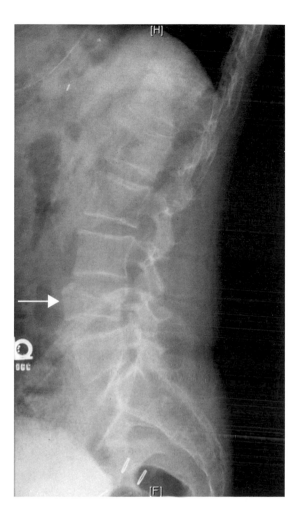

Figure 28.5
Lumbar compression fracture. Lateral radiograph of the lumbar spine demonstrating a compression fracture of the L4 vertebra, with probable retropulsion of bony fragments. *Courtesy*: Kathryn Stevens, MD.

Emergent computed tomography (CT) or magnetic resonance imaging (MRI) are indicated in patients with a history, physical examination, or prior tests that strongly suggest a serious cause for back pain. These include cauda equina syndrome, AAA (Figure 28.6), infection, or tumor. Non-contrast CT is indicated when bony abnormalities (i.e., fracture, degenerative changes) are suspected, or when MRI is contraindicated. Radiologists favor MRI for suspected radiculopathy compared with CT, as it provides better resolution, no ionizing radiation, and superior ability to diagnose other inflammatory, malignant, or vascular conditions (Figure 28.7). For patients with sciatica likely due to a herniated disc or spinal stenosis, and who lack major neurologic abnormalities,

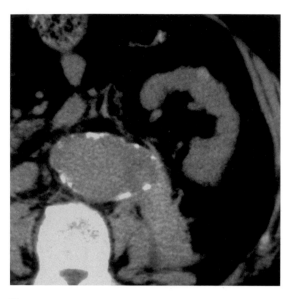

Figure 28.6
Non-contrast CT of ruptured AAA. Note high attenuation left peri-aortic hemorrhage adjacent to calcified AAA. *Courtesy*: R. Brooke Jeffrey, MD.

imaging can be deferred 4–8 weeks as the majority of these patients improve with conservative therapy.

The clinical significance of any abnormalities detected on imaging studies must be carefully interpreted in the context of the patient's presenting symptoms. It is well known that plain films, CT and MRI may reveal abnormalities such as lumbar disc degeneration, spondylosis (osteophytes), facet joint arthritis, lumbar disc herniation, spinal stenosis, and spondylolisthesis (anterior displacement of the vertebra) in asymptomatic patients. This is especially true in older subjects.

General treatment principles

In the majority of patients without red flags, the principles of therapy include analgesia and return to normal activity as quickly as possible, with lifting modifications and instructions on correct

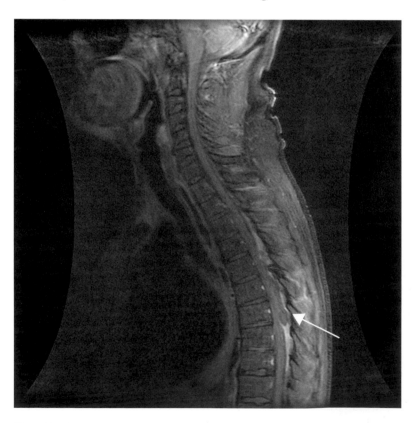

Figure 28.7
Epidural abscess. Sagittal T1 weighted MRI (post-gadolinium) reveals epidural enhancement and abscess collection (see arrow). *Courtesy*: Mahesh Jayaraman, MD.

posture, lifting techniques, and simple exercises. Table 28.6 provides initial treatment recommendations for several serious causes of LBP.

Table 28.6 Diagnosis and treatment of serious causes of low back pain

Disease	Initial treatment and consultation
Abdominal aortic aneurysm	Two or more large bore IVs. Six units of blood for crossmatch. Immediate vascular surgery consultation, routine age-appropriate preoperative laboratories, including hematocrit and creatinine.
Cancer	Aggressive analgesia, CBC, CXR (looking for metastases), CT or MRI to determine extent of disease.
Cauda equina or cord compression syndromes	Immediate neurosurgical consultation. Imaging with MRI or CT myelography. High dose steroids: 30 mg/kg methylprednisolone bolus then 5.4 mg/kg/hours infusion for 20 hours if symptoms started <8 hours ago (this treatment is common but controversial, and may result in more harm than help). Routine age-appropriate preoperative laboratories.
Epidural abscess or spinal infection	Blood cultures × 3. IV antibiotics, generally a combination of anti-staphylococcal and aminoglycoside agents. Neurosurgical consultation. Routine age-appropriate preoperative laboratories.
Fractures	Appropriate analgesia, generally CT scanning to define the extent of the fracture. Orthopedic or neurosurgical consultation (often institution-specific). Additional work-up needed if fractures are atraumatic.

CBC: complete blood count; CT: computed tomography; CXR: chest X-ray; IV: intravenous; MRI: magnetic resonance imaging.

Analgesia

Analgesia should be adequate to allow patients to comfortably return to normal activity as quickly as possible. Analgesia should be given on a timed interval initially, then on an "as required" basis as the pain resolves. Hydrocodone/acetaminophen combinations are commonly used and generally effective: one or two tablets of 5/500 strength every 4 hours for short courses may be effective. For mild pain, acetaminophen alone in doses of 15 mg/kg is an excellent medication. Tylenol with codeine is generally a poor choice, since it has many GI side effects and little efficacy over acetaminophen alone. Musculoskeletal back pain is rarely inflammatory; therefore, non-steroidal anti-inflammatory drugs (NSAIDs) such as ibuprofen do not offer any particular advantage. However, doses of 400–600 mg every 6 hours of ibuprofen may provide some relief. Any prescription for NSAIDs should be for short courses, because GI ulceration and hemorrhage is an increasingly recognized side effect (especially in the elderly), even after relatively short exposure.

Muscle relaxants

There is no doubt that many patients with uncomplicated back pain have muscle spasm. However, there is controversy as to the effectiveness of muscle relaxants. While diazepam at doses of 2–10 mg every 4–6 hours may be effective, many other choices exist. The addictive potential of diazepam, other muscle relaxants, and narcotics is real, but when used for acute pain and for short durations, the risk of addiction is small.

Steroids

Although corticosteroids are prescribed for patients with low back pain (especially with radiculopathy), evidence supporting their use is lacking.

Other therapies

Early ambulation and avoidance of activities that provoke pain should be encouraged. Patients should avoid prolonged sitting or standing and should get up at regular intervals to walk and move their backs. Bed rest should be limited to periods of severe pain, and never for more than a few days at a time.

Evidence recommending routine heat or cold therapy, physical therapy, or chiropractic manipulation is lacking. Since most episodes of acute low back pain resolve in 2–4 weeks, these therapies are best reserved for patients not responding to initial conservative management.

Prevention

Back exercises during the acute phase should be avoided, as they may exacerbate symptoms.

However, education on specific back strengthening exercises and proper lifting techniques may reduce subsequent episodes of pain or injury. In general, the best prevention is the maintenance of an appropriate body mass index (i.e., weight loss for most patients), exercise promoting cardiovascular fitness (without specific back exercises), and smoking cessation (this probably does not reduce back pain episodes substantially but is good for overall health and reduces the risk for lung cancer). Abdominal core muscle strengthening is helpful in minimizing low back pain as well.

Special patients
Elderly

Back pain at the extremes of age should always cause concern. Elderly patients with back pain can harbor multiple pathologies, including AAA and cancer. The most immediately life-threatening condition is AAA. Cancer in this age group is frequently a subsequent diagnosis in a patient who initially presents without an obvious mechanism of injury.

Pediatric

In children, controversy exists about the seriousness of acute low back pain. Some authors note it is a rare complaint, suggesting significant pathology, while others have demonstrated the opposite. Suspect serious pathology when children complain of nocturnal pain or limit their activity secondary to pain. All children who remain undiagnosed following their ED visit need close follow-up and reevaluation.

Athletes

Athletes of all ages involved in hyperextension sports (e.g., baseball pitchers, golfers, gymnasts) can develop pars interarticularis fractures and subsequent spondylolisthesis. These injuries are more likely found in those involved at the competitive level. In this case, referral to an orthopedist or neurosurgeon is recommended.

Pregnancy

Back pain in pregnancy is an extremely common complaint. There are many potential causes of back pain in pregnancy, resulting from changes in maternal weight, center of gravity, posture, and ligamentous stability. While pregnant patients are not immune from serious causes of low back pain, it is generally true that most pain resolves following delivery. Due to the potential effects of ionizing radiation and medications on the growing fetus, additional consideration should be given prior to diagnostic imaging or therapy in these patients.

Malingering

The patient who embellishes medical history, exaggerates pain, or provides inconsistent responses on physical examination can be particularly challenging. "Pain behaviors" such as amplified grimacing, distorted gait or posture, moaning, and rubbing of painful body parts may cloud medical issues and evoke responses from the clinician. Rather than interpreting these inconsistencies or pain behaviors as malingering, the clinician should view them as a plea for help or an attempt to enlist the practitioner as an advocate. In patients with recurrent back problems, these behaviors and inconsistencies may simply be habits learned during previous medical evaluations. In working with these patients, the clinician should attempt to identify psychologic or socioeconomic pressures that might influence the presentation. The overall goal should always be to facilitate the patient's recovery and return to work or normal activities, without the development of chronic low back disability.

Disposition

Patients with uncomplicated back pain can generally be discharged home. Patients with severe pain or social circumstances that make self-care difficult may require a short hospital or skilled nursing facility stay until pain is controlled. Discharge instructions should include encouragement to return to usual activites and the appropriate use of analgesia. Serious or worsening symptoms (fever, progressive unremitting pain, loss of bowel or bladder function, and progressive impairment of neurologic function such as sensory loss that expands or motor weakness that progresses up or down nerve roots) should prompt a return visit.

Patients with serious etiologies of their back pain should be admitted to the appropriate inpatient service with rapid consultation. AAA is a vascular emergency; the vascular surgeon should be called as soon as the diagnosis is suspected. Cauda equina syndrome, other spinal cord syndromes, and spinal infections require immediate neurosurgical consultation and admission. While some lumbar spine fractures are stable, it is generally safest to have an orthopedic or neurosurgical consultant assist with treatment and disposition. Cancer is a serious cause of back pain, although not all cancer patients require admission. Cancer patients who are candidates for discharge include those without evidence of neurologic involvement, whose pain is controlled, and for whom rapid outpatient follow-up can be obtained. This plan, of course, assumes that an appropriate consultation has been arranged to follow the patient and expedite further evaluation.

Pearls, pitfalls, and myths

Perhaps the most common pitfall in caring for back pain patients is the failure to recognize the small portion of patients with serious disease. The frequency with which these patients are seen and the relatively infrequent serious pathology identified can create a false sense of security for clinicians and make them less thorough than is appropriate.

Another common problem for emergency practitioners is to view back pain patients as drug-seeking. While there may be a small number of patients with back pain complaints whose true objective is to obtain narcotic analgesia, it is likely a small percentage. Making this assumption can be dangerous. Indeed, a patient with a narcotic problem that prompts him or her to seek emergency care for back pain may also be at high risk for serious conditions, like an epidural abscess. The best approach is to rapidly relieve pain, search for reversible disease, and make multidisciplinary referrals if questions about narcotic abuse exist.

References

1. Atlas SJ, Nardin RA. Evaluation and treatment of low back pain: an evidenced-based approach to clinical care. *Muscle Nerve* 2003;27:265–284.
2. Bigos S, et al. Acute Low Back Problems in Adults. *Clinical Practice Guidelines No 14.* Agency For Health Care Policy and Research (AHCPR) Publication 95-0642, December 1994.
3. Cherkin DC, Deyo RA, Battié M, Street J, Barlow W. A comparison of physical therapy, chiropractic manipulation, and provision of an educational booklet for the treatment of patients with low back pain. *New Engl J Med* 1998;339: 1021–1029.
4. Cherkin D, et al. Comparison of physical therapy, chiropractic manipulation and provision of an educational booklet for the treatment of patients with low back pain. *New Engl J Med* 1998;339(15):1021.
5. Daltroy LH, et al. A controlled trial of an educational program to prevent low back injuries. *New Engl J Med* 1997;337(5):322.
6. Della-Giustina D, Kilcline BA, Denny M. Back pain: cost-effective strategies for distinguishing between benign and life-threatening causes. *EM Practice* 2000; 2(2) December.
7. Deyo R, et al. What can the history and physical examination tell us about low back pain. *J Am Med Assoc* 1992;268(6):760.
8. Faas A, et al. A randomized trial of exercise therapy in patients with acute low back pain. Efficacy on sickness absence. *Spine* 1995;20(8):941.
9. Kristiansson P, et al. Back pain during pregnancy. A prospective study. *Spine* 1996;21:702.
10. Lahad A, et al. The effectiveness of four interventions for the prevention of low back pain. *J Am Med Assoc* 1994;272(16):1286.
11. Meade TW, et al. Randomized comparison of chiropractic and hospital outpatient management for low back pain: results from extended follow up. *Br Med J* 1995;311(7001):349.
12. Micheli LJ, et al. Back pain in young athletes: significant differences from adults in causes and patterns. *Arch Ped Adol Med* 1995;149(1):15.
13. Rodgers KG, Jones JB. Back pain. In: Marx JA (ed.). *Rosen's Emergency Medicine: Concepts and Clinical Practice*, 5th ed., St. Louis: Mosby, 2002.
14. Tawney PJW, et al. Thoracic and lumbar pain syndromes. In: Tintinalli JE (ed.). *Emergency Medicine: A Comprehensive Study Guide*, 5th ed., McGraw Hill, 2000.
15. Turner PG, et al. Back pain in children. *Spine* 1989;14(8):812
16. Wright MD. Acute low back pain. In: Hamilton GC (ed.). *Emergency Medicine: An Approach to Clinical Problem-Solving*, 2nd ed., Philadelphia: W. B. Saunders, 2001.

29 Pelvic pain

Peter G. Kumasaka, MD

Scope of the problem

Pelvic pain is a common emergency department (ED) condition, and is the second most common gynecologic complaint. The pain may be acute or chronic, vague or defined, and occasionally referred to other parts of the body. Etiologies of pelvic pain may be reproductive, gastrointestinal (GI), vascular or urinary. Though specific causes of pelvic pain often do not require emergent diagnosis or treatment, other diagnoses may pose a threat to life (e.g., ectopic pregnancy) or may have serious reproductive sequelae, such as infertility (e.g., salpingitis).

Anatomic essentials

Pelvic pain may originate from the reproductive organs (uterus, fallopian tubes, ovaries) or local organs, such as the appendix, ureters, bladder, sigmoid colon or rectum (Figure 29.1).

Visceral pelvic pain is usually caused by distention of hollow organs by fluid or gas, or capsular stretching of solid organs secondary to edema, blood, cysts or abscesses. Less commonly it is caused by ischemia or inflammation. It is often the earliest manifestation of a particular disease process. The discomfort is often poorly characterized and hard to localize, varying from a steady ache or vague discomfort to excruciating or colicky pain. Examples include distention of the fallopian tube in ectopic pregnancy, uterine contractions in dysmenorrhea, or stretch of the round ligament with advancing stages of pregnancy.

Parietal (somatic) pelvic pain is caused by irritation of the parietal peritoneum. This is usually caused by infection, chemical irritation, or other inflammatory processes. This type of pain is typically sharp, knife-like and constant. Parietal pain, in contrast to visceral pain, can be localized to the dermatome directly above the painful stimulus. Parietal pain is responsible for the physical examination findings of tenderness to palpation, guarding, rebound and rigidity. Examples include salpingitis and endometritis.

Referred pain is defined as pain felt at a distance from the involved organ. Pelvic pain may be referred to the buttocks, back, groin, perineum, legs, or upper abdomen.

History

Clues gleaned from a careful history direct the examination and subsequent diagnostic testing. Patients should always be asked about their sexual history and the possibility of pregnancy. Personal questions should be asked in a nonjudgmental manner and in strict privacy. Spouses, parents,

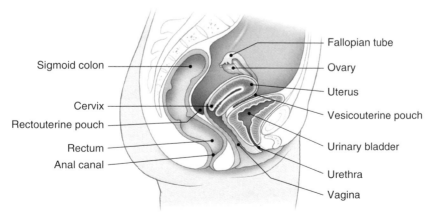

Figure 29.1
Pelvic anatomy (sagittal).

Sigmoid colon

Cervix

Rectouterine pouch

Rectum

Anal canal

Fallopian tube

Ovary

Uterus

Vesicouterine pouch

Urinary bladder

Urethra

Vagina

friends or significant others should be asked to leave the room. This will encourage patients to provide honest answers to questions. Even so, be aware that some patients may still not be truthful in their responses.

How did the pain begin? How long have you had it? Have you had it before? Is there a pattern to it?

Sudden onset of pain may indicate a disease with significant morbidity and mortality, such as perforation of a hollow viscus, intrapelvic hemorrhage or vascular compromise (ovarian torsion). Chronic or recurrent pain can be associated with endometriosis, recurrent ovarian cysts, or a persistent ovarian mass. It is important to determine why the patient came in to seek help if she complains of chronic pain. The answer may reveal a new problem or a significant change of a chronic ailment. It is helpful to ascertain if the pain follows a cyclical pattern, and its relationship to the menstrual cycle. The pain of endometriosis usually accompanies the onset of menses, whereas pain associated with ovulation (Mittelschmerz) typically occurs during midcycle.

How would you describe the pain?

Pain that is sharp is more likely to be related to peritoneal irritation, whereas dull or crampy pain suggests contraction of an organ (e.g., uterus) or obstruction of a viscus (fallopian tube or ureter). Steady, progressive pain is associated with inflammatory or neoplastic causes.

Where is the pain?

The ability to localize the pain can be extremely helpful. Lateral pelvic pain can often be traced to the fallopian tube or ovary; central pelvic pain suggests a process involving the bladder or uterus. Diffuse pain can occur with pelvic inflammatory disease (PID) or peritonitis.

How severe is the pain?

Pain severity is subjective and not always helpful in directing the work-up. The patient complaining of "severe" pain whom you see laughing with a friend is clearly not the same as the patient grimacing and in tears. Pain can wax and wane, however, and different individuals assess, tolerate, and respond to pain differently.

Does the pain radiate?

Pain radiating to the low back may indicate ovarian or uterine pathology; radiation to the flanks may be due to ureteral problems. Radiation of pain to the rectum can be caused by blood or fluid collecting in the cul-de-sac.

Does the pain occur during intercourse?

Sudden onset of pain during intercourse often accompanies a ruptured ovarian cyst. Most other causes of *dyspareunia* can be evaluated as an outpatient. These include gynecologic tumors, pelvic adhesions, adenomyosis, endometriosis, fibroids and uterine retroversion.

Are you pregnant? When was your last normal menstrual cycle? Describe any previous (especially abnormal) pregnancies?

The possibility of pregnancy may significantly alter the differential diagnosis, as well as raise concern for possible adverse effects of diagnostic testing or therapeutic intervention. Assume that all women of childbearing age may be pregnant despite claims of celibacy, the use of birth control (including tubal ligation) and reports of "normal" menstrual periods. If pregnant, risk factors for ectopic pregnancy should be identified (Table 29.1).

Table 29.1 Risk factors for ectopic pregnancy and pelvic inflammatory disease (PID)

Risk factor	Ectopic pregnancy	PID
Previous ectopic pregnancy	Yes	No
History of PID	Yes	Yes
Tubal surgery	Yes	No
Prior abdominal surgery or inflammatory condition (e.g., appendectomy or inflammatory bowel disease)	Yes	No
Endometriosis	Yes	No
Multiple sexual partners	Yes	Yes
Presence of IUD	Yes	Yes
Assisted fertility	Yes	No
IUD: intrauterine device.		

What is your sexual history?

Obtaining a good sexual history, including a history of sexually transmitted illnesses (STIs), birth control devices, and sexual partners is imperative. Keep in mind that a monogamous patient does not mean a monogamous partner.

Do you have any vaginal bleeding and/or discharge?

In the nonpregnant patient, bleeding may be associated with a number of conditions including dysmenorrhea, dysfunctional uterine bleeding or cancer (cervical or uterine). In the pregnant patient, think of the ectopic pregnancy first. Other etiologies include spontaneous miscarriage, threatened abortion or later complications of pregnancy, such as placenta previa or abruption. Vaginal discharge is associated with PID, cervicitis and vaginitis.

Associated symptoms

Fever, nausea, vomiting, syncope, or urinary complaints

Presence of a fever suggests an infectious cause of pain such as PID. Nausea or vomiting is more common with GI processes, but may also be seen in ureteral stones and ovarian torsion. Syncope should raise the suspicion for blood loss (e.g., ruptured ectopic pregnancy or hemorrhagic ovarian cyst), volume depletion, or sepsis (e.g., PID or perforated appendix). Dysuria or other urinary tract symptoms may point to a simple cystitis or STI; however, these symptoms may also result from irritation of the bladder as a consequence of free peritoneal fluid or an ectopic pregnancy.

Past medical

A medical history is imperative, and should detail any past pregnancies including associated problems. A history of abdominal or obstetric-gynecologic operations should be elicited. Systemic diseases also need to be reviewed. Recent procedures or surgeries raise concern for iatrogenic problems. The diabetic or immunocompromised patient may not be able to mount a normal response to an illness or infection. More liberal laboratory testing and imaging studies should be used in evaluating these patients than for patients with normal immune status.

Medications

Antibiotic (recent or current) or steroid use may influence the patient's presentation by masking infectious processes. Birth control pills do not preclude pregnancy, and many patients do not consider oral contraceptives as medications.

Social

Alcoholics are relatively immunocompromised, unreliable for follow-up, and may be coagulopathic. Smokers have an increased risk of cancer and vascular disease (e.g., mesenteric ischemia and aneurysms). Patients with drug addiction may be human immunodeficiency virus (HIV) positive, have lifestyles that put themselves at risk for STIs, and may be unreliable for follow-up.

Physical examination

General appearance

Begin your physical examination upon walking into the room. Always start by evaluating the Airway, Breathing and Circulation (ABCs). Again, if you deem the patient unstable, or are unsure, seek help immediately. If the patient can comfortably talk to you, then her airway and breathing are adequate. Feel the patient's pulse as you talk with her. Can you feel one? Is it thready? Is it fast? Does the patient look pale, pasty or diaphoretic? Is she mentating properly? These findings may suggest that she is in shock. Does she feel hot? If the oral temperature is normal, check a rectal temperature when you are concerned about a fever.

Vital signs

Attention to the patient's *vital* signs should be noted on initial evaluation of the patient. Significant tachycardia or hypotension in a patient with pelvic or abdominal pain, or vaginal bleeding should prompt aggressive measures, such as starting intravenous (IV) fluids immediately. Paradoxically, the patient may be bradycardic in the presence of intraperitoneal bleeding. When in doubt about the patient's stability, seek assistance immediately.

Abdomen

A detailed discussion of the abdominal examination is found in Chapter 9. Key aspects of the examination with respect to pelvic pain are described below.

Inspection

Is the abdomen distended or gravid-appearing? Any ecchymoses? Grey Turner's sign (flank ecchymoses) or Cullen's sign (periumbilical ecchymoses) may indicate retroperitoneal or intraperitoneal bleeding. Check for the presence of hernias. If the patient is pregnant, observe for fetal movement.

Auscultation

Listen for abdominal bruits, bowel sounds, or fetal heart tones if the patient is pregnant.

Palpation

Can the pain be localized to a specific area? You may be able to palpate masses (gravid uterus or distended bladder) or hernias. The patient may need to valsalva or cough to make a hernia apparent.

Pelvic

Male and female physicians are equally advised to have a chaperone present during the pelvic examination. Allow the patient to empty her bladder or remove a tampon prior to the examination. Position and drape the patient in such a manner that allows her to see you during the examination. Explain and describe to the patient each step of the examination and let her know what she may feel. Ask the patient to mention if the examination is different or more painful than previous pelvic examinations. Monitor the patient's reaction and behavior to the pelvic examination. Always be gentle and describe in advance what you are going to do.

Equipment

You should have good lighting, a vaginal speculum of appropriate size, water-soluble lubricant and materials for bacteriologic studies and wet mount prior to starting the examination.

External genitalia

Inspect the external genitalia for any evidence of inflammation, trauma, ulceration, discharge, swelling or nodules. A Bartholin cyst may present as a vulvar mass or swelling. A vesicular rash may represent genital herpes. Gently insert your finger into the patient's vagina and milk the urethra from the inside outward. Culture any discharge from the urethral orifice.

Speculum

Warming of a speculum under a stream of warm water helps avoid the shock and discomfort of a cold speculum. Lubricate the speculum prior to insertion. Begin by rotating the speculum obliquely, such that the handle hangs at about 4 or 8 o'clock, and then slowly and gently advance the speculum in a slightly posterior direction while rotating the speculum to allow the handle to hang straight down. Take care to avoid the more sensitive anterior vaginal wall and urethra. Open the blades gently, and note the cervix. If the cervix is not visible, try repositioning the speculum by slowly withdrawing it; often this maneuver allows the cervix to "drop" into view.

Note the appearance of the cervix. In pregnancy, the cervix may have a bluish hue (Chadwick's sign). The cervix and the cervical os should be inspected for blood, polyps, masses, inflammation, ulceration, signs of infection and the presence of an intrauterine device (IUD). The presence and description of any discharge in the cervix should be noted. Is it bloody, frothy, purulent or mucoid? Samples of any discharge or tissue should be sent for appropriate testing.

In the presence of bleeding and early pregnancy, assess the patency of the cervical os. Gently insert the ring forceps into the os. If the forceps can be inserted more than a centimeter or so, the internal os may be open, indicating an incomplete or inevitable miscarriage. If a patient in her third trimester presents with vaginal bleeding, do <u>not</u> attempt to assess if the cervical os is open. Severe hemorrhage may result if placenta previa is present.

Prior to and while slowly withdrawing the speculum, inspect the vagina for signs of infection, trauma, lesions or foreign bodies, as well as blood, tissue or discharge.

Bimanual

Next, perform a bimanual examination. Though the diagnostic accuracy of this examination has been questioned, every woman with pelvic pain should have a bimanual examination. Gently insert a lubricated middle and index finger into the patient's vagina. Palpate the anterior vaginal wall to differentiate bladder or urethral problems from gynecologic etiologies. Likewise, palpation of the posterior wall may identify rectal or sphincter pathology. With two fingers in the vaginal vault and one hand on the pubic region, palpate the uterus for size, tenderness or masses. Place the cervix between the two fingers in the vault, and gently move it side to side. Exquisite pain or discomfort from this maneuver is known as *cervical motion tenderness* (CMT), producing the "chandelier sign" (denoting the patient jumping off the table to grab the chandelier with movement of the cervix). Though CMT has classically been associated with PID, its presence is nonspecific and may represent irritation from an inflamed appendix, ruptured cyst or ectopic pregnancy. Importantly, CMT is also an insensitive finding, as it may be mild or absent in patients with PID.

Next, sweep the fingers to the adnexal regions. Start by examining the nontender side. With the external hand, pull the fingertips firmly but gently downward and feel for any adnexal masses and tenderness. Adnexal masses include ovarian cysts, tumors, or swollen fallopian tubes associated with PID or tubal pregnancy. In a patient with severe discomfort, adnexal palpation may be facilitated by the administration of an analgesic (e.g., morphine).

Lastly, a rectovaginal examination is performed with one digit in the vagina and one in the rectum. Sweep these fingers back and forth in a horizontal plane to feel for any masses, fullness or areas of discomfort. The rectovaginal examination allows for the evaluation of the posterior wall of the uterus, the posterior cul-de-sac (ovarian masses) and the ureterosacral ligaments (metastatic nodules or ectopic endometriosis).

Rectal

The rectal examination can reveal the presence of gross blood, nodularity or mass in the rectum. Ask the patient if the examination was painful or just uncomfortable.

Breast

Breast engorgement or tenderness may indicate pregnancy or a change related to menstrual cycle.

Lymph

Femoral and inguinal nodes should be evaluated for size and tenderness.

Differential diagnosis

Common gynecological sources of pelvic pain are shown in Figure 29.2 and described in Table 29.2. Non-gynecological sources are listed below.

Gastrointestinal etiologies

- Appendicitis
- Mesenteric ischemia
- Bowel obstruction
- Diverticulitis
- Inflammatory bowel
- Volvulus
- Cancer
- Constipation
- Gastroenteritis/enteritis
- Mesenteric adenitis

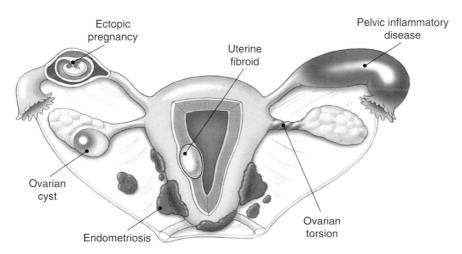

Figure 29.2
Common gynecologic sources of pelvic pain.

Table 29.2 Differential diagnosis of pelvic pain

Diagnoses	Symptoms	Signs	Work-up
Cancer Ovarian Uterine Cervical	Typically would not present with symptoms until late in course. Vague bloating/cramping. With or without abnormal bleeding. Dyspareunia.	Ascites. Pelvic mass.	Work-up to exclude other etiologies of pain. CT scan for staging. If ascites present, paracentesis for fluid analysis.
Degeneration of uterine fibroids	Acute, severe pain. Poorly localized. May have history of dysfunctional uterine bleeding/fibroids.	Large uterus on pelvic examination.	US or CT scan. IV hydration. Pain control.
Dysmenorrhea	Crampy pain around and during menses. Cyclical occurrence.	Stable. Nontender or nonspecific tenderness.	Test for pregnancy; otherwise, no other testing necessary.
Ectopic pregnancy	Pain and/or vaginal bleeding within 10–12 weeks gestation (though dates can be off and misleading). Pain lateralizes to one of the adnexal regions, but can be anywhere in the abdomen. May become lightheaded or weak with significant hemorrhage.	Normal vitals to significant tachycardia (may exhibit paradoxical bradycardia) and hypotension. Tenderness with or without mass in adnexal region. May have peritoneal signs and/or CMT.	Beta-HCG lower than expected for dates, but needed for interpretation of US. Transvaginal US shows complex adnexal mass and absence of IUP, unless heterotopic pregnancy. Recent research into progesterone as a marker of abnormal and normal pregnancy may change current practice. Immediate Ob/Gyn consultation.
Endometriosis	Cyclical pain that can occur anywhere in the abdomino-pelvic region. Worse around the time of menses. Dyspareunia.	Pain localized to the sites of endometriomas, which may be palpable on pelvic examination. Otherwise, may have a normal examination.	No specific testing. Clinical history and response to hormonal therapy may be diagnostic. Laparoscopy can be diagnostic and/or therapeutic.
Endometritis	Fever, significant pelvic pain, with or without discharge. Nausea and vomiting.	Tender uterus. May be enlarged. Foul-smelling, with or without bloody discharge.	History may include recent delivery, uterine manipulation/procedure (including IUD, D and C). Triple antibiotic therapy. Pain medication. Ob/Gyn consultation. May need D and C if retained products.
Labor	Cramping, intermittent pain, with or without rush of fluid (rupture of membranes).	Uterine contractions. Cervix examination shows dilation and effacement. Crowning. Noting fetal descent into canal.	Tocodynamometry shows regular contractions. Sterile pelvic examination. Vaginal fluid pH ~ 7; presence of *ferning*. Prepare for delivery. Follow fetal heart rate for evidence of distress. Transfer to labor and delivery if not imminently delivering.
Miscarriage/threatened abortion	Crampy pain. Vaginal bleeding. May be passing tissue.	Rarely associated with significant vital sign abnormalities. Uterine tenderness.	US varies from an IUP to no evidence of pregnancy, to blighted ovum. Check Rh status if bleeding present.

(continued)

Table 29.2 Differential diagnosis of pelvic pain (*cont*)

Diagnoses	Symptoms	Signs	Work-up
Mittelschmerz	Vague, aching pain 2 weeks before menses.	Stable. Tender on examination, lateralizing to one adnexal region.	Test for pregnancy; otherwise, no other testing necessary.
Ovarian cyst – ruptured	Sudden onset of severe pain. May have had pain prior to this related to cyst (see below). Lightheaded/syncope if severe and hemorrhage is present. Localizes to one side. Corpus luteal cysts rupture around 6–8 weeks from last menses.	Hemodynamically stable, unless severe hemorrhage. Tachycardic, but may be paradoxically bradycardic. Unilateral tenderness on pelvic examination, but may be confused by peritoneal signs. CMT.	IV fluids. Pain control. Type and screen/cross. Transabdominal US can assess for intra-abdominal fluid. Transvaginal US shows ruptured cyst.
Ovarian cyst – unruptured	Aching pain, typically cyclical with periods.	Hemodynamically stable, but may present with tachycardia due to pain. If palpable, examination will show ovarian fullness/mass.	US not necessary, unless to rule out other problems (e.g., torsion).
Ovarian torsion	"Classic" symptoms: acute (59%), crampy (44%), severe pain in lower quadrant (90%). Patient will find the position of most comfort. May have had several similar occurrences. Nausea and vomiting.	Stable vitals. Pelvic examination reveals unilateral tenderness. Mass may or may not be noted (47%).	High index of suspicion needed. Often missed as diagnosis. US shows an adnexa without blood flow. Often a mass (especially cyst) in the involved ovary, but presence of mass is not necessary. Doppler US to evaluate ovarian blood flow. Ob/Gyn consult for surgery to preserve ovary.
Pelvic congestion	Cyclical. About 7–10 days before menses. Worse with upright positioning. Often with musculoskeletal symptoms (e.g., back and leg pain).	Uterine tenderness.	No testing needed except to exclude other etiologies (e.g., PID). NSAIDs are treatment.
PID with or without tubo-ovarian abscess	Vaginal discharge, abdominal pain. Multiple sexual partners.	Fever. Hypotension may be present if septic. Discharge present. May have CMT.	IV fluids, cervical cultures, antibiotics and pain medication. US may be needed to assess for TOA. Ob/Gyn consult if TOA.
Placental abruption	Third-trimester pregnancy. Crampy pain, usually accompanied by bleeding. History of trauma, hypertension, cocaine use.	Vital signs may show cardiovascular collapse due to bleeding, but may be normal as well. Patient can exsanguinate into the uterus without any external evidence of bleeding (concealed hemorrhage). Enlarging abdomen. Evaluate for contractions and fetal distress. Petechiae or other evidence of DIC. Fetal heart rate may drop (indicating stress).	Hemoglobin may be normal to very low. As large amounts of bleeding consume up coagulation products, the picture of DIC develops (elevated INR, D-dimer and fibrin degradation products; low fibrinogen). US shows hemorrhage between placenta and uterine wall, but may be normal. Immediate Ob/Gyn consultation.
Round ligament pain	Mid-pregnancy, aching, nonspecific pain. May be unilateral or bilateral.	Stable vitals. No bleeding/discharge. Relatively unremarkable pelvic examination.	No work-up needed except to exclude other etiologies of pain.

(*continued*)

Table 29.2 Differential diagnosis of pelvic pain (*cont*)

Diagnoses	Symptoms	Signs	Work-up
Septic abortion	Fever. Severe pain.	Peritonitis. Foul smelling, bloody discharge.	US shows retained products. IV hydration through large bore catheter. Broad-spectrum antibiotics. Immediate Ob/Gyn consultation for D and C.
Septic thrombophlebitis	Pain and fever (if develops from infection). Lower extremity swelling/pain indicating DVT. Any symptoms that may indicate PE.	Fever. May have CMT/uterine tenderness. Peri-adnexal masses (abscesses) may present with fullness on examination.	History may suggest DVT, especially surgical or puerperal. Evidence of pelvic infection. CT scanning/ US may help define infections or thrombosis (contrast CT). MRI has been used to document pelvic DVT. Heparin. IV antibiotics.
Uterine fibroids	Intermittent pain that is cyclical. Associated with heavy bleeding.	Pelvic examination reveals a uterus that is enlarged.	US not necessary, but will reveal discrete masses within the uterine myometrium.
Uterine perforation	Abdomino-pelvic pain. Fever if infection present.	Peritonitis. Uterine/adnexal tenderness. Fever.	History of recent uterine procedure (e.g., D and C). Antibiotics for infection. CT or US for evaluation of abdomino-pelvic pathology. Ob/Gyn consultation.

Beta-HCG: beta-human chorionic gonadotropin; CMT: cervical motion tenderness; CT: computed tomography; D and C: dilation and curettage; DIC: disseminated intravascular coagulation; DVT: deep venous thrombosis; INR: international normalized ratio; IUD: intrauterine device; IUP: intrauterine pregnancy; IV: intravenous; NSAIDs: non-steroidal anti-inflammatory agents; Ob/Gyn: obstetrics/gynecology; PE: pulmonary embolism; PID: pelvic inflammatory disease; TOA: tubo-ovarian abscess; US: ultrasound.

- Colitis
- Hernias

Urinary tract etiologies

- Pyelonephritis
- Ureteral stone
- Cystitis
- Urethral syndrome

Toxic/metabolic etiologies

- Lead toxicity
- Acute porphyria
- Diabetic ketoacidosis

Vascular/other etiologies

- Aneurysm (aortic, iliac, femoral)
- Deep vein thrombosis (pelvic veins)
- Mesenteric vein thrombosis
- Sickle cell anemia

Diagnostic testing

Laboratory studies

Pregnancy test

This test should be ordered for any female patient of childbearing potential presenting with pelvic pain. The history of birth control use, tubal ligation and abstinence should not dissuade you from testing for pregnancy. Although infrequent, failure may occur with all forms of birth control. Quantitative beta-human chorionic gonadotropin (beta-HCG) testing may be helpful when the presence of a normal intrauterine pregnancy (IUP) is in question. In early pregnancy, the level of beta-HCG normally (approximately) doubles every 48 hours.

Progesterone level

Several studies have examined the use of a progesterone level to rule out ectopic pregnancy. One strategy involves using a two-tiered cutoff, with low levels (<5 ng/ml) associated with an abnormal pregnancy (but not specifically ectopic pregnancy); levels above 25 ng/ml indicate a normal IUP with a high degree of specificity (however, levels less than this can be found in normal pregnancies). This still leaves the gray area between these cutoffs, where there is insufficient sensitivity and specificity to differentiate normal from abnormal pregnancy. In such cases, a common strategy is to combine the beta-HCG level or US result with the progesterone level. Currently, there does not appear to be consistent agreement about the utility of progesterone levels in the ED, and they are not often readily available.

Urinalysis

Virtually all patients with pelvic pain should have a urinalysis, although further confirmatory testing should be guided by clinical suspicion. Hematuria has been noted in patients with several conditions, including AAA and kidney stones. Pyuria (presence of white cells) can be present in inflammatory conditions adjacent to the bladder or ureter (e.g., appendicitis), as well as in urinary tract infections.

Complete blood count

Though the white blood cell (WBC) count is often ordered, many studies have shown that this test has limited clinical utility. The value of the WBC count is not useful, except if it is extremely high or extremely low. The hemoglobin and hematocrit may be helpful in patients who are bleeding heavily or showing evidence of hemodynamic compromise. Take note, however, that these values may not reflect changes due to acute hemorrhage, and may not adequately reflect the patient's current circulating blood volume.

Electrolytes

Electrolytes will only occasionally aid the work-up of a patient with pelvic pain. Knowing the blood urea nitrogen (BUN) and creatinine may be helpful for diagnostic testing purposes (e.g., contrast-enhanced CT scan).

Cervical cultures

Cultures for *Gonorrhea* and *Chlamydia*, as well as a wet prep for *Trichomonas*, *Gardnerella vaginalis* and yeast should be obtained when suspecting PID or if the patient complains of a vaginal discharge.

Other

Some patients will require blood products, and anticipating this by ordering appropriate laboratories is helpful. *Type and crossmatch* of blood is needed in the patient exhibiting vital sign instability, whereas *type and screen* may be indicated for patients who are bleeding and may need blood on short notice. *Rh factor* should be ordered in all patients who are pregnant and bleeding. Some institutions require checking the Rh factor on all pregnant patients with vaginal bleeding even when the patient claims to know their Rh status or records are available with the patient's Rh status. This policy may reduce medical error in the rare instance of obtaining the wrong patient's record. Additionally, in some EDs, the misuse of someone else's identification card is not uncommon. DIC profiles should be ordered for the patient with suspected placental abruption. Protime and partial thromboplastin time should be ordered for patients with bleeding disorders, those taking anticoagulants, in cases of suspected DIC or the potential to develop DIC, or patients who are hemodynamically unstable.

Radiologic studies

Pelvic ultrasound

US can be very helpful in the work-up of pelvic pain. Transvaginal US is the test of choice to evaluate for IUP, ovarian lesions, ovarian torsion and TOA (Figure 29.3). Furthermore, it can provide information on the presence of pelvic fluid, uterine masses, or retained products of conception.

Of note, for first-trimester bleeding, the usefulness of US must be assessed in conjunction with the patient's clinical situation and laboratory values. Transvaginal US can typically detect the presence of an IUP at a beta-HCG level of approximately 1500 mIU/ml (around the 5th to 6th week by dates). This *discriminatory zone* varies by institution, and may lie between 1000 and 2000 mIU/ml. At levels above the discriminatory zone, a viable IUP should be visible by transvaginal US; if an IUP is not visualized, then it is likely a non-viable pregnancy, ectopic pregnancy or inevitable miscarriage. Although rare, an ectopic pregnancy may coexist with an IUP (*heterotopic pregnancy*), especially if the patient has undergone assisted fertilization. The incidence of heterotopic pregnancy is typically cited at 1 in 30,000. However, recent data suggest it may be 1 in 3000–7000, and much higher (1 in 100) if infertility medications or *in vitro* fertilization has been used. Clinical suspicion should

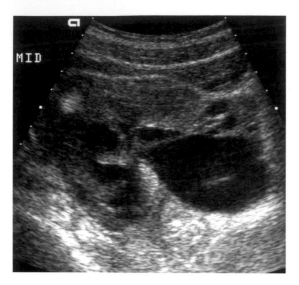

Figure 29.3
Tubo-ovarian abscess. Transverse sonogram reveals complex fluid collection posterior to uterus in the cul-de-sac. More discrete abscess located along left pelvic sidewall. *Courtesy*: R. Brooke Jeffrey, MD.

guide your work-up in these patients. At levels below the discriminatory zone, if an IUP is not seen on transvaginal US, then a normal pregnancy, threatened miscarriage or ectopic pregnancy is likely. Consult with the Ob/Gyn service if the clinical suspicion for an ectopic pregnancy is high. Otherwise, have the patient follow-up for a repeat beta-HCG in 48 hours. An explanation of indications for the patient to return immediately to the ED (e.g., syncope, heavy bleeding, fever, or severe pain) is important.

Computed tomography

CT is another modality for assessing the abdominal and pelvic structures. CT can identify ureteral stones, AAA, as well as areas of inflammation (e.g., pelvic abscesses or appendicitis). Some of the studies may require IV contrast, which may limit use in patients with renal failure or allergies to IV contrast dye. Oral and/or rectal contrast may be needed as well, and its ability to pass through the GI tract may affect the quality of the images.

Though the use of CT is increasing as a result of increasing availability and improved sensitivity and specificity, US is generally considered the imaging study of first choice in patients with pelvic pain. This is especially true in young or pregnant patients, because CT will expose the pelvis to significant amounts of radiation. US can delineate most of the true pelvic inflammatory

conditions, may demonstrate appendicitis, and can give information regarding blood flow to the ovaries if ovarian torsion is a concern.

General treatment principles

Stabilization

As with any patient, assessment and stabilization of airway, breathing and circulatory status are the first duties of the emergency physician. This may necessitate the need for intubation, IV fluids, or the use of blood products.

Intravenous access/fluids

Two large bore IVs should be placed in patients exhibiting hemodynamic compromise, or when there is a strong suspicion of significant hemorrhage or sepsis (e.g., ectopic pregnancy, endometritis). Patients unable to tolerate oral fluids and those who need to be kept NPO may benefit from IV fluids. Furthermore, patients who require multiple doses of parenteral medication, blood and blood products, or IV contrast require an IV.

Pain relief

Relieving pain is one of the primary responsibilities of emergency physicians. Often, narcotic analgesics are used to alleviate a patient's pain. Their administration does not interfere with making the diagnosis. Withholding pain medications is inhumane and this practice should be condemned.

Other medications such as non-steroidal anti-inflammatory drugs (NSAIDs) may help. NSAIDs help relieve prostaglandin-mediated pain, such as that created by smooth muscle contraction (e.g., uterine cramping). If the patient is unable to tolerate fluids, or needs to be NPO, then ketorolac may be useful. Studies do not show a faster or stronger effect from ketorolac via intramuscular (IM) injection versus ibuprofen; however, this has not been examined when ketorolac is given IV.

Antibiotics

The diagnosis, patient condition and other patient-related issues guide antibiotic coverage and routes of administration as well as the decision for inpatient versus outpatient treatment. Factors that influence the specific therapy chosen include the patient's condition, comorbid conditions, likelihood of patient compliance, local resistance patterns, pregnancy status, patient age and medication allergies.

Antibiotic selection for treating STIs should cover *N. gonorrhoeae* and *C. trachomatis*. For simple cervicitis, one time oral regimens are available and often given in the ED. PID can be managed as an outpatient if the patient's pain can be controlled, peritoneal signs are absent, adequate follow-up is ensured, and the patient can tolerate oral medications. Otherwise, parenteral antibiotics and admission are indicated. Unlike a simple cervicitis, PID appears to be a polymicrobial disease. Organisms other than *N. gonorrhoeae* and *C. trachomatis* may cause PID, including streptococci, Gram-negative organisms, anaerobes and *Trichomonas*. A choice of broad-spectrum antibiotics or combination of antibiotics such as a third-generation cephalosporin plus doxycycline, or

Table 29.3 Antibiotic selection for pelvic infections

Diagnosis	Pathogen	Antibiotic
Bacterial vaginosis	*G. vaginalis* Generally a disruption of normal vaginal flora	Metronidazole 500 mg PO BID × 7 days *or* Metronidazole gel 0.75%, 1 applicator intravaginally qD × 5 days *or* Metronidazole 2 g PO × 1 dose *or* Clindamycin cream 2%, 1 applicator (5 gm) intravaginally qHS × 7 days *or* Clindamycin 300 mg PO BID × 7 days *or* Clindamycin ovules 100 mg intravaginally qHS × 3 days *In pregnancy* Metronidazole 250 mg PO TID × 7 days *or* Clindamycin 300 mg PO BID × 7 days
Mucopurulent cervicitis	*N. gonorrhea /C. trachomatis*	Cefixime 400 mg PO × 1 dose *or* Ceftriaxone 125 mg IM × 1 dose *or* Levofloxacin 250 mg PO × 1 dose *or* Spectinomycin 2 gm IM × 1 dose *Plus* Azithromycin 1 gm PO × 1 dose *or* Doxycyline 100 mg PO BID × 7 days *or* Ofloxacin 300 mg PO BID × 7 days *or* Levofloxacin 500 mg PO qD × 7 days *or* Erythromycin base 500 mg PO QID × 7 days *or* Amoxicillin 500 mg PO TID × 7 days
Pelvic inflammatory disease (Oral regimen)	*N. gonorrhea /C. trachomatis, M. hominis,* anaerobes, *Enterbacteriaceae*	Ofloxacin 400 mg PO BID × 14 days *or* Levofloxacin 500 mg PO qD × 14 days *or* Ceftriaxone 250 mg IM × 1 dose *or* Cefoxitin 2 gm IM × 1 dose + Probenecid 1 gm PO × 1 *Plus/minus* Metronidazole 500 mg BID × 14 days
Pelvic inflammatory disease (Parenteral regimen)	*N. gonorrhea /C. trachomatis, M. hominis,* anaerobes, *Enterbacteriaceae*	Cefotetan 2 gm IV q12 hours *or* Cefoxitin 2 gm IV q12 hours *Plus* Doxycycline 100 mg PO/IV q12 hours *or* Clindamycin 900 mg IV q8 hours *Plus* Gentamicin 2 mg/kg load IV then 1.5 mg/kg q8 hours IV
Trichomoniasis	*T. vaginalis*	Metronidazole 2 gm PO × 1 dose *or* Metronidazole 500 mg PO BID × 7 days *In pregnancy* (treat only if symptomatic) Metronidazole 2 gm PO × 1 dose

BID: twice a day; *C. trachomatis*: *Chlamydia trachomatis*; *G. vaginalis*: *Gardnerella vaginalis*; IM: intramuscular; IV: intravenous; *M. hominis*: *Mycoplasma hominis*; *N. gonorrhoeae*: *Neisseria gonorrhoeae*; PO: per os; qD: once daily; qHS: every night at bedtime; QID: four times a day; TID: three times a day; *T. vaginalis*: *Trichomonas vaginalis*.

fluoroquinolone (not ciprofloxacin) plus metronidazole is appropriate. Inpatient, parenteral therapy is indicated if the patient is immunocompromised, pregnant or has failed outpatient therapy (Table 29.3).

Other pelvic infections, such as endometritis, require broad coverage of Gram-negative, Gram-positive and anaerobic organisms. Broad-spectrum antibiotics include regimens such as a synthetic penicillin/beta-lactamase inhibitor (e.g., ticarcillin/clavulanate) plus doxycycline, or clindamycin plus a third-generation cephalosporin.

Blood products

A blood transfusion is indicated in the patient who is hemodynamically unstable from hemorrhage and unresponsive to crystalloid boluses. A type and screen or crossmatch should be sent for those patients who are resuscitated, or whom you suspect may become unstable. Fresh frozen plasma (FFP) is given if the patient develops DIC. DIC can develop in septic patients and those with severe hemorrhage from placental abruption. FFP may be needed for patients on warfarin (coumadin). Platelets may be needed for thrombocytopenic states such as idiopathic thrombocytopenic purpura (ITP).

Rh immune globulin (Rho-GAM)

Rho-GAM is indicated for the Rh-negative pregnant patient who presents with vaginal bleeding, suspected or proven placental abruption, and trauma with the potential for fetal–maternal transfusion or proven fetal–maternal transfusion (by *Kleihauer–Betke* testing). Dosing is based on gestational age. Low dose Rho-GAM (MicRho- GAM) is given for miscarriages, abortion or ectopic pregnancy termination to Rh-negative mothers when between 0 and 12 weeks gestational age. This dose is 50 mcg. Beyond 12 weeks and for threatened miscarriage at any gestational age, full dose Rho-GAM (300 mcg) is given. In the situation of fetal–maternal hemorrhage, 300 mcg is given for every 15 ml of fetal red blood cells (or 30 ml of fetal whole blood) that the mother has been exposed to based on Kleihauer–Betke testing.

Medications

Other than analgesics and antibiotics, other medications may be needed to treat the patient. Antiemetics are useful for intractable or problematic nausea and vomiting. Methotrexate can be used in selective patients for the treatment of ectopic pregnancy. Misoprostol has been used in patients with incomplete or inevitable miscarriages.

Special patients
Pediatric

The physician must be diligent to search for a cause of pelvic pain in the young patient. Due to social, cultural and parenteral pressures, these patients and their parents may be scared or embarrassed to answer questions about their sexuality and genitalia, much less undergo a pelvic examination. Any child that is perimenarchal should be assumed pregnant until proven otherwise.

Prepubertal children are most likely to present with pelvic pain secondary to vaginal foreign body, urinary tract infection or sexual abuse. A pelvic examination is still indicated in these patients to assess for evidence of abuse. A modified approach can be used, but a full pelvic examination may be required under conscious sedation or general anesthesia. Proper collection of samples and precise documentation are required for evidence if a criminal case is suspected. Most local police departments have developed a sexual assault kit for these purposes. Child protective services should be consulted in cases of suspected or proven abuse or STI.

All states allow minors to consent to evaluation and treatment of STIs and drug abuse without parental consent. There is also the legal status of the *emancipated minor* and the *mature minor*, which varies from state to state. These statutes allow minors certain rights, including seeking and consenting to medical care without the authorization and notification of their parents. Keep in mind that any emergent care deemed necessary should supercede any parental rights.

Geriatric

The older patient may not be willing or able to communicate her problems. Nursing home workers, paramedics and family, as well as the patient's medical chart may be extremely useful, particularly if they provide information on any associated signs or symptoms. In general, the older patient is relatively immunocompromised and is more likely to have other comorbid problems that can affect the presentation and the work-up. Older patients with pelvic pain need a complete gynecologic examination. Often, the geriatric patient will not present with the "classic" symptoms of an acute inflammatory process such as appendicitis or diverticulitis. They may not develop a fever, mount an increased WBC count, or have peritoneal signs. As a result, the morbidity and mortality of abdomino-pelvic complaints in the elderly patient is significant.

The physiologic drop in estrogen levels with age can cause vaginal irritation and thinning of the mucosa. On the other hand, unopposed estrogen levels secondary to decreased progesterone can lead to endometrial hyperplasia and possibly endometrial cancer. Uterine prolapse is common, as are cystoceles, rectoceles and urethroceles. Furthermore, the normal ovary should not be palpable 5 years after menopause; any enlargement is abnormal and mandates further investigation.

Chemically dependant or impaired

Patients who are intoxicated can present with pain that may be overlooked. Their ability to relate a coherent history may likewise present problems for the clinician. Despite these issues, such patients may be at higher risk to develop certain diseases (e.g., STIs, ectopic pregnancy) and at the same time are less likely to be able to schedule a follow-up appointment, purchase or take their medications, or return if the problem worsens.

Assisted reproductive therapy

Today, more patients are undergoing some form of assisted reproductive therapy (ART). This has raised the incidence of *ovarian hyperstimulation syndrome* (OHSS), as well as the presence of multiple gestations. OHSS can be mild to severe. In its mild form, patients may feel some distension and pain; when it becomes severe, the patient may present with extremely large ovaries (over 10 cm) and large amounts of free fluid in the abdomen. Electrolyte abnormalities, hypotension, pleural effusions and oliguria may ensue.

The use of ART has increased the prevalence of multiple gestation pregnancies. Along with the rise in multiple gestations, the risk for *heterotopic pregnancy* has increased as well. The presence of an ectopic pregnancy should be considered even if an IUP is present by US.

Other

Patients who are unable to communicate clearly (e.g., language barrier or mentally handicapped)

deserve a thorough and sensitive investigation. Even a mentally-challenged patient can contract STIs and develop ectopic pregnancies. The non-English speaking patient may also be more of a challenge due to cultural issues or anatomic problems (e.g., female circumcision).

Disposition

Obstetric/gynecologic consultation

Ob/Gyn should be consulted for all ectopic pregnancies. If a definitive IUP is not identified and the possibility of an ectopic pregnancy exists, consultation should also occur; definitive follow-up should be arranged for a repeat evaluation and beta-HCG determination. Other cases requiring consultation include ovarian torsion, TOA, ruptured ovarian cyst with hemodynamic compromise, placental abruption, placenta previa (these patients typically do not have pain) and active labor. All of these patients generally require admission. Patients also require admission for other significant pelvic infections, uncontrolled pain and inability to tolerate fluids or oral medications.

Ob/Gyn should be contacted for a patient with problematic ovarian cysts, follow-up of pelvic infections, any complications of pelvic procedures, and ongoing/threatened miscarriage. The patient may not need to be seen immediately, but input from the Ob/Gyn consultant should be obtained and follow-up arranged.

Admission

Admission is the general rule for acute life- or fertility-threatening diseases. The patient who is at risk for failing outpatient therapy due to noncompliance, chemical dependency, social situations, comorbid diseases or associated conditions (e.g., vomiting) should be deemed a candidate for inpatient treatment.

Discharge

Many patients may be managed on an outpatient basis with close Ob/Gyn follow-up and strict instructions to return for appropriate indications. Returning to the ED is a viable alternative if unable to follow-up in Ob/Gyn clinic. The alternative of losing a patient to follow-up with a resultant adverse outcome is unacceptable. For example, outpatient medical treatment of selected ectopic pregnancies with methotrexate is possible if the patient is hemodynamically stable, has adequate pain control, tolerates fluids by mouth, is reliable, and can follow-up appropriately. This patient should return to the ED if she develops intractable nausea, severe pain, fever, severe weakness, lightheadedness, or has syncope.

Pearls, pitfalls, and myths

- All women of childbearing age should be considered pregnant until proven otherwise.
- Do not rely on the patient's beta-HCG to decide whether to order a pelvic US when considering ectopic pregnancy. Ectopic pregnancies produce beta-HCG at an abnormal rate. A beta-HCG level above the discriminatory zone only helps to determine if a viable IUP should be visible on transvaginal US. Therefore, use the beta-HCG to assist with interpretation of the pelvic US.
- Heterotopic pregnancy has a reported incidence as low as 1:100 in patients undergoing ART. Therefore, it must be considered even with confirmed IUPs. Patients not undergoing ART still have a possibility of heterotopic pregnancy, although the likelihood is much lower. Clinical suspicion should guide the work-up.
- Empirically treat suspected PID and STIs before laboratory results return. These often will not be back before the patient's disposition from the ED, and major life- or fertility-threatening sequelae may occur (e.g., abscess, sepsis, infertility). Many patients at greatest risk of developing these diseases are of limited financial resources, suffer from substance abuse, or have other problems limiting their access to care and follow-up.
- Several diagnoses can be missed without full consideration of other diagnostic possibilities (e.g., ovarian torsion). An ovarian cyst or mass may predispose a patient to ovarian torsion. These may not be appreciated on pelvic examination despite their presence. In fact, some question the diagnostic value of the pelvic examination, especially in the obese patient.
- Consider sexual/physical abuse in patients, especially if they present with nonspecific complaints or inconsistent findings. Often, the only way to uncover this history is to directly ask the patient in a private setting. Therefore, it is prudent to ask any friends, spouses, boyfriends, girlfriends or family members to leave the room when obtaining this history.
- Consider non-pelvic etiologies for a patient's pelvic pain. Furthermore, pain may be the result of some catastrophic conditions, which must be considered and aggressively managed if present.

References

1. Bates B, Bickley LS, Hoekelman RA. Female genitalia. In: *A Guide to Physical Examination and History Taking*, 6th ed., Philadelphia, PA: J. B. Lippincott Company, 1995. pp. 377–400.
2. Behrman AJ, Shepherd SM. Pelvic inflammatory disease. In: Tintinalli JE, et al. (eds). *Emergency Medicine: A Comprehensive Study Guide*, 5th ed., New York, NY: McGraw-Hill, 2000. pp. 719–723.
3. Dart R. Acute pelvic pain. In: Marx JA, Hockberger RS, Walls RM, et al. (eds). *Rosen's Emergency Medicine*, 5th ed., St Louis, MO: Mosby, 2002. pp. 219–226.
4. Dart R, Ramanujam P, Dart L. Progesterone as a predictor of ectopic pregnancy when the ultrasound is indeterminate. *Am J Emerg Med* 2002;20(7):575–579.
5. Houry D, Abbott JT. Ovarian torsion: a fifteen-year review. *Ann Emerg Med* 2001;38:156–159.
6. Krause RS, Janicke DM. Ectopic pregnancy. In: Tintinalli JE, et al. (eds). *Emergency Medicine: A Comprehensive Study Guide*, 5th ed., New York, NY: McGraw-Hill, 2000. pp. 686–693.
7. Kuhn GJ. Emergencies during pregnancy and the postpartum period. In: Tintinalli JE, et al. (eds). *Emergency Medicine: A Comprehensive Study Guide*, 5th ed., New York, NY: McGraw-Hill, 2000. pp. 694–702.
8. Lipscomb GH, Stovall TG, Ling FW. Nonsurgical treatment of ectopic pregnancy. *New Engl J Med* 2000;343:1325–1329.
9. Maradiegue A. Minor's rights versus parental rights: review of legal issues in adolescent health care. *J Midwifery Womens Health* 2003;48(3):170–177.
10. Moellman JJ, Bocock JM. Acute pelvic pain. In: Hamilton G, et al. (eds). *Emergency Medicine: An Approach to Clinical Problem-Solving*, 2nd ed., Philadelphia, PA: W.B. Saunders, 2003. pp. 659–676.

11. Morrison L, Spence J. Vaginal bleeding and pelvic pain in the nonpregnant patient. In: Tintinalli JE, et al. (eds). *Emergency Medicine: A Comprehensive Study Guide*, 5th ed., New York, NY: McGraw-Hill, 2000. pp. 669–680.

12. Rapkin AJ. Pelvic pain and dysmenorrhea. In: Berek JS, Adashi EY, Hillard PA (eds). *Novak's Gynecology*, 12th ed., Baltimore, MD: Williams & Wilkins, 1996. pp. 399–428.

13. Reardon RF, Jehle DVK. Pelvic ultrasonography. In: Tintinalli JE, et al. (eds). *Emergency Medicine: A Comprehensive Study Guide*, 5th ed., New York, NY: McGraw-Hill, 2000. pp. 737–748.

14. Ringo PM, Gynecologic causes of abdominal pain. In: Harwood-Nuss AL, et al. (eds). *The Clinical Practice of Emergency Medicine*, 3rd ed., Philadelphia, PA: Lippinicott, Williams & Wilkins, 2001, pp. 379–383.

15. The CDC 2002. Guidelines for the treatment of sexually transmitted diseases: implications for women's health care. *J Midwifery Women Health* 2003; 48(2):96–104.

30 Rash

Jamie Collings, MD and Brigham Temple, MD

Scope of the problem

The skin is the body's most visible organ system and its main protection against the environment. It is not surprising that skin complaints account for 4–10% of all emergency department visits annually in the US. Skin disease can represent a wide array of disease processes, from a local dermatologic disease to the manifestation of an underlying systemic illness. The majority of rashes that present to the emergency department (ED) involve infections, irritants, and allergies.

While most of these rashes are benign and self-limited, cutaneous lesions are often the first clinical sign of serious systemic disease. Dermatologic findings can be associated with serious infectious diseases including meningococcemia, gonococcemia, cellulitis, toxic shock syndrome, staphylococcal scalded skin syndrome, disseminated herpetic infections, and Rocky Mountain spotted fever. Other potentially life-threatening skin diseases (Stevens–Johnson syndrome (SJS), toxic epidermal necrolysis (TEN), and urticaria with anaphylaxis) can result from medications. Carcinomas and other inflammatory skin diseases (pustular psoriasis, pemphigus, pemphigoid, and lupus) also have the potential to be life-threatening (Table 30.1).

Table 30.1 Life-threatening dermatoses

Behcet's syndrome
Brown recluse spider bite
Bullous pemphigoid
Cutaneous T-cell lymphoma
Disseminated gonococcemia
Disseminated herpes or zoster
Generalized exfoliative erythroderma
Hematologic disorders
Kaposi sarcoma
Kawasaki disease
Malignant melanoma
Meningococcemia
Pemphigus vulgaris
Pustular psoriasis
Rocky Mountain spotted fever
Staphylococcal scalded skin syndrome
Stevens–Johnson syndrome
Systemic lupus erythematosus
Toxic epidermal necrolysis
Toxic shock syndrome
Urticaria with anaphylaxis

Anatomic essentials

The skin is divided into three layers. The outer layer is the *epidermis*, which serves as the outer most protective barrier against the environment. Underneath the epidermis, the vascularized *dermis* provides support and nutrition for the cells in the epidermis. Other important skin structures are also found in the dermal layer, including nerves, sweat glands, hair follicles, and sebaceous glands. The inner most layer is the *subcutaneous tissue*.

History

A complete history of the eruption is essential and should include the duration, rate of onset, and location of the current eruption. Symptoms including pruritus, pain, and fever should be noted.

When did the rash begin?

Sudden onset of a rash is more concerning than a rash that has been present for days. Sudden onset of rash while eating shellfish most likely represents an allergic reaction, which may signal the beginning of anaphylaxis. A rash that develops after three days of fever in a 12-month-old child is likely roseola infantum, a benign condition which resolves spontaneously.

Where on your body did you first notice the rash, and did it spread?

Identifying the location the rash first appeared helps further differentiate its etiology. Rashes that present on the scalp and then erupt on the elbows may represent psoriasis. Rocky Mountain spotted fever starts on the wrists and ankles, then spreads to the trunk.

Have you had this rash before?

Rashes that are recurrent are more likely to represent an underlying dermatitis or non-infectious systemic illness, such as a recurring rash on the face from seborrheic dermatitis.

Did you have a fever or recent fever?

In both children and adults, fever associated with rash often signifies the presence of an infection.

For example, a young child with fever and sore throat that presents with a diffuse, red, sandpaper-like rash on the trunk, back, and extremities is likely to have scarlet fever. Fever with sudden onset of a petechial rash in a college student is meningococcemia until proven otherwise.

Does the rash itch?

Rashes that itch indicate an inflammatory reaction in the skin with histamine release. Pruritus represents an intradermal inflammatory response that can be from a local exposure to an irritant or a systemic reaction, such as an allergic reaction to shellfish. The patient who presents with pruritus and linear eruptions on his hands or legs after a recent hiking trip likely has contact dermatitis from poison ivy exposure. Intense pruritis is often associated with scabies or urticaria.

Is the rash painful?

A history that the rash is associated with pain may be significant. With herpes zoster, pain often precedes the rash. In patients with necrotizing fasciitis, the pain may be out of proportion to physical examination findings.

Did you use any new soaps, perfumes, lotions, or detergents?

Many commercially-sold products contain chemicals that can produce a local inflammatory reaction. The patient who presents with a new rash on their trunk and arms after changing laundry detergent brands likely has contact dermatitis. Many lotions for dry skin contain alcohol, which may exacerbate eczema or contact dermatitis.

Did you use any medications for the rash?

There are many over-the-counter medications available to the public, from antihistamines to topical steroid ointments. Use of such medications prior to seeking medical attention may indicate a partially- or under-treated medical condition. Furthermore, some of these therapies may exacerbate instead of alleviate the rash, such as topical steroid use on a cutaneous fungal infection.

What medications do you take regularly? Any new medications?

Rashes associated with medications can range from mild allergic eruptions to anaphylaxis or other life-threatening systemic complications. Therefore, a complete history of past and current medications, dosages, duration of therapy, and prior history of allergic or adverse reactions to these medications must be elicited. Recent immunizations may account for an allergic eruption or exanthem. It is also essential to review patient use of over-the-counter medications, herbals, dietary supplements, and vitamins.

Do you have any known environmental allergies or exposures?

Home or work exposure to chemicals that may be irritants may cause a contact dermatitis. Exposure to animal dander, insects bites, and plants may represent allergic contact dermatitis. A history of recent sun exposure may represent sunburn, atopic dermatitis, or an allergic reaction.

Associated symptoms

Respiratory

Ask about nasal discharge, sore throat, shortness of breath, and cough. Viral infections often present with upper respiratory symptoms and help signal an infectious etiology of the rash. Children are more likely to have viral exanthems, such as hand–foot–mouth disease and measles. Adult viral infections such as influenza and adenovirus are rarely associated with rashes. Bacterial sources, such as *Streptococcus*, should also be considered. Wheezing and shortness of breath are often associated with urticaria.

Gastrointestinal

Ask about abdominal pain, nausea, vomiting, and diarrhea. Gastrointestinal (GI) symptoms are present in 90% of patients with Henoch–Schonlein purpura. Other viral etiologies may also have GI symptoms.

Neurologic

Ask about altered mental status, headache, seizures, and other neurologic symptoms. Meningitis may first present with fever and rash; encephalitis is associated with herpes and varicella viruses.

Genitourinary

Ask about pregnancy, sexual history, and any prior GU lesions. Syphilis may not be recognized until the secondary stages, when a rash is involved. Many etiologies of rash have few side effects on the typical patient, but can be devastating to an unborn fetus or immune compromised individual.

Past medical

A history of previous and recurrent eruptions along with other systemic disease (e.g., diabetes, systemic lupus erythematosus (SLE), and cancer) is helpful in order to identify the cause of the rash. Environmental and chemical exposures should be considered by reviewing the patient's occupational history and hobbies.

Family

Family history of rashes and certain systemic illnesses, such as SLE, should be considered. Allergies to medications and foods in family members should be identified, and may be helpful.

Physical examination

Although the history may help narrow the differential diagnosis, the ability to identify, interpret, and describe what is observed is more important. Rashes are classified using specific nomenclature (Tables 30.2 and 30.3).

Further descriptors for shape are used, including serpiginous, arcuate, annular, discoid, target, dermatomal, and confluent.

Physical examination of patients with a rash should be performed from head-to-toe with the patient completely disrobed in a well-lit examination room. The practitioner should allow plenty of time for a thorough physical examination of the skin.

General appearance

The general appearance of the patient will often suggest the severity of underlying disease causing the rash in question. Patients who have viral exanthems may be well-appearing or sick-appearing depending on the severity of infection. Patients with serious bacterial infections are likely to appear ill. Patients with urticarial rash associated with anaphylaxis will exhibit signs of respiratory distress or anxiety if the oropharynx or respiratory tract is involved. Severely pruritic rashes often cause patients to feel restless and agitated. For the most part, however, the majority of patients presenting with rash appear well, although uncomfortable.

Table 30.2 Primary skin lesions

Term	Definition
Macule	Flat, non-palpable discoloration, <1 cm in size. May be brown, blue, red, or hypopigmented
Patch	Flat non-palpable discoloration, >1 cm in size
Papule	Solid, raised, palpable lesion up to 0.5 cm diameter, may become confluent (plaque)
Plaque	Circumscribed, elevated, superficial, solid lesion, >0.5 cm in diameter
Nodule	Circumscribed, rounded, raised, palpable lesion, >0.5 cm in diameter. A large nodule is a tumor
Vesicle	Well-circumscribed, raised, and fluid-filled lesion, <0.5 cm in size
Bulla	Well-circumscribed, fluid-filled, raised lesion, >0.5 cm in diameter
Wheal (hive)	Firm, edematous, transient plaque resulting from infiltration of the dermis with fluid

Table 30.3 Secondary and other skin lesions

Term	Definition
Scales	Excess dead epidermal cells that are produced by abnormal keratinization and shedding
Crust	Collection of dried serum and cellular debris (scab)
Erosion	Focal loss of epidermis that does not penetrate the dermis (no scar)
Ulcer	Focal loss of epidermis and dermis (scar)
Excoriation	Erosion caused by scratching (often linear)
Lichenification	Area of thickened epidermis induced by scratching; surface looks like a washboard
Petechiae	Round, pinpoint, flat purplish spots secondary to intradermal or subdermal hemorrhage, <0.5 cm diameter
Purpura	Blue or purple in color; secondary to hemorrhage in the skin, >0.5 cm diameter

Vital signs

Fever is often used as a marker for infection and may indicate a viral or bacterial cause for the rash. Conversely, the afebrile patient may still have a rash secondary to an infectious cause. Patients with petechial or purpural lesions, and signs of sepsis (tachycardia and hypotension) are presumed to have a bacterial infection with bacteremia and should be aggressively resuscitated.

Other vital signs may be helpful in diagnosing an infectious systemic process or an acute allergic reaction with anaphylaxis. However, most infectious causes of rash do not affect the heart rate, blood pressure, or respiratory rate, unless accompanied by severe dehydration, sepsis, or airway compromise.

Head and neck

Inspection of the head and neck should focus on identifying signs of infection. The scalp and mucosa should be inspected for rash or lesions. Erythema or lesions may indicate a systemic viral infection, such as Koplik's spots in the buccal mucosa which occur with measles infection. Examine the soft palate for petechiae, which may indicate an underlying streptococcal infection. When an allergic reaction is suspected, look for soft palate and uvular edema. Examine the neck for signs of infection, including reactive lymph nodes, swollen glands, and nuchal rigidity. Auscultate the neck for stridor if an allergic reaction is suspected.

Genital

Rashes in the groin and on the genitalia necessitate a thorough examination. A pelvic examination may be indicated if disseminated gonococcal infection is possible, or staphylococcal toxic shock syndrome secondary to a retained foreign body (i.e., tampon) in the vaginal canal is suspected. Tests for sexually transmitted infections (STIs) like syphilis (Figure 30.1) and gonorrhea should be performed.

Skin

The skin should be examined in a systematic and orderly process noting the distribution, pattern, arrangement, and morphology of the rash. Many rashes have a predilection for certain areas of the body, so the patient should have a thorough examination.

The pattern of the rash should be noted. A rash only on skin exposed to the environment or a particular object points to reactions associated with

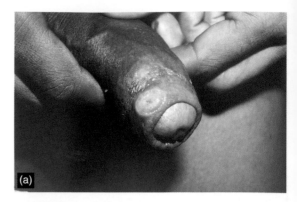
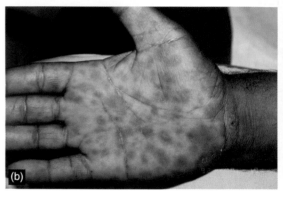

Figure 30.1
(a) Chancre of primary syphilis: round to oval indurated plaques eroded not ulcerated. (b) Secondary syphilis: macular erythematous to brown lesions nonconfluent. *Courtesy*: Steven Shpall, MD.

sun exposure, jewelry (nickel), or lotions. Pityriasis rosea is typically localized to the trunk and proximal extremities (Figure 30.2). The lesions of hand–foot–mouth disease are located where the name implies. Erythema nodosum and Henoch–Schonlein purpura (Figure 30.3) have a predilection for the lower extremities.

Lesion arrangement, which refers to both the symmetry and configuration, should be noted. Rashes that are bilaterally symmetric often signify systemic disease or uniform external exposure. Configuration refers to the relationship between multiple lesions, such as the linear pattern in a poison ivy exposure and the Christmas-tree distribution of pityriasis rosea (Figure 30.2).

Recognition of the primary lesion is vital in establishing the diagnosis. The primary lesion can be altered by secondary issues, including excoriation, healing, or complications of infection. Once the primary lesion is noted and its morphology determined, the differential diagnosis of the most likely causes can be made (Table 30.4).

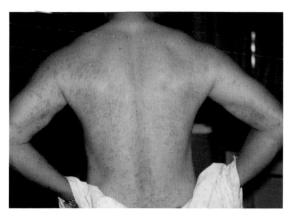

Figure 30.2
Pityriasis rosea. Round to oval spots with an inner collarette of scale (scale inside the lesion, not at its edge) distributed along skin lines. *Courtesy:* Steven Shpall, MD.

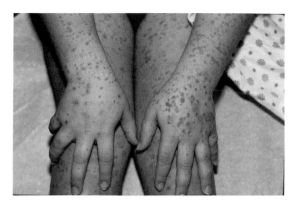

Figure 30.3
Henoch-Schonlein purpura. Palpable purpura with small hemorrhagic (purple) macules and papules, usually on the extensor surface of the extremities. *Courtesy:* Steven Shpall, MD.

Table 30.4 Differential diagnosis of primary and secondary lesions

Morphology	Differential considerations
Bullae	Bullous impetigo, bullous pemphigoid, pemphigus vulgaris, toxic epidermal necrolysis, thermal burn, toxicodendron dermatitis
Crusts	Eczema, tineas, impetigo, contact dermatitis, insect bite
Erosions	Candidiasis, tineas, eczema, toxic epidermal necrolysis, toxic-infectious erythemas, erythema multiforme, primary blistering diseases (bullous pemphigoid, pemphigus vulgaris), brown recluse spider bite
Macules	Drug eruption, rheumatic fever, erythema multiforme, cellulitis, lice infestation, secondary syphilis, viral exanthems, early meningococcemia
Nodules	Basal cell carcinoma, melanoma, lipoma, warts
Papules	Atopic dermatitis, acne, folliculitis, psoriasis, eczema, urticaria, toxicodendron dermatitis (poison ivy, oak, or sumac), insect bites
Petechiae	Gonococcemia, leukocytoclastic vasculitis, meningococcemia
Plaques	Eczema, pityriasis rosea, tinea corporis and versicolor, psoriasis, urticaria, erythema multiforme
Purpura	Platelet abnormalities, Rocky Mountain spotted fever, scurvy, senile purpura
Pustules	Folliculitis, acne, gonococcemia, herpetic infections, impetigo, psoriasis
Scales	Psoriasis, pityriasis rosea, toxic-infectious erythemas, secondary syphilis, tineas
Ulcers	Aphthous lesions, chancroid, decubitus, thermal injury, subacute/chronic ischemia, malignancy, chancre, primary blistering disorders, pyoderma gangrenosum, stasis
Vesicles	Herpetic infections, toxic epidermal necrolysis, toxicodendron dermatitis, thermal burn, bullous pemphigoid, pemphigus vulgaris
Wheals	Angioedema, hives, urticaria, erythema multiforme

Differential diagnosis

Tables 30.5, 30.6, 30.7, 30.8 and 30.9 describe the differential diagnosis of various causes of rash.

Table 30.5 Differential diagnosis of viral etiologies of rash

Diagnosis	Epidemiology	Symptoms/signs of rash	Work-up/treatment
Erythema infectiosum or Fifth disease	• Childhood rash, primarily age 5–14 years • 50% of adults have serologic evidence of past infection • Caused by parvovirus B19	• Characterized by erythematous plaques on cheeks • *Slapped cheek appearance* • Asymptomatic infection is common, but severe complications can be seen in pregnant, anemic, or immunocompromised patients • Women (not men) can have acute polyarthropathy that can last 2 weeks to 4 years	• Diagnosis is made clinically • Laboratories not indicated • Treatment usually only supportive care
Hand–foot–mouth disease	• Largely a disease of childhood • Caused by coxsackie B virus	• Characterized by ulcerative oral lesions, primarily on soft palate, and rash on palms and soles of feet • Rash is macular and quickly has pustular eruptions which crust over	• Diagnosis is made clinically • Laboratories not indicated • Treatment usually only supportive care
Herpes simplex virus eruption	• Two most common serotypes 1 and 2 • Most common in children and young adults	• Grouped vesicles on an erythematous base • On keratinized skin and mucous membranes • Usually on cheeks, lips, mouth, fingers, and genitalia	• Tzanck smear if diagnosis in question • Viral cultures • HSV antibody serologies • Acyclovir used for both treatment and prevention of eruptions • Prednisone may decrease acute pain, but increases complications
Herpes zoster (Shingles) (Figure 30.4)	• Nearly 100% of US adults are seropositive for anti-VZV antibodies by third decade of life • Two-thirds of cases occur in patients >50 years old	• Rash erupts as papules and transforms to vesicles or bullae in 24 hours • Vesicles become pustules in 48 hours and crusts by day 7 • Erupts in dermatomal pattern (pathognomonic) • Typically does not cross midline unless patient is immunocompromised	• Diagnosis made by history and physical examination • Tzanck smear if diagnosis in question • Laboratories only indicated if severe secondary infection suspected • Treatment with Acyclovir and pain medication
Measles	• Highly contagious disease of childhood • Rarely seen in children in the US due to immunization • Outbreaks may be seen in third decade of life in the US	• Characterized by fever, cough, and coryza • Rash on face, neck, and shoulders • *Koplik's spots* in mouth are bluish-white papules with erythema on the buccal mucosa (pathognomonic)	• Diagnosis is made clinically • Laboratories not indicated • Treatment usually only supportive care

(continued)

Table 30.5 Differential diagnosis of viral etiologies of rash (*cont*)

Diagnosis	Epidemiology	Symptoms/signs of rash	Work-up/treatment
Roseola infantum	• Affects infants between 6 and 24 months of age • Caused by human herpes virus 6 and 7	• Characterized by sudden appearance of rash after defervescence of a high fever • Infant usually appears well despite fever • Rash is small pink macules and papules that become confluent and fade	• Diagnosis is made clinically • Laboratories not indicated • Treatment usually only supportive care
Rubella (German measles)	• Benign childhood infection • Rarely seen in the US due to immunization	• Pink papules that start on forehead and spread to face, trunk, and extremities • Characteristic 3-day course after which the rash fades completely • Infection during pregnancy can result in congenital defects	• Diagnosis is made clinically • Laboratories not indicated • Treatment usually only supportive care • Infection during pregnancy – therapeutic abortion or passive immunization
Varicella (chicken pox)	• Nearly 95% occurs before the age of 10 years • 3–4 million cases annually in the US • Decreasing prevalence due to vaccine • Transmitted by both direct contact and airborne droplets	• Highly pruritic • Begins as a papular eruption that evolves into vesicles • Vesicles become pustules and crust over a 12-hour period • Continual eruptions over 4–5 days; infectious while vesicles are present • *Dewdrop-on-a-rose-petal* • Beware of severe complications (pneumonia, meningitis, encephalitis)	• Diagnosis made by a history of viral prodrome and recent exposure • Laboratories not indicated • Oral acyclovir may decrease severity of outbreak if started within 24 hours of first eruptions

HSV: herpes simplex virus; VZV: varicella zoster virus.

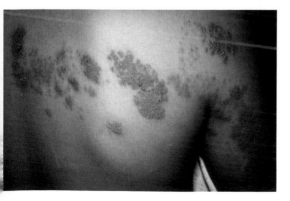

Figure 30.4
Herpes Zoster (Shingles). Erythematous macules and papules developing into vesicles on an erythematous plaque, and finally into crusts, distributed over one or two dermatomes. *Courtesy*: Steven Shpall, MD.

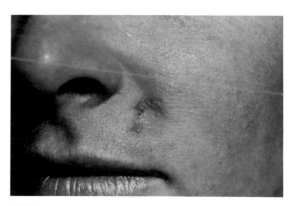

Figure 30.5
Impetigo. Honey colored crusts often on erythematous base. *Courtesy*: Steven Shpall, MD.

Table 30.6 Differential diagnosis of bacterial etiologies of rash

Diagnosis	Epidemiology	Symptoms/signs of rash	Work-up/treatment
Erysipelas	• Occurs at any age • Most frequently in children <3 years old and older individuals • Commonly caused by Group A Strep	• Characterized by red, hot, and tender area of skin • High fever and chills associated with Group A Strep • Pus or clear discharge at site of entry into the skin	• Gram's stain of discharge if present. Blood cultures are very low yield • Treatment with penicillin G, dicloxacillin, or equivalent
Impetigo (Figure 30.5)	• Primary infections most common in children • Secondary infections in patients with underlying dermatoses • Caused by *S. aureus* and Group A Strep	• Superficial bacterial infection of the epidermal skin • Rash appears as a golden yellow-crusted erosion • Commonly seen on face around mouth and on cheeks	• Diagnosis is made clinically • Laboratories not indicated • Treatment with oral and/or topical antibiotics, such as 2% mupirocin ointment, dicloxacillin, first generation cephalosporins, or azithromycin
Meningo-coccemia	• Occurs at any age • Most common in teenage and college-age individuals • 50–88% develop meningitis	• Rash is maculopapular with petechiae • High fever, tachycardia, tachypnea, and hypotension • Patient appears acutely ill with marked prostration	• Immediate antibiotic treatment that penetrates the CSF blood–brain barrier (penicillin G, ceftriaxone, cefotaxime, ampicillin, or chloramphenicol) • CBC, Chem7, clotting studies • Blood and CSF cultures • Isolation and admission to the hospital
Scarlet fever (Figure 30.6)	• Seen primarily in children with pharyngitis • Usually caused by Group A Strep • Rarely caused by *S. aureus*	• Rash appears 1–3 days after onset of infection • Scarlatiniform rash is a finely punctate erythema on the upper trunk, with a sandpaper-like feel • Progresses to neck, back, groin, and axilla • Spares palms and soles • Pharynx is beefy red with *strawberry tongue*	• Rapid direct antigen test to screen for Group A Strep • Oral swab for bacterial culture • ASO titer if diagnosis in question • Treatment with penicillin G or equivalent
Staphylococcal scalded skin syndrome (Figure 30.7)	• Most common in neonates <3 months old • Caused by toxin-producing *S. aureus* • Infections of umbilical stump or nares	• Widespread detachment of the superficial layers of the epidermis • Ranges from localized bullous impetigo to extensive epidermolysis • Desquamation of the affected area is common	• CBC and blood cultures • Bacterial cultures of wound are not indicated • Oral or intravenous antibiotics based on severity (erythromycins, penicillinase-resistant penicillins, or cephalosporins) • Hospital admission for severe cases
Streptococcal toxic shock syndrome	• Usually caused by Group A beta-hemolytic Strep • Increasing frequency in recent years • Mortality may be as high as 30%	• Generalized erythroderma with or without bullae either before or concomittent with the onset of the full-blown syndrome • May have fever, hypotension, cerebral dysfunction, renal failure, respiratory distress syndrome, toxic cardiomyopathy, hepatic dysfunction, and hypocalcemia • Desquamation follows the rash • Infection in the soft tissues or skin and bacteremia often present	• Blood and wound cultures • Intravenous antibiotics, such as oxacillin, cefoxitin, vancomycin, and clindamycin • May require operative debridement

(continued)

Table 30.6 Differential diagnosis of bacterial etiologies of rash (*cont*)

Diagnosis	Epidemiology	Symptoms/signs of rash	Work-up/treatment
Syphilis (Figure 30.1a, b)	• *Treponema pallidum* • Called the "great masquerader" because of the variety of presentations of rash • Rash starts 9–90 days after chancre	• Generalized, painless and non-pruritic • Distributed on skin and mucous membranes • Follows skin cleavage lines • Discrete, scaly, red–brown papules and plaques • Associated with headache, sore throat, malaise, and generalized arthralgias	• Laboratory testing with VDRL or RPR necessary to make diagnosis • Dark-field examination of scrapings may be beneficial • Treatment is with penicillin G or equivalent
Toxic shock syndrome	• Most common in women age 20–30 years • Primarily caused by toxin-producing *S. aureus* • Risk factors: vaginal tampons, surgical packing, postpartum wounds	• Generalized scarlatiniform erythroderma most intense around infected area • Edema of face, hands, and feet are common • Criteria for diagnosis: fever >38.9°C, erythroderma, mucous membrane involvement, signs of sepsis, particularly hypotension	• Blood cultures and wound cultures (often negative) • CBC, chemistries, and liver panel • Intravenous antibiotics with Staph coverage, such as oxacillin, cefoxitin, vancomycin, and clindamycin • Hospitalization and fluid resuscitation

ASO: anti-streptolysin; CBC: complete blood count; CSF: cerebrospinal fluid; *S. aureus*: *Staphylococcus aureus*; Strep: *streptococcus*; RPR: rapid plasma reagin; VDRL: venereal disease research laboratory.

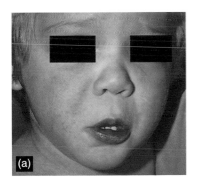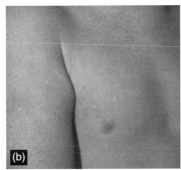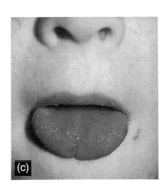

Figure 30.6
Streptococcal Scarlet Fever. (a) The patient has a flushed face and perioral pallor; (b) a diffuse, blanching, erythematous rash that has a sandpapery consistency on palpation; (c): the characteristic red strawberry tongue with glistening surface and prominent papillae. Reprinted from Atlas of Pediatric Physical Diagnosis, 4th ed., Eds Zitelli BJ, Davis HW. Copyright 2002, with permission from Elsevier.

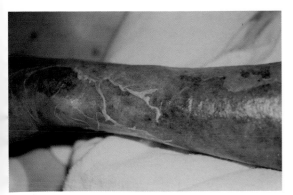

Figure 30.7
Staphylococcal scalded skin syndrome. Erythema in which a superficial split in the epidermis develops, leading to widespread exfoliation of large sheets of the upper epidermis. *Courtesy*: Steven Shpall, MD.

Table 30.7 Differential diagnosis of fungal etiologies of rash

Diagnosis	Epidemiology	Symptoms/signs of rash	Work-up/treatment
Tinea capitis	• Mostly children 6–10 years old • Increased rural prevalence • Blacks > whites • Risk factors include debilitation, malnutrition, and chronic disease	• Inflammatory type associated with pain, tenderness, and/or alopecia • With non-inflammatory infection, scaling, pruritis, diffuse or circumscribed alopecia, and lymphadenopathy	• Wood's lamp • Cultures • Topical antifungals are not effective • Systemic treatment with griseofulvin, terbinafine, fluconazole, or ketoconazole
Tinea pedis	• 20–50 year old • Males > females • Predisposing factors include hot, humid weather, occlusive footwear, or excessive sweating	• May be dry and scaly or macerated, peeling, and associated with fissures between 4th and 5th toes • Other forms include well-demarcated erythema with minute papules, vesicles or bullae, or ulcerations	• Scrapings to detect hyphae • Wood's lamp • Fungal culture • Treatment with topical or oral antifungals, such as terbinafine, naftifine, or fluconazole
Tinea corporis	• Occurs in all age groups • Higher incidence in animal workers and individuals with pets • Dermatophyte infection of the dermis	• Characterized by small to large scaling, sharply demarcated plaques • Lesions have peripheral enlargement and central clearing • Most lesions have an annular configuration	• Diagnosis by KOH slide preparation • Wood's lamp can assist with diagnosis • Treatment with topical azole cream is usually effective • Systemic antifungal treatment for large infections or if refractory to topical creams
Tinea cruris	• Predisposing factor is a warm, moist environment • Males > females	• Lesions are often bilateral and begin in skin folds • Half moon-shaped plaque with well-defined scaly border	• Treatment with topical antifungals, such as clotrimazole, miconazole, naftifine, or terbinafine

KOH: potassium hydroxide.

Table 30.8 Differential diagnosis of infestations and bites

Diagnosis	Epidemiology	Symptoms/signs of rash	Work-up/treatment
Lyme disease (Figure 27.3)	• Tick-borne illness • Caused by the spirochete *Borrelia burgdorferi* • Predominantly seen in eastern US during summer months	• Initial erythematous macule or papule that expands with distinct red border with central clearing (ECM) • Other symptoms include malaise, fever, chills, arthralgias, myalgias, sore throat, and anorexia	• Skin biopsy of ECM lesion (spirochetes in up to 40%) • Serology studies • Borrelia culture from skin biopsy • Oral antibiotics (penicillin G, doxycycline, amoxicillin, or azithromycin) and close outpatient follow-up

(continued)

Table 30.8 Differential diagnosis of infestations and bites (*cont*)

Diagnosis	Epidemiology	Symptoms/signs of rash	Work-up/treatment
Rocky Mountain spotted fever (Figure 30.8)	• Incidence highest 5–9 years old, 600 cases/year • Fatality highest in males • *Rickettsia rickettsii* • Transmitted by ticks • Occurs mainly in northern climates in the spring, later in southern climates	• Prodrome of anorexia, irritability, malaise, fever, and chills • Followed by abrupt fever, severe headache, generalized myalgias, rigors, photophobia, and prostration • Rash can start on the 1st day (14%) up to the 6th day (20%), or not appear at all (13%) • Rash begins on wrists, forearms, and ankles • Early lesions are 2–6 mm pink, blanchable macules which evolve to deep red papules and then become hemorrhagic over 1–4 days	• Diagnosis depends on clinical symptoms and history of potential or confirmed tick exposure, because laboratory confirmation cannot occur before 10–14 days • Treatment with tetracycline, doxycycline, and chloramphenicol
Scabies	• Microscopic mite • *Sarcoptes scabiei* • White, transparent creature <0.5 mm long • Transmitted by close personal contact • Mite life-span is 30 days	• Pruritic, worse at night • Papulovesicular dermatitis • Distribution predominately volar wrists, medial palms, interdigital web spaces, and axillary folds • Usually spares face and scalp, except in infants • Skin burrows seen	• Skin scrapings may demonstrate mites, eggs, or feces • Treatment includes washing all clothes and bed linens • Rx with lindane, permethrin, or crotamiton

ECM: erythema chronicum migrans.

Table 30.9 Differential diagnosis of dermatitis and inflammatory disorders

Diagnosis	Epidemiology	Symptoms/signs of rash	Work-up/treatment
Allergic contact dermatitis	• Often associated with plants • Termed *allergic phytodermatitis* • Poison ivy/oak are the most common causes	• Primarily on hands and exposed extremities • Begins as erythematous areas that evolve into edematous papules, nodules, and plaques • Often in a linear arrangement	• Topical corticosteroids are effective for small areas with non-bullous lesions • Systemic steroids are indicated for large areas of exposure or if blisters present
Atopic dermatitis	• Begins in the 1st year of life in 60% of patients • May have association with aeroallergens (dust mites) and foods (peanuts, milk, eggs) • Exacerbated skin dehydration from frequent showers and hand washing • Usually a personal or family history of atopy (asthma or allergic rhinitis)	• Patients have dry skin • Pruritus is the hallmark of atopic dermatitis • Scratching leads to lichenification of the skin, which causes the skin to become more dried out • Predilection for flexure surfaces, sides of the neck, face, wrists, and dorsum of the feet	• Bacterial cultures for possible secondary infection with *S. aureus* • Viral culture to rule out HSV in crusted lesions • Check serum IgE levels • Treatment: oral antihistamines, topical steroids, and skin hydration with emollient creams

(*continued*)

Table 30.9 Differential diagnosis of dermatitis and inflammatory disorders (*cont*)

Diagnosis	Epidemiology	Symptoms/signs of rash	Work-up/treatment
Bullous pemphigoid	• Autoimmune disorder • Occurs in sixth to eighth decade of life • Complement activation leading to inflammatory cascade response • Due to circulating IgG auto-antibodies	• Erythematous, papular, or urticarial-type lesions followed by bullae formation • Contain serous or hemorrhagic fluid • Bleeding is sometimes a problem • Found predominantly on axillae, groin, abdomen, and lower legs	• Neutrophils at dermal–epidermal junction on light microscopy • Serum tests for circulating auto-antibodies • IV fluid replacement • Oral steroids with azathioprine or dapsone
Erythema multiforme (Figure 30.9)	• Occurs at any age, but 50% under the age of 20 years • Associated primarily with HSV infection • 50% of cases from unknown etiology • More frequent in men than women	• Vesicle and bullae in the center of a papule • Peripheral clearing produces a distinct target lesion • Most common on the palms, soles, forearms, elbows, and knees	• Diagnosis confirmed by biopsy showing perivascular mononuclear infiltrate • Treatment with oral acyclovir may prevent recurrent EM • Steroids are often used, but not proven effective
Henoch–Schonlein purpura (Figure 30.3)	• Children 2–10 years of age • Peaks in winter • No clear etiology • Some association with Group A beta-hemolytic Strep and viruses • Acute vasculitis with IgA deposits • Male/female 2 : 1	• Palpable purpura on buttocks and lower extremities • May begin as urticaria • In severe cases hemorrhagic vesicles • Association with arthritis in two-thirds of cases • May be associated with intussusception	• Increased WBC, mild anemia, and thrombocytopenia can be seen • 40% will have proteinuria and hematuria • Blood cultures may be necessary to rule-out sepsis • Supportive care • Hydration • Prednisone, NSAIDs
Irritant contact dermatitis	• Caused by exposure of the skin to chemicals or other irritants • Hands are the most commonly affected area • Most cases are caused by chronic exposure	• Symptoms of itching, burning, and stinging are usually the only manifestations • Dry skin with erythema and chapping common • Severe cases produce a caustic burn with vesiculation	• Patch testing can be done by dermatologist for possible allergic etiology • Avoidance of caustic agents is treatment of choice • Topical corticosteroid and barrier creams are effective
Kawasaki's disease (Figures 23.1, 23.2)	• Peak onset at 1 year of age, mean age 2.5 years • Slight male and Asian predominance • Acute febrile illness of infants and children • Unknown etiology • Systemic vasculitis of microvessels • 2000–4000 cases/year	• Cutaneous and mucosal erythema and edema with subsequent desquamation • Lesions appear 1–2 days after onset of fever • Rash first noted on palms and soles, then spreads to trunk and extremities • Edema of hands and feet develop after rash • Oropharynx becomes erythematous • Complications are predominately coronary, including aneurysms, CHF, MI, dysrhythmias, and valvular insufficiency; also hydrops of the gallbladder	• Clinical diagnosis includes fever for at least 5 days and skin changes • Laboratories: WBC >18K common • LFTs are abnormal • Thrombocytosis and elevated ESR after 10th day of illness • Urine may show sterile pyuria • Treatment with high-dose aspirin and IVIG • Admission to hospital required

(continued)

Table 30.9 Differential diagnosis of dermatitis and inflammatory disorders (*cont*)

Diagnosis	Epidemiology	Symptoms/signs of rash	Work-up/treatment
Pemphigus vulgaris	• Autoimmune disorder • Occurs in fourth to sixth decade of life • Loss of normal cell-to-cell adhesion in the epidermis • Due to circulating IgG autoantibodies	• Starts in the oral mucosa • Skin lesions are round, or vesicles and bullae with serous content • *Nikolsky's sign* positive (slight thumb pressure causes the skin to wrinkle, slide laterally, and separate from the dermis) • Found predominantly on scalp, face, chest, axilla, and groin	• Immunofluorescence of skin biopsy reveals IgG deposits • IV fluid replacement necessary • Systemic steroids and immunosuppressive therapy required
Pityriasis rosea (Figure 30.2)	• Occurs between first and fourth decades of life • More common in the spring and fall months • Possibly due to human herpes virus 7	• Begins with a single truncal lesion or *herald patch* (2–5 cm diameter salmon-colored, single oval scaly patch) • Secondary eruption 1–2 weeks later usually on the trunk and proximal aspects of extremities • Lesions are erythematous macules or papules • "Christmas-tree" pattern	• Diagnosis made by skin biopsy and light microscopy • Self-limited with spontaneous remission in 6–12 weeks • Treatment with oral antihistamines and topical steroids
Psoriasis	• Peak incidence in 20–30 years of age • Chronic disease without cure	• Pruritus is common • Silver, scaly rash on an erythematous base • Located on scalp, extensor surfaces, and groin area • May produce arthritis in distal joints	• Should be managed by a dermatologist due to need for "shifting" therapies • Treatment with topical steroids, tar-based shampoos, and vitamin D analogues
Stevens–Johnson syndrome (SJS) (Figure 30.10)	• Occurs at any age but most common in adults >40 years • 50% are associated with drug exposure • Drugs most frequently implicated: sulfa, aminopenicillins, carbamazepine, phenytoin and allopurinol • Also caused by viral infections, *Mycoplasma pneumoniae*	• Prodrome with fever and flu-like symptoms • 1–3 days later develop mucocutaneous lesions • Skin rash is EM which is brightly erythematous with bullae • Fever is common • Secondary infection may occur, making diagnosis more difficult • Anemia, lymphocytopenia and neutropenia may occur	• Diagnosis is confirmed by biopsy • IV fluids critical to replace fluids lost from wounds • Treatment is similar to that of burns, supportive mostly • Early diagnosis and withdrawal of suspected drugs critical • Systemic steroids have not been proven helpful
Toxic epidermal necrolysis (Figure 30.11)	• Occurs at any age but most common in adults >40 years • 80% are associated with drug exposure • Drugs most frequently implicated: sulfa, aminopenicillins, carbamazepine, phenytoin and allopurinol	• Skin rash is EM which is brightly erythematous with bullae • >30% epidermal detachment • Fever is common and typically higher than in SJS • Secondary infection may occur, making diagnosis more difficult • *Nikolsky's sign* positive	• Diagnosis confirmed by biopsy • IV fluids critical to replace fluids lost from skin • Treatment is similar to that of burns, consider transfer to a burn center • Early diagnosis and withdrawal of suspected drugs critical • Systemic steroids have not been proven helpful

(*continued*)

Table 30.9 Differential diagnosis of dermatitis and inflammatory disorders (*cont*)

Diagnosis	Epidemiology	Symptoms/signs of rash	Work-up/treatment
Urticaria (Figure 11.1)	• Most common skin rash for which acute care is sought • Mast cell degranulation and histamine release causes hives • Majority of etiologies unknown • May result from infection, medications, foods, autoimmune diseases, and malignancies	• Benign and self-limited usually • Raised erythematous borders with serpiginous edges and blanched centers • Diameter ranges from a few millimeters to 30 cm • Pruritic • Lasts for a few minutes to several hours	• Laboratory tests not usually indicated • Consider Strep screen or culture • Symptomatic treatment with antihistamines • Prednisone short course preferred over taper • Epinephrine if severe associated reaction

CHF: congestive heart failure; EM: erythema multiforme; ESR: erythrocyte sedimentation rate; HSV: herpes simplex virus; IV: intravenous; IVIG: intravenous immunoglobulin; LFTs: liver function tests; MI: myocardial infarction; NSAIDs: non-steroidal anti-inflammatory drugs; Rx: treatment; SJS: Stevens–Johnson syndrome; WBC: white blood cell.

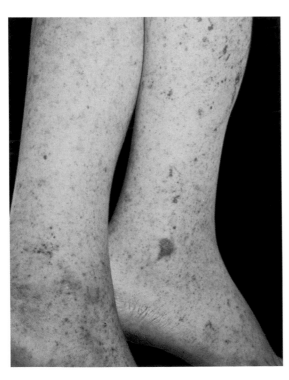

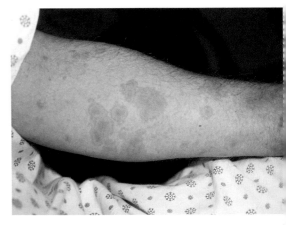

Figure 30.9
Erythema multiforme. Target lesions, erythematous patches or plaques with dusky central areas which can develop into bullae. *Courtesy*: Steven Shpall, MD.

Figure 30.8
Rocky Mountain spotted fever. A generalized petechial eruption that involves the entire cutaneous surface, including the palms and soles. Permission granted from Habif, TP; Reprinted from Clinical Dermatology, 4th ed., Habif TP, page 525, Copyright 2004, with permission from Elsevier.

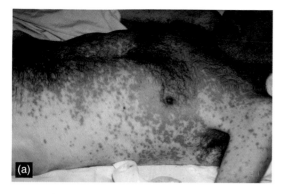

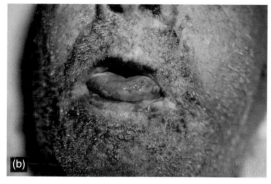

Figure 30.10
Stevens–Johnson syndrome. Atypical or incomplete target lesions that coalesce and can develop into bullae. The mucous membranes usually are involved with erosions and crusting. *Courtesy:* Steven Shpall, MD.

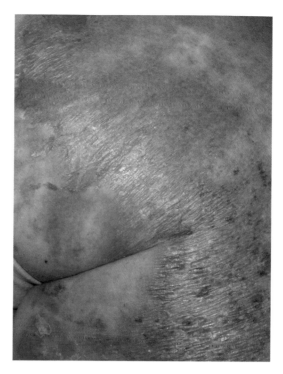

Figure 30.11
Toxic epidermal necrolysis. Erythema in which a full thickness split below the epidermis develops, leading to widespread exfoliation of large sheets of epidermis. *Courtesy:* Steven Shpall, MD.

Diagnostic testing

Traditional laboratory tests are generally non-diagnostic and of little use in diagnosing most rashes. Specific tests for viral infections, such as the Tzanck smear for herpetic eruptions, can be performed when the diagnosis is in question. Patients presenting with severe bacterial infections or signs of cardiovascular collapse, as in sepsis, require appropriate testing, which includes the following: complete blood count (CBC) with differential to look for signs of hemolysis, leukocytosis and demarginization; prothrombin time/partial thromboplastin time (PT/PTT) to look for etiologies of petechiae or purpura; Gram's stain to identify organisms; blood cultures for identification of bacteremia; and chemistries to look for signs of renal failure or electrolyte abnormalities. Lyme serologies, VDRL testing for syphilis, or erythrocyte sedimentation rate (ESR) testing for vasculitis should be obtained if indicated.

For rashes from non-infectious causes, laboratories should be directed towards identification

Table 30.10 Methods of diagnostic testing

Diascopy	A glass slide pressed firmly against a red lesion will determine if it is due to capillary dilation (blanchable) or to extravasation of blood (non-blanchable)
KOH preparation	Scrape scales from the skin, hair, or nails. Add 10% KOH solution to dissolve tissue material. Identification of septated hyphae indicates fungal infection; pseudohyphae and budding spores indicate yeast infection
Tzanck preparation	Scrape the base of a vesicle and smear cells on a glass slide. Multinucleated giant cells are associated with herpes simplex, zoster, and varicella infections
Scabies preparation	Scrape skin of a burrow and place on a slide. Mites, eggs, or feces seen in scabies infections
Wood's lamp	Examination under a long-wave ultraviolet light ("black" lamp). Tinea capitis will fluoresce green or yellow on the hair shaft

of an immunologic or hematologic etiology. Specific tests, such as the Tzanck smear for herpetic eruptions, can be performed when the diagnosis is in question (Table 30.10). Results for such testing may not be available immediately and should be done in conjunction with the appropriate follow-up physician.

General treatment principles

The treatment of rashes varies greatly based on the cause of the eruption and the severity of the illness. The main goal of treatment is largely supportive and symptomatic, aimed at relieving pain and pruritus. Usually only those patients with severe systemic illness from overwhelming infection, fluid losses, and severe pain require inpatient care.

Volume repletion

Patients with signs of sepsis, as in toxic shock syndrome, or with severe fluid losses, as in toxic epidermal necrolysis, should be aggressively resuscitated with intravenous crystalloid fluid. The rate of repletion is based on the patient's degree of hypovolemia as evidenced by the vital signs and physical examination.

Pruritis and pain control

Patients often present complaining not just of rash, but also of pruritus and pain. Use of antihistamines (oral and topical) for symptomatic relief coupled with topical steroid agents or systemic corticosteroids as indicated provide the patient with significant relief. Non-steroidal anti-inflammatory drugs (NSAIDs) and narcotics should be used judiciously for pain control. For example, adults with zoster should be given high doses of NSAIDs with or without narcotics for pain and inflammation. NSAIDs are to be avoided in children with varicella or chickenpox due to the risk of Reye's syndrome.

Emollients

Emollient creams and lotions restore water and lipids to the epidermis. Preparations that contain urea or lactic acid have special lubricating properties, and may be the most effective. Creams are thicker and more lubricating than lotions, and many lotions contain alcohol to ease

application. As petroleum jelly and mineral oil contain no water, water should be added to the skin prior to application.

Topical corticosteroids

Topical steroids are the most powerful tool for treating dermatologic diseases. There are many products, and new ones are introduced frequently. Steroids are divided by potency, from Group I to Group VII (I is the strongest, VII is the weakest). Their effects result in part from their ability to induce vasoconstriction of small vessels in the dermis. It is this degree of vasoconstriction that determines a steroid's grouping. Lowering the concentration of the drug would not necessarily decrease the vasoconstriction; many have the same vasoconstriction despite different concentrations (0.25%, 0.5%, 1%). Generic substitutes are not necessarily equivalent (most important for potent steroids), and adequate potency and treatment length are important considerations when prescribing. Physicians should avoid prescribing a weaker, "safe" preparation that fails to give the desired anti-inflammatory effect and prolongs the disease, often leading to secondary infection. The base determines the rate at which the active ingredient is absorbed through the skin. Creams are somewhat greasy, usable in most areas, cosmetically most acceptable, and best for intertriginous areas. Ointments are translucent, greasy, more lubricating, have greater penetration than creams, and are too occlusive for use in acute eczematous inflammation or intertriginous areas. Gels are clear and useful for acute exudative inflammation, such as poison ivy, and in the hair because they result in less "matting" of the hair. Lotions are clear or milky, most useful for the scalp, and may result in stinging and drying when applied to intertriginous areas. The amount of cream dispensed is important; 1 g of cream covers 10 cm $\times$ 10 cm of skin, 20–30 g covers the entire skin of most adults. For ointments, the amount that fits on your fingertip typically covers the equivalent of the front and back of the hand.

Antivirals and antibiotics

Viral exanthems do not require antibiotics. However, the use of *antivirals* in varicella, zoster, and herpetic eruptions may change the duration of symptoms, decrease the incidence of post-herpetic neuralgia, or decrease future outbreaks. For bacterial infections, topical antibiotic ointments in superficial cutaneous infections or intravenous antibiotics in patients with systemic infections are necessary. Antibiotics should be targeted to cover the likely bacterial pathogens.

Antifungals

The newest class of antifungal agents, the allylamines (e.g., terbinafine), have been shown to produce higher cure rates and more rapid responses in dermatophyte infections than older agents. Some of the oral medications (fluconazole) are effective in weekly dosing patterns, which may increase compliance. Since most fungal infections require long treatment courses (2–12 weeks or more), lack of compliance is frequently associated with treatment failure. Other side effects, such as hepatic injury, have been associated with ketoconazole and less frequently griseofulvin. Because of this, monitoring liver enzymes is advised.

Immunosuppressants

Autoimmune-mediated disorders may require the use of systemic steroids or other medications to produce immunosuppression. Immunosuppressant medications should be given only after consultation with the appropriate specialist. Such medications carry with them severe adverse effects, and often need close monitoring to prevent iatrogenic disease.

Special patients

Elderly

Geriatric patients are often on more medications than children and adults. Therefore, reviewing medications and recent changes is extremely important in this population, as allergic reactions may occur in addition to drug–drug interactions. Furthermore, the geriatric population may not tolerate treatment recommendations, like antihistamines or analgesics.

Pediatric

Many of the viral exanthems occur only in childhood and are self-limited. Exanthems were previously consecutively numbered according to their historical appearance and description:

- First disease: measles
- Second disease: scarlet fever
- Third disease: rubella
- Fourth disease: "Dukes" disease (probably coxsackie virus or echovirus)
- Fifth disease: erythema infectiosum
- Sixth disease: roseola infantum.

Immune compromised

Patients who are immunocompromised are more susceptible to infection and secondary infection when the integrity of the skin barrier has been compromised. Suspected bacterial infections in this group should be treated aggressively with appropriate antibiotics and observation in the hospital if systemic illness is feared.

Disposition

Dermatologic consultation

The majority of patients with complaints of rash do not require an emergent consultation with a dermatologist. Emergency physicians and primary care physicians can adequately treat and care for most disease processes. In patients with severe dermatologic disease or in cases where the diagnosis remains in question, dermatologic consult is required for possible biopsy and analysis.

Admission

Most patients with complaints of a rash do not require inpatient care. Such care is reserved for those with systemic bacterial infection, signs of sepsis, severe dehydration, and intractable pain. Patients who require admission should first be adequately resuscitated in the ED with appropriate therapies initiated. A dermatology or infectious disease consultation can be obtained in association with the admission.

Discharge

After a thorough evaluation in the ED, many patients can be discharged home with supportive care instructions. Follow-up should be scheduled for these patients within 1–2 days to ensure that no other signs or symptoms of systemic illness or secondary infection have begun, and to evaluate their response to outpatient therapy. Referral to a dermatologic specialist should be made in those patients who have severe disease or a chronic dermatologic process. Pregnant women exposed to a patient with rubella, varicella or fifth disease are at risk for fetal complications, and therefore need expeditious follow-up with appropriate healthcare professionals.

Pearls, pitfalls, and myths

- Most rashes are benign and self-limited, requiring only supportive care. A few can be life-threatening and should not be overlooked (Table 30.1).
- History and physical examination is vital to diagnose a rash or identify its cause.
- Toxic epidermal necrolysis and staphylococcal scalded skin syndrome look similar; however, the first requires removal of the offending agent (often an antibiotic) and the second requires treatment with an antibiotic.
- The rash of toxic shock syndrome can be indistinct and should be considered in patients with fever and volume depletion associated with a rash.
- The early rash of meningococcemia may be macular, maculopapular, or petechial; early identification is important and potentially life-saving.
- Extensive work-ups with laboratory studies are often unnecessary and should be discouraged in the ED evaluation of most rashes.
- Urticarial skin lesions may be the first sign of infection, infestation, or systemic disease which requires further investigation.
- While the disease causing the rash may be benign, patients who are immune compromised or pregnant may have higher risks of complications.

References

1. Edwards, L. *Dermatology in Emergency Care*, 1st ed., Churchill Livingstone, 1997.
2. Fitzpatrick, Johnson, et al. (eds). *Color Atlas and Synopsis of Clinical Dermatology*, 4th ed., McGraw Hill, 2000.
3. Fleisher AB (ed.). *Emergency Dermatology: A Rapid Treatment Guide*, 1st ed., McGraw Hill, 2002.
4. Habif TP (ed.). *Clinical Dermatology: A Color Guide to Diagnosis and Therapy*, 4th ed., St. Louis: Mosby, 2003.
5. Harwood-Nuss A (ed.). *The Clinical Practice of Emergency Medicine*, 3rd ed., Philadelphia: Lippincott Williams & Wilkins, 2001.
6. Marx JA (ed.). *Rosen's Emergency Medicine: Concepts and Clinical Practice*, 5th ed., St. Louis: Mosby, 2002.
7. Tintinalli JE (ed.). *Emergency Medicine: A Comprehensive Study Guide*, 6th ed., McGraw Hill, 2003.

31 Scrotal pain

Jonathan E. Davis, MD

Scope of the problem

One of the most challenging presentations to the emergency department (ED) is a male with acute testicular pain. This complaint causes a high level of patient and health care provider anxiety, owing to the highly sensitive nature of the male genitalia, and the often associated fear of embarrassment on behalf of the patient with problems localized to this region.

Precise diagnosis of acute scrotal problems is not always straightforward; however, differentiating true genitourinary (GU) emergencies requiring prompt evaluation from urgent conditions safe for outpatient management takes precedence over definitive diagnosis. The vast majority of cases of acute testicular pain can be attributed to three diagnostic entities: testicular torsion, epididymitis and appendage torsion. Identification of testicular torsion is of paramount importance

as it may threaten testicular viability and future fertility if not managed swiftly and appropriately. Similarly, early identification and aggressive management of necrotizing fasciitis of the perineum (Fournier's disease) is critical.

Anatomic essentials

The male genitalia is composed of the *penis* (contains the paired erectile bodies and penile urethra), as well as the *scrotum* (encases the testes, epididymis and vas deferens) (Figure 31.1). There are several fascial planes which collectively comprise the *perineum*, providing protection and stability to the enclosed structures. However, these anatomic layers may also provide a conduit for the rapid spread of infection in certain cases.

The scrotal wall contains several layers deep to the epidermis, many of which are contiguous with

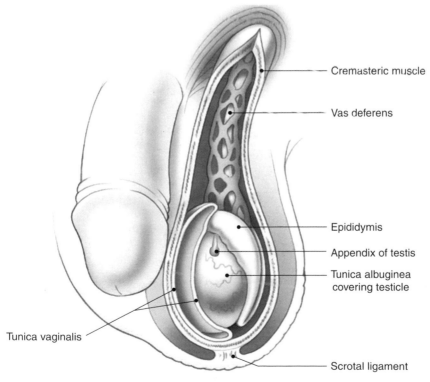

Cremasteric muscle

Vas deferens

Epididymis

Appendix of testis

Tunica albuginea covering testicle

Tunica vaginalis

Scrotal ligament

Figure 31.1
Anatomy of the scrotum.

the penis, perirectal region and anterior abdominal wall. The paired testes are each encapsulated within a dense connective tissue layer termed the *tunica albuginea*. A break in the integrity of this thick connective tissue represents a "ruptured" testicle, as may occur with direct trauma. External to the testicular parenchyma and tunica albuginea is the *tunica vaginalis*, which envelops each testicle and fastens it to the posterior scrotal wall. Providing additional stability is the *scrotal ligament* (gubernaculum), which anchors each testicle inferiorly. The tunica vaginalis consists of both visceral (contiguous with the tunica albuginea) and parietal leafs, with an interposed potential space. The significance of this potential space is that a lack of firm attachment of the testicle to the posterior scrotal wall makes the testes prone to rotation in a horizontal plane about the spermatic cord within the tunica vaginalis, a condition termed *testicular torsion*. The spermatic cord contains both the blood supply to each testicle (via the gonadal vessels) and the vas deferens (described below). Interruption of blood flow to the testes by twisting the spermatic cord, as occurs in testicular torsion, can lead to rapid ischemia and subsequent infarction of the affected testicle. The *appendix testes* are embryologic remnants with no known physiologic function located at the uppermost pole of the testes. This appendage is prone to torsion as well, leading to self-limited localized necrosis of the appendage. This results in pain which can be confused with pain due to torsion of the testicle.

The *epididymis* is a fine tubular structure which adheres closely to the posterolateral aspect of each testicle. It is involved in promoting sperm maturation and motility. Similar to the appendix testes, the *appendix epididymis* is an embryologic remnant with no known function attached to the head of each epididymis. This, too, is prone to torsion, similarly leading to localized necrosis of the appendage. The *vas deferens* is a tubular structure involved in sperm transit, extending from the epididymis distally to the prostatic portion of the urethra proximally.

History

A diligent and focused history in the patient presenting with acute scrotal pain is the key to formulating an appropriate differential diagnosis and management plan. Acute scrotal complaints will often include a component of patient embarrassment and apprehension; this is especially true in children and adolescents. In any situation where a patient presents with a family member or friend, it is important to offer to speak with the patient alone to ensure patient confidentiality and, in some cases, facilitate a more accurate history.

How did the pain begin (sudden versus gradual onset)?

Pain that begins abruptly and severely is concerning for testicular torsion. The sudden twisting of the spermatic cord characteristic of torsion leads to rapid diminution of blood supply to the affected testicle, causing ischemic pain. This is in contrast to the more indolent and smoldering pain of epididymitis, a gradually progressive inflammatory process. Long-standing inguinal hernias often present with isolated genital pain that is of prolonged duration. However, incarcerated (unable to reduce) or strangulated (ischemia and infarction of herniated bowel) hernias may present in a more dramatic fashion.

Is the pain "constant and progressive" or "intermittent and colicky"?

Constant and progressive pain is likely the result of a progressive inflammatory process (such as acute appendicitis); intermittent and colicky pain is more consistent with rapid onset and offset conditions, such as irritation and spasm of hollow structures (renal and biliary colic) or a twisting mechanism (testicular torsion). As epididymitis is a progressive inflammatory condition, pain follows in a constant and progressive manner. Patients may exhibit pain with ambulation and movement as a result of the inflammation. Pain of testicular torsion, on the other hand, may be intermittent and colicky, as the spermatic cord may spontaneously torse and detorse.

What were you doing when the pain began?

Testicular torsion is often accompanied by an inciting history of minor trauma, leading to rotation of the testicle (and twisting of the spermatic cord) within the tunica vaginalis. However, testicular torsion may occur in the absence of such events, and may occur during sleep. It is critical to elicit a history of any blunt or penetrating trauma to the scrotum, penis or surrounding structures, as the differential must then include injuries directly related to such traumatic events.

How long has the pain been present?

The pain of acute testicular torsion often develops over minutes, whereas pain associated with more indolent inflammatory conditions such as epididymitis develops over several hours to days. Testicular masses, such as testicular cancer, usually progress over several weeks to months. However, a patient with a long-standing testicular tumor may develop acute pain secondary to hemorrhage within the tumor, given the rich vascular supply of such lesions.

How would you characterize the pain (dull, aching, sharp, stabbing, throbbing)?

The patient's description of the pain may be helpful in differentiating potential etiologies. Pain associated with epididymitis is often described as dull and aching. Early in the course, pain may be mild, but increases in severity commensurate with worsening inflammation. The sudden pain associated with testicular torsion, however, is often described as sharp, stabbing or throbbing.

How would you rate the pain on a scale of 0–10, ten being the worst pain you could ever imagine and zero being no pain at all?

Patients with testicular torsion often complain of severe pain owing to resultant testicular ischemia. Unfortunately, the patient's quantification of pain is often inconsistent and generally unreliable in narrowing a differential diagnosis. Indeed, a majority of queried patients convey a "10 out of 10" response, especially in a highly sensitive region such as the genitalia. Given these limitations, pain associated with epididymitis and appendage torsion is often less severe in nature when compared with that of testicular torsion.

Have you ever had similar episodes of pain?

Patients with testicular torsion may have had prior episodes of similar pain which resolved prior to seeking medical care as a result of spontaneous detorsion. Also, pain of long-standing conditions such as hernias, hydroceles, varicoceles and tumors may present with subacute or chronic pain with intermittent exacerbations.

Are there any alleviating or exacerbating factors?

Pain resulting from inflammatory processes, such as epididymitis, may be temporarily relieved by rest and scrotal elevation with supportive undergarments, such as a "jock-strap." Similarly, inflammatory pain is often exacerbated by movement and activity. In contrast, patients

exhibiting the symptoms of testicular torsion often writhe in pain and cannot find a position of comfort.

Point with one finger and show me exactly where the pain is located?

It is essential to delineate the precise anatomic region(s) where the pain is localized. Pain may be due to structures within or adjoining that particular region, or may be referred from other areas. The majority of patients with the complaint of acute testicular pain will have a problem isolated to the genitalia. Etiologies of referred testicular pain include abdominal aortic aneurysm (AAA), renal colic and pyelonephritis.

Does the pain move anywhere?

It is common for patients with acute scrotal pain from a variety of causes to complain of lower abdominal, proximal lower extremity (i.e., inner thigh, groin) or back/flank pain. Likewise, it is important to consider acute GU pathology in any male patient presenting with seemingly isolated pain to the aforementioned anatomic regions. For instance, always consider GU conditions in any male presenting with abdominal pain.

Associated symptoms

Systemic

It is critical to ask about "systemic" findings in any patient with an acute scrotum. As a general rule, males with testicular torsion are more ill-appearing, with associated systemic signs and symptoms of illness such as nausea and emesis. In comparison, patients with appendage torsion or uncomplicated epididymitis have less severe symptoms. While patients with epididymitis may present with a low-grade fever, nausea and malaise, patients with a more advanced degree of infection (known as epididymo-orchitis) often have higher fever and more "systemic" involvement.

Urinary

Always inquire about changes in urination, including urgency, frequency, dysuria, hesitancy and hematuria. Urinary symptoms may accompany many causes of acute testicular pain. Classically, epididymitis may be accompanied by urinary complaints. Eliciting the inability to void is also important, as this may indicate urethral obstruction or severe volume depletion.

Genital

Ask about reproductive tract symptoms, such as erectile function, penile discharge and ejaculatory changes. A yellow-green penile discharge may provide clues to the diagnosis of urethritis or epididymitis, often caused by *Gonorrhea* and *Chlamydia* species in sexually active males. Hematospermia may be present in cases of epididymitis, as the inflammatory process leads to breaches in the integrity of the vascular endothelium and spilling of blood into the seminal fluid.

Gastrointestinal

Ask specifically about abdominal or flank pain, nausea, vomiting, distention and bowel changes. One important consideration in the patient with GU complaints and abdominal findings such as pain, distention and constipation/obstipation is an incarcerated or strangulated inguinal hernia. Also remember that patients with a retroperitoneal abdominal process, such as renal colic, pyelonephritis or ruptured AAA, may present with pain referred to the ipsilateral testicle with or without associated flank or abdominal pain.

Physical examination

General appearance

The general appearance of a patient provides important diagnostic clues. Most often, patients with testicular torsion are more ill-appearing than patients with other common etiologies of acute scrotal pain. In addition, patients with testicular torsion and renal colic tend to writhe in pain, as they cannot find a position of comfort. In contrast, patients with progressive inflammatory conditions such as epididymitis or epididymo-orchitis tend to minimize activity, as even minimal movement may exacerbate their discomfort.

Vital signs

Inflammatory and infectious conditions such as epididymitis, scrotal abscess and Fournier's disease tend to present with fever. However, fever is a very nonspecific finding, as it may be present in varying degrees in a variety of conditions. Abnormalities of other vitals signs may be helpful in uncovering more advanced stages of disease progression. Hypotension and tachycardia may be the result of dehydration, sepsis or blood loss (as in the case of a ruptured AAA). Tachycardia and tachypnea may occur as a consequence of substantial pain, or may signify more ominous physiologic derangements.

Abdominal

A complete abdominal examination is crucial in any patient presenting with acute scrotal pain. Many abdominal processes present with a component of, or even isolated, testicular pain. Always assess for costovertebral angle (CVA) tenderness. CVA tenderness is often present in retroperitoneal processes, such as pyelonephritis, renal colic, and expanding or ruptured AAAs. All of these conditions may present with testicular pain. In addition, it is important to assess for lower abdominal tenderness or masses, which may be present in cases of acute appendicitis, inguinal hernias, GU malignancies, traumatic injuries and spreading infections (i.e., Fournier's disease).

Genital

It is important to examine the male genitalia while the patient is standing and supine. Exercise caution, however, when examining a standing patient as some males may experience a strong vagal response to scrotal (or prostate) stimulation, leading to pre-syncope or syncope. Also, examination of the testes and epididymis may cause significant discomfort even in the absence of pathology. As many patients will have unilateral localization of pain, always examine the unaffected side first. This serves as a control and will help the patient gain confidence and trust (which may rapidly wane after examination of a swollen and painful scrotum).

Inspection

Visual examination of the genitals may reveal cutaneous rashes or lesions, abnormal testicular symmetry or position, edema (evident by loss of scrotal skin folds) or masses. Key visual features of testicular torsion include a high-riding testicle and a transverse lie of the affected testicle, both resulting from twisting of the spermatic cord (Figure 31.2). It is also important to look for evidence of scrotal or perineal erythema or ecchymoses in older male patients with scrotal pain. These may be clues to the presence of Fournier's disease, a necrotizing fasciitis of the perineum (Figure 31.3a and b). Fournier's disease most often affects diabetic or other immunocompromised patients. A prominent feature of early necrotizing fasciitis is significant pain in the absence of pronounced physical findings.

Palpation

Differentiating between the etiologies of acute scrotal pain is challenging, as various scrotal conditions may present in a similar fashion: unilateral (or bilateral) scrotal swelling and testicular enlargement with blurring of the distinction between the testicle and epididymis as a result of swelling. Often confounding the problem is the exquisite pain and discomfort elicited by the examination itself. However, there are some findings which, if present, may facilitate a more accurate diagnosis.

If isolated swelling and tenderness of the epididymis is present, epididymitis is the likely diagnosis (Figure 31.4). The natural progression of this infection is first to affect only the epididymis, and then progress to affect the ipsilateral testicle as well (epididymo-orchitis). Isolated nodularity at the superior pole of either the testicle or epididymis is often the result of appendage torsion,

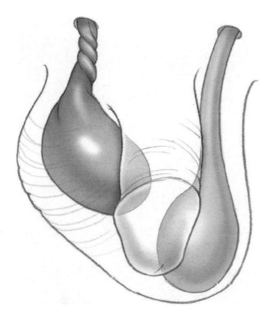

Figure 31.2
Testicular torsion.

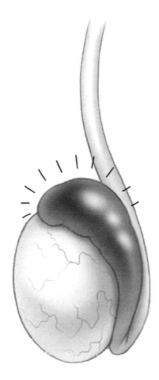

Figure 31.4
Epididymitis.

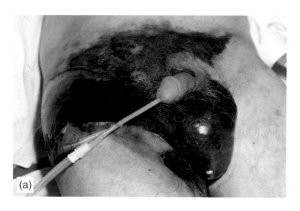

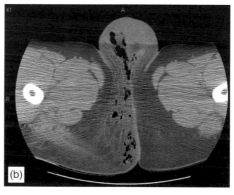

Figure 31.3
(a) Advanced Fournier's disease. *Courtesy:* Knowledge and Skills Website RCS, Edinburgh. (b) Axial CT section through the groin, showing gas within the scrotum and right perineal region, consistent with necrotizing fasciitis (Fournier's gangrene). *Courtesy:* GM Garmel, MD.

given the anatomic location of these structures. Isolated testicular swelling may result from testicular torsion, orchitis or vasculitis (i.e., Henoch-Schonlein Purpura). Swelling in the inguinal region is common in inguinal hernias. Swelling surrounding the testicle may be due to a hydrocele or hematocele. Hydroceles result from fluid accumulation (or blood in the case of hematoceles) in the tunica vaginalis. A varicocele is an abnormal engorgement of the gonadal venous plexus, classically described as a "bag of worms" and appreciated on palpation of the spermatic cord superior to the testicle. Any testicular nodularity or firmness is assumed carcinoma until proven otherwise.

Rectal

A digital rectal examination provides information on the prostate and prostatic portion of the urethra. Exquisite prostate tenderness may indicate acute infection (prostatitis). Prostate firmness and enlargement is a finding in benign prostatic hypertrophy; nodularity is concerning for prostate carcinoma. These conditions may present with varying GU symptoms.

Special signs/techniques

There are several commonly employed adjuncts to the traditional examination in assessing the male GU tract. Certain signs, if present, may aid in the proper identification of male genital pathology.

The absence of an ipsilateral *cremasteric reflex* is highly sensitive for the diagnosis of testicular torsion (Figure 31.5). This reflex is elicited by stroking the ipsilateral inner thigh which should result in a reflex elevation of the testicle greater than 0.5 cm

through contraction of the cremaster muscle. Some authors report a high association between an absent cremasteric reflex and the diagnosis of testicular torsion; however, many exceptions exist. *Prehn's sign*, relief of pain with scrotal elevation, was previously thought to help differentiate epididymitis (relieved with scrotal elevation) from testicular torsion (no change in symptoms with elevation). However, this sign has been found to be unreliable in distinguishing these two disorders, and its use for this purpose is not recommended.

In cases of suspected appendage torsion, assess for the pathognomonic *blue dot sign* (Figure 31.6). As appendage torsion is most common in the prepubescent age group, visualization of the infarcted appendage (the "blue dot") is seen through thin, non-hormonally stimulated pre-pubertal skin. *Scrotal transillumination* should be performed in cases of suspected hydrocele. The scrotal contents will transilluminate when filled with light-transmitting fluid, as is the case of a hydrocele. Transillumination, however, is insensitive and not specific for the diagnosis of hydrocele.

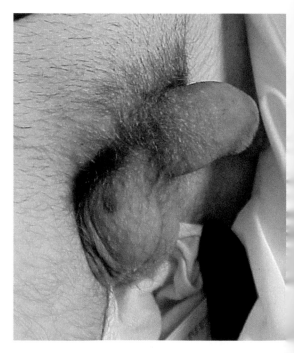

Figure 31.6
Blue dot sign. *Courtesy*: Selim Suner, MD.

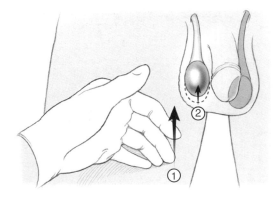

Figure 31.5
Cremasteric reflex.

Differential diagnosis

Table 31.1 describes causes of scrotal pain.

Table 31.1 Differential diagnosis of scrotal pain

Diagnosis	Symptoms	Signs	Work-up
Abdominal aortic aneurysm	Constant or intermittent flank, abdomen or GU pain	Tachycardia, hypertension (prior to rupture) or hypotension (post rupture); abdominal and/or CVA tenderness	US or CT; immediate surgical consultation
Acute appendicitis	Fever, nausea/vomiting, anorexia, RLQ pain	RLQ tenderness classic; may have associated abdominal rebound/guarding	CBC, urinalysis; CT or US; surgical consultation
Appendage torsion	More indolent onset of symptoms compared with testicular torsion; rarely "systemic" symptoms such as nausea and vomiting	Tender nodule at head of testicle or epididymis; "blue dot sign" pathognomonic	Imaging to ensure normal intratesticular blood flow (and therefore exclude the possibility of testicular torsion)
Epididymitis	More indolent onset of symptoms compared with testicular torsion	*Early*: firmness and nodularity isolated to epididymis. *Late*: with progression, inflammation becomes contiguous with testicle (epididymo-orchitis)	Testicular US (or radionucleotide imaging) reveals preserved (or increased) blood flow to affected testicle
Epididymo-orchitis	Often more "systemic" findings compared with isolated epididymitis	Large, swollen scrotal mass. Indistinct border between testicle and epididymis	Same as epididymitis
Fournier's disease	Perineal pain, swelling, redness, bruising; fever, vomiting, lethargy/weakness ("systemic" signs of illness)	Paucity of local findings in early stages (pain "out of proportion" to physical findings); may rapidly progress to fulminant sepsis and shock	Emergent surgical consultation for debridement; broad-spectrum antibiotics (covering Gram positive, Gram negative and anaerobic species)
Hematocele	Large, painful scrotal mass; often antecedent history of trauma	Ecchymoses of scrotal skin; testicular tenderness	US
Hernia	Unilateral inguinal/scrotal swelling and pain	Reducible, incarcerated and strangulated forms; latter two often more tender on examination	Surgical consultation in ED if incarcerated or strangulated; surgical referral if reducible
Hydrocele	Gradual onset of swelling	Transillumination may be helpful	US examination identifies fluid-filled cavity
Orchitis	Gradual onset of unilateral (or bilateral) testicular swelling and pain	Swelling and tenderness isolated to testicle (or testes); no epididymal involvement	Often seen in conjunction with other systemic diseases; therefore treatment is disease-specific
Scrotal skin disorders	Variable depending on cause	Must distinguish between lesions localized to scrotal wall versus those contiguous with deeper structures	US (or CT) may be helpful in determining extent of deeper structure involvement
Testicular torsion	Sudden and severe onset of pain; often associated with nausea and emesis ("systemic" symptoms)	High-riding testicle and transverse lie of testicle; ipsilateral cremasteric reflex often absent	Emergent urology consultation in high-probability cases; consider US (or radionucleotide) imaging if diagnosis uncertain
Trauma	History of blunt or penetrating mechanism of injury	Highly variable depending on mechanism	Urology consultation

(continued)

Table 31.1 Differential diagnosis of scrotal pain (*cont*)

Diagnosis	Symptoms	Signs	Work-up
Tumor	Gradually progressive testicular mass; often painless	May appreciate mass, firmness or induration	US
Varicocele	Gradual onset of unilateral swelling; often painless	Abnormally enlarged spermatic cord venous plexus (described as a "bag of worms" on palpation)	US
Vasculitis (i.e., HSP)	Testicular swelling and pain	Associated vasculitis findings (such as buttock/lower extremity purpura and renal involvement in case of HSP)	Laboratory evaluation, including renal function tests; may necessitate admission

CBC: complete blood count; CT: computed tomography; CVA: costovertebral angle; ED: emergency department; GU: genitourinary; HSP: Henoch-Schonlein purpura; RLQ: right lower quadrant; US: ultrasound.

Table 31.2 Differentiating characteristics of testicular torsion and epididymitis/epididymo-orchitis

	Testicular torsion	Epididymitis and epididymo-orchitis
Age	Incidence peaks in neonatal and adolescent groups, but may occur at any age	Primarily adolescents and adults
Risk factors	Undescended testicle (neonate), rapid increase in testicular size (adolescent), failure of prior torsion surgical repair	Sexual activity/promiscuity, GU anomalies, GU instrumentation
Pain onset	Sudden	Gradual
Prior episodes of similar pain	Up to 30%	Rare
History of trauma	Possible	Possible
Nausea/vomiting	Common	Rare
Dysuria	Rare	Common
Pyuria	Rare	Common
Fever	Rare	Common in epididymo-orchitis
Location of swelling/tenderness	Testicle, progressing to global involvement	Epididymis, progressing to global involvement
Cremasteric reflex	Absent	Present
Testicle position	High-riding testicle with transverse alignment	Normal position and vertical alignment

GU: genitourinary.

Diagnostic testing

The key to managing acute scrotal pain is the timely recognition of fertility-threatening, testicular viability-threatening or life-threatening conditions. Of the potential diagnoses, recognition of true testicular and scrotal emergencies takes precedence. As testicular torsion produces end-organ ischemia, rapid detorsion (often accomplished in the operating room) must occur in order to prevent subsequent infarction and necrosis. Most routine diagnostic aids (such as blood or urine testing) add little to distinguish between the common etiologies of acute scrotal pain.

Rather, they may actually detract from patient outcome by causing delays in diagnosis. If the history and examination suggest the diagnosis of testicular torsion, immediate urology (or general surgery) consultation and plans for surgical exploration should be obtained without delay. A patient of appropriate age with classic historical and examination findings of testicular torsion does not require diagnostic or confirmatory tests. With less distinct circumstances, a confirmatory radiologic study (ultrasound or radionucleotide imaging) is indicated. In cases of Fournier's disease, delays in recognition and definitive surgical debridement can be life-threatening. Early consultation and administration of broad-spectrum antibiotics is indicated in all suspected cases.

Laboratory studies

Urinalysis

Findings suggestive of a urinary tract infection (pyuria, bacteruria, positive nitrites, positive leukocyte esterase) may be present in cases of epididymitis.

Complete blood count

An elevated systemic white blood cell (WBC) count may be present in cases of inflammation as well as infection. Thus, this finding is rather non-specific and does little to narrow the differential. Moreover, obtaining and awaiting results of such studies often delays diagnosis and definitive management. However, patients with advanced infections (scrotal abscess, epididymo-orchitis and Fournier's disease) may have a markedly elevated WBC count or granulocyte predominance.

Radiologic studies

Ultrasound

A color-flow duplex Doppler ultrasound may be helpful in indeterminate cases of acute scrotal pain. The classic finding suggestive of testicular torsion is diminished intratesticular blood flow (Figure 31.7). In epididymitis, perfusion will be normal (or possibly increased due to the vasodilatory action of inflammatory mediators on local vascular beds). An infarcted appendage may be visualized on ultrasound as well, if appendage torsion is responsible for the painful presentation. Ultrasonography may also identify hydroceles, hematoceles, varicoceles, hernias, tumors, abscesses and gonadal vasculitis.

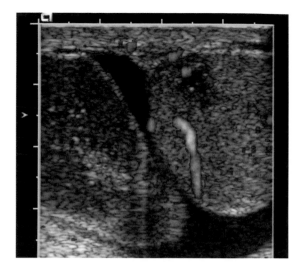

Figure 31.7
Transverse color Doppler sonogram of both testes revealing right testicular torsion. Note enlarged hypoechoic right testis with no intrinsic color flow. Normal flow and echogenicity are seen in left testis. Torsion with infarction of right testis was confirmed surgically.
Courtesy: R. Brooke Jeffrey, MD.

Radionucleotide imaging

Given the widespread availability and expertise with ultrasound technology, and the inherent risks associated with radiation exposure, radionucleotide procedures are falling out of favor at many centers. With this technique, findings suggestive of testicular torsion include diminished radionucleotide uptake due to compromised blood flow. Likewise, appendage torsion and epididymitis result in preserved (or even increased) uptake compared with the unaffected testicle.

Computed tomography

Computed tomography (CT) may be helpful in assessing the degree of extension in cases of GU abscess or Fournier's disease.

General treatment principles

As with any patient presenting to the ED, priorities begin with attention to the airway, breathing and circulation (ABCs). The primary goals of treatment are physiologic stabilization, symptom relief, administration of antibiotics when indicated and, in some cases, preparation for surgical intervention.

Pain relief

Acute scrotal problems encountered in the ED commonly present with a significant (and often distressing) component of pain. The greatest priority is identifying GU pathology that necessitates rapid surgical intervention. Therefore, initial pain relief should be administered intravenously (IV) or intramuscularly (IM) in order to keep the patient ready for possible surgical intervention. Under no circumstances should analgesia be withheld pending consultation. If the likelihood of surgical intervention is low, and the pain is mild to moderate on presentation, a trial of oral medications can be offered. Agents used most frequently are narcotic analgesics, non-steroidal anti-inflammatory drugs (NSAIDs) and acetaminophen. In addition, the pain of testicular torsion may be relieved by *manual detorsion* of the affected testicle. As the testes most frequently torse in a lateral to medial fashion, it follows that detorsion is accomplished by rotation of the affected testicle from medial to lateral. The end point of the detorsion procedure is relief of pain. Scrotal elevation may be beneficial in patients with inflammatory conditions such as epididymitis. This is easily accomplished by a towel roll. In addition, ice may reduce edema and provide a mild degree of analgesia.

Antibiotics

Antimicrobial agents are indicated in cases of suspected or proven infectious processes. Early broad-spectrum antibiotic therapy is imperative in all cases of suspected Fournier's disease. Suggested regimens include extended-spectrum penicillin/beta-lactamase inhibitors (such as ampicillin/sulbactam, ticarcillin/clavulanate, piperacillin/tazobactam), a 3rd generation cephalosporin plus clindamycin, or vancomycin plus flagyl in penicillin-allergic patients. Antibiotics are the cornerstone of therapy for epididymitis. Antimicrobial selection is guided by patient demographics: younger, sexually-active males are treated with agents to cover *Neisseria gonorrhoeae* and *Chlamydia trachomatis*, such as ceftriaxone IM with oral doxycycline, or oral ofloxacin alone. Males older than 35 years are treated with agents such as oral fluoroquinolones to cover common "urinary" pathogens (*Escherichia coli* and *Klebsiella* species) most frequently encountered in this demographic group. Also, consider broader coverage for both coliform and fungal species in males who practice anal-insertive intercourse. Epididymitis may occur in pre-pubescent males.

In this case, the inflammation is often caused by reflux of sterile urine into the epididymis (often the result of minor congenital GU anomalies). Treatment of the resulting "chemical" (non-infectious) inflammation is with prophylactic oral trimethoprim/sulfamethoxazole.

Special patients

Elderly

Evaluation and management of elderly males with acute scrotal pain follows the same guidelines as other patients, with a few notable exceptions. First, accurate historical information may be elusive in patients with age-related cognitive impairment. Also, family members and caretakers may be unaware of complaints and findings associated with a "private" region. In addition, geriatric patients have relatively limited physiologic reserve, which present management challenges (i.e., effects of administered narcotics, antiemetics, IV fluids), challenges in surgical preparation (i.e., need for medical clearance) and diminished resistance to rapid progression of various disease states. Institutionalized or sedentary patients may present with acute symptomotology of chronic GU pathology (such as strangulation of a chronically-incarcerated hernia or coagulopathy-induced bleeding into a hydrocele cavity). An important consideration in any older male patient with testicular discomfort is pain referred from a retroperitoneal process, such as an expanding or ruptured AAA.

Immune compromised

Diabetic and other immunocompromised patients are at increased risk for infections. Be especially wary of Fournier's disease in these patients. Fournier's presents with significant perineal pain (both resting and on palpation of perineal structures) in the absence of notable scrotal skin pathology, termed pain "out of proportion" to physical findings. GU examination revealing scrotal erythema, ecchymoses or subcutaneous emphysema (the result of gas-forming organisms) may indicate end-stage disease.

Pediatric

Evaluation and management of the pediatric population presents unique challenges. Pre-verbal children may be unable to express the location and nature of their pain. Completely undress all patients with an unclear presentation or uncertain diagnoses. In infants, acute scrotal pain from conditions such as testicular torsion may be responsible for inconsolable crying. Also, consider sexual abuse in pre-pubescent males presenting with sexually transmitted infections or GU trauma, such as human "bite" marks or contusions to the scrotum or perineum. In addition, care must be taken to respect and address privacy issues, especially in the adolescent age group. Likewise, parents may be uncomfortable discussing their child's problem. A useful approach to facilitating a more comprehensive history and examination is to first interview, examine and discuss with the teenage male alone, then offer to speak with all parties in concert.

Disposition

There are several urologic emergencies which require immediate evaluation by an appropriate specialist (i.e., urologist or general surgeon) in the ED. Emergent conditions discussed in this chapter include known or suspected cases of testicular torsion, Fournier's disease, and AAA. In addition, maintain a very low threshold for consultation in any case of GU trauma (blunt or penetrating).

Patients with acute scrotal pain who have been ruled-out for conditions necessitating emergent consultation can be referred for urgent primary care or specialty follow-up. Whenever in doubt, err on the side of caution and obtain appropriate consultation while the patient remains in the ED. Another approach is to obtain urgent follow-up in an appropriate clinic by discussing the case with the on-call specialist.

Always address pain issues by providing options for adequate analgesia, whether this includes over-the-counter analgesics or prescription medications. Also, be certain to provide prescriptions for outpatient antimicrobials when indicated.

Patients with unclear diagnoses, intractable pain or vomiting, unreliable follow-up or an unstable social situation may require inpatient management by either a primary care provider (internist, pediatrician, family practitioner) or appropriate specialist.

Pearls, pitfalls, and myths

1. In cases of suspected torsion, emergent specialist consultation is imperative. Remember that "time is testicle," so be careful to avoid "castration by procrastination."

2. Maintain a high index of suspicion for testicular torsion in all age groups, even though its peak incidence occurs in adolescents and neonates.

3. Any asymptomatic testicular mass, firmness or induration is a malignancy until proven otherwise.

4. Ultrasound examination is widely available and extremely useful at differentiating between etiologies of acute testicular pain.

5. The appearance of overt physical findings in Fournier's disease may be a harbinger of terminal disease progression. The hallmark of this disease is pain "out of proportion" to physical findings in any high-risk (i.e., diabetic or other immunocompromised) patient.

6. Always consult a urologist in cases of GU trauma to help guide decision-making and disposition.

References

1. Freeman L. Male genitourinary emergencies: preserving fertility and providing relief. *Emerg Med Prac* 2000;2(11):1–20.
2. Galejs LE, Kass EJ. Diagnosis and treatment of the acute scrotum. *Am Fam Physician* 1999;59(4):817–824.
3. Garmel GM. Non-traumatic male genitourinary emergencies. *Hosp Physic Emerg Med Board Rev Manual* 1998;4(4):1–15.
4. Hals GD, Dietrich T, Ford D. Diagnosis and Emergency Department management of urologic emergencies in the male patient. *Emerg Med Rep* 2002;23(2):17–28.
5. Kadish HA, Bolte RG. A retrospective review of pediatric patients with epididymitis, testicular torsion, and torsion of testicular appendages. *Pediatrics* 1998;100(1):73–76.
6. Kass EJ, Lundak B. The acute scrotum. *Pediatr Clin N Am* 1997;44(5):1251–1266.
7. Knoop KJ, Stack LB, Storrow AB. *Atlas of Emergency Medicine*. McGraw Hill, 1997.
8. Samm BJ, Dmochowski RR. Urologic emergencies – trauma injuries and conditions affecting the penis, scrotum and testicles. *Postgrad Med* 1996;100(4):187–200.
9. Schneider RE. Male genital problems. In: Tintinalli JE et al. (eds). *Emergency Medicine: A Comprehensive Study Guide*, 5th ed., McGraw Hill, 1999;631–640.
10. Swartz MH. *Textbook of Physical Diagnosis, History and Examination*, 3rd ed., WB Saunders, 1998.

32 Seizures

Stephen R. Hayden, MD

Scope of the problem

Seizures are common presenting complaints to the emergency department (ED). One in twenty of the population will have a seizure during their lifetime. This increases to one in eleven if the patient reaches the age of 80 years. Adults presenting to the ED with a first-time seizure account for nearly 1% of ED visits annually. Seizures have a bimodal distribution, declining in older childhood until age 60, when the incidence increases again. Febrile seizures occur in approximately 3% of children and account for approximately 30% of all childhood seizures. Noncompliance with anticonvulsant medications is the most common cause for seizures in adults less than 60 years of age. The most common cause of seizures in the age group over 60 years is stroke, followed by malignancy. The mortality rate from seizures is reported between 1% and 10%. The highest mortality is with status epilepticus. Seizures can cause permanent neurologic sequelae as well.

Pathophysiology

A seizure occurs when there is excessive, abnormal cortical activity. The clinical manifestations depend on the specific area of the brain cortex involved. A distinction is often made between primary and secondary seizures. *Primary seizures* are seizures recurring without consistent provocation or cause. *Secondary seizures* occur as a response to certain toxic, metabolic, or environmental events (Table 32.1). *Generalized seizures* occur from an electrical event that simultaneously involves both cerebral hemispheres and is accompanied by loss of consciousness. These can be convulsive (grand mal seizures) or nonconvulsive (absence seizures). *Partial seizures* involve one cerebral hemisphere, and can be divided further into those in which consciousness is maintained (simple partial), and those in which consciousness is abnormal (complex partial).

Proposed mechanisms for a seizure include the disruption of normal anatomical cortex structure or disruption of local metabolic or biochemical function of neuronal cells. Either of these mechanisms can produce sustained depolarization of neuronal cells, creating an ictogenic focus, followed by recruitment of adjacent cells. When the electrical discharge extends below the cortex to the reticular activating system, consciousness may become impaired. Most commonly, seizures

Table 32.1 Etiology of secondary seizures

Metabolic causes
- Hypoglycemia
- Hyponatremia/hypernatremia
- Hypocalcemia/hypomagnesemia
- Renal failure/dialysis complications
- High anion gap acidosis
- Thyroid disease

Infectious causes
- Meningitis
- Encephalitis
- CNS abscess
- HIV disease
- Syphilis
- Toxoplasmosis
- Neurocysticercosis

Degenerative CNS disease
- Alzheimer's disease
- Neurofibromatosis
- Tuberous sclerosis
- Multiple sclerosis

Drugs and toxins
- Noncompliance with anticonvulsants
- Withdrawal of EtOH/sedative/hypnotic
- Cocaine
- Methamphetamines
- PCP
- Anticholinergic agents (including tricyclic antidepressants)
- Salicylates
- Lithium

Anatomic causes
- Post-traumatic
- CNS neoplasms
- CNS vasculitis (SLE, polyarteritis)
- Arteriovenous malformation
- CVA (stroke)

Miscellaneous causes
- Febrile seizures
- Eclampsia
- Cerebral arterial gas embolism
- Pseudoseizures

CNS: central nervous system; CVA: cerebrovascular accident; EtOH: ethanol; HIV: human immunodeficiency virus; PCP: phencyclidine; SLE: systemic lupus erythematosus.

are self-limited with the sustained electrical activity resolving spontaneously. *Status epilepticus* is defined when the abnormal electrical activity is sustained for more than 30–60 minutes without an opportunity for recovery between seizure episodes, which may occur with any type of seizure.

History

Do you have a prior history of seizures?

The work-up for a patient with an established seizure disorder differs significantly from a patient who presents with a first-time seizure. New onset seizures require a more extensive work-up to evaluate for conditions identified in Table 32.1.

How long did the seizure last? How many seizures did you have?

This information may need to come from witnesses of the event. It may be helpful to ask the patient "What is the last thing you remember clearly before the event?," and "What is the very next thing you remember clearly after the event?" This may give an estimate of the elapsed time. The duration of the event and whether the seizures were recurrent provide important information to assess the severity of the seizure. Seizures that last more than 30 minutes, or recur without clearing of mental status between successive seizures, define *status epilepticus.*

Has there been a recent change in your seizure pattern?

A significant change in seizure pattern would require a work-up similar to that for first-time seizures.

Did you hit your head prior to having a seizure?

It is important to distinguish between a patient who sustains head trauma followed by a seizure from a patient who has a seizure, then falls and has head trauma. Even in patients with known seizure disorders, there is higher incidence of significant abnormalities on head computed tomography (CT) in those who hit their head first and immediately have a seizure.

What medications are you taking?

Many medications are associated with seizures at toxic doses. Furthermore, it is important to know if the patient is taking any anti-seizure medications in order to assess medication levels. Noncompliance with anticonvulsants is the most common cause of recurrent seizures in known epileptics. Use of anticoagulants such as coumadin increases suspicion for intracranial bleeding.

Did you have an aura or premonition prior to the event?

Many patients will describe symptoms of paresthesias, flashing lights, or other visual symptoms immediately prior to having a seizure.

Do you remember what you were doing immediately preceding your loss of consciousness?

Retrograde amnesia of activities preceding the event is more indicative of a seizure.

Did you bite your tongue? Were you incontinent of urine?

These are important questions to ask as these findings are more likely associated with a seizure.

How long did you feel confused after the event?

A postictal period of around 30 minutes is not unusual after a seizure. If possible, obtain history from the paramedics or other witnesses of the event. Try to determine if tonic or clonic motor activity occurred, if the patient maintained consciousness during the event, and if there was focality to the neurologic symptoms.

Do you drink daily, regularly, or heavily?

If the answer to any of these is yes, then ask *"When was your last drink?"* Seizures are a common manifestation of alcohol withdrawal. Furthermore, patients who drink regularly are at greater risk for falls resulting in chronic subdural hematomas or hyponatremia.

Do you use street/recreational drugs?

Common drugs of abuse such as cocaine, crystal methamphetamine, phencyclidine (PCP), and ecstasy may induce seizures.

Associated symptoms

Associated symptoms often include hypertension, tachycardia, muscle soreness, and headache. Elicit symptoms of pain or soreness after the seizure. A posterior shoulder dislocation, often not discovered until several days after the event, is commonly missed following a prolonged tonic–clonic seizure.

Past medical

It is important to ascertain a prior history of renal or liver disease, malignancy, diabetes, cardiovascular disease, hypertension, human immunodeficiency virus (HIV) risk factors, drug or alcohol abuse, recent trauma, degenerative central nervous system (CNS) diseases, prior neurosurgery, psychiatric history, family history of seizures, and pregnancy, as they all are associated with secondary seizures.

Physical examination

The primary purpose of the physical examination is to evaluate for focal neurologic deficits or other signs that might suggest a secondary cause for seizures.

General appearance

Many times the physical examination is normal in the seizure patient. Of primary importance in the immediate postictal period is to evaluate whether the patient is adequately protecting the airway. Level of consciousness will often be depressed; therefore, evaluate and maintain patency of the airway. On occasion, patients may bleed profusely from oral trauma, requiring that the airway be secured. Also take note if the patient was incontinent of urine, as this may support the diagnosis of a seizure.

The postictal state is often characterized by decreased responsiveness, disorientation, amnesia, and headache. The mental status examination should slowly improve over time, ranging from a few moments to an hour or more. This may not be consistent between patients or even between seizures in the same patient. If mental status does not improve appropriately, this should prompt further investigation. Some patients in nonconvulsive status are mistakenly assumed to be postictal instead of actively seizing.

Vital signs

Following a seizure, patients are frequently hypertensive, tachycardic, tachypneic, and may have lowered oxygen saturation. These abnormalities should improve as the patient recovers. Mild hyperthermia may occur, but a significantly elevated temperature or persistently abnormal vital signs should prompt further investigation for a secondary cause of the seizure.

Head and neck

Head and neck examination should focus on identifying signs of head trauma such as cephalohematoma, depressed skull fracture, lacerations and abrasions, and hemotympanum. Pupils should be evaluated for reactivity and symmetry, and cranial nerve abnormalities should be sought. Anisocoria may suggest impending herniation through the foramen magnum. Nystagmus, especially rotary, is associated with certain drugs such as PCP. Persistent eye deviation may indicate ongoing seizure activity. The oropharynx must be examined for signs of oral trauma. The presence of a bite mark to the lateral tongue strongly suggests that a seizure occurred. The finding of oral thrush may suggest that the patient is immunocompromised. *Automatisms* (repetitive actions such as lip smacking, swallowing, or chewing) are frequent in complex partial seizures and may be the only indication of ongoing seizure activity. The cervical spine should be palpated for midline tenderness or deformity. If there is no evidence of neck trauma, the neck should be evaluated for meningismus.

Pulmonary

Pulmonary examination should assess symmetry and character of breath sounds, looking for aspiration that may have occurred during the seizure. Neurogenic pulmonary edema can occur following a seizure, but is usually mild and self-limited. It is characterized by diffuse crackles, hypoxia, and the absence of signs of congestive heart failure.

Cardiovascular

Cardiac examination may reveal a heart murmur and might indicate subacute bacterial endocarditis (SBE) with resultant embolization as the cause of the seizure. An irregular heart rate or carotid bruits may accompany a stroke, which is a common cause of new-onset seizures in the elderly.

Neurologic

A detailed neurologic examination must be performed. The patient should be carefully assessed for focal motor or sensory deficits, and abnormalities of cerebellar function. Postictal paralysis (Todd's paralysis) may follow generalized or partial seizures. This is typically characterized by weakness of one extremity or complete hemiparesis. Symptoms may persist for up to 24 hours. Todd's paralysis indicates a higher likelihood of an underlying structural cause for the seizure, and should therefore be investigated. Tremulousness of the extremities and tongue, in conjunction with other stigmata of ethanol abuse, suggest an alcohol withdrawal seizure.

Extremities

Examination of the extremities may demonstrate evidence of trauma. Particular attention should be paid to identifying shoulder dislocations (seizures are a common cause of posterior shoulder dislocations).

Skin

The skin should be examined for lesions consistent with infections, such as meningococcemia or SBE (splinter hemorrhages, Janeway lesions, Osler's nodes). Evidence of underlying liver disease or coagulopathy should be sought. Similarly, skin lesions such as axillary freckling, café au lait spots, port wine nevi, or subcutaneous nodules may indicate a neurocutaneous disorder. Needle tracks indicate IV drug use, which may indicate a toxicologic or infectious etiology for seizures.

Differential diagnosis

Even when witnessed, other abnormal states of consciousness can produce twitching or jerking movements that can be difficult to distinguish from a seizure. In 40–50% of cases of vasovagal syncope (fainting), brief twitching movements occur. Generally the tonic or clonic movements associated with a seizure are much more forceful and prolonged, and associated with a postictal state, urinary incontinence, and tongue biting that does not typically occur in fainting.

Other causes of sudden loss of consciousness that resemble a seizure include hyperventilation syndrome, prolonged breath-holding spells in infants, numerous toxic and metabolic states, transient ischemic attack (TIA)/cerebrovascular accident (CVA), narcolepsy, and causes of syncope (Table 32.2). Extrapyramidal reactions,

Table 32.2 Differential diagnosis of seizure

Diagnosis	Classic symptoms	Signs	Work-up
Breath-holding spells in infants	Usually brought on by anger, fear, frustration Pallor or cyanotic spells Apnea or bradycardia	Normal neurologic examination	ECG to check QT interval EEG during spells
Extrapyramidal reactions	Tongue deviation Torticollis Jerking, random limb movements History of taking phenothiazines/butyrophenones	Level of consciousness usually maintained	Clinical diagnosis in setting of taking specific medications
Hyperventilation syndrome	Shortness of breath followed by paresthesias, carpopedal spasm and loss of consciousness	Increased respiratory rate Normal neurologic examination	Typically clinical diagnosis, ABG may be useful
Psychogenic seizures	May closely mimic symptoms of true seizure Often in the setting of emotional distress	Usually quick return to normal mental status post-event	Continuous EEG monitoring during events
TIA/CVA	Sudden onset of weakness, difficulty speaking, or walking	Abnormal neurologic findings	Head CT, ECG, laboratories
Vasovagal syncope	Brief twitching movements Classic prodrome of lightheadedness, tunnel vision	No postictal state Lack of tongue biting	ECG, glucose testing, pregnancy test

ABG: arterial blood gas; CT: computed tomography; CVA: cerebrovascular accident; ECG: electrocardiogram; EEG: electroencephalogram; TIA: transient ischemic attack.

especially in children, may be confused with seizure activity. Psychogenic states, in particular pseudoseizures, may be difficult to differentiate from true seizure activity. Continuous EEG monitoring during such episodes may be necessary to make a correct diagnosis.

Diagnostic testing

The diagnostic work-up for patients presenting to the ED with seizures depends on whether it was a first-time seizure, what underlying conditions the patient may have, and whether a clear seizure precipitant (hypoglycemia, hypoxia, intoxication, withdrawal state) is identified (Figure 32.1).

Laboratory studies

Complete blood count

The complete blood count (CBC) is rarely useful in a seizure patient. The white blood cell (WBC) count is often elevated from demargination during the seizure. However, a CBC is often ordered in patients presenting with a seizure when the mental status is not returning to normal, the patient has HIV or is immunosuppressed (to determine the absolute neutrophil count), and in patients with platelet disorders or coagulation abnormalities. In febrile patients, including young children with a febrile seizure, a CBC may be ordered as part of the evaluation for the underlying source of infection.

Electrolytes

Electrolytes, especially sodium, calcium, and magnesium, are indicated for patients with a first-time seizure, or alcoholics who likely have nutritional deficiencies. Additionally, any patient in which the mental status is not returning to normal after a seizure should have electrolytes checked as part of the work-up. Children less than 1 year of age who have had a seizure in the absence of fever should also have electrolytes checked.

Glucose

All patients presenting with a seizure should have rapid glucose determination performed.

Cerebrospinal fluid analysis

A lumbar puncture (LP) is indicated in a seizure patient when the mental status fails to return to normal after seizure, if a subarachnoid hemorrhage is suspected (sudden onset of worst headache in conjunction with a seizure), or when a CNS infection is suspected (patients with fever, headache, or stiff neck). In addition, cerebrospinal fluid (CSF) analysis may be helpful for HIV or immunocompromised patients who are at risk for opportunistic CNS infections that may only be diagnosed by analyzing the CSF. CSF analysis may also be helpful for the evaluation of a febrile infant who has had a seizure. Traditionally, an LP was recommended for a febrile seizure in the age group less than 12 months. However, newer evidence-based guidelines suggest that for infants with a febrile seizure, if the infant otherwise appears well and there is no history of recent antibiotic use, a routine LP is not indicated. If the child appears ill, or the mental status is not returning to normal, an LP should be performed.

Anticonvulsant levels

Anticonvulsant levels are indicated in seizure patients who report taking medications for which a therapeutic level can be determined.

Toxicology screening

Toxicology screening should be performed when the mental status is not returning to normal after a seizure. In the setting of specific toxic exposures for which toxin levels can be determined (e.g., carbon monoxide), toxicologic screening may also be useful. For first-time seizures, if the patient can provide an appropriate history, routine toxicology screening is of little value.

Creatine phosphokinase

Creatine phosphokinase (CPK) levels may be important to determine in patients with status epilepticus, seizures resulting from toxic ingestions (especially sympathomimetics), or a prolonged downtime before coming to the ED.

Pregnancy testing

Pregnancy testing should be performed in any woman of childbearing age in whom the mental status does not return to baseline after the seizure. Additionally, pregnancy testing may be performed prior to initiating any new medications if there is a possibility the patient may be pregnant.

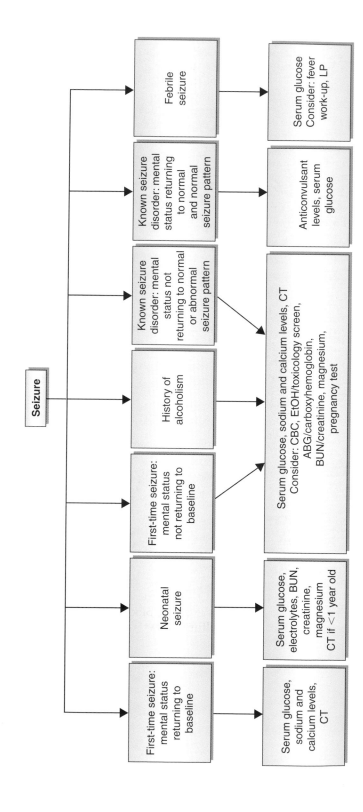

Figure 32.1

Algorithm for the evaluation of the patient with seizures. Adapted from Bradford JC, Kyriakedes CG. Evaluation of the patient with seizures: an evidence based approach. *Emerg Med Clin North Am* 1999; 17(1):203–220. ABG: arterial blood gas; BUN: blood urea nitrogen; CBC: complete blood count; CT: computed tomography; EtOH: ethanol; LP: lumbar puncture.

Coagulation

Coagulation studies should be performed if the patient with a seizure has a known coagulation disorder, is on anticoagulant medication, or has any condition that might be expected to alter coagulation parameters (i.e., liver disease or alcoholism).

Radiologic studies

Computed tomography

CT should be performed in any patient with a first-time seizure, a patient in whom the mental status fails to return to normal post-seizure, in the setting of neonatal seizures without fever, seizures following head trauma, patients with coagulation disorders or on anticoagulants, malignancy, or patients with an abnormal neurologic examination. Appropriate timing of the head CT is discussed in a subsequent section.

Other studies

An electroencephalogram (EEG) can be performed as part of the work-up of a seizure as an outpatient for first-time seizures, or more emergently at the bedside when the mental status does not return to normal (to evaluate for nonconvulsive status epilepticus). EEG is necessary in the setting of refractory status epilepticus requiring general anesthesia and paralysis or barbiturate coma.

An electrocardiogram (ECG) should be performed if the seizure is believed to be due to drug or toxin exposure, or if the patient has underlying comorbid conditions that increase the risk of coronary artery disease or dysrhythmias.

Summary of diagnostic considerations for certain types of seizures

For *first-time seizures* without an obvious cause, with mental status returning to normal, current evidence-based guidelines suggest that serum glucose, sodium and calcium levels be obtained, and a head CT be performed. An LP needs to be performed only if an adult has a fever without an obvious source, or to evaluate for possible subarachnoid hemorrhage. The question arises whether the head CT needs to be performed during the ED visit. The decision must be based on the patient's current condition, access to medical care, reliability of follow-up and their ability to understand the nature of their medical condition and follow-up instructions. It is often expeditious to perform a head CT in the ED. If the mental status does not return to normal, then the above work-up should also include a CBC, alcohol/toxicology screening, blood urea nitrogen (BUN)/ creatinine, magnesium level, ECG, pregnancy test, and arterial blood gas (ABG)/carboxyhemoglobin level if clinically warranted. In this case, a head CT should be performed urgently in the ED. Although unlikely, an EEG may be performed if available.

For patients with a *known seizure disorder*, typical seizure pattern, and mental status returning to normal, rapid glucose testing and serum anticonvulsant levels are recommended. For a known seizure patient that has an abnormal seizure pattern or mental status that does not return to normal, the work-up is the same as for a first-time seizure patient whose mental status is not returning to normal.

For a known *alcoholic* in whom an alcohol withdrawal seizure is suspected and mental status is returning to baseline, rapid glucose determination and anticonvulsant levels may be performed if the patient takes such medications. Routine laboratory testing is usually unnecessary unless performed for a more generalized health status evaluation or if the patient has significant comorbidities. If there is concomitant evidence of head trauma, a head CT is indicated. If the mental status is not returning to normal, the work-up should proceed as for a first-time seizure patient whose mental status is not returning to normal.

Febrile seizures in the pediatric population are relatively common occurrences, especially if there is a history of febrile seizures in a first-degree relative. For an otherwise healthy, well-appearing child with a febrile seizure, serum glucose testing should be obtained, and other diagnostic tests to evaluate for an occult source of fever (CBC, blood cultures, urinalysis (UA) and culture, chest radiography, and stool studies) should be considered. Traditionally, some authorities have recommended LP for children less than 12 months old, and as an option in children less than 18 months. *Current evidence-based guidelines, however, do not recommend routine LP for febrile seizures unless the patient has a history of recent antibiotic use.* If a child appears ill or mental status is not improving after the febrile seizure, a comprehensive fever work-up including LP is warranted in addition to consideration for the tests outlined for a first-time seizure patient whose mental status is not returning to normal.

Neonatal seizures without fever need to have a variety of diagnostic tests performed, including serum glucose, electrolytes, BUN/creatinine, calcium/magnesium levels, and head CT if the child is less than 1 year old.

A number of conditions deserve special consideration in the setting of a seizure. If the patient has a history or findings of coagulopathy, platelet disorders, or is taking anticoagulant medication, the work-up should include a CBC, coagulation studies, and head CT. In patients with history of renal failure, BUN/creatinine and electrolytes should be tested. Patients who are known or suspected HIV positive or immunosuppressed should have a CBC, head CT, and LP performed. For toxic exposures or ingestions, consider an ECG, specific drug, alcohol, and acetaminophen/salicylate levels, and toxicology screens. Patients with a history of malignancy or recent head trauma should have a head CT performed.

General treatment principles

Status epilepticus

Status epilepticus is a life-threatening emergency with potential for airway compromise, severe hypoxia, and neurologic injury. Whether the seizure activity is continuous or recurrent without clearing of the mental state, assume the airway is compromised. Active measures should be taken to secure it. Placing the patient in the left lateral decubitus position, removing dentures, and carefully suctioning vomit and saliva are appropriate initial steps. If the airway cannot be adequately protected by these simple measures, endotracheal intubation may be necessary. A rapid-acting benzodiazepine (such as midazolam) is a good choice as the induction agent, as it may terminate seizure activity. If tonic activity or trismus prevents adequate opening of the mouth, paralytics may be necessary. Bear in mind that once the patient is paralyzed, tonic–clonic activity will cease but the abnormal cortical neuronal activity may continue (i.e., the patient continues to seize without the muscular activity). Second- or third-line anticonvulsants may be necessary, and EEG monitoring will be required as soon as practical.

Status epilepticus is often the result of a secondary cause for seizures (Table 32.1). These conditions may be rapidly reversible and must be diagnosed early and corrected immediately (i.e., hypoglycemia, hyponatremia, and hypoxia). Structural abnormalities (i.e., subarachnoid or intracranial hemorrhage) and toxic states may be present; these conditions should be considered early and appropriate management instituted (e.g., isoniazid (INH) overdose would be managed with pyridoxine). Concomitant with the work-up for these diseases, abortive therapy may be instituted using the medications indicated below.

Pharmacologic abortive seizure therapy

In general, the first-line medication for terminating seizure activity in the ED is intravenous (IV) or intramuscular (IM) benzodiazepines (Table 32.3). IV access must be established if not already accomplished. It should be noted that diazepam can be administered via an endotracheal tube, rectally, or through an interosseus line. Benzodiazepines enhance gamma amino butyric acid (GABA)-mediated inhibition and are effective in terminating seizures in 80–90% of cases. Diazepam, lorazepam, and midazolam are common medications used in the ED to abort seizures because of their rapid onset and efficacy. There have been no compelling studies in an ED population that clearly establish the superiority of one of these medications over the other.

Common second-line pharmacologic agents used in the ED for seizures include phenytoin (or the pro-phenytoin drug fosphenytoin) and phenobarbital. Phenytoin suppresses neuronal recruitment around the seizure focus. The propylene glycol diluent with phenytoin may cause hypotension and cardiac dysrhythmias if administered too rapidly IV. Fosphenytoin can be administered quickly IV without deleterious effect, and has the additional advantage of IM administration if IV access is a problem. The cost differential, however, may keep fosphenytoin from replacing phenytoin as a second-line agent. Phenobarbital is a CNS depressant that decreases neuronal electrical activity at the seizure focus as well as terminates recruitment. Most experience with phenobarbital as a second-line agent to terminate seizures is in the pediatric population. Barbiturates have the adverse effects of significant sedation, hypotension, and respiratory depression; therefore, patients must be monitored closely.

If seizure activity is not suppressed by the above measures, additional therapeutic options in the ED include using valproate, barbiturate coma, or

Table 32.3 Pharmacologic treatment of seizures

Drug	Adult dose	Pediatric dose
Diazepam	5–10 mg IV every 5–10 minutes	0.2–0.5 mg/kg IV/PR/ETT/IO
Lorazepam	2–4 mg IV every 5–10 minutes	0.05–0.1 mg/kg IV (maximum 4 mg)
Midazolam	2.5–15 mg IV or IM (unpredictable absorption IM)	0.15 mg/kg IV then drip 2–10 mcg/kg/minute or 0.15 mg/kg IM (unpredictable absorption)
Phenytoin	1 gm IV load at 50 mg/minute	20 mg/kg IV at 1 mg/kg/minute
Fosphenytoin	15–20 mg PE/kg IV/IM single loading dose	10–20 mg PE/kg IV/IM single loading dose
Phenobarbital	10–20 mg/kg IV at 60–100 mg/minute	10–20 mg/kg IV × 1, then 5–10 mg/kg IV every 15–30 minutes
Pentobarbital	10–15 mg/kg IV first 1–2 hours then 1 mg/kg/hour IV	10–15 mg/kg IV first 1–2 hours then 1 mg/kg/hour IV
Valproate	20 mg/kg PR or 15 mg/kg IV (maximum 250 mg)	20 mg/kg PR or 15 mg/kg IV (maximum 250 mg)

ETT: endotracheal tube; IM: intramuscular; IO: interosseous; IV: intravenous; PE: phenytoin equivalents; PR: per rectum.

general inhalational anesthesia. Valproate may be administered rectally, and a parenteral form exists (Depacon). A recent meta-analysis, however, found that there are certain risks associated with IV Depacon, including neurotoxicity, and it must be administered over 60 minutes. This review concluded that the evidence is too limited to routinely recommend IV valproate unless it is not desirable to induce a barbiturate coma or begin inhalational anesthesia.

The typical agent used to induce barbiturate coma is pentobarbital. Pentobarbital suppresses all cortical neuronal activity, decreases intracranial pressure (ICP), and increases cerebral perfusion. It also induces respiratory depression/arrest and causes hypotension, so patients must be intubated and monitored closely.

Isoflurane inhalational anesthesia is another option for seizure activity that does not respond to first- or second-line agents, or treatment for underlying conditions. Isoflurane suppresses electrical seizure foci and is titratable. It is preferred that patients are intubated to protect their airway before instituting isoflurane anesthesia to terminate seizures. Inhalational anesthesia is usually reserved for patients admitted to the intensive care unit (ICU) or operating room unless there will be a significant delay in transferring the patient to these settings.

Special patients
Pediatric

The work-up of a child with a febrile seizure has been discussed. Remember that febrile seizures are associated more with the rapidity of temperature rise, not the absolute temperature. In determining what work-up to do for a child with febrile seizure, the clinician should be guided by the general appearance of the child, and consider the underlying cause of the fever. Generally, anticonvulsant therapy is not instituted for simple febrile seizures. It is important to educate parents on appropriate temperature control measures, including alternating doses of acetaminophen (15–20 mg/kg/dose orally (PO) or per rectum (PR) every 4–6 hours) and ibuprofen (5–10 mg/kg/dose PO every 4–6 hours). Additionally, the child can have frequent sponge baths with tepid water, as this is a very effective cooling measure.

In children with afebrile seizures, many of the same diagnostic and therapeutic considerations are present as with adults. Two special causes of childhood seizures are worth mentioning. The first is the "morning after" seizure caused by drinking alcohol left within reach of children at a party, leading to hypoglycemia and seizures. Another cause of hypoglycemia-induced seizures in children is

Table 32.4 Pediatric seizures in children

Seizure type	Clinical findings	Work-up and management
Febrile seizure	Age less than 5 years Well appearing Lack of signs of serious bacterial illness Normal neurologic examination	CBC, blood cultures, UA, CXR if indicated to evaluate for underlying infection LP if recent antibiotic course (some recommend LP routinely for age <1 year)
Morning after seizure	Ambulatory child drinks leftover alcohol from a party and becomes hypoglycemic and seizes	History is key, parental education
Ketotic hypoglycemia	Children 6–18 months Periods of caloric deprivation lead to profound hypoglycemia	Rapid glucose testing Urine dipstick for ketones Consider chemistry panel
Absence seizures	Staring episodes Automatisms Appear awake but are not responsive No postictal period	Electrolytes, glucose Head CT (or MRI) EEG
Infantile spasms	History of congenital abnormality or perinatal brain injury Myoclonic seizures in clusters Development delay Age less than 1 year	Head CT (or MRI) Electrolytes, glucose EEG (high voltage chaotic slowing, hypsarrythmia)
Status epilepticus	Seizure activity for >30 minutes Series of seizures, mental status does not return to normal between events	Head CT, electrolytes, glucose, CBC, toxicology screening, ECG and EEG

CBC: complete blood count; CT: computed tomography; CXR: chest X-ray; ECG: electrocardiogram;
EEG: electroencephalogram; LP: lumbar puncture; MRI: magnetic resonance imaging; UA: urinalysis.

ketotic hypoglycemia. Periods of caloric depriva-tion cause abnormally low blood glucose levels and seizures. This occurs in young children between 6 and 18 months of age when the inter-val between feedings is increased. The diagnosis is suggested in the ED when typical symptoms occur, and hypoglycemia and ketonuria are pres-ent (Table 32.4).

Alcoholic

Chronic alcohol use stimulates GABA enhance-ment. Alcohol withdrawal seizures may have onset 6 hours or more after abrupt cessation of drinking. They are typically generalized and recurrent. With each episode of alcohol cessation, the seizure threshold may decrease, increasing the risk and severity of seizures. Other symp-toms include those associated with autonomic instability, such as tachycardia, hypertension, mild hyperthermia, and CNS activation includ-ing tremor and jerking movements. If the patient's mental status is significantly altered or confused, *delirium tremens* ensues. This carries a mortality rate as high as 20–30% in some series.

Alcoholics are at risk for other secondary causes of seizures, such as hypoglycemia, intracranial bleeding, other drugs/toxins, and electrolyte disturbances (especially hypomagnesemia or hypocalcemia). Treatment of alcohol withdrawal seizures includes benzodiazepines (often in high doses), which substitute for the GABA-enhancing effect of ethanol. Most patients with alcohol withdrawal seizures do not need second-line treatments such as phenytoin.

Pregnant

Seizures in pregnancy are generally of two cat-egories: *gestational,* in which underlying seizure disorder or anticonvulsant levels are adversely impacted by hormonal and metabolic changes of pregnancy; and *eclampsia,* which is associated with hypertensive encephalopathy, proteinuria, edema, and seizures. Eclampsia generally occurs after the 20th week of pregnancy. The likelihood decreases after delivery, though seizures may occur days to weeks after delivery. It may not be obvious, however, that a woman is more than 20 weeks pregnant, so all women of childbearing age presenting in status epilepticus should be evaluated for pregnancy. The treatment of seizures in the setting of eclampsia is controversial; specialists in obstetrics or perinatology should be consulted early. In addition to the same management considerations for patients in status epilepticus previously outlined, high-dose parenteral magnesium sulfate therapy (4 g IV bolus followed by 2 g/hour infusion) has traditionally been used to help control seizure symptoms. Careful monitoring of respiratory status and reflexes is essential when giving magnesium.

Cerebral arterial gas embolism (CAGE)

When the cerebral circulation is showered with air bubbles, a common manifestation is the abrupt onset of a seizure. In self-contained underwater breathing apparatus (SCUBA) divers, rapid ascent from depth while holding their breath may lead to pulmonary overinflation, tear of the bronchoalveolar sheath and air entering the pulmonary venous system, return of air to the left side of the heart and systemic embolization of air bubbles. The hallmark of cerebral arterial gas embolism (CAGE) is the abrupt loss of consciousness with the onset of seizures or other neurologic symptoms upon surfacing. On the other hand, decompression sickness typically has a latent period before the development of neurologic symptoms and does not usually present with seizures. Other causes of CAGE include pulmonary overinflation from positive pressure ventilation, air entry during catheterization or other vascular procedures, brain surgery, cardiac surgery, and cardiopulmonary bypass. There have even been reports of CAGE from inhaling directly from a helium tank and vaginal insufflation during pregnancy. The abrupt appearance of any new neurologic symptoms, including seizures, during any of the above activities or procedures should prompt investigation for pulmonary overinflation injury and CAGE. The definitive treatment for CAGE is hyperbaric oxygen therapy. The patient should be placed on 100% oxygen until arrangements can be made with the hyperbaric consulting service.

Pseudoseizures

It can be difficult at times to differentiate between true seizures and pseudoseizures. Events often occur in the setting of emotional distress. Pseudoseizures are characterized by palpitations, choking sensations, dizziness, malaise, sensory disturbances, crying, and alterations in consciousness with or without motor manifestations. Unlike true seizures, motor activity generally consists of side-to-side head movements, opisthotonus, pelvis thrusting, trembling, and random asynchronous movements. Urinary incontinence and postictal somnolence may occur; however, the postictal period is often short. Pseudoseizures tend to be more gradual in evolution and longer in duration. Some patients can be very skilled at mimicking the tonic–clonic activity of a seizure. In a few cases, patients can be startled out of pseudoseizure activity or may respond to noxious stimuli such as ammonia capsules. Ultimately, pseudoseizures are diagnosed when normal EEG activity is documented during apparent seizure activity.

Disposition

Patients with status epilepticus, mental status examinations that do not return to normal, or seizures associated with serious underlying medical conditions should be admitted to a monitored setting and given first- and often second-line medications to suppress seizures. Most other seizure patients can be managed in the outpatient setting, with close follow-up and support from family or friends.

Patients with a first-time seizure in whom the work-up does not identify a serious underlying medical condition can be discharged with close follow-up. The question arises whether to institute anticonvulsant therapy after a first-time seizure. Factors that increase the risk of recurrent seizures include EEG abnormalities (though this diagnostic test is infrequently obtained in the ED), partial versus generalized seizures, recurrent seizures in the ED, history of intracranial surgery or head trauma, and persistent neurologic abnormality such as Todd's paralysis. These patients might be candidates for initiating seizure medications after a first episode. This is often done in consultation with an on-call neurologist or the patients' primary care provider, if available.

The side effects of anticonvulsants are numerous; some patients cannot tolerate them, and many drug interactions may occur. In the absence of factors that are likely to predict recurrent seizures, and if provoking factors are easily managed (i.e., hypoglycemia), anticonvulsant therapy after a first-time seizure is not indicated. In patients with a known seizure disorder, anticonvulsant levels should be checked and managed appropriately in consultation with the physician responsible for those medications, if possible.

Many states have mandatory reporting laws for any episode of sudden lapse of consciousness, including seizures. Physicians should follow state laws regarding this, and advise patients not to drive or engage in activities that might be hazardous if a seizure were to recur. It is reasonable to document that this activity was reported.

Pearls, pitfalls, and myths

- The most common cause of recurrent primary seizures is subtherapeutic anticonvulsant levels; check anticonvulsant levels in a patient with a history of seizures.
- Since the most common cause of secondary seizures is hypoglycemia, rapid glucose determination is important for all seizure patients.
- Benzodiazepines are the first-line treatment for seizures or status epilepticus in the ED. They can be administered via multiple routes.
- Urgent neuroimaging is recommended for patients with first-time seizures, suspicion of head trauma or increased ICP, intracranial mass or history of cancer, persistently abnormal mental status, focal neurologic deficit, underlying HIV or other immunocompromising diseases, or in patients taking anticoagulant medications.
- For otherwise healthy, well-appearing children with a febrile seizure, some authorities recommend LP for all children less than 12 months old; however, current evidence-based guidelines suggest that an LP is necessary only if there is clinical suspicion for a CNS infection, or if the child has a history of recent antibiotic use.
- It is not always easy to distinguish a seizure from syncope. Seizure activity is suggested by retrograde amnesia, preceding aura, bowel or bladder incontinence, tongue biting, and a prolonged postictal state.

- Alcoholics are at higher risk of falls, electrolyte abnormalities, and hypoglycemia. Patients with alcohol withdrawal and a seizure must be carefully evaluated for these secondary conditions before concluding that the seizure is simply the result of the withdrawal state.
- Patients that have required intubation and neuromuscular blockade may still be seizing at the neuronal level. Further investigation must be performed to determine if seizure activity continues, such as a bedside EEG.
- The appearance of new neurologic symptoms or seizure activity in a SCUBA diver, a patient who is intubated on positive-pressure ventilation, or after vascular procedures should prompt investigation for CAGE.
- Follow mandatory reporting laws for all patients experiencing any episode of loss of consciousness, including a seizure.

References

1. American College of Emergency Physicians. Clinical policy for the initial approach to patients presenting with a chief complaint of seizure who are not in status epilepticus. *Ann Emerg Med* 1997; 29:706–724.
2. Bradford JC, Kyriakedes CG. Evaluation of the patient with seizures: an evidence based approach. *Emerg Med Clin North Am* 1999; 17(1): 03–220.
3. David P, Smith-Coggins R. Seizure, adult. In: Rosen, et al. (eds). *The Five Minute Emergency Medicine Consult*. Philadelphia, PA: Lippincott Williams & Wilkins, 1999. pp. 1018–1019.
4. Pollack CV, Pollack ES. Seizures. In: Marx JA, et al. (eds). *Rosen's Emergency Medicine*, 5th ed., St. Louis, MO: Mosby, 2002. pp. 1445–1456.
5. Upshaw GL. Seizure, pediatric. In: Rosen, et al. (eds). *The Five Minute Emergency Medicine Consult*. Philadelphia, PA: Lippincott Williams & Wilkins, 1999. pp. 1020–1021.

33 Shortness of breath in adults

Sharon E. Mace, MD

Scope of the problem

Dyspnea is the perception of uncomfortable breathing and is synonymous with the terms "shortness of breath" or "breathlessness." Other terms patients may use to describe dyspnea include "labored," "heavy," "difficult," or "uncomfortable" breathing. Dyspneic patients often say they feel like they are being smothered, cannot catch their breath, or are unable to get enough air.

Dyspnea is a symptom associated with many disorders, from nonurgent to life-threatening. Like the perception of pain, dyspnea is subjective and its severity does not necessarily correlate with the seriousness of the underlying pathology.

The chief complaint "shortness of breath" is encountered in about 3% of all emergency department (ED) patients. Approximately two-thirds of these patients have an underlying cardiac or pulmonary disorder. Specific data on the general prevalence of dyspnea is not available, although in the Framingham study, 6–27% of the adult population reported experiencing dyspnea. In some patient populations (e.g., oncology patients), the prevalence of dyspnea may be much higher.

Pathophysiology

In general, breathing is a well-synchronized, unconscious, quiet and effortless process. Dyspnea results when ventilatory demand exceeds respiratory function. Although the exact mechanism responsible for dyspnea is unknown, abnormalities or alterations of gas exchange, pulmonary circulation, cardiovascular function, respiratory mechanics, or the oxygen (O_2) carrying capacity of blood may result in dyspnea.

Respirations are generally "automatic" and under the control of the respiratory centers in the central nervous system (CNS) (e.g., medulla/pons). Respirations are regulated by various afferent input from *mechanoreceptors* in the lungs, airways and respiratory muscles, as well as *chemoreceptors* in the blood (e.g., aortic and carotid bodies) and brain. These chemoreceptors sense changes in the blood pH, partial pressures of O_2 (PO_2) and carbon dioxide (PCO_2), then transmit signals back to the central respiratory center. Here, the rate of ventilation is adjusted to maintain blood gas and acid–base homeostasis. Feedback from mechanoreceptors regarding the mechanical status and function of the ventilatory pump and respiratory muscles leads to adjustment of the level and pattern of breathing. The efferent nerve pathway to the muscles of respiration starts in the brainstem (medulla/pons), crosses over and then travels in the contralateral spinal cord to reach the spinal motor neurons.

Respirations are also subject to voluntary control through input from the cerebral cortex to the respiratory centers in the medulla/pons. Of all the vital signs, respiratory rate is the only vital sign which can be influenced by voluntary control, although to a limited extent.

During "normal" respiration, the main work of breathing is done by the diaphragm and intercostal muscles. When a patient experiences respiratory distress, contraction of the intercostal muscles becomes more forceful and visible to the observer. This condition is referred to as "intercostal retractions" or "retractions." In this situation, the patient is said to be "retracting." Retractions may also occur in the supraclavicular and substernal areas. When there is increased work of breathing or respiratory distress, other muscles are recruited in an effort to maintain the movement of air in the lungs. When the neck muscles are recruited, their contractions become evident. This is described as "accessory muscle use" (of respiration). Similarly, "abdominal breathing" or "see-saw" respirations occur when the abdominal muscles are recruited. Marked movements of the abdomen and paradoxical chest wall motion may also occur.

History

If dyspnea is not due to an immediate life-threat, the history and physical examination can proceed in an orderly fashion. Immediate resuscitation must occur if the shortness of breath is from respiratory failure, shock with inadequate tissue perfusion, or hypoxia at a cellular level. The history is critical in the evaluation of dyspnea in order to differentiate life-threatening from benign causes, and in determining its etiology.

How did the shortness of breath begin (sudden or gradual onset)?

The acute onset of dyspnea raises concern for disorders such as spontaneous pneumothorax, pulmonary embolism (PE), acute coronary syndrome (ACS), acute pulmonary edema, or anaphylaxis. Gradual onset of shortness of breath in a patient may represent pneumonia, congestive heart failure (CHF), reactive airway disease (RAD), or malignancy. However, variation occurs in these classic presentations.

Have you had shortness of breath before?

Previous episodes of dyspnea suggest a chronic cardiac or pulmonary disorder such as asthma, chronic obstructive pulmonary disease (COPD), or CHF. Asthma is the most likely diagnosis in a child or nonsmoking adult who experiences chronic symptoms of shortness of breath which wax and wane, especially if wheezing is present. COPD should be considered in an adult smoker with recurrent episodes of dyspnea. In an adult with dyspnea and bilateral lower extremity edema, CHF should be considered.

A patient with "chronic" shortness of breath (for months or years) may present with an acute exacerbation of dyspnea. This is often the case with COPD or CHF. The physician needs to determine what caused the sudden worsening of symptoms, such as medication noncompliance, pulmonary infection in a COPD patient, change in diet (e.g., increased salt intake in a CHF patient), or cardiac ischemia or myocardial infarction (MI).

Does anything make the shortness of breath better or worse?

Orthopnea is dyspnea that is worse with lying down and better with sitting or standing. Typically, CHF and pulmonary edema are associated with orthopnea. Orthopnea is also one of the earliest findings in patients with diaphragmatic weakness from neuromuscular disorders. *Paroxysmal nocturnal dyspnea* (PND) refers to the patient waking up suddenly at night with acute shortness of breath. In patients with CHF, this is due to the accumulation of fluid in the lungs while the patient lays flat and sleeps. As a result of PND or orthopnea, patients may sleep sitting in a chair or with multiple pillows under their head

in order to avoid becoming dyspneic. *Trepopnea* is dyspnea associated with a unilateral recumbent position, and may occur in patients with unilateral lung disease, ball-valve airway obstruction, diaphragmatic paralysis, or COPD.

Do you have chest pain?

Chest pain associated with dyspnea suggests a serious underlying disorder, such as ACS or PE. Sharp chest pain worsened by breathing but not by movement suggests a PE or spontaneous pneumothorax.

Do you have palpitations or feel an abnormal heartbeat?

Palpitations or an irregular heartbeat felt by the patient generally signifies a cardiac etiology for the dyspnea, particularly if new. A dyspneic patient who complains that "my heart was beating fast," "slow," "skipped a beat," or "beating funny" suggests a dysrhythmia.

Do you have swelling of the lower extremities?

Is it difficult for the patient to put on their shoes because of edematous feet? Bilateral lower extremity edema may occur with right-sided CHF, while unilateral lower extremity swelling with calf pain is suspicious for a deep vein thrombosis (DVT). Patients with a DVT in the lower extremity may have pain and swelling in that calf. Dyspnea in a patient with a known DVT or unilateral leg swelling is worrisome for a clot that has broken off from the leg and embolized to the lung (PE).

Do you feel faint or did you pass out?

A dyspneic patient who passed out (syncope) or almost passed out (near-syncope) may have significant cardiac (ACS, MI, dysrhythmias, valvular disease, and cardiomyopathy) or pulmonary disease, such as PE. However, syncope/near-syncope may result from other causes, such as gastrointestinal (GI) hemorrhage or volume depletion from dehydration caused by excessive fluid loss or inadequate oral fluid intake.

Do you have any upper respiratory symptoms?

Patients with pulmonary infections (pneumonia or acute bronchitis) resulting in shortness of breath may also have a cough, purulent sputum, fever and/or chills, and possibly prodromal upper respiratory tract (URI) symptoms. URI or "cold" symptoms include rhinorrhea and generalized myalgias. Dyspnea with symptoms such as drooling, hoarseness, aphonia, and "muffled voice" suggest upper airway problems, specifically airway obstruction, such as epiglottitis or foreign body.

Are you coughing up blood?

Hemoptysis may occur with pulmonary or upper airway tumors/malignancies, pulmonary infections, tuberculosis, and vasculitis. Frothy blood-tinged sputum is a classic sign of acute pulmonary edema.

Any tarry or bloody stools?

Patients with severe anemia (whether from GI bleeding or other causes) may experience dyspnea because of decreased O_2 delivery to the tissues or secondary to limited O_2 carrying capacity from lack of red blood cells (RBCs).

Have you been vomiting?

Vomiting can lead to electrolyte abnormalities, which may result in dyspnea, or can be due to diabetic ketoacidosis, with dyspnea secondary to a compensatory respiratory alkalosis from metabolic abnormalities.

Have you had recent unintentional weight loss?

This could be due to malignancy, especially lung cancer in a smoker.

Past medical

A history of previous PE, DVT, or clotting disorder in a dyspneic patient suggests PE. Recent surgery (especially abdominal or pelvic surgery), atrial fibrillation, pregnancy, malignancy, and prolonged immobility are predisposing factors (Table 33.1).

A previous history of any neurologic or muscular disorders may provide a clue to the etiology of dyspnea, as patients with such conditions may experience respiratory muscle weakness and develop respiratory failure. CNS disorders that affect the respiratory centers in the medulla could lead to respiratory failure from loss of the central respiratory drive. Traumatic injury or disease of the cervical spine that affects C3/C4/C5 could

Table 33.1 Predisposing conditions for pulmonary embolism

- Birth control pills and/or estrogens
- Cardiac disease: atrial fibrillation, congestive heart failure
- Clotting disorders
- Family history
- Immobility
- Malignancy
- Pregnancy
- Previous pulmonary emboli or deep vein thrombosis
- Recent past surgery: esp. abdominal/pelvic

result in paralysis of the diaphragm. Injury or illness to either phrenic nerve can cause paralysis of the diaphragmatic muscles.

Oncology patients, patients on immunosuppressive agents, or patients with autoimmune disorders are especially prone to dyspnea. This may be due to infection or severe anemia secondary to bone marrow suppression.

Female patients on birth control pills or estrogens are at risk for PE. Medicines can have dangerous side effects and can be a clue to any underlying diseases. Allergies should be noted in case patients need therapy for their dyspnea, or if a particular medication is causing the dyspnea.

Social

Tobacco, alcohol, and illicit drugs

A significant smoking history points towards COPD or lung cancer. A patient without a smoking history is unlikely to have COPD. An intoxicated patient with shortness of breath, cough, and fever may have aspiration pneumonia. Patients inhaling illegal drugs may get a pneumonitis from the adulterants used to "cut" the drugs. Intravenous drug abusers can contract human immunodeficiency virus (HIV) infection from an infected needle, and may present with *Pneumocystis carinii* pneumonia (PCP) as a manifestation of acquired immune deficiency syndrome (AIDS).

Review the patient's occupational history or any acute or chronic exposures to toxins

An acute hypersensitivity reaction or toxic lung injury may occur in workers who inhale various particulates. A dyspneic patient exposed to a fire may have smoke inhalation or a hypersensitivity reaction from burning chemicals or toxins. A dyspneic patient with the gradual onset of symptoms exposed to toxins at work over years may have asbestosis, silicosis, berylliosis, or "coal worker's" pneumoconiosis.

Physical examination

Physical examination may be instrumental in diagnosing the etiology of dyspnea, as well as in determining which patients are critically ill and need immediate therapy (even resuscitation).

General appearance

The patient's general appearance is a critical part of the physical examination. A patient who is sitting upright and leaning forward on the hands (the "tripod" position) is urgently attempting to maintain an open airway and improve ventilation. Pursing of the lips, intercostal retractions, or the use of accessory muscles are other methods to facilitate air entry into the lungs. A patient who can speak in full sentences does *not* have significant respiratory distress; a patient who can speak only a few words has moderate respiratory distress. A patient who is too short of breath to even answer with a few words is experiencing severe respiratory distress. An anxious appearance or agitation suggests hypoxia. Somnolence suggests hypercarbia.

Vital signs

Fever is nonspecific and may occur with respiratory infections or other etiologies, such as PE. Although a fever is typically found in patients with respiratory infections, they may have a normal temperature or hypothermia. Patients with PE rarely have temperatures >102°F.

Hypotension can occur secondary to dehydration, sepsis, shock, or hemorrhage. The combination of hypotension and dyspnea should raise concern for PE, cardiac disease, and tension pneumothorax. Increased respiratory effort and rate, especially if prolonged, may contribute to dehydration due to increased insensible losses from the airway and lungs.

Tachycardia usually accompanies respiratory distress, although exceptions may occur in patients taking beta- or calcium channel blockers. These medications may blunt the patient's heart rate (HR) response to respiratory distress.

The respiratory rate can be a clue to underlying respiratory problems. In an attempt to improve oxygenation and ventilation, there is a compensatory increase in the respiratory rate. An abnormally low respiratory rate (*bradypnea*) is an ominous sign, usually signifying impending respiratory failure. Although a normal respiratory rate generally suggests that respiration is not impaired, this finding can be tragically misleading and must be viewed in the context of the patient's presentation. For example, an asthmatic in respiratory distress will initially increase their respiratory rate in order to improve their oxygenation and ventilation. However, they can maintain this compensation for only a finite period of time. When they begin to tire from the additional work of breathing, their respiratory rate starts to drop. They may fall into the normal range of respiratory rates during this period of decompensation before they become bradypneic and have a respiratory arrest.

All patients complaining of shortness of breath should have pulse oximetry measured. Although pulse oximetry has a few technical limitations, a pulse oximetry <90% indicates hypoxia and requires immediate evaluation (Table 33.2).

Table 33.2 Clinical signs of respiratory distress

- Abnormal vital signs
  - Heart rate: tachycardia
  - Respiratory rate: tachypnea or bradypnea
  - Abnormal respiratory pattern: periodic, Biot's, Cheyne-Stokes, apnea
- Cyanosis
- Pursed lips
- Grunting
- Nasal flaring
- Intercostal retractions
- Use of accessory muscles of the neck
- Abdominal breathing
- Paradoxical motion of chest

Head, eyes, ears, nose, and throat

Signs of respiratory distress include nasal flaring, pursing of the lips, grunting, and perioral cyanosis. Any facial abnormalities or asymmetry secondary to masses, tumors, infections, or edema that could result in an obstructed airway should be identified. Drooling or inability to handle secretions is worrisome for upper airway obstruction. Stridor may accompany upper airway obstruction.

If signs of airway obstruction are present, allow the patient to remain sitting upright or in the position they find maximally comfortable, since this may help keep the upper airway open. Do not force the patient to lie flat or tilt their head backwards. Do not insert a tongue blade into the mouth, since this may worsen airway obstruction and convert a partial airway obstruction into a complete obstruction. Most patients in respiratory distress prefer the upright position, as the work of breathing is greater when lying flat because the supine position requires breathing against the weight of the abdomen.

If the patient has no signs of airway obstruction and is stable, examine the oropharynx for masses, edema, infections, and bleeding. The presence of oral thrush suggests an immunocompromised host, such as an HIV-positive individual, and raises concern for opportunistic infections like PCP.

Neck

Examine the neck for asymmetry, masses, swelling, and jugular venous distention. Listen for bruits over the carotid arteries consistent with vascular disease. Jugular venous distention on inspiration (*Kussmaul's sign*) may occur in pericardial tamponade, PE, or pneumothorax.

Pulmonary

Examination of the lungs is mandatory in the evaluation of any patient with dyspnea, and often reveals the etiology of the patient's dyspnea.

Inspect the chest for symmetric chest rise, deformities, or paradoxical movement. Paradoxical chest movement refers to chest contraction during inspiration and the abnormal part of the chest fluttering out during expiration; this is the opposite of normal chest wall motion. Intercostal, supraclavicular, and substernal retractions (the use of accessory muscles of respiration) are indicators of respiratory distress.

Palpate the chest for any areas of tenderness, masses, or crepitus (subcutaneous air is suggestive of pneumothorax).

Auscultate both lung fields for wheezing, rales, and rhonchi. Unilaterally decreased breath sounds suggest pneumothorax, atelectasis, pleural effusion, or pneumonia. Wheezing usually is secondary to bronchospasm, which most often occurs in pulmonary diseases such as asthma, COPD, bronchiolitis, and occasionally acute bronchitis. Wheezing may also occur with CHF ("cardiac asthma"), foreign bodies, and PE. Rales may be present due to underlying cardiac disease (pulmonary edema or CHF) or pulmonary disease (pneumonia). Rhonchi may be present with pneumonia or bronchitis.

Hyperresonance on percussion occurs with a pneumothorax; dullness on percussion suggests a pleural effusion, infiltrate, hemothorax, or chylothorax.

Cardiac

Feel the precordium for a precordial bulge, a hyperdynamic heart, or thrills. Auscultate for abnormal heart sounds such as an S3 or S4, rubs, clicks, or murmurs. An S3 gallop or S4 may occur with CHF. A pericardial friction rub is sometimes heard with a pericardial effusion. A click suggests valvular disease. A murmur may be present with valvular disease or other cardiac disorders, or may be physiologic.

Palpate the pulses for strength, equality, and regularity. A weak or thready pulse occurs in shock.

Abdomen

Inspect for abdominal distention, pregnancy, or ascites, which can limit movement of the diaphragm and interfere with respiration. Identify the "see-saw" respirations of abdominal breathing. Hepatosplenomegaly can occur with right-sided CHF. The presence of hepatojugular reflux (distention of the neck veins with firm palpation of the liver) indicates heart failure.

Neurologic

A generalized muscular disorder with peripheral muscle weakness may also have respiratory muscle weakness, leading to respiratory distress or failure.

Extremity

Inspect for cyanosis, edema, clubbing, cords, venous distention, changes of peripheral vascular disease, infection, or nicotine stains. Clubbing indicates longstanding hypoxia. The presence of unilateral leg swelling and dyspnea suggests PE.

Skin

Examine the skin for color (pallor, cyanosis), temperature and moisture (cold/clammy or warm/dry). The skin should also be examined to assess capillary refill, identify rashes (suggesting infection) or petechiae (indicating a hematologic disorder, vasculitis, or infection such as meningococcemia), or track marks (denoting IVDA).

Differential diagnosis

Although the differential diagnosis of dyspnea is extensive (Table 33.3), the majority of dyspneic patients have a cardiopulmonary etiology. Most

Table 33.3 The etiology and differential diagnosis of dyspnea

I. **Respiratory system**
   1. Airway obstruction
      - Foreign body
      - Mass: tumor/malignancy
      - Angioedema
      - Infections: epiglottitis, retropharyngeal abscess, parapharyngeal abscess, croup, bacterial tracheitis, bronchitis
      - Tracheomalacia, tracheal stenosis (congenital or acquired – often post-intubation)
      - Bronchiectasis
   2. Lungs (pulmonary parenchyma)
      - Asthma
      - Chronic obstructive pulmonary disease
      - Infections: pneumonia, lung abscess
      - Trauma: pulmonary contusion, pulmonary hemorrhage
      - Pulmonary edema (non-cardiogenic)
      - Atelectasis
      - Pulmonary fibrosis
      - Environmental/occupational lung disease: coal worker's pneumoconiosis, asbestosis, silicosis, berylliosis
      - Adult respiratory distress syndrome
      - Rheumatologic/autoimmune disorders: sarcoidosis, lupus
      - Hemorrhagic: Goodpasture's syndrome
      - Mass: tumor, malignancy (primary or metastatic)
   3. Pleura
      - Trauma: hemothorax, pneumothorax (tension, simple)
      - Atraumatic: spontaneous pneumothorax
      - Infections: empyema, pyothorax
      - Chylothorax
      - Pleural effusion
      - Pleural adhesions
      - Mass: pleural tumor, malignancy
   4. Chest wall
      - Trauma: flail chest, fractured ribs, other chest wall injury
      - Bony abnormalities: pectus excavatum, kyphoscoliosis
   5. Decreased lung volume due to interference with chest expansion
      - Abdominal distention
      - Abdominal mass
      - Diaphragm injury
      - Ruptured diaphragm
      - Paralysis of diaphragm

II. **Cardiac**
   1. Myocardium
      - Coronary artery disease: ischemia, infarction
      - Myocarditis/cardiomyopathy
      - Rheumatologic/immunologic disorders: lupus, sarcoid (any disease that infiltrates or destroys myocardium)
   2. Pericardium
      - Pericarditis
      - Pericardial tamponade
   3. Valvular
      - Aortic, mitral, tricuspid, pulmonic regurgitation or stenosis
   4. Cardiac shunts
      - Atrial septal defect
      - Ventricular septal defect
      - Patent ductus arteriosus
   5. Outflow obstruction
      - Left ventricular outflow tract obstruction: hypertrophic obstructive cardiomyopathy, critical aortic stenosis
      - Myxoma
   6. Congenital heart disease
      - Cyanotic congenital heart disease: tetralogy of Fallot, hypoplastic heart, Eisenmenger's syndrome
      - Shunts: atrial septal disease, ventricular septal disease, ostium primum, patent foramen ovale, patent ductus arteriosus
      - Coarctation of aorta

(continued)

Table 33.3 The etiology and differential diagnosis of dyspnea (*cont*)

    7. Dysrhythmias
    8. Decreased cardiac output
       • Shock, myocarditis, dysrhythmias
    9. Heart failure

III. **Vascular**
    1. Emboli
       • Pulmonary, air, fat, amniotic fluid
    2. Pulmonary hypertension
    3. Veno-occlusive disease
    4. Sickle cell disease
    5. Vasculitis (rheumatologic/collagen, vascular diseases)
    6. Arteriovenous fistula

IV. **Neurologic/muscular**
    1. Neurologic
       • Central nervous system
          – Cerebrovascular accident, traumatic injuries, infections, multiple sclerosis, amyotrophic lateral sclerosis, botulism, organophosphate poisoning
       • Spinal cord
          – Trauma (e.g., spinal cord injury above C3 affects nerves C3, C4, C5 to diaphragm which results in paralysis of diaphragm)
          – Spinal cord diseases: poliomyelitis, amyotrophic lateral sclerosis, spinal muscular atrophies
       • Peripheral nerves:
          – Peripheral neuropathies: Guillain–Barré syndrome, tetanus, tick paralysis
    2. Muscle
          – Myopathies: myasthenia gravis, polymyositis, muscular dystrophy, some glycogen storage diseases, periodic paralysis (some forms)

V. **Cardiac output**
    1. Shock
    2. Low cardiac output

VI. **Metabolic/renal**
    1. Diabetic ketoacidosis
    2. Metabolic acidosis
    3. Renal disease: renal tubular acidosis, renal failure

VII. **Endocrine**
    • Thyroid disease: hyperthyroidism, hypothyroidism, Cushing's

VIII. **Hematologic**
    1. Anemia
    2. Methemoglobinemia

IX. **Gastrointestinal**
    1. Gastrointestinal reflux
    2. Abdominal loading: ascites, obesity, pregnancy

X. **Toxins/poisons/drugs**
    1. Carbon monoxide poisoning
    2. Drugs: beta-blockers in patients with asthma/chronic obstructive pulmonary disease

XI. **Psychologic**
    1. Hyperventilation syndrome
    2. Anxiety
    3. Panic disorder

XII. **Deconditioning**

Note: Some disorders may affect multiple areas of the nervous system and thus could be listed under several areas. For example, amyotrophic lateral sclerosis affects motor neurons in the spinal cord, brainstem and corticospinal tracts.

Table 33.4 Symptoms, signs, evaluation and specific treatments for common and life-threatening causes of dyspnea

Diagnosis*	Classic symptoms*	Signs*	Work-up**	Specific treatment
Acute Exacerbation COPD	Wheezing Shortness of breath Chest pain	Respiratory distress ↓ Breath sounds Wheezing Prolonged I/E ratio Barrel chest Clubbing	O_x, peak expiratory flow (often pre/post treatment to compare) CXR: r/o pneumonia or PTX as exacerbating factors	O_2, (monitor for ↑PCO_2 but do not withhold O_2 if needed; start low FiO_2 if possible). Beta-agonists, anticholinergics, corticosteroids. If severe, NIPPV, intubation
Airway obstruction	Drooling	Respiratory distress Sitting up/leaning forward to open airway "Tripod" position	Secure airway first if critical or potentially unstable. Diagnosis: laryngoscopy, CT scan of neck, soft tissue X-rays of neck; ENT consult	O_2; secure airway: intubate, cricothy-rotomy, tracheostomy if potentially unstable; heliox in some. Treat underlying cause: aerosolized epinephrine for edema, remove foreign body
Asthma	Wheezing Shortness of breath Chest pain	Respiratory distress Prolonged I/E ratio Wheezing (if severe, there may not be wheezing – the "quiet" chest → no air flow)	O_x, peak expiratory flow (often pre/post treatment to compare), CXR (hyperinflation ± infiltrate), ABG (possibly)	O_2, beta-agonists, corticosteroids, anti-cholinergics, anti-microbials if infection present. If severe, NIPPV, intubation
Congestive heart failure	Shortness of breath (Chest pain if CAD also present)	Respiratory distress L-sided CHF: rales, JVD. R-sided CHF: hepatomegaly, splenomegaly, lower extremity edema	O_x, CXR, ABG, BNP, cardiac enzymes if precipitated by CAD	O_2, Diuretics, Nitroglycerin, ACE inhibitors. If severe, NIPPV, intubation
Pneumonia	Cough Shortness of breath Chest pain Sputum Hemoptysis	Respiratory distress Rales Egophony Fever	O_x, ABG (possibly) CBC: ↑WBC, ±left shift. CXR: infiltrate (may not be visible if dehydrated or early)	O_2, Antimicrobials if bacterial etiology suspected. If severe, NIPPV, intubation
Pneumothorax	Abrupt onset Shortness of breath Pleuritic chest pain	Decreased breath sounds on affected side Hyperresonance to percussion Subcutaneous emphysema	O_x, CXR	100% O_2 Tube thoracostomy Needle thoracostomy if tension
Pulmonary embolism	Abrupt onset Shortness of breath Chest pain (usually sharp pleuritic) Syncope Cough	Respiratory distress (if large PE); ↑RR, ↑HR, loud P_2 (if small, VS may be normal); Leg swelling (if DVT), (clots may be from pelvis or lower extremity); Low-grade fever	O_x, ABG, D-dimer, V/Q scan, helical CT scan, pulmonary angiogram, lower extremity ultrasound	O_2 Anticoagulation

ACE: angiotensin converting enzyme; ABG: arterial blood gas; BNP: B-natriuretic peptide; CAD: coronary artery disease; COPD: chronic obstructive pulmonary disease; CXR: chest X-ray; DVT: deep vein thrombosis; HR: heart rate; JVD: jugular venous distention; NIPPV: non-invasive positive pressure ventilation; O_x: pulse oximetry; PE: pulmonary embolism; PTX: pneumothorax; VS: vital signs.
*Classic symptoms and signs may or may not be present in any given patient.
**Work-up varies depending on patient, test availability, and conditions.

clinicians approach the differential diagnosis in terms of organ systems, especially respiratory (both pulmonary and extrapulmonary), cardiac, and other causes. However, some physicians consider the etiology in terms of acute versus chronic processes. Table 33.4 lists the presentation, work-up, and treatment for a number of causes of dyspnea.

Diagnostic testing

Since the majority of patients with dyspnea have cardiopulmonary disease, the two most common diagnostic tests are the chest radiograph and electrocardiogram (ECG). These two tests are easy to perform, noninvasive, inexpensive, safe, and can quickly confirm or exclude many common diagnoses. Other commonly utilized adjunctive studies are also discussed.

Radiologic studies

Chest X-ray

Since pulmonary disorders are the most common etiology of dyspnea (about half in one study of adults in a clinic setting), the chest X-ray may be the most useful test in dyspneic patients of all ages. Posteroanterior (PA) and lateral chest films provide the most information. However, in very ill patients, a portable anteroposterior (AP) film can be performed at the bedside and interpreted immediately. Additionally, this prevents a potentially unstable patient from leaving the ED. The chest film can reveal abnormalities such as an infiltrate, may distinguish CHF from COPD, and can exclude a clinically significant pneumothorax (Figure 33.1). A normal chest X-ray in the presence of unexplained hypoxemia is worrisome for PE. Patients with mild exacerbations of asthma or COPD who respond to emergent therapy do not need routine chest X-rays.

Electrocardiogram

An ECG is warranted in dyspneic patients with known or suspected CAD, and in patients with both dyspnea and chest pain. Dyspnea may represent an "anginal equivalent," especially in elderly patients or diabetics. The incidence of "silent" myocardial infarction (MI) is estimated to be about 20% of all MIs. The ECG may also be helpful for detecting cardiopulmonary diseases other than ACS that present with dyspnea, including CHF, pericarditis, cardiomyopathy,

and dysrhythmias. The ECG is rarely helpful in the diagnosis of pulmonary emboli. The classic finding of "$S_1Q_3T_3$" is neither sensitive nor specific. Sinus tachycardia and right ventricular strain are more commonly present.

Laboratory studies

Arterial blood gas

Arterial blood gases (ABGs) are not routinely necessary in all dyspneic patients. They may be useful in patients with unexplained dyspnea, altered mental status, suspected acidosis, and serious illness. An ABG can detect hypoxemia ($PO_2 < 90$–95), hypercarbia ($PCO_2 > 45$), metabolic acidosis (bicarb < 20), acidosis ($pH < 7.35$), or alkalosis ($pH > 7.45$). Renal disease and metabolic disorders can lead to acidosis that may result in compensatory hyperventilation and dyspnea.

The ABG may be used to calculate the alveolar–arterial gradient (A–a gradient). This is the calculated difference between the alveolar and arterial O_2, representing the difference in the PO_2 between the alveolus and the blood.

The alveolar oxygen tension, PAO_2, is calculated from the alveolar gas equation FIO_2 = inspired oxygen fraction, PB = barometric pressure, PH_2O = water vapor pressure (which is 47 at sea level), and RQ = respiratory quotient, which is the rate of CO_2 production/rate of oxygen consumption (a constant which is 0.8).

$$PAO_2 = FIO_2 (PB - PH_2O) - PaCO_2/RQ.$$

Thus, in room air with FIO_2 of 0.21 and a $PCO_2 = 40$, the alveolar oxygen tension is:
$$\begin{aligned} PAO_2 &= 0.21(760 - 47) - (PCO_2 \times 1.25) \\ &= 0.21(713) - (PCO_2/0.8) \\ &= 150 - (40/0.8) \\ &= 150 - 50 \\ &= 100 \end{aligned}$$

The A–a gradient is merely the difference between the alveolar and arterial blood PO_2, or $PAO_2 - PaO_2$. Normally, this difference is between 2–10 mmHg.

This value normally increases with age, and may be as high as 30 mmHg in elderly patients. Abnormal A–a gradients may be found in conditions such as PE, although this is neither sensitive nor specific.

D-dimer

The D-dimer is a product of blood clot breakdown and is typically elevated in patients with thromboembolic disease. The D-dimer is nonspecific and

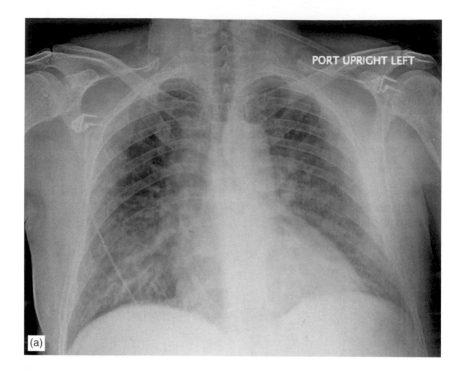

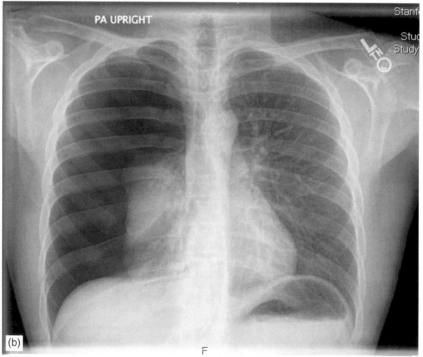

Figure 33.1
(a) Congestive heart failure. AP chest radiograph demonstrating cardiomegaly,
peribronchial cuffing and early airspace disease consistent with pulmonary edema
(b) Pneumothorax. PA chest radiograph demonstrating a large spontaneous
pneumothorax on the right, with almost complete collapse of the underlying lung.
Courtesy: Kathryn Stevens, MD.

may be elevated in conditions other than PE, such as pneumonia, chronic inflammatory states, and neoplastic conditions. In patients with low clinical risk for PE, a negative D-dimer assay makes the diagnosis very unlikely.

Cardiac enzymes

Cardiac enzymes (Troponin, CK-MB, and Myoglobin) should be ordered if an ACS is a possible cause of the dyspnea. Dyspnea is a common presentation of ACS in the elderly and in diabetics. Furthermore, prolonged dyspnea, hypoxia, and increased work of breathing may result in cardiac ischemia.

B-type natriuretic peptide

B-type natriuretic peptide (BNP) levels may be helpful in the diagnosis of CHF in patients with undifferentiated dyspnea. BNP is a good screening tool because of its high sensitivity and high negative predictive value. BNP levels are generally increased in patients presenting with CHF, whereas a level <100 pg/ml is very accurate in excluding CHF as the cause of dyspnea. BNP may be falsely elevated in some patients without CHF, so the BNP level needs to be interpreted in the context of the patient's clinical presentation.

White blood cell

Although an elevated white blood cell (WBC) count and/or left shift can occur with many infections, malignancies, and inflammatory processes, patients with a pulmonary infection such as pneumonia may have a normal WBC and differential. However, a WBC count with differential can be helpful in certain situations. A markedly elevated WBC and/or a significantly abnormal differential suggests an infectious pulmonary process or malignancy, especially in combination with an abnormal chest X-ray. An abnormal peripheral smear showing immature forms or blasts is suggestive of malignancy. A markedly decreased WBC raises the possibility of immunosuppression and increased susceptibility to infection. A patient with an infiltrate on chest X-ray and a very low absolute neutrophil count (ANC) is at greater risk for opportunistic infectious complications; this will undoubtedly influence the choice of antibiotics.

Hematocrit/hemoglobin

The hematocrit (Hct)/hemoglobin (Hgb) may also be helpful in the evaluation of dyspnea. A markedly low Hct/Hgb can cause dyspnea due to inadequate delivery of O_2 to the cells or tissue from lack of RBCs. Conversely, a markedly elevated Hct/Hgb can occur in patients with cyanotic congenital heart disease or polycythemia, who may present with dyspnea.

Electrolytes

Serum electrolytes may be indicated in patients who have dyspnea or tachypnea to evaluate for metabolic acidosis, diabetic ketoacidosis, or significant dehydration.

Glucose

A dextrostix, accucheck, or bedside glucose test (confirmed by a serum glucose) is indicated when hyperglycemia or diabetic ketoacidosis is suspected as the cause of the dyspnea or tachypnea.

Pregnancy test

In women of childbearing age, a pregnancy test may be indicated. Pregnant women have an increased risk of pulmonary emboli and preeclampsia, two life threatening disorders that can present with dyspnea. A positive pregnancy test may influence the choice of diagnostic tests. A ventilation/perfusion (V/Q) scan is preferred over computed tomography (CT) of the chest in pregnant women with suspected PE because there is less radiation exposure. A half-dose perfusion scan without the ventilation component can be done in order to reduce radiation exposure to the fetus. Placing a lead apron over the uterus during the chest roentgenogram will also decrease fetal radiation exposure.

Other laboratories

In patients for whom ACS or PE is a likely cause of dyspnea, baseline prothrombin time (PT) and partial thromboplastin time (PTT) tests are indicated if anticoagulation is being considered. Liver function tests may be done if ascites or hepatomegaly is present. In some patients with pulmonary infections, other studies such as blood cultures, sputum Gram's stain and sputum culture may be warranted. In patients in whom a pulmonary malignancy is a concern, sputum for cytology may be sent for evaluation.

Additional specialized studies

Chest computed tomography

Helical chest CT has emerged as the modality of choice for the diagnosis of PE (Figure 33.2). Chest CT has the advantage over V/Q scan in that it may identify pulmonary or thoracic abnormalities in addition to PE.

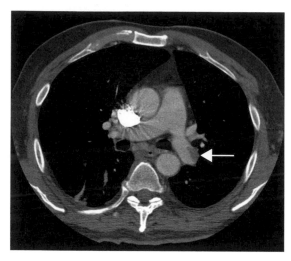

Figure 33.2
Axial CT section through the thorax following intravenous contrast, showing a large thrombus within the left main pulmonary artery. *Courtesy*: S.V. Mahadevan, MD.

Ventilation/perfusion scans

Ventilation/perfusion (V/Q) scans were once commonly ordered to diagnose PE, despite the test's several limitations. In patients with an abnormal chest X-ray, there is a high incidence of indeterminate readings. Similarly, up to 40% of patients with a high pretest probability of PE but low probability V/Q scan have a PE. Recognizing these limitations, the V/Q scan is currently reserved for patients with contrast allergies, renal insufficiency (creatinine > 1.5), or pregnancy (Figure 33.3).

Echocardiogram

The echocardiogram may be useful to diagnose a pericardial effusion or cardiac tamponade. In less critical situations, the echocardiogram may help diagnose heart failure, valvular disease, congenital heart disease, hypertrophic obstructive cardiomyopathy (HOCM), cardiac tumors, or PE.

Peak expiratory flow rate

The peak expiratory flow rate (PEFR), also called the peak flow (PF), can be useful to monitor a patient's response to bronchodilator therapy. Measurements of PF are commonly obtained in ED patients since it is noninvasive, easy to obtain, and cost-effective. The results are dependent on patient cooperation and effort, and

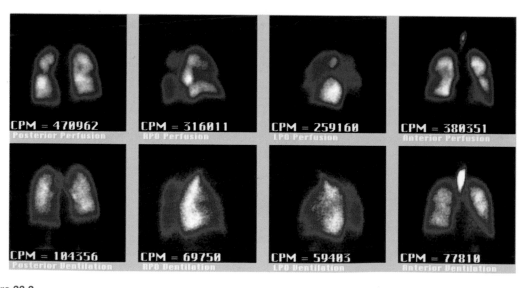

Figure 33.3
Lung ventilation/perfusion (V/Q) scan. The bottom row shows different views of the ventilation study. The top row shows the same views of the perfusion study. Heterogeneous perfusion is observed in both lung fields, with multiple peripheral wedge-shaped defects present with preserved ventilation (mismatched defects), consistent with high probability for pulmonary embolism. *Courtesy*: Carina Mari Aparici, MD and Sanjiv Gambhir MD, PhD.

cannot be used in critically ill patients. Trends in PEFR may be more useful than absolute values in many cases.

General treatment principles

The general appearance of the patient is key to determining which patients need immediate lifesaving measures (Table 33.5). The first priority is to determine whether the patient is in respiratory distress, respiratory failure, or shock. If this is the case, treatment must be instituted immediately, before the entire history is obtained and the physical examination is completed.

Table 33.5 Treatment for the dyspneic patient

- Airway, breathing, circulation
- Maintain the airway
- Give O_2 (even if chronic obstructive pulmonary disease is present)
- Apply pulse oximetry with continuous monitoring
- Continuous monitoring of HR, BP, ECG
- May try NIPPV in some patients
- Emergency airway management, if needed: endotracheal or nasotracheal intubation, laryngeal mask airway, transtracheal jet ventilation, cricothyrotomy (surgical)
- Sit patient upright (↓ work of breathing, may ↓ pulmonary congestion in CHF) if no acute cervical spine injury
- If possible airway obstruction: do not lie patient flat, lean head backward, or use a tongue blade in mouth

Evaluation of the airway, breathing, and circulation (ABCs) is the first priority. Does the patient have a patent airway? Is the patient in respiratory failure? Does the patient have respiratory distress and/or shock requiring emergent treatment?

Rules when treating patients with dyspnea include maintaining the airway and keeping it open, and providing supplemental O_2. Pulse oximetry should be placed in order to detect hypoxia and monitor therapy. Patients in the ED being evaluated for significant, life-threatening causes of dyspnea should be placed in a monitored bed with continuous HR, blood pressure (BP), and ECG monitoring, in addition to the continuous pulse oximetry.

Administer supplemental O_2 to any patient who suffers from hypoxia, respiratory distress, respiratory failure, or shock, even if the patient has COPD. It is more important to provide O_2 to the tissues than to be concerned about suppressing the hypoxic respiratory drive in COPD patients. After the administration of supplemental O_2, allow the patient to sit upright, unless there are contraindications such as an acute cervical spine injury. The upright position makes it easier for the patient to breathe by decreasing the work of breathing. This position decreases the "abdominal breathing," aids accessory muscle use, and decreases pulmonary congestion in patient with heart failure.

Noninvasive positive pressure ventilation (NIPPV), bilevel positive airway pressure (BiPAP), or continous positive airway pressure (CPAP) may be tried in some patients with respiratory distress. The physician should be prepared to intubate a patient in respiratory distress if the patient fails a brief trial of NIPPV.

If bradypnea or apnea occurs, ventilation may be assisted with bag-valve-mask prior to definitive airway management. Emergent airway management may be indicated if airway obstruction, altered mental status, shock, inability to speak, or inadequate ventilation is present. Intubation is the definitive airway of choice, with laryngeal mask airway (LMA), fiberoptics, cricothyrotomy, or transtracheal jet ventilation serving as alternatives in the event of unsuccessful intubation. Emergent airway management is discussed in detail in Chapter 2.

Acute asthma excacerbation

Pharmacologic agents that are used for the treatment of an acute asthmatic episode are known as "rescue medications." The inhaled beta-2-selective agonists are the initial therapeutic agents for all exacerbations. Inhaled beta-2-selective agonists cause bronchial smooth muscle relaxation and bronchodilation. The most commonly used beta-agonist in this sympathomimetic class of drugs is albuterol. Inhaled beta-agonists are generally preferred over other routes of administration (such as subcutaneous) because of fewer side effects and better efficacy. Anticholinergic agents, such as ipratropium, cause bronchodilation via inhibition of vagal tone from blocking muscarinic receptors in the airway smooth muscle. The beta-agonist albuterol and the anticholinergic ipratropium can be given in combination. Corticosteroids are used because of their anti-inflammatory effects. These include blocking the release of inflammatory mediators (which attract polymorphonuclear leukocytes), blocking increased capillary permeability, and increasing the "receptiveness" and thus "availability" of beta-adrenergic receptors. High-doses of corticosteroids for short durations are used initially for moderate to severe exacerbations, and in mild exacerbations in poorly-controlled or steroid-dependent asthmatics. Inhaled corticosteroids are prophylactic treatment for essentially all patients with asthma. Antibiotics are given only in the presence of a bacterial infection. With severe asthma or status asthmaticus, medications such as magnesium, epinephrine, and heliox are sometimes administered in addition to those discussed.

Acute exacerbation of chronic obstructive pulmonary disease

The mainstay of therapy for acute exacerbation of COPD is the same as for asthma: inhaled beta-adrenergic agents, anticholinergic bronchodilators, and corticosteroids. The need for corticosteroids is even more apparent in patients with COPD. Antibiotics are more often initiated in patients experiencing COPD exacerbations, as bacterial infections are more likely.

Pneumonia

Specific therapy depends on the underlying etiologic agent causing the pneumonia. Bacterial infections are treated with antibiotics. The choice of antimicrobial therapy is influenced not only by the suspected causative organism, but also by age, comorbidity, and clinical severity. Empiric antibiotic therapy is based on whether the pneumonia is "community-acquired" or "hospital-acquired." Aspiration pneumonias are particularly difficult to treat, and often occur in debilitated patients, alcoholics, patients with changes in consciousness, and those who cannot protect their airway. Pneumonia in an HIV-positive patient differs from pneumonia in a geriatric nursing home patient with numerous comorbidities (such as diabetes, CHF, COPD, renal failure, or risk of aspiration). An atypical pneumonia in an otherwise healthy young adult has a relatively benign (often outpatient) course. Supportive treatment is generally the rule for viral pneumonia, although amantadine can be used for severe pneumonia due to influenza. Ribavirin is optional therapy for severe respiratory syncytial virus (RSV) pneumonia.

Congestive heart failure

Emergency treatment of CHF includes removal of the precipitating factor(s), identification and correction of the underlying etiology, as well as redistribution and removal of excess fluid in the lungs. Three common mnemonics to help remember therapies used in the treatment of CHF are provided in Table 33.6 (these treatment modalities are not listed in particular order of use).

Table 33.6 Mnemonic therapies used in the treatment of CHF

UNLOAD ME
U   upright position
N   nitrates/nitroprusside/nesiritide
L   Lasix
O   oxygen
A   ACE inhibitors and aspirin
D   dopamine/dobutamine

M   morphine sulfate
E   endotracheal intubation (if needed)

MOIST AND DAMP
M   morphine sulfate
O   oxygen
I   inotropic support
S   sitting upright, salt restriction
T   tourniquets (rotating)

A   aspirin
N   nitrates/nitroprusside/nesiritide
D   diuretics (dialysis if appropriate)

D   digoxin
A   ACE inhibitors
M   monitors (cardiac, pulse ox, BP)
P   positive pressure ventilation, phlebotomy

LMNOP
L   lasix
M   morphine
N   nitrates/nitroprusside/nesiritide
O   oxygen
P   position (upright), positive pressure ventilation

In the setting of acute pulmonary edema, 100% O_2 must be provided, often delivered under positive pressure. The patient is maintained in the upright sitting posture, with legs dangling if possible to assist with fluid redistribution away from the lungs.

Many of the clinical manifestations of CHF result from hypervolemia and expansion of the interstitial fluid volume. Commonly used pharmacologic agents in the treatment of CHF include diuretics to control excessive fluid. They contribute to excess fluid removal and redistribution. In acute emergencies, loop diuretics (e.g., furosemide) are administered IV. This route results in rapid and reliable absorption, resulting in increased venous capacitance (venodilation), which decreases venous return, in addition to reducing circulating blood volume by its renal diuretic effect. The usual starting dose for furosemide is 20–80 mg IV, depending on prior exposure, chronic therapy, and renal function (larger doses are required in patients with renal insufficiency).

Nitroglycerin may be administered sublingually or IV to decrease pulmonary congestion and peripheral resistance through veno- and arteriodilation. This also causes afterload reduction and redistributes fluid from the lungs. In acute emergencies, when systolic blood pressure (SBP) is high due to increased sympathetic tone and intense vasoconstriction, sodium nitroprusside may be administered IV. Patients receiving nitroprusside must have continuous monitoring, preferably using an arterial line. Nesiritide is a recombinant human brain natriuretic peptide that has been studied regarding its use in patients in CHF. It is promoted as having vasodilatory, natriuretic, and diuretic effects. Nesiritide is contraindicated in patients who are hypersensitive to any of its components. It should not be used in patients with cardiogenic shock or in those with SBP <90 mmHg, and should be avoided in patients with suspected or known low cardiac filling pressures.

Morphine sulphate decreases adrenergic vasoconstrictor stimuli to arteriolar venous beds. It also reduces anxiety. Caution is warranted, as it may cause CNS and respiratory depression.

Dopamine and dobutamine have a limited role in the acute management of CHF exacerbations. These inotropic agents may be necessary when patients present in acute respiratory distress and hypotension, and are not responding to other therapeutic agents. Dopamine (which increases renal blood flow in low doses according to some authorities), can increase peripheral tone if a patient is hypotensive and needs support. Dobutamine has been demonstrated to improve cardiac contractility and output, which may assist with fluid redistribution. However, dobutamine can cause tachycardia and dysrhythmias, and should be used with caution.

Angiotensin-converting enzyme (ACE) inhibitors cause peripheral vasodilation, decreasing systemic pressure that may lead to regression of left ventricular hypertrophy (LVH). The effect of ACE inhibitors may be partly due to a decrease in myocardial angiotensin II production and to cardiac remodeling. The role of ACE inhibitors in the acute management of CHF remains controversial. Some emergency physicians advocate sublingual ACE inhibitor administration in acute presentations of CHF. Angiotensin II receptor blockers (ARBs) promote regression of LVH due to hypertension. Contraindications to the use of ACE inhibitors include pregnancy, prior ACE inhibitor-induced angioedema, or hyperkalemia.

Bronchodilators, such as beta-2-agonists, may be of limited benefit in patients presenting in acute pulmonary edema, as there is often mild to moderate bronchospasm secondary to fluid congestion. Caution is warranted, however, as these agents may increase HR, agitation or anxiety, thereby worsening dyspnea.

Digoxin has no definitive role in the acute management of CHF. Digitalis glycosides are commonly used in chronic therapy to increase myocardial contractility and improve ventricular emptying. Digoxin toxicity should be considered with acute or chronic digoxin therapy, especially in association with concomitant dehydration and renal insufficiency.

Beta-blockers slow the HR (increasing the time available for coronary flow and filling of the left ventricle), decrease myocardial O_2 demand, and lower the BP (causing a regression of LVH). The use of beta-blockers in acute CHF is extremely controversial; most authorities do not recommend their use in the ED unless diastolic dysfunction is known to exist, or if tachycardia or excess catecholamines is causing the CHF exacerbation, not a response to it. When needed, short-acting beta-blockers (such as esmolol) are recommended. Chronic beta-blocker therapy has been shown to improve LV function and long-term survival. Contraindications include bradycardia or known atrioventricular (AV) block, severe lung disease or bronchospasm, and previous adverse response to beta-blockers. They should be used with extreme caution in asthmatics and patients with COPD.

For patients on dialysis with chronic renal failure, presentations of acute CHF exacerbations due to fluid overload with resultant respiratory distress are common. Emergent dialysis may be the only treatment that can successfully remove the fluid responsible for respiratory distress.

It should be noted that not all of these drugs are used for every patient presenting in CHF. The choice of pharmacologic agent/s depends on many variables, including the clinical situation, vital signs, comorbid conditions (angina, hypertension, diabetes), and whether the heart failure is due to systolic or diastolic dysfunction.

In addition to pharmacologic therapy, lifestyle modification is recommended for CHF patients. These include smoking cessation, decreasing alcohol intake, salt restriction, water restriction if hyponatremic, weight reduction, and cardiac rehabilitation if stable.

Pulmonary embolism

Therapy for PE is anticoagulation. The standard anticoagulant regimen is the simultaneous initiation of heparin (either unfractionated or low-molecular weight) and oral warfarin in stable patients. Major side effects of heparin are bleeding and heparin-induced thrombocytopenia (HIT), often associated with thrombosis. IV thrombolytic therapy may be used for PE that causes hemodynamic compromise or respiratory distress. Thrombolytics accelerate clot lysis, but their use is associated with an increased risk of intracranial and GI bleeding. Contraindications to their use include patients at very high risk of bleeding or unstable patients needing immediate intervention, such as surgery or insertion of a vena cava filter.

Central airway obstruction

Management of central or upper airway obstruction entails ensuring ventilation and oxygenation. Following this, determining the treatment depends on the etiology. If an allergic or anaphylactic reaction is suspected, then epinephrine (aerosolized, subcutaneous, or IV), IV diphenhydramine, IV corticosteroids, and sometimes IV H_2-blockers are used. If the cause is a bacterial infection (epiglottis, retropharyngeal abscess) then antibiotics are warranted. With epiglottitis, management may vary depending on age and severity. Pediatric patients and critically-ill adults generally go to the operating room (OR) for emergent securing of the airway. In selected stable adult epiglottitis patients, admission to an intensive care unit (ICU) with close monitoring for airway obstruction and IV antibiotics can be done. Some patients with retropharyngeal abscess may need surgical drainage in the OR, depending on the amount of airway compromise. If the etiology is a foreign body, removal via laryngoscopy or bronchoscopy is indicated. If a mass is responsible for the obstruction, then surgery, radiation therapy, or chemotherapy are possible treatment options. Rapid involvement of specialists is often mandatory and may be life-saving in these circumstances.

Special patients
Elderly

Cardiopulmonary causes of dyspnea increase in incidence with advancing age. Typically, older patients have multiple comorbidities (e.g., COPD and CHF) limiting their cardiopulmonary reserve so that an additional disorder such as pneumonia is poorly tolerated. Any physiologic stress on the heart or lungs may result in increased morbidity and mortality. It is usually more difficult to diagnose the causes of dyspnea in the elderly for many reasons. Signs and symptoms may be nonspecific, mild, and even absent. Diagnostic tests are less likely to be abnormal or specific. Elderly patients may have an acute MI without chest pain. Their baseline ECG is often abnormal with hypertrophy, previous MI, or a bundle branch block, so that diagnosing an acute MI by ECG alone may be difficult. Laboratory studies may have an abnormal baseline. For example, in patients with renal failure, the troponin is often elevated even if an acute MI is not present. If an elevated troponin is present, whether or not it is from cardiac or renal disease (or both) may be difficult to determine.

Pediatric

The etiologies of dyspnea in children vary from those in adults. ACS is not a common cause of dyspnea in children. Cardiac causes of dyspnea in pediatric patients include myocarditis or myocardiopathy, congenital heart disease, and pericarditis. Although asthma occurs in both children and adults, other chronic lung disease is uncommon in children with the exception of cystic fibrosis. In comparison, chronic lung disease is fairly common in adults, especially COPD or pneumoconiosis from occupational or environmental exposure. In terms of incidence, pulmonary disorders (asthma, pneumonia, bronchitis, other respiratory infections, congenital disorders, and acquired diseases) make up a greater percentage of dyspnea than cardiac disorders in pediatric patients when compared to adults (Chapter 34).

Pregnant

Dyspnea is extremely common in pregnancy and occurs in three-fourths of pregnant women by 30-weeks gestation. This physiologic dyspnea of pregnancy occurs gradually, usually with exertion, and is not severe. The cause of dyspnea during pregnancy is due to the physiologic effects of an elevated diaphragm and postural-dependent alterations in blood flow. Also, hyperventilation from increased circulating progesterone and an increased sensitivity to CO_2 results in dyspnea. The physiologic dyspnea of pregnancy rarely increases in severity during the final weeks before delivery. However, dyspnea during pregnancy that is acute, severe, progressive, occurs at rest, or occurs with other symptoms or signs of cardiopulmonary disease is abnormal and deserves further evaluation. Pregnant women are at increased risk for two life-threatening causes of dyspnea: PE and preeclampsia.

Patients who are pregnant, postpartum, have had a recent miscarriage or abortion, or have had recent gynecologic or pelvic surgery are at increased risk for PE. Additionally, women who have a history of multiple episodes of fetal demise (e.g., multiple miscarriages) may have a coagulopathy that predisposes them to miscarriage and PE. When any pregnant patient presents with shortness of breath or chest pain, PE is a diagnostic possibility that warrants consideration.

Do not let unrealistic concerns over potential fetal harm from radiation exposure dissuade you from doing appropriate radiologic studies when warranted. Limiting fetal exposure can be accomplished by:

1. Shielding the abdomen when doing the chest X-ray
2. Doing a V/Q scan instead of a chest CT scan
3. Doing a half-dose perfusion scan without the ventilation component.

Disposition

Patients requiring supplemental O_2 to maintain adequate oxygenation, and those with respiratory distress need admission. Disposition generally depends on the underlying etiology and response to therapy. For example, a dyspneic patient with asthma, COPD, or CHF who responds to therapy in the ED and is no longer dyspneic (or returns to his or her baseline if suffering from chronic dyspnea), has acceptable pulse oximetry, a normal respiratory rate and no signs of respiratory distress may be discharged home on appropriate therapy with close follow-up. If any of the above are abnormal (dyspnea remains, hypoxia, increased work of breathing, PF significantly below baseline) then admission is warranted. Admission is also indicated in a patient with dyspnea secondary to ACS, such as unstable angina or acute MI, even if he or she responds to therapy in the ED and is no longer dyspneic.

Disposition may be affected by the clinical situation and comorbidities. In an otherwise healthy young adult without respiratory distress and normal vital signs, pneumonia is generally well-tolerated, and the patient can be safely discharged home. A geriatric patient with COPD or CHF has limited cardiopulmonary reserve, and pneumonia in such a patient is not well-tolerated. Admission for initial therapy and observation is indicated. Similarly, an asthmatic child with a poor social situation and unreliable caregivers, who may not receive his or her discharge medications, should be considered for admission.

Pearls and pitfalls

- Patients with apparently normal breathing (e.g., normal respiratory rate and respirations) may have a serious etiology for their dyspnea.
- A normal pulse oximetry and ABG do not rule out significant disease. For example, patients with dyspnea secondary to PE or ACS may have a normal pulse oximetry and PaO_2.
- Absence of chest pain does not rule out ACS or PE in patients with dyspnea.
- Dyspnea and hypotension or shock is an ominous combination. These patients need emergent evaluation and immediate treatment.
- Dyspnea and chest pain in adults usually has a cardiopulmonary etiology and deserves further evaluation.
- Dyspnea during pregnancy is common. However, pregnant women with acute or unexplained severe dyspnea deserve further evaluation, especially for PE.
- In pregnant women, do not avoid studies that are indicated. Remember, a chest X-ray can be done with shielding of the abdomen. A V/Q scan has less fetal radiation exposure than a chest CT scan. A half-dose perfusion scan without the ventilation component can be done.
- Psychogenic dyspnea is a diagnosis of exclusion. Other diagnoses should be

considered and ruled out by history, physical examination, and testing as indicated.

- Do not assume hysterical patients have psychogenic dyspnea. Patients with life-threatening causes of dyspnea may be hysterical because of their hypoxia.
- All patients with dyspnea deserve an evaluation that includes a thorough history, physical examination, and simple diagnostic tests. Specifically, pulse oximetry, a chest X-ray, and an ECG (if cardiac disease is a concern).
- Do not assume that just because a patient has a history of a chronic cardiopulmonary disease that his or her acute episode of dyspnea is due to chronic disease. For instance, patients with CHF can develop PE, COPD patients can have acute pneumonia, and asthmatics can have a pneumothorax.
- Ambulation is a functional "test" which can provide tremendous information about a patient's respiratory status. Vital signs and the amount of dyspnea should be evaluated following ambulation and compared to baseline, if possible.

References

1. Castro M. Control of breathing. In: Berne RM, Levy MN (eds). *Principles of Physiology.* St. Louis: Mosby, 2000. pp. 343–353.
2. DePaso WJ, Winterbauer RG, Lusk JA, et al. Chronic dyspnea unexplained by history, physical examination, chest roentgenogram, and spirometry: analysis of a 7-year experience. *Chest* 1991;100:1293–1299.
3. Dyspnea. Mechanisms, assessment, and management: a consensus statement. American Thoracic Society. *Am J Respir Crit Care Med* 1999;159:321–340.
4. Fedullo AJ, Swinburne AJ, McGuire-Dunn C. Complaints of breathlessness in the emergency department. The experience at a community hospital. *NYS J Med* 1986;86(1):4–6.
5. Kline JA. Dyspnea: fear, loathing, and physiology. *Emerg Med Prac* 1999;1(3):1–20.
6. Mace SE. Acute epiglottitis in adults. *Am J Emerg Med* 1985;3(6):543–550.
7. Mace SE. Asthma therapy in the observation unit. *Emerg Med Clinic North Am* 2001;19(1):169–185.
8. Mace SE. BiLevel positive airway pressure (BiPAP) ventilation. *J Clin Outcomes Manage* 1999;6(9):41–48.
9. Mace SE. Cricothyrotomy. *Am J Emerg Med* 1988;6:309–319.
10. Mace SE, Hedges JR. Cricothyrotomy and translaryngeal jet ventilation. In: Roberts JR, Hedges JR (eds). *Procedures in Emergency Medicine.* Philadelphia: WB Saunders, 2003, C.6.
11. Mace SE. Laryngeal mask airway. *Res Staff Phys* 2001;47(1):30–40.
12. Mace SE. Noninvasive respiratory monitoring: pulse oximetry and capnography. *Pediatr Med Rep* 2003 (In press).
13. Mace SE. Pneumonia in infants and children: systematic assessment and outcome – effective treatment guidelines. *Emerg Med Rep* 1998;19(20):203–218.
14. Mace SE. The pediatric patient with acute respiratory failure. Clinical diagnosis and pathophysiology. *Pediatr Emerg Med Rep* 2001;6(1):21–32.
15. Manning HL, Schwartzstein RM. Pathophysiology of dyspnea. *Neth J Med* 1995;333(23):1547–1553.
16. Martinez FJ, Stanopoulos I, Acero R, et al. Graded comprehensive cardiopulmonary testing in the evaluation of dyspnea unexplained by routine evaluation. *Chest* 1994;168–174.
17. Pratter MR, Curley FJ, Dubois J, et al. The spectrum and frequency of causes of dyspnea. *Arch Intern Med* 1989;149:2277–2282.
18. Regulation of respiration. In: Guyton AC, Hall JE (eds). *Textbook of Medical Physiology.* Philadelphia: WB Saunders Co. 2000. pp. 474–483.

34   Shortness of breath in children

Lance Brown, MD, MPH and Steven M. Green, MD

Scope of the problem

Difficulty breathing is one of the most common reasons for children to visit the emergency department (ED). In the US, tens of thousands of children are hospitalized for respiratory problems each year. In the winter, most emergency physicians will likely evaluate several children with difficulty breathing a day. The needed interventions can be as simple as reassurance for a head cold to intubation for respiratory failure. The outcomes vary considerably. Although most children recover completely from episodes of difficulty breathing, permanent lung or brain injury and death may occur, typically in very young infants or chronically-ill children.

Anatomic essentials

Infants and young children have relatively narrow airways, with high resistance. If the diameter of these small airways is decreased, the work of breathing can increase dramatically. The airways can narrow due to inflammation (e.g., asthma, chemical pneumonitis, bacterial tracheitis, croup), bronchospasm (e.g., asthma, bronchiolitis), extrinsic compression (e.g., esophageal foreign body, retropharyngeal abscess), excessive mucus and secretions with airway plugging (e.g., bronchiolitis, bacterial tracheitis, pneumonia) or mechanical obstruction (e.g., aspirated foreign body). Infants have a pliable chest wall and immature diaphragm which also contribute to respiratory fatigue and failure. Increased work of breathing may cause a child to be unable to feed with resultant dehydration or respiratory muscle fatigue leading to respiratory failure and mechanical ventilation.

History

Conditions that cause difficulty breathing in children have many similar features. Many are preceded by rhinorrhea, low-grade fever, and other symptoms of upper respiratory tract infection. This can make differentiating between conditions difficult. The history, however, can be used to modify the overall likelihood of some diagnoses.

How old is this child?

The likelihood of some disorders depends greatly on age. For example, pertussis is primarily seen in infants less than 6 months of age who are partially immunized. Croup is a disease of young children, such as toddlers and preschool groups. Bronchiolitis is generally not diagnosed past the age of 2 years. Infants who do not yet crawl, usually less than 9 months of age, seldom aspirate foreign bodies.

How long have these symptoms been going on?

The time course of the illness may be helpful. Abrupt-onset conditions include foreign body aspiration and chemical pneumonitis from hydrocarbon ingestion. Disorders such as bacterial tracheitis and epiglottitis may present after a few days of mild upper respiratory tract symptoms and then have a rapid worsening. Croup tends to begin with mild coughing for a day or two before the parents notice a relatively severe barking cough late in the evening. Bronchiolitis and asthma exacerbations typically worsen over a few days. Pertussis is usually associated with 7–10 days of rhinorrhea and upper respiratory tract symptoms, followed by 2–4 weeks of a relatively severe staccato cough often accompanied by posttussive vomiting and periods of cyanosis.

Have there been any fevers or ill contacts?

Fever or ill contacts tend to suggest an infectious etiology. Retropharyngeal and peritonsilar abscesses typically present with fever. Bronchiolitis usually presents with a fever while an asthma exacerbation does not (unless the aggravating factor is an upper respiratory tract infection). Bacterial tracheitis and epiglottitis tend to have higher fevers than croup and upper respiratory tract infections, although the recent administration of antipyretics or the presence of an immune-compromising condition may affect the presenting temperature. Ill contacts may suggest a highly infectious agent such as pertussis or respiratory syncytial virus (RSV).

Does the child have a cough? What does it sound like?

Some conditions cause children to have distinctive features to their cough. A seal-like, barking cough in a toddler is characteristic of croup and can be seen in bacterial tracheitis. Pertussis is suggested if a young infant has coughing that comes in bursts or paroxysms followed by periods that are relatively free of coughing. A persistent, repetitive cough with an abrupt onset may be due to an aspirated foreign body. A cough that is associated with bilateral wheezing suggests a bronchospastic process such as asthma or bronchiolitis.

How is the child feeding/urinating?

It is important to assess the hydration status of a young child with difficulty breathing. Something as simple as nasal congestion in a young infant who is an obligate nasal breather can result in serious dehydration. Some children are simply breathing too fast to feed. The increased work of breathing, tachypnea, and fluid losses from the lungs may contribute to dehydration. Other findings such as sweating with feeds, suggestive of congestive heart failure, may be helpful in making a diagnosis. A history of feeding honey to a young infant may suggest botulism.

How is the child handling their secretions?

Although all young infants leave some drool on their toys and parents' shirts, excessive drooling may suggest epiglottitis, retropharyngeal abscess, or an esophageal foreign body. These conditions typically inhibit swallowing to some degree and present with excessive drooling.

Where was this child when you noticed a problem?

Being in the garage, under the sink, or out of sight may suggest a chemical ingestion or foreign body aspiration. Being near water (even in a tub or bucket) may suggest near-drowning.

Past medical

There are several conditions which may alter the likelihood of certain diagnoses. If a child has a history of atopy, including eczema, environmental allergies, or asthma, an exacerbation of asthma is highly likely if the child is wheezing. Many children with a history of prematurity and intubation in the neonatal intensive care unit have bronchopulmonary dysplasia and are prone to lung infections that can become severe. Children with known cardiac defects may wheeze when they are in congestive heart failure, or have a cardiac cause to their difficulty breathing. Children with laryngo- or tracheomalacia may become more acutely ill with croup than other children. Clinicians should inquire about chronic lung conditions such as cystic fibrosis.

Medications

One of the most common complaints in the ED is that "cough medicine" does not work. Many cough medicines given to children are expectorants that actually make children cough more than they would otherwise. Other medications, particularly for chronic conditions such as asthma, may give some indication of the severity of the child's underlying health. A child with asthma who has used inhaled beta-agonists a few times in their life may respond to a respiratory infection more robustly than a child with severe asthma who is frequently on oral steroids in addition to beta-agonists.

Immunizations

Although perhaps important as a general marker of the overall health care that a child has been receiving, the presence of complete immunization seldom has a significant impact on the identification or management of children with difficulty breathing. Due to herd immunity, infections with *Haemophilus influenzae* type b (Hib) are uncommon even in unimmunized children. A child who has not received the pneumococcal vaccine may be more likely to have pneumonia due to an invasive strain of the organism, but ED management is not impacted by this. Pertussis is now typically seen in young infants who are incompletely immunized at the time of infection because of their young age, even though they are immunized according to published schedules.

Family

Some conditions run in families, such as asthma. Occasionally a family history will prove helpful.

Social

Occasionally a social history will be revealing. A history of homelessness may suggest tuberculosis. Foster mothers who have just received a child may not know much of the medical history. Day care attendance may expose children to a greater number of viral respiratory illnesses, but the importance of this in the ED is seldom significant. Smoke exposure in the home may exacerbate chronic conditions such as asthma.

Physical examination

General appearance

An assessment of the degree to which a child is having difficulty breathing can be made upon entering the examination room. Infants should be removed from car seats or infant carriers and all young children should be undressed at least from the waist up initially. There are three main components to the initial general assessment: the work of breathing, the degree of dehydration, and the mental status. An experienced clinician can assess these three components in a matter of seconds.

Work of breathing

Assessing the work of breathing is perhaps the key to assessing difficulty breathing in children. This assessment does not require a stethoscope and can be made upon entering the patient's room. A happy, playful, well-appearing child generally has a normal work of breathing. Signs of increased work of breathing include retractions, grunting, nasal flaring, head bobbing, sitting forward to maintain an open airway, and tachypnea (respiratory rates may approach 100 breaths per minute in young infants). When the child can no longer sustain the increased work of breathing, the child will characteristically appear fatigued, develop altered mental status, and have periods of apnea or irregular respirations. Experienced clinicians make this vital assessment within seconds of seeing the child.

Degree of dehydration

The degree of dehydration may indirectly indicate the overall impact that increased work of breathing is having on the child. A child who is working too hard or is too sick to feed requires more aggressive fluid resuscitation than a child who is feeding well. A decrease in the number of wet diapers per day may indicate dehydration. Other signs and symptoms of dehydration include a sunken fontanel or eyes, dry tongue and mouth, tachycardia, and either irritability or lethargy.

Mental status

A child's mental status can be rapidly assessed by simply watching the child interact with the parent, play with a toy, interact with the environment (i.e., pull things off the wall, climb around the room), or by interacting with the patient. A bright, alert, interactive, smiling, playful child can be readily differentiated from a listless, limp, disinterested, tired-appearing child.

Vital signs

There are five main vital signs that should be assessed in children with difficulty breathing.

Respiratory rate

Although there are published tables of normal respiratory rates for children, these values are seldom helpful in the ED. The respiratory rate is quite variable and can depend on several factors that may change rapidly. Crying, fever, anxiety, hypoxia, increased work of breathing, shock, dehydration, and pain can make a child breathe faster than normal. Counting the respiratory rate for only a few seconds and then using a multiple of that count to generate breaths per minute may inaccurately reflect the true respiratory rate. Rough guidelines for tachypnea suggest that a normal respiratory rate during the first couple of months of life is in the 30–60 breaths per minute range. Respiratory rates greater than 60 for a sustained period of time while calm are nearly always abnormal. Very rapid rates in the 80–100 range may be seen. As infants age, the normal respiratory rate decreases. Older infants and toddlers typically have normal respiratory rates in the 20–40 range. School-aged children usually have respiratory rates in the 20s at most. More ominous than tachypnea is bradypnea, or slow respirations. Bradypnea typically signals respiratory fatigue that may require prompt intubation and mechanical ventilation. Young infants in the first couple months of life should not be breathing slower than about 30 breaths per minute. Young children should not breathe more slowly than about 20 breaths per minute. Adolescents can be assessed like adults.

Heart rate

The heart rate is variable in the same way as the respiratory rate. Multiple transient factors may result in tachycardia. These include crying, fever, anxiety, increased work of breathing, shock, dehydration, and pain. In young infants who have difficulty breathing, a heart rate of about 200 beats per minute is not uncommon. Supraventricular tachycardia is suggested by very rapid heart rates of at least 220 beats per minute and more often in the high 200s. Persistent tachycardia while calm and relaxed most commonly represents dehydration, but may also be seen in early shock and myocarditis.

Pulse oximetry

Using a non-invasive sensor that attaches to the finger, a painless assessment of the child's oxygenation can be performed with a bedside pulse oximeter. This "fifth vital sign" should be routinely assessed in all children with respiratory complaints. Subtle alterations in oxygenation that are not typically picked up on physical examination may be appreciated with pulse oximetry. Pulse oximetry has several limitations, however. It cannot be used to exclude respiratory conditions such as pneumonia. Due to the small digits and vasoconstriction in acutely ill infants, the pulse oximeter may have difficulty picking up a signal and generating useful output. The pulse oximeter frequently false alarms when there is excessive movement, the device fails to sense the pulse, or the probe falls off. Typically, young children have pulse oximetry readings in the high 90s or 100% at sea level or in the low 90s at significant elevation. The value that constitutes clinically significant hypoxia requiring oxygen administration and admission to the hospital is unknown. Many physicians will select a value in the low 90s as their threshold for administering oxygen.

Temperature

A good deal of fever phobia exists among parents and health care providers. In the setting of difficulty breathing, a fever typically suggests an infectious etiology. Foreign bodies, for example, do not usually present with a fever.

Blood pressure

Although blood pressure measurements are commonly obtained on patients in the ED, the role of blood pressure measurement in young infants is controversial. Young children often have transiently elevated blood pressures in the ED that have no clinical significance. Low blood pressures are seen in critically ill patients. Young children do not exhibit low blood pressure even when they are in early shock due to their excellent capacity to peripherally vasoconstrict.

Head, eyes, ears, nose, and throat

Head

In young infants, a sunken fontanel may suggest dehydration.

Eyes

The concurrent presence of conjunctivitis in the setting of clinical pneumonia is suggestive of an infection with *Mycoplasma pneumoniae* and may indicate that a macrolide antibiotic (e.g., erythromycin) is indicated.

Ears

An ear examination is seldom helpful in examining a child with difficulty breathing. The inappropriate diagnosis otitis media ("soft call") may lead to the inappropriate use of antibiotics in the setting of a viral upper respiratory tract infection.

Nose

Copious rhinorrhea is most consistent with upper respiratory tract infections. Rhinorrhea in the setting of wheezing is consistent with asthma exacerbated by a viral upper respiratory tract infection and bronchiolitis. Significant rhinorrhea is not typically seen in cases of peritonsillar or retropharyngeal abscess. Nasal flaring can be seen in young infants in respiratory distress.

Throat

The oropharyngeal examination may be particularly helpful in identifying cases of peritonsillar abscess. Dryness of the mucous membranes may indicate dehydration. Physicians who practiced in the 1980s are familiar with the general principle that no child with suspected epiglottitis should have an oropharyngeal examination due to the potential for the child's tenuous airway to close. In contemporary practice this concern has essentially been eliminated due to the introduction of the Hib vaccine and increased emphasis on pediatric airway management by emergency physicians (including rapid sequence intubation).

Neck

Asymmetric cervical adenopathy is typically seen with peritonsillar abscesses.

Pulmonary

The vast majority of information about the pulmonary examination is obtained without a stethoscope while assessing the general appearance and work of breathing (see above). The features of the chest to specifically note include the presence or absence of retractions, asymmetry of breath sounds when the right and left sides are compared, a prolonged expiratory phase or wheezing suggesting bronchospasm, and the presence of rales. Palpation and percussion have no appreciable role in the chest examination of an infant or young child.

Breath sounds

The physical examination should include an assessment of stridor, wheezing, and abnormal or asymmetric breath sounds. Conditions that partially occlude the upper airway (epiglottitis, esophageal foreign body, croup, and bacterial tracheitis) typically cause stridor. *Stridor* is an abnormal sound made during inspiration. Conditions that partially occlude the lower airways, such as asthma and bronchiolitis, typically cause wheezing and a prolonged expiratory phase. *Wheezing* is an abnormal sound made during expiration. Localized lung involvement as seen in pneumonia or aspirated foreign bodies may simply cause one side of the chest to sound different than the other. Rales can be heard in chemical pneumonitis, near-drowning, and less commonly in congestive heart failure. With poor air exchange, there may be few or no breath sounds (the "quiet" wheezer).

Cardiac

There are two main objectives in performing a cardiac examination on a child who is having difficulty breathing: identifying pathologic murmurs and identifying rate-related problems. Heart murmurs are quite common in young children; many have a known murmur that is of no clinical significance. Benign murmurs may also be heard in the setting of fever and shock. These "flow murmurs" are typically heard in systole, do not last for its entire duration, and are decrescendo in pattern. Pathologic murmurs that may be acquired or newly-discovered congenital problems have subtle and not-so-subtle features. Subtle features that have been described but may be difficult to assess in a loud ED on a tachycardic, ill child include an S3 and the absence of a split S1 sound. Not-so-subtle features, such as a loud, blowing, holosytolic murmur, are unlikely to be missed.

Abdomen

A meaningful abdominal examination on a child who is having difficulty breathing can be very difficult. Depending on the work of breathing, a young child with respiratory distress may preferentially sit up to breath. A brief and somewhat gross examination may be performed on the child in a seated position. If forced to lie down, these children typically fight to sit back up, strain their abdominal muscles, and provide no opportunity for a meaningful examination. A reasonable exam may be possible in young infants and children who are either moribund or in little distress.

Extremities

Capillary refill is quite dependent on the ambient temperature. An abnormal capillary refill is usually defined as greater than 2 seconds duration. Although capillary refill prolongation may represent shock, peripheral vasoconstriction due to an infant being cold will also manifest as prolonged capillary refill. Cyanotic extremities may be seen in hypoxic children.

Neurologic

The neurologic examination performed on a child with difficulty breathing is typically brief and global. The physician should immediately be able to note how the child interacts with his or her environment. A child who is lying down with obviously labored breathing who looks tired can be easily distinguished from a child who is playing, smiling, and, if old enough, sitting up and talking comfortably. As a child tires from a prolonged increase in the work of breathing, mental status typically deteriorates. The child will appear tired, less interactive, and may stare somewhat blankly forward no longer seeming to recognize or care about the environment. Altered mental status in a child with difficulty breathing can result from related concurrent conditions. For example, a child with pneumonia may develop sepsis. This may progress to septic shock causing tachypnea initially and then respiratory depression and altered mental status. Children seem to tolerate modest degrees of hypoxia, but if acutely and severely hypoxic, mental status may be depressed. Fluid losses typically occur from the inability to feed, insensible losses with exhalation, and increased work of breathing. These fluid losses may lead to dehydration that can result in depressed mental status. This is especially true if dehydration progresses to hypovolemic shock.

Differential diagnosis

Table 34.1 describes causes of shortness of breath in children.

Table 34.1 Differential diagnosis of shortness of breath in children

Diagnosis	Clinical presentation	Evaluation
Aspiration/ chemical pneumonitis (e.g., hydrocarbon ingestion)	Coughing and gagging at the time of ingestion followed by wheezing and tachypnea. Cyanosis may be present as well as hypoxia assessed by pulse oximetry. Mental status may be depressed. Fever may develop. Accidental and small volume ingestions predominate in young children. Adolescents may present after intentional, large volume ingestions.	Prevent spontaneous emesis if possible and do not induce emesis. Avoid activated charcoal to further decrease the risk of vomiting and aspiration. Attempt to identify the exact compound ingested and contact a poison control center. A chest X-ray should be obtained looking for bronchovascular markings, bibasilar infiltrates, and perihilar infiltrates.
Asthma	Wheezing and respiratory distress are the hallmarks of an asthma exacerbation. Fever may be present if an infection is the trigger for the exacerbation. Sitting upright with a hyperexpanded chest is common. Severe cases may have an absence of wheezing due to poor air exchange. A known history of asthma, hay fever, and/or eczema (i.e., atopy) is typical. Most will have a prior history of wheezing or asthma.	Pulse oximetry may reveal hypoxia. Response to bronchodilators may be helpful. In cases where there is poor air exchange, wheezing may become much more prominent *after* albuterol. Chest X-ray may be helpful if there is fever to assess for concurrent lobar pneumonia.
Bacterial tracheitis	In many ways, the presentation of bacterial (or membranous) tracheitis is like severe croup. The same age group as croup (toddlers and preschoolers) is typically affected. A prodrome of rhinorrhea and a barking cough is common. Bacterial tracheitis, however, presents with a high fever, ill appearance, and sometimes a productive cough. Children usually require prompt intubation.	Bacterial tracheitis is a clinical diagnosis; there is no specific laboratory or radiographic workup. If obtained for other reasons, a lateral neck X-ray may demonstrate an exudate within the trachea.
Bronchiolitis	The hallmark of bronchiolitis is wheezing. The typical age group is less than 24 months. The degree of respiratory distress ranges from minimal (a "happy wheezer") to severe with respiratory fatigue and failure requiring prompt intubation. Apnea may be the first sign seen in a small number of very young infants. Some infants seem to improve with beta-agonist therapy while others do not.	Bronchiolitis is a clinical diagnosis and is the most common diagnosis made in infants who are wheezing for the first time. A test for the RSV is available as a nasal washing. This test is primarily used for hospitalized infants to identify those needing respiratory isolation from other children. About half of the cases of bronchiolitis are positive for RSV. A chest X-ray may be normal or may reveal peribronchial cuffing or bilateral hyperexpanded lung fields.

(continued)

Table 34.1 Differential diagnosis of shortness of breath in children (*cont*)

Diagnosis	Clinical presentation	Evaluation
Croup	Most commonly affects toddlers and preschool children. Prodrome of a few days of rhinorrhea and cough. Barky cough and stridor develop. In mild cases, the stridor is present only when the child is agitated or crying. More severe cases have stridor at rest. Low-grade fever is common. Marked improvement after exposure to cool night air (usually on the way to the ED) is common. Typically, these children have a non-toxic appearance.	In general, the diagnosis of croup is made on clinical grounds and no diagnostic workup is indicated. Neck X-rays may be used to assess for esophageal or tracheal foreign body. Children with croup will usually have a narrowed tracheal shadow ("steeple sign").
Epiglottitis	Nearly eliminated in developed countries due to the widespread use of the *Haemophilus influenzae* type b vaccine. Most commonly affected are preschool and young school-aged children. Abrupt onset of fever with dysphagia, drooling, refusal to speak, muffled voice, and sitting upright in the "sniffing" position are common features.	Minimal agitation of the patient. Lateral neck X-ray should demonstrate an enlarged epiglottitis. Be prepared for airway obstruction – be ready to intubate (likely to be very difficult) or use needle cricothyroidotomy jet ventilation. Emergent ENT consultation for direct visualization of the epiglottis in the operating room is indicated.
Foreign body aspiration (Figure 34.1)	The presentation of a child with a foreign body in the airway can be quite subtle or very dramatic. The most common symptoms are choking, coughing, a sense of breathlessness, and wheezing. Abrupt onset of symptoms while eating would be expected in many cases as peanuts and other foods are the most commonly identified aspirated objects. About 80% of foreign body aspirations occur in toddlers and preschoolers.	The workup depends on the severity of symptoms. Children with severe respiratory distress and impending airway obstruction are best managed in the operating room by a bronchoscopist. Aspirated foreign bodies are seen on chest X-ray less than 20% of the time. Inspiratory/expiratory or decubitus X-rays may be needed to show air trapping and unilateral hyperexpansion, suggestive of aspirated foreign body.
Esophageal foreign body (Figure 34.2)	Esophageal foreign bodies that are in the upper esophagus may compress the airway "from behind" and cause respiratory distress. Symptoms may include drooling and stridor. An abrupt onset of symptoms and the absence of fever are common.	Coins are the most commonly identified esophageal foreign bodies and are visible on X-ray.
Muscle weakness (e.g., infant botulism, Guillain–Barré syndrome)	Muscle weakness in a previously-well child is an uncommon event. Difficulty breathing arises when the respiratory muscles no longer can sustain the work of breathing. The onset is usually gradual and progressive. However, when the point at which the work of breathing can no longer be sustained is reached, respiratory failure and the need for intubation arise suddenly.	There is no specific workup for this set of conditions in the ED. Ventilatory support is the primary concern and focus. Elevated PCO_2 on a blood gas may occur too late to be of any clinical utility.
Myocarditis and congestive heart failure	Acquired congestive heart failure in children is a relatively rare event. A history of a recent viral infection is possible but nonspecific. Tachycardia that fails to improve or worsens with the administration of IV fluids is suggestive of congestive heart failure. Rales, pedal edema, and jugular venous distention commonly seen	An enlarged cardiac silhouette and cephalization on chest X-ray may be seen. Although uncommonly performed on children in the ED, echocardiography would be helpful in identifying cardiac dysfunction. The role of laboratory studies more commonly used in adults with heart disease (e.g., troponin, B-type natriuretic peptide) is unclear in children.

(*continued*)

Table 34.1 Differential diagnosis of shortness of breath in children (*cont*)

Diagnosis	Clinical presentation	Evaluation
	in adults are atypical for young children. More typical symptoms include an enlarged liver and sweating during feedings. Fever may or may not be present.	
Near-drowning	Presentation varies with patient severity. The child may be initially asymptomatic and develop shortness of breath and cough over a few hours. Alternatively, the child may present in a coma due to anoxic brain injury and be intubated by the paramedics at the scene.	In the awake, well-appearing child a chest X-ray should be obtained to look for developing infiltrates. A second X-ray obtained a few hours later may show progressively worsening infiltrates. In the more critically-ill child, the initial chest X-ray may show florid pulmonary edema and interstitial infiltrates.
Peritonsillar abscess	Sore throat that progressively worsens in severity is common. This is typically seen in older children. Drooling is uncommon. A muffled voice may be present. This diagnosis is usually made by examining the posterior pharynx and seeing asymmetric swelling next to the tonsils and uvular deviation away from the swelling.	There is no specific workup. Diagnosis is initially made by visual inspection of the posterior oropharynx. Diagnosis is confirmed by needle aspiration or during incision and drainage.
Pertussis	Presentation is primarily based on age. The classic presentation has been described in young children and consists of mild rhinorrhea and cough followed by severe paroxysms of cough (with a characteristic "whoop") associated with vomiting. Immunizations have made this classic presentation of whooping cough rare. Young infants present with fever and repetitive paroxysms of cough and may have associated seizures, pneumonia, or encephalopathy.	The definitive test is the culture of the etiologic agent, *Bordetella pertussis* from nasopharyngeal mucus. This does not help with ED management as the test takes about 2 weeks. The repetitive nature of a cough in a young infant suggest the diagnosis. Chest X-ray may identify associated pneumonias.
Pneumonia	A wide range of clinical presentations can be seen in children with pneumonia. An otherwise well-appearing child may present with a mild cough and fever. Alternatively, the child may present in septic shock with respiratory failure.	The hallmark of pneumonia is an infiltrate on chest X-ray. The combination of cough and fever with an infiltrate on chest X-ray is indicative of pneumonia.
Retropharyngeal abscess (Figure 34.3)	Younger children (less than 3 years of age) typically develop the abscess in the setting of suppurative cervical lymphadenopathy. An older child may fall with something in his mouth and develop an abscess following penetration of the posterior oropharynx.	Diagnosis can be difficult. A lateral neck X-ray may show prevertebral soft tissue swelling. Confirmation with a neck CT is usually necessary.
Upper respiratory tract infection/ nasal congestion	Although not usually a problem in toddlers and school-aged children, nasal congestion can lead to difficulty breathing in young infants since they are obligate nasal breathers.	The diagnosis is clinical and made on examination of the child.

CT: computed tomography; ED: emergency department; ENT: ear, nose and throat; IV: intravenous; PCO_2: partial pressure of carbon dioxide; RSV: respiratory syncytial virus.

Diagnostic testing

Radiologic studies

Chest X-ray

Lobar or interstitial infiltrates suggest pneumonia. Unilateral hyperexpansion suggests an aspirated foreign body (Figure 34.1). Symmetric hyperexpansion can be seen in asthma and bronchiolitis. An esophageal foreign body may be discovered or confirmed (Figure 34.2). Serial chest X-rays may show the progression of disease in conditions such as chemical pneumonitis and near-drowning. Special chest X-rays such as bilateral decubitus or inspiratory and expiratory films may identify unilateral hyperexpansion suggestive of an aspirated foreign body. Additional findings such as pneumothorax, pnuemomediastinum, and masses can be seen. Chest X-rays are typically unnecessary unless there is reasonable clinical suspicion of one of the above diagnoses.

Neck X-rays

Soft tissue neck X-rays may be helpful in identifying the cause of shortness of breath. They should be ordered selectively to identify prevertebral soft tissue swelling suggestive of a retropharyngeal abscess (Figure 34.3) or an upper esophageal foreign body (usually a coin). A narrowed tracheal shadow may be noted in cases of croup, but is not used to make the diagnosis. Exudate visible in the trachea on X-ray is suggestive of bacterial tracheitis.

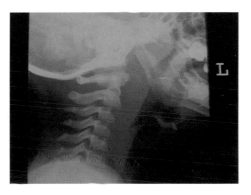

Figure 34.3
A child with a retropharyngeal abscess. Note the prevertebral soft tissue swelling.

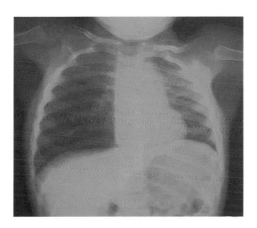

Figure 34.1
Right lung hyperexpansion. This child has aspirated a right-sided radiolucent foreign body.

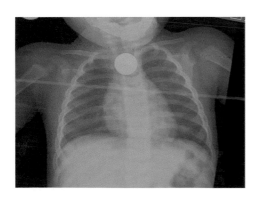

Figure 34.2
An esophageal coin. This child presented with the abrupt onset of difficulty breathing and drooling.

Laboratory studies

Specific testing

Some tests may identify the etiologic agent, although the utility of these tests in the ED is questionable. There is a nasal wash test for RSV, the organism identified in about 50% of bronchiolitis cases. This test is performed on nasopharyngeal mucus, and results can be returned within an hour in most hospitals. Since RSV is highly infectious, the primary purpose of this test is to detect infected children prior to hospitalization, and place them in respiratory isolation. The use of this test for children treated as outpatients is controversial. There is also a nasopharyngeal swab test for pertussis. This test is also performed on nasopharyngeal mucus but it takes nearly two weeks to get the results.

Arterial blood gas

An arterial blood gas is rarely indicated for infants and children with difficulty breathing. If carbon monoxide poisoning is suspected, as in smoke inhalation, an arterial blood gas with co-oximetry can be used to determine the percent carboxy-hemoglobin. It may also be used to guide management. If methemoglobinemia is suspected, as seen in teething gel ingestion, co-oximetry can be used to determine the percent methemoglobinemia, and may guide therapy with respect to administering methylene blue. Arterial blood gases may also be used after intubation to evaluate and appropriately adjust ventilator settings. In the vast majority of cases, pulse oximetry and the clinical examination are used to monitor the patient and guide therapy. The degree to which a child has respiratory fatigue determines when to intubate a child with respiratory distress, *not* the partial pressure of carbon dioxide ($PaCO_2$) from an arterial blood gas.

Peak flow

Peak flow is a bedside test in which a child is asked to blow as hard as they can with their lips around an L-shaped tube. One portion of the tube has a sliding gauge that is moved by the child's breath. The numeric output from these peak flow meters has been advocated for the home assessment of chronic asthma. The role of the peak flow meter in young children is controversial. Infants and young children who cannot forcefully exhale on command cannot use peak flow meters. The numeric output is effort-dependent, and even older school-aged children who are unfamiliar with the peak flow meter may not perform adequately to give useful information in the ED. Experienced older school-aged asthmatics may provide useful information from peak flow assessment in the ED. Reliance on peak flow performance in other children is problematic at best and may be misleading.

Treatment principles

There are several general treatment principles that apply to all children with difficulty breathing.

General treatment

- Oxygenation
- Respiratory support
- Anticipate dehydration
- Identify cases that require a procedure

Oxygenation

Ensuring adequate oxygenation is an important principle in managing children with difficulty breathing. Oxygenation can be assessed non-invasively using pulse oximetry. Oxygen delivery can be achieved in a relatively non-threatening manner with the parent holding oxygen tubing near the patient's face ("blow by"). Alternatively, infant and child-sized oxygen delivery tubing and masks can be used.

Respiratory support

Although a child may have adequate oxygenation, this is not the same as adequate ventilation. The child may not be able to overcome excessive work of breathing and may fatigue. In these instances, although the pulse oximetry readings may be adequate, the carbon dioxide level is rising. This rise in carbon dioxide may lead to mental status changes, decreased respiratory rate, and finally bradycardia and apnea. If a child presents in respiratory failure or is apneic, immediate ventilatory assistance with a bag-valve-mask is indicated. If a child is more slowly deteriorating, a trial of non-invasive ventilatory support such as nasal continuous positive airway pressure (CPAP) or a bi-level positive airway pressure (BiPAP) mask may be tried. Ultimately, a child in respiratory failure will need to be endotracheally intubated and placed on mechanical ventilation. If at all possible, the emergency physician should have all appropriate personnel and equipment for intubation readily available in anticipation of respiratory failure.

Anticipate dehydration

A child who has an increased work of breathing will have increased fluid losses from the lungs. These children typically have difficulty feeding and taking in adequate fluid volume. In general, children become dehydrated more rapidly than adults due to higher metabolic demands and decreased intake. IV access should be obtained early in the ED course unless discharging the child home is considered after the initial evaluation. If the child appears to be in shock, volume support with 20 ml/kg boluses of normal saline is indicated.

Identify cases that require a procedure

Identifying foreign bodies may be straightforward or subtle. Once identified, all aspirated foreign bodies and most high esophageal coins will need removal usually by a consultant. Retropharyngeal abscesses are usually drained by ENT consultants. Young infants are obligate nasal breathers and typically feed with a nipple in their mouth for several minutes without interruption. Nasal passage narrowing from nasal mucus or a viral upper respiratory tract infection may disrupt feeding and cause a surprising degree of distress in a neonate or young infant. Bulb suctioning the nose may be helpful in clearing secretions and may result in dramatic improvement in the ease of breathing and feeding for these babies.

Specific treatment

Asthma

Asthma has been increasing both in prevalence and severity for the past few decades. There are several treatments for acute exacerbations of asthma that can be life-saving. The two major pathophysiologic components of acute asthma exacerbations are bronchospasm and airway inflammation. The primary treatments are directed toward these features. Bronchospasm is currently treated with albuterol, a relatively beta-2 specific bronchodilator. There are two main methods of delivery that seem to have similar efficacy. Albuterol may be administered as a nebulized solution or as an inhaler with a spacer (and mask in young infants). Published doses are controversial. In a sense, children will drive the dosing through their pulmonary tidal volume. Inflammation is primarily treated with steroids. Commonly administered steroids include prednisone, prednisolone, methylprednisolone, and dexamethasone. The dosing is typically 2 mg/kg/day once daily (or divided into two equal doses) for 5 days for outpatients, except dexamethasone which is dosed from 0.15 to 0.6 mg/kg/dose for 2 days. It is commonly thought that in patients who can take oral medications, oral steroids are as effective as IV steroids.

Bronchiolitis

Bronchiolitis is a clinical syndrome that comprises a group of presumed viral lung infections in children. Although many cases are thought to be due to RSV, a substantial percentage of clinically indistinguishable cases test negative. As bronchiolitis is not a uniform disease, treatment responses are variable and the literature is varied with regard to treatment recommendations. Options include steroids, beta-agonists, and nebulized epinephrine.

The effectiveness of steroids is thought to be highest in cases where the child has underlying reactive airway disease (usually bronchopulmonary dysplasia or asthma). For a child with allergies and eczema, steroids may be effective therapy if he or she has bronchiolitis. The dosing of the steroids is the same as for asthma: 2 mg/kg/day once daily (or divided into two equal doses) for 5 days. Beta-agonists seem to work for some children and not for others. A trial of two or three nebulized albuterol treatments may be undertaken in the ED. If effective, treatment may be continued as an outpatient using an inhaler with a spacer and mask or as an inpatient with a nebulizer. If ineffective, further treatments are not usually helpful. The use of nebulized epinephrine is currently controversial. Clinical experience suggests that some children respond well to nebulized epinephrine (at least transiently) while others do not. However, recently performed, well-designed studies have failed to show a significant benefit. Antiviral treatment (e.g., with ribavirin) has no role in the ED.

Croup

The treatment of croup is based on the severity of symptoms. A child with only a history of a barky cough with no demonstrable cough in the ED is typically discharged for observation at home. A child with a demonstrable barky cough and no stridor at rest is treated with steroids as an outpatient. Historically a single dose of dexamethasone has been given. There is great controversy over the dosing and route of administration of dexamethasone for croup. In all likelihood, this controversy exists because the dosing and route of administration do not matter. Dosing ranges from 0.15 to 0.6 mg/kg, and the routes include oral, intramuscular, and nebulized. Based on studies from the late 1980s and early 1990s, 0.6 mg/kg of dexamethasone has been given intramuscularly. Other routes and dosing are clearly acceptable. If a child has a demonstrable barky cough and stridor at rest, nebulized epinephrine may be administered in addition to dexamethasone. The dose of nebulized solution is 0.05 ml/kg (up to 0.5 ml) of 2.25% racemic epinephrine diluted in 3 ml of normal saline. Since only half of the racemic epinephrine solution is biologically active and 1:1000 epinephrine is available in every "crash cart", nebulized 1:1000 epinephrine is now being used at a dose of 0.5 ml/kg (up to 5 ml) diluted in 3 ml of normal saline. If there is no prompt resolution of the stridor at rest, admission is typically warranted. If the stridor at rest resolves after a nebulized epinephrine treatment, the child is usually observed in the ED for 2–3 hours. If stridor at rest returns, the child requires admission. If stridor at rest does not return, discharge home from the ED is usually appropriate. Although cool mist has been advocated and used historically, clinical efficacy is doubtful and a recent, well-designed study suggested no demonstrable benefit. There has been concern that children treated with nebulized epinephrine would "rebound" and substantially worsen after an initial period of clinical improvement; this is now considered a myth.

Pneumonia

The treatment of pneumonia in children is primarily based on the likely etiology given the age of the child. Children rarely produce sputum, blood cultures are rarely positive in children with pneumonia, and the specific etiology of pneumonia in children is rarely determined by microbiologic means. In neonates, pneumonia is treated like all potentially serious bacterial infections with intravenous ampicillin (100 mg/kg per dose) and cefotaxime (100 mg/kg per dose) and admission to the hospital. In young infants, particularly those with minimal temperature elevation, repetitive coughing, and a history of conjunctivitis, *Chlamydia* is the presumed etiology, and treatment is with IV or oral erythromycin (10 mg/kg per dose four times per day). For children between the first few months of life and 5 years of age, the most likely bacterial etiology of lobar pneumonia is *Streptococcus pneumoniae*. Treatment for this age group is with IV cefuroxime (50 mg/kg per dose) for children admitted to the hospital or oral amoxicillin (45 mg/kg per dose twice daily) for children discharged home from the ED. Presumed viral pneumonia (clinically indistinguishable from bacterial and along the spectrum of bronchiolitis) is not treated with antibiotics. So-called "atypical" pneumonia is most common in children older than 5 years of age, and macrolide antibiotics (such as azithromycin 10 mg/kg on day 1 – not to exceed 500 mg – and 5 mg/kg once daily for 4 subsequent days – not to exceed 250 mg per day) are appropriate. The most common reason for children outside the neonatal period to be admitted is hypoxia. The pulse oximetry threshold that determines clinically significant hypoxia warranting admission is unknown. It has been suggested that children with room air pulse oximetry readings below 90–92% should be admitted to the hospital.

Special patients
Bronchopulmonary dysplasia

Former premature infants, particularly those with lung disease identified in the neonatal intensive care unit and those with prolonged mechanical ventilation, may have bronchopulmonary dysplasia. These children have reactive airways and often wheeze when they get upper respiratory tract infections. If they develop bronchiolitis, particularly if they test positive for RSV, they can have particularly severe disease and may progress to respiratory failure. Similarly, pneumonia that is well-tolerated by other children may make children with bronchopulmonary dysplasia critically ill.

Cystic fibrosis

Although systemic and genetic, cystic fibrosis primarily manifests as a lung disorder. These children have frequent lung infections and may have relatively unusual pneumonias caused by Gram-negative organisms including *Pseudomonas aeruginosa*.

Sickle cell disease

A child with sickle cell disease may develop *acute chest syndrome*. These children typically present with fever, cough, and chest pain. They may or may not be hypoxic. In most instances, it is difficult to distinguish lung infarction from a bacterial pneumonia; the two conditions may co-exist. These children are usually admitted to the hospital for hydration, analgesia and pain control, and parenteral antibiotics.

Children with tracheostomies

Children with tracheostomies may have mechanical complications. Tracheostomy dislodgment may lead to cardiopulmonary arrest. Plugging of the tracheostomy tube with mucus may occur and lead to profound respiratory distress.

Disposition
Consultation

Subspecialty consultation is infrequently needed in cases of children with difficulty breathing. Consultation (usually from an ENT specialist or a pediatric surgeon) for the removal of aspirated or esophageal foreign bodies is usually indicated

ENT surgeons are usually consulted to drain retropharyngeal abscesses in the operating room. Emergency physicians often perform needle drainage of peritonsillar abscesses in the ED.

Monitoring

For moderately-ill children, it is sometimes difficult to predict whether they will improve or deteriorate. Close monitoring with frequent re-examinations and continuous pulse oximetry is prudent. Anticipating and responding to respiratory distress is a key management principle.

Intensive care unit admissions

Any child who is endotracheally intubated will be admitted to an intensive care setting. Other children in whom it is desirable to aggressively treat without intubation (particularly asthmatics) may also be appropriate for the intensive care unit. Any case where impending airway compromise is a serious consideration (e.g., epiglottitis, retropharyngeal abscess, bacterial tracheitis) should be admitted to the intensive care unit. Cases in which the condition is worsening but may not progress to respiratory failure (e.g., hydrocarbon aspirations and near-drowning) may also be appropriate for the intensive care unit.

Ward admissions

Children who are dehydrated and require IV fluids should be admitted to the hospital. Children with croup and stridor at rest 2 hours after treatment with nebulized epinephrine should be admitted. Children with pneumonia who are suspected of being septic should be admitted to the hospital. Young children with bronchiolitis who are slowly worsening should be admitted. Asthmatic children who require nebulized beta-agonist therapy more frequently than every 3 or 4 hours should strongly be considered for admission to the hospital. Due to a risk of apnea, an infant with a history and examination consistent with pertussis should be admitted for observation. Although the specific pulse oximetry value which constitutes clinically significant hypoxia is controversial, in general, hypoxic children should be given oxygen and admitted to the hospital.

Discharges

Most children with difficulty breathing can be discharged home after treatment in the ED, a prescription for medicine to take at home, and reassurance. Croup that is improving and does not produce stridor at rest can typically be discharged home. Most asthmatics can be treated with oral steroids and beta-agonist therapy and discharged home. Children with esophageal coins in or distal to the stomach can be discharged home. Most children with bronchiolitis can be treated as outpatients. If a near-drowning patient has a clear chest X-ray and normal oxygenation after several hours of observation, discharge home with close parental supervision is usually appropriate.

Pearls, pitfalls, and myths
Pearls
RSV bronchiolitis in young infants may initially present with apnea

Before the onset of wheezing, infants in the first few months of life may present after a brief period of apnea.

Inspiratory/expiratory and decubitus chest X-rays may help identify cases of foreign body aspiration

More than 80% of aspirated foreign bodies are not directly visible on X-ray. Indirect findings should be sought. Due to a ball-valve mechanism, air trapping occurs on the side with the foreign body. Unilateral hyperexpansion may be seen on the chest X-ray and this phenomenon may be exaggerated in an expiratory or decubitus film.

A child in moderately severe respiratory distress should be allowed to assume a position of comfort unless you are ready to aggressively manage the airway

Although we often remove children from their parents' arms to perform parts of the physical examination, agitating a child with a tenuous airway may lead to airway occlusion. Aggressive and prompt airway management may be required. If not prepared to immediately manage the airway of a young infant, keep the child in a position of comfort until a definitive management plan is in place.

Severe asthma may present without wheezing due to poor air exchange

In order to make the musical sound of wheezing, enough air has to pass through the airways. No air movement, no sound.

A decrease in pulse oximetry does not necessarily indicate a worsening clinical condition in an asthmatic just starting bronchodilator therapy in the ED

As bronchodilator therapy is initiated, areas of lung that were previously "shut down" open up. There is a lag between the time when the blood flow normalizes in a region of lung and when the airways open up. A transient ventilation–perfusion mismatch develops and the patient's oxygenation may actually fall briefly before improving.

Pitfalls

Slowing respirations may imply getting better or getting worse

As a patient improves, tachypnea usually normalizes. However, if a patient is worsening and developing respiratory fatigue, their respiratory rate will also fall. A slower respiratory rate has to be assessed in relation to the overall clinical appearance of the child.

Vomiting and hydrocarbon ingestion

Hydrocarbons in the stomach and intestines are usually well-tolerated. Hydrocarbons in the lungs can cause a devastating chemical pneumonitis. Vomiting offers another chance for the hydrocarbon to go into the lungs.

Myths

Wheezing means asthma

A frequently repeated mantra is that "all that wheezes is not asthma." Other conditions such as aspirated foreign bodies, chemical pneumonitis, bronchiolitis, and gastroesophageal reflux often cause wheezing.

All wheezing children need albuterol

A trial of a bronchodilator is a reasonable intervention in young children with wheezing and respiratory distress. However, if the cause is not asthma, bronchodilators are often ineffective. If a child improves with a bronchodilator, it is reasonable to continue with additional doses. If a child has a foreign body or chemical pneumonitis, repeated doses of bronchodilators are not indicated. Although commonly administered, the effectiveness of bronchodilators in many cases of bronchiolitis is unclear.

References

1. Brown K. Bronchiolitis. In: Strange GR, Ahrens WR, Lelyveld S, et al. (eds). *Pediatric Emergency Medicine: A Comprehensive Study Guide*, 2nd ed., New York, NY: McGraw-Hill, 2002. pp. 215–218.
2. Brown K. Pneumonia. In: Strange GR, Ahrens WR, Lelyveld S, et al. (eds). *Pediatric Emergency Medicine: A Comprehensive Study Guide*, 2nd ed., New York, NY: McGraw-Hill, 2002: pp. 219–225.
3. Harley JR, Ochsenschlager DW. Near drowning. In: Barkin RM, Caputo GL, Jaffe DM, et al. (eds). *Pediatric Emergency Medicine: Concepts and Clinical Practice*, 2nd ed., New York, NY: Mosby, 1997. 474–481.
4. Schunk JE. Foreign body – ingestion/aspiration. In: Fleisher GR, Ludwig S, Henretig FM, et al. (eds). *Textbook of Pediatric Emergency Medicine*, 4th ed., Philadelphia, PA: Lippincott Williams and Wilkins, 2000. pp. 267–273.
5. Shih RD. Hydrocarbons. In: Goldfrank LR, Flomenbaum NE, Lewin NA, et al. (eds). *Goldfrank's Toxicologic Emergencies*, 6th ed., Stamford, Connecticut: Appleton and Lange, 1998. pp. 1383–1398.
6. Strange GR, Cooper A, Gausche M, et al. (eds). Respiratory distress. In: *APLS: The Pediatric Emergency Medicine Course*, 3rd ed., Dallas, TX: American College of Emergency Physicians, 1998. pp. 3–16.
7. Swischuk LE. The chest. In: Swischuk LE (ed.). *Emergency Imaging of the Acutely Ill or Injured Child*, 3rd ed., Philadelphia, PA: Williams and Wilkins, 1994. pp. 1–150.
8. Weiner DL. Respiratory distress. In: Fleisher GR, Ludwig S, Henretig FM, et al. (eds). *Textbook of Pediatric Emergency Medicine*, 4th ed., Philadelphia, PA: Lippincott Williams and Wilkins, 2000. pp. 553–564.

35 Syncope

Amal Mattu, MD

Scope of the problem

Syncope is defined as a transient loss of consciousness and postural tone caused by an abrupt decrease in cerebral perfusion, with subsequent spontaneous recovery. When recovery occurs prior to complete loss of consciousness, the episode is referred to as pre- or near-syncope. Syncope and pre-syncope are generally considered the same condition at different points along a continuum. Therefore, the emergency department (ED) evaluation and work-up for both is similar.

Syncope is a common presenting complaint in the ED. It accounts for approximately 1–3% of ED visits and 1–6% of hospital admissions. As much as $750 million per year is spent in the US to diagnose and treat syncope. The differential diagnosis of syncope includes both benign and life-threatening etiologies. Emergency physicians must have a sound knowledge of diagnostic considerations in order to perform an adequate and cost-effective work-up and make appropriate disposition decisions.

Pathophysiology

Consciousness is maintained through the proper functioning of the cerebral hemispheres and the reticular activating system (RAS). Syncope occurs when there is dysfunction of either both cerebral hemispheres or the RAS. Proper function of these structures depends on cerebral metabolism and delivery of oxygen and glucose. Disruption of this metabolism can occur because of generalized systemic hypoperfusion (e.g., cardiac dysrhythmia, hypovolemia with orthostasis), localized cerebral hypoperfusion (e.g., transient ischemia attack, stroke), systemic hypoxia, or hypoglycemia.

History

Syncope has many causes, some benign and others life-threatening. As many as 45% of cases of syncope remain undiagnosed after a standard work-up. However, most diagnoses that *are* made are established during the initial work-up in the ED. Only a minority of cases are diagnosed during inpatient admission. Therefore, a thorough history, physical examination, and work-up in the ED are crucial in order to maximize the chances of properly identifying the cause of syncope.

What were you doing when you "passed out?"

A sudden change in position from supine to standing suggests syncope due to orthostatic hypotension (orthostatic syncope). However, syncope while supine indicates a cardiac etiology or a seizure (not a true cause of syncope, but generally included in the differential diagnosis). Syncope during exertion may also indicate orthostatic syncope, but may instead be caused by cardiac outflow obstruction (e.g., hypertrophic cardiomyopathy or aortic stenosis). Syncope associated with sudden head-turning, tight neck collars, or shaving the neck may be caused by carotid sinus hypersensitivity. Syncope that occurs shortly after exposure to pain or that is associated with strong emotions (e.g., fear, anxiety) is usually known as vasovagal or vasomotor syncope. Forceful prolonged coughing, defecation, micturition, and weight-lifting (Valsalva maneuvers) can induce syncope by increasing intrathoracic pressure, leading to decreased venous return to the heart and decreased cardiac output.

What symptoms do you remember just before you "passed out?" What symptoms did you experience after you woke up?

Severe headache around the time of the syncopal episode suggests intracranial bleed, especially subarachnoid hemorrhage. Chest pain, palpitations, or dyspnea suggest cardiovascular etiologies, such as acute coronary syndrome (ACS), dysrhythmia, pericardial tamponade, or aortic dissection; or a pulmonary cause, such as pulmonary embolism (PE). Aortic dissection is often accompanied by upper back pain. Abdominal or low back pain may indicate a ruptured abdominal aortic aneurysm (AAA) or ectopic pregnancy. A sense of progressive lightheadedness, weakness, and "tunnel vision" just prior to the syncopal episode is often associated with vasomotor and orthostatic syncope, although this prodrome does not exclude more life-threatening causes. In contrast, the absence of any prodromal symptoms is often associated with a dysrhythmia. If the patient describes an aura, a seizure is the probable cause of the episode. Patients reporting a prodrome of lightheadedness, nausea, diaphoresis, and tremulousness should be evaluated for hypoglycemia.

Were there any witnesses?

Witnesses to the episode can be helpful in distinguishing between some causes of syncope. Witnesses should be questioned regarding the duration of unconsciousness. True syncope is generally associated with unconsciousness lasting no more than seconds to minutes. Prolonged unconsciousness before waking is more likely due to a seizure (postictal state) or drug effects (e.g., alcohol). Witnesses may report "seizure" activity. Tonic–clonic movements lasting for several seconds are common in cases of syncope; however, if the movements last more than 20–30 seconds, a seizure is the more likely cause. Witnesses should also be questioned regarding the mental status of the patient after waking. Seizures are associated with postictal confusion lasting more than 5 minutes. Syncope, on the other hand, is associated with a rapid return to a normal level of consciousness. Witnesses may also be helpful in describing the patient's activities and complaints immediately before and after the syncopal episode.

Have you been feeling ill lately?

Recent nausea, vomiting, anorexia, or diarrhea may suggest orthostatic syncope due to intravascular volume depletion. If the patient has had abdominal pain, vomiting, or diarrhea, specific questions pertaining to hematemesis or melena may indicate gastrointestinal blood loss as a cause of orthostatic syncope. Anemia from chronic blood loss is associated with a more prolonged sense of fatigue, malaise, and dyspnea with exertion. Recent episodes of chest pain or palpitations may indicate a cardiac cause of syncope. Recent abdominal or back pain during the days preceding the syncopal episode may suggest an expanding AAA or ectopic pregnancy prior to rupture.

What medications have you been taking? Any drugs or alcohol?

Many medications have been implicated in inducing syncope (Table 35.1). The primary

Table 35.1 Drugs associated with syncope

| Antiarrhythmics |
| Anticonvulsants |
| Antidepressants |
| Antiparkinsonism agents |
| Antipsychotics |
| Benzodiazepines |
| Beta-adrenergic blocking agents |
| Calcium channel blocking agents |
| Diuretics |
| Hypnotics |
| Narcotics |
| Nitrates |
| Phenothiazines |

Source: Hunt M. Syncope. In: Rosen P, et al. (eds). *Emergency Medicine: Concepts and Clinical Practice.* St. Louis: Mosby-Year Book, 1998.

mechanism through which medication-induced syncope occurs is from excessive bradycardia or vasodilation. Patients that abuse illicit drugs and alcohol may also report that they "passed out." The period of unconsciousness associated with these drugs and alcohol is more prolonged before recovery than most other causes of syncope. Alchohol consumption, even in moderation, causes vasodilation and therefore predisposes individuals to syncope from other causes as well.

Has this ever happened before? Did you see a doctor? Was there any work-up?

Many types of benign syncope have a repeated pattern of occurrence. However, some of the life-threatening causes of syncope can also be associated with prior episodes, including dysrhythmias, hypertrophic cardiomyopathy, and aortic stenosis. Information from prior work-ups helps rule in or exclude some life-threatening etiologies (e.g., prior echocardiography results will provide information regarding hypertrophic cardiomyopathy or aortic stenosis; prior cardiac catheterization results will help risk-stratify patients for suspected ACS).

Has any member of your family died suddenly?

Some of the life-threatening causes of syncope including hypertrophic cardiomyopathy, Jervel Lang–Nielson, Romano–Ward and the Brugada syndromes are associated with a family history of sudden death. Also, there may be a family predilection for subarachnoid hemorrhage (SAH)

Emergency physicians should have a lower threshold to perform a more extensive work-up in patients who report this family history.

Associated symptoms

Cardiopulmonary

Chest or upper back pain prior to or following the syncopal episode warrant strong consideration for ACS, aortic dissection, PE, or pericardial tamponade. Acute dyspnea also warrants consideration of PE and pericardial tamponade. Palpitations suggest a dysrhythmia.

Neurologic

The presence of a headache (especially of abrupt onset) prior to the syncopal episode suggests the possibility of intracranial hemorrhage, most commonly SAH. The presence of a headache after recovery is less specific, as many patients will report a post-syncopal (or post-seizure) headache. However, if the headache is severe or persistent, intracranial hemorrhage should be ruled out. Diplopia, dysarthria, ataxia, or vertigo prior to or after the syncopal episode indicates a posterior circulation stroke or transient ischemic attack (TIA). Any neurologic complaint that is accompanied by chest or upper back pain should be considered an aortic dissection until proven otherwise.

Gastrointestinal

The presence of nausea, vomiting, anorexia, or diarrhea may suggest orthostatic syncope due to intravascular volume depletion. Hematemesis or blood in the bowel movements indicates gastrointestinal blood loss causing orthostatic syncope. Abdominal or low back pain may indicate a ruptured AAA.

Gynecologic

Ruptured ectopic pregnancy can cause sufficient blood loss to induce orthostatic syncope. The abrupt pain from a ruptured ectopic pregnancy can also cause vasomotor syncope. Clues to the diagnosis of ruptured ectopic pregnancy include known or suspected first-trimester pregnancy, irregular vaginal bleeding, and abdominal, pelvic, or low back pain. Frequent and heavy vaginal bleeding can induce severe anemia and also lead to orthostatic syncope.

Extremities

Leg pain or swelling suggests deep venous thrombosis (DVT) and syncope due to PE. Leg pain may also be caused by acute vascular insufficiency, often associated with aortic dissection or AAA. Unilateral extremity weakness suggests a cerebrovascular cause of syncope.

Past medical

Cardiovascular

Cardiac risk factors increase the likelihood of cardiac causes of syncope, especially ACS and dysrhythmia. Hypertension and atherosclerotic coronary vascular disease also predispose to aortic dissection and AAA, respectively.

A history of previous dysrhythmias warrants work-up for recurrent atrial or ventricular dysrhythmias. A history of Wolff–Parkinson–White syndrome should also prompt strong consideration of tachydysrhythmia-induced syncope.

Aortic stenosis is associated with exertional syncope. Advanced aortic stenosis can cause syncope with even minimal exertion. Valvular rupture or worsening incompetence may cause syncope from decreased cardiac output.

Pulmonary

Patients who report recent surgeries, recent or current pregnancy, or other risk factors for thromboembolism should be evaluated for possible PE. Prior episodes of DVT or PE also predispose individuals to recurrent PE.

Physical examination

A comprehensive physical examination should be performed in all patients with syncope. Emphasis should be placed on the cardiovascular and neurologic examinations.

General appearance

If the patient appears pale, ashen, or diaphoretic at the time of presentation, consider a life-threatening cause of syncope. Intravascular volume depletion with shock due to a ruptured AAA or ectopic pregnancy, aortic dissection, gastrointestinal bleeding, sepsis, or severe dehydration are diagnostic possibilities. Shock may also be caused by an ACS or persisting dysrhythmia.

Vital signs

Hypotension indicates significant intravascular volume depletion or cardiogenic shock due to ACS or dysrhythmia. The heart rate can also indicate the presence of a brady- or tachy-dysrhythmia. A rapid heart rate may be caused by a dysrhythmia, or it may be a compensatory response to shock. Tachypnea is nonspecific, but may be a marker for PE or shock. A fingerstick glucose and pulse oximetry should be obtained as part of the routine vital sign assessment in patients with syncope as well. If the fingerstick glucose is noted to be low during the initial evaluation, hypoglycemia-induced syncope is suggested. This diagnosis should only be made if the history is supportive (the patient exercised without eating for many hours, for example). Unconsciousness due to insulin-induced hypoglycemia is unlikely to resolve without administration of exogenous glucose. Hypoxia noted on pulse oximetry suggests PE. Orthostatic vital signs are often checked in patients with syncope. However, they have poor sensitivity and specificity for intravascular volume depletion, especially in elderly patients. Up to 30% of cardiac-related syncope cases will have positive orthostatic vital sign changes (heart rate increase of more than 30 beats per minute or systolic blood pressure fall of more than 20 mmHg). Fever or mild hypothermia may occur in sepsis. Low-grade fevers may also occur in patients with PE.

Head and neck

The head and neck should be assessed for signs of trauma that may have occurred during the syncopal episode. Pupillary or facial asymmetry may indicate a cerebrovascular cause of syncope. On the other hand, bilateral pupillary constriction or dilation may indicate a medication effect or drug ingestion; most narcotics induce pupillary constriction, whereas anticholinergics and sympathomimetics may cause pupillary dilation. Carotid pulses should be assessed for symmetry and bruits. Some authors have suggested carotid sinus massage (CSM) to assess for carotid sinus hypersensitivity. However, this should only be done in patients who have a history suggestive of this diagnosis (e.g., syncope while shaving) and in whom the risk of carotid atherosclerotic plaques is negligible. The mouth should be assessed for evidence of tongue-biting, more commonly discovered after seizures than syncope.

Cardiovascular

The cardiac examination is the most important part of the examination in patients presenting with syncope. The ventricular rate should be assessed, and may indicate the presence of a tachy- or bradydysrhythmia. The regularity of the heart rhythm should also be assessed. An irregular rhythm suggests atrial fibrillation, premature complexes, or second-degree atrioventricular (AV) block. Beware, however, that a normal heart rate and rhythm does not exclude the possibility that the patient's episode of syncope was caused by a transient dysrhythmia. Carefully auscultate for murmurs. Aortic stenosis is associated with a crescendo–decrescendo systolic murmur, heard loudest at the upper sternal border and radiating to the carotid arteries. Hypertrophic cardiomyopathy is also associated with a systolic murmur, but the intensity is greatest at the lower sternal border or apex. The intensity of the murmur of hypertrophic cardiomyopathy generally increases with Valsalva maneuvers and decreases with Trendelenburg positioning and squatting. The vascular examination is crucial as well. Assess for equal upper and lower extremity pulses. Unequal pulses in the upper extremities may suggest aortic dissection in the right clinical scenario.

Pulmonary

Abnormal lung sounds suggest a pulmonary cause of syncope. Rales can be caused by pulmonary edema due to myocardial ischemia or infarction. Focal wheezes can be caused by PE. Diffuse wheezes may be due to multiple pulmonary emboli or pulmonary edema.

Abdomen

The abdomen should be assessed for tenderness. Consider a ruptured AAA or ectopic pregnancy in the patient with syncope who has abdominal tenderness. An enlarged pulsatile abdominal aorta is sometimes appreciated in cases of aortic aneurysm.

Pelvic

The pelvic examination is useful in the patient in whom ruptured ectopic pregnancy is a consideration. Any female patient of childbearing age with syncope who reports pelvic or abdominal pain, vaginal bleeding, or is known to be pregnant in the first- or second-trimester should have a pelvic examination to assess for vaginal bleeding, adnexal masses, or adnexal and uterine tenderness.

Rectal

The rectal examination should be considered a routine part of the physical examination for a patient with syncope. Gross blood or melena is suggestive of significant gastrointestinal bleeding causing syncope. The presence of occult blood may indicate chronic gastrointestinal blood loss and anemia.

Neurologic

A detailed neurologic examination should be performed on all patients who present after a syncopal episode. A depressed level of consciousness may be caused by persistent shock, hypoxia, hypoglycemia, seizure (postictal state), stroke, intracranial bleed, or drug/medication effect. Vertigo, ataxia, dysarthria, or any focal neurologic deficits indicate a stroke or intracranial hemorrhage. Neurologic symptoms or signs that are accompanied by chest or upper back pain should be considered an aortic dissection until proven otherwise.

Differential diagnosis

Table 35.2 lists a number of causes of syncope.

Table 35.2 Differential diagnosis of syncope

Causes of syncope	Symptoms	Signs	Work-up
Acute coronary syndrome	Chest pain or other "anginal equivalent" is usually present. Elderly patients and diabetics are prone to more atypical and painless presentations.	Patients usually appear uncomfortable; signs of heart failure (hypoxia, rales) may accompany ACS.	ECG and cardiac enzyme testing is warranted. Patients should be admitted. Isolated syncope with neither anginal symptoms nor ECG abnormalities is very unlikely due to ACS.
Aortic dissection	Classically, patients with AD present with sudden onset of "ripping" or "tearing" chest pain with radiation to the upper back. Up to 15% will present with syncope, but the majority will have preceding or post-syncope chest or upper back pain.	Although classically these patients are severely hypertensive, two-thirds will be normotensive or hypotensive. Suggestive findings include unequal pulses in the extremities or associated neurologic deficits.	CXR is neither sensitive nor specific enough to be a definitive test for the diagnosis. If the diagnosis is suspected based on history and physical examination, CT of the great vessels with IV contrast should be obtained. Alternatively, emergent aortography or TEE can be performed with equal or greater sensitivity, although they are usually less available in the ED.
Aortic stenosis	Syncope in patients with AS usually occurs with exertion. Severe AS may produce syncope with even mild amounts of exertion. Patients are usually elderly.	The main physical examination finding is a systolic crescendo–decrescendo murmur heard best at the upper sternal border that radiates to the carotid arteries.	The diagnosis of AS is established during echocardiography. The ECG usually demonstrates left atrial and left ventricular enlargement, but these are nonspecific findings.
Carotid sinus hypersensitivity	Syncope is associated with maneuvers that result in direct pressure applied to the carotid sinus (e.g., shaving, tight-fitting collar), and sudden turning of the neck.	The vital signs and examination after recovery is normal. CSM may reproduce syncope, but this maneuver is reserved for patients that have negligible risk of carotid atherosclerotic disease.	No specific work-up is indicated, although patients should be warned about the factors associated with recurrence.

(continued)

Table 35.2 Differential diagnosis of syncope (*cont*)

Causes of syncope	Symptoms	Signs	Work-up
Dysrhythmia	The classic presentation is an abrupt onset of syncope without prodrome. On the other hand, palpitations or chest pain may precede the syncopal episode.	Tachycardia, bradycardia, or irregular pulses are typical. Signs of heart failure may be present if the dysrhythmia is severe or persistent.	The ECG may show an obvious dysrhythmia or more subtle findings, including signs of WPW (short PR interval, wide QRS interval, and delta-wave) or prolonged QT interval; the ECG may also be completely normal. Admission for cardiac monitoring is recommended.
Hypertrophic cardiomyopathy	Syncope in these patients often occurs with exertion, but may occur at rest as well. Patients are often young athletes, although the average age at diagnosis is 30–40 years.	Examination is usually notable for a systolic murmur heard best at the lower sternal border or apex. The murmur intensity increases with maneuvers which decrease venous return, such as Valsalva or standing; and decreases with maneuvers which increase venous return, such as Trendelenburg or squatting.	The diagnosis of hypertrophic cardiomyopathy is definitively established during doppler echocardiography.
Intracranial hemorrhage	Patients usually report the presence of a severe or sudden headache prior to the syncopal episode, or a severe persistent headache after the episode. Some patients may report neurologic abnormalities as well.	A detailed neurologic examination may reveal subtle or overt neurologic deficits. Subarachnoid hemorrhage, however, may be associated with a normal examination.	CT of the head is diagnostic of intraparenchymal hemorrhage and will detect more than 90% of subarachnoid hemorrhages. Lumbar puncture should be performed in patients who have a headache associated with syncope when the CT is negative.
Medication effects	Syncope may occur in a fashion similar to orthostatic syncope. Associated weakness and lightheadedness tend to be more persistent. However, patients usually report a recent change in or addition to their medication regimen.	Orthostatic hypotension or persistent bradycardia is common. Toxicity due to anticholinergic medications may be associated with warm, dry, erythematous skin and dilated pupils. Narcotic toxicity is associated with persistent decreased level of consciousness and miosis.	Signs of medication toxicity, especially medications that have a type IA antiarrhythmic effects, often manifest abnormalities on the ECG; therefore, an ECG should always be obtained. Medication levels should be obtained when appropriate.
Orthostatic syncope	This type of syncope, associated with intravascular fluid depletion (dehydration, acute or chonic blood loss) occurs when there are abrupt changes in body position from supine to standing or with walking.	Intravascular fluid depletion may be associated with tachycardia and/or hypotension. Orthostatic vital sign changes are common, though not 100% sensitive or specific. Signs of blood loss may be present.	Serum electrolyte testing is indicated if the patient reports ongoing vomiting or diarrhea. Hemoglobin testing is indicated if the patient reports blood loss (e.g., hematemesis, melena, heavy vaginal bleeding) or if there is evidence of blood loss on the examination (e.g., fecal occult blood).

(continued)

Table 35.2 Differential diagnosis of syncope (*cont*)

Causes of syncope	Symptoms	Signs	Work-up
Pulmonary embolism	PE is associated with syncope in 10–15% of cases. Patients usually complain of dyspnea or pleuritic chest pain. If the source of the embolism is from a DVT, the patient may also complain of leg pain or swelling.	The majority of patients will have tachypnea (respiratory rate $\geqslant$ 20/minute). Approximately half will also have tachycardia. Lung sounds are variable; wheezing is common, but the lungs may be clear.	CXR is often obtained to evaluate for alternative diagnoses. Further work-up for PE varies between physicians. Testing may involve CT of the lungs with IV contrast, V/Q scanning, D-dimer testing, or any combination of the above. Pulmonary angiography is generally considered the gold standard test.
Pericardial tamponade	Patients typically complain of dyspnea. Chest pain associated with pericarditis may precede the development of tamponade.	Tachycardia and hypotension is very common. The lungs are usually clear. Jugular venous distension is typical unless the patient is hypovolemic.	The ECG often shows evidence of low voltage or *electrical alternans*. CXR typically shows massive cardiomegaly. Definitive diagnosis is made with emergent echocardiography (diastolic collapse of the right atrium and right ventricle).
Ruptured ectopic pregnancy	Syncope occurs in patients with ruptured ectopic pregnancy in 10–15% of cases. Patients usually report abdominal pain, pelvic pain, low back pain, or vaginal bleeding.	Hypotension may be present if significant blood loss has occurred. The examination may be notable for abdominal and adnexal tenderness with vaginal blood on the pelvic examination.	Any woman of childbearing age who presents with syncope in association with abdominal, low back or pelvic pain, or with vaginal bleeding should have immediate pregnancy testing. If the test is positive, obtain an immediate pelvic ultrasound as well as a quantitative serum hCG level, type and Rh, and "pre-op labs."
Ruptured abdominal aortic aneurysm	As many as 10–15% of patients with ruptured AAA present with syncope. These patients usually complain of abdominal or low back pain prior to or after the syncopal episode.	Classic findings include hypotension and an enlarged, palpable pulsatile abdominal aorta. However, more than one-third of patients are normotensive, and more than two-thirds of patients do not have an enlarged palpable aorta noted on initial examination. Femoral pulses may be unequal, but this finding is not sensitive.	If a ruptured AAA is suspected, surgical consultation should be obtained immediately. Bedside ultrasound is helpful in evaluating for the presence of an aneurysm. If a bedside ultrasound is not available, abdominal CT with IV contrast can be obtained. However, if the patient is hemodynamically unstable and the diagnosis is highly suspected, surgical intervention is warranted.
Stroke or transient ischemic attack	Stroke/TIA are rare causes of syncope. A stroke that induces a loss of consciousness (disrupting perfusion to the bilateral cerebral hemispheres or RAS) is unlikely to be associated with a normal level of consciousness and normal neurologic examination after recovery.	Syncope due to stroke will invariably be associated with neurologic deficits associated with the posterior circulation of the brain.	CT of the head should be performed in patients with syncope who have neurologic deficits on regaining consciousness. However, if a detailed neurologic examination is normal, the yield of CT is extremely low and not warranted.

(*continued*)

Table 35.2 Differential diagnosis of syncope (*cont*)

Causes of syncope	Symptoms	Signs	Work-up
	One exception is the posterior circulation stroke or TIA, which is associated with dysarthria, diplopia, ataxia, or vertigo. In the absence of these symptoms, stroke and TIA are unlikely.		
Seizure	Patients with seizures often report a preceding aura. No other self-reported symptoms are particularly helpful in distinguishing seizures from true syncope.	If the patient presents during the postictal period, seizure is most easily diagnosed based on the confusion that slowly resolves. Another characteristic that has been shown to be more specific for seizure (vs. true syncope) is evidence of tongue-biting. Loss of bowel/bladder control is fairly nonspecific.	Patients with a first-time seizure usually have an extensive ED work-up, including laboratory testing, drug and alcohol screening, and CT of the head. Patients with a history of prior seizures who have a recurrent uncomplicated seizure followed by a brief postictal period usually require nothing more than anticonvulsant level testing.
Vasomotor (also sometimes referred to as "vasovagal" or "vasodepressor" syncope)	Includes episodes associated with emotional factors (e.g., sudden exposure to fear or anxiety) and situational factors (e.g., micturition). The episode is usually preceded by a prodrome of progressive lightheadedness and tunnel vision. Recovery occurs quickly after the patient assumes a supine position.	If the heart rate is obtained at first onset of symptoms, transient bradycardia is usually noted. Patients are often diaphoretic, cold, and clammy during the first few minutes after recovery, but the remainder of the examination is normal.	No specific work-up is indicated aside from the thorough history and physical examination.

AAA: abdominal aortic aneurysm; ACS: acute coronary syndrome; AD: aortic dissection; AS: aortic stenosis; CSM: carotid sinus massage; CT: computed tomography; CXR: chest X-ray; DVT: deep venous thrombosis; ECG: electrocardiogram; hCG: human chorionic gonadotropin; PE: pulmonary embolism; RAS: reticular activating system; TEE: transesophageal echocardiography; TIA: transient ischemic attack; V/Q: ventilation–perfusion; WPW: Wolff–Parkinson–White syndrome.

Diagnostic testing

A routine "shotgun" approach to diagnostic testing in the patient with syncope wastes valuable time and resources. The electrocardiogram (ECG) is perhaps the only diagnostic test that is routinely indicated in these patients. All other tests should be obtained based on concerns raised during the detailed history and physical examination.

Electrocardiogram

The ECG should be considered a routine part of the ED evaluation of the patient presenting with syncope. The emergency physician should evaluate the ECG for evidence of tachydysrhythmias, bradydysrhythmias, and AV blocks. The presence of any of these abnormalities suggests a dysrhythmia as the cause of the syncopal episode. The ECG should also be evaluated for evidence of acute myocardial ischemia (ST-segment elevation or depression, inverted T-waves, or new intraventricular conduction abnormalities or bundle branch blocks). PE may be associated with an assortment of ECG abnormalities, including sinus tachycardia, inverted T-waves (especially in the right precordial leads), a rightward axis, Q-waves in lead III, and tall R-waves in lead V_1 (Figure 35.1). The ECG may have *none* of these findings. Pericardial tamponade is suggested by the combination of tachycardia plus low QRS voltage or electrical alternans (Figure 35.2). Close attention should be paid to the ECG intervals. A short PR interval in combination with a slightly prolonged QRS interval and delta-waves is diagnostic of Wolff–Parkinson–White syndrome (Figure 35.3) and increases the likelihood of tachyarrhythmias. Prolongation of the QT interval, which may be congenital, or caused by electrolyte abnormalities or medications, predisposes to polymorphic ventricular tachycardia. Less common syndromes

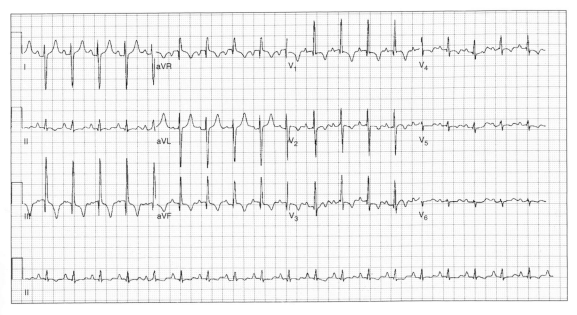

Figure 35.1
ECG in a patient with pulmonary embolism demonstrating the classic $S_1Q_3T_3$ pattern and rightward axis shift. T wave inversions in leads V_1–V_3 are indicative of right heart strain.

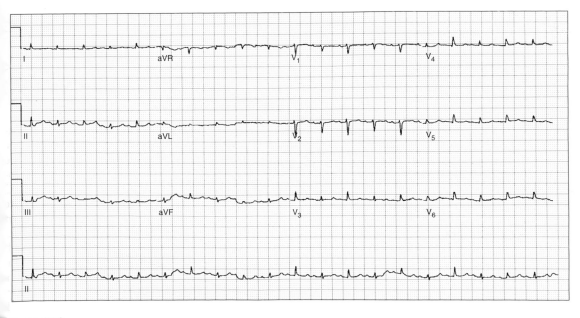

Figure 35.2
ECG in a patient with cardiac tamponade demonstrating low QRS voltages and electrical alternans.

that predispose to ventricular tachyarrhythmias include hypertrophic cardiomyopathy and the Brugada syndrome. Hypertrophic cardiomyopathy is identified on the ECG when large-amplitude QRS complexes, tall R-waves in the right precordial leads, and deep narrow Q-waves in the inferior or lateral leads are present (Figure 35.4). The Brugada syndrome is identified on the ECG by the presence of a complete or incomplete right bundle branch block pattern with ST-segment elevation in the

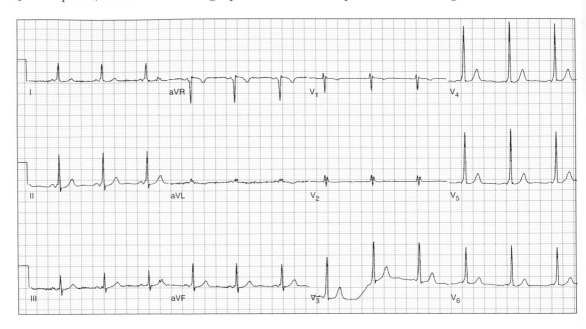

Figure 35.3
ECG in a patient with Wolff–Parkinson–White (pre-excitation) syndrome demonstrating short PR intervals and delta waves.

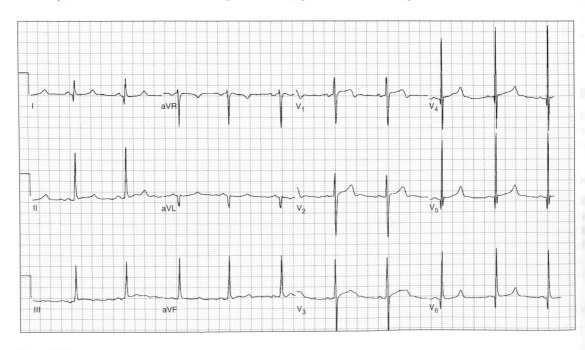

Figure 35.4
ECG in a patient with hypertrophic cardiomyopathy demonstrating high QRS voltage reflecting LVH and "pseudo-infarct pattern" of Q waves in V₄–V₆.

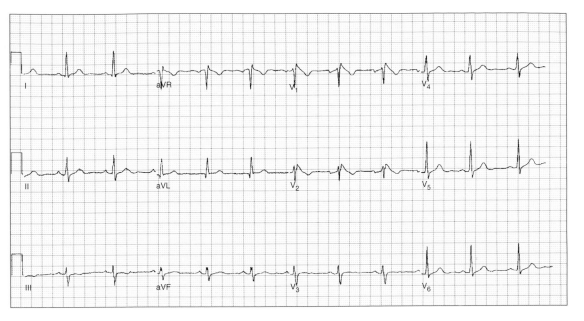

Figure 35.5
ECG in a patient with Brugada syndrome demonstrating coved ST segment elevation in leads V_1 and V_2, and right bundle branch pattern (absence of terminal S waves in leads I and V_6).

right precordial leads (Figure 35.5). Hypertrophic cardiomyopathy and the Brugada syndrome are confirmed with Doppler echocardiography and electrophysiologic testing, respectively. Non-specific ECG abnormalities, such as premature atrial or ventricular complexes, sinus tachycardia, and first-degree AV block, have no diagnostic significance.

Laboratory studies

In general, laboratory studies should only be ordered when the history or physical examination suggests a likely abnormality.

Glucose

Routine serum glucose testing is of low yield if the patient is asymptomatic on arrival to the ED. However, in the patient with persistent light-headedness, nausea, tremulousness, or diaphoresis, or a patient with diabetes, a fingerstick glucose is warranted.

Complete blood count

The complete blood count (CBC) is rarely helpful in evaluating patients with syncope. The white blood cell count is nonspecific. Hemoglobin and hematocrit testing are useful when the history or physical examination suggests blood loss (most commonly from a gastrointestinal or vaginal source). Patients with renal failure, human immunodeficiency virus, sickle cell anemia, and other chronic diseases may be predisposed to anemia and warrant routine CBC testing.

Electrolytes

Routine electrolyte testing is rarely helpful in the evaluation of the patient with syncope. However, patients who use diuretics or have protracted vomiting and/or diarrhea probably warrant electrolyte testing. Emergency physicians should have a low threshold for obtaining electrolytes in elderly patients, as they are more likely to have significant abnormalities.

Pregnancy test

Female patients of childbearing age who present with abdominal or pelvic pain, low back pain, or vaginal bleeding should be tested for pregnancy. However, in the absence of any of these symptoms, pregnancy testing is unlikely to be helpful.

Radiologic studies

Routine radiologic imaging for patients with syncope is not indicated. However, the history and physical examination will help determine which patients require imaging.

Chest radiography

Routine chest radiography is not cost-effective and rarely leads to a definitive diagnosis. Patients who complain of dyspnea, chest pain, or upper back pain, or who are noted on examination to be hypoxic, tachypneic, or have abnormal lung sounds should receive chest radiography to evaluate for signs of PE. The most common findings in PE include elevation of a hemidiaphragm, atelectasis, and small pleural effusions; less common findings include pulmonary infiltrates and peripheral oligemia. The chest radiograph may also display evidence of congestive heart failure (CHF) associated with ACS, large pericardial effusions (massive cardiomegaly, water bottle-shaped heart), and aortic dissection in patients with chest or upper back pain (widened mediastinum, left pleural effusion, blurring of the aortic knob, rightward tracheal deviation, pleural cap).

Computerized tomography of the chest

Patients with suspected aortic dissection or PE based on history and physical examination should have diagnostic imaging of the great vessels or lungs, respectively. Computerized tomography (CT) is emerging as the diagnostic test of choice for both conditions, in part due to the accessibility of CT in most EDs. However, emergency physicians should remember that the test is not 100% sensitive; therefore, if clinical suspicion of either diagnosis is high, further testing may be indicated even after a negative CT.

Computerized tomography of the brain

Patients who experience syncope after recent head trauma should receive CT of the brain. Emergency physicians should also consider CT of the brain in patients who experience head trauma during the syncopal episode, although studies evaluating the utility of the test in this situation are lacking. Any patient with syncope who experiences a severe headache prior to or after the syncopal episode should have brain CT. Also, patients who experience new seizures, report focal neurologic symptoms, or have new focal neurologic deficits on examination should have emergent CT of the brain. Overall, neurologic causes of syncope are rare, especially in the patient without

focal neurologic symptoms or deficits. Routine brain CT is not indicated in such patients.

Echocardiography

Emergent echocardiography is indicated only in cases of suspected pericardial tamponade. Echocardiography may also be helpful in evaluating wall motion abnormalities in cases of ACS or right heart strain in cases of massive PE; however, the test is rarely required for diagnosis of either condition in the ED. Echocardiography is also diagnostic for aortic stenosis and hypertrophic cardiomyopathy, but obtaining the test emergently for either condition is rarely necessary.

General treatment principles

Due to the many life-threatening etiologies of syncope, treatment should begin with assessment of the Airway, Breathing, and Circulation (ABCs). Once initial stabilization has occurred, further treatment will be guided by the presumed etiology. Patients with an uncertain diagnosis should be monitored and observed in the ED. Bed rails should be maintained in an upright position in the event of a seizure, and placement of an IV line is prudent in case emergent medications are required.

Special patients
Elderly

Geriatric patients are well known to present with atypical symptoms and signs, even in the presence of deadly diseases. A majority of patients more than 75 years of age present with a chief complaint of dyspnea rather than chest pain when they experience ACS. Some geriatric patients will also experience painless aortic dissection. Geriatric patients are more likely than younger patients to have many of the cardiovascular causes of syncope: ACS, dysrhythmias, aortic dissection, ruptured AAA, and aortic stenosis. Vital sign assessment can be misleading; cardiac medications may blunt the expected tachycardic response to acute blood loss, and this population is prone to false-positive and false-negative orthostatic vital signs. Polypharmacy is common in this population as well, increasing the likelihood of medication-related syncope. Elderly patients are more likely to have electrolyte abnormalities, anemia, and intracranial abnormalities. Elderly patients also experience a much higher mortality from their causes of syncope. As a result, emergency physicians must maintain a low threshold to order laboratory studies (including cardiac), obtain CT of the brain, and admit geriatric patients who present after a syncopal episode.

Pacemakers

Patients with artificial cardiac pacemakers that present with syncope should generally have at least 24 hours of cardiac monitoring and evaluation for pacemaker malfunction. This usually requires admission and cardiologist consultation.

Pregnant

Patients who are pregnant, especially during their second and third trimester, are prone to vasomotor and orthostatic syncope. However, pregnancy also increases the risk for PE. Therefore, pregnant patients who present with or after syncope should be evaluated for PE if they are tachypneic, hypoxic, or report chest pain.

Pediatric

Syncope in pediatric patients is rare. The most common causes are vasomotor syncope and syncope related to dehydration. Adolescents who report exertional syncope should be assessed for hypertrophic cardiomyopathy.

Disposition

Admission

All patients with a suspected cardiovascular, pulmonary, or neurologic cause of syncope should be admitted. Patients with cardiac risk factors should be considered for admission for cardiac monitoring. Although there is no specific age cutoff for routine admission of patients experiencing syncope, most authors recommend that patients more than 45–50 years of age should be strongly considered for routine admission in order to monitor for an ACS or dysrhythmia. It should be noted, however, that patients with isolated syncope and no other symptoms, signs, or ECG findings suggestive of ACS are extremely unlikely to have positive cardiac enzymes during their admission. Clinical rules have been studied to determine those patients with syncope who are at risk for serious short-term outcomes. Although

these decision rules were derived from a cohort in whom not all studies were obtained, they have been prospectively validated and make excellent sense (Table 35.3).

Table 35.3 Syncope rules to predict short-term serious outcomes

FED 30 90
F   Failure (congestive heart failure) E   ECG abnormalities D   Dyspnea (shortness of breath) 30 Hematocrit < 30% 90 Systolic blood pressure < 90 mmHg (at any time)
* Modification of San Francisco Syncope Rules from Quinn JV, Stiell IG, McDermott DA, Sellers KL, Kohn MA, Wells GA. Derivation of the San Francisco Syncope Rule to predict patients with short-term serious outcomes. *Ann Emerg Med.* 2004 Feb;43(2): 224–32. Modified by GM Garmel.

Immediate surgical/obstetric consultation

Patients with suspected aortic dissection, ruptured AAA, and pericardial tamponade warrant immediate surgical consultation. Patients with suspected ectopic pregnancy should have immediate obstetric consultation. All patients with surgical causes of syncope should receive two large-bore IV lines, a broad panel of "pre-op labs," and a type and cross for at least 4 units of blood.

Discharge

The most common cause of syncope in young patients with a normal physical examination is vasomotor syncope. Patients with this benign condition can be discharged for outpatient follow-up. These patients should be counseled to maintain adequate hydration, as hypovolemia increases the likelihood of syncope. Patients should also be counseled to immediately lie down if they begin to experience a similar prodrome as that which preceded their syncopal episode. In general, all patients who are discharged after a syncopal episode should follow-up with a primary-care physician or cardiologist for reevaluation within 1 week. In addition, patients should be counseled to avoid swimming, playing sports, driving, or operating any heavy machinery until further evaluation by their physician. Patients who have an uncomplicated recurrence of a chronic seizure disorder should be counseled to maintain proper compliance with medications, and to follow-up with their physician for reassessment of their medication regimen.

Pearls, pitfalls, and myths

Pearls

- Abrupt onset of syncope without any prodromal symptoms should prompt strong suspicion of a dysrhythmia.
- Up to 30% of cardiac-related syncope cases have positive orthostatic vital sign changes.
- The ECG is useful not only for evaluation of myocardial ischemia and dysrhythmias, but also for evaluation of Wolff–Parkinson–White syndrome, pericardial tamponade, prolonged QT syndrome, hypertrophic cardiomyopathy, and the Brugada syndrome.

Pitfalls

- Gastrointestinal bleeding may be missed because of failure to perform a rectal examination.
- Hypertrophic cardiomyopathy may be missed because of failure to detect a murmur (or changes in the murmur with provocative maneuvers) in a young patient.
- PE is commonly undiagnosed as a cause of syncope.

Myths

- CT of the head should be performed on all patients that present after syncope.
- Serum electrolyte and CBC testing must be performed on all patients who present after syncope.
- Orthostatic vital sign abnormalities are highly specific for dehydration and rule out cardiac causes of syncope.

References

1. Atkins D, Hanusa B, Sefcik T, et al. Syncope and orthostatic hypotension. *Am J Med* 1991;91:179–187.
2. Benditt D, Lurie K, Fabian W. Clinical approach to diagnosis of syncope: an overview. *Cardiol Clin* 1997;165–176.
3. Elpidoforos SS, Evans JC, Larson MG, et al. Incidence and prognosis of syncope. *New Engl J Med* 2002;347:878–885.
4. Fenton AM, Hammill SC, Rea RF, et al. Vasovagal syncope. *Ann Int Med* 2000;133:714–725.
5. Forman D, Lipsitz L. Syncope in the elderly. *Cardiol Clin* 1997;15:295–311.
6. Georgeson S, Linzer M, Griffith J, et al. Acute cardiac ischemia in patients with syncope. *J Gen Int Med* 1992;7:379–386.
7. Hauer KE. Discovering the cause of syncope. *Postgrad Med* 2003;113:31–38, 95.
8. Henderson MC, Prabhu SD. Syncope: current diagnosis and treatment. *Curr Probl Cardiol* 1997;22:242–296.
9. Hunt M. Syncope. In: Rosen P, et al. (eds). *Emergency Medicine: Concepts and Clinical Practice.* St. Louis: Mosby-Year Book, 1998.
10. Kapoor WN. Syncope. *New Engl J Med* 2000;343:1856–1862.
11. Maisel WH, Stevenson WG. Syncope – getting to the heart of the matter. *New Engl J Med* 2002;347:931–933.
12. Meyer MD, Handler J. Evaluation of the patient with syncope: an evidence based approach. *Emerg Med Clin North Am* 1999;17:189–201.
14. Quinn JV, Stiell IG, McDermott DA, Sellers KL, Kohn MA, Wells GA. Derivation of the San Francisco Syncope Rule to predict patients with short-term serious outcomes. *Ann. Emrg. Med.* 2004 Feb;43(2): 224–32.
13. Zurcher R. Syncope. In: Hamilton GC (ed.). *Presenting Signs and Symptoms in the Emergency Department: Evaluation and Treatment.* Baltimore: Williams & Wilkins, 1993.

36 Toxicologic emergencies

Steven A. McLaughlin, MD

Scope of the problem

The American Academy of Poison Control Centers (AAPCC) reports over 2 million toxic exposures each year across the US. The demographics of human poisoning show two peaks of exposure. The first peak is in children from 1 to 3 years of age reflecting accidental ingestions. The second peak is in the elderly due to the increased risk of toxicity from multiple prescription drugs. Intentional overdose for abuse or suicidal intent is seen throughout the adolescent and adult populations.

The most common exposures are cleaning agents and over-the-counter analgesics (acetaminophen (APAP), ibuprofen, etc.). The agents responsible for the most fatalities are analgesics, antidepressants, cardiovascular agents, and drugs of abuse. Carbon monoxide (CO) and drugs of abuse are responsible for many deaths that are never reported to a poison control center (PCC). Data show that analgesics, antidepressants, and cardiovascular agents are also associated with significant morbidity and mortality.

Most patients who are poisoned will recover with supportive care alone. However, some may require specific antidotes or other therapeutics under the guidance of a regional PCC or medical toxicologist. The identification and treatment of poisoning emergencies is part of the unique and specialized knowledge of emergency medicine physicians and medical toxicologists. Emergency physicians are on the front line of caring for these patients and must be familiar with the principles of common poisoning diagnosis and management.

Pathophysiology

There are three basic physiologic concepts required to understand the effects of toxic agents on the human body: absorption, distribution, and elimination. In addition, each toxic substance has specific mechanisms of toxicity and effects on organ systems which will not be described in this chapter but can be found in several of the references.

Absorption is defined as the process by which a drug or chemical enters the body. Drugs can be absorbed through a variety of different pathways, including the lungs, skin, muscle tissue, oral mucosa, stomach, intestine, rectal mucosa, and eyes. The route of absorption directly affects its rate and extent. Absorption is also affected by the formulation of the agent and by host factors, such as skin thickness or gastric motility.

Distribution is the process by which a drug or chemical that has reached the bloodstream is transported to peripheral tissues. Distribution is a complex process with a large number of variables. Volume of distribution (V_d) is the apparent volume into which a drug distributes. It reflects the distribution of the drug into all of the body tissues. A drug that is distributed only in the plasma will have a V_d near that of total body water (between 0.6 and 1 L/kg). Drugs that are heavily concentrated in the body fat will have a V_d much greater than total body water.

Elimination is the removal of a drug or chemical from the body. Elimination can occur either by excretion or through biotransformation to one or more metabolites. The lungs, kidneys, and liver are responsible for the majority of drug elimination. Elimination is affected by integrity of organ systems, age, saturation of key enzyme processes, and the specific properties of the drug.

History

The primary goal of the history is to identify if a poisoning occured and which toxic agents are responsible. This can range from a simple to extremely complex process depending on the ability and willingness of the patient to answer historical questions and the extent to which corroborating information is available. Historical information should be solicited from the patient, family members, companions, friends, emergency medical services (EMS), law enforcement, or any other available witnesses.

For the patient

What drugs or pills did you take or what chemicals were you exposed to?

In a cooperative patient this may be your quickest way to a diagnosis and plan. The question can be phrased to reflect what you know about the patient's history. For example, you could ask: What pills did you take? What did the pills look like? What chemicals were you working with at your job? What drugs were you injecting? The core of this question is to get the patient's best description of what agent(s) he or she was exposed to in whatever context is appropriate. Recognize that poisoned patients may not be reliable historians either from altered level of consciousness or due to suicidiality, and additional history should be obtained from other sources.

What time did the ingestion occur?

Timing of exposure is critical in order to determine expected signs and symptoms based on the natural history of the exposure. It also helps guide therapy such as gastric decontamination. For agents that can be measured in the blood, such as APAP, time of ingestion is essential to interpret drug levels. The patient's response can be corroborated by family, friends, time last seen well, or other sources.

How and why did the exposure occur?

Patients may come into contact with toxic agents for a variety of reasons. The exposure may be a suicide attempt or gesture, a medication error, or an accidental, work-related, or environmental exposure. Understanding the reason for the exposure may significantly influence your plan of management, the classic example being the need for psychiatric evaluation of the suicidal patient.

What symptoms have you had since the exposure?

Initially, open-ended questions can be used to find out the patient's symptoms, which can be followed up with specific questions looking for clinical features of the likely exposures. In many cases, treatment of an exposure is based on the severity of the patients' symptoms.

For the family, friends, emergency medical services, and law enforcement

What drugs, pills, or chemicals did the patient ingest or was the patient exposed to? What time did the ingestion occur? How and why did the exposure occur?

These questions should always be asked to family, friends, EMS, or other witnesses to confirm

the patient's history and to provide additional details or a different perspective. In patients with an altered level of consciousness, history of seizure, or concern about suicidiality, this additional history is extremely important.

What other medications, agents, drugs, chemicals were noted at the scene? Did you bring in any pill bottles or containers?

In the situation where the type of exposure, quantity of drug or other details are missing, having EMS or law enforcement bring pill bottles, chemical containers, material safety data sheets (MSDS), or other objects from the scene can be very helpful in providing needed information.

What other pills, drugs, agents, or herbals does the patient have access to in the home, from family members, friends, etc.?

A complete list of agents that the patient takes or has access to is invaluable in narrowing your differential and interpreting diagnostic tests. Frequently, patients may provide inaccurate information regarding the types of medications or doses, and a list of possible agents allows the provider to look for signs/symptoms and laboratory findings that do not fit with the patient's reported exposure. Certain drugs such as lithium or digoxin, if available to the patient, may prompt additional laboratory testing.

What did the home or scene look like?

In addition, a description of the scene may provide clues to the cause of exposure, the patient's state of mind or symptoms prior to the exposure.

How has the patient's condition changed over time? What signs or symptoms have you noticed since the exposure?

These two questions again provide a picture of the patient's clinical course since ingestion, which may help with diagnosis, triage, and assessment of the severity of exposure. They may also indicate possible required interventions.

Additional sources of information include the patient's pharmacy, workplace for MSDS, and regional PCCs. Key items from the previous medical history include prior exposures, psychiatric illnesses, prior suicide attempts, social history including drugs of abuse, occupational history, general medical problems, and allergies.

Questions related to dosing, signs and symptoms, or other features of the patient's clinical course may be indicated in certain overdose situations and should be discussed with your regional PCC.

Physical examination

The physical examination may provide valuable clues to the diagnosis as well as severity of symptoms. The examination initially focuses on key areas for supportive care: the airway, breathing, and circulation (ABCs). Repeated examination of the ABCs and neurologic status is essential to identify early changes and anticipate increasing toxicity.

General appearance

The poisoned patient should be examined for evidence of trauma, general level of consciousness, and ability to maintain adequate airway and breathing. Odors can also provide valuable clues to possible exposures. Some classic examples of odors that may be found in poisoned patients include: bitter almonds with cyanide, fruity smell of ketoacidosis from any cause, garlic from organophosphates, and rotten eggs from hydrogen sulfide.

Vital signs

Vital signs are critical to establish the severity and stability of the poisoning at any point in time. In addition, specific constellations of vital signs can provide clues to the diagnosis (Table 36.1).

Eyes

The size of the pupils can provide additional diagnostic clues in the poisoned patient. Miosis (small pupils) can be caused by opioids, organophosphates, clonidine, phenothiazines, and sedatives. Mydriasis (large pupils) can be caused by sympathomimetics, cocaine, many hallucinogens and anticholinergics. Horizontal nystagmus can be caused by lithium, ethanol, carbamazepine, phenytoin, and other anticonvulsants. Phencyclidine (PCP) causes a vertical or rotatory nystagmus which is not typically seen with other ingestions.

Cardiovascular

Examination of the heart should be performed to search for bradycardia from cardiotoxic overdose or tachycardia from a variety of exposures. A new murmur in a patient with a history of intravenous (IV) drug use may represent endocarditis. Abnormal rhythms found on examination should be further defined with a 12-lead electrocardiogram (ECG). The peripheral pulses and skin should be examined for signs of shock, including mottling, delayed capillary refill, or weak or absent distal pulses.

Pulmonary

The respiratory system should be examined through inspection of respiratory rate, depth, and effort. Auscultation of the lung fields should be performed to assess for symmetry and abnormal sounds. Drugs such as opioids, tricyclic antidepressants (TCAs), and cholinergic agents may produce pulmonary edema that can be heard with a careful pulmonary examination. Wheezing or rales may also be heard in patients following aspiration of hydrocarbons or exposure to irritant toxic gases. Toxic agents producing a metabolic acidosis will cause a compensatory increase in respiratory rate and depth, which can be seen on examination.

Table 36.1 Important toxicologic causes of abnormal vital signs

Bradycardia/hypotension	Beta blockers, calcium channel blockers, clonidine, digoxin, organophosphates, ethanol, opioids, other sedatives
Tachycardia/hypertension	Sympathomimetics, cocaine, anticholinergics, theophylline, nicotine, thyroid hormone
Hyperthermia	Salicylates, anticholinergics, sympathomimetics, sedative withdrawal, neuroleptic malignant syndrome, serotonin syndrome
Tachypnea	Salicylates, metabolic acidosis, paraquat, chemical pneumonitis
Bradypnea	Sedatives, ethanol, opioids

Neurologic

A complete neurologic examination looking for focal findings of the cranial nerves or extremities is extremely important to rule out structural brain injury in any patient with altered mental status. Toxicologic causes of altered mental status less frequently cause focal neurologic deficits. Other important findings include muscle rigidity (serotonin syndrome, neuroleptic malignant syndrome or strychnine), tremors (lithium, sympathomimetics and sedative withdrawal), and fasciculations (organophosphate poisoning).

Skin

A careful skin examination can provide important diagnostic information. Survey the entire skin surface looking for needle track marks, nail changes with heavy metal poisoning, spider or snake bites, trauma, or paint residue from "huffing." The oral cavity can provide clues if residual pill fragments, odors, burns from caustic exposures, or bite marks from seizure activity are identified. Very dry skin is seen with anticholinergic poisoning, while diaphoretic skin is seen with sympathomimetics, organophosphates, and salicylates.

Abdomen

A thorough abdominal examination is important to look for other diagnoses in your differential and complications of caustic ingestions. In the poisoned patient, hyperactive bowel sounds can be heard with organophosphate poisoning. Diminished bowel sounds can help make the diagnosis of anticholinergic poisoning.

Pelvic, genital and rectal

If there is any suspicion of a foreign body or drug packets, a rectal and pelvic examination should be performed to search for these potentially dangerous objects.

Differential diagnosis

The correct diagnosis of a patient with a toxic exposure is most often found in the history using directed questions and alternative sources. When the history does not provide a diagnosis, look at the patients' signs and symptoms to identify the possible exposure. Classic constellations of signs and symptoms linked with particular poisonings are called *toxidromes*. These can be very helpful in single overdoses with a classic clinical picture. In cases with multiple exposures or with complications related to timing, or underlying illness, classic toxidromes may be of limited value. Four common toxidromes are from cholinergic, anticholinergic, sympathomimetic, and opioid agents (Table 36.2). A common mnemonic for cholinergic poisoning which helps with recollection of the toxidrome is SLUDGE: Salivation, Lacrimation, Urination, Defecation, Gastric Emptying. In other words, patients are "leaky." For anticholinergic exposures, ANTI-SLUDGE can be used (the opposite of cholinergic symptoms), but the mnemonic "blind as a bat, mad as a hatter, hot as a hare, looney as a toon, red as a beet, and dry as a bone" has been used by many. Other less common toxidromes exist. Important poisonings to recognize which have identifiable clinical findings are salicylates, non-steroidal anti-inflammatory drugs (NSAIDs), TCAs, digoxin, beta and calcium channel blockers, lithium, and hypoglycemic agents.

Table 36.2 Common toxidromes

	Pupils	Skin/ENT	Cardiovascular	Pulmonary	CNS	GI/GU
Cholinergic	Miosis	Diaphoresis Salivation Lacrimation	Bradycardia	Increased secretions	Coma Seizures	Emesis Diarrhea Urination
Anticholinergic	Mydriasis	Dry skin	Tachycardia	Variable	Delirium	Decreased motility Urinary retention
Sympathomimetic	Mydriasis	Diaphoresis	Tachycardia Hypertension	Variable	Agitation Seizures	Variable
Opioid	Miosis	Variable	Bradycardia Hypotension	Hypo-ventilation	Hypnosis Coma	Decreased motility

Diagnostic testing

Although laboratory testing can be helpful in diagnosing, defining and treating acute toxic exposures, the most important therapeutic decisions are those regarding airway management, circulatory support, and decontamination, which do not depend on ancillary testing. Treatment of critically-ill patients should proceed based on the clinician's best judgment, and should not be delayed while awaiting the results of ancillary testing.

Electrocardiogram

The ECG may be helpful in both diagnosis and prediction of toxicity in acute overdose. A 12-lead ECG is suggested in any cardiotoxic overdose including digoxin, other antidysrhythmics, phenothiazines, beta blockers, calcium channel blockers, cocaine and other sympathomimetics, and TCAs. It can be helpful in an unknown overdose to look for cardiotoxic agents.

TCAs have characteristic ECG changes that help with diagnosis and as well as suggest an increased risk of complications. In TCA overdose, the ECG commonly shows a sinus tachycardia from anticholinergic effects, which alone does not predict serious toxicity. ECG findings of a QRS interval of more than 100 milliseconds or a large terminal R wave in aVR in a TCA-poisoned patient predict an increased risk of both seizures and ventricular tachycardia (Figures 36.1 and 36.2).

Radiologic studies

There are no routine radiologic studies for patients with toxic ingestions or exposures. A KUB (kidneys, ureters, bladder) film can be helpful in visualizing radio-opaque drugs, drug packets, and other foreign bodies. "Body stuffers" ingest single packets of drugs to avoid detection; these are rarely seen on plain radiographs. "Body packers" ingest large numbers of well-wrapped drug packets as a technique to transport drugs without detection; these large numbers of packets are usually seen on a KUB. Other agents can be seen occasionally depending on quantity, concentration, and time of ingestion. These potentially visible agents can be remembered by the mnemonic "CHIPES" (Table 36.3). A KUB can be helpful in iron ingestions both for initial detection of the ingestion as well as following the progress of gastrointestinal (GI) decontamination. Chest radiographs are indicated in patients with potential aspiration of hydrocarbons or other agents that can cause chemical pneumonitis.

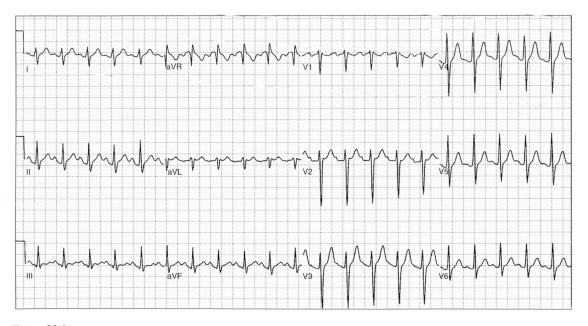

Figure 36.1
Electrocardiogram of tricyclic antidepressant poisoned patient showing tachycardia, a widened QRS, a rightward QRS axis and a large terminal R wave in aVR. *Courtesy:* Amal Mattu, MD.

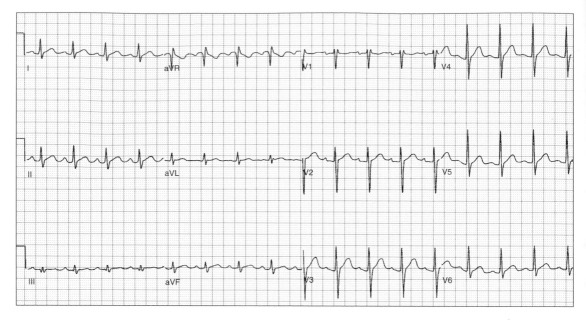

Figure 36.2
Electrocardiogram of the same patient following administration of 3 ampules of Sodium bicarbonate showing resolution of abnormalities. *Courtesy*: Amal Mattu, MD.

Table 36.3 CHIPES

C	Chloral hydrate, calcium carbonate
H	Heavy metals
I	Iron, iodinated compounds
P	Psychotropics, potassium preparations, packets of drugs
ES	Enteric-coated and Slow-release formulations

Table 36.4 Differential diagnosis of an anion gap metabolic acidosis using the "MUDPILECATS" mnemonic

M	Methanol, metformin
U	Uremia
D	Diabetic ketoacidosis
P	Paraldehyde, phenformin
I	Iron, isoniazid
L	Lactic acidosis
E	Ethylene glycol
C	Cyanide, carbon monoxide
A	Alcoholic ketoacidosis
T	Toluene
S	Salicylates, seizure

Laboratory tests

Laboratory testing in ingestions should include a urine pregnancy test in females of childbearing age and blood chemistries. The electrolytes, blood urea nitrogen (BUN), creatinine, and glucose can be used to search for metabolic acidosis, renal insufficiency, and significant sodium or potassium abnormalities. All of these potentially impact the management of a poisoned patient. In a patient with a metabolic acidosis, the electrolytes can be used to calculate the anion gap and help to narrow the differential diagnosis.

Anion gap = Na − (Cl + bicarbonate)

Normal range is 8–12 meq/L.

The differential diagnosis of an anion gap metabolic acidosis can be remembered using the mnemonic "MUDPILECATS" (Table 36.4).

The calculated osmolal gap can narrow the differential diagnosis even further in a patient with a metabolic acidosis. An elevated osmolal gap is suggestive of poisoning with methanol, ethylene glycol, mannitol, or isopropanol. The utility of this test is limited by the fact that it does not reveal the specific cause of the increased gap, and a normal osmolal gap does NOT rule out poisoning with any of these agents.

Osmolar Gap = Measured osmoles[a] − 2Na + (Glucose/18) + (BUN/2.8) + (EtOH/4.6)
[a]: Freezing point depression technique; Na: Sodium; BUN: Blood urea nitrogen; EtOH: Ethanol. Normal osmolal gap range is <10 mOsm.

APAP is a common over-the-counter medication, contained in a variety of combination products. It may be described by patients as "aspirin" or "pain killers." In addition, APAP toxicity is initially clinically silent; treatment must be started before the patient manifests signs of hepatic toxicity (Figure 36.3). Therefore, measurement of serum APAP levels is indicated in any suspected overdose or unknown exposure.

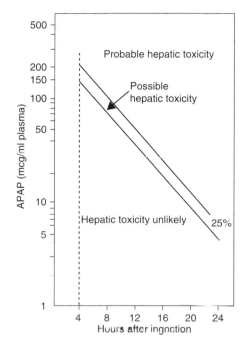

Figure 36.3
Acetaminophen toxicity nomogram. The Rumack-Matthew nomogram, relating expected severity of liver toxicity to serum acetaminophen concentrations. *Source*: From Smilkstein MJ, Bronstein AC, Linden C, et al. Acetaminophen overdose: a 48-hour intravenous *N*-acetylcysteine treatment protocol. *Ann Emerg Med* 1991;20(10):1058, with permission.

Controversy exists regarding the use of routine salicylate levels in overdose patients. Salicylate toxicity typically produces recognizable signs and symptoms in serious overdose, including tachypnea, tinnitus, and diaphoresis, so screening levels may not routinely be indicated. However, because this is a common, potentially life-threatening ingestion, with subtle early signs of toxicity, routine salicylate levels may be appropriate in some situations.

Quantitative levels of specific drugs such as carbamazepine, lithium, phenobarbitol, carbon monoxide, and digoxin are indicated in patients when there is a clinical suspicion of exposure based on the history or physical. They should not be ordered routinely as screening tests.

Qualitative urine drug screens, often referred to as "tox screens," generally test the urine for the presence of multiple drugs or their metabolites. These tests most commonly identify drugs of abuse including opioids, benzodiazepines, cocaine, amphetamines, barbiturates, marijuana, and PCP. The test will be positive with "therapeutic" levels or with significant ingestions. The amount of drug present cannot be inferred from the result of the test. Qualitative drug screens are only useful for identifying the presence or absence of this limited group of drugs. In several studies, these tests have been shown to have limited impact on the management plan in an unknown overdose and are not routinely recommended in overdose patients. Recognizing these limitations, drug screens can be used to determine which drugs a patient has been exposed to recently, and may be helpful in creating an accurate differential diagnosis or in arranging for appropriate psychiatric follow-up or substance abuse counseling.

General treatment principles

There are four main components of treatment for the poisoned patient: supportive care, antidotes, gastric (and other) decontamination, and enhanced elimination. These can be remembered using the mnemonic "SAGE".

S	Supportive care: ABCs and the "coma cocktail".
A	Antidotes: specific therapy for certain exposures.
G	Gastric (and other) decontamination: removal from stomach, skin, eyes.
E	Enhanced elimination: includes dialysis, urinary excretion, hemofiltration.

Supportive care

The majority of patients with toxic exposures will survive with supportive care, which includes airway management, supplemental oxygen and ventilation, and normalization of blood pressure using IV crystalloid fluids and inotropes or vasopressor agents (if necessary). Every overdose patient should be monitored initially with continuous cardiac, non-invasive blood pressure and pulse oximetry monitoring. IV access should be established in all patients. Patients with unstable vital signs or potentially serious ingestions require two large-bore IVs. Patients can deteriorate rapidly, especially in cases of TCA overdose, and early airway management with rapid sequence intubation as needed can be lifesaving.

During the initial evaluation of any patient with altered mental status, consideration should be given to using the "coma cocktail." The coma cocktail typically consists of naloxone to reverse opioid toxicity, a fingerstick glucose and supplemental dextrose if hypoglycemia is found, and thiamine to prevent or treat Wernicke's encephalopathy. In patients with a reversible overdose such as opioid intoxication from heroin, the patient should be oxygenated and ventilated with a bag-valve-mask device until naloxone can be administered and take effect.

Naloxone is a specific opioid antagonist which lasts 60–90 minutes. When given IV, intramuscular (IM), subcutaneous (SQ), intranasally, by nebulizer or via an endotracheal tube, it will result in a rapid return to consciousness and spontaneous ventilation in the opioid-poisoned patient. The initial dose of naloxone ranges from 0.1 mg for a chronic opioid abuser to 0.4 mg for the general acute overdose. Naloxone should be titrated to adequate spontaneous ventilation and mental status alert enough to provide a medical history. The dose may be increased up to 2–10 mg in patients who fail to respond to the initial dose if the clinical suspicion of opioid intoxication remains high. The only significant side effect from naloxone in adults is acute opioid withdrawal, which is non-life threatening but may cause discomfort for the patient.

There are no good data to support the use of thiamine in all patients with altered mental status, and it does not need to be given before glucose. Treatment of hypoglycemia takes priority. Risk factors for thiamine deficiency include malnutrition, alcoholism, extreme diets, or a history of a previous deficiency. Such patients should be given thiamine during the first 12 hours or immediately if they have altered mental status. The usual adult dose of thiamine is 100 mg IV or IM.

Flumazenil, which is a reversal agent for benzodiazepines, is not part of this "cocktail." Flumazenil can cause seizures in patients with some ingestions, including TCAs, cocaine, and sympathomimetics, and can cause acute withdrawal in patients who are tolerant to benzodiazepines. In addition, benzodiazepine overdose can be safely managed with supportive care. Therefore, flumazenil is not recommended as part of the coma cocktail.

Antidotes

Antidotes are an exciting part of toxicology, despite being of limited utility in most cases. It is important to be aware of the toxins that may need antidote therapy so that appropriate consideration can be given to this treatment modality. A list of important toxins and their antidotes is provided (Table 36.5).

Table 36.5 Important toxic substances and antidotes

Toxic substance	Antidote
Acetaminophen	N-acetylcysteine
Beta blockers	Glucagon
Calcium channel blockers	Calcium, glucagon, insulin/dextrose
Carbon monoxide	Oxygen, Hyperbaric oxygen
Cyanide	Cyanide kit – amyl nitrate, sodium nitrite, sodium thiosulfate
Digoxin	Digibind Fab-fragments
Hydrofluoric acid	Calcium
Iron	Deferoxamine
Methanol/ethylene glycol	Ethanol or Fomepizole
Opioids	Naloxone
Organophosphates	Atropine and pralidoxime
Sulfonylureas (oral hypoglycemics)	Glucose, Octreotide
Tricyclic antidepressants	Sodium bicarbonate and hypertonic saline

Gastric and other decontamination

Decontamination of the GI system after an oral exposure, or the skin and eyes after a dermal exposure is critical to reduce the amount of absorbed drug and reduce potential toxicity. Appropriate protective gear should be used when indicated in order to protect health care providers from possible exposure.

Skin decontamination begins with the removal of all of the patient's clothing. Any dry powder or debris can be brushed off. The skin is then washed with warm soapy water until no evidence of contamination remains. In an ocular exposure, the eyes should be irrigated with generous amounts of normal saline until symptoms are relieved and pH returns to normal (in the case of an acid or alkali exposure.)

There are four basic techniques for decontamination of the GI system: induced emesis using syrup of ipecac, gastric lavage, activated charcoal, and whole bowel irrigation. A significant amount of ingested toxic material may remain in the GI tract even with optimal application of these techniques. Given the limited effectiveness of gastric decontamination, the trend in recent years has been to use safer and less invasive techniques.

Syrup of ipecac induces vomiting through local irritation of the stomach and activation of the chemotactic trigger zone in the central nervous system. Ninety percent of patients begin to vomit within 30 minutes, and symptoms usually resolve by 2 hours. Due to a lack of evidence to support its effectiveness, and the potential risk of aspiration from persistent vomiting in a seizing or comatose patient, syrup of ipecac is no longer recommended for use in health care facilities. There may be a limited role for home-use of this agent with very specific ingestions and guidance from a PCC.

Gastric lavage involves placing a large plastic tube (36–40 French in adults) through the mouth into the stomach. The stomach is emptied and lavaged with warm normal saline until the lavage effluent is clear. Activated charcoal is then placed down the tube into the stomach and the lavage tube is removed. Significant risks from this procedure include aspiration, esophageal perforation, and hypoxia. It should not be performed following caustic or hydrocarbon ingestion, minor ingestions, or in patients who are unable to protect their own airway. The evidence suggesting a benefit from this procedure is limited. In an optimal scenario of small pill fragments, ingestion within an hour, and aggressive lavage, the best mean recoveries have been from 36% to 50% of ingested material. Balancing these significant risks with minimal benefits, this procedure is usually recommended in patients who present within 1 hour of life-threatening ingestions and have had their airway protected by endotracheal intubation. Even in highly selected patients, there is no evidence that it improves outcomes.

Activated charcoal has become the mainstay of GI decontamination in recent years. It is a highly effective treatment for a variety of ingestions and has a very good safety profile. Activated charcoal works by adsorbing the toxin, thereby making it less available for absorption from the gut into the bloodstream. It is most effective if given within one hour of ingestion, although its use is suggested in patients presenting up to 12–24 hours from ingestion if they continue to be symptomatic or have potentially delayed absorption from decreased intestinal motility, delayed-release products, or concretions. It is typically given in a dose of 1 g/kg, although larger doses are occasionally indicated. Patients can drink the activated charcoal through a straw, or it can be given via nasogastric (NG) or lavage tube. The first dose of charcoal is often given with sorbitol or magnesium citrate as a cathartic to reduce GI transit time. Multiple doses of activated charcoal are indicated for certain ingestions and may be done in consultation with a PCC. Contraindications to activated charcoal are an inability to protect the airway, ingestion of a caustic agent, hydrocarbons, or other agent not bound to charcoal, or planned endoscopy.

Whole bowel irrigation (WBI) involves placing an NG tube or having the patient drink a balanced solution of polyethylene glycol and electrolytes at a rate of 1–2 L/hour. The goal is to mechanically flush out the GI tract, reducing the absorption of certain ingested agents. Treatment should be continued until the patient has clear rectal effluent and no further evidence of progressive toxicity. It can cause vomiting, diarrhea, and abdominal pain and it should not be used in patients with intestinal obstruction or absent bowel sounds. WBI may be beneficial for decontamination in selected cases of drug bezoars, iron ingestions, sustained-release preparations of drugs such as calcium channel blockers, and ingested drug packets.

Enhanced elimination

There are two primary methods of enhancing the elimination of a toxin from the body: urinary alkalinization and hemodialysis. These techniques are useful only for a limited number of substances, and should be guided by advice from a PCC.

Urinary alkalinization works by "trapping" agents that are weak acids in the renal tubules and increasing their excretion in the urine. The urine can be alkalinized by administration 1 meq/liters of IV sodium bicarbonate. The patient is given a bolus of sodium bicarbonate and then a drip (prepared with three ampules of sodium bicarbonate added to 1 L of D5W with 40 meq of KCl) is infused at 150–200 ml/hour. The goal is a urine pH of 7.5–8.0. A normal serum pH should be maintained during this process. The administration of adequate potassium is essential to prevent paradoxical aciduria from occurring due to hypokalemia. Complications include volume overload, hypokalemia, and changes in serum pH. Urinary alkalinization may be indicated for symptomatic ingestions of salicylates, chlorpropamide, and phenobarbital.

Hemodialysis is effective at removing small, water soluble substances with low protein binding and small V_d. Commonly dialyzable toxins include salicylates, theophylline, barbiturates, lithium, methanol, isopropanol, and ethylene glycol. This invasive procedure requires placement of a large central venous access device. Hemodialysis can be life-saving in a number of these overdoses, and should be considered with the guidance of a PCC and a consulting nephrologist. The role of newer continuous arterial or venous filtration techniques in the treatment of toxic exposures has not been clearly defined.

Special patients
Pediatric

The approach to pediatric poisonings is very similar to that in adults. Children make up a significant proportion of toxic exposures in the US. In general, supportive care and gastric decontamination with activated charcoal will be critical factors in treatment. Small doses (a single pill or taste) of TCAs, cardiotoxic agents, Lomotil®, oral hypoglycemics, methylsalicylate, camphor, Visine®, and methanol can be fatal in children. Children with serious or potentially serious ingestions should be managed in a pediatric intensive care unit (PICU) setting. For accidental exposures, educate the parents or caregivers to prevent future incidents. Cases of suspected abuse or neglect should trigger mandatory referral to child protective services or police authorities.

Elderly

Geriatric patients are at high risk for complications of toxic exposure due to underlying cardiovascular, pulmonary, renal, hepatic, and other systemic diseases. Patients on large numbers of medications are also at risk for adverse reactions from dosing errors, wrong medications or medication interactions. Medication complications such as chronic salicylism should be considered in geriatric patients presenting with hypotension, bradycardia, altered mental status, weakness, nausea or vomiting, and acidosis. Depression is also common in elderly patients, and appropriate screening should occur if there is a suspicion of an intentional overdose.

Immune compromised

Patients with human immunodeficiency virus (HIV), acquired immune deficiency syndrome (AIDS), or malignancy may be on a large number of toxic medications and should be carefully screened for medication-related causes of any presenting complaint. The patient's primary care provider or specialist as well as the PCC can provide guidance on the clinical presentation and treatment of toxicity from any unusual medications. An appropriate psychiatric history should be taken to look for signs or symptoms of depression and suicidal ideation.

Pregnancy

In general, appropriate treatment of the mother for her overdoses will also benefit the fetus. Life-saving therapy should not be withheld from the mother because of concerns for fetal toxicity. Depression is also common in this group and should be screened for in any suspected intentional overdose. CO poisoning, APAP and iron ingestions are good examples of serious exposures where the antidote given to the mother is safe and also protects the fetus from toxicity.

Disposition

Asymptomatic patients with potentially serious exposures should have appropriate diagnostic studies and be watched for at least 6 hours. In most cases, if they remain asymptomatic at the end of 6 hours, they can be safely discharged. Every patient with suspected suicidiality should receive an appropriate evaluation by a mental health professional.

Certain medications with delayed onset of symptoms or prolonged clinical toxicity may require 12–24 hours observation in an emergency department (ED) or short-stay unit. These agents are methadone, Lomotil®, oral hypoglycemics, lithium, sustained-release calcium channel blockers, and theophylline. In every case of toxic exposure, be familiar with the expected time course of symptoms.

Patients who have more than minor symptoms, develop toxicity during the 6 hour observation period, or who have evidence of toxicity on diagnostic testing should be admitted to the appropriate subacute care or ICU setting.

PCCs are the single best source for information about diagnosis, management and disposition of patients with toxic exposures. They can provide consultation with a toxicologist, follow-up for patients discharged home, locations of medical centers that may accept transfers of patients with special therapeutic needs, and assist with monitoring of hospitalized patients.

Pearls, pitfalls, and myths

- Poisoning is common in the US. The most common serious exposures are from analgesics, antidepressants, cardiovascular drugs, CO, and drugs of abuse.
- History from the patient may not be reliable and should be confirmed through different sources if possible.
- The physical examination may occasionally lead to a diagnosis through classic signs and symptoms of common poisonings called toxidromes.
- A fingerstick glucose and oxygen saturation should be checked in every patient with altered mental status, and consideration should be given to the immediate administration of naloxone and thiamine.
- Antidotes, although occasionally helpful, are secondary to general supportive care in the management of most toxic exposures.
- Gastric lavage is rarely performed, except on intubated and critically-ill patients. There is essentially no role for syrup of ipecac in a hospital setting. The mainstay of gastric decontamination is activated charcoal.
- Pediatric patients are at high risk for accidental exposures and may have serious effects or death even from small doses or single tablets of certain medications and chemicals.
- Geriatric and immunocompromised patients are at high risk for drug toxicity from dosing errors, wrong medications, or medication interactions. Intentional ingestions should be considered in these groups.
- Asymptomatic patients should be watched in the ED for at least 6 hours. Patients with exposures to long-acting agents or agents with a delayed onset of action may need 12–24 hours observation.
- The PCC is the best source of information on diagnosis and management of toxic exposures and should be consulted on essentially every case that presents to a health care facility.

References

1. Bateman DN. Gastric decontamination – a view for the millennium. *J Accid Emerg Med* 1999;16:84–86.
2. Doyon S, Roberts JR. Reappraisal of the "coma cocktail": dextrose, flumazenil, naloxone and thiamine. *Emerg Med Clin North Am* 1994;12:301–316.
3. Erickson TB, Aks SE, Gussow L, Williams RH. Toxicology update: a rational approach to managing the poisoned patient. *Emerg Med Pract* 2001;3(8):1–28.
4. Frommer DA, Kulig KW, Marx JA, Rumack B. Tricyclic antidepressant overdose. *J Am Med Assoc* 1987;257:521–526.
5. Gibb K. Serum alcohol levels, toxicology screens, and the use of the breath alcohol analyzer. *Ann Emerg Med* 1986;15:349–353.
6. Goldfrank LR, Flomenbaum NE, Lewin NA, Weisman RS, Howland MA, Hoffman RS. *Goldfrank's Toxicologic Emergencies*, 6th ed., Appleton and Lange, Stanford, CT, 1998.
7. Groleau G, Jotte R, Barish R. The electrocardiographic manifestations of cyclic antidepressant therapy and overdose: a review. *J Emerg Med* 1990;8:597–605.
8. Hack JB, Hoffman RS. General management of poisoned patients. In: Tintinalli JE (ed.). *Emergency Medicine: A Comprehensive Study Guide*, 5th ed., McGraw Hill, NY, 2000. pp. 1057–1063.
9. Haddad LM, Shannon MW, Winchester JF. *Clinical Management of Poisoning and Drug Overdose*, 3rd ed., W.B. Saunders, Philadelphia, PA, 1998.
10. Kulig K, Bar-Or D, Cantrill SV, Rosen P, Rumack BH. Management of acutely poisoned patients without gastric emptying. *Ann Emerg Med* 1985;14:562–567.
11. Kulig K. Initial management of ingestions of toxic substances. *New Engl J Med* 1992;326:1677–1681.
12. McLaughlin SA, Crandall CS, McKinney PE. Octreotide: an antidote for

sulfonyurea-induced hypoglycemia. *Ann Emerg Med* August 2000;36: 133–138.

13. Mills KC. Tricyclic antidepressants. In: Tintinalli JE (ed.). *Emergency Medicine: A Comprehensive Study Guide*, 5th ed., McGraw Hill, NY, 2000. pp. 1063–1071.

14. Savitt DL, Hawkins HH, Roberts JR. The radiopacity of ingested medications. *Ann Emerg Med* 1987;16:331–339.

15. Smilkstein MJ. Reviewing cyclic antidepressant cardiotoxicity: wheat and chaff. *J Emerg Med* 1990;8:645–648.

542   Primary Complaints

37 Urinary-related complaints

Fred A. Severyn, MD

Scope of the problem

Urinary-related complaints are found in many patients presenting to the emergency department (ED). The wide variety of complaints can be staggering, overshadowed only by their cost to the health care system. Careful evaluation may uncover undiagnosed congenital abnormalities threatening future renal function, serious infections, or disease complications. Identification of urosepsis allows prompt treatment to prevent subsequent morbidity and mortality.

This chapter focuses on dysuria, hematuria, nephrolithiasis, urinary tract infection (UTI), and acute urinary retention. These categories alone account for billions of health care dollars, and several million ED visits annually. As such, it is important for practitioners to have knowledge of anatomy, evaluation, and treatment.

Anatomic essentials

Urologic anatomy is essentially identical from renal unit to bladder in both sexes (Figure 37.1). It differs from bladder to meatus in obvious ways. The renal unit and the gonads have a similar embryologic origin, so pain in one location is often referred to the other. The kidneys themselves are retroperitoneal organs, relatively protected by the inferior ribs posteriorly.

After formation of urine in the glomerular unit, urine travels into the renal calyces which merge to form the renal pelvis. This renal pelvis cones down to form the ureter. The ureter travels caudally and arises out of the posterior pelvic brim as it crosses over the iliac vessels, then inserts into the bladder itself through a small narrowed intramural portion. It is in these anatomic points of narrowing that calculi of the renal system can potentially lodge. A significant percentage of cases of ureteral obstruction cause pain from distention and dilation of the upper ureter and renal pelvis (hydronephrosis).

Normal micturition is a very complicated neuromotor process, with a micturition control center located in the spinal cord at the S2–S4 level. Autonomic control of various muscle groups allows for coordinated voiding via a balance between parasympathetic and sympathetic innervation. Any interruption of this sacral reflex arc from a lower motor neuron lesion will lead to loss of sensation of bladder fullness, resulting in an atonic bladder that fails to empty. This may occur via traumatic mechanisms, as in lumbar vertebral fractures or disc herniation, or from atraumatic mechanisms, such as epidural abscess or tumor metastasis. Unfortunately, up to 5–10% of carcinomas (especially cancers of the breast, lung, prostate, and kidney) show predilection for epidural metastasis. Upper motor neuron lesions

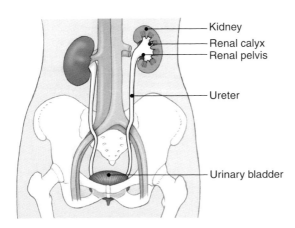
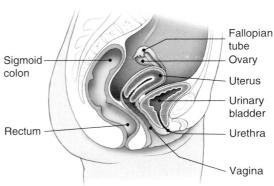

Figure 37.1
Female urinary tract anatomy (a) anteroposterior (AP) view (b) sagittal view.

above T11 may result in a spastic bladder that fails to allow for adequate urine storage.

Normal urinary flow through the bladder with its subsequent bladder washout is the primary host defense mechanism against infection. Bacteria from the perineum can migrate up the urethra. Hence, the shorter female urethra predisposes females to more frequent UTIs, especially in infants, children, and sexually-active women. Predominance shifts towards males as they get older, when incomplete emptying of the bladder due to prostatic enlargement becomes a problem. Some authors comment upon a "milking" action which occurs to the female urethra during sexual intercourse. This has led to the observation that prompt voiding following intercourse lessens the frequency of UTI. Certain bacteria, however, have evolved very efficient mechanisms over time to attach to bladder's epithelial and mucosal surfaces, bypassing normal washout defense mechanisms.

From bladder to meatus, the anatomy differs greatly between genders. The female anatomy includes a short urethral distance to the actual meatus. However, the nearby vagina, cervix, uterus, and parametrial structures complicate disease processes as well as evaluation.

The male urethra exits the bladder and is enveloped by the prostate gland (Figure 37.2). The male urethra is longer anatomically than the female urethra, and as such is more prone to strictures over its caliber and length. These may occur as a result of prior instrumentation (indwelling foley catheter), trauma, or as a sequelae of urethritis. The striated muscle in the urogenital diaphragm that is distal to the prostate itself forms the external sphincter. Benign prostatic hypertrophy or hyperplasia (BPH) is extremely common as males age; autopsy studies show that upwards of 50–60% of men over 50 years of age have some element of BPH.

History

The history in the patient with urinary complaints is extremely important, as there are generally no specific external findings associated with the common causes of urinary complaints. A careful history also helps identify clues that can be used to guide clinical investigation. One needs to determine if the ailment involves the urinary or reproductive tract, and investigate accordingly.

How did your symptoms begin?

It is typically a sudden change in normal voiding pattern that brings the patient to see a physician. The time course, time of day that symptoms occur, and alleviating or irritating factors should be ascertained. Sudden onset of pain is often

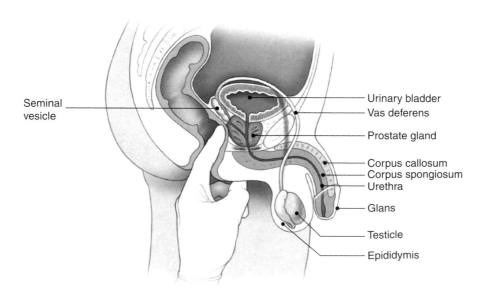

Seminal vesicle —
Urinary bladder
Vas deferens
Prostate gland
Corpus callosum
Corpus spongiosum
Urethra
Glans
Testicle
Epididymis

Figure 37.2
Male urinary tract anatomy: sagittal view.

characteristic of acute obstruction. Progressive symptoms such as dribbling and increased nocturia frequently accompany slow enlargement of the prostate (BPH) that tends to develop over time.

Can you describe the pain?

Many urologic presentations have some component of associated pain. This may be irritative pain during micturition, lower abdominal pain in the suprapubic region or perineum associated with the bladder or prostate, or flank pain associated with ureteral or renal disease. Renal colic is typically abrupt in onset, although some irritative symptoms may be noted preceding the abrupt onset of colic. It may radiate towards the groin, testicles, or ovaries.

Are you unable to spontaneously void?

Inability to void is typically an acute presentation, and the patient presents with an urgent need for relief. It is key to inquire about obstructive symptoms, such as slowly worsening hesitancy, decrease in stream force or caliber, and post-void dribbling. These clue the examiner to a slowly progressive obstruction with an acute endpoint, as opposed to an acute process with a different etiology. With acute presentations, think of infection, clot retention, medication, or toxicologic causes.

Is your urinary elimination normal?

Micturition-associated symptoms include frequency, urgency, dysuria, post-void fullness, incontinence, and suprapubic pain. Careful questioning of the patient as to when the symptoms occur may help localize the inflammatory process. Do the symptoms predominate before voiding, at the initiation of the voiding stream, during the mid-stream phase, or after the voiding act itself? This line of questioning can help differentiate bladder from urethral symptoms. The presence of gas bubbles in association with the urinary stream can help identify an abnormal communication between the gastrointestinal (GI) and genitourinary (GU) tracts, often associated with colonic diverticula (colovesicle fistula).

Is the urine discolored?

Not all discolored urine is secondary to hematuria. Gross hematuria and clot formation are easily identified, but abnormally-pigmented urine may be from blood, abnormal chromagens such as bile, nutritional sources, and dyes themselves. Cloudy urine usually occurs from protein or crystals, not from cells. One should also ask about the timing of the hematuria in relation to the urinary stream. Bleeding from the anterior urethra to the trigone, or the bladder and proximal structures, can present with initial, terminal, or total stream hematuria, respectively.

Are you having other abnormal symptoms associated with either elimination or the perineum?

Abnormalities of the micturition reflex arc tend to have other neurologic manifestations, such as bowel dysfunction with either incontinence or retention. The patient may also complain of anesthesia in a saddle distribution, if specifically asked. A sexual history can be very helpful, for the same autonomic innervation is important for both male and female sexual function. Abnormal pain, anesthesia, or inability to achieve an erection (impotence) may help identify neurologic pathology.

Have you had any genitourinary problems in the past?

Many urologic conditions are chronic in nature, and the patient may be able to relate symptoms to prior disease presentations. A history of kidney stones, urologic malignancies, prior surgical instrumentation of the urinary tract, and prior infections can help clinicians narrow down the differential diagnosis. Abrupt flank pain in the elderly hypertensive patient without a history of stone disease could be related to nephrolithiasis, but acute aortic disease must have higher diagnostic consideration. Prior instrumentation of the urethra from indwelling foley catheters may lead to urethral strictures. A careful sexual history can also identify risk factors for sexually transmitted infections (STIs), such as a history of abnormal discharge, genital pain or lesions, or unprotected sexual activity with multiple partners.

Are you taking any prescription or over-the-counter medications?

Recent antibiotic use can help identify the potential for antibiotic resistance if an infection is present. Many medications have anticholinergic side effects, which can cause bladder outlet obstruction and acute urinary retention. A common example is the over-the-counter antihistamine used for a variety of unrelated symptoms. Other medications or foods can cause urinary discoloration, and at times burning.

Associated symptoms

A history of fever or chills may serve as an indirect marker of infection, especially in the afebrile patient who may have recently taken non-steroidal anti-inflammatory drugs (NSAIDs) or acetaminophen for pain relief. Ureterolithiasis may cause intermittent pallor, nausea, diaphoresis, and vomiting; a relative bradycardia is not uncommon with kidney stone presentations. Flank pain with shoulder radiation usually reflects a sub-diaphragmatic process such as hemorrhage or abscess. One should ask about cardiopulmonary symptoms such as cough, dyspnea, and chest pain that may cause pain referred to the flanks. Renal disease may stimulate the celiac ganglion that serves both kidney and stomach, producing classic nausea and vomiting. The inability to keep down oral fluids or medications can help with patient disposition. Diarrhea in the female patient can easily colonize the urethra and bladder with coliform bacteria, causing UTI. Gynecologic symptoms such as menses, vaginal discharge and/or bleeding, abnormal pelvic pain, and contraception practices can help establish a differential diagnosis.

Physical examination

A focused physical examination may help differentiate upper tract disease from lower tract disease, but may be normal. The clinician must first look at the entire patient, starting with the general appearance.

General appearance

The general appearance of a patient with urinary complaints may vary from minimal to no discomfort to severe pain. Patients may appear pale, diaphoretic, cool, and/or clammy. They may be actively vomiting and writhing in pain, or be very comfortable reading a magazine. Hydration status of the patient can also be quickly gleaned at this time.

Renal colic tends to cause the patient to writhe about, restless on the examination table, with neither relief nor exacerbation upon movement. Peritonitis, on the other hand, is classically much worse with patient movement; most patients with peritoneal pathology lie still to avoid exacerbating their pain.

Vital signs

Vital signs are a key component of every patient encounter. Hemodynamic instability can be inferred from tachycardia, hypotension, and signs of inadequate tissue perfusion, such as altered mental status. An accurate temperature is essential, especially in the context of infection. A relative bradycardia may be associated with nephrolithiasis.

Cardiopulmonary

Cardiopulmonary examination may identify comorbid conditions. Lower lobe pulmonary disease, such as infiltrates, pleural collections, and pulmonary infarctions can cause pain referred to the flank. Rales, decreased breath sounds, pleural rubs, or isolated wheezing can give the clinician clues to these diseases. Cardiac auscultation can identify fibrillation that may predispose to the production of emboli. Abnormal valvular murmurs raise suspicion for infectious endocarditis, which may result in renal infarction.

Abdomen

On abdominal examination, the kidneys are generally not palpable. However, with polycystic disease or significant hydronephrosis, one may actually palpate them as deep structures in the upper abdomen. One must examine the patient for other masses, such as a pulsatile abdominal aortic aneurysm (AAA), pregnant uterus, or distended bladder. Auscultation of abnormal abdominal bruits may suggest vascular disease.

Back

Here, the kidneys are relatively protected in the bony confines of the costovertebral angles. Fist percussion may elicit flank pain, and careful finger palpation separates this from midline musculoskeletal causes. Renovascular disease may cause posteriorly-located bruits.

Perineum

Examination of the external meatus may reveal irritation and/or discharge. Examine the labia and/or scrotum for additional pathology, such as subcutaneous air or cutaneous discoloration associated with necrotizing fasciitis. Prompt identification of this disease allows timely surgical debridement in the operating room (OR) and proper administration of intravenous (IV) antibiotics. Lesions should be identified anywhere in or surrounding the perineum, which may be the cause of pain or suggest alternate etiologies.

Rectal

A careful examination investigates not only for rectal pathology, but also documents the integrity of the micturition reflex arc. Perianal sensation and "normal" sphincter tone may be subjective, but an intact bulbocavernosus reflex is objective evidence that a complete reflex arc integrating the sensory nerves, spinal cord, and motor fibers exists. The bulbocavernosus reflex is tested by inserting a finger into the patient's rectum and then gently tugging on an indwelling foley catheter or lightly squeezing the glans or clitoris. Normally, this will induce contraction of the anal sphincter and verify integrity of spinal cord segments S2–S4. The anal wink reflex (S2–S5) is tested by scratching the perianal skin which normally induces anal sphincter contraction.

Prostate

The digital examination of the prostate assesses for hypertrophy, tenderness, and masses. A normal digital examination does not rule out internal urethral compression from asymmetric prostate lobe enlargement. Often one may find a loss of the "normal" median sulcus on digital examination with significant prostate enlargement, and the superior boundary of the prostate may be beyond reach of the examining digit. Abnormal pain or "bogginess" is a sign of prostatic infection. One must take care not to massage a tender or boggy prostate; bacteremia may occur as a result, complicating the patient's course.

Pelvic

Often, the history alone in the female patient cannot differentiate between a urologic or gynecologic cause of symptoms. A careful speculum and bimanual examination can identify gynecologic etiologies such as cervicitis, ovarian pathology, or urinary frequency associated with pregnancy. From a practical standpoint, it also allows a "quick-cath" urine sampling during the examination.

Differential diagnosis

Table 37.1 Differential diagnosis of urinary-related complaints

Dysuria
Bladder calculus
Cervicitis
Cystitis
Prostatitis
Urethral obstruction
• Stricture
• Foreign body
• Extrinsic compression
Urethritis
Urolithiasis
Vaginitis
Hematuria
Bleeding dyscrasias
Exercise
Infection – parasites, bacteria, renal tuberculosis
Glomerulonephritis
Myoglobinuria (positive dipstick, negative RBCs)
Neoplasia – from kidney, bladder, prostate to urethra
Polycystic kidney disease
Renal infarction – vascular disease, sickle cell disease
Trauma – from renal parenchyma to urethral orifice
Urolithiasis
Urinary retention
Benign prostatic hypertrophy (BPH)
Clot retention – from trauma, neoplasia, renal origin
Myelitis
Paraplegia/cauda equina syndrome
Prostatitis
Urethral irritation – HSV infection, candida, chlamydia
Urethral or bladder neck calculus
Urethral stricture
Urethral trauma – Iatrogenic vs. mechanical

HSV: herpes simplex virus; RBC: red blood cell.

Diagnostic testing

Laboratory studies

Urine collection

One must obtain and study a clean sample of urine for patients with urologic complaints. This is often problematic during the ED visit. Long waiting times often preclude adequate and timely sampling from patients able to produce an adequate specimen. The verbal presentation of diagnostic bladder catheterization to parents or patients is often met with fear.

In the pediatric population, a bag specimen is generally not accepted for identification of infection and culture. Eighty-five percent or more of positive urine collections obtained via bag collection are false positives, prompting unnecessary and potentially harmful treatment and imaging studies that follow. Females and uncircumsized males need adequate urine obtained by a one-time "in-and-out" bladder catheterization, which has less than a 1% chance of inducing a UTI. Some literature argues for the usefulness of a spontaneously voided mid-stream sample in a circumsized pediatric male, but waiting with a cup next to an uncomfortable patient is challenging at best, and futile in practice.

Adult males for the most part can provide a clean catch, mid-stream urine collection. This may be impossible in a debilitated patient unable to comply with instructions. Proper cleansing is important, as well as wasting the initial portion of urine into the toilet before collecting the sample.

Urine collection in the sexually-active adult female relies on the absence of vaginal discharge which can contaminate the urinary stream. History may or may not be accurate, making a pelvic examination important (especially in the adolescent female). If there are no gynecologic complaints or discharge, a correctly obtained clean-catch urine sampling should suffice. Have the patient sit backwards on the toilet, cleanse the external genitalia, void a small amount into the toilet, and then collect a sample into the cup.

Urinalysis

Once an adequate urine sample is obtained, debate between dipstick testing versus formal laboratory urinalysis (UA) occurs. Time of testing, cost, and local practice trends all contribute to the widespread variation between the actual test used. Urine dipstick testing (a 30 cent test that takes a few minutes to perform at the bedside) has a high positive predictive value, but is not without limitations. Up to 5% of patients with normal dipsticks have abnormal microscopy. Leukocyte esterase will pick up white blood cells (WBCs) associated with infection, but will also identify WBCs associated with any inflammation. Nitrite examination has a high positive predictive value (96%) for UTI, but a low negative predictive value. Nitrate is converted to nitrite via bacterial metabolism; however, bladder incubation is a prerequisite. Nitrite testing is best performed on the first void of the day, after overnight incubation in the bladder has allowed for nitrite production. Bacterial counts will double every hour at room temperature, and double more quickly at body temperature. Once obtained, perform a dipstick analysis promptly or send the urine to the laboratory. The lab typically takes over an hour to process the specimen and provide results. Delayed evaluation of a urine specimen (e.g., urine obtained from the patient in the waiting room and left sitting for hours before actually going to the laboratory) may lead to falsely-positive results.

The dipstick method for blood will look for hemoglobin-like compounds. It does not differentiate between hemoglobin from red blood cells (RBCs) and myoglobin from skeletal muscle breakdown. Positive dipsticks should have confirmatory microscopy to quantitate the degree of hematuria. There is no correlation between red cells on microscopy and the degree of obstruction seen with renal calculi. Occasionally, one may have complete obstruction of the ureteter without RBCs on initial UA. Subsequent follow-up UAs may reveal hematuria.

Urinary pH is obtained via dipstick, and helps differentiate infections from intrinsic metabolic conditions. Alkaline urine (pH > 7.5) typically results from urea-splitting bacterial infections such as those caused by *Proteus* or *Pseudomonas*. Acidic urine (pH < 5.5) effectively rules out renal tubular acidosis (RTA) as a cause for nephrolithiasis.

If the preliminary testing is suggestive of UTI, the next question is: does the patient need a urine culture? Multiple studies have shown the ineffectiveness and wasted expense of urine cultures in the management of simple, uncomplicated patients. High-risk groups mandating culture include immunocompromised, age extremes, pregnant, obstructed, and treatment failures.

Additional studies

If a pelvic examination has been performed, standard practice is to send off cultures looking for STIs such as gonorrhea and chlamydia. The actual test varies with institution, but often uncovers silent STIs. The female patient of childbearing age should also have a pregnancy test performed.

Gross hematuria may also prompt hematologic testing. A baseline hematocrit can identify anemia and help with follow-up care, but is often unnecessary with simple hematuria. Historical questions such as prior bleeding problems or easy bruising can usually uncover bleeding tendencies, as in inherited coagulation disorders. Laboratory investigation of coagulation profiles may be helpful in the patient currently treated with coumadin, but there is no indication for routine testing in the patient with hematuria. An International Normalized Ratio (INR) may be indicated to uncover drug interactions between oral anticoagulants and antibiotics (such as sulfon-amides or quinolones) that prolong the INR, even if there has not been a change to a patient's anti-coagulation dose.

Routine investigation of renal function via crea-tinine levels promotes controversy. Older forms of urologic imaging that utilized contrast radiogra-phy often required assessment of creatinine levels before the administration of the IV contrast. Prolonged ureteral obstruction can cause irre-versible renal damage and creatinine elevation; however, not every patient with a kidney stone needs a baseline creatinine. Practice variations do occur, but most urologists request a baseline creati-nine for any stone greater than 5 mm in size, as these stones may not pass spontaneously.

Radiologic studies

Radiologic imaging for urinary complaints is utilized for complicated infections, anatomic abnormalities, or obstruction. Options include ultrasound, plain films, intravenous pyelograms (IVPs) and computerized tomography (CT).

US is very useful in delineating bladder dis-tention, and a carefully performed study often can show fluid fluid interfaces between urine and retained clot. Renal ultrasound may show hydronephrosis from obstruction, but the degree of hydronephrosis depends upon many factors which may lead to inconsistencies in interpreta-tion. Shadowing may occasionally be seen from renal parenchymal stones, but ureteral stones are often not visualized with US.

The kidney–ureter–bladder (KUB) film, if prop-erly performed, can be helpful in the identification of radiopaque structures such as ureteral or blad-der calculi. The urologist can identify stone loca-tion and follow progress towards spontaneous elimination. One may also diagnose emphysema-tous pyelonephritis from gas-forming organisms.

The IVP utilizes injected contrast to image the renal unit via excretion of dye into the collecting system and transit to the bladder. This procedure places the patient at risk for ionic contrast medium reactions that range from increased pain from the contrast load to fatal anaphylaxis. If pos-tive for high-grade obstruction, a properly per-ormed study requires delayed films that may ake hours. IVPs can, however, generate valuable anatomic and functional data, and are the pre-erred test of many urologists.

A newer advance in urinary imaging, espe-ially for calculus disease, is the non-contrast CT scan. This study may reveal the obstructing

calculus as well as the degree of resulting hydronephrosis (Figure 37.3). Perhaps more importantly, the scan can identify an alternative etiology for the patient's symptoms. If the CT is positive for obstruction, the urologist may ask for a confirmatory KUB film to identify the stone's loca-tion in two dimensions in relation to radiographic structures, such as a transverse process or the pelvic brim. This is a more cost-effective method of following stone progress through the collecting system, when compared to a repeat CT scan or IVP.

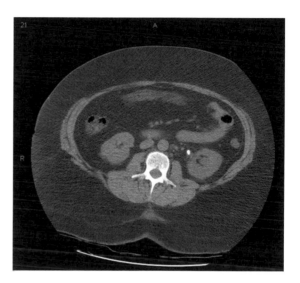

Figure 37.3
Kidney stone. Axial CT scan demonstrating a calcific opacity adjacent to the left kidney, consistent with a calculus in the proximal ureter. *Courtesy:* Gus Garmel, MD.

Calculous disease is often diagnosed clinically, and confirmed with radiologic imaging or even-tual stone passage. These modalities allow the cli-nician to accurately measure the size and precise anatomic location of the obstruction. Calculi siz-ing is very important in prognosis, as <4–5 mm sized-stones pass spontaneously greater than 90% of the time. This rate of spontaneous passage falls dramatically with increasing stone size; only 10% of 8 mm calculi will pass spontaneously.

The time from diagnosis to actual stone pas-sage also varies with stone size and initial stone location, among other things. Gravel-sized cal-culi up to 2 mm typically pass in 5–8 days. Larger 2–4 mm calculi often require 7–14 days for spon-taneous passage. These are rough estimations at best, and individual time to passage varies with the clinical situation, the stone's location, and the patient's anatomy.

Overall, distal calculi are more likely to pass spontaneously than calculi causing proximal obstruction that have already lodged. Right-sided calculi are more likely to pass spontaneously compared to left-sided calculi. The three most common sites for ureteral obstruction include the junction of the ureter with the renal pelvis, the deflection of the ureter over the iliac vessels, and the uretero-vesicle junction (UVJ), the most common site of obstruction.

General treatment principles

Specific treatment of urologic disorders encountered in the ED varies by etiology. It is easiest to divide these into infection treatment, obstruction relief, and pain control. The majority of urinary tract complaints have a combination of symptoms for clinicians to address.

Infection treatment

Infectious disorders need antimicrobial therapy directed against typical uropathogens. Most causative organisms are from colonization of the perineum, which helps direct therapy. There are many effective drugs for the typical uropathogen, but one must balance cost, local resistance to a particular agent, and unique patient characteristics, such as pregnancy and age, when choosing specific treatment.

Recommended therapy for UTIs, both complicated and simple, is not without controversy. Advocates for all types of therapy try to balance cost of therapy with local bacterial resistance patterns in order to come up with specific treatment recommendations. Problematic to this is the fact that antimicrobial resistance is often difficult to characterize, because empiric therapy without urine culture is commonplace. Some locales are showing increasing bacterial resistance to anti-microbials.

Bacterial resistance to drugs and cost recommendations specific to a hospital's formulary are best handled by referring to your particular hospital or region's bacterial sensitivity patterns. Some regions have abnormally high bacterial resistance to cephalosporins or sulfonamide drugs. In these regions, quinolone therapy may be a more expensive yet practical choice for therapy. The potential for quinolone-directed osseous and cartilage damage prevents its use in the pediatric population. Sulfa-based medicines have worked well in the pediatric population in the past, attacking bacteria by inhibiting folate metabolism. This class of drugs poses special concerns to the pregnant patient and fetus in the first trimester, however, when folate is so important in organogenesis. Third trimester use of sulfonamides may also lead to *kernicterus*, to the fetus, the deposition of bili-rubin pigments in the fetal brain.

For uncomplicated UTIs, a 3-day course of trimethoprim–sulfamethoxazole (TMP–SMX) results in a bacteriologic cure within 7 days in 94% of women (Table 37.2). Even where bacterial resistance rates are as high as 30%, cure rates of 80–85% in women are still possible. The concern resistance has prompted various authors to recommend of flouroquinolones in place of TMP–SMX for the treatment of UTIs. Fluoroquinolones are bioavailable, often allowing for single daily dosing and higher patient compliance. However, they are Class C agents (with regard to pregnancy) and are more expensive. The Infectious Diseases Society of America recommends initial use of TMP–SMX except in areas where resistance exceeds 10–20%. Care must be exercised with some of the newer quinolone formulations on the market, for they have little or no renal penetration, limiting their effectiveness against urinary pathogens.

Table 37.2 Uncomplicated UTIs

Agent	Dosing
TMP–SMX	160/800 PO bid for 3 days
Ciprofloxacin	250 mg PO bid for 3 days
Levofloxacin	250 mg PO q day for 3 days
Nitrofurantoin monohydrate	100 mg PO bid for 7 days

BID: twice a day; PO: per os;
TMP–SMX: Trimethoprim–Sulfamethoxazole.

There can be simple as well as complicated UTIs. This differentiation can be difficult to make clinically, for 30–50% of women with isolated lower tract symptoms have subclinical pyelonephritis. Prior treatment, microabscess formation, retained calculi, indwelling catheters, and urine obstruction and stasis all create complicated infections in otherwise immunocompetent hosts. Altered anatomy, such as progesterone-induced ureteral dilation with subsequent stasis found in pregnant patients, warrants prolonged treatment for a 7–14 days (Table 37.3). As many pediatric UTIs are also accompanied by anatomic

Table 37.3 Complicated UTIs

Agent	Dosing
Initial therapy – flouroquinolone	
Levofloxacin	250 mg PO q day for 10–14 days
Ciprofloxacin XR	500 mg PO q day for 10–14 days
Second-line therapy	
TMP–SMX	160/800 PO bid for 10–14 days
Amoxicillin/clavulanate	500 mg PO tid, 875 mg PO bid for 10–14 days
Ceftriaxone–parenteral	1–2 grams IV q day
Gentamycin–parenteral	3–5 mg/kg/day IV divided tid (according to renal function)
Unasyn–parenteral	3 grams IV q 6 hours

BID: twice a day; IV: intravenous; PO: per os; TID: three times a day; TMP–SMX: Trimethoprim–Sulfamethoxazole.

abnormalities, a longer treatment regimen with continued prophylaxis until the child has had urologic imaging is often recommended (Table 37.4). Patients at age extremes not uncommonly suffer from transient bacteremia, making aggressive therapy important in these patient populations.

Table 37.4 Treatment of pediatric UTIs

Agent	Dosing
Amoxicillin	30–50 mg/kg/day PO divided tid
Amoxicillin/clavulanate	45 mg/kg/day PO divided bid
TMP–SMX	8–10 mg/kg/day PO divided bid
Cephalexin	25–50 mg/kg/day PO divided qid

BID: twice a day; PO: per os; QID: four times a day; TID: three times a day; TMP–SMX: Trimethoprim–Sulfamethoxazole.

Other clinical factors for the clinician to consider are the patient's hydration status and his or her ability to maintain hydration following discharge. Failure to keep even the most powerful and expensive antibiotic in the GI system renders it ineffective. If hydrated, discharge instructions for the patient with a simple UTI often encourage forcing fluids" and acidifying the urine. Forcing fluids should ensure adequate hydration, and contributes to bladder washout. However, large volumes of dilute urine will decrease the concentration of antibiotic in the urine. It is probably more important to emphasize frequent and complete bladder emptying. Urine acidification, often through cranberry juice ingestion, can result in a relative reduction of bacterial loads in infected urine. Some of this may be related to interference with bacterial adherence to uroepithelial cells via an unknown mechanism.

If the patient has infection concomitant with ureteral obstruction, this creates a proximal renal unit abscess. Antibiotics start therapy, but prompt renal pelvis emptying via either ureteral stent or directed nephrostomy drainage will be required in most cases. Urologic consultation is important in these complicated patients.

Obstruction relief

Bladder obstruction requires urinary drainage or diversion. Any mechanical instrumentation to relieve such obstruction poses iatrogenic risks to the patient, either via transient bacteremia or creation of a false urethral passage. Lubrication, topical anesthetics, patience, and practice help prevent iatrogenic problems. The most common approach to bladder obstruction is placement of a Foley catheter. Another specialized urinary catheter regularly used in the ED setting is the coudé catheter, which has a relatively fixed curve to the distal few centimeters of the catheter. This feature allows the catheter to deflect off an enlarged prostate lobe at the bladder neck and pass through the prostatic urethra. Another option for urinary diversion is the placement of a suprapubic catheter, bypassing the prostate and urethra completely. A urologist may also attempt to instrument the urethra through the use of urethral sounds, filiforms and followers, or fiber-optic instruments and seldinger wire passage. These techniques are beyond the scope of emergency physician practice.

After satisfactory Foley catheter placement in the setting of acute urinary retention, the question arises as to how fast to empty the bladder. Theoretical complications include intramural hemorrhage and hematuria from rapid decompression, as well as potential for post-obstructive diuresis and high-output renal failure after any drainage procedure. One must balance such theoretical concerns (e.g., rare, usually inconsequential bleeding) with genuine patient concerns such as pain from continued retention. If more than 800 ml of urine is obtained, it is prudent to leave the catheter in place and remove it at a later time. Otherwise, bladder atony will likely lead to a subsequent episode of urinary retention, as will continued obstruction secondary to prostatic enlargement. Transient hypotension following catheterization, perhaps related to vagal stimulation, has been reported in the literature.

Pain control

Pain management with urinary complaints is directed at either irritative or obstructive symptoms. Irritative symptoms may require only acetaminophen or NSAID, and occasional use of urinary anesthetics such as pyridium. Typically, only a few days of therapy are required for relief of irritative symptoms. Side effects of pyridium include urine discoloration and the potential for hemolysis and methemoglobinemia, especially in susceptible patients with unknown glucose-6-dehydrogenase (G6PD) deficiency who are also treated with sulfonamides.

Ureteral obstruction from calculi creates intermittent episodes of complete obstruction, hydronephrosis, and pain. Some clinicians use either spasmolytic or anticholinergic drugs to reduce pain and frequency of these colicky episodes, but the medical literature has not supported this practice. Newer investigations have revealed that much of the pain is mediated by ureter-released prostaglandins in response to obstruction. These prostaglandins increase peristalsis, which is an attempt by the ureter to move the stone down for spontaneous passage. NSAIDs, such as ketorolac or ibuprofen, are very effective in relieving the pain, nausea, and vomiting associated with colic. Their use is not without caution, however, as canine models have demonstrated decreased renal blood flow and acute, transient renal failure.

Narcotics are also effective at blunting pain in the ED. Incremental IV dosing is effective at pain reduction, and allows further titration of medication without the additional discomfort of intramuscular (IM) injections. Narcotic medication for a short course of therapy is usually prudent upon patient discharge, often in addition to a prescription for NSAIDs.

Special patients

Elderly

The elderly patient is likely to present with comorbidity, but may also be unable to give an accurate history to the clinician. It is not uncommon for UTIs to cause altered mentation, which must be considered in the differential diagnosis for behavioral changes. The nursing home patient presents several unique challenges; not only does this patient population tend to be colonized with antibiotic-resistant organisms, but indwelling catheters predispose to bladder colonization and resultant ascending infections. A unique problem in the elderly male patient is extension of organisms into the prostate itself, with subsequent obstruction of prostatic drainage from an indwelling catheter. This patient needs prompt urologic consultation and suprapubic urinary diversion.

Pregnant

Urinary tract symptoms are relatively common throughout pregnancy. Conditions ranging from asymptomatic bacteriuria to complicated upper tract disease (pyelonephritis) can have adverse effects on both mother and fetus, and are important for clinicians to consider. Hormone-induced changes of the renal collecting system, primarily from elevated progesterone levels, lead to reduced ureteral and bladder tone and physiologic hydroureter of pregnancy. Pregnant women also have increased bladder capacity which, combined with urinary stasis, predisposes to bacterial overgrowth and proliferation.

Asymptomatic bacteriuria is a relatively common entity, found in up to 9% of first trimester gestations. Untreated disease can progress to pyelonephritis in 20 to 40% of patients in some studies, with its associated risks (sepsis, preterm delivery, and potential intrauterine fetal growth retardation) to both mother and fetus. Symptomatic cystitis in pregnancy deserves empiric treatment, with the additional caveat that a urine culture be sent. Up to 15% of pregnant patients with cystitis will develop relapses during their pregnancy, and the culture and sensitivity helps guide follow-up therapy. Ascending upper tract infection in the form of pyelonephritis poses significant risk to pregnant women, both from a medical as well as an obstetrical standpoint. Up to 20% of such patients have been shown to develop severe complications, such as urosepsis or preterm delivery.

Outpatient management of asymptomatic bacteriuria and uncomplicated cystitis in pregnancy is directed at the typical uropathogens, with E. coli responsible for up to 2/3 of all cases. Cephalosporins, amoxicillin, or sulfonamide therapy for a 3-day course is appropriate (Table 37.5). Use of sulfonamides in pregnant women at term

Table 37.5 Treatment of UTI during pregnancy

Agent	Dosing
Amoxicillin	500 mg PO tid
Cephalexin	500 mg PO qid
TMP–SMX (2nd trimester only)	160/800 PO bid
Nitrofurantoin monohydrate	100 mg PO bid
Ceftriaxone–parenteral therapy	1–2 grams IV q day

BID: twice a day; PO: per os; QID: four times a day; TID: three times a day; TMP–SMX: Trimethoprim–Sulfamethoxazole.

or mothers nursing infants younger than 2 months of age is not advised as sulfonamides may promote the displacement of bilirubin from plasma proteins leading to kernicterus. Flouroquinolones should never be used in the pregnant patient due to their actions on growing cartilage. Nitrofurantoin for a seven-day course of therapy is also an effective agent for uncomplicated disease.

Pyelonephritis may complicate up to 2% of all gestations. The non-pregnant patient often responds to outpatient therapy, but the pregnant patient may require admission by the obstetrical service for IV hydration and antibiotics. Cephalosporins are typically chosen for therapy, but local resistance patterns as well as obstetrical preferences in caring for this population should be considered. It is prudent to involve the obstetrical service in the care plan. If discharge occurs, a 10–14 day course of antibiotic therapy is typical.

Pediatric

Pediatric patients, like the elderly, often cannot localize pathology via an adequate history. One must consider a urinary source of infection in all febrile infants. When obtaining urine samples via bladder instrumentation, it is advised to send off a culture to ensure proper treatment when follow-up is arranged. Following a single infection in a high-risk pediatric patient, many authors recommend outpatient urologic imaging to identify possible anatomic anomalies, so prompt follow-up is crucial.

Immune compromised

There are several important points to remember when clinicians encounter an immunocompromised patient. Often, the organisms causing infection can be atypical in nature, so culture is important to document the organism and antibiotic sensitivities. If the patient is immunocompromised, one must have a much lower threshold for admission. If the patient is post-renal transplant, it is very important to carefully examine the transplanted kidney during the abdominal examination. The transplanted organ typically lies in the right lower quadrant, and excessive pain upon palpation can signify either rejection or complicated pyelonephritis. In such cases, consultation with the patient's nephrologist is required.

Disposition

The ultimate patient disposition depends upon several factors, including disease process, co-morbidities, and ability to follow directed therapy. Urinary obstruction with concomitant infection predisposes to renal abscess formation, so admission with urinary drainage to bypass the obstruction is mandatory. Pain that is not well controlled by oral agents, as well as persistent nausea and vomiting that prevent adequate hydration are also considerations for hospital admission. An immunocompromised state, a problem with a solitary kidney, and a painful high-grade obstruction are relative indications for hospital admission, as are complicated social situations and pregnancy.

Patients with intermittent obstruction secondary to calculi need proper follow-up arranged. One pitfall in management is the erroneous conclusion that the absence of pain means the absence of obstruction. Irreversible renal damage can be seen in as little as 2 weeks, so prompt patient follow-up is imperative. Confirmation of calculi passage is the gold standard. Instruct patients to strain their urine after discharge from the ED. This is much easier for the male patient to accomplish, using either a strainer or urinating onto coffee filters. Upon passage, the patient is instructed to bring the stone to their primary care provider. Crystallographic analysis of the stone is often difficult to arrange, costly to the patient, and helpful only in genetic- or metabolic-induced nephrolithiasis.

Pearls and pitfalls

1. UA is the cornerstone for diagnosing patients with urologic disease, yet false negatives do occur. Negative dipstick analysis carries a 5% chance of abnormal urinary sediment on

microscopy. Nephrolithiasis with complete ureteral obstruction may have a completely normal UA due to flow down of the unaffected ureter.

2. Though nephrolithiasis is a common clinical diagnosis, resist the temptation to discharge the patient without an analysis of the urine. An infection in the presence of obstruction is a true urologic emergency, often called "pus under pressure."

3. Cost-effective emergency care should be a goal of all clinicians, but the total elimination of urine cultures should not be part of this goal. Culture the high-risk patient (immuno-compromised, elderly, infants, and pregnant) as well as those patients with prior treatment failures.

4. Though quinolones are increasingly being utilized as excellent monotherapy in urologic infections, clinicians must consider quinolone-related drug interactions, especially when prescribing these medications to the elderly. Always investigate such potential drug interactions to prevent iatrogenic complications, such as bleeding or elevated INR in the patient taking anticoagulants.

References

1. Barker LR (ed.). *Principles of Ambulatory Medicine*, 5th ed., Philadelphia: Lippincott Williams and Wilkins, 1999.

2. Cantrill SV (ed.). *Cost-Effective Diagnostic Testing in Emergency Medicine: Guidelines for Appropriate Utilization of Clinical Laboratory and Radiology Studies*. Dallas: American College of Emergency Physicians, 2000.

3. Demetriou E, et al. Dysuria in adolescent girls: urinary tract infection or vaginitis? *Pediatrics* 1982;70(2):299.

4. Fihn S. Acute uncomplicated urinary tract infections in women. *New Engl J Med* 2003;349:259–266.

5. Gupta K, et al. Antimicrobial resistance among uropathogens that cause community acquired urinary tract infections in women: a nationwide analysis. *Clin Infect Dis* 2001;33:89.

6. Harwood-Nuss A (ed.). *The Clinical Practice of Emergency Medicine*, 3rd ed., Philadelphia: Lippincott Williams and Wilkins, 2001.

7. Lowe FC, et al. Cranberry juice and urinary tract infections: what is the evidence? *Urology* 2001;57(3):407.

8. Marx J (ed.). *Rosen's Emergency Medicine: Concepts and Clinical Practice*, 5th ed., St. Louis: Mosby, 2002.

9. Miller OF, et al. Time to stone passage for observed ureteral calculi: a guide for patient education. *J Urology* 1999;162:688.

10. Nyman MA, et al. Management of urinary retention: rapid versus gradual decompression and risk of complications. *Mayo Clin Proc* 1997;72:951.

11. Preminger GM, et al. Urolithiasis: detection and management with unenhanced spiral CT – a urologic perspective. *Radiology* 1998;207(2):308.

12. Rachner H, et al. Prevalence of bacteriuria in febrile children. *Pediatr Infect Dis* 1987;6(3):239.

13. Schwartz G (ed.). *Principles and Practice of Emergency Medicine*, 4th ed., Baltimore: Williams and Wilkins, 1999.

14. Stamm WE, et al. Treatment of the acute urethral syndrome. *New Engl J Med* 1981;304(16):956.

15. Taube M, et al. Trial without catheter following acute retention of urine. *Brit J Urol* 1989;63(2):180.

16. Tintinalli J (ed.). *Emergency Medicine: A Comprehensive Study Guide*, 5th ed., New York: McGraw Hill, 2000.

17. Warren JW, et al. Guidelines for antimicrobial treatment of uncomplicated acute bacterial cystitis and acute pyelonephritis in women. *Clin Infect Dis* 1999;29:745.

38   Vaginal bleeding

Pamela L. Dyne, MD and Rita Oregon, MD

Scope of the problem

A common emergency department (ED) complaint is vaginal bleeding, accounting for up to 10% of ED visits in many centers. The differential diagnosis for vaginal bleeding is relatively short, with the most serious condition being ectopic pregnancy, and the most common conditions being threatened miscarriage in the pregnant patient and abnormal uterine bleeding (AUB) in the non-pregnant patient. According to the Centers for Disease Control and Prevention (CDC-P), there were 108,000 ectopic pregnancies reported in the US in 1992. Ectopic pregnancies account for approximately 2% of reported pregnancies. Threatened miscarriage occurs in 20–30% of all pregnancies, and up to 50% of those threatened will go on to spontaneously abort. Septic abortions and gestational trophoblastic disease must also be considered in the differential diagnosis of vaginal bleeding in a pregnant woman, accounting for 0.4–0.6 per 100,000 spontaneous miscarriages and 0.1–1% of pregnancies, respectively. An understanding of the definitions of the different classifications and management options for non-viable gestations is important for effective management in the ED and for communication with consultants. Second- and third-trimester bleeding and postpartum vaginal bleeding are not discussed in this chapter because these patients are routinely evaluated in labor and delivery areas and infrequently cared for by emergency physicians.

Not all women with vaginal bleeding are pregnant. In the reproductive years, AUB is defined as bleeding from the uterus that is irregular in amount, timing, or duration. Prior to menarche or following menopause, any uterine bleeding is considered abnormal. Dysfunctional uterine bleeding (DUB) is a subset of AUB, and is defined as abnormal bleeding unrelated to pregnancy, exogenous gonadal steroids (such as oral contraceptives and hormone replacement), intrauterine contraceptive devices (IUDs), other medical conditions, or structural uterine pathology. DUB is estimated to affect up to 20% of reproductive-aged women. While diagnosis and ultimate treatment may be left to specialists, the acute care practitioner should have an understanding of the various causes of AUB so that the appropriate acute intervention is offered.

Pathophysiology

Physiology of menstruation

Normal menstrual bleeding results from the cyclical withdrawal of estrogens and progesterone that occurs, on average, 14 days following ovulation in the absence of pregnancy (Figure 38.1). Menses typically last 4 or 5 days, with a normal range of 2–7 days. Flow is usually heaviest in the first 2–3 days and tapers to spotting in the last 2–3 days. The normal volume of blood lost in a single menses averages 30–40 ml; >80 ml is considered excessive. For the typical woman of reproductive age, depletion of iron stores occurs when monthly blood loss exceeds 60 ml. The term *menorrhagia* means excessive menstrual blood flow. Menses are normally predictable, with a cycle (first day of one menses to the first day of the next) that ranges from 21 to 35 days.

The regulation of menses is dependent upon a number of hormonal factors that result in the process of ovulation. If ovulation does not occur, as in anovulation associated with polycystic ovarian syndrome, the endometrium is exposed solely to the proliferative effects of unopposed estrogen. This endometrium will eventually build to the point of instability and result in heavy, asynchronous bleeding, termed *metrorrhagia*. Following ovulation, the Graafian follicle that expelled the ovum becomes the corpus luteum (CL), which produces abundant estradiol and progesterone. These hormones exert profound effects on the endometrium causing it to be receptive to implantation for a short period of time. In the absence of pregnancy, the CL involutes resulting in withdrawal of the effects of estradiol and progesterone on the endometrium, culminating in sloughing and bleeding that comprises menstrual flow.

The next steps in the menstrual process are all directed at establishing hemostasis and subsequent regeneration of the endometrium's superficial layer. The endometrium is unique in that platelets have relatively little role in the process

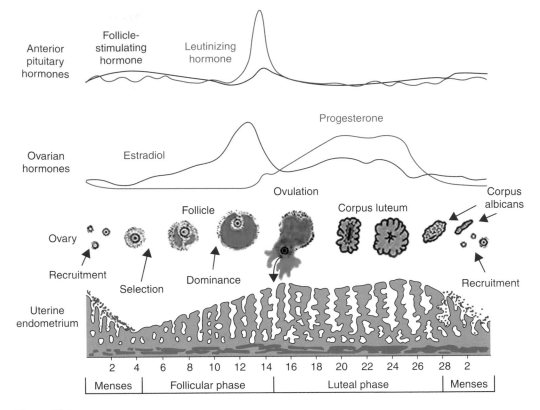

Figure 38.1
Normal menstrual cycle, including ovulation and menses. Used with permission, John Parrish, University of Wisconsin-Madison.

of hemostasis. Instead, endometrial hemostasis relies first upon the presence of local vasoconstrictors, then on factors of the extrinsic and intrinsic clotting cascades that result in the formation of a vascular clot. Once hemostasis has been achieved, the processes of endometrial angiogenesis and re-epithelialization rebuild the endometrium, thereby preparing it for implantation should fertilization occur in the next cycle. The factors involved in the initiation of angiogenesis are unclear, but appear to be associated with rising estrogen levels.

Fertilization, implantation, and embryology

For pregnancy to occur, fertilization must take place after ovulation. This generally occurs in the ampullary region of the fallopian tube. The ovum, fertilized or not, then moves by ciliary transport along the tube towards the uterine endometrial cavity. Implantation of the fertilized ovum in the endometrium occurs at about 7 days post-fertilization, which is approximately 3 weeks

after the last menstrual period (LMP). The developing embryo is surrounded by the trophoblast, which gives rise to the placenta and secretes human chorionic gonadotropin (hCG). It is hCG which prevents the degeneration of the CL, which continues to secrete adequate progesterone levels to maintain the developing gestation.

Ectopic pregnancy results from implantation of the fertilized ovum in a location other than the endometrium. Greater than 95% of ectopic pregnancies implant in the fallopian tube. Of these 80% implant in the ampullary portion, 12% in the isthmus, 5% in the fimbriated end of the tube, and 2% at the junction of the fallopian tube and uterus. The latter site of implantation is often referred to as an interstitial or cornual ectopic pregnancy. Interstitial ectopic pregnancies deserve special consideration, because they are both rare (accounting for only 2–3% of ectopic pregnancies) and dangerous, with a mortality rate more than twice that of other tubal pregnancies (2.2% vs. <1%). Additional sites of ectopic implantation include the abdomen, the cervix, and the ovary. Once tubal implantation has occurred, there are four potential outcomes: the ectopic may erode through the tube leading to tubal rupture with associated intra-abdominal hemorrhage; the ectopic may persist within an intact tube with or without an associated tubal hematoma and/or intra-abdominal hemorrhage; the ectopic may abort out the fimbriated end of the fallopian tube; or the ectopic may spontaneously involute.

History

Are you pregnant?

This is the key question, as the entire thought process for caring for and diagnosing patients with vaginal bleeding is contingent on whether or not they are pregnant. While many patients know they are pregnant, many do not. Sixty-three percent of the time a woman who thinks she may be pregnant is correct. However, about 11% of ED patients who deny pregnancy are pregnant, and about 7% who report a normal menstrual history and deny sexual contact are pregnant. Therefore, a negative history for pregnancy is unreliable. All women of childbearing age (12–55 years old) with vaginal bleeding should have a pregnancy test, regardless of menstrual history.

When was your last normal menstrual period, and are your periods usually regular?

Despite the above discussion, it is useful to identify approximately when the patient's LMP was to attempt to date the pregnancy, should it be confirmed. The most common reason for amenorrhea (cessation of menses) is pregnancy. This is also important information in the non-pregnant vaginal bleeding patient, as the pattern of her periods and current bleeding history are important to establish whether her abnormal bleeding is ovulatory (bleeding is cyclic and predictable) or anovulatory (neither cyclic nor predictable).

When did the bleeding start, is the bleeding more than a usual period in quantity, is the blood clotted or not, and are you dizzy with position change?

These questions help provide a feel for how much blood has been lost. A recent onset of bleeding may be more consistent with potentially life-threatening conditions, such as ectopic pregnancy and miscarriage, whereas more prolonged or insidious bleeding is more suggestive of hormonal dysfunction. The actual amount of blood lost is usually difficult for a patient to quantify specifically, so comparing the amount of blood lost to the woman's usual menstrual flow may be helpful. Menstrual blood does not usually clot because of fibrinolysis that occurs in the endometrium. However, clots in the menstrual flow indicate relatively heavy bleeding, because the blood does not remain in the uterus long enough for fibrinolysis to occur. The clinical significance of the bleeding (such as symptomatic anemia) is key since this helps guide ED management and resuscitation, if necessary.

Have you passed any tissue?

The passage of fetal tissue may be helpful in excluding ectopic pregnancy in the right clinical context. However, without products of conception to look at for confirmation by the clinician, the information is too unreliable to be of much value. Additionally, large clots or a decidual cast from the endometrium can also be passed and mimic products of conception in ectopic pregnancies, which may confuse the clinical scenario.

What medications do you take? Are you on hormones or using some type of birth control?

Exogenous gonadal steroids (estrogens and progesterones) can be associated with AUB. These hormones may be being used for contraception or hormone replacement therapy (HRT), depending on the woman's age. Non-hormonal IUDs being used for contraception have also been associated with heavy menses and AUB secondary to changes in the prostaglandin milieu of the endometrium. Becoming pregnant despite the use of an IUD is a risk factor for ectopic pregnancy.

Any history of trauma?

Vaginal bleeding in the setting of abdominal or pelvic trauma expands the differential diagnosis to include uterine rupture and placental abruption in the pregnant patient. The trauma patient will generally be evaluated and resuscitated more urgently because of the potential for rapid hemodynamic compromise. Pregnant women are at risk for non-accidental abdominal and pelvic trauma from current or prior partners, which should be kept in mind during patient evaluation.

Associated symptoms

Nausea and vomiting

Gastrointestinal (GI) upset or distress may be the first symptom of early pregnancy in a woman who is having AUB. Thus, it is important to rule-in or rule-out pregnancy at the beginning of an evaluation of nausea or vomiting. Pyelonephritis also commonly presents with nausea and vomiting, and management of the pregnant patient with pyelonephritis may differ from the non-pregnant patient.

Fever or "flu"

Pelvic inflammatory disease (PID) may present with AUB secondary to concomitant endometritis. Septic abortion, which is any abortion (spontaneous or induced) accompanied by infection, may also present with these symptoms.

Urinary tract infection

Dysuria is a common complaint in women with gynecologic (GYN) pathology, but hematuria from a urinary tract infection (UTI) or pyelonephritis may present with what is mistaken as vaginal bleeding and urinary symptoms.

Dizziness, lightheadedness, syncope, or near-syncope

Does the patient have symptomatic anemia? Has the patient lost enough blood volume that she now has orthostatic hypotension? These symptoms suggest the clinician begin immediate fluid resuscitation, decide upon blood product replacement, and closely monitor vital signs.

Past medical

Obstetrical

By convention, the number of pregnancies, regardless of their result, is termed *gravida*, the number of live births is termed *para*, and the number of pregnancies that did not result in a live birth is termed *abortions*. These terms are short handed into G–P–Ab, such that a woman who has been pregnant five times, with three live births, one miscarriage and one therapeutic abortion would have her obstetrical history summarized by $G_5P_3Ab_{1,1}$.

Prior sexually transmitted infection, pelvic inflammatory disease, previous ectopic pregnancy, tubal surgery, smoking, frequent (daily) douching, current intrauterine contraceptive devices, or infertility with or without treatment

The most common cause of ectopic pregnancy is damage to the mucosa of the fallopian tube, which prevents transport of the fertilized ovum to the endometrial cavity. Mucosal damage is most often a result of tubal infection. Tubal surgery and diethylstilbesterol exposure have been demonstrated to play a role in other causes, as well as defects in tubal motility. Defects in the fertilized ovum itself may contribute to increased ectopic pregnancy risk due to impaired implantation prior to arrival in the endometrial cavity. Hormonal factors have also been associated with an increased risk of ectopic pregnancy. Supraphysiologic levels of estradiol or progesterone have been demonstrated to inhibit tubal migration, which may account for the increased incidence of ectopic pregnancies in patients on ovulation-induction agents (fertility agents, such as Clomid). There has been an association of smoking and daily douching with ectopic pregnancy as well, assumed to be due to abnormal ciliary transport.

Risk factors for ectopic pregnancy are important to elicit, as 50% of women with ectopic pregnancy will have one or more of these risk factors (Table 38.1). However, depending on the population, 25% of women with threatened abortion will have one or more risk factors for ectopic. It is important to note that the presence of one or more of these risk factors is helpful, but ectopic pregnancy is still possible in their absence.

Table 38.1 Ectopic pregnancy risk factors

- Previous ectopic pregnancy
- Tubal infection
- Tubal or pelvic surgery
- Intrauterine contraceptive device usage
- Infertility for >2 years, treated or untreated
- Diethylstilbesterol exposure
- Smoking
- Frequent (daily) douching

Previous treatment for abnormal uterine bleeding, oligomenorrhea, or amenorrhea

Oligomenorrhea is a decreased frequency of menstrual periods, and amenorrhea is the cessation of menses. Such history would lead one to suspect anovulation and possibly DUB as the cause for the abnormal bleeding.

Hirsuitism, obesity, acne, heat or cold intolerance, diarrhea, constipation, weight loss or gain, or galactorrhea

Signs of androgen excess commonly associated with polycystic ovarian syndrome may point to a cause of AUB. Other endocrinopathies, such as thyroid dysfunction (mainly hypothyroidism) and hyperprolactinemia can cause AUB and would be relevant to the work-up if there were such a history.

Easy bruising, excessive bleeding, or familial bleeding tendencies that may warrant investigation of a coagulopathy

Vaginal bleeding might be the presenting sign of a coagulopathy, such as idiopathic thrombocytopenic purpura (ITP) or von Willebrand's disease.

Medications

Use of platelet inhibitors such as aspirin or Plavix, or other anticoagulants like warfarin or low-molecular-weight heparin would be important to elicit, because the vaginal bleeding might be iatrogenic. Use of ovulation-induction agents are crucial because of the increased risk for ectopic and twin gestations with these agents. Additionally, concomitant intrauterine and ectopic pregnancies, termed *heterotopic pregnancy*, can occur with significantly increased frequency in women using these agents. This fact impacts the diagnostic accuracy of conventional tests used for excluding ectopic pregnancy, including pelvic ultrasound and quantitative β-hCG levels.

Physical examination

General appearance

One should immediately assess if the patient appears to be in distress secondary to pelvic or abdominal pain. A pale, diaphoretic patient is worrisome for hemoperitoneum and requires more urgent and aggressive intervention than the patient who appears well.

Vital signs

Blood pressure and pulse are key vital signs to assess. However, young healthy patients may become symptomatic from significant blood loss (dizzy or near-syncopal) before their vital signs

become abnormal. Elevated temperature may imply an infectious etiology for the patient's symptoms.

Abdomen

The abdomen should be evaluated thoroughly for signs of hemoperitoneum. Distention, rigidity, rebound, and guarding, as well as localization of pain should be assessed.

Pelvic

A speculum examination is an essential part of the assessment of AUB of any type. However, there is much information to be obtained by visual inspection of the external genitalia prior to the insertion of the speculum. Assess the vulva, anus, and urethra for non-uterine sources of bleeding and areas of infection or inflammation. Upon speculum insertion, a vaginal wet mount, cervical gonorrhea and chlamydia cultures should be obtained. While these are collected, evaluate for foreign bodies, masses, vaginal synechiae, or lacerations and note the quality and quantity of blood or clots in the vaginal vault. Bright red blood implies ongoing bleeding, whereas brownish discharge is more consistent with bleeding that has already stopped. Inspect the cervix as well for evidence of trauma, active bleeding, expulsion of tissue, or mass arising from the cervix. If the cervix is difficult to visualize due to bleeding or discharge, a ringed forceps with a small gauze may be gently inserted to clean the area.

A careful bimanual examination is a routine component of the evaluation of a woman with vaginal bleeding. It is performed in order to assess the uterus and adnexae for size and for tenderness, as well as the status of the internal cervical os in the pregnant patient. The external cervical os may remain slightly open to fingertip in any woman who has delivered a baby. However, the internal cervical os only opens (dilates) when uterine contents are in the process of being expelled. The internal os is examined by inserting the index finger through the external os. If there is the sensation that the finger in the opening enters without resistance, the internal os is open. If the finger is stopped by closed tissue, then the internal os is closed. After assessing for patency, the cervix should be held between the second and third fingers of the examining hand and gently moved from side to side to assess for cervical motion tenderness (CMT). This may be found in conditions that involve peritoneal or pelvic floor inflammation or irritation, although it is a nonspecific finding. Next, the uterus is palpated between the examiner's intravaginal hand and the hand on the patient's suprapubic area. The uterine size, shape, position, and contour are assessed, as well as its degree of tenderness. Uterine size may be estimated by comparison to common standard-sized objects, such as a golf ball (normal, non-pregnant), baseball (4–6 weeks gestational age), or softball (6–8 weeks gestational age). Lastly, the adnexae are palpated to assess for ovarian size, tenderness, and masses. The ovaries are normally non-palpable in post-menopausal women, and are the size of walnuts in pre-menopausal women.

In order to maximize the yield from the pelvic examination, the patient should be as comfortable as possible. If the patient is in significant distress with abdominal or pelvic pain, it is prudent to medicate the patient with appropriate analgesia before attempting to perform this examination. The choice of analgesic agent should take into consideration whether the patient is pregnant or lactating, and avoidance of agents that alter clotting function (aspirin and non-steroidal anti-inflammatory agents, such as ketorolac and ibuprofen) is wise. While there are not studies specifically addressing the safety and efficacy of premedicating a woman in distress before pelvic examination, there is literature to support this practice in patients with abdominal pain before abdominal examination. Thus, appropriate analgesia should not be withheld. Additionally, while a bimanual examination is routine in this setting, there are data that suggest poor inter-examiner reliability of the bimanual pelvic examination, which questions the utility of this portion of the examination in the non-pregnant female.

Auscultation for fetal heart tones

Fetal heart tones (FHTs) should be heard using a hand-held Doppler on the suprapubic area if the fetus is at least 12 weeks estimated gestational age (EGA). FHTs may be audible at 10 weeks EGA, but there is no cause for concern unless they are not present at 12 weeks EGA, provided a woman's dates are accurate. A normal fetal heart rate is between 120 and 160 bpm. It is important to document the presence, rate, and location of the FHTs if the patient is >12 weeks EGA, as it is both a verification of dates and viability of the gestation at that point in time.

Differential diagnosis

Table 38.2 Differential diagnosis of vaginal bleeding in first-trimester pregnancy

Diagnosis	Symptoms	Signs	Work-up
Blighted ovum (anembryonic gestation, embryonic failure)	Varied	Internal cervical os open or closed	Serum β-hCG (declining or plateau, if there is a previous level for comparison), CBC, EVUS (gestational sac too big to not have embryo >20 mm), Type and Rh, Urinalysis
Completed abortion	Vaginal bleeding ± abdominal pain	Benign examination, internal cervical os closed	Serum β-hCG (declining, if there is previous level for comparison), CBC, EVUS (empty uterus), Type and Rh, Urinalysis
Ectopic pregnancy	Varied: vaginal spotting or bleeding, and/or abdominal pain, syncope or orthostatic hypotension possible	Varied: benign pelvic and abdominal examination, or tachycardia, hypotension, abdominal rigidity, rebound and/or guarding, adnexal mass and/or tenderness	Serum β-hCG (level correlates with EVUS findings), CBC, EVUS (varied: normal with empty uterus, or adnexal or intrauterine findings consistent with ectopic pregnancy), Type and Rh
Embryonic demise (missed abortion)	Varied	Internal cervical os closed	Serum β-hCG (declining or plateau, if there is a previous level for comparison), CBC, EVUS (embryo lacking cardiac activity with CRL >5 mm), Type and Rh, Urinalysis

(continued)

Table 38.3 Differential diagnosis of vaginal bleeding in first-trimester pregnancy (*cont*)

Diagnosis	Symptoms	Signs	Work-up
Gestational trophoblastic disease	Vaginal bleeding or spotting, nausea/vomiting	Tremor, tachycardia	Serum β-hCG (may be greater than expected for EGA), Serum TSH, EVUS ("snowstorm" appearance)
Implantation bleeding	Minimal vaginal spotting at or about the timing of the missed period	Benign examination	Serum β-hCG, CBC, EVUS (empty uterus seen if EGA 3–5 weeks), Type and Rh, Urinalysis
Incomplete abortion	Vaginal bleeding or spotting and/or abdominal pain	Benign or tender pelvic examination, internal cervical os open or closed	Serum β-hCG (declining or plateau, if there is a previous level for comparison), CBC, EVUS (thickened, irregular endometrium >5 mm double stripe), Type and Rh, Urinalysis
Inevitable abortion (abortion in progress)	Vaginal bleeding or spotting and/or abdominal pain	Benign or tender pelvic examination, internal cervical os open	Serum β-hCG (declining or plateau, if there is a previous level for comparison), CBC, EVUS (retained POC), Type and Rh, Urinalysis
Septic abortion	Varied: vaginal bleeding or spotting, fever, abdominal pain, foul vaginal discharge	Internal cervical os open or closed, abdominal tenderness, peritoneal signs, CMT, foul cervical discharge	Serum β-hCG (declining or plateau, if there is a previous level for comparison), CBC, Blood and cervical cultures, EVUS (thickened, irregular endometrium >5 mm double stripe), Type and Rh, Urinalysis
Threatened abortion	Vaginal bleeding or spotting and/or abdominal pain	Internal cervical os closed, pelvic and abdominal examination benign or mild-moderately tender	Serum β-hCG, CBC, EVUS (embryo with cardiac activity or empty gestational sac (5–6.5 weeks), empty uterus (3–5 weeks), or subchorionic hemorrhage with any of the above), Type and Rh, Urinalysis

CBC: complete blood count; CMT: cervical motion tenderness; CRL: crown-rump length; EGA: estimated gestational age; EVUS: endovaginal ultrasonography; hCG: human chorionic gonadotropin; POC: products of conception; TSH: thyroid-stimulating hormone.

Table 38.3 Differential diagnosis of non-pregnant vaginal bleeding

Diagnosis	Symptoms	Signs	Work-up
Abnormal uterine bleeding due to exogenous gonadal steroids (estrogens, progestins, and/or androgens, and combined estrogen/progestin preparations for OCP and HRT)	Breakthrough bleeding with first three cycles of using OCP preparations. HRT preparations: (a) Cyclic progestin component – predictable and cyclic withdrawal bleeding starting at end of progestin phase. (b) Continuous progestin regimens – bleeding in first 3 months, then eventual amenorrhea. (c) Progestin-only contraceptives – irregular bleeding. Post-coital emergency contraception: irregular bleeding or delayed menses. Menorrhagia Metrorrhagia Oligomenorrhea	Benign examination, though orthostatic hypotension or symptomatic anemia may result if bleeding is prolonged or heavy	Urine qualitative pregnancy test, CBC (if clinically indicated)

(*continued*)

Table 38.3 Differential diagnosis of non-pregnant vaginal bleeding (*cont*)

Diagnosis	Symptoms	Signs	Work-up
Abnormal uterine bleeding due to IUD	Menorrhagia Metrorrhagia Oligomenorrhea (if progestin-impregnated IUD)	Benign examination, though orthostatic hypotension or symptomatic anemia may result if bleeding is prolonged or heavy	Urine qualitative pregnancy test, CBC (if clinically indicated)
Dysfunctional uterine bleeding (anovulatory)	Irregular vaginal bleeding in timing and in quantity, including oligomenorrhea or amenorrhea (no menses for 6 months), metro-rhagia, history of psychologic stress, weight gain, weight loss	Acne, obesity, hirsuitism	Urine qualitative pregnancy test, CBC, Estrogen level, 17-OH progesterone level, Free testosterone level, Prolactin level, TSH
Dysfunctional uterine bleeding (ovulatory)	Cyclic and predictable heavy menstrual bleeding (menorrhagia), fatigue	Anemia	Urine qualitative pregnancy test, CBC
Endometrial hyperplasia and carcinoma of the vulva, vagina, cervix, and endometrium	Menorrhagia Metrorrhagia Oligomenorrhea Constitutional symptoms (if carcinoma is etiology)	Benign examination or mild pelvic tenderness	Urine qualitative pregnancy test, CBC (if clinically indicated), EVUS, Endometrial sampling
Uterine leiomyoma	Menorrhagia Metrorrhagia	Benign examination or mild pelvic tenderness, orthostatic hypo-tension or symptomatic anemia if bleeding excessive or prolonged	Urine qualitative pregnancy test, CBC (if clinically indicated), EVUS
Vaginal trauma	Vaginal bleeding, pain, spotting, discharge	Vaginal laceration or foreign body	Urine qualitative pregnancy test, CBC (if clinically indicated)
Vaginitis/cervicitis	Vaginal bleeding or spotting, especially after intercourse, insertion of diaphragm, or pelvic examination, discharge	Cervical or vaginal wall friability	Urine qualitative pregnancy test, Cervical cultures, Wet mount

CBC: complete blood count; EVUS: endovaginal ultrasonography; HRT: hormone replacement therapy. IUD: intrauterine contraceptive device; OCP: oral contraceptive pills; TSH: thyroid-stimulating hormone.

Diagnostic testing

Laboratory studies

Urine pregnancy test

A urine qualitative pregnancy test is absolutely necessary in the work-up of *any* woman of reproductive age with abnormal bleeding. The sensitivity for diagnosing pregnancy is 99.4%, so it is an extremely useful test for ruling-out pregnancy by approximately the same date that a woman misses her period, or possibly a few days before, when the serum β-hCG is >25 mIU/ml. False negative tests occur when the serum β-hCG is between 10 and 50 mIU/ml, and also when the urine is dilute (specific gravity <1.015). This may be overcome by using 20 drops of urine instead of the usual 5 drops to super-concentrate the hormone on the test diaphragm. The urine pregnancy test establishes the patient as pregnant, and should be ordered for all patients with vaginal bleeding, regardless of the patient's menstrual history.

Urinalysis

A urinalysis with urine culture should be ordered in all pregnant patients with vaginal bleeding to diagnose UTI, regardless of symptoms. Generally, a catheterized specimen is best in this setting, given the difficulty in obtaining a true "clean catch" in a woman with vaginal bleeding. It has been well-described that UTIs are an etiologic risk factor for miscarriage. Also, asymptomatic bacturia and pyuria are relatively common in pregnancy, occurring in 2–11% of pregnant women. Up to one-fourth of these asymptomatic women will go on to develop upper-tract infections. Thus, UTIs in pregnant patients should be looked for and treated to potentially prevent miscarriage.

Rh type

Routine screening for Rhesus (Rh) status in the pregnant vaginal bleeding patient is controversial. It has been well-established that completed abortion, ectopic pregnancy, antepartum hemorrhage and trauma are associated with possible fetomaternal transfusion, and thus potential for Rh isoimmunization if the mother is Rh-negative and the fetus is Rh-positive. Literature support for the same concept in threatened abortion is equivocal. However, ED patients may not have access to or seek follow-up if they complete their miscarriage, and it would be unfortunate if such a patient became Rh-sensitized without prophylaxis. It is thus standard of care to give Rh immune prophylaxis to Rh-negative, pregnant women with vaginal bleeding. If the gestational age is <12 weeks, a dose of 50 mcg Rhogam intramuscularly is sufficient. However, as pregnancy dating is difficult and often inaccurate, it is recommended that all unsensitized Rh-negative women with vaginal bleeding receive 300 mcg of Rh immune globulin in the first or second trimester. This should be given before the patient leaves the ED, but protection occurs if it is administered within 72 hours of bleeding. It is not necessary to repeat the dosage at subsequent ED or clinic visits for continued or repeat bleeding before 20 weeks gestation. A subsequent 300 mcg dose should be administered in the third trimester or prior to delivery.

Complete blood count

A complete blood count (CBC) is routinely obtained in bleeding patients in order to estimate how much they have bled prior to arrival in the ED. A baseline hematocrit (HCT) is also useful for comparison if serial HCTs are obtained during the patient's course due to changes in hemodynamic status.

Serum quantitative beta-human chorionic gonadotropin

The serum quantitative β-hCG is a measure of trophoblastic tissue activity, a marker for the volume of living trophoblastic tissue. It is a function of renal clearance. Both ectopic and intrauterine pregnancies (IUPs) produce β-hCG, though they usually differ in the rate at which the quantitative β-hCG level increases. Patients with ectopic pregnancy tend to have a lower quantitative β-hCG than those with viable IUPs given the same gestational age. Abnormal IUPs may also have lower β-hCGs than normal IUPs. Due to the large range of acceptable β-hCG levels for each stage of embryonic development, a single value of β-hCG is not useful for differentiating between normal IUP, abnormal IUP, and ectopic pregnancy. Variation in the expected rate of rise of the β-hCG level can be helpful. For levels <10,000 mIU/ml, the β-hCG normally doubles in 1.9 ± 0.5 days. Also, an increase of ≥ 66% over 48 hours is seen in 85% of normal IUPs. An abnormal increase is thus <66% over 48 hours, which is 75% sensitive and 93% specific for an abnormal gestation of some variety. Additionally, 85% of ectopic pregnancies and 15% of normal IUPs have an abnormal rate of rise of β-hCG. Declining β-hCG levels indicate fetal non-viability, either ectopic or intrauterine. The rate of fall of the β-hCG has been found to differ significantly between these two entities. The half-life of the β-hCG is >7 days in ectopic pregnancy, whereas it is <1.4 days in failing IUPs. A falling β-hCG does not exclude the possibility of tubal rupture, and there is no minimum value of β-hCG that precludes rupture.

Radiologic studies

Ultrasound

The value of pelvic endovaginal ultrasonography (EVUS) in the evaluation of a pregnant vaginal bleeding patient is principally to confirm the presence of an IUP, which ostensibly excludes the diagnosis of ectopic pregnancy. An understanding of what is necessary to make the sonographic diagnosis of an IUP is important for the clinician to optimally use the information. The hormones of pregnancy cause an early uterine decidual reaction that may be seen soon after a missed menses by ultrasound. This is nonspecific and occurs with both IUPs and ectopic pregnancies, however. The earliest sonographic landmark consistent with an IUP is the gestational sac. With endovaginal ultrasound, this can be visualized as early as 4.5 weeks after the LMP, reliably by 5 weeks. The gestational sac lies eccentrically within the decidua of the endometrium, and is seen to have two distinct layers sonographically: the decidua capsularis and decidua parietalis. These two layers give a sonographic appearance of two rings, called the "double ring sign," that is diagnostic of an intrauterine gestational sac. The yolk sac seen within the gestational sac is the next sonographic landmark of the developing pregnancy, seen reliably by the end of the 5th week (Figure 38.2). The embryo and cardiac activity are seen concurrently and reliably adjacent to the yolk sac by 6.5 weeks gestation using endovaginal ultrasound. Table 38.4 lists the sonographic findings of early pregnancy development with their corresponding gestational ages and discriminatory levels of β-hCG.

The sonographic finding that is most reassuring for a favorable prognosis is the presence of embryonic cardiac activity. For women under 35 years of age at 8 weeks EGA, the sonographic presence of cardiac activity suggests a rate of spontaneous abortion of only 3–5% overall. This increases to about 8% for women over 35 years of age. Sonographic findings that foreshadow a poor outcome include a slow embryonic heart rate (<90 bpm), small gestational sac for the size of the embryo, and large yolk sac (>6 mm).

Differentiation between complete and incomplete abortion can be challenging if the cervical os is closed, bleeding is not heavy, and the patient is not appreciably tender on examination. In this setting, ultrasound is a reliable and useful adjunct to making the diagnosis of completed abortion based on the presence of an empty uterus.

Specific findings suggestive or diagnostic of ectopic pregnancy will be identified by ultrasound in up to 79% of ED cases (Figure 38.3). Intrauterine findings suggestive of ectopic pregnancy include the intrauterine decidual reaction. This can be problematic because 10–20% of the time it can form a cystic shape resembling a sac. This is referred to as a "pseudogestational sac," which is thought to represent blood surrounded by decidual cast. The finding of an empty uterus in a pregnant woman is present in up to 20% of cases of ectopic pregnancy. Extrauterine findings on EVUS may also be consistent with ectopic pregnancy; the most common finding is a complex adnexal mass, seen in 60–90% of cases. Other findings seen include free fluid in the cul-de-sac (20–40%) and an ectopic embryo (25–35%).

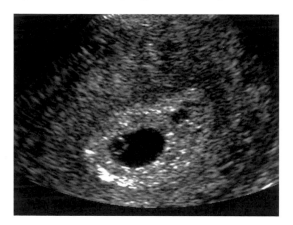

Figure 38.2
Normal intrauterine pregnancy. Sagittal endovaginal US of normal first trimester pregnancy. Note echogenic gestational sac within the uterus containing a yolk sac.

Table 38.4 Sonographic embryology in early pregancy

Sonographic landmarks of early pregnancy	EGA (weeks)	Serum quantitative beta-hCG (mIU/ml)
Gestational sac	4.5	>1500
Yolk sac	5.5	1000–7500
Embryo with cardiac activity	6.5	7000–23,000

EGA: estimated gestational age; hCG: human chorionic gonadotropin.

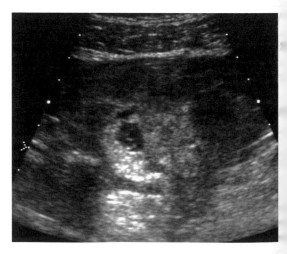

Figure 38.3
Ecotopic pregnancy. Transverse scan of right adnexa demonstrating echogenic gestational sac containing a yolk sac within an ectopic pregnancy. *Courtesy*: R Brooke Jeffrey, MD.

A completely normal pelvic ultrasound in seen in approximately 20% of all patients with proven ectopic pregnancies.

When EVUS is neither diagnostic of an IUP nor suggestive of an ectopic pregnancy, it is characterized as indeterminate. Interpretation of this result requires consideration of the clinical context. Depending on their clinical status and β-hCG level, these patients will need to be followed closely by a gynecologist in order to have their β-hCG level re-checked in 48 hours along with a reassessment of their clinical status.

In the non-pregnant woman with vaginal bleeding, an EVUS is a useful adjunct to the physical examination, particularly if an adequate pelvic examination cannot be performed or the patient has an abnormal pelvic examination (i.e., adnexal mass, enlarged uterus).

In post-menopausal women who are not on HRT with AUB, EVUS can be utilized to measure the endometrial thickness. An endometrial stripe thickness of <4 mm can reliably exclude endometrial neoplasm as an etiology of the bleeding, which obviates the need for endometrial biopsy.

General treatment principles

As with all ED patients, treatment begins with a general assessment of the patient's hemodynamic status. Patients with vaginal bleeding present with varying clinical states, which may change during their evaluation period in the ED. While any such patient may be or become hemodynamically compromised, pregnant vaginal bleeding patients have the greatest potential for rapid change in volume status. Hence, frequent reassessment of these patients is prudent.

Volume repletion

Not all patients with vaginal bleeding require intravenous (IV) access or IV fluid replacement. However, most first trimester pregnant vaginal bleeding patients will undergo a work-up for ectopic pregnancy, a potentially life-threatening condition due to exsanguination. Therefore, such patients should have an IV placed upon initial assessment. The degree of volume replacement required will vary depending on the patient's clinical status. Crystalloids (normal saline) are appropriate as initial resuscitation fluids, adding packed red blood cell transfusion if the patient's clinical status deteriorates despite aggressive

volume replacement. As most of these patients are young and otherwise healthy, they should be able to tolerate significant anemia (e.g., down to a HCT of 20%) before blood transfusion is needed. For women with history or risk factors for cardiac ischemia, significant anemia is akin to a cardiac stress test and may not be well-tolerated. Thus a different standard for transfusion is prudent in such patients.

Patients diagnosed with or suspected of having septic abortion should receive broad spectrum IV antibiotics as soon as possible.

Ectopic pregnancy

A reasonably thorough understanding of the non-surgical management options for patients diagnosed with ectopic pregnancy in the ED is important for emergency physicians, because these options involve discharging a patient from the ED with a potentially life-threatening surgical emergency. Medical management is with methotrexate, a folic acid antagonist that prevents the synthesis of amino acids, ribonucleic acid (RNA), and deoxyribonucleic acid (DNA), thereby eradicating rapidly developing trophoblastic tissue. The criteria for methotrexate therapy are:

- Hemodynamic stability
- EVUS showing an unruptured ectopic pregnancy with greatest diameter <4 cm (<3.5 cm if cardiac activity present)
- No active bleeding or free fluid on ultrasound
- Stable or rising β-hCG titer <5000 mIU/ml
- β-hCG increasing after curettage
- Desired future fertility
- Patient does not desire surgical therapy
- Patient willingness and ability to return for weekly follow-up
- Some cases of cervical and cornual pregnancy.

The contraindications to methotrexate therapy are hepatic or renal dysfunction, active peptic ulcer disease, or blood dyscrasias. The protocol for management with methotrexate involves a single intramuscular (IM) injection of 50 mcg/m² body surface area, with close GYN follow-up and serial β-hCG levels. The success rate for this protocol is 85–100% for resolving the ectopic pregnancy without surgical intervention. However, it takes between 20 and 44 days for the β-hCG levels to become undetectable. The main complication of methotrexate therapy is tubal rupture, which occurs in about 4% of cases. Methotrexate has a variety of side effects, the most common of which is increased abdominal pain in up to 60% of patients. This is problematic, as this symptom is indistinguishable from tubal rupture if severe in nature. Patients who have been treated for ectopic pregnancy with methotrexate and complain of increasing abdominal pain should have an immediate ultrasound and GYN consultation to evaluate for this potentially serious complication. Other side effects are nausea, vomiting, and diarrhea, which occur in 5–20% of cases.

Surgical management of ectopic pregnancy is reserved for patients who do not fall into the medical management group described above. This is generally done either by tube-sparing laparoscopic salpingotomy, salpingectomy, or through open laparotomy, which may be required for patients in extremis or with significant hemoperitoneum.

Abnormal uterine bleeding

Gonadal steroids are the first-line therapeutic option for vaginal bleeding in the non-pregnant patient. Immediate therapy for severe symptomatic bleeding for patients hemodynamically compromised requiring hospital admission may consist of high dose conjugated estrogens. Starting doses of 25 mg IV every 4 hours for up to 48 hours usually results in the desired response within the first 5 hours. For more stable patients, oral treatment with medroxyprogesterone 60–120 mg on day one followed by 20 mg daily for 10 days is effective in halting AUB. Another alternative, especially for pre-menopausal patients, is combined estrogen and progestin oral contraceptive pills (OCP). A monophasic pill preparation (constant dosage throughout the pill-pack month) with at least 35 mcg of ethinyl estradiol is utilized in the following manner: 3 pills/day for 3 days, then 2 pills/day for 2 days, then 1 pill/ day and continue until the package is finished. This regimen is termed the "OCP taper." Women should skip the placebo pills in the first pack and start the next pack of 1 pill/day to avoid withdrawal bleeding so soon after the previous bleeding episode. Ideally, estrogen therapy should not be initiated on patients until the diagnosis of endometrial carcinoma has been excluded. A general guideline is that for women over the age of 40, endometrial sampling should be obtained either prior to or within a week of initiating hormone therapy. Additionally, OCPs and estrogens are in general not recommended for women who have hypertension or smoke, so their use in this setting should only be with caution and in consultation with the patient's gynecologist.

Disposition

First-trimester vaginal bleeding

Patients for whom the diagnosis of ectopic pregnancy is made conclusively by EVUS require immediate GYN consultation, because they must initiate either surgical or medical management. This depends on the patient's hemodynamic stability, and if she meets criteria for methotrexate usage.

Patients with first-trimester bleeding, a β-hCG below 1500 mIU/ml, and an indeterminate EVUS may be sent home from the ED with a diagnosis of "possible ectopic pregnancy" if they remain hemodynamically stable. These patients require close follow-up and a repeat β-hCG measurement in 48 hours by their OB/GYN physician. It is appropriate for these follow-up arrangements to be made prior to ED disposition in order to ensure compliance with the recommendation. When discharging patients from the ED, it is essential that they comprehend the potentially life-threatening nature of the condition and understand specific instructions for when to return to the ED in advance of their scheduled follow-up. These indications include dizziness or syncope, increased abdominal pain or heavy vaginal bleeding greater than one pad per hour, and fever. They should also be advised to remain at pelvic rest (nothing inside the vagina). There is no evidence that bed rest is necessary.

Patients diagnosed with inevitable or septic abortion require immediate GYN consultation for surgical intervention.

Patients with threatened and completed abortion do not require GYN consultation in the ED. In these patients for whom ectopic pregnancy has been excluded, follow-up with their OB/GYN in 1–2 weeks is appropriate, with careful discharge instructions recommending return precautions described above.

Patients with incomplete and missed abortions are managed differently in different practice environments, and in some cases, depending on patient preference. Some gynecologists and patients prefer expectant management with arranged follow-up in 1–2 weeks for possible elective dilation and curettage (D&C), while others prefer to perform semi-urgent D&C at the time of initial diagnosis. The literature does not favor either management style, so patient and physician preferences should be taken into account.

It is important to discuss the common nature of spontaneous miscarriage with the patient, emphasizing to the patient (and her partner, if appropriate) that she did nothing to precipitate the situation. Many patients will have a significant emotional response to having a miscarriage, and a few minutes of reassurance and correct information from a caring provider can frame the situation in a way that facilitates emotional healing. Additionally, keep in mind that pregnant women are at increased risk for being victims of intimate partner violence.

Non-pregnant abnormal uterine bleeding

Generally patients with AUB do not require urgent GYN consultation unless they require admission to the hospital due to severe anemia or acute hemorrhage. Women over 40 years of age for whom hormone therapy is indicated should have endometrial sampling either prior to or within 1 week of hormone initiation. Since this procedure generally falls outside of the scope of emergency physician practice, specific follow-up should be arranged from the ED. Patients under 40 years of age may begin outpatient management as discussed above, and have follow-up arranged for 1–2 weeks with a gynecologist. Specific ED return precautions include symptoms of severe anemia (excessive fatigue, orthostasis, syncope) or increased bleeding. Patients should contact and follow-up with their gynecologist or primary care provider if the bleeding does not improve within 3–5 days of initiation of therapy.

Pearls, pitfalls, and myths

- Obtain a pregnancy test on *every* woman of childbearing age with abdominal and/or pelvic complaints. A negative history for pregnancy and/or sexual activity is unreliable, and the differential diagnosis is very different whether the patient is or is not pregnant.
- Every patient with first-trimester bleeding without a documented IUP must have ectopic pregnancy ruled-out. This should include a quantitative β-hCG and EVUS in the ED, and appropriate follow-up for those with indeterminate results. There is no minimum β-hCG level below which one should no

longer consider ectopic pregnancy or not obtain an ultrasound. Keep in mind that over 80% of patients with ectopic pregnancy have a β-hCG <1000 mIU/ml, and 79% of ED patients with first-trimester bleeding will be diagnosed in the ED by EVUS.
- Patients diagnosed with ectopic pregnancy by EVUS may be candidates for methotrexate treatment if they meet strict criteria and do not have contraindications. However, the decision to treat the patient with methotrexate should be made by the consulting gynecologist.
- Patients treated with methotrexate must be able to return to the ED immediately should they experience increased abdominal pain, because methotrexate does not alter the 4% risk for rupture of the ectopic pregnancy in the short term (approximately 1 week). When these patients return to the ED with increased abdominal or pelvic pain, a EVUS and gynecology consultation should be obtained immediately to rule-out a ruptured ectopic.
- Patients on ovulation-induction agents are at significantly increased risk for heterotopic pregnancy, up to 1:34 pregnancies. Thus it is essential to specifically ask the patient if she has taken these medications.
- Patients diagnosed with intrauterine fetal demise do not require an emergent D&C. It is appropriate to manage these patients expectantly, if desired by the patient and the consulting gynecologist.
- Patients with possible septic abortion should receive prompt IV broad-spectrum antibiotics, even before the confirmatory EVUS is obtained or specialist consultation arrives, as these infections may progress very rapidly.

References

1. Abbott J, Emmans LS, Lowenstein SR. Ectopic pregnancy: ten common pitfalls in diagnosis. *Am J Emerg Med* 1990;8: 515–522.
2. Bradford JC, Kyriakedes CG. Vaginal bleeding. In: Rosen, et al. (eds). *Rosen's Emergency Medicine.* Mosby publishers, 2001.
3. Brennan DF. Ectopic pregnancy – Part I: Clinical and laboratory diagnosis. *Acad EM* 1995;2(12):1081–1089.

4. Brennan DF. Ectopic pregancy – Part II: Diagnostic procedures and imaging. *Acad EM* 1995;2(12):1090–1097.

5. Brenner PF. Differential diagnosis of abnormal uterine bleeding. *Am J Obstet Gynecol* 1996;175:766–769.

6. Brewster GS, Herbert ME, Hoffman JR. Medical myth: analgesia should not be given to patients with an acute abdomen because it obscures the diagnosis. *Western J Med* 2000;172:209–210.

7. Cartwright PS. Diagnosis of ectopic pregnancy. *Obstet Gyn Clin North Am* 1991;18:19–37.

8. Close R, Sachs C, Dyne P. Reliability of bimanual pelvic examinations performed in emergency departments. *Western J Med* 2001;175:240–244.

9. Current trends ectopic pregnancy – United States, 1990–1992. *Morb Mort Week Rep* 1995;44:46–48.

10. Dart RG, Kaplan B, Cox C. Transvaginal ultrasound in patients with low beta-human chorionic gonadotropin values: How often is the study diagnostic? *Ann Emerg Med* 1997;30:135–140.

11. Hopkins C, Krisanda T. Vaginal bleeding. In: Hamilton, et al. (eds). *Emergency Medicine: An Approach to Clinical Problem-Solving*, 2nd ed., WB Saunders publishers, 2002.

12. Munro MG. Abnormal uterine bleeding in the reproductive years: Part 1, pathogeneis and clinical investigation. *J Am Assoc Gyn Lap* 1999;6(4):393–416.

13. Newton E, Henderson S. Vaginal bleeding in early pregnancy. In: Harwood Nuss, et al. (eds). *The Clinical Practice of Emergency Medicine*, 5th ed., Lippincott, Williams and Wilkins, 2001.

14. Pearlman MD, Tintinalli JE (eds). *Emergency Care of the Woman*. New York: McGraw-Hill, 1999.

15. Pearlman MD, Tintinalli JE, Dyne PL (eds). *Obstetric and Gynecologic Emergencies*. New York: McGraw-Hill, 2003.

16. Speroff L, Glass RH, Kase NG. *Clinical Gynecologic Endocrinology and Infertility*, 6th ed., Maryland: Lippincott, Williams and Wilkins, 1999.

17. Stovall TG, Ling FW. Ectopic pregnancy: Diagnostic and therapeutic algorithms minimizing surgical intervention. *J Reprod. Med* 1993;38:807–812.

39 Vomiting

Jennifer A. Oman, MD

Scope of the problem

Vomiting is a common presenting complaint to the emergency department (ED), accounting for nearly 2 million annual visits. It has no age or gender predilection, and has many etiologies. The most common causes of vomiting are acute gastroenteritis, febrile systemic illness, and drug-related effects. The emergency physician's main responsibility is differentiating the emergent and life-threatening causes of vomiting from those caused by more benign entities. The remainder of ED management is targeted toward symptom alleviation and rehydration.

Pathophysiology

Vomiting is induced by physical stimulation of the back of the throat (gag reflex), mucosal irritation of the upper digestive tract, stimulation of the vomiting center in the medulla oblongata, stimulation by biochemical emetic stimuli on the chemoreceptor trigger zone in the area postrema, or by severe emotion. Nausea frequently precedes vomiting and is marked by reduced gastric tone and peristalsis. Regurgitation, by contrast, is the passive retrograde movement of esophageal contents into the mouth, as in gastroesophageal reflux.

True vomiting refers to the rapid ejection of gastric contents. The abdominal muscles rapidly contract, while the cardia of the stomach, esophagus, and throat remain open with the glottis closed. Copious salivation usually precedes vomiting, and serves to lubricate the digestive tract and dilute the gastric acid. Repeated contractions of the abdominal muscles against a relaxed stomach produce retching. The repetitive abdominal contractions build up a pressure gradient in the stomach prior to vomiting. This allows gastric contents to move to the upper portion of the stomach. Retching may also occur without expulsion of gastric contents, and is referred to as "dry heaves."

Repeated vomiting can lead to hypovolemia, metabolic alkalosis, and hypokalemia. A forceful episode of vomiting or retching can lead to gastrointestinal (GI) bleeding (Mallory–Weiss tear) or esophageal perforation (Boerhaave's syndrome).

History

What did you vomit (food, blood, mucus)?

The composition of the vomitus is important for determining both the etiology of vomiting and treatment. If the vomitus is coffee-ground material, this most often represents blood that has been exposed to the stomach's acidic environment. If the blood is bright red, an esophageal or vascular source of bleeding is likely. It is important to determine the volume of blood and whether it occurred initially with vomiting or after several episodes of vomiting. Mallory–Weiss tears generally occur following several episodes of forceful vomiting, and can also be a source for blood in the vomitus. Vomitus containing undigested food may be seen with gastric outlet obstruction, gastric retention, and psychogenic vomiting. Vomitus with mucous must be differentiated from coughing or spitting up phlegm. Other potential contents of vomitus include bile and stool, both of which portend a serious etiology.

Was there anything that preceded or is associated with the vomiting (coughing, abdominal pain)?

Vomiting does not mean the same thing to all people. Frequently, patients will cough, which evokes a gag reflex causing them to "vomit." Vomiting as a consequence of severe coughing is known as post-tussive emesis. Abdominal pain may follow vomiting; this may be related to forceful abdominal muscle contraction. Vomiting which follows the development of abdominal pain is nonspecific; however, pain relieved by vomiting may suggest gastric outlet obstruction. A report of vomiting prior to chest pain is an ominous sign, and is likely due to a non-GI cause.

How many times did you vomit?

Although the exact answer is not necessary, this provides an indication of whether the vomiting occurred only once or several times. If the patient has been vomiting several times, it may increase the likelihood of dehydration or underlying pathology (e.g., Mallory–Weiss tear), in addition to suggesting the cause.

When did the vomiting occur?

Vomiting in the morning is more common during pregnancy and uremia. Vomiting associated with increased intracranial pressure may be more frequent when intracranial pressure is higher, such as in the morning or with bending movements. Vomiting less than 1 hour after eating may be related to gastroparesis or gastric outlet obstruction.

Have you been able to tolerate liquids or fluids between the vomiting episodes?

This question helps to assess the patient's hydration status.

Associated symptoms

Gastrointestinal

Ask about abdominal pain, diarrhea, constipation, or inability to pass gas. If constipation or the inability to pass gas accompanies vomiting in a patient with prior surgeries, bowel obstruction must be considered. Vomiting preceded by abdominal pain has a broad differential. Abdominal pain temporarily relieved by vomiting suggests delayed gastric emptying, as with gastroparesis from diabetes or gastric outlet obstruction. When vomiting is associated with diarrhea, a GI infectious etiology is likely responsible.

Neurologic

Ask about headache, dizziness, vertigo, weakness, numbness or tingling of the extremities. Serious causes of vomiting include subarachnoid hemorrhage and increased intracranial pressure from obstruction, tumor, or infection. Any cause of increased intracranial pressure can cause vomiting with or without preceding nausea by direct interaction on vomiting centers in the area postrema. Causes of vertigo, such as labyrinthitis and Ménière's disease, produce vomiting by stimulation of the vestibular nuclei and subsequent stimulation of brainstem nuclei. Vomiting is a common symptom of migraine headache. A sudden-onset severe or atypical headache may represent a subarachnoid hemorrhage. Meningitis may also present as headache and fever associated with vomiting.

Genitourinary (in females)

Ask about dysuria, back pain, vaginal discharge, vaginal bleeding, lower abdominal cramping, sexual history, sexually transmitted illness (STI) history, and pregnancy. Vomiting is associated with pyelonephritis, pelvic inflammatory disease, tubo-ovarian abscess, ovarian torsion, ectopic pregnancy and normal first-trimester pregnancy.

Genitourinary (in males)

Ask about testicular or groin pain. Testicular torsion or an incarcerated inguinal hernia can present with vomiting and groin or testicular pain.

Cardiopulmonary

Ask about chest pain, cough and fever. Vomiting can be associated with myocardial infarction. Remember not all vomiting is true vomiting; the patient may have phlegm production from pneumonia.

Other

Ask about other symptoms. These include recent chemotherapy if the patient has cancer, ingestions if the patient is depressed or suicidal, other family members who may be vomiting if the illness is acute, recent trauma to the abdomen or head, what the patient ate (home canned goods, raw fish, food at a picnic), and atypical hobbies (foraging for wild mushrooms).

Past medical

The patient's medical history is an important adjunct to determining the source of vomiting. Common conditions associated with vomiting include hypertension, liver disease, cholelithiasis, excessive alcohol use, previous surgeries, recent head or abdominal trauma, thyroid disorders, renal insufficiency or failure, chemotherapy, diabetes, current pregnancy, cardiac disease, or peripheral vascular disease. A thorough medication list of all current and recent previous medications, including all over-the-counter, herbal, and "natural" medicines must be obtained.

Physical examination

A thorough physical examination must be performed, as several etiologies of vomiting are not isolated to one anatomic system. The current and past medical history, plus associated symptoms will help guide which portions of the examination need increased attention.

General appearance

The patient's general appearance can range from normal to severe distress from discomfort, continued vomiting, dehydration, or the underlying cause of vomiting.

Vital signs

Special attention to the patient's pulse and blood pressure are essential in determining the patient's hydration status. However, the absence of tachycardia does not exclude significant dehydration or disease. The blood pressure is especially concerning if it is abnormally low or high. Changes in orthostatic blood pressure are mostly of historical significance and do not aid in determining the patient's volume status. If the patient becomes dizzy or lightheaded with standing, this may indicate significant fluid loss. If the patient is pregnant, fetal heart tones should be obtained if possible.

The presence of a fever may indicate an infectious or inflammatory response, or a toxic ingestion, and requires prompt evaluation.

Head, eyes, ears, nose, and throat

Head

Examine the head for hematomas and bruising.

Eyes

Visual acuity should be determined for patients with vomiting and visual complaints to screen for conditions such as acute angle closure glaucoma. A close examination of the pupils should be performed to look for symmetry and normal reactivity. A funduscopic examination is necessary to look for papilledema, which may indicate a brain tumor. Visual fields should also be tested to determine the presence of a deficit. Extraocular movements should be evaluated and any nystagmus noted.

Nose

The nose should be inspected for evidence of bleeding if the patient is complaining of vomiting blood.

Mouth

Examine the mucus membranes for dryness and evidence of bleeding.

Abdomen

The abdominal examination will often be the most important examination; a complete examination must be performed on every vomiting patient.

On inspection of the abdomen, the presence of previous surgical scars should be noted and inquired about to determine their etiology. The abdomen should be observed for peristaltic waves when an obstruction is suspected. Abdominal distention should be noted and may be due to excess fluid or air within the peritoneal cavity.

Bowel sounds should be assessed. The presence of high-pitched, rushing bowel sounds (borborygmi) may indicate an obstruction. Normal or absent bowel sounds are unhelpful in elucidating the etiology of vomiting.

Localized tenderness is helpful and may guide therapy and diagnostic studies. The abdominal examination may be difficult to interpret if the patient has had several episodes of emesis. Serial examinations or return for re-evaluation may be necessary to determine the etiology of vomiting.

Genital

Tenderness of the lower abdominal area of female patients mandates a pelvic examination to identify cervical motion tenderness, adnexal masses, pus from the cervical os, and vaginal bleeding. Male patients with persistent vomiting require a testicular examination to palpate for masses or tenderness, and to assure normal lie and size.

Rectal

A digital rectal examination should be performed on patients to look for the presence of stool, bleeding, or mass.

Neurologic

A complete neurologic examination, including assessment of mental status, motor strength, sensation, cranial nerves, cerebellar function, and gait should be performed on all patients with headache associated with vomiting.

Extremity

Distal pulse presence, amplitude, and symmetry should be noted. Any edema of the lower extremities should be noted and recorded.

Skin

Assess the patient's skin turgor when evaluating volume status, and note jaundice, paleness, temperature, or flushing.

Differential diagnosis

Table 39.1 Differential diagnosis for vomiting

Diagnosis	Symptoms	Signs	Work-up
Acetaminophen toxicity	Anorexia, nausea, vomiting, and malaise. Psychiatric history not always apparent.	May have normal physical exam or RUQ pain.	Serum acetaminophen level at 4 hours after ingestion. Poison control consultation.
Acute appendicitis	Epigastric or periumbilical pain migrates to RLQ over 8–12 hours (50%). Later presentations associated with higher perforation rates. Pain, low-grade fever (15%), and anorexia (80%) common, vomiting less common (50–70%).	Mean temperature 38°C (100.5°F). Higher temperature associated with perforation. RLQ tenderness (90–95%) with rebound (40–70%) in majority of cases. Rectal tenderness in up to 30%.	WBC usually elevated or may show left shift. Urine may show sterile pyuria. CRP sensitive, but accuracy varies. CT is sensitive and specific. US may have a role in women or children with RLQ pain.
Acute gastroenteritis	Nausea and vomiting usually begin before pain. Pain usually poorly localized. Diarrhea is a key element in diagnosis, usually large volume, watery.	Abdominal examination usually nonspecific without peritoneal signs. Watery or no stool noted on rectal examination. Fever is usually present.	Usually symptomatic care with antiemetics and volume repletion. Key is not assuming this diagnosis and missing more serious disease.
Acute pancreatitis	Mid-epigastric or LUQ pain that is constant, boring and often radiates to the back, flanks, chest, or lower abdomen. Usually severe but may be mild. Supine position exacerbates pain. Nausea and vomiting are common.	Patient usually in moderate distress. Low-grade fevers and tachycardia are frequently present. Patients may present in hypovolemic shock. Abdominal examination is notable for epigastric tenderness. Cullen's sign, a bluish discoloration around the umbilicus, and Grey-Turner's sign, a bluish discoloration of the flanks are late signs of hemorrhagic pancreatitis.	Serum lipase is the best test used to diagnose pancreatitis. Serum amylase is neither sensitive nor specific, but more readily available.
Aspirin intoxication	Altered mental status, headache, tinnitus, abdominal pain, nausea and vomiting.	Tachypnea, abdominal tenderness.	Chemistry panel, LFTs, CBC, coagulation profile. Aspirin and acetaminophen levels should be sent.
Biliary tract disease	Crampy RUQ pain radiates to right subscapular area. Prior history of pain is common.	Temperature normal in biliary colic, RUQ tenderness.	US shows anatomy, stones, or duct dilatation. Hepatobillary scintigraphy demonstrates gallbladder function.
Boerhaave's syndrome	Acute, severe, unrelenting, and diffuse pain in the chest, neck and abdomen with radiation to the back and shoulders. Back pain may be the predominant symptom. Pain is often exacerbated by swallowing after 6–12 hours.	Patients appear ill. Tachycardia and tachypnea, abdominal rigidity with hypotension and fever often occur early. Cervical subcutaneous emphysema or a Hamman's crunch (air in the mediastinum being moved by the beating heart) can sometimes be auscultated.	Initiated based on clinical suspicion of the diagnosis. CXR and water-soluble contrast esophagography most often make the diagnosis. Endoscopy and CT of the chest are useful adjuncts. Thoracentesis may identify GI contents, but not recommended.

(continued)

Table 39.1 Differential diagnosis for vomiting (*cont*)

Diagnosis	Symptoms	Signs	Work-up
Bowel obstruction	Clinical presentation depends on the site of obstruction. Most patients have abdominal pain. The pain is generally described as crampy, intermittent and usually referred to the periumbilical area. Pain may be episodic, usually lasting a few minutes at a time. Bilious vomiting is often present if the obstruction is proximal. Inability to have a bowel movement or pass flatus is common.	Abdominal tenderness may be minimal and diffuse or localized and severe. Abdomen may be tympanitic to percussion with active, high pitched bowel sounds with occasional "rushes" on auscultation.	Acute abdominal series usually yields the diagnosis. If AAS is unclear, a CT may be ordered. Laboratory work includes a CBC and electrolytes but these are not sensitive nor specific for the diagnosis.
Cholecystitis	RUQ pain that initially is persistent, not colicky, beyond 6 hours. Associated nausea, vomiting, and anorexia. History of fever and/or chills is not uncommon. Patients may have either a history of similar attacks or documented gallstones.	Moderate to severe distress with signs of systemic toxicity including tachycardia and fever. The abdomen is tender in the RUQ. Generalized peritonitis is rare. Murphy's sign (worsened pain or inspiratory arrest resulting from deep, subcostal palpation on inspiration) is generally present.	WBC count, serum bilirubin, alkaline phosphatase and aminotransferase levels are often normal. Serum amylase and lipase to rule out pancreatitis. Urine pregnancy test in females. Urinalysis to look for other cause of abdominal pain. US is the diagnostic modality of choice.
Diabetic ketoacidosis	Preceding polyuria and polydipsia. Unexplained nausea, vomiting, and abdominal pain are frequently seen, especially in children.	Abnormal vital signs may be the only physical findings at the time of presentation. Tachycardia and either orthostasis or hypotension are usually present. Kussmaul respirations with severe acidemia. Characteristic fruity odor on the breath found in some patients. Diffuse abdominal tenderness may also be present.	Serum glucose determination, chemistry panel, ABG or VBG to determine degree of acidemia. Work-up to determine concomitant infection or myocardial infarction. Fluid hydration and repletion of potassium.
GI bleed (Mallory–Weiss tear, peptic ulcer disease, erosive gastritis and esophagitis, esophageal and gastric varices). Peptic ulcer disease is the most common etiology.	Hematemesis, coffee-ground emesis, melena, or hematochezia. Vomiting and retching, followed by hematemesis, is suggestive of a Mallory–Weiss tear. A history of an aortic graft should suggest the possibility of an aortoenteric fistula. Alcohol, NSAIDs, and GI bleed history should be determined.	Altered mental status, hypotension, tachycardia decreased pulse pressure or tachypnea. Paradoxical bradycardia can occur in the face of profound hypovolemia. Petechiae and purpura suggest an underlying coagulopathy. Tenderness, masses, ascites, or organomegaly on abdominal examination. Digital rectal examination needed to detect the presence of bright red, maroon, or melanotic stool.	The most important laboratory test is to type and crossmatch blood. CBC, electrolytes, coagulation studies are also indicated.
Intussusception	6–18 month old previously healthy infant. Intermittent episodes of severe abdominal pain. Vomiting is rare in the first few hours but usually develops after 6–12 hours.	Fever can occur and even rise to 41°C (106°F). Respirations may be shallow and grunting in nature. Apathy or lethargy may be the only presenting sign in up to 10% of cases. Classic "currant jelly" stool is	Diagnosis considered on the basis of the history. AAS may reveal a mass or filling defect in the RUQ of the abdomen. Thirty percent of X-rays are normal. US may

(*continued*)

Table 39.1 Differential diagnosis for vomiting (*cont*)

Diagnosis	Symptoms	Signs	Work-up
Intussusception (*cont*)		a late manifestation of the disease and is present in only 50% of cases. Examination between attacks may reveal sausage-shaped mass in the right side of the abdomen in 66%.	identify mass. Barium or air-contrast enema may be necessary, and possibly therapeutic.
Mesenteric ischemia	Severe pain, colicky, starting in periumbilical region and becomes diffuse. Often associated with vomiting and diarrhea.	Early examination can be remarkably benign in the presence of severe ischemia. Bowel sounds often still present. Rectal examination is important because mild ischemia may present with only hemoccult-positive stools.	Pronounced leukocytosis usually present. Elevations of amylase and creatine phosphokinase levels can be seen. Metabolic acidosis due to lactic acidemia is often seen with infarction. Plain films of limited benefit until late. CT, MRI, and angiography are accurate to varying degrees.
Myocardial infarction	Chest pain, shortness of breath, or abdominal discomfort predominate. Associated symptoms such as nausea, vomiting, diaphoresis, dyspnea, light-headedness, syncope, and palpitations may be present. A detailed history is essential.	The patient may appear well or exhibit signs of shock. An S3 is present in 15–20% of patients and may imply a failing myocardium. A new systolic murmur may signify papillary muscle dysfunction, a flail leaflet of the mitral valve with resultant MR, or a VSD. Rales are associated with LV dysfunction and left-sided CHF. JVD, HJR, and peripheral edema suggest right-sided CHF.	The standard 12-lead ECG is the single best test to identify patients with AMI. Cardiac enzymes (CK-MB and troponin) should also be obtained.
Ovarian torsion	Acute, severe, and unilateral pain, felt in the lower abdomen and pelvis; may be related to a change in position. May be intermittent. Nausea and vomiting are common.	Possible palpation of a mass on bimanual pelvic examination.	Pelvic US, CBC, urine pregnancy test.
Pelvic inflammatory disease	Abdominal pain, pain with intercourse. Nausea and vomiting are common.	Fever should be present. Lower abdominal tenderness common. Discharge from cervical os likely present. Cervical motion tenderness pronounced.	Cervical cultures for GC and Chlamydia, CBC. IV hydration, pain medication, and antibiotics. Pelvic US to exclude a tubo-ovarian abscess.
Pregnancy	Nausea and vomiting, breast pain, weight gain.	May be normal. On pelvic examination, uterus is larger than normal.	Urine pregnancy test.
Pyloric stenosis	Infant (older than 1 week but less than 3 months) with non-bilious projectile vomiting. Vomiting usually becomes projectile within a week of symptom onset. Vomiting occurs just after or near the end of feeding; patient	Hungry infant who has failed to gain weight over the past several weeks or has lost weight and is dehydrated or lethargic. Peristaltic waves can sometimes be seen passing from left to right across the upper abdomen,	Abdominal US is recommended as well as a serum chemistry panel and CBC. IV hydration and glucose administration especially if ill-appearing.

(continued)

Table 39.1 Differential diagnosis for vomiting (*cont*)

Diagnosis	Symptoms	Signs	Work-up
Pyloric stenosis (*cont*)	re-feeds as if never fed.	just prior to an episode of vomiting. May palpate an "olive" (pyloric tumor near the lateral margin of the right rectus muscle just below the liver edge).	
Subarachnoid hemorrhage	Sudden onset of a severe constant headache that is often occipital or nuchal. "Sentinel hemorrhage" in 15–31% of cases. Vomiting often with onset of headache. Cerebellar hemorrhage: sudden onset of dizziness, vomiting, marked truncal ataxia, and inability to walk.	Awake to lethargic. Markedly elevated BP. Contralateral hemiplegia, hemianesthesia, and aphasia or neglect (depending on the hemisphere involved). Cerebellar hemorrhage: gaze palsies and increasing stupor; patients may rapidly progress to coma.	Fingerstick glucose, non contrast head CT, ECG. LP if CT negative. Laboratory tests may be indicated.
Testicular torsion	History of an athletic event, strenuous physical activity, or trauma just prior to the onset of scrotal pain. Also awaking from sleep with unilateral testicular pain. Severe pain felt in lower abdominal quadrant, inguinal canal, or the testis.	Involved testis is aligned along a horizontal rather than a vertical axis. The axis of alignment can be determined only with the patient in an upright position. Diminished or absent cremasteric reflex on involved side.	If testicular torsion cannot be excluded by history and physical examination, emergency scrotal exploration is the definitive diagnostic test and procedure of choice. In patients with indeterminate clinical presentations, color-flow duplex. Doppler US and radionuclide scintigraphy may be used.
Ureteral colic	Acute onset of flank pain radiating to groin. Nausea and vomiting are common. Patient usually writhing in pain. May have bloody urine.	Vital signs usually normal. CVAT with percussion; benign abdominal examination	UA usually shows hematuria. Helical or spiral CT (CT urogram) performed without contrast has become common, replacing the IVP as the test of choice.
Vertigo	Sudden or gradual onset of sensation of room spinning (depending on etiology), associated with nausea and vomiting. May be related to head position in peripheral vertigo. Peripheral vertigo may involve tinnitus, ear ringing, buzzing, or headache. Other neurologic symptoms may be present in central vertigo.	Vertigo sensation may be reproduced depending on the patient's position. Nystagmus may be present with vertigo symptoms. For peripheral vertigo, other neurologic abnormalities should not be present.	Peripheral: Symptomatic therapy. Central: CT head and neurologic consultation warranted.
Volvulus (Duodenal stenosis or atresia)	Bilious vomiting, with or without abdominal distention, and streaks of blood in the stool. In older children, pain is usually constant, not colicky.	In newborns, the sudden onset of an acute abdomen and shock. May be pale and have grunting respirations. Approximately 33% of infants will appear jaundiced.	AAS, CBC, chemistry panel, and fluid rehydration.

AAS: acute abdominal series; ABG: arterial blood gas; AMI: acute myocardial infarction; BP: blood pressure; CBC: complete blood count; CHF: congestive heart failure; CK-MB: creatine kinase muscle band; CRP: C-reactive protein; CT: computed tomography; CVAT: costovertebral angle tenderness; CXR: chest X-ray; DKA: diabetic ketoacidosis; ECG: electrocardiogram; GC: gonorrhea; GI: gastrointestinal; HJR: hepatojugular reflux; IV: intravenous; IVP: intravenous pyelogram; JVD: jugular venous distention; LFTs: liver function tests; LUQ: left upper quadrant; MR: mitral regurgitation; MRI: magnetic resonance imaging; NSAID: non-steroidal anti-inflammatory drug; RLQ: right lower quadrant; RUQ: right upper quadrant; US: ultrasound; VBG: venous blood gas; VSD: ventricular septal defect; WBC: white blood cell.

Diagnostic testing

The history and physical examination should determine which laboratory studies will aid in determining the etiology of vomiting.

Laboratory studies

Bedside glucose

A bedside glucose should be performed on patients who look ill and complain of vomiting.

Complete blood count

A complete blood count (CBC) is not usually helpful unless blood loss is suspected.

Chemistry panel

In an otherwise healthy young adult with vomiting for less than a day, a chemistry panel will add little. In patients with an underlying disease, especially diabetes, or tenuous health status, more comprehensive laboratory testing guided by history and suspected diagnosis may be beneficial. The likelihood of an abnormality increases due to decreased compensatory mechanisms.

Urinalysis

A urinalysis should also be ordered to evaluate urine concentration and identify urinary tract infection (UTI).

Pregnancy test

A urine or serum pregnancy test should be ordered on all females of child-bearing age.

Other tests

Liver function tests (LFTs) are of equivocal value in the evaluation of the patient with suspected gallbladder disease. However, they are useful if hepatitis is suspected. A serum amylase and lipase should be ordered if pancreatitis is suspected. If the patient has liver disease and is vomiting blood, a prothrombin time/International Normalized Ratio (PT/INR) and type and crossmatch should be ordered. If cardiac ischemia is suspected as the etiology of vomiting, cardiac enzymes should be obtained.

Electrocardiogram

All patients with presumed cardiac-induced vomiting need an electrocardiogram (ECG).

Radiologic studies

Plain films

A kidney, ureter, bladder (KUB) X-ray series is not indicated in the evaluation of vomiting. An acute abdominal series (AAS) is indicated for patients with previous surgeries, the presence of a hernia on physical examination, suspected ingestion of radiopaque drugs, tympany, or high suspicion for bowel obstruction. A chest X-ray (CXR) may be indicated if the "vomiting" is actually a gag reflex evoked by coughing.

Computed tomography

Computed tomography (CT) of the brain should be performed on any patient with suspected increased intracranial pressure, intracranial bleeding, head trauma, or intracranial pathology (brain tumor or cysts). An abdominal CT is indicated for patients over the age of 55 years with an unclear vomiting etiology, or those with persistent symptoms such as abdominal pain, history of abdominal trauma, suspicion of appendicitis or mass which is not obvious on physical examination.

Ultrasound

If one suspects gallbladder pathology, a right upper quadrant (RUQ) ultrasound should be performed. A pelvic ultrasound should be performed on female patients in whom there is suspicion for ovarian torsion, tubo-ovarian abscess, or an undocumented pregnancy. A testicular ultrasound should be obtained whenever testicular torsion or mass is suspected.

Other

If the patient is vomiting blood, a nasogastric (NG) tube should be placed to determine the quantity and intensity of bleeding.

General treatment principles

Volume repletion

Regardless of the etiology of vomiting, the Airway, Breathing, and Circulation (ABCs) must first be addressed and stabilized. If the patient is in circulatory collapse, venous access with two large bore peripheral IVs must be established and a fluid bolus of normal saline administered.

The administration of fluids to the vomiting patient can be accomplished in several ways. Sometimes, oral rehydration may be attempted, especially in children. Depending on the underlying etiology of the vomiting, IV rehydration may be more efficient. An IV also allows access for the administration of medications.

Antiemetics

Most vomiting patients are treated symptomatically by relieving the nausea and vomiting. However, this may not be possible if the underlying cause is metabolic or neurologic; these cases require treatment of the underlying disease to treat the vomiting.

There are several types of medications used to alleviate vomiting (Table 39.2). If the vomiting is

Table 39.2 Antiemetic medications for vomiting

Agent	Route of administration	Indications	Side effects
Meclizine	25–50 mg PO every 6 hours.	Labyrinthitis, motion sickness, vestibular causes.	Sedation.
Diphenhydramine	25–50 mg (or 5 mg/kg/day divided every 4–6 hours for peds) PO/IM/IV every 4–6 hours.		
Scopolamine	1.5 mg disc transdermal every 3 days.		
Prochlorperazine	5–10 mg PO/IM/IV or 25 mg PR (not recommended IV in children).	GI irritation, gastritis, appendicitis, biliary disease, gastroenteritis, DKA, intracranial pathology, digoxin or theophylline toxicity, chemotherapy-related, vertigo, motion sickness.	Sedation, akathisia, dystonia.
Promethazine	12.5–25 mg PO/IM/PR every 6 hours. IV use not approved but common (0.25–0.5 mg/kg PO/IM/PR every 6 hours in children).		
5-HT antagonists:			
Ondansetron	4–32 mg PO/IV GI irritation, gastritis, appendicitis, biliary disease, gastroenteritis, DKA, intracranial pathology, digoxin or theophylline toxicity, chemotherapy-related, vertigo, motion sickness.		Sedation less than with phenothiazines.
Granisetron	10 mcg/kg/IV or 1 mg PO BID for 1 day only.	Refractory vomiting.	
Dolasetron	12.5 mg IV in adults or 0.35 mg/kg IV in children.		
Metoclopramide	10 mg IM/IV every 2–3 hours 10–15 mg PO QID	Exerts both anti-emetic and prokinetic effects. Gastroparesis and gastroesophageal reflux.	Adverse effects appear common in young children and the elderly, and include fatigue and extrapyramidal phenomena (dystonia, dyskinesia, akathisia, opisthotonos and oculogyric crises). Chronic use of metoclopramide also induces hyperprolactinemia, which may result in gynecomastia and galactorrhea.

BID: two times a day; DKA: diabetic ketoacidosis; GI: gastrointestinal; IV: intravenous; IM: intramuscular; PO: per os; PR: per rectum; QID: four times a day.

due to a labyrinthine disorder, agents such as meclizine or diazepam may be used to alleviate symptoms.

Most vomiting may be relieved by a single dose of prochlorperazine or promethazine, commonly used agents to treat vomiting of unknown etiology. The newer 5-HT$_3$ antagonists such as ondansetron, dolasetron, or granisetron are particularly effective at reducing chemotherapy-associated or refractory nausea and vomiting.

The primary side effect of all antiemetics is sedation. Therefore, the patient must have a ride home and be cautioned not to drive for the following day or when taking the medication (if discharged with a prescription). Possible side effects of the phenothiazine antiemetics and metoclopramide are akathisia and dystonia. Akathisia is a condition of restlessness that can include nervousness, anxiety, and a feeling that one's skin is "crawling." This can be treated with diphenhydramine or a benzodiazepine. A dystonic reaction can be far more serious, and may include rhythmic contractions of the neck and back as well as repetitive protrusion of the tongue. A dystonic reaction requires treatment with diphenhydramine or benztropine for 48 hours and possible hospital admission if severe. No further doses of antiemetics that may cause dystonia should be given.

Special patients
Pediatric

Vomiting can represent a benign, self-limited illness or a severe underlying illness in a child. A history of bilious vomiting in a young child is an ominous finding and suggests malrotation of the gut or intussusception until proven otherwise. Causes of vomiting in infants and children include infectious (acute gastroenteritis, otitis media, pneumonia), metabolic (diabetic ketoacidosis), mechanical (obstruction), and neurogenic (increased intracranial pressure). The most common cause of vomiting in an older child or adolescent is infectious gastroenteritis. Evaluation of a child's hydration status is particularly important. Vital signs may be normal despite significant dehydration; dry mucus membranes, decreased urine output and mental status changes may be more indicative of dehydration. Moderate to severe dehydration should be treated with an initial IV normal saline bolus of 20 ml/kg. If vomiting has been protracted, a bedside glucose should also be obtained as part of the initial evaluation. Further evaluation and treatment is aimed at determining if a serious underlying cause of vomiting is present.

Elderly

The general evaluation and treatment principles for vomiting also apply to the geriatric population. The response of geriatric patients to dehydration may be blunted by their chronic illnesses or medications; vital signs may not demonstrate hypotension or tachycardia despite severe dehydration. In the elderly, a serious cause of vomiting is found more frequently than in younger adult populations. The laboratory evaluation and diagnostic work-up is typically more extensive, as the cause of vomiting in this population is rarely benign. Attention to the ABCs remains critical in this population. Aggressive rehydration may be complicated by underlying illness and cardiac disease.

Pregnant

Pregnant patients commonly present to the ED with significant nausea and vomiting (sometimes referred to as "morning sickness"). These patients should be aggressively hydrated, as they are at increased risk of miscarriage if they are volume-depleted. Antiemetics should be selected with pregnancy risk categories in mind. Despite the Class C classification for many of these agents, physicians commonly use them in the treatment of pregnant women who need relief from vomiting. Close follow-up with the patient's obstetrician is essential.

Disposition

A majority of patients will not have their cause of vomiting diagnosed in the ED, and will only receive symptomatic therapy.

Admission

All patients with life-threatening causes of vomiting or serious illness related to the vomiting should be admitted to the hospital.

Consultation

Consultation of a specialist will depend on the underlying etiology of the vomiting.

Discharge

In order to assure continued hydration, the patient's ability to keep down a small amount of fluid (water) without vomiting should be assessed prior to discharge. This is known as a "PO challenge." If the patient receives adequate IV hydration in the ED, an oral fluid challenge is not essential for the final disposition. Occasionally, patients without serious causes of vomiting who have received IV fluids and feel better may go home despite being unable to tolerate PO fluids. Most patients with simple vomiting due to a benign etiology and without signs of significant dehydration or metabolic derangement may be discharged home provided liquids are tolerated in the ED and follow-up can be assured.

Pearls, pitfalls, and myths

Pearls

Patients may confuse coughing or spitting up phlegm with true vomiting. The history and physical examination usually help determine the cause of the vomiting. Although the etiology of vomiting is not always identified in the ED, therapy should not be withheld.

Pitfalls

Regardless of the cause of the vomiting, the evaluation of these patients should focus on the ABCs. Resuscitation of the markedly dehydrated individual, regardless of the etiology of vomiting, needs to be addressed in an urgent fashion.

Treatment of life-threatening etiologies must often be initiated prior to establishing a firm diagnosis.

References

1. Baraff LJ, Schriger DL. Orthostatic vital signs: variation with age, specificity, and sensitivity in detecting a 450-ml blood loss. *Am J Emerg Med* 1992;10(2):99–103.
2. Harwood-Nuss A (ed.). *Clinical Practice of Emergency Medicine*. Philadelphia: Lippincott Williams and Wilkins, 2001. pp. 1206–1208.
3. Marx JA (ed.). *Rosen's Emergency Medicine: Concepts and Clinical Practices*, 5th ed., St Louis: Mosby, 2002. pp. 178–185.
4. McCaig LF, Ly N. *National Hospital Ambulatory Medical Care Survey: 2000 Emergency Department Summary*. Advance Data from Vital and Health Statistics; No. 326, Hyattsville, Maryland: National Center for Health Statistics. 2001.
5. Quigley E, Hasler W, Parkman H. American Gastroenterological Association Practice Guidelines; AGA technical Review on Nausea and Vomiting. *Gastroenterology* 2001;120(1).
6. Tintinalli JE (ed.). *Emergency Medicine: A Comprehensive Study Guide*, 5th ed., Philadelphia: Lippincott Williams and Wilkins, 2001. pp. 567–569.
7. Vinson DR, Drotts DL. Diphenhydramine for the prevention of akathisia induced by prochlorperazine: a randomized, controlled trial. *Ann Emerg Med* 2001;37(2).

40 Weakness

R. Jason Thurman, MD and Kristy Self Reynolds, MD

Scope of the problem

On almost a daily basis, emergency physicians encounter at least one patient with the chief complaint of "weakness." In contrast to most other presentations, the true meaning of the patient's complaint may sometimes be difficult to ascertain. What symptoms are the patient and/or his or her family trying to convey?

On the one hand, the patient may be complaining of a sensation of global lack of energy, extreme fatigue, lightheadedness, or simply feeling "ill." In this regard, the differential diagnosis extends from fairly benign etiologies (mild dehydration, viral syndrome, hypothyroidism, mild depression) to life-threatening emergencies requiring immediate intervention (acute myocardial infarction (AMI), sepsis, pericardial effusion with tamponade). Other clues may be present to help make the correct diagnosis, but the isolated complaint of "weakness" may be associated with any of these pathologies in isolation or combination, or a myriad of other possible etiologies.

On the other hand, the patient may present complaining of a specific distribution of weakness associated with a true impairment of motor function. Patients with the chief complaint of motor weakness present in a number of different ways. They may present with hemiparesis (weakness of one side of the body without complete paralysis) or hemiplegia (complete paralysis of one side of the body) indicating probable vascular occlusion in a cervicocerebral arterial distribution and ongoing ischemic stroke or transient ischemic attack (TIA). Patients may also present with a pattern of symmetric ascending paresis or paralysis (Guillain–Barré syndrome (GBS)), focal peripheral motor weakness (carpal tunnel syndrome), symmetric proximal muscle weakness (polymyositis), weakness in a bulbar muscle distribution causing diplopia or ptosis (myasthenia gravis (MG), botulism), or even a combination of the above findings (multiple sclerosis (MS)).

This chapter focuses primarily on the patient presenting with the complaint of weakness associated with true objective impairment of motor function. Acute ischemic stroke (AIS) and TIA are discussed in detail, as these are the most important disease processes causing motor weakness that the emergency physicians encounter. The importance of acute stroke cannot be overemphasized, as this disease alone accounts for approximately 1 million hospitalizations per year in the US, and it is the third leading cause of death and the number one cause of adult disability in this country. The emergency physician must also be prepared to identify and manage other selected etiologies of motor weakness.

Anatomic essentials

Accurate diagnosis and effective treatment planning for the patient with motor weakness hinges upon the emergency physician's ability to identify the underlying lesion(s) responsible for the patient's disability. First, physicians must determine whether the patient's weakness arises from a central nervous system (CNS) or peripheral nervous system (PNS) problem, or in the muscles themselves.

Central nervous system

CNS disturbances result in a constellation of signs and symptoms due to the specific underlying lesion(s) present. Most often, acute weakness caused by a lesion in the CNS is the result of an acute cervicocerebral vascular occlusion depriving brain parenchyma in a given dependent area of oxygenated blood. When examining cerebral blood flow, the vascular distributions may be divided into the anterior circulation (carotid artery distribution) and the posterior circulation (vertebrobasilar distribution). In the anterior circulation, the carotid terminus divides into the anterior cerebral artery (ACA) and the middle cerebral artery (MCA). Occlusions of the ACA cause sudden onset of contralateral upper and lower extremity weakness and numbness, with the lower extremity being affected greater than the upper extremity. There may also be associated gait apraxia (clumsiness), incontinence, and slowed mentation (Table 40.1). Occlusions of the MCA result in the acute onset of contralateral upper

Table 40.1 Clinical stroke syndromes and site of arterial occlusion

Syndrome	Arterial occlusion site	Clinical manifestations
Anterior cerebral artery occlusion	Anterior cerebral artery	Contralateral upper and lower extremity motor weakness and sensory loss, with lower extremity more affected than upper, apraxia, incontinence, slowed mentation
Central midbrain syndrome (Tegmental syndrome)	Paramedian branches of basilar artery	(A) Ipsilateral oculomotor nerve palsy, (B) Hemichorea of contralateral limbs, (C) Contralateral loss of cutaneous sensation and proprioception
Dorsal midbrain syndrome (Parinaud syndrome)	Usually caused by compression by extra-axial lesion (pinealoma)	Paralysis of upward gaze
Lateral inferior pontine syndrome	Anterior inferior cerebellar artery	(a) Ipsilateral limb ataxia, (b) Ipsilateral loss of facial cutaneous sensation, (c) Hiccup, (d) Ipsilateral Horner's syndrome, (e) Nausea/vomiting/nystagmus, (f) Contralateral loss of pain and temperature sensation, (g) Ipsilateral facial paralysis, (h) Deafness and tinnitus, (i) Ipsilateral gaze paralysis
Lateral medullary syndrome (Wallenburg syndrome)	Posterior inferior cerebellar artery (often lesion in vertebral artery)	(a) Ipsilateral limb ataxia, (b) Ipsilateral loss of facial cutaneous sensation, (c) Hiccup, (d) Ipsilateral Horner's syndrome, (e) Nausea/vomiting/nystagmus, (f) Contralateral loss of pain and temperature sensation, (g) Dysphagia, (h) Hoarseness with ipsilateral vocal cord paralysis, (i) Loss of ipsilateral pharyngeal reflex
Lateral mid-pontine syndrome	Short circumferential artery	(a) Ipsilateral limb ataxia, (b) Ipsilateral loss of facial cutaneous sensation, (c) Hiccup, (d) Ipsilateral Horner's syndrome, (e) Nausea/vomiting/nystagmus, (f) Contralateral loss of pain and temperature sensation, (g) *Trigeminal nerve impairment*: Chewing difficulty (bilateral lesions) or ipsilateral jaw deviation with mouth opened (unilateral lesions)
Lateral superior pontine syndrome	Superior cerebellar artery	(a) Ipsilateral limb ataxia, (b) Ipsilateral loss of facial cutaneous sensation, (c) Hiccup, (d) Ipsilateral Horner's syndrome, (e) Nausea/vomiting/nystagmus, (f) Contralateral loss of pain and temperature sensation, (g) Absence of specific cranial nerve signs
Locked-in syndrome	Basilar artery occlusion causing bilateral ventral pontine lesions	Complete quadriplegia, inability to speak, and loss of all facial movements despite normal level of consciousness; patients may communicate with eye or eyelid movements
Medial inferior pontine syndrome	Paramedian branches of basilar artery	(A) Contralateral hemiparesis, (B) Contralateral loss of proprioception and vibratory sensory function, (C) Ipsilateral limb ataxia, (D) Ipsilateral gaze paralysis, (E) Ipsilateral lateral rectus paralysis, (F) Gaze-evoked nystagmus
Medial medullary syndrome	Paramedian branches of basilar artery	(A) Contralateral hemiparesis, (B) Contralateral loss of proprioception and vibratory sensory function, (C) Ipsilateral limb ataxia, (D) Ipsilateral tongue weakness
Medial superior pontine syndrome	Paramedian branches of basilar artery	(A) Contralateral hemiparesis, (B) Contralateral loss of proprioception and vibratory sensory function, (C) Ipsilateral limb ataxia, (D) Internuclear ophthalmoplegia, (E) Palatal myoclonus
Middle cerebral artery occlusion, dominant hemisphere	Middle cerebral artery, usually left	Contralateral upper and lower extremity motor weakness and sensory loss, with upper extremity more affected than lower, contralateral facial droop, homonymous hemianopsia, gaze deviation to side of lesion. Language disturbances (expressive, receptive, and/or global aphasia)
Middle cerebral artery occlusion, nondominant hemisphere	Middle cerebral artery, usually right	Contralateral upper and lower extremity motor weakness and sensory loss, with upper extremity more affected than lower, contralateral facial droop, homonymous hemianopsia, gaze deviation to side of lesion. Hemineglect
Ventral midbrain syndrome (Weber syndrome)	Paramedian branches of basilar artery	(A) Contralateral hemiparesis, (B) Contralateral supranuclear facial paresis, (C) Ipsilateral oculomotor nerve palsy

and lower extremity weakness and numbness, with the upper extremity being affected greater than the lower extremity. A contralateral facial droop is usually present with hemiparesis of the extremities. Contralateral homonymous hemianopsia (visual field disturbance) is also often present, and conjugate gaze may be affected with the eyes pointing towards the side of the lesion. Depending on which cerebral hemisphere is affected, further deficits also occur. If the dominant hemisphere (usually the left brain) is deprived of blood flow, aphasia is commonly present. The aphasia may be *expressive* (the patient knows what he wants to say but cannot get the words out), *receptive* (the patient cannot understand what is being communicated to them), or *global* (both expressive and receptive aphasia present). If the nondominant hemisphere is affected (usually the right brain), hemineglect (the patient unconsciously ignores the affected side of the body) may be present (Table 40.1).

Vertebrobasilar arterial occlusions result in a constellation of symptoms that may include ipsilateral cerebellar dysfunction (severe vertigo, nausea and vomiting, tinnitus and deafness, ataxia, and nystagmus), cranial nerve (CN) dysfunctions, and hemiparesis and/or hemisensory deficits. The variety of findings observed by the emergency physician depends on the specific arterial distribution affected. Table 40.1 includes descriptions of various uncommon stroke/TIA syndromes resulting from posterior cerebrovascular occlusions.

Some CNS disturbances are caused by inflammatory or demyelinating disorders. Demyelinating disorders may cause a confusing variety of signs and symptoms, such as the combination of unilateral visual disturbance and variable motor weakness seen in patients with MS.

Peripheral nervous system

PNS dysfunction may cause motor weakness as a result of pathophysiologic processes involving the neuromuscular junction or the peripheral nerves themselves. Disruption of neuromuscular junction causes motor weakness by inhibiting the normal physiology of motor end plate stimulation to facilitate muscle contraction. This may be the result of a toxin-mediated process (botulism) or abnormal antibodies attacking the motor end plate (MG). Dysfunction of the neuromuscular junction also occurs iatrogenically with the use of drugs that act at the neuromuscular junction

(succinylcholine, vecuronium). Peripheral nerve malfunction that impairs motor strength may result from direct damage to peripheral nerves (GBS), toxins (tick paralysis, arsenic poisoning), compressive neuropathies (carpal tunnel syndrome), or peripheral vascular occlusions.

Primary muscle dysfunction

Primary muscle dysfunction resulting in motor weakness may be caused by an inflammatory myopathy (polymyositis, dermatomyositis) or abnormalities in ion channels found in skeletal muscles (hypokalemic periodic paralysis).

History

Obtaining an accurate and complete history can be quite challenging in the patient presenting with acute weakness. Many patients have difficulty pinpointing the exact timing of their weakness. In addition, some stroke and TIA patients suffer an accompanying aphasia and are unable to relay their history. With nondominant hemispheric strokes and TIAs, the patient may be completely unaware that a large neurologic deficit even exists. The use of family or bystanders is critical to the emergency physician's ability to procure a thorough history.

What is the distribution of motor weakness?

The distribution of motor weakness corresponds to the underlying anatomical lesion(s) present. Hemiparesis is indicative of stroke, TIA, or possible mimics. Isolated extremity weakness is likely the result of a compressive radicular or peripheral neuropathy, or peripheral vascular occlusion. When bilateral weakness is encountered, further historical points must be explored. GBS is associated with a symmetric ascending paralysis initially involving the lower extremities, then progressing in a cephalad direction. Motor weakness encompassing both cranial and peripheral nerve distributions is likely the result of inflammatory (MS), toxic/metabolic (botulism), or autoimmune processes (MG). When bilateral weakness is associated with a discrete sensory level (below which the patient has loss of sensation) and/or bladder dysfunction, a lesion in the spinal cord is suspected. Bilateral weakness that affects the proximal musculature to a greater degree than distal motor strength is indicative of myopathy (polymyositis, dermatomyositis). In these patients, difficulty ascending stairs, rising from a chair, or problems with personal grooming commonly arise.

Was the onset of weakness sudden or gradual?

The sudden onset of motor weakness implies a vaso-occlusive etiology. Ischemic strokes and TIAs are the result of thrombotic or embolic occlusion of a cervicocerebral artery, and in general occur with sudden onset. This may be difficult for the patient to identify, as they may be unaware of the symptoms. In addition, the patient may have been asleep when the stroke or TIA began, making the determination of onset impossible. The sudden onset of extremity weakness caused by the abrupt occlusion of a major artery supplying that extremity will likely be accompanied by paresthesias, pain, pallor, and pulselessness.

Patients presenting with the gradual onset of progressive motor weakness probably suffer from a nonvascular pathophysiologic process. Subacute motor weakness is more likely associated with inflammatory disorders of the nervous system (MS, transverse myelitis) or musculoskeletal system (polymyositis, dermatomyositis), compression neuropathies (carpal tunnel syndrome), autoimmune disorders (MG, GBS), or toxic/metabolic processes (botulism, hypokalemic periodic paralysis).

Were there any significant events surrounding the onset of weakness?

Many stroke mimics are associated with easily identifiable conditions that accompany the onset of weakness. Seizures preceding the onset of weakness may imply postictal (Todd's) paralysis. Ongoing migraine headache in a young female associated with motor weakness might indicate a complicated migraine. Severe sudden headache with motor weakness should alarm the examiner of a possible subarachnoid hemorrhage. Weakness in the setting of trauma could indicate a subdural or epidural hematoma. Severe migratory chest or neck pain accompanying motor weakness should alert the physician to the possibility of arterial dissection syndromes.

Is there a temporal pattern to the weakness?

Patients who complain of weakness worsening with repetitive motions may be exhibiting symptoms of neuromuscular junction pathology (such as MG). These patients may report difficulty with blinking, chewing, typing, or other motor tasks requiring frequent repeated movements. Increased clinical suspicion for dyskalemic periodic paralysis occurs when the patient complains of sudden episodic resolving motor weakness.

When did the weakness begin?

Emergent stroke therapy is extremely time-dependent. The option of intravenous (IV) thrombolytic therapy for AIS is available only within a strict (and brief) time window of 3 hours from symptom onset. It is therefore critical that the emergency physician extract from the patient or witnesses the exact time of symptom onset.

Associated symptoms

Headache

Ischemic stroke and TIA are not usually associated with severe headache initially. Acute motor weakness accompanied by a significant headache is worrisome for subarachnoid hemorrhage, arterial vascular malformation, or epidural/subdural hematoma. When headache occurs concomitantly with ischemic stroke, the evaluating physician must consider the possibility of increased intracranial pressure. Stroke symptoms accompanying a migraine-type headache may indicate complicated migraine, classically a disease of young adult females.

Visual changes

Double vision (diplopia) of acute onset may be associated with a posterior circulation stroke. In isolation, this complaint usually implies a process affecting the neuromuscular junction. Monocular visual complaints may be exhibited with optic neuritis of new-onset MS.

Nausea and vomiting

The presence of nausea and vomiting may also be a warning sign of increased intracranial pressure. Careful evaluation for intracranial lesions and cerebral edema is warranted. Severe vomiting and/or diarrhea may predispose the patient to electrolyte imbalances leading to motor weakness.

Chest or neck pain

The presence of ongoing migratory chest or neck pain may indicate the presence of an acute arterial dissection (thoracic aorta or carotid/vertebral artery dissection). Appropriate radiologic studies should be emergently executed when arterial dissection is suspected. AMI may also be associated with AIS.

Abdominal and/or back pain

Abdominal and/or back pain accompanied by lower extremity weakness could signify dissection of an abdominal aortic aneurysm (AAA) with concomitant spinal cord infarction. Back pain with unilateral lower extremity weakness may indicate herniated lumbar disk with nerve root impingement. Back pain with bilateral lower extremity weakness, sensory level, and priapism in the setting of significant trauma is worrisome for spinal cord injury. Similar symptoms without a history of trauma should alert the physician to the possibility of acute cauda equina syndrome, primary spinal cord lesions, or compressive spinal cord lesions such as epidural hematoma or abscess.

Musculoskeletal pain and tenderness

Musculoskeletal pain and diffuse muscular tenderness associated with motor weakness (especially proximal weakness) is suggestive of myopathy (polymyositis, dermatomyositis). Severe muscular pain coupled with dark urine or oliguria and motor weakness may indicate acute rhabdomyolysis.

Rash

The complaint of rash, particularly in the periorbital region, is associated with dermatomyositis.

Past medical

When eliciting a patient's history in the setting of acute motor weakness, the emergency physician must focus on identifying risk factors for the suspected etiology of weakness. When AIS or TIA is suspected, the physician should inquire about risk factors (Table 40.2). A recent history of viral

Table 40.2 Risk factors for acute ischemic stroke or transient ischemic attack

History of transient ischemic attack	Old age
History of stroke	African–American race
Cigarette smoking	Hypertension
Atrial fibrillation	Diabetes mellitus
Hyperlipidemia	Coronary artery disease
Carotid stenosis	Male gender

illness accompanied by the acute onset of ascending bilateral motor weakness is classic for GBS. Occupational exposures to heavy metal toxins (arsenic poisoning) or to repetitive hand motions, such as hammering or typing (carpal tunnel syndrome) may provide clues to the diagnosis. Social history should include questions about possible cocaine use in the setting of stroke, suspected subarachnoid hemorrhage, or TIA. Heavy alcohol use accompanies alcohol-induced myopathies. Family history may be positive for familial causes of weakness (hypokalemic periodic paralysis).

A complete list of the patient's current medications should be carefully reviewed. The use of corticosteroid therapy as well as some lipid-lowering agents may induce drug-related myopathy. Although not usually a cause of true motor weakness, medication use in the elderly is commonly attributed to the subjective complaints of weakness and dizziness.

Physical examination

The primary aim of the physical examination is to both localize and quantify the extent of neurologic deficit(s) present. The distribution and extent of weakness often lend important clues to the underlying lesion(s) and aid in the diagnosis and management of the patient.

General appearance

As with all ED patients, global assessment of the airway, breathing, and circulation takes first priority. Fortunately, most patients presenting with motor weakness do not have major issues in these areas. Exceptions are patients suffering from large intracranial hemorrhage who may need immediate airway assistance. Patients with advanced GBS may have extremely poor respiratory effort secondary to paralysis of their breathing musculature, and may need emergent mechanical ventilation. Trauma patients with spinal cord injuries may suffer spinal shock and require interventions to correct circulatory collapse.

Vital signs

As a general rule, most patients presenting with acute motor weakness will not exhibit major vital sign abnormalities. Patients with AIS often present with elevated blood pressure (BP), as underlying uncontrolled hypertension is very common among stroke victims. Wide fluctuations in BP and heart rate may reflect autonomic instability associated with GBS. The presence of fever may suggest an infectious etiology associated with acute motor weakness (epidural abscess), or may contribute to the precipitation of motor weakness with underlying disease (MG).

Head, eyes, ears, nose, and throat

The head and neck are inspected for signs of trauma that may be associated with epidural or subdural hematoma, or carotid dissection. Carotid auscultation is performed to identify the presence of carotid bruits, which may signify underlying carotid stenosis. Abnormalities of the thyroid gland prompt the examiner to search for thyroid dysfunction as a potential contributor to weakness.

Cardiopulmonary

The heart is auscultated to evaluate rhythm and to detect murmurs. An irregularly irregular rhythm is present with atrial fibrillation, an important risk factor for embolic stroke. The presence of a murmur alerts the examiner of the possibility of valvular heart disease and the potential for emboli.

Extremities

Unequal pulses may be present in acute arterial dissection syndromes, which may cause acute motor weakness secondary to distal ischemia to either a limb or the CNS.

Skin

The presence of a periorbital violaceous rash may be present with dermatomyositis. Careful examination for the presence of a tick should take place in the at-risk patient with motor weakness.

Neurologic

A careful and thorough neurologic examination is of critical importance in the evaluation of the patient with acute motor weakness. The essential neurologic examination consists of six major areas: mental status, CNs, motor function, sensory function, deep tendon reflexes, and cerebellar function.

Mental status

First the examiner performs an overall assessment of the patient's level of awareness. Level of consciousness and degree of orientation to person, place, time, and situation are assessed. Concurrent with the mental status examination, the emergency physician learns of any deficiencies of speech that may be present. Dysarthria (slurred speech) is readily detected, as are more profound language deficits, such as receptive aphasia (the patient cannot understand what is being said) or expressive aphasia (the patient cannot get his or her words out).

Cranial nerves

A quick, systematic assessment of CN function follows the mental status examination. The emergency physician tests for visual field deficits by confrontation (examiner faces the patient and slowly brings moving fingers in from the sides until the patient detects them), examines pupillary light reflexes, then tests all extraocular movements (CN II, III, IV, VI). The examiner has the patient smile and looks for facial palsy (droop), and also tests facial sensation (CN V, VII). Testing swallowing and symmetrical palate rise (CN IX, X), shoulder shrugging (CN XI), and tongue deviation while the tongue protrudes from the mouth (CN XII) completes the CN examination.

Motor function

The strength examination assesses strength in all four extremities. Marked strength deficits may be detected on examination and are graded according to a 5-point scale (Table 40.3). Subtle strength deficits may be more difficult to elicit. Evaluation for the presence of *pronator drift* may be helpful to

Table 40.3 Strength scale 0–5

Grade	Description
0	No discernable movement
1	Trace movement detected
2	Movement with force of gravity taken away by assistance
3	Movement against gravity
4	Movement against added resistance but less than normal strength
5	Normal strength

Table 40.4 Deep tendon reflex scale (0–4)

Grade	Description
0	Reflexes are absent
1	Reflexes are diminished but present
2	Normal reflexes
3	Reflexes are increased
4	Clonus present

detect very mild strength deficits of the proximal upper extremities. The examiner has the patient hold both arms out 90° with palms up and eyes closed and watches for slight pronation of either forearm.

An overall assessment of function is also helpful to the examiner. Subtle deficiencies of motor strength may be identified with somewhat more difficult motor tasks, such as tiptoe walking, heel walking, or rapid alternating movements. Difficulty rising from a chair or stool or with brushing hair may identify proximal muscle weakness associated with myopathies. Fatigability of a particular motor function (with initially normal strength) points to a disturbance at the neuromuscular junction (MG).

Sensory function

The sensory examination is arguably the least important component of the emergency neurologic examination; therefore, the examiner need not spend an inordinate amount of time testing sensation. A brief assessment of fine touch suffices in the emergent setting. If deficits are detected, more time may be taken to delineate exact distributions of sensory disturbances. If time allows, assessment of vibratory sensation, 2-point discrimination, and sharp/dull discrimination may be performed but is usually not essential in the emergent setting.

Reflexes

The emergency physician's assessment of deep tendon reflexes (DTRs) should include reflex testing in both upper and lower extremities. Reflexes are graded on a 0–4 point scale (Table 40.4). Absence of lower extremity reflexes in the setting of acute bilateral lower extremity weakness is a hallmark of GBS. Peripheral reflexes of a particular myotome may be diminished or absent in a peripheral neuropathy or radiculopathy compression syndrome. Asymmetric hyperreflexia and/or clonus (extreme hyperreflexia with the presence of repetitive contraction of a muscle group) may be seen with CNS lesions. *Babinski's sign* (dorsiflexion of the great toe and fanning of the other toes when the plantar aspect of the foot is stroked) may be present in CNS lesions as well.

Cerebellar function

Finally, the emergency physician should examine the patient for cerebellar dysfunction. Coordination tests such as finger-to-nose coordination and heel-to-shin coordination are performed. In the able patient, standard gait is assessed along with heel-to-toe walking. Difficulty in coordination may be quite apparent on examination of rapid alternating movements (dysdiadochokinesia).

The National Institutes of Health Stroke Scale (NIHSS)

In the AIS patient, an adjunct to the standard neurologic examination may be used. The National Institutes of Health Stroke Scale (NIHSS) is a 42-point scale which focuses on and grades level of consciousness, visual function, motor function, sensation and neglect, language, and cerebellar integrity (Table 40.5). It therefore closely mirrors the standard neurologic examination already discussed. As can be seen from the scale, the higher the score, the worse the neurologic deficit associated with ongoing stroke. The NIHSS can provide insight into the location and severity of underlying ischemic stroke, and has been shown to be a strong initial predictor of overall clinical outcome. Perhaps most important, its use provides emergency physicians a powerful and accurate means of communication with the stroke team or neurology consultants.

Table 40.5 The National Institutes of Health Stroke Scale

	Category	Description	Score
1a	Level of consciousness (LOC)	Alert Drowsy Stuporous Coma	0 1 2 3
1b	LOC questions (month, age)	Answers both correctly Answers one correctly Incorrect on both	0 1 2
1c	LOC commands (open/close eyes, show thumb)	Obeys both correctly Obeys one correctly Incorrect on both	0 1 2
2	Best gaze (follow finger)	Normal Partial gaze palsy Forced deviation	0 1 2
3	Best visual (visual fields)	No visual loss Partial hemianopia Complete hemianopia Bilateral hemianopsia	0 1 2 3
4	Facial palsy (show teeth, raise brows, squeeze eyes shut)	Normal Minor Partial Complete	0 1 2 3
5	Motor arm left[a] (raise 90°, hold 10 seconds)	No drift Drift Cannot resist gravity No effort against gravity No movement	0 1 2 3 4
6	Motor arm right[a] (raise 90°, hold 10 seconds)	No drift Drift Cannot resist gravity No effort against gravity No movement	0 1 2 3 4
7	Motor leg left[a] (raise 30°, hold 5 seconds)	No drift Drift Cannot resist gravity No effort against gravity No movement	0 1 2 3 4
8	Motor leg right[a] (raise 30°, hold 5 seconds)	No drift Drift Cannot resist gravity No effort against gravity No movement	0 1 2 3 4
9	Limb ataxia	Absent Present in one limb Present in two limbs	0 1 2
10	Sensory (fine touch to face, arm, leg)	Normal Partial loss Severe loss	0 1 2
11	Extinction/neglect (double simultaneous testing)	No neglect Partial neglect Complete neglect	0 1 2
12	Dysarthria (speech clarity to "mama, baseball, huckleberry, tip-top, fifty-fifty")	Normal articulation Mild to moderate dysarthria Near to unintelligible or worse	0 1 2
13	Best language[b] (name items, describe pictures)	No aphasia Mild to moderate aphasia Severe aphasia Mute	0 1 2 3
	Total (0–42)		

[a] For limbs with amputation, joint fusion, etc. score a "9" and explain.
[b] For intubation or other physical barrier to speech, score a "9" and explain.

Differential diagnosis

Tables 40.6 and 40.7. provide diagnostic possibilities and suggested evaluations for patients with weakness.

Table 40.6 Differential diagnosis of acute ischemic stroke or transient ischemic attack

Diagnosis	Symptoms	Signs	Work-up
Arterial dissection syndromes	Patients usually present with focal motor weakness accompanied by severe tearing pain in the anterior neck and jaw (carotid dissection), posterior neck and back of head (vertebral dissection), chest and/or back (thoracic aortic dissection), or abdomen and/or back (abdominal aortic dissection).	Hypertension is frequently present. Focal motor weakness follows distribution of artery(ies) affected and may involve an entire cerebrovascular distribution. Asymmetric BP and/or unequal pulses in extremities may be present with aortic dissection.	BP measurement in all four extremities for aortic dissection. CT scanning of chest and/or abdomen with IV contrast (vascular surgeon should be emergently consulted prior to imaging if clinical suspicion high). Angiography preferred for suspected carotid or vertebral dissection, as MRA may miss some dissections.
Bell's palsy	Patients complain of unilateral facial droop, eye pain (from dry eyes), hyperacusis (extreme sensitivity to noise), taste abnormalities, and sometimes retroauricular pain. History of recent upper respiratory infection may be obtained.	Peripheral 7th (facial) nerve palsy is found on examination (ipsilateral upper and lower facial motor weakness present). Conjunctivitis/keratitis may be present on affected side.	Diagnosis of Bell's palsy is clinical. Appropriate treatment and urgent referral are important to initiate from the ED.
Complicated migraine headache	Patients are often young peripartum females with history of migraine headaches. Patients present with symptoms of migraine headache (with or without pain, photophobia, phonophobia, nausea or vomiting) plus neurologic deficit.	Neurologic deficit may consist of focal motor weakness, sensory abnormality, aphasia, ataxia, or all of the above and may perfectly mimic a hemispheric stroke.	Diagnosis of exclusion. Demographic information provides clue. Subarachnoid hemorrhage must be ruled out in patients without history of complicated migraines.
Epidural/ subdural hematoma	Classic history for epidural hematoma is head trauma with loss of consciousness followed by lucid period, then declining mental status with eventual comatose state. Subdural hematoma usually a subacute process following head injury or repeated trauma. Headache, nausea, vomiting, and other symptoms of increase ICP may be present.	Focal neurologic deficit may be present depending on location of hematoma. When hematoma is large enough to cause mass effect, Cushing's response may be observed. Abnormal pupil examination may be helpful in comatose patient.	CT scan of head is very sensitive for acute epidural and subdural hematoma. Epidural hematoma appears as a convex blood collection between dura and skull which does not cross suture lines. Subdural hematomas have a more concave or flattened appearance and may cross sutures lines.
Encephalitis/ meningitis	Patients may complain of fever, severe headache, neck pain/ stiffness, photophobia, and general malaise. History of recent infectious illness may be present. With acute encephalitis, patients may present with altered mental status.	Fever, nuchal rigidity, and photophobia may be found on examination. Petechial rash may be seen with meningococcus. In severe cases seizures may be observed. Stupor and coma may be present. Focal motor weakness/aphasia may be present but are uncommon.	In all patients with suspected meningitis or encephalitis, diagnostic lumbar puncture is essential. Antibiotics/ antiviral agents should be administered as soon as possible.

(continued)

Table 40.6 Differential diagnosis of acute ischemic stroke or transient ischemic attack (*cont*)

Diagnosis	Symptoms	Signs	Work-up
Hyperglycemia	Antecedent polyuria, polyphagia, and polydipsia may be elicited on history. General malaise and extreme thirst with dehydration may be present. Often patients are elderly diabetics with difficulty caring for themselves.	Variable and similar to hypoglycemia. Focal neurologic deficits are uncommon but hyperglycemia should be considered in the patient with focal weakness. Fever may be present from concurrent infectious illness contributing to poor glycemic control.	Immediate bedside serum glucose measurement is warranted in all patients with altered mental status or focal neurologic deficits.
Hypertensive encephalopathy	Patients present with symptoms of diffuse cerebral dysfunction and may be confused or comatose. When lucid, patients often complain of headache, visual problems, and/or focal neurologic deficits. Shortness of breath may be present secondary to pulmonary edema.	Severe hypertension is present with diastolic pressure typically greater than 130 mmHg. Focal neurologic deficits may be found on physical examination. Signs of CNS dysfunction such as stupor, coma, or seizures may be present.	Hypertensive encephalopathy is a clinical diagnosis in the setting of severe hypertension. Ongoing intracerebral hemorrhage should be sought with head CT. Cocaine-induced sympathomimetic toxidrome should be considered.
Hypoglycemia	Variable: patient may present along spectrum from agitated to comatose, with global weakness to a focal neurologic deficit. May perfectly mimic virtually any neurologic illness.	Also variable; focal or generalized weakness may be found on examination. Seizure activity may occur. Hypothermia may be present. Diaphoresis is common.	Immediate bedside serum glucose measurement is warranted in all patients with altered mental status or focal neurologic deficits.
Hyponatremia/ uremia	Symptoms vary from paresthesias to diffuse weakness/fatigue to focal motor weakness. History of renal failure may be offered.	Variable presentation. Focal motor findings are less common than subjective weakness and paresthesias but may be present.	Electrolyte panel with renal function in the appropriate clinical setting confirms the diagnosis.
Intracerebral hemorrhage	Severe headache usually of sudden onset. History of poorly-controlled hypertension common. Patient may present obtunded with sonorous respirations.	Hypertension is frequently present. Focal motor weakness may be found and coincides with affected hemorrhagic distributions. With large hemorrhage causing mass effect, Cushing's response may be observed.	CT scan of head is very sensitive for acute intracerebral hemorrhage. Lumbar puncture should follow a negative head CT in patients with suspected SAH.
Neoplasm	Patients may present with acute or subacute weakness and give a history of long-standing headaches. Acute severe headache with weakness may occur with sudden neoplastic hemorrhage. Symptoms of increased ICP may be present.	Signs are largely variable. When motor weakness is present, distribution may follow along hemispheric pattern depending on location of tumor. Cranial nerve impairment often present with brainstem tumor. Signs of increased ICP may be present.	CT scan of head fairly helpful in detecting major neoplasm, but further radiographic evaluation such as MRI usually needed to delineate mass. CT head very sensitive for hemorrhagic neoplasms.
Psychiatric	*Variable*: history of psychiatric illness or prior similar presentation helpful. Secondary gain may be an issue or patient may not be consciously producing symptoms (conversion disorder).	*Variable*: physical examination "tricks" useful to delineate true motor weakness from psychogenic weakness. Conversion disorder very difficult to identify.	High index of suspicion with psychiatric history helpful. Always a diagnosis of exclusion when stroke symptoms are mimicked.

(continued)

Table 40.6 Differential diagnosis of acute ischemic stroke or transient ischemic attack (*cont*)

Diagnosis	Symptoms	Signs	Work-up
Septic embolus with bacterial endocarditis	Patients may present with fever, general malaise, and focal weakness. A history of valvular heart disease and/or IV drug abuse may be elicited.	Classic findings in acute bacterial endocarditis include fever, heart murmur, Roth's spots, splinter hemorrhages, Janeway lesions, and Osler's nodes. CNS emboli give rise to hemispheric strokes and resulting focal motor weakness and/or hemiparesis.	Work-up includes head CT, which may demonstrate multiple infarctions caused by showering of emboli. Diagnosis made based on three sets of positive blood cultures and transesophageal echocardiography in the appropriate clinical setting. Urinalysis often abnormal.
Todd's (postictal) paralysis	The key is the history of having had a seizure. Following seizure, patient presents with focal neurologic deficit(s).	Any array of neurologic deficits may be present including focal motor weakness, sensory loss, ataxia, aphasia, or all of those listed, mimicking hemispheric stroke. Postictal decreased level of consciousness may be present.	Diagnosis of exclusion and based on history. Traumatic brain injury with or without epidural or subdural hematoma must be considered in patient with unknown history. Drug levels should be sent to ensure therapeutic levels, and other causes of seizure should be entertained.
Toxocologic	*Variable*: depends on particular toxin.	*Variable*: depends in particular toxin. Focal motor weakness may be observed with a number of toxins.	When toxin suspected, toxicology screens and/or specific toxin levels are ordered.
Trauma	*Variable*: depends on injuries present.	*Variable*: depends on injuries present. Focal neurologic deficits may be present with peripheral arterial/nerve injuries, while hemispheric deficits may be seen with intracranial injuries. Spinal cord injuries may present with profound sensory/motor deficit at level of lesion, or may demonstrate central cord syndromes.	A thorough work-up of any trauma patient with neurologic deficits is essential. Emergent head CT, peripheral angiography, or spinal MRI may be needed depending on specific injuries/deficits noted.

BP: blood pressure; CNS: central nervous system; CT: computed tomography; ED: emergency department; ICP: intracranial pressure; IV: intravenous; MRA: magnetic resonance angiography; MRI: magnetic resonance imaging; SAH: subarachnoid hemorrhage.

Table 40.7 Differential diagnosis: other selected causes of motor weakness

Diagnosis	Symptoms	Signs	Work-up
Acute transverse myelitis	Patients may present with rapidly developing paraparesis and sensory level deficit with or without severe acute back pain. Accompanying bladder and bowel dysfunction is common. Acute onset implies a vascular etiology, while subacute onset may indicate cord compression syndrome from underlying neoplasm.	*Variable examination findings may be seen*: signs similar to spinal cord injury predominate including paraparesis/paraplegia, sensory level deficit, diminished rectal tone, and combinations. Examination consistent with complete cord transection uncommon.	Diagnosis suggested by clinical presentation. Emergent MRI essential to identify underlying compressing lesions such as epidural abscess, epidural hematoma, tumor, or herniated disk. Cord infarction may also be identified on MRI. Work-up for MS as etiology indicated if other work-up does not identify cause. *(continued)*

Table 40.7 Differential diagnosis: other selected causes of motor weakness (*cont*)

Diagnosis	Symptoms	Signs	Work-up
Amyotrophic lateral sclerosis	Hallmark of ALS is exhibition of UMN and LMN symptoms in progressive severity over time. Patients may complain of progressive stiffness, slowed speech, and explosive laughter (UMN symptoms) and/or muscle weakness, muscle wasting, cramping, and fasciculations (LMN symptoms). Ocular and sensory complaints uncommon.	Muscle weakness with hyper-reflexia may be observed. Muscle atrophy and asymmetric weakness may be seen on examination. In advanced cases, respiratory distress from involvement of breathing musculature may be observed. Babinski sign may be present. Sensation usually preserved.	Diagnosis of ALS is based on clinical presentation with gradual severe progression over time and UMN and LMN signs present.
Botulism	Presentation depends on type: *Infantile botulism*: patient is less than 1-year old and presents with poor feeding, constipation, weakness, and failure-to-thrive. This form of botulism is associated with the child's ingestion of honey contaminated with the infectious spores of the bacteria *C. botulinum*. *Food-borne botulism*: associated with ingestion of inadequately sterilized home-canned vegetables. Patients present with visual disturbances, dysarthria, dysphonia, dysphagia, and a severe symmetric descending limb paralysis. *Wound botulism*: presents similarly; patients have a history of a wound, often a history of IV drug abuse.	Patients generally exhibit normal mentation with multiple CN abnormalities (diplopia, ptosis, absent pupillary light reflex) along with profound descending bilateral motor weakness. DTRs are usually intact. Weakness of the neck muscles is common. In severe cases respiratory distress may be present.	Diagnosis suspected with historical factors of honey ingestion in the infant and home-canned vegetables in others. Large numbers of patients presenting with symptoms and signs of botulism should prompt alert of terrorist activity. Diagnosis may be confirmed with identification of botulinum toxin in serum, stool, food, or with stool cultures positive for *C. botulinum*. With wound botulism, serum studies are useful, as are wound cultures positive for the bacteria.
Dermatomyositis	Presenting complaints are similar to those with polymyositis with the addition of rash.	Similar findings to polymyositis with presence of rash. Classic rash is reddish-purple discoloration of the upper eyelids (heliotrope rash) associated with periorbital edema. Scaly erythematous plaques and papules may be seen, especially over the knuckles (Gottron's papules).	Diagnosis confirmed with same testing for polymyositis. Concomitant malignancy should be considered.
Dyskalemic periodic paralysis	Patients may present with localized or generalized motor weakness. Attacks may occur after carbohydrate-laden meal, during rest after strenuous exercise, or during sleep with weakness apparent on awakening. Cold weather may also provoke motor weakness. Attacks may last	Generalized or focal motor weakness may be observed. Diminished or absent DTRs are found on examination. Respiratory difficulties and CN abnormalities are not commonly seen.	With primary (inherited) disorders, a family history of similar episodic weakness is highly suggestive of dyskalemic periodic paralysis. Serum potassium levels may be low, normal, or high, but hypokalemic periodic paralysis is most common.

(continued)

Table 40.7 Differential diagnosis: other selected causes of motor weakness (*cont*)

Diagnosis	Symptoms	Signs	Work-up
Dyskalemic periodic paralysis (*cont*)	less than an hour or for several days. With generalized attacks, the weakness usually spreads from proximal to distal. Typically patients present with their first attack in their first or second decade of life.		Potassium-wasting processes and thyrotoxicosis must be ruled out. The administration of glucose and insulin may provoke an attack within 2–3 hours.
Guillain–Barré syndrome	Ascending paralysis is the hallmark symptom. Patients usually in third or fourth decade of life. Antecedent viral illness 2–3 weeks prior to GBS may be reported. Numbness or tingling in lower extremities may precede ascending weakness. GI infection with *Campylobacter jejuni* may precede illness by 1–3 weeks. Shortness of breath may be a complaint in severe cases. *Miller–Fischer variant* presents as descending paralysis with ataxia/ophthalmoplegia.	Bilateral motor weakness of the lower extremities in ascending pattern over time (may be unilateral). Absence of lower extremity DTRs is a key finding. Sensory deficits may occur but motor findings predominate. CN abnormalities may be present in severe disease. Respiratory distress may be seen in severe cases.	Clinical picture largely makes the diagnosis. CSF studies may demonstrate markedly elevated protein levels without pleocytosis; may not be abnormal early in disease course. FVC and NIF used at bedside to predict impending respiratory failure.
Heavy metal toxicity	Presentation usually vague; high clinical suspicion needed. Patients may complain of generalized motor weakness with abdominal pain, muscle aches, memory loss, peripheral edema, and skin rash on hands and feet.	Patients may exhibit sensory loss in a stocking-glove distribution, hyperpigmentation of palms and soles, and delirium on physical examination.	High clinical suspicion needed. Abdominal radiograph may demonstrate radiopaque metallic flecks. Laboratories may show anemia, leukopenia, eosinophilia, and basophilic stippling. Hair and nail clippings may be evaluated for arsenic levels (the most common acute metal poisoning). In acute poisoning urine arsenic levels may be measured.
Lambert–Eaton syndrome	Variant of myasthenic syndrome most commonly seen in patients with underlying malignancy, usually small-cell lung cancer. Weakness in the limbs and girdle musculature predominates with relative sparing of the bulbar musculature. Dysphagia may be seen. Autonomic dysfunction commonly causes symptoms of dry mouth, taste abnormalities, and impotence.	In contrast to MG, bulbar musculature largely spared. Fatigability less prominent. On examination, strength may actually increase with prolonged contraction. Weakness of pharyngeal musculature may be observed. Reflexes may be decreased or absent.	EMG demonstrates increased response of muscle to each stimulation (in contrast to MG). Tensilon test has no effect, and serology testing for Ach receptor antibodies is negative.
Multiple sclerosis	Monocular visual disturbances common initial complaint (optic neuritis is initial sign in up to 30% of MS patients); diplopia may also be present. Patients may present with a	Many different neurologic abnormalities may be present on examination depending on anatomical pathology of disease. Afferent pupillary defect may be observed with	Diagnosis is suggested by historical data. Symptoms tend to present with exacerbations followed by recovery with progression of disease. Optic findings

(*continued*)

Table 40.7 Differential diagnosis: other selected causes of motor weakness (*cont*)

Diagnosis	Symptoms	Signs	Work-up
Multiple sclerosis (*cont*)	variety of neurologic symptoms including motor weakness, spasticity, paresthesias, and dysautonomic symptoms such as sexual dysfunction and GI/GU symptoms. MS is strongly suggested by two or more prolonged episodes of neurologic dysfunction with intermittent recovery followed by worsening over a period of months. Symptoms commonly worsen with increased ambient temperature, exercise, and fever.	ophthalmoplegia and/or nystagmus. Abnormalities of the optic disk may be observed on fundoscopy. Decreased strength, increased tone, hyperreflexia, and sensory abnormalities may be present in affected distribution. The patient may complain of electrical shock-like pain down the back and into extremities upon neck flexion (Lhermitte's sign).	without other explainable etiologies highly suggestive of MS. CSF studies may demonstrate discrete oligoclonal bands in gamma globulins. Increased latency in visual-evoked potentials may be observed. T2-weighted imaging of MRI often reveals plaques.
Myasthenia gravis	Most common initial symptoms are double vision and/or ptosis causing blurred vision, especially after hours of reading. Complaint of weakness or extreme muscle fatigue with repetitive use is common, especially jaw weakness after prolonged chewing. Dysarthria and dysphagia may be present. Limb weakness predominates in the upper extremities. Symptoms may be temporally related to heat, pregnancy, emotional stress, and infection.	Ptosis and ophthalmoplegia may be observed. On physical examination, extended gaze testing often exacerbates muscle fatigue. Pupillary light reflexes and DTRs are preserved. Hallmark is fluctuating weakness that resolves with rest. *Ice testing* on patient's ptosis (ice packs applied to eyelids for 2–3 minutes resulting in improvement) may aid in diagnosis.	*Tensilon test*: 1–2 mg of edrophonium IV is given. Onset of action is about 30 seconds and its effects last about 5 minutes. If no change or problems are observed, an additional 8 mg is infused (may be given in 4 mg increments). For patients in myasthenic crisis, this maneuver results in increased amounts of Ach at the neuromuscular junction and results in improvement in motor function. EMG and serologic testing for Ach receptor antibodies also aid in diagnosis.
Polymyositis	Patients primarily complain of weakness largely in proximal muscle groups. This may be expressed with difficulties rising from a chair, climbing stairs, brushing hair or teeth, and lifting objects over one's head. Proximal muscle pain may also be present. Patients may complain of dysphagia.	Symmetric motor weakness is observed by testing the functions described (e.g., standing from sitting position). DTRs and sensation are intact. Muscle tenderness may be present.	Serum creatinine kinase and erythrocyte sedimentation rate are increased. Diagnosis is confirmed with EMG studies and muscle biopsy. Concomitant malignancy should be considered.
Tick paralysis	Patients generally present in late spring and early summer in tick-prone areas. Patients may complain of symmetric ascending muscle weakness or difficulties with coordination. Paralysis usually develops 4–7 days after tick attaches. History of camping or hiking in this time frame may be elicited.	Patients may demonstrate profound ascending flaccid paralysis with dysphagia and dysarthria. DTRs may be diminished or absent. Mental status is preserved. The tick is usually still attached and must be searched for in all patients presenting with this clinical picture, especially in high-risk environments.	Diagnosis may be obvious in high-risk patient with attached tick. Clinically, syndrome is difficult to distinguish from GBS without presence of tick, but CSF should be normal in tick paralysis patient. Removal of tick is curative in 24–48 hours and confirms the diagnosis.

Ach: acetylcholine; ALS: amyotrophic lateral sclerosis; *C. botulinum*: *Clostridium botulinum*; CN: cranial nerve; CNS: central nervous system; CSF: cerebrospinal fluid; DTR: deep tendon reflex; EMG: electromyography; FVC: forced vital capacity; GBS: Guillain–Barré syndrome; GI: gastrointestinal; GU: genitourinary; IV: intravenous; LMN: lower motor neuron; MG: myasthenia gravis; MRI: magnetic resonance imaging; MS: multiple sclerosis; NIF: negative inspiratory force; UMN: upper motor neuron.

Diagnostic testing

Laboratory studies

Serum glucose measurement

The most common and convincing stroke or TIA mimic is hypoglycemia. Hypoglycemia must be considered immediately in all patients presenting with acute motor weakness. It should be quickly identified and treated with IV dextrose. Treatment of hypoglycemia usually results in the immediate resolution of neurologic deficits if hypoglycemia is the cause.

Complete blood count

A complete blood count (CBC) is useful for screening for polycythemia-induced hyperviscosity. In addition, the CBC is used to identify patients with thrombocytopenia (an important consideration for thrombolytic treatment in AIS). Certain leukemic or myelodysplastic syndromes may increase a patient's risk for TIA/AIS.

Electrolyte panel

Electrolyte and renal function panels are important for identifying uncommon stroke mimics such as uremia and hyponatremia. Calcium, magnesium, and phosphorus levels should also be routinely checked in the patient with acute motor weakness. Dyskalemic syndromes (most commonly hypokalemic periodic paralysis) may be identified on an electrolyte panel, although serum potassium may be normal.

Coagulation studies

Coagulation studies including International Normalized Ratio (INR) are important in patients taking warfarin, and must be known prior to initiation of thrombolytic or additional anticoagulation therapy.

Creatine kinase

Elevations in serum creatine kinase (CK) may be seen in patients with myopathies such as polymyositis and dermatomyositis. CK levels should be measured in all patients with diffuse motor weakness, especially when proximal muscle weakness or muscle tenderness is present.

Cardiac enzymes

Not uncommonly, AMI occurs concomitantly with AIS and TIA. Embolic strokes may occur as a result of clots arising from the heart, as focal myocardial hypokinesis gives rise to local stasis and clot formation. All AIS patients should therefore be screened for ongoing myocardial infarction.

Erythrocyte sedimentation rate

Erythrocyte sedimentation rate (ESR) is a non-specific marker for inflammatory processes. It may also be elevated in the presence of neoplasm. An elevated ESR may be seen in many disorders causing acute motor weakness, including polymyositis, dermatomyositis, or Lambert–Eaton syndrome (LES).

Cerebrospinal fluid studies

Abnormalities in cerebrospinal fluid (CSF) studies may be used to aid in the diagnosis of some etiologies of acute motor weakness. Markedly elevated CSF protein levels are often detected with GBS. CSF in patients with MS may demonstrate oligoclonal bands in the gamma-globulin region. Patients with transverse myelitis have CSF abnormalities including a markedly elevated white blood cell (WBC) count (>50–100/hpf) along with elevated protein.

Heavy metals

Heavy metal levels are generally not helpful in the acute setting, as most results are not rapidly available to emergency physicians. Therefore, diagnosis of toxicity must be based largely on clinical suspicion. Diagnosis is confirmed with elevated serum levels of the causative agents (i.e., arsenic, lead).

Electrocardiogram

An electrocardiogram (ECG) and cardiac enzyme studies are used to search for concurrent cardiac ischemia. An ECG is also important for the identification of underlying dysrhythmias, especially atrial fibrillation or atrial flutter, which predispose a patient to stroke or TIA. Imbalances of calcium, magnesium, and potassium may be detected on an ECG before laboratory values are obtainable.

Radiologic studies

Head computed tomography

Emergent computed tomography (CT) of the head is by far the most important radiographic study in the evaluation of a patient with AIS. As thrombolytic therapy for ischemic stroke is extremely time-dependent, rapid CT scanning of the head is the highest priority. All efforts should be made towards getting the patient to the scanner and having the CT interpreted as quickly as possible. Thrombolytic therapy treatment algorithms hinge on the presence or absence of intracranial blood on head CT, and this critical determination must be made within 3 hours of onset of the patient's symptoms. Emergent head CT also helps to rule out nonvascular lesions of the brain (neoplasm, subdural hematoma), which may present similarly to stroke or TIA.

In patients presenting with AIS beyond thrombolytic therapeutic time windows, CT scanning of the head remains a useful screening tool for nonvascular lesions, and also helps delineate the anatomical distribution and extent of the stroke. Vasogenic edema or mass effect associated with large ischemic strokes may be seen on head CT and help identify patients at risk for dangerous rises in intracranial pressure.

CT scanning is of little use in patients presenting with generalized weakness. When patients present with signs and symptoms of peripheral neuropathy or radiculopathy, head CT can be avoided.

CT angiography may play an important role in the future of emergent stroke management, but at present remains under investigation.

Carotid duplex scanning

Carotid duplex scanning does not have an important role in the emergent diagnostic work-up of AIS. However, carotid studies may be extremely valuable in the emergent work-up of TIA by identifying patients with significant carotid stenosis amenable to surgical carotid endarterectomy. Since current literature demonstrates that patients with TIA are at great immediate risk for AIS (approximately 10.5% stroke risk at 90 days, 5.3% within 48 hours), it is essential to identify those at greatest risk and those for whom intervention may prevent future stroke. The recommendation of these authors is that carotid duplex studies be performed on all patients presenting with anterior circulation (carotid distribution) TIA before discharge from the hospital.

Echocardiography

Echocardiography is useful to identify cardiac thrombi as a potential origin of embolic cerebral ischemic events. All patients with ischemic stroke or TIA and evidence of cardiac dysrhythmia (e.g., atrial fibrillation) or cardiac ischemia should undergo echocardiography as a part of their work-up.

Magnetic resonance imaging or angiography

Magnetic resonance imaging (MRI) has limited utility in the emergent evaluation of AIS. Availability of emergent MRI is limited at most institutions, and the test is very time-consuming. MRI or magnetic resonance angiography (MRA) is very useful in the evaluation of acute TIA. Subtle changes not identified on CT scanning may be discovered, and MRA adds sensitivity to carotid duplex studies to identify carotid lesions. MRA is essential in the evaluation of posterior circulation TIA, and is the preferred method to evaluate the vertebrobasilar circulation. Newer modalities such as diffusion-weighted MRI are under investigation and may play a greater role in the future evaluation of AIS and TIA.

MRI is of great value in patients presenting with signs and symptoms consistent with acute myelopathy. Acute cord compression syndromes related to epidural abscess, epidural hematoma, mass lesion, or herniated vertebral disk are readily identified on spinal MRI. Spinal cord edema resulting from acute transverse myelitis may also be identified with MRI scanning.

MRI of the brain is useful in the diagnosis of MS. On T2-weighted imaging, discrete white matter lesions (plaques) are visible in greater than 85% of patients with MS.

Other studies

Tensilon test

The tensilon test is specifically used in making the diagnosis of MG. To perform this test, the physician administers 1–2 mg of edrophonium (a short-acting acetylcholinesterase inhibitor) IV and watches for signs of improvement in the patient's weakness. The onset of action of edrophonium is about 30 seconds and its effects last about 5 minutes. If no change or problems are observed, an additional 8 mg is infused (may be given in 4 mg increments). For patients in myasthenic crisis, this maneuver results in increased amounts of acetylcholine (Ach) at the neuromuscular junction and results in improvement in motor function. Caution must be used with the tensilon test, as significantly increased amounts of Ach may result in cholinergic crisis with life-threatening bradycardia, atrioventricular block, bronchorrhea, and other symptoms (diarrhea, salivation, lacrimation). Atropine may be used to reverse toxicity. In patients with MG who are already on cholinesterase inhibitor therapy, even greater caution must be used as these patients may present with weakness resulting from underlying medication-induced cholinergic crisis.

Pulmonary function testing

Though not commonly utilized by emergency physicians, bedside pulmonary function testing (forced vital capacity (FVC), negative inspiratory force (NIF)) may be useful in the patient with motor weakness contributing to marked respiratory difficulty. In the patient with severe GBS or MG, progressive respiratory failure may require emergent mechanical ventilation. The decision of whether to intubate the patient may be difficult, as these patients are usually able to compensate well with tachypnea and accessory musculature use.

The use of routine measures of respiratory function such as pulse oximetry and arterial blood gases generally does not render an accurate picture of the degree of respiratory failure in these patients. By the time a drop in pulse oximetry and rise in PCO_2 are detected, the patient may be well beyond the need for mechanical assistance. The need for mechanical intervention may be identified earlier with the measurement of FVC and NIF by a respiratory therapist. Generally, an FVC below 10 ml/kg or NIF below 20 cmH₂O indicates the need for emergent mechanical ventilation.

Swallowing studies

Aspiration pneumonia is a major contributor to the morbidity and mortality of stroke patients. All patients with AIS/TIA should undergo formal swallowing evaluation before oral intake of any kind is allowed.

General treatment principles
Airway, breathing, circulation (ABCs)

In general, most patients presenting to the ED with AIS or TIA do not have problems with airway, breathing, or circulatory status. Exceptions arise in patients who present 2–5 days after a large ischemic stroke, when ischemia-related cerebral edema begins to exert mass effect.

Acute ischemic stroke
Oxygen

No benefit has been observed with the routine administration of oxygen to patients with AIS. Conversely, some evidence exists which suggests that supranormal oxygenation may worsen outcome. Therefore, supplemental oxygen should be reserved for patients with hypoxia in the setting of AIS.

Hyperthermia

Hyperthermia should be treated in all stroke patients, as elevated core temperature is known to be harmful in the setting of AIS. Conversely, there are studies that have demonstrated a decrease in infarct size with lower core temperatures. The presence of fever in the setting of stroke should prompt emergency physicians to consider and investigate concurrent infectious conditions.

Glucose control

Hypoglycemia in the setting of acute motor weakness requires immediate treatment with IV dextrose, which usually resolves ongoing symptoms rapidly. Some studies have found that hyperglycemia may worsen overall stroke outcome by aggravating ongoing neuronal ischemia. Therefore, serum glucose levels greater than 300 mg/dl should be treated with insulin.

Hypertension

The management of hypertension in the setting of AIS is somewhat controversial. There is general agreement that elevated BPs should not be aggressively lowered in patients with ongoing AIS or TIA. Many stroke/TIA patients have underlying chronic hypertension and limited autoregulatory capabilities of cerebral circulation. In ischemic situations, the acute lowering of BP may decrease cerebral perfusion and collateral circulation further, leading to infarct extension and acceleration of neuronal injury.

Special situations such as ongoing AMI, hypertensive encephalopathy, aortic dissection, congestive heart failure, acute renal failure, and thrombolytic therapy for ischemic stroke may be present and call for careful hypertensive control in the setting of stroke. In these situations, easily titratable pharmacologic agents are preferred (Table 40.8), and medications that precipitously drop BP should be avoided. The management of hypertension in candidates for thrombolytic therapy is quite different from these other conditions.

Table 40.8 Pharmacologic agents recommended for BP control in non-thrombolytic candidates

DBP > 140 mmHg	Sodium nitroprusside (0.5 mcg/kg/minute). Carefully reduce pressure by 10–20%
SBP > 220 or DBP > 121–140 or MAP > 130 mmHg	Labetalol 10–20 mg IV push over 1–2 minutes. May repeat or double every 10 minutes to maximum dose of 150 mg. Enalapril 1.25 mg IV push may also be used
SBP < 220 DBP ≤ 120 or MAP < 130 mmHg	Antihypertensive therapy indicated only if ongoing AMI, severe CHF, aortic dissection, acute renal failure, hypertensive encephalopathy

AMI: acute myocardial infarction; CHF: congestive heart failure; DBP: diastolic blood pressure; IV: intravenous; MAP: mean arterial pressure; SBP: systolic blood pressure.

Aspirin

The role of antiplatelet medications in the treatment of AIS remains under debate. In the large International Stroke Trial, aspirin treatment provided no significant benefit with regard to death or disability at 2 week or 6 month outcome measures. However, in the same trial there was significant reduction in the recurrence rate of ischemic stroke. Based on this finding and other data, it is currently recommended that aspirin therapy following AIS begin within 48 hours of stroke onset to help prevent recurrent ischemic stroke.

Aspirin use before the administration of thrombolytics is not a contraindication to thrombolytic therapy; however, the theoretical increase in hemorrhage risk precludes the routine use of aspirin in thrombolytic candidates. Aspirin is held for 24 hours following the administration of thrombolytic therapy before being added back to the patient's daily regimen (50–325 mg). Oral aspirin should be withheld to avoid aspiration until formal swallowing evaluation is completed.

Anticoagulation

The use of unfractionated and low-molecular weight heparins (LMWH) for the initial management of AIS is somewhat controversial. The current literature, most notably the International Stroke Trial, does not support the administration of unfractionated heparins, as no published data demonstrate sustained improved in clinical outcome for ischemic stroke with their use.

LMWH has been studied as well; similarly, there has been no sustained improved clinical outcome for AIS to date with the use of LMWH. Many clinical trials have shown a significant decrease in the incidence of deep venous thrombosis (DVT) and pulmonary embolism (PE) following AIS with the use of LMWH, and its use should be considered for thromboembolic complications of bedridden stroke victims.

Thrombolytics

Background

A discussion of thrombolytic therapy for AIS is incomplete without mention of the landmark study that propelled IV tissue plasminogen activator (t-PA) into the stroke care provider's armamentarium. In 1995, the National Institute of Neurological Disorders and Stroke (NINDS) Study Group published the results of the NINDS trial of t-PA for AIS. Using recombinant t-PA (rt-PA) under a specific set of guidelines, the NINDS investigators demonstrated a significant improvement in clinical outcome at 3 months for patients with AIS.

The NINDS trial consisted of two major parts. Part I enrolled 291 patients and appraised the efficacy of rt-PA based on a 4-point improvement in NIHSS score or complete resolution of neurologic deficit at 24 hours following treatment. Although Part I did not demonstrate significant improvement in 24 hours, there was a statistically significant benefit found at 3 months for the treatment group in four separate outcome measures (NIHSS, modified Rankin scale, Glasgow outcome scale, and Barthel Index). Part II of the NINDS trial followed, enrolling 333 patients and confirming significant clinical improvement at 3 months for AIS patients found in Part I. In a later publication, the significant improvement in clinical outcome was sustained at 1-year follow-up. Overall, AIS patients treated with rt-PA within the strict parameters of the NINDS trial were found to be 30% more likely to have minimal or no disability compared to the placebo group at 3 months and 1 year outcome measures.

The most feared complication of thrombolytic therapy for stroke is symptomatic intracerebral hemorrhage. In the NINDS trial, the incidence of symptomatic intracerebral hemorrhage (ICH) occurred ten-fold times higher in the treatment group compared to placebo (6.4% vs. 0.6%). However, there was no significance difference in mortality at 3 months between the treatment and placebo groups in the trial (17% and 21%, respectively) and no increase in the severely disabled group was observed.

Since 1996 there have been other trials in the US and Canada that have attempted to reproduce the results of the NINDS trial. Research continues to further determine the optimal pharmacotherapy for AIS. At present, there remains only one therapy approved by the FDA. Based on the available data, the treatment of AIS with thrombolytic therapy carries the Grade A recommendation of the Stroke Council of the American Heart Association and currently provides the best hope for an improved outcome for stroke patients.

Administration of intravenous tissue plasminogen activator for acute ischemic stroke

Having made the diagnosis of AIS, the emergency physician should consider thrombolytic therapy with the help of neurology or stroke team consultants. The therapeutic window for IV t-PA lies within 3 hours from stroke symptom onset. This window must be strictly adhered to in order to optimize outcome and minimize the incidence of ICH. The inclusion and exclusion criteria for thrombolytic therapy are reviewed (Table 40.9). Extensive discussion with the patient and family must take place to provide all available information necessary to make an informed decision. Primarily, this conversation revolves around the potential benefits the patient may have with thrombolytic therapy, as well as the risks the patient will be exposed to by thrombolytic administration. After these discussions take place and the individual risk/benefit profile of the patient is assessed, the decision whether to treat with thrombolytic therapy is made. The dose of IV t-PA for AIS is 0.9 mg/kg (90 mg maximum dose) with 10% of total dose given IV over 1–2 minutes and the remaining 90% infused over 1 hour.

T-PA may also be given intra-arterially (IA t-PA) at the site of the vaso-occlusive clot by skilled interventional neuroradiologists in specialized centers with this capability. The therapeutic window for IA t-PA extends out to 6 hours

Table 40.9 Indications and contraindications to thrombolytic therapy in acute ischemic stroke

Indications
- Acute ischemic stroke within 3 hours from symptom onset.
- Age greater than 18 years (recombinant tissue plasminogen activator has not been studied in pediatric stroke).

Contraindications
- Evidence of intracranial hemorrhage on pretreatment evaluation.
- Suspicion of subarachnoid hemorrhage.
- Recent stroke, intracranial or intraspinal surgery, or serious head trauma in the past 3 months.
- Major surgery or serious trauma in the previous 14 days[*].
- Arterial puncture at a noncompressible site or lumbar puncture in the last 7 days[*].
- Major symptoms that are rapidly improving or only minor stroke symptoms[*].
- History of intracranial hemorrhage.
- Uncontrolled hypertension at the time of treatment.
- Seizure at the stroke onset.
- Active internal bleeding.
- Intracranial neoplasm, arteriovenous malformation, or aneurysm.
- Known bleeding diathesis including but not limited to:
  - Current use of anticoagulants or an International Normalized Ratio >1.7 or Prothrombin time >15 seconds.
  - Administration of heparin within 48 hours preceding the onset of stroke and an elevated activated partial thromboplastin time at presentation.
  - Platelet count <100,000 mm³.

[*] In the National Institute of Neurological Disorders and Stroke trial; not present in current package insert.

following ischemic stroke onset according to present research. If this therapy is available either in the treating emergency physician's institution or a nearby referral center, IA t-PA should be carefully considered as possible therapy for AIS.

Management of hypertension in thrombolytic candidates requires special attention, as uncontrolled hypertension is a contraindication to thrombolytic therapy. Before treatment with t-PA can be considered, the pretreatment BP must be gently lowered to a systolic pressure less than 185 mmHg and a diastolic pressure less than 110 mmHg. Recommendations for the management of hypertension in the thrombolytic candidate are based on Advanced Cardiac Life Support (ACLS) guidelines (Table 40.10). If aggressive means are required to hold the patient's BP within the accepted guidelines, consideration of thrombolytic therapy must be aborted as uncontrolled

Table 40.10 Emergent antihypertensive therapies in acute ischemic stroke (for thrombolytic candidates)

Pretreatment	
SBP > 185 mmHg or DBP > 110 mmHg	Labetalol 10–20 mg IVP, 1–2 doses or nitroglycerin paste 1–2" or enalapril 1.25 mg IVP
Post-treatment[*]	
DBP > 140 mmHg	Sodium nitroprusside (0.5 mcg/kg/minute)
SBP > 230 mmHg or DBP 121–140 mmHg	Labetalol 10–20 mg IVP and consider a labetalol drip at 1–2 mg/minute
SBP 180–230 mmHg or DBP 105–120 mmHg	Labetalol 10 mg IVP, may repeat and double up to a maximum dose of 150 mg

DBP: diastolic blood pressure; SBP: systolic blood pressure; IVP: intravenous push.

[*]Monitor vitals every 15 minutes × 2 hours, then every 30 minutes × 6 hours, then every hour × 16 hours;

hypertension is associated with a greatly increased risk of intracranial hemorrhage.

Post-treatment considerations

Admission to a specialized neurointensive care unit should occur as soon as possible following thrombolytic therapy. Neurologic exams and BP monitoring must be performed at regular intervals. If such monitoring is unavailable, transfer to an appropriate facility should be considered.

Transient ischemic attack

There is no specific emergency treatment for acute TIA. Most importantly, the emergency physician must recognize the immediate significant risk for imminent AIS that TIA represents. Recent literature suggests that the risk of AIS following TIA is approximately 10.5% within 3 months, with about half of these ischemic strokes occurring within the first 48 hours following TIA. A complete work-up with neurology consultation and advancement of antiplatelet therapy is recommended. If the patient is already on a maximum antiplatelet regimen (aspirin plus clopidogrel, aspirin plus dypyridamole, etc.) then anticoagulation with warfarin is considered. For TIA patients in whom a critical carotid stenosis is discovered on carotid duplex studies, surgical carotid endarterectomy should be considered.

Guillain–Barré syndrome

In patients with GBS, special attention should be paid to identify involvement of the respiratory muscles. Ventilatory assistance is necessary when the patient's FVC falls below 1 liter. Respiratory failure requiring mechanical ventilation occurs in nearly 20% of patients with GBS.

Further therapy, generally initiated on an inpatient basis, involves immunosuppression because of the immune and inflammatory components of the disease. Such treatment continues to be studied and includes plasma exchange with the removal of 200–250 ml/kg over 7–10 days. Intravenous immunoglobulin (IVIG) may also be given at 0.4 g/kg/day for 5 days. Both plasma exchange and IVIG should be started early, as they have been shown to stop progression of the symptoms and accelerate recovery. CSF filtration is currently being studied, but remains controversial at this time. DVT prophylaxis is warranted, as thromboembolism causes significant morbidity and mortality in patients with GBS. There is no evidence supporting the use of corticosteroid therapy in GBS.

Myasthenia gravis

The emergency physician must recognize and manage the acute deterioration of a patient with MG based on clinical findings. As with GBS, observing the patient for respiratory compromise is of the utmost importance. Intubation is usually required if FVC falls below 1 liter. If endotracheal intubation is necessary, depolarizing paralytic agents should be avoided.

Once the airway is appropriately managed, further therapy is considered. In a known MG patient in myasthenic crisis, reasons for the exacerbation need to be determined and appropriately managed. This includes identifying and treating any source of infection, reducing elevated environmental and body temperatures, and controlling emotional stress. Once a patient is found to be in myasthenic crisis with a positive tensilon test, drugs designed to increase the amount of Ach at the neuromuscular junction can be initiated. Acetylcholinesterase inhibitors are the primary agents used; they act to increase available Ach thereby reaching a critical threshold of activated Ach receptors needed to enhance muscle activity and improve strength. Pyridostigmine can be used at an initial dose of 60 mg every 4–6 hours per os (PO). If patient is intubated or is nulla per os (NPO), IV pyridostigmine can be used at one-thirteenth the dose. Neostigmine is an alternate acetylcholinesterase inhibitor and can be administered at the dose of 0.5 mg IV or 15 mg PO. Both of these medications may cause increased airway resistance in patients with concomitant asthma or chronic obstructive pulmonary disease (COPD). The use of inhaled ipratropium may help prevent this side effect. If patients are not responding to acetylcholinesterase inhibitors, steroids are added. However, they may take weeks to have an effect and are not practical in the acute setting. Other therapies available outside of the ED include thymectomy, plasma exchange, and IVIG. The reason for improvement in MG patients after a thymectomy is still unclear, but interestingly 75% of patients are noted to have an abnormal thymus gland upon diagnosis.

The emergency physician should also be aware that a myasthenic crisis might result from the use of certain drugs in treatment of other diseases. Medications that can precipitate a crisis should be avoided unless they are emergently necessary.

Cholinergic crises may be treated with incremental doses of atropine but should be managed conservatively if mild. Acetylcholinesterase therapy is temporarily discontinued.

Lambert–Eaton myasthenic syndrome

There is no specific treatment for LES, but the syndrome usually does not lead to respiratory or bulbar muscle failure.

Multiple sclerosis

In the acute care setting, effort should be directed at eliminating exacerbating conditions such fever and infectious processes. Respiratory compromise should be managed aggressively. An increased risk of aspiration is present when endotracheal intubation is required for MS patients due to decreased gastric motility. Due to vesicourethral dysfunction, MS patients are at a higher risk of urinary tract infections, especially if the post-void residual exceeds 100 ml. High-dose methylprednisolone and adrenocorticotropic hormone (ACTH) may shorten MS exacerbations. Consultation with a neurologist and admission are usually required.

Acute transverse myelitis

There is no proven effective treatment for inflammatory transverse myelitis, but corticosteroids are often administered in the acute setting to reduce inflammation. Up to one-third of patients suffering from transverse myelitis recover spontaneously. For acute episodes resulting from compressive lesions, emergent surgical consultation is required for immediate decompression.

Polymyositis or dermatomyositis

Treatment involves supportive care along with immunosuppressive therapy with steroids or methotrexate, as well as extensive physical and occupational therapy.

Hypokalemic periodic paralysis

Treatment involves supportive care and oral potassium replacement or IV potassium administration if necessary. Acetazolamide 125–1500 mg/day is used for prophylaxis.

Botulism

Treatment of botulism consists mainly of supportive care with special attention to respiratory status. Gastrointestinal decontamination should be considered in food-borne and infantile botulism. Infantile botulism should generally not be treated with antibiotics, as this may lead to further lysis of *Clostridium botulinum* in the gut and increase the infant's toxin load. A trivalent antitoxin is available but its use should be generally reserved for severe cases. Botulism antitoxin is equine-derived, making acute allergic reaction and serum sickness a concern. The antitoxin should be avoided in infantile botulism; human botulism immunoglobulin (BIG) is available.

Heavy metals

Treatment is withheld until definitive diagnosis is established. Dimercaptosuccinic acid (DMSA) and dimercaprol (BAL) are heavy metal chelators used in arsenic poisoning. BAL chelation is the preferred therapy for acute poisoning and is given intramuscularly at the dose of 3–5 mg/kg every 4 hours initially. DMSA (10 mg/kg) may be given orally every 8 hours.

Tick paralysis

Treatment simply involves removing the tick, which results in full recovery in 24–48 hours.

Evaluation of any patient with the acute onset of motor weakness should include examining for the presence of a tick, especially in high-risk geographical regions.

Special patients

As with many other disease processes, special consideration should be given to very young children and elderly patients with generalized acute motor weakness, as mild progression of disease may lead to rapid respiratory decompensation. Patients with sickle cell disease are at high risk for cerebrovascular events even at young ages. Pay careful attention to symptoms of underlying major depression in patients carrying a diagnosis involving long-term progressive motor weakness such as ALS or MS, and ensure that adequate resources are made available to the patient. In addition, make an effort to ensure that the family members and other direct caregivers of these patients are exposed to outside resources and are given the chance for respite if needed, as these people themselves are quite special.

Disposition

Although controversial, these authors feel that all patients presenting to the ED with AIS should be admitted to the hospital. Whether or not the patient receives thrombolytic therapy, coordinated inpatient efforts should occur to maximize the patient's opportunity for improved outcome. Occupational and physical therapy teams should be involved with the stroke patient's care, as well as speech therapy when appropriate. Rehabilitation efforts should be initiated as early as possible, and special attention should be given to watch for signs of depression, a significant co-morbidity of ischemic stroke. Swallowing evaluations help prevent aspiration pneumonia, and DVT prophylaxis should be initiated if patients are bedridden. Some patients may be able to be discharged home after a short hospital stay, but many require extended care in rehabilitation facilities.

For TIA, virtually all patients should be admitted for a complete work-up as previously outlined. The only exceptions are patients in whom a complete work-up, including head CT, laboratory studies, carotid Doppler imaging, and MRI/MRA along with formal neurology consultation can be carried out from the emergency care area in a timely fashion. Since such an expedited work-up and consultation is rarely possible, admission for appropriate work-up and pharmacotherapy determination is recommended.

In the case of other etiologies of acute motor weakness, the emergency physician's assessment of overall respiratory function is the key to appropriate patient disposition. All patients in whom moderate to severe respiratory compromise is either observed or anticipated require admission to an intensive care unit. Others with the potential for respiratory compromise should be admitted and adequately monitored. As a general rule, patients with a new diagnosis of an acute cause of motor weakness should probably be admitted for observation and education. If urgent neurology consultation and prompt follow-up are available, less severe cases may be sent home if the patient and family members are comfortable with this arrangement. However, discharge home should only be considered in cases where rapid progression of disease is unlikely and only after thorough patient education has occurred.

Pearls and pitfalls

- There is no substitute for a careful and thorough neurologic examination. Ample time practicing and reviewing the proper and complete technique helps determine the diagnosis, treatment, and disposition.
- A complete neurologic examination should be performed and documented, including mental status, CNs, motor strength in all extremities, gross sensation, DTRs, and cerebellar function in *any* patient presenting to the ED with the complaint of weakness, dizziness, headache, or visual problems. "Neuro WNL (within normal limits)" does not suffice!
- AIS care is extremely time-dependent. Protocols designed to streamline acute stroke patients into the optimal care scenario *before* the patient arrives are warranted.
- Consider TIA as "unstable angina of the brain," and treat these patients with the proper urgency. Patients with true TIA should not be discharged without adequate work-up *and* initiation or advancement of antiplatelet therapies.
- When the diagnosis is in doubt, always obtain formal neurologic consultation for the patient with true acute motor weakness. If consultation and/or the proper imaging

techniques are unavailable, admit or transfer the patient as the situation dictates.

References

1. Adams HP, Brott TG, Crowell RM, et al. Guidelines for the management of patients with acute ischemic stroke: a statement for healthcare professionals from a Special Writing Group of the Stroke Council, American Heart Association. *Stroke* 1994;25:1901–1914.

2. Adams HP, Brott T, Furlan AJ, et al. Guidelines for thrombolytic therapy for acute stroke: a supplement to the guidelines for the management of patients with acute ischemic stroke: a statement for health care professionals from a Special Writing Group of the Stroke Council, American Heart Association. *Circulation* 1996;94:1167–1174.

3. Adams HP, Davis PH, Leira EC, et al. Baseline NIH Stroke Scale strongly predicts outcome after stroke: a report of the Trial of Org 10172 in Acute Stroke Treatment (TOAST). *Neurology* 1999;53:126–131.

4. Albers GW, Amarenco P, Easton JD, Sacco RL, Teal P. Antithrombotic and thrombolytic therapy for ischemic stroke. *Chest* 2001;119:300S–320S.

5. Albers GW, Bates VE, Clark WM, et al. Intravenous tissue-type plasminogen activator for treatment of acute stroke: the Standard Treatment with Alteplase to Reverse Stroke (STARS) study. *J Am Med Assoc* 2000;283:1145–1150.

6. American Heart Association. *2001 Heart and Stroke Statistical Update*. Dallas, Texas: American Heart Association, 2000.

7. American Heart Association. *Textbook of Advanced Cardiac Life Support*. Dallas, TX: American Heart Association, 1997.

8. Asimos AW. Weakness: a systematic approach to acute, non-traumatic, neurologic and neuromuscular causes. *Emerg Med Pract* 2002;4(12).

9. Bennet JC, Moreland LW. Miscellaneous forms of arthritis. From *Cecil Essentials of Medicine*, 4th ed., Philadelphia: W.B. Saunders Company, 1997. pp. 630.

10. Broderick J, Brott T, Barsan W, et al. Blood pressure during the first minutes of focal cerebral ischemia. *Ann Emerg Med* 1993;22:1438–1443.

11. Brott T, Bogousslavsky J. Treatment of acute ischemic stroke. *New Engl J Med* 2000;343:710–722.

12. Burns TM. Neuroendocrine lung tumors and disorders of the neuromuscular junction. *Neurology* 1999;52(7):1490–1491.

13. Culebras A, Kase CS, Masdeu JC, et al. Practice guidelines for the use of imaging in transient ischemic attacks and acute stroke: a report of the stroke council, American Heart Association. *Stroke* 1997;28:1480–1497.

14. Furlan A, Higashida R, Wechsler L, et al. Intra-arterial prourokinase for acute ischemic stroke: the PROACT II study: a randomized controlled trial. *J Am Med Assoc* 1999;282:2003–2011.

15. Goldsweig CD. Infectious colitis excluding *E. coli* 0157:H7 and *C. difficile*. *Gastroenterol Clin North Am* 2001;30(3):704–733.

16. Grau AJ, Hacke W. Is there still a role for intravenous heparin in acute stroke? Yes. *Arch Neurol* 1999;56:1159–1160.

17. Gresham GE, Alexander D, Bishop DS, et al. American Heart Association Prevention Conference. IV. Prevention and rehabilitation of stroke: rehabilitation. *Stroke* 1997;28:1522–1526.

18. Grotta J. Should thrombolytic therapy be the first-line treatment for acute ischemic stroke? t-PA the best current option for most patients. *New Engl J Med* 1997;337:1310–1313.

19. International Stroke Trial Collaborative Group. The International Stroke Trial (IST): a randomized trial of aspirin, subcutaneous heparin, both, or neither among 19,435 patients with acute ischemic stroke. *Lancet* 1997;349:1569–1581.

20. Jauch E. Ischemic anterior circulation stroke. From the *Foundation for Education and Research in Neurological Emergencies Presentation at the SAEM Conference*. Atlanta, GA, 2001.

21. Jauch EC, Kissela B, McNeil P. *Acute Stroke Management from Neurology/Neuro-vascular Diseases*. Sited from eMedicine.com, Inc., eMedicine Journal. 2001.

22. Johnston SC, Gress DR, Browner WS. Short-term prognosis after emergency department diagnosis of transient ischemic attack. *J Am Med Assoc* 2000;284(22):2901–2906.

23. Kandel ER, Schwartz JH, Jessell TM. *Principles of Neural Science*, 3rd ed.,

New York: Elsevier Science Publishing Co., Inc., 1991. pp. 724–729.

24. Kanter D, Kothari R, Pancioli A, et al. The greater cincinnati t-PA experience after the NINDS trial: does a longer time to treatment within the current three-hour window reduce efficacy? *Stroke* 1999;30:244 (abstract).

25. Kothari R, Pancioli A, Brott T, Broderick J. Thrombolytic therapy for cerebral infarction. *Acad Emerg Med* 1996;3:881–892.

26. Kwiatkowski TG, Libman RB, Frankel M, et al. Effects of tissue plasminogen activator for acute ischemic stroke at one year. *New Engl J Med* 1999;340:1781–1787.

27. Latov N. Use of intravenous gamma globulin in neuroimmune disease. *J Allergy Clin Immunol* 2001;108(suppl. 4):s12632.

28. Moore P, James O. Guillain–Barre' syndrome: incidence, management, outcome, and major complications. *Crit Care Med* 1981;9:549.

29. Plum F. Infectious and inflammatory disorders of the nervous system. In: *Cecil Essentials of Medicine*, 4th ed., Philadelphia: W.B. Sauders Company, 1997. pp. 905.

30. Sandercock P. Is there still a role for intravenous heparin in acute stroke? No. *Arch Neurol* 1999;56:1160–1161.

31. Seybold M. Myasthenia gravis: a clinical and basic science review. *J Am Med Assoc* 1983;250:2516.

32. Sloan EP. Chronic neurologic disorders. In: Tintanelli, et al. (eds) *Emergency Medicine: A Comprehensive Study Guide*, 5th ed., New York: McGraw-Hill, 2000. pp. 1478–1480.

33. The National Institute of Neurological Disorders and Stroke. *Proceedings of the National Symposium on Rapid Identification and Treatment of Acute Stroke*. In: Marler JR, Winter-Jones P, Emr M (eds). Bethesda, MD: National Institutes of Health, NIH Publication No. 97-4239, 1997. pp. 157–158.

34. The National Institute of Neurological Disorders and Stroke rt-PA Stroke Study Group. Tissue plasminogen activator for acute ischemic stroke. *New Engl J Med* 1995;333:1581–1587.

35. Thurman RJ, Jauch EC. Acute ischemic stroke: emergent evaluation and management. *Emerg Med Clin North Am* 2002;20:609–630.

36. Wollinsky KH. Drain the roots: a new testament for Guillain–Barré syndrome. *Neurology* 2001;57(5):753–754, 774–780.

Unique Issues in Emergency Medicine

41 Child abuse, elder abuse, intimate partner violence

Carolyn J. Sachs, MD, MPH

Scope of the problem

Emergency physicians are specialists in dealing with violence-related problems. Emergency physicians treat both victims and perpetrators of violence, often on a daily basis. Additionally, emergency department (ED) staff may become the target of violence at the hands of their patients or their patient's families and associates. This chapter covers ED treatment of patients suffering from child abuse, intimate partner violence (IPV), and elder abuse. Management of the violent patient is covered in Chapter 10.

In the US, over 3000 children, women, and elders die yearly from abuse. Additionally, there are 3 million reports of child abuse, 2 million cases of elder abuse, and 2–4 million cases of IPV each year. Emergency physicians are in a unique position to identify abusive situations before they result in permanent physical or psychologic disability or death. A Kansas City study found that the majority of family violence homicide victims were seen in local EDs or other health care settings in the year before they were killed.

Due to the relative isolation of many victims, a visit to the ED may be the only opportunity for abuse detection. Recognition of victimized individuals often requires a high degree of examiner suspicion. Although physical injuries may be the presenting complaint of many abused patients, these victims (or their caretakers) rarely disclose the true mechanism of injury. Victims may fear retaliation by the perpetrator or ambivalence about separation. Caretakers may not disclose the abuse because they themselves are the abusers, or because they are unaware of the abuse by another person. Furthermore, the majority of reported cases of child and elder abuse involve neglect, which may present with medical problems resulting from poor nutrition, poor hygiene, or lack of needed medications and care.

Elder neglect is defined as the refusal or failure of a caregiver to fulfill his or her obligations or duties to an elderly person, including (but not limited to) providing food, clothing, medicine, shelter, supervision, medical care, and services that a prudent person would deem essential for the well-being of another.

Intimate partner violence is defined as a pattern of assault or coercive behavior of one intimate partner by the other, including physical, sexual, and psychologic abuse. IPV is repetitive (victims typically suffer six episodes per year) and often escalates. Women comprise the vast majority of IPV victims, although physicians must consider the possibility of male victims in the appropriate setting. IPV victims are at higher risk for chronic pain, substance abuse, depression, and suicide attempts, which makes IPV a significant public health issue. Over a lifetime, at least one out of three women in the US will be physically assaulted by a partner. Approximately 2% of female patients presenting to the ED are seeking care for injuries inflicted by their partners. Unlike children and dependent adults, victims of IPV are by and large considered competent adults; therefore, the definition does not include *neglect*.

The following discussion focuses on the four main goals that emergency staff must have when interacting with victims of violence: identification, treatment, documentation, and referral.

Identification

According to current research, patients presenting to EDs support routine questioning by doctors and nurses about violence. Most cases require investigation on the physician's part, as victims rarely disclose abuse without prompting. Patients may feel embarrassed or guilty about their situation. Victims often feel that they deserve the physical violence, as this is what the parent, caretaker, or intimate partner has repeatedly told them.

In addition, victims may worry about the consequences of legal intervention. Abusers may be arrested and incarcerated. Victims of child and elder abuse may be removed from the home and placed in foster care or an institution. Victims may also worry about further abuse from the perpetrator for having disclosed an abusive situation.

Preverbal children or demented elders may be unable to provide any history.

Although inquiring about abuse may seem difficult at first, recognizing that it is important, legitimate, potentially lifesaving, and often legally mandated should help clinicians overcome their initial resistance. Clinicians can help patients feel more comfortable disclosing abuse by framing questions in ways that let patients know that they are not alone, that the provider takes this issue seriously, that the provider is comfortable hearing about abuse, and that help is available. With practice, each clinician will develop his or her own style of asking questions about abuse. Patients must be questioned about abuse independently (i.e., without family members or friends present).

1. *Framing questions.* Sometimes it is awkward to introduce the subject of abuse. The following are examples of ways providers can introduce the topic:
   - "Because violence is common in patient's lives, I now ask every patient in my practice about violence."
   - "I don't know if this is a problem for you, but many patients are dealing with abusive relationships. Some are to afraid or uncomfortable to bring it up themselves, so I've started asking about it routinely."
   - "Some patients think they deserve abuse because they have not lived up to someone else's (parent's, caregiver's, or partner's) expectations. No matter what someone has or hasn't done, no one deserves to be abused. Have you ever been hit or threatened because of something you did or didn't do?"
   - "Because so many patients I see in my practice are involved with someone who hits them, threatens them, continually puts them down, or tries to control them, I now ask all my patients about abuse."
   - Specifically for caregivers: "It must be difficult to care for such an active child or an elder relative who needs so much attention. How do you cope when you feel frustrated? What sources of respite do you use?"
2. *Direct questions.* However one initially raises the issue of violence, it is also important to include direct and specific questions:
   - "Did someone hit you? Are you comfortable telling me who did this to you? Are you comfortable telling the police about it?"

- "Has your caregiver, parent, partner, or ex-partner ever hit you or physically hurt you? Has she/he ever threatened to hurt you or someone close to you?"
- "I'm concerned that your symptoms may have been caused by someone hurting you. Has someone been hurting you?"
- "Does your caregiver, parent, or partner ever try to control you by threatening to hurt you or your family?"
- "Has your partner ever forced you to have sex when you didn't want to? Has he ever refused to practice safe sex?"
- "Has your caregiver ever touched you in places that made you feel uncomfortable?"
- "Has your partner tried to restrict your freedom or keep you from doing things that were important to you, like going to school or work, or visiting your friends or family?"
- "Does your parent, caregiver, or partner frequently belittle you, insult you, and blame you?"
- "Do you feel controlled or isolated by your caregiver or partner?"
- "Do you ever feel afraid of your caregiver, parent, or partner? Do you feel you are in danger? Is it safe for you to go home?"

History
Child abuse

Children presenting with injuries that seem incompatible with the given history or with injuries that have no logical explanation should raise a red flag for abuse. Although the majority of injured children seen in the ED are not victims of abuse, ED staff must maintain a high index of suspicion to identify the approximately 10% of injured children who are abused. To encourage disclosure, examiners must obtain the history in a nonaccusatory manner. If the child is verbal, a separate history should be obtained from the child and the caretaker when each is alone (i.e., without other family members or friends present). It may be helpful for an examiner to simply explain that he/she is concerned about the child's safety without blaming any specific person, and will need to call in another person to help with the evaluation (i.e., child protective services or a social worker). Any child who presents with a change in mental status or seizures must raise concern for intracranial injury from abuse. The most common form of head injury from abuse is due to "shaken baby syndrome," the forcible shaking of an infant resulting in subdural hematomas, retinal hemorrhages, and diffuse brain injury.

Elder abuse

In elderly patients, female gender, cognitive impairment, and increased dependency are universally considered risk factors for abuse. Certain chief complaints commonly encountered in maltreated elderly include injuries, pressure ulcers, falls, dehydration, and functional decline. All of these may be a sign of abusive behavior or neglect.

Intimate partner violence

Although not well-proven in prospective studies, experts consider the following historical factors suggestive of intimate partner abuse: frequent physician visits for trauma, chronic pain syndromes or gastrointestinal (GI) complaints, delays in seeking medical treatment after an injury, an overprotective partner, injuries during pregnancy, a history of depression or suicide attempts, and a history of prior abuse or abuse in the family. The presence of any of these factors should heighten a clinician's suspicion for violence as an etiology for the visit. Clinicians should be especially diligent in questioning patients who present with depression, anxiety, substance abuse, or symptoms lacking a clear etiology.

Physical examination

The majority of injuries seen in pediatric ED patients are not due to abuse, as active children sustain many injuries unintentionally. These injuries are often termed "accidental" injuries. Most educators prefer the adjective "unintentional" to "accidental" when describing these injuries, as "accidental" implies that nothing could have been done to prevent the injury. In fact, many unintentional injuries can be prevented with safety precautions, such as making sure that the water heater is set below 104°F to avoid scald injuries in the bathtub.

Intentionally-inflicted injuries (those from abuse) frequently differ significantly from the unintentional injuries seen during usual activity. Toddlers learning to walk almost universally display unintentional bruises or cuts to the forehead from frequent collisions with furniture or the floor. Conversely, common physical injuries from abuse include bruises without a logical explanation, burns, fractures, lacerations, abrasions, and significant head injury. Perpetrators of abuse may purposely injure victims in areas that are usually covered by clothing. Hence, patients must be completely disrobed to identify possible injuries. In children and dependent adults, physical manifestations of neglect may be uncovered during the examination. These include failure to grow and/or reach developmental milestones, dehydration, malnutrition, late-stage bedsores, inappropriate clothing, and improper administration of medications. Table 41.1 lists various childhood injuries indicative of abuse.

Table 41.1 Physical indicators of child abuse

- Any unexplained change in mental status should raise concern for occult head injury and "shaken baby syndrome"
- Metaphyseal fractures (Figure 41.8)
- Posterior rib fractures
- Unexplained retinal hemorrhages
- Symmetric extremity injuries
- Multiple injuries at different stages of healing
- Scapular fractures
- Spinous process fractures
- Sternal fractures
- Vertebral body fractures
- Multiple skull fractures
- Circumferential immersion burns (Figure 41.6a)
- Buttock burns
- Cigarette burns
- Evidence of poor care or failure-to-thrive
- Blunt instrument marks (belts, bats, rods)
- Patterned burns
- Human hand marks
- Bite marks

Any injury without a logical explanation in adult patients should raise suspicion for abuse. Many of the same injuries described in Table 41.1 should raise red flags for IPV and elder abuse when found in adults. While unintentional injuries may occur anywhere (given a credible history), certain locations are more difficult to injure accidentally and warrant careful scrutiny for abuse. Unintentional injuries tend to occur in a distal and/or lateral anatomic distribution, as these areas have greater exposure and are more likely to be injured while running into objects. Distal and lateral body parts (e.g., outstretched arms, knees, and shins) generally provide protection when you fall. Therefore, central injuries to the face, neck, breasts, and abdomen should raise suspicion for intentional trauma. Unintentional injuries also tend to be unilateral. It is rare to sustain symmetrical bruises from an unintentional mechanism. It is always important to consider the history in context of the injury. Examples of intentionally-inflicted bilateral injuries include finger tip grab marks on both arms, bruises on the medial aspect of upper arms from having them pinned down by the perpetrator's knees, and inner thigh bruises from forced sexual assault.

Any injury to the genital or rectal area should raise suspicion for sexual assault and abuse. Unintentional injuries to this area, termed *straddle injuries*, are rare. Straddle injuries to the female genitalia usually result in trauma to the anterior portion around the urethra. In females, genital injuries from assault are likely to be found more posteriorly, in the posterior fourchette, fossa navicularis, hymen, and labia minora, but may be found anywhere (Figure 41.1). Females and males may display anal injuries after abuse from sodomy or attempted sodomy (Figure 41.2). Oral injuries may be found after forced oral copulation of children, intimate partners, or adults. Emergency physicians must examine the oral cavity for lacerations, petechiae, and contusions in all suspected cases. Intentionally abused victims often display defensive injuries, such as scratch marks from trying to pry off the perpetrator's hands, injuries to dorsum of hands when victim tries to protect his or her

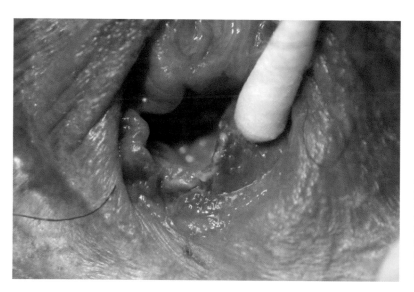

Figure 41.1
Genital injury from assault. The patient was a 15 year old female (previously non-sexually active) who presented 10 hours post sexual assault. The photo demonstrates hymenal trauma with a posterior rim tear and wound necrosis. *Courtesy:* Malinda Waddell-Wheeler, RN, MN, CFNP.

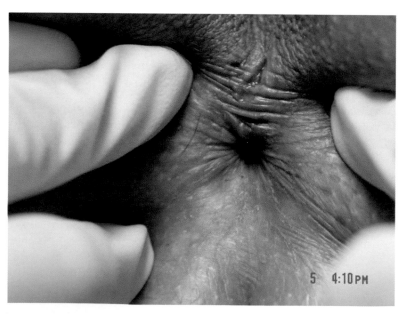

Figure 41.2
Anal injury following sodomy. *Courtesy:* Malinda Waddell-Wheeler, RN, MN, CFNP.

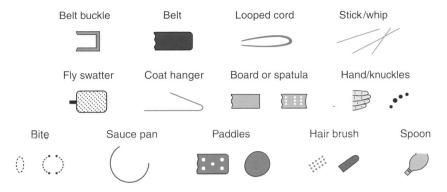

Figure 41.3
Patterns of marks from objects. Reprinted from Pediatric Clinics of North America,
37(4): 791–814. Johnson CF. Inflicted injury versus accidental injury. Copyright 1990,
with permission from Elsevier.

face, or forearm contusions and fractures (termed "nightstick" fractures).

In patients of any age, "patterned" injuries should raise suspicion for intentionality. Patterned injuries reflect the shape of objects used to inflict intentional injuries (Figure 41.3). They usually have sharper edges and are more geometric than the typical unintentional injury. Common objects which leave patterned injuries include hands, rods, belts, and cords (Figure 41.4). After being slapped, a bruise in the shape of the entire digits may be left, with "fingers" visible. Slaps more often result in parallel linear bruises from capillaries breaking at skin areas between fingers.

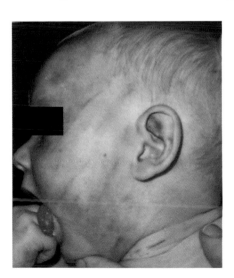

Figure 41.4
The characteristic pattern of parallel lines that results from blows with a belt. Reprinted from Atlas of Pediatric Physical Diagnosis, 4th ed., Eds Zitelli BJ, Davis HW. Copyright 2002, with permission from Elsevier.

Burn patterned injuries are common in child abuse, but may also be found in IPV and elder abuse. (Figure 41.5). These burns occur by three mechanisms: contact burns (i.e., clothes or curling irons), liquid burns (sharply demarcated burns to the wrists or ankles (Figure 41.6) or burns to the genital area inflicted during toilet training), and friction burns (on the torso from being dragged over the ground or on the wrists and ankles from being tied up).

Diagnostic tests

In cases of suspected child and elder abuse, emergency physicians must evaluate for injuries from prior episodes of abuse. In children, this includes a "skeletal survey," consisting of radiographs of the entire body to detect old or healing fractures (Figures 41.7 and 41.8). Suspected shaken baby syndrome mandates evaluation for intracranial injury with brain computed tomography (CT) or magnetic resonance imaging (MRI), as well as a detailed ophthalmologic evaluation for retinal hemorrhages. Laboratory studies are rarely helpful in the evaluation of suspected abuse. In specific clinical situations involving multiple bruises of an unknown origin, coagulation studies and platelet testing may help exclude the possibility of a bleeding disorder.

Occasionally, geriatric patients experience such severe abuse and neglect that they are severely dehydrated, or possibly septic, from a urinary tract infection (UTI). In this scenario, a comprehensive evaluation, including serum chemistries, urinalysis, and radiographs should be obtained.

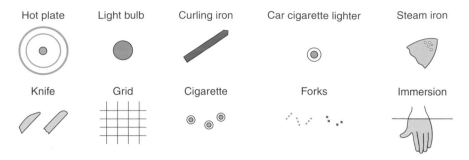

Figure 41.5
Patterns of burns from objects. Reprinted from Pediatric Clinics of North America, 37(4): 791–814. Johnson CF. Inflicted injury versus accidental injury. Copyright 1990, with permission from Elsevier.

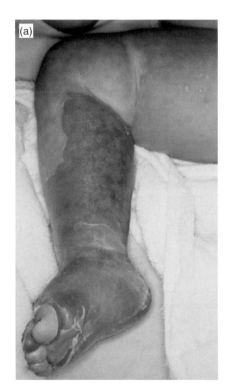

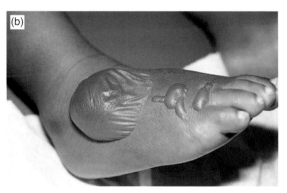

Figure 41.6
(a) Intentional scald. This toddler was dipped in scalding water (as an object lesion following a toileting accident) resulting in severe second-degree burns of the foot and lower leg. *Courtesy*: Dr. Thomas Layton. (b) Accidental scald. The splash-and-droplet pattern of an accidental scald is evident on the foot of a toddler who grabbed a hot cup of tea from the table while sitting on his grandmother's lap. Reprinted from Atlas of Pediatric Physical Diagnosis, 4th ed., Eds Zitelli BJ, Davis HW. Copyright 2002, with permission from Elsevier.

Treatment

Child abuse

Most institutions have written protocols for treating victims of child abuse. Emergency physicians should know where to locate these protocols and how to utilize them. Hospitalization may be indicated for injuries, as well as to allow time for child protective services (CPS) to investigate the source of the injury and whether or not the child is safe at home. When there are other children at home, the safety of these children must also be considered.

Appropriate identification of minor abusive trauma and subsequent parental education has the potential to prevent future abuse.

Elder abuse

If the patient no longer has the capacity to make reasonable decisions for him- or herself, law enforcement or adult protective services (APS) should be contacted. APS agencies, established by state statutes, have the ability to assist with immediate evaluation, provide counseling, and suggest relocation in suspected cases of elder

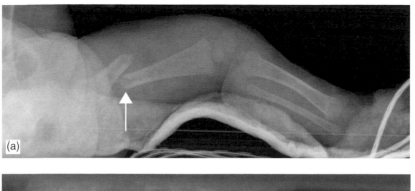

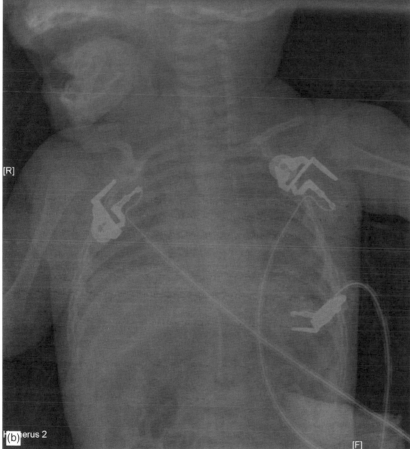

Figure 41.7
(a) Lateral radiograph of the left femur of 6 month old infant revealing a displaced, rotated mid-shaft femoral fracture resulting from child abuse. (b) Chest radiograph of the same child demonstrates healing rib fractures bilaterally. *Courtesy*: S.V. Mahadevan, MD.

mistreatment. In some cases of neglect, APS may provide needed assistance to caregivers so that further neglect is avoided and the patient may remain at home. In other cases, APS may establish a court-ordered guardianship or conservatorship to arrange shelter, finances, and care. The

physician should carefully document the findings of mistreatment or self-neglect and the reasons for declaring the patient incapable of acting in his or her own best interest.

When a patient agrees to intervention, a variety of options can be exercised depending on the type

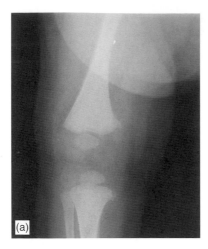
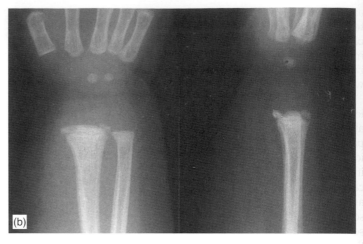

Figure 41.8
Metaphyseal fractures. (a) Metaphyseal "chip" fractures involving the medial aspects of the distal right femur and proximal tibia were found in this infant whose mother confessed to repeated episodes of shaking, after which she would throw the baby down onto a bed or couch. Note the subperiosteal new bone along the lateral aspect of the femur and medial margins of the tibia. (b) Metaphyseal chips are seen on either side of the radial metaphysis in the AP view along with a faint central metaphyseal lucency. In the lateral projection, metaphyseal chips of both radius and ulna are evident. Subtle rims of subperiosteal new bone are present along the diaphyses of both bones. Reprinted from Atlas of Pediatric Physical Diagnosis, 4th ed., Eds Zitelli BJ, Davis HW. Copyright 2002, with permission from Elsevier.

of abuse. If the situation involves physical abuse, severe neglect, or abandonment, and no immediate solution can be arranged, hospital admission is warranted. Admission provides the opportunity for necessary medical treatment and additional time to activate the appropriate social support resources. It also separates the victim from the abuser. Most often, medical complications for a specific problem (i.e., decubiti or dehydration) warrant admission independent of the abuse itself.

In non-life-threatening situations, a solution can be tailored to fit individual circumstances. Even though the caregiver may be the source of abuse, she/he is also likely to provide the greatest amount of support for the victim. Whenever possible, treatment includes crisis intervention with family members. Options for support should be provided to the family in an attempt to diffuse the stress and anxiety that preceded the abuse. Examples include home health aides, respite services, day programs, or transportation assistance if the caregiver is overburdened or ill-equipped to deal with the patient's needs.

Intimate partner violence

Victims of IPV often present with traumatic injuries or medical conditions requiring treatment. Physical symptoms should not be minimized nor ascribed solely to IPV. The majority of

treatment will focus on treating the victim's psyche. Brief supportive counseling by physicians may result in a dramatic catharsis for a victim who until then has been suffering in silence. It is very important for the physician to let a victim know that the abuse and violence is *not* her or his fault. Victims universally feel that they did something to deserve the abuse. Abusers repeat this message to their victim with every beating. A few kind supportive words from an authority figure such as a physician goes a long way in alleviating some of the guilt and shame a victim feels once her abuse has been revealed.

Several comforting phrases to use after any type of abuse is uncovered are listed below:

1. "No one deserves to be physically abused. It doesn't matter what you did or he said you did, you do not deserve to be hit."
2. "You are not the only one who has suffered this kind of abuse. Family violence is a common problem."
3. "You don't have to deal with this alone. We have people here (or in the community) who can help you."

Documentation

Most states provide specific reporting forms for child abuse, child sexual abuse, sexual assault and elder abuse. Some states also provide forms to document IPV and other violent injuries. Most of these forms are available in the ED. Practitioners must be familiar with these forms and the organizations (i.e., CPS, APS, and law enforcement) where these forms must be sent.

Documentation of family violence in the medical chart may be the only written evidence of abuse, and may play a crucial role in aiding the patient. Appropriate documentation by the physician can be crucial in subsequent legal proceedings against the perpetrator or in child custody cases. Many district attorney offices file charges against perpetrators of family violence based solely on carefully documented medical, protective service, and police records, and do not require that the victim press charges or testify in court against the perpetrator. Clear physician documentation can make or break a case in these circumstances.

Guidelines for effective documentation include the following:

1. Record what the patient and/or caretaker tells you using exact words in quotations.
2. Spontaneous utterances such as "He said he was going to beat me until he killed me" can be used in court and for danger assessment.
3. Record prior incidents of abuse, including use of or access to a weapon.
4. Specific threats made by the perpetrator should be recorded in quotations.
5. Record any inconsistencies that lead you to suspect abuse despite caretaker or patient denial.
6. Record the name and relationship of alleged perpetrator and time, date, and place of assault using the exact address if possible.
7. Record details of the injury and identify its location on a body map.
8. Record old injuries as well as new ones.
9. Document the services provided during the visit, either in the physician note or the social worker/victim advocate note. These include CPS or APS reports made, physical evidence given to police, photographs taken, referrals given, assessment of the patient's safety, and subsequent medical care offered or recommended.

Photography

Carefully obtained photographs of injuries provide victims and protective authorities with permanent evidence of the assault, even after the injuries have healed. As with appropriate written documentation, photographs can make a difference in subsequent legal proceedings.

Clinicians have several options for photographing injuries; the best method depends on what is available in each setting. Instant photography (i.e., Polaroid) is convenient and used most often in EDs. Photographs can be affixed to the chart and are extremely valuable in court. Other types of photography (35-mm film, digital, slide film, or video) can be used as long as a secure chain of evidence can be established. Every step of the process, from picture taking to film developing and return, should be accounted for and signed over on a written form. Most institutions that utilize colposcopy for sexual assault examinations have a formal protocol for dealing with photographic evidence. It often involves handing over the film or digitally-recorded images to law enforcement at the end of the examination. These protocols can be easily adapted to family violence photography.

Although not mandated by all states, consent for photography is required by most institutions in competent patients. In children and dependent adults when the legal guardian is the suspected perpetrator, most state laws allow photographs and evidence collection without guardian consent. Clinicians must be knowledgeable of their own state and institutional policies regarding this.

Photographs should include a standard, such as a ruler, so the size of the injury can be easily determined. With proper photographic documentation, forensic experts can comment on the likelihood that a particular person or a given weapon caused a particular injury. Retrospectively, properly photographed and measured bite marks can often be matched to potential perpetrator. At least one photograph that includes the patient's face with the injury is recommended so the identification of the injured person cannot be challenged. All photographs should be labeled with patient information, date, time, location, and photographer's name.

Physical evidence

Victims of family violence who are also recent victims of sexual assault must be offered an evidentiary examination and the standard physical evidence collection per state protocol. In typical cases of family violence, physical evidence, when applicable, should also be collected and turned over to police using the format stipulated by sexual assault protocols. Appropriate specimens include torn or bloody clothing, saliva from bite marks, and bullet, glass, or other weapon fragments. All evidence should be placed in paper (not plastic) bags to avoid bacterial overgrowth and decomposition of the specimen. As with photographs from sexual assaults, transfer of this material must be documented through a written "chain of evidence."

Referral

After identification of abuse, referral is perhaps the physician's most crucial intervention for dealing with victims of family violence. Identification, documentation, and treatment of injuries mean little unless a victim or caretaker is given the resources needed to change the situation. In some cases, government agencies remove the victim from the dangerous situation. These agencies may take legal action against the perpetrator so others will not suffer similar abuse.

In general, emergency physicians have neither the time nor the expertise to comprehensively counsel a victim or caretaker. Referral services fulfill this important obligation. The level of referral depends on the nature of the abusive situation and, in competent adults, the victim's desire for intervention. Many hospitals and clinics have a dedicated social worker on staff to respond to the ED, and often have a specific team of clinicians that help evaluate suspected cases of child abuse, sexual assault, and elder abuse. Many EDs have an affiliation with a victim's group or local woman's shelter that will assist in caring for victims of IPV. Under some circumstances, these groups will dispatch a representative to the medical setting for immediate counseling, legal advocacy, and placement (if necessary).

The revelation of abuse in the medical setting often comes at a time of crisis. This creates a window of opportunity for intervention, at a time when a victim or caretaker is more likely to agree to or desire a change in their situation. Immediate contact with experienced advocates often makes a tremendous difference. Medical personnel may be unaware of these services within their institution or community. The names and numbers of these local services must be included in a written ED protocol. In fact, the Joint Commission on Accreditation of Healthcare Organizations (JCAHO) and several state laws mandate a written protocol for treatment and referral of victims of family violence. Web-based information often provides links to local resources in the user's area.

Furthermore, information on state laws pertaining to abuse can be found through each state's legislative web site.

Child and elder abuse hotlines are available in all locations, but vary by jurisdiction. These numbers should be readily available in all EDs. They can be found in the phone book or from calling information. The US national IPV hotline (800-799-SAFE) can be used by victims and practitioners 24 hours a day, and will automatically direct callers to local shelter services. For hearing-impaired victims of IPV, the TTY number is 800-787-3224.

Safety assessment

All victims of child or elder abuse must receive a safety assessment by either the hospital social worker, abuse team, or protective services. In situations of a competent adult without other resources, a physician or nurse may perform safety assessments. Experts feel that danger increases with increasing numbers of positive answers on the safety screen. The danger assessment screen developed by Campbell after decades of research in IPV homicide may be used for this purpose (Figure 41.9). Physician assessment of safety should also include an assessment of suicide and homicide risk by the victim. Suicide risk increases in the presence of IPV, and homicide of the batterer is possible if the victim feels that this is her or his only way out. Acutely suicidal or homicidal victims warrant immediate psychiatric consultation and admission.

Reporting

Child abuse

All 50 states mandate reporting of any suspected child abuse and neglect by medical professionals to local CPS. Failure to report suspected abuse may result in fines, jail time, and successful civil suit against practitioners. Forms to report abuse and agencies which accept these reports vary by jurisdiction.

Elder abuse

Presently, 47 states require reporting of elder abuse to APS or law enforcement. Abuse suffered by nursing home patients should be reported under the national Omnibus Budget Reconciliation Act of 1987 (OBRA 1987). This law established state run nursing home ombudsman programs which

DANGER ASSESSMENT

Several risk factors have been associated with increased risk of homicides (murders) of women and men in violent relationships. We cannot predict what will happen in your case, but we would like you to be aware of the danger of homicide in situations of abuse and for you to see how many of the risk factors apply to your situation.

Using the calendar, please mark the approximate dates during the past year when you were abused by your partner or ex-partner. Write on that date how bad the incident was according to the following scale:

1. Slapping, pushing; no injuries and/or lasting pain
2. Punching, kicking; bruises, cuts, and/or continuing pain
3. "Beating up", severe contusions, burns, broken bones
4. Threat to use weapon; head injury, internal injury, permanent injury
5. Use of weapon; wounds from weapon

(If **any** of the descriptions for the higher number apply, use the higher number.)

Mark **Yes** or **No** for each of the following. ("He" refers to your husband, partner, ex-husband, ex-partner, or whoever is currently physically hurting you.)

_____ 1. Has the physical violence increased in severity or frequency over the past year?

_____ 2. Dose he own a gun?

_____ 3. Have you left him after living together during the past year?
    3a. (If have *never* lived with him, check here_____)

_____ 4. Is he unemployed?

_____ 5. Has he ever used a weapon against you or threatened you with a lethal weapon?
    (If yes, was the weapon a gun?_____)

_____ 6. Does he threaten to kill you?

_____ 7. Has he avoided being arrested for domestic violence?

_____ 8. Do you have a child that is not his?

_____ 9. Has he ever forced you to have sex when you did not wish to do so?

_____ 10. Does he ever try to choke you?

_____ 11. Does he use illegal drugs? By drugs, I mean "uppers" or amphetamines, speed, angel dust, cocaine, "crack", street drugs or mixtures.

_____ 12. Is he an alcoholic or problem drinker?

_____ 13. Does he control most or all of your daily activities? For instance: does he tell you who you can be friends with, when you can see your family, how much money you can use, or when you can take the car? (If he tries, but you do not let him, check here: _____)

_____ 14. Is he violently and constantly jealous of you? (For instance, does he say "If I can't have you, no one can.")

_____ 15. Have you ever been beaten by him while you were pregnant? (If you have never been pregnant by him, check here: _____)

_____ 16. Have you ever threatened or tried to commit suicide?

_____ 17. Has he ever threatened or tried to commit suicide?

_____ 18. Does he threaten to harm your children?

_____ 19. Do you believe he is capable of killing you?

_____ 20. Does he follow or spy on you, leave threatening notes or messages on the answering machine, destroy your property, or call you when you don't want him to?

_____   Total "Yes" Answers

**Thank you. Please talk to your nurse, advocate or counselor about
what the Danger Assessment means in terms of your situation.**

Figure 41.9

Danger assessment. *Source*: From Campbell JC et al. Risk factors for femicide in abusive relationships: results from a multi-site case control study. *Am J Public Health* (in press).

receive and respond to reports of neglect or abuse in nursing homes. Nursing home residents must have access to a designated ombudsman for that facility. Physicians who suspect abuse in institutionalized elderly must report suspicions of abuse to the state ombudsman, APS, or law enforcement.

Intimate partner violence

Few states have statutes addressing medical treatment of IPV specifically, but IPV reporting falls under other state statutes. Currently, all but five states require some reporting of injured victims of IPV under laws which require reporting of any injured person. Forty-two states require health providers to report injuries resulting from firearms, knives, or other weapons to law enforcement. Additionally, 23 states require reports of injuries resulting from "crimes" or "violently-inflicted injuries." A complete list of state reporting laws pertaining to injured patients can be found in the references section.

Conclusion

The entire ED staff plays a critical role in the identification of abused children, intimate partners, and dependent elders. Their role continues to be critical in documenting, treating, and referring these patients. ED staff must be comfortable questioning patients about abuse, and must be aware of community resources available to aid these victimized populations. It is best to remain an advocate for these patients, and to arrange an appropriate safety assessment following a complete history and physical examination; ensure detailed documentation and careful evidence collection before considering discharge from the ED.

References

1. Abbott J, Johnson R, Koziol-McLain J, Lowenstein SR. Domestic violence against women: incidence and prevalence in an emergency department population. *J Am Med Assoc* 1995;273:1763–1767.

2. American Academy of Pediatrics: Committee on Child Abuse and Neglect. Shaken baby syndrome: rotational cranial injuries – technical report. *Pediatrics* 2001;108:206.

3. Feldhaus KM, Koziol-McLain J, Amsbury HL, Norton IM, Lowenstein SR, Abbott JT. Accuracy of 3 brief screening questions for detecting partner violence in the emergency department. *J Am Med Assoc* 1997;277(17):1357–1361.

4. Hazzard W. Elder abuse: definitions and implications for medical education. *Acad Med* 1995;70:979–981.

5. Houry D, Sachs CJ, Feldhaus KM, Linden J. Violence-inflicted injuries: reporting laws in the fifty states. *Ann Emerg Med* 2002;39(1):56–60.

6. Kleinschmidt KC, Krueger P, Patterson C. Elder abuse: a review. *Ann Emerg Med* 1997;30:463–472.

7. Lachs M, Pillemer K. Abuse and neglect of elderly persons. *New Engl J Med* 1995;332:437–443.

8. Little K. Screening for domestic violence: identifying, assisting, and empowering adult victims of abuse. *Postgrad Med* 2000;108(2):135–141.

9. Nagler J. Child abuse and neglect. *Curr Opin Pediatr* 2002;14(2):251–254.

10. Nimkin K, Kleinman PK. Imaging of child abuse. *Radiol Clin North Am* 2001;39:843–864.

11. Policy Statement: American College of Emergency Physicians. Management of elder abuse and neglect. *Ann Emerg Med* 1998;31:149–150.

12. Slep AM, O'Leary SG. Examining partner and child abuse: are we ready for a more integrated approach to family violence? *Clin Child Fam Psychol Rev* 2001;4(2):87–107 (review).

13. Wadman MC, Muelleman RL. Domestic violence homicides: ED use before victimization. *Am J Emerg Med* 1999;17(7):689–691.

HEAT ILLNESS

Ken Zafren, MD

Scope of the problem

In the US from 1979 to 1995, heat stroke was the stated cause of death in nearly 400 people each year. However, 10 times that number of elderly patients with underlying cardiopulmonary disease are thought to die annually from heat-related complications.

The two major heat illnesses are heat exhaustion and heat stroke.

- *Heat exhaustion* is a syndrome characterized by volume depletion. The core temperature is generally <40.5°C. Mental status is normal.
- *Heat stroke* is a medical emergency characterized by a core temperature >40.5°C and altered mental status.

A number of minor heat illnesses have also been described, including heat cramps, heat edema, heat syncope, heat tetany, and prickly heat. Malignant hyperthermia is characterized by very high core temperature and altered mental status, but is not considered an environmental illness.

- *Heat cramps* are painful muscle cramps which generally occur after exercise in unacclimatized individuals who sweat freely and replace sweat losses with large amounts of water or other hypotonic fluids. Hyponatremia may also occur in this scenario.
- *Heat edema* is a benign condition, most often found in the elderly, in which swelling occurs in the feet and sometimes the hands during the first few days in a hot environment.
- *Heat syncope* is a self-limited condition usually found in unacclimatized persons. Prolonged standing causes venous pooling in the legs which, combined with peripheral vasodilation and volume loss, causes orthostatic hypotension and fainting.
- *Heat tetany* is caused by hyperventilation after brief exposure to intense heat.
- *Prickly heat*, also known as heat rash, lichen tropicus, or miliaria rubra is a maculopapular or vesicular erythematous pruritic rash found in areas of the body covered by clothing. It is caused by obstruction of sweat ducts.

Pathophysiology

Body temperature regulation is a balance between heat production and heat loss. Basal heat production is approximately 40–60 kcal/m^2 body surface area/hour. Voluntary exercise can increase heat production up to 20 times. Metabolism may also be increased by hyperthyroidism or by ingestion of sympathomimetic drugs. Environmental heat adds to the heat load and can interfere with heat dissipation.

Heat is lost by radiation, conduction, convection, and evaporation. Radiation is the exchange of radiant energy with the surrounding environment. Conduction is the exchange of heat by direct contact with a cooler object. Convection is the transfer of heat to (or from) gas or liquid, such as air and water moving by the body. Evaporation is the conversion of liquid to gas, such as sweat to water vapor, which requires energy and removes heat from the body. In hot conditions, conduction, convection, and radiation often transfer heat to the body; the evaporation of sweat is the dominant mechanism of heat loss. Evaporation of 1 L of sweat removes approximately 600 kcal of heat.

Heat loss in a hot environment can impose large metabolic demands on the body. Skin blood flow may increase from <0.5 to 7–8 L/minute in a hot environment. Exercising in a hot environment may be associated with sweat losses of 1–2 L/hour. Peripheral vasodilation and fluid losses from sweating reduce stroke volume. The heart typically compensates with an increased rate if possible.

Acclimatization is the adaptation of the body to heat stress. After daily exercise in a hot environment for 1–2 weeks, sweating increases, occurs at lower core temperatures, and contains less sodium chloride. Peripheral blood flow increases. Increased plasma volume leads to higher stroke volume and a lower heart rate resulting in increased exercise tolerance. Acclimatization is lost over about 1 week in the absence of continued exposure to heat.

Heat exhaustion is a poorly-defined clinical syndrome characterized by volume depletion. Various combinations of water and salt depletion can be found depending on the amount of water and electrolytes used to replace fluid losses. Symptoms are similar whether the lost volume has not been replaced ("water depletion") or replaced using water with inadequate salt ("salt depletion"). The terms "water depletion" and "salt depletion" are misleading, since in both cases volume (not free water only) has been lost.

Heat stroke is a life-threatening condition in which the thermoregulatory mechanisms fail, allowing extremely high core temperatures. The brain is particularly vulnerable to damage, but multiple organ systems are affected. Coagulation abnormalities, as well as damage to the liver or kidneys are common. Cellular damage depends more on the duration of exposure than on the maximum core temperature. In the past, the absence of sweating was considered important to the diagnosis of heat stroke. However, patients with early heat stroke may still sweat. Traditionally, a distinction has been made between "exertional" heat stroke, caused by exercise in a hot environment with increased heat production, and "non-exertional" (classic) heat stroke, due to increased exogenous heat gain and decreased ability to lose heat. This difference has little clinical significance.

History

Does the patient have a reason for heat illness?

The diagnosis of heat illness is usually straightforward. Predisposing factors fit into three broad categories:

- increased heat gain from the environment
- increased internal heat production
- decreased ability to dissipate excess heat.

Does the patient have an associated condition predisposing to heat illness or caused by heat illness?

Heat illness may coexist with other diagnoses, such as fever or trauma. Heat illness may cause trauma due to an altered level of consciousness or syncope.

Is the patient predisposed to heat illness by not being acclimatized?

Risk of heat illness is highest in late spring or early summer, during heat waves, and in persons who have recently arrived at warmer climates.

Does the patient have weakness, fatigue, headache, light-headedness, vertigo, nausea, vomiting, or myalgias?

These are symptoms of both heat exhaustion and heat stroke, and do not distinguish between the two.

Has the patient had hallucinations?

Hallucinations suggest heat stroke.

Does the patient have vomiting or diarrhea?

These are common in heat stroke, but uncommon in heat exhaustion.

Increased heat gain from the environment

Does the patient have a reason for increased heat gain from the environment?

Exposure to high temperatures and high humidity may lead to heat illness. During heat waves, lack of access to air conditioning is a risk factor for heat stroke. Even during less extreme periods, there are many microclimates that can create considerable heat stress. These include indoor or outdoor areas exposed to direct sun, upper floors of buildings, car interiors, boiler rooms, hot tubs, and saunas.

Increased internal heat production

Does the patient have a reason for increased internal heat production?

Has he or she been exercising in a hot environment?

Has the patient been using medications, alcohol, or illicit drugs which increase heat production?

Salicylates increase heat production by uncoupling oxidative phosphorylation. The use of certain drugs can cause increased activity or combative behavior, drug withdrawal, seizures, or neuroleptic malignant syndrome. Drugs with sympathomimetic properties, such as cocaine or amphetamines, cause increased muscle activity. Drugs such as phencyclidine (PCP) and lysergic acid diethylamide (LSD) increase metabolism by central nervous system (CNS) effects. 3,4-methylenedioxymethamphetamine (MDMA or "ecstasy") is a drug used at dance parties ("raves"). The prolonged activity may lead to heat stroke. MDMA can also cause a clinical picture similar to the syndrome of inappropriate antidiuretic hormone (SIADH), resulting in high urine sodium and osmolality despite hypotonic hyponatremia and normal blood volume. Participants in rave parties are often aware of the danger of heat stroke and have been told to drink plenty of water. This response exacerbates hyponatremia, which can cause seizures.

Does the patient have a febrile illness causing increased heat production?

The presence of cough, meningismus, or shaking chills suggest a febrile illness due to an infectious etiology.

Does the patient have another metabolic condition causing increased heat production, such as hyperthyroidism or pheochromocytoma?

This will be identified by abnormal hormone levels.

Decreased ability to dissipate excess heat

Is the patient dehydrated or volume depleted?

Lack of appropriate fluids to replace increased losses in a hot environment can reduce the ability to lose heat through sweating and peripheral vasodilation.

Has the patient been using alcohol or other drugs that increase fluid losses or interfere with behavioral responses to heat exposure?

Alcohol predisposes to dehydration by inhibiting antidiuretic hormone. The use of alcohol and other drugs may decrease one's level of consciousness or alter judgment and interfere with the behavioral response of seeking shelter away from hot microclimates. Alcohol and other drugs, especially phenothiazines, may also limit

thirst. Any mind-altering substance can interfere with the ability to obtain and drink fluids to replace losses.

Was the patient wearing clothing that decreased heat loss?

Clothing that is too warm, especially vapor barrier clothing worn by those trying to lose weight, can markedly decrease heat loss.

Past medical

Cardiovascular disease

Patients with cardiovascular disease may be unable to compensate for changes induced by heat stress, resulting in heat stroke or cardiac complications.

Skin and systemic diseases

Skin diseases that decrease the ability to sweat include eczema, psoriasis, burns, or heat rash. Systemic diseases affecting the ability to sweat include ectodermal dysplasia, scleroderma, and cystic fibrosis.

Medications

Anticholinergic agents decrease sweating. Phenothiazines impair central thermoregulation and have anticholinergic effects. Cardiovascular drugs such as beta-blockers, calcium-channel blockers, and alpha-agonists decrease the heart's ability to compensate for the effects of heat and decrease peripheral blood flow. Sympathomimetics limit skin vasodilation.

Physical examination

The primary goals of the physical examination are to distinguish heat exhaustion from heat stroke, to identify diseases or underlying conditions which may have caused or contributed to heat illness, and to identify other conditions or injuries which require treatment. The emphasis here is on heat stroke, because heat exhaustion is not a life-threatening illness.

General appearance

The patient with heat stroke appears ill, and most likely will not be sweating. Other than body temperature, alteration of consciousness is the main feature which distinguishes heat stroke from heat exhaustion.

Vital signs

Core temperature is the temperature of internal organs. Its measurement is key to the evaluation and treatment of heat illness. In heat illness, brain temperature is of particular importance, because prolonged exposure to high temperatures may cause permanent brain damage. In heat exhaustion, core temperature is generally <40°C. If altered mental status is present, or the core temperature is >40.5°C, the patient should be diagnosed with heat stroke. Core temperature may be <40°C in heat stroke if there is a delay of several hours after the acute event, but these patients are generally comatose.

The best method of measuring core temperature, especially in intubated patients, is with an esophageal probe. Brain temperature can be accurately measured using an epitympanic probe, which contacts the tympanic membrane. This differs from infrared tympanic temperature measurement, which is unreliable. Unfortunately, epitympanic probes are not yet being marketed in North America.

Rectal probe thermometers have been traditionally used, but rectal temperature changes significantly lag core temperature changes. Bladder temperature is less reflective of core temperature than rectal temperature. Oral temperature varies with respiration and is a poor reflection of core temperature.

In heat stroke, expect tachypnea, tachycardia, and normal to low blood pressure. Pulse pressure may be widened. Deviations from this may provide clues to underlying diagnoses. For example, excessive tachypnea may indicate salicylate toxicity. Relative bradycardia may suggest certain infectious diagnoses, such as typhoid fever, or reflect cardiac drugs, such as beta- or calcium-channel blockers. High blood pressure may be a clue to thyroid storm or pheochromocytoma. Heat exhaustion also presents with tachycardia.

Neurologic

Any neurologic sign may be found in heat stroke. Dysarthria and ataxia are common, but agitation, stroke-like symptoms, posturing, seizures, and coma can all be identified. Miosis is often present.

Skin

At the time of collapse from heat stroke, most patients will be sweating profusely. By the time of arrival in the emergency department (ED), the skin is often hot and dry. The presence of heat rash is a risk factor for heat stroke. Purpura indicates coagulation abnormalities, which implies a poor prognosis.

Differential diagnosis

If body temperature is >40.5°C, rapid cooling measures must be initiated immediately. If cardiovascular parameters improve and mental status returns to normal, most other diagnostic possibilities are eliminated. If the core temperature does not decrease or the mental status does not improve, other etiologies must be investigated (Table 42.1).

Unlike heat stroke, most febrile states which produce altered mental status are associated with normal hepatic transaminases. Reye's syndrome causes encephalopathy and elevated transaminases without fever.

Table 42.1 Differential diagnosis of heat illness

Diagnosis	Symptoms	Signs	Work-up
Anticholinergic toxicity	Blurred vision	Mydriasis	Clinical diagnosis
Brain abscess, cerebral hemorrhage	Variable – may be identical	Neurologic abnormalities including altered mental status	CT scan
Cerebral (falciparum) malaria	Shaking chills	Variable – may be identical to heat stroke	CT scan, thin and thick smears of blood looking for parasites
Delirium tremens	Anxiety	Tremors	Careful history

(continued)

Table 42.1 Differential diagnosis of heat illness (*cont*)

Diagnosis	Symptoms	Signs	Work-up
Diabetic ketoacidosis	Thirst	Kussmaul breathing	Electrolytes, renal function, serum ketones, ABG or VBG
Meningitis, encephalitis	Headache, vomiting often prominent	Meningismus, altered mental status	LP with CSF analysis; other adjunctive studies
Neuroleptic malignant syndrome, malignant hyperthermia	Nonspecific	May be identical to heat stroke	Clinical diagnosis based on medication history, response to dantrolene
Other infections	Depending on infection	Depending on infection	History, physical, laboratory work as indicated
PCP, cocaine, amphetamine toxicity	Mood disturbances	Variable	History, urine toxicology screen
Salicylate toxicity	Tinnitus	Tachypnea	Salicylate level, electrolytes, renal function
Sepsis	May be identical to heat stroke – sepsis can cause heat stroke	May be identical to heat stroke	Search for source of infection
Status epilepticus	Seizures	May be identical to heat stroke	Usually clinical diagnosis; CT scan usually indicated; EEG may be necessary
Thyroid storm	May be nonspecific	Altered mental status; associated stigmata of hyperthyroidism	Thyroid function studies
Typhoid fever	Fever, headache, anorexia, cough, constipation or diarrhea	Relative bradycardia	Blood and stool cultures

ABG: arterial blood gas; CSF: cerebrospinal fluid; CT: computed tomography; EEG: electroencephalograph; LP: lumbar puncture; PCP: phencyclidine; VBG: venous blood gas.

Diagnostic testing

Laboratory studies

Complete blood count, comprehensive metabolic panel, and coagulation profile

Complete blood count (CBC), comprehensive metabolic panel (CMP), and coagulation profile are helpful in detecting organ damage and in excluding associated diagnoses. Hemoconcentration is almost always present. Hypoglycemia is common, as are hypokalemia and hypernatremia. Renal failure may occur. Hepatic transaminases are usually elevated. Coagulation abnormalities imply a poor prognosis.

Creatine kinase

Creatine kinase should be measured to assess for rhabdomyolysis. No discrete cutoff exists, but values of >1000 U/L (approximately 5 times normal) are considered diagnostic. As the rise in CK begins 2–12 hours after muscle injury, early diagnosis and treatment may prevent renal damage.

Amylase and lipase

Both are likely to be elevated if pancreatitis is present.

Urinalysis

Urinalysis (UA) should reveal maximally concentrated urine.

Urine toxicology

Urine toxicology screens may be helpful in identifying drugs of abuse contributing to hyperthermia.

Salicylate level

Abnormal salicylate levels can make the diagnosis of salicylism.

Thyroid profile

Thyroid profile should be obtained if thyroid storm is suspected.

Cerebrospinal fluid

Cerebrospinal fluid (CSF) studies may be indicated if meningitis is suspected as a cause of altered mental status.

Electrocardiogram

An electrocardiogram (ECG) should be obtained to rule out associated diagnoses, including myocardial infarction and drug toxicity.

Radiologic studies

Computed tomography (CT) of the head may be necessary as part of the evaluation of altered mental status.

General treatment principles

As with all emergency patients, treatment begins with Airway, Breathing, and Circulation (ABCs). The main goal of treatment is rapid cooling. Only after stabilizing measures have been initiated should a more detailed diagnostic work-up be undertaken.

Airway, Breathing, Circulation

The airway must be controlled, which includes intubation of the unconscious patient. Supplemental oxygen should be administered. Intravenous (IV) access should be established, but aggressive volume resuscitation is usually unnecessary since cooling can be expected to decrease peripheral vasodilation. This decreases the demands on the heart and raises blood pressure. Fingerstick glucose may reveal hypo- or hyperglycemia. Continuous cardiac, pulse oximetry, and temperature monitoring should be established. Cardiac monitor electrodes can be attached to the patient's back if they will not stick to the chest. A Foley catheter should be placed and urine output monitored. Urine temperature can be measured with a Foley catheter probe if other methods are not available.

Cooling

The patient should be immediately undressed. Ice packs can be placed in the axillae and groin. Evaporative cooling is the method of choice at most institutions. Spraying lukewarm water over the patient and blowing room temperature or even heated air over the skin prevents cutaneous vasoconstriction and minimizes shivering. As shivering causes undesired heat production, it can be treated with IV medications, such as chlorpromazine 25 mg or meperidine 100 mg. Hypotension is a concern with these drugs.

Immersion cooling in ice water is also used in some circumstances, but has a number of practical drawbacks and may not be safe in patients who are neither young nor healthy. Cardiopulmonary bypass is another alternative but is rarely necessary. It has been used successfully in the treatment of malignant hyperthermia. Peritoneal lavage is also a possibility to decrease core temperature. Venous catheter heat exchangers have been used to produce controlled hypothermia and are less invasive than cardiopulmonary bypass. They are as yet untested for treatment of heat stroke. Cooling blankets are not effective.

Cooling measures should be discontinued when body temperature reaches 39°C in order to avoid hypothermia.

Antipyretics such as acetaminophen and nonsteroidal anti-inflammatory drugs (NSAIDs) are effective only in the event of fever and should not be used in heat stroke. Dantrolene is indicated in malignant hyperthermia or neuroleptic malignant syndrome, and has no effect on hyperthermia due to other causes.

Supportive care

Volume status, glucose and electrolyte abnormalities, coagulopathies, seizures, and other complications are managed in the standard fashion.

Special patients
Elderly

Geriatric patients have decreased cardiovascular reserve and a decreased ability to sweat. Elderly patients may be further limited by cardiac and vascular disease, complicating the management of heat stroke. They are often taking medications, such as beta-blockers, which decrease an individual's ability to dissipate heat.

Pediatric

Children have a greater surface area-to-mass ratio than adults, allowing for greater exogenous heat gain. They have a higher metabolic rate, increased heat production, and less ability to sweat than adults, limiting their ability to lose excess heat by evaporative cooling.

Obese

Obese patients have a decreased surface area-to-mass ratio and decreased skin blood flow. The physical effects of adipose tissue predispose obese people to heat illness.

Disposition

Patients with minor heat illnesses and most patients with heat exhaustion can safely be discharged home in the company of a reliable adult, with close outpatient follow-up. Infants and the very elderly, individuals with underlying conditions predisposing to heat illness, those who are significantly volume depleted, and patients with end-organ damage due to heat illness should be admitted.

All patients with heat stroke should be admitted. Patients who are unstable should be admitted to an intensive care setting. This may require transfer to a hospital offering a higher level of care.

Pearls, pitfalls, and myths
Pearls

- Heat stroke presents with altered level of consciousness.
- Consider heat syncope in a syncope work-up.
- Obtain as much history as possible about what the patient was doing and the environmental conditions during the time when the patient collapsed or had changes in behavior.

- Aggressive fluid resuscitation is usually not necessary. Aggressive immediate cooling is imperative.

Pitfalls

- Not considering the diagnosis of heat stroke.
- Not measuring core temperature as soon or as often as possible, or using suboptimal methods, such as oral or tympanic thermometers.
- Not considering associated diagnoses, such as trauma or sepsis.
- Not instituting cooling measures promptly.
- Using antipyretics to cool a patient suffering from heat stroke.
- Giving excess fluids to a patient on MDMA, which can worsen hyponatremia and cause seizures.

Myths

- A patient who is sweating cannot have heat stroke.
- A patient in the ED who has a normal core temperature and normal transaminases cannot have heat stroke. (The patient may have cooled off; transaminases may rise only after 24–48 hours.)

References

1. Bouchama A, Knochel JP. Heat stroke. *New Engl J Med* 2002;346:1978–1988.
2. Gaffin SL, Moran DS. Pathophysiology of heat-related illnesses. In: Auerbach P (ed.). *Wilderness Medicine*, 4th ed., St. Louis: Mosby, 2001. pp. 240–289.
3. Moran DS, Gaffin SL. Clinical management of heat-related illnesses. In: Auerbach P (ed.). *Wilderness Medicine*, 4th ed., St. Louis: Mosby, 2001. pp. 290–316.
4. Walker JS, Barnes SB. Heat emergencies. In: Tintinalli JE (ed.). *Emergency Medicine: A Comprehensive Study Guide*, 5th ed., McGraw Hill: New York, 2000.
5. Yarbrough B, Vicario S. Heat illness. In: Marx JA (ed.). *Rosen's Emergency Medicine: Concepts and Clinical Practice*, 5th ed., St. Louis: Mosby, 2002. pp. 1997–2009.

HYPOTHERMIA

Ken Zafren, MD

Scope of the problem

Hypothermia is defined as a core temperature <35°C (95°F). It can occur at any place and any time. Hypothermia is the stated cause of over 700 deaths annually in the US. About half of these deaths occur in patients over 65 years of age.

Primary hypothermia affects otherwise healthy patients exposed to cold environmental conditions. *Secondary hypothermia* is caused by a variety of diseases. Primary hypothermia is a disease of wars throughout history. During peacetime, it is most common in urban areas in association with homelessness and the use of alcohol and other drugs. Also at risk are participants in outdoor activities, such as skiing, hunting, climbing, sailing, swimming, and diving. Secondary hypothermia is associated with sepsis, trauma, and diseases such as hypoendocrine states, which decrease metabolic rate, as well as conditions which affect hypothalamic function such as tumors and stroke. Elderly and ill patients are often found indoors in well-heated houses, which may confuse the diagnosis. *Iatrogenic hypothermia* may be induced by resuscitation with room temperature fluids or refrigerated blood products.

Pathophysiology

Body temperature regulation is a balance between heat production and heat loss. Heat production can be increased by increasing the metabolic rate, shivering, or voluntary activity. Increased metabolic rate is mediated by thyroid and adrenal glands.

Heat is lost by radiation, conduction, convection, and evaporation. These mechanisms are explained in the section on Heat illness. Wet clothing increases the rate of heat loss up to fivefold, while immersion in water increases the rate as much as 25–30 times. Wind and moving water further increase heat loss by disrupting the warm microclimate, which can otherwise protect against heat loss from skin. Evaporation of water from the skin surface and from respiration may also cause significant heat loss.

Heat loss can be limited by vasoconstriction and behavioral responses. Humans are adapted to tropical environments and have a limited ability to decrease heat loss by physiologic means. The most important responses are usually behavioral, such as putting on warm clothing and seeking refuge from cold environments. If these mechanisms are somehow limited, the risk of hypothermia markedly increases.

History

History may be straightforward, especially in primary hypothermia, or may be difficult to obtain, as in an unconscious patient found indoors.

Where was the patient found? What was he or she doing?

Patients found outdoors in cold conditions have one reason for being hypothermic, but there may be predisposing causes for hypothermia, such as trauma or intoxication with alcohol or other drugs.

Does the patient have an immobilizing condition or injury?

The patient may have become hypothermic due to the inability to reach shelter.

Does the patient have a metabolic cause for hypothermia?

Metabolic causes include hypothyroidism, hypoadrenalism, hypopituitarism, and hypoglycemia, which lead to decreased metabolic rates.

Does the patient have another cause of hypothalamic dysfunction?

These include head trauma, tumor, stroke, or Wernicke's syndrome.

Is the patient intoxicated?

The use of alcohol and other sedative-hypnotics predisposes to hypothermia by interfering with adaptive behavorial responses to cold. Alcohol causes cutaneous vasodilation, which increases heat loss from the skin.

Could the patient be septic or in diabetic ketoacidosis?

Hypothermia in sepsis carries a grave prognosis. Diabetic ketoacidosis (DKA) also interferes with thermoregulatory mechanisms.

Has the patient been resuscitated with room temperature fluid or chilled blood?

Iatrogenic hypothermia is of particular importance in trauma patients receiving volume replacement therapy. All trauma patients should receive IV fluids warmed to 40°C.

Has the patient received drugs that decrease shivering?

These include phenothiazines, meperidine, and buspirone. Chlorpromazine is commonly used in treatment of heat stroke to abolish shivering. In mildly hypothermic patients, shivering is a major mechanism to increase core temperature.

Past medical

Use of phenothiazines is a risk factor for hypothermia. Burns or exfoliating skin conditions predispose patients to increased heat loss.

Physical examination

The primary goals of the physical examination are to establish the degree of hypothermia, to identify diseases or underlying conditions which may have caused or contributed to hypothermia, and to identify associated injuries which require treatment.

Airway, Breathing, Circulation

As with all patients, the ABCs are of primary importance. These may be difficult to assess in a severely hypothermic patient, because respiratory rate and heart rate may be extremely slow. Respirations are often very shallow, and pulses are likely to be weak and difficult to palpate through cold skin. It is often hard to make cardiac monitor leads adhere to cold, moist skin, and pulse oximeters do not work on cool, vasoconstricted extremities.

Level of consciousness

Alert patients generally have only mild hypothermia. Patients with alterations of consciousness must have etiologies other than hypothermia considered as their cause of impaired consciousness.

Vital signs

Core temperature is the temperature of the key internal organs, primarily the heart. Precisely measuring the core temperature is key to the evaluation and treatment of hypothermia.

Standard clinical thermometers may record temperatures only as low as 34°C. In case of a low reading, an electronic thermometer with an esophageal probe should be used. In mild hypothermia, a rectal temperature may be adequate. If a glass thermometer is used, it must be a "low reading" type. Rectal probe temperatures have been used traditionally, but rectal temperature changes significantly lag changes in core temperature. Bladder temperature is even less reflective of core temperature than is rectal temperature. Oral temperatures are notoriously inaccurate.

As the patient cools, the initial response is tachycardia, after which there is progressive bradycardia. The heart rate is about 50% of normal at a core temperature of 28°C. If the heart rate is faster than expected at a given temperature, other causes of tachycardia should be suspected, including hypovolemia, hypoglycemia, or drug ingestions. Blood pressure and respiratory rate also initially increase before declining, as hypothermia becomes more severe. Inappropriate respiratory rates should suggest metabolic acidosis or a CNS lesion.

Abdomen

Decreased intestinal motility may lead to abdominal distention or rigidity, and may mimic or mask an acute abdomen.

Neurologic

Dysarthria and ataxia may be found in mild hypothermia. These are likely to increase in severity at lower core temperatures. Reflexes are initially increased, and then decrease before eventually disappearing as core temperature decreases. Muscle tone increases in the preshivering phase. Shivering is maximal at about 35°C, and gradually decreases until the core temperature is about 31°C, at which point shivering disappears entirely.

Differential diagnosis

Hypothermia is diagnosed by measuring core temperature. However, conditions other than environmental exposure can cause hypothermia. While not truly differential diagnoses, associated diagnoses should be considered in hypothermic patients. Table 42.2 is a partial list of etiologies to consider.

Table 42.2 Differential diagnosis of hypothermia

Diagnosis	Symptoms	Signs	Work-up
Acute spinal cord transection	Lack of peripheral sensation	Paralysis, vasodilation	Neurologic examination, X-ray, CT, MRI
Alcohol, drugs, and other toxic exposures, including benzodiazepines, barbiturates, phenothiazines, and carbon monoxide	Depends on agent(s)	Specific toxidromes may be identified	Drug levels, urine toxicology screen; consider naloxone, flumazenil (acute, isolated benzodiazepine OD only), and high-flow (or hyperbaric) oxygen
CNS lesions (trauma, CVA, mass), hypothalamic dysfunction (including Wernicke's syndrome)	Variable	Signs of trauma, abnormal neurologic examination	CT scan, thiamine administration
Endocrine dysfunction (hypoglycemia, thyroid, adrenal or pituitary insufficiency)	Often nonspecific	Typical signs of endocrine abnormalities may be present	Laboratory studies, fingerstick glucose, steroid administration
Iatrogenic (fluid resuscitation, exposure in ED, OR and radiology suite, drug administration, heat stroke cooling, emergency delivery)	Nonspecific	Nonspecific	Diagnosed by history
Infection, including meningitis, encephalitis, pneumonia, sepsis	Variable	Tachycardia, hypotension	Search for source of infection (CXR, UA, blood cultures, CSF)
Myocardial infarction	Chest pain may be present; additional symptoms include dyspnea, dizziness, syncope, weakness, confusion, or other nonspecific symptoms	May include low cardiac output	ECG, cardiac markers
Pancreatitis, peritonitis	Abdominal pain	Abdominal rigidity, peritoneal signs	Laboratories, CT scan
Skin lesions or diseases	Nonspecific	Burns, exfoliative dermatitis	Consider Dermatology consult/biposy

CNS: central nervous system; CSF: cerebrospinal fluid; CT: computed tomography; CVA: cerebrovascular accident; CXR: chest X-ray; ECG: electrocardiogram; MRI: magnetic resonance imaging; OR: operating room; OD: overdose; UA: urinalysis.

Diagnostic testing

Laboratory studies

Complete blood count

Hematocrit increases about 2% with every 1°C decrease in temperature. A moderately or severely hypothermic patient with a "normal" hematocrit is actually anemic. White blood cell and platelet counts are depressed by sequestration.

Metabolic profile

Potassium levels are independent of temperature. However, hypothermia increases the toxic effects of hyperkalemia. Blood glucose is increased in hypothermia, because endogenous insulin is inactive at temperatures <30–32°C.

Coagulation studies

Hypothermia induces a coagulopathy, although coagulation studies are insensitive in the hypothermic patient.

Creatine kinase

Rhabdomyolysis is a potential complication of immobility, which may be associated with hypothermia.

Arterial blood gas

Although blood gas values which are "corrected" for temperature are available, they should not be used. Uncorrected blood gas values should be used to guide treatment at all temperatures. Using "corrected" blood gas values will cause pH abnormalities.

Electrocardiogram

Numerous ECG changes can be found in the hypothermic patient. Prolongation of PR, QRS and QT intervals is usual; T wave inversion may be seen. Muscle tremor artifacts may make obtaining an adequate ECG difficult. The Osborne (J) wave, a slow deflection at the junction of the QRS complex and the ST segment, is a common finding (Figure 42.1). These waves are usually upright in left-sided precordial leads. Dysrhythmias may include sinus tachycardia in mild hypothermia, sinus bradycardia, atrial fibrillation or flutter, atrioventricular (AV) block, nodal rhythms, premature ventricular contractions (PVCs), ventricular fibrillation (VF), or asystole. Atrial fibrillation is the most common dysrhythmia other than rate disturbances of sinus origin.

Radiologic studies

If trauma is suspected, cervical spine, chest, and pelvis films may be appropriate. Other X-rays and CT scans are indicated based on clinical presentation.

General treatment principles

As with all patients, treatment begins with the ABCs. After the emergency physician secures these, an appropriate method of rewarming must be initiated, and volume status and electrolyte fluxes must be managed.

Initial resuscitation

Endotracheal (ET) intubation is mandatory unless the patient is alert and protecting the airway. The patient should have continuous cardiac and vital sign monitoring. Pulse oximetry is seldom possible (or reliable) in the hypothermic patient due to peripheral vasoconstriction. Both a nasogastric (NG) tube and indwelling urinary catheter should be gently inserted. Monitor the temperature continuously using an esophageal probe. Insulate the patient to protect against further heat loss.

If the heart is in ventricular fibrillation (VF) or asystole, cardiopulmonary resuscitation (CPR) should be initiated. If VF is present, three attempts should be made to defibrillate the patient, according to Advanced Cardiovascular Life Support (ACLS) guidelines. However, defibrillation is seldom successful if the patient's core temperature is <28–30°C. Start CPR if the patient does not have a perfusing rhythm. Atrial dysrhythmias resolve with rewarming and do not require treatment.

Obtain IV access: Catheters inserted into the heart or pulmonary artery are contraindicated. Hypothermic patients are generally volume depleted. Replace volume with D5NS initially. All IV fluids should be heated to 40–42°C to prevent further heat loss.

Pharmacology

The IV route is the only effective route of administration for medications, but most drugs are not active at temperatures <30°C. Protein binding of drugs increases in hypothermia, further limiting their effects. Medications given in the hypothermic patient are generally ineffective until rewarming takes place, after which they suddenly become effective and possibly toxic. Thiamine and glucose should be given empirically.

Rewarming

Following initial stabilization, the emergency physician must choose a rewarming method. *Passive rewarming* refers to methods which use heat generated by the patient. *Active rewarming* methods add heat to the patient from other sources. Mildly hypothermic patients (core temperature 32–35°C) can be treated with passive external rewarming, utilizing their own body heat and shivering to rewarm. In practice, most of these patients will receive active external rewarming with warm blankets or forced heated air. Hypothermic patients with body temperatures <32°C, with cardiovascular instability, or with underlying conditions predisposing to hypothermia require active core rewarming; this refers to methods that preferentially heat the central

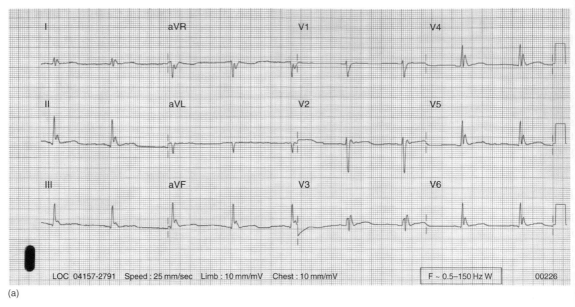

(a)

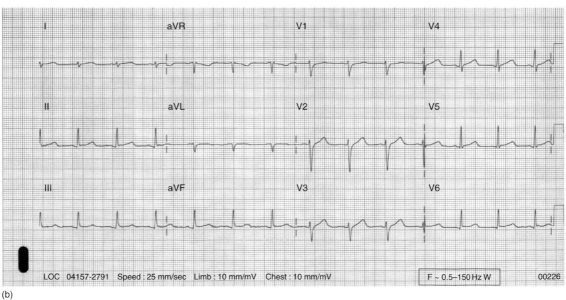

(b)

Figure 42.1
Resolution of Osborne J waves in a patient with (a) hypothermia and (b) rewarming. *Courtesy*: Joel Levis, MD.

organs. While there are many methods of active core rewarming, the most common are peritoneal lavage and various blood rewarming techniques. Blood rewarming techniques include arteriovenous or venovenous rewarming, hemodialysis, and cardiopulmonary bypass. The choice of specific rewarming techniques is complex and depends on institutional resources. Obtaining assistance from the nephrology, cardiac, or trauma surgery services may prove life-saving.

Further management

During rewarming, electrolyte and volume status fluxes require active management. Coagulopathies may pose special problems. Also during this time, underlying diseases and traumatic injuries need to be addressed. Close cardiopulmonary monitoring and continued reassessment of neurologic status are crucial.

Special patients

Elderly

Geriatric patients are more prone to hypothermia, tend to have more underlying diseases, and generally have less physiologic reserve than younger adults. They often require more aggressive treatment for hypothermia and its complications. Geriatric patients with hypothermia should generally be treated as if they are septic.

Pediatric

Neonates require aggressive volume resuscitation in addition to the usual treatment of hypothermia. Unless cold exposure is the clear cause of hypothermia, pediatric patients should be evaluated and treated for sepsis.

Immune compromised

Sepsis may be an important cause of hypothermia in immunocompromised patients. If there is any doubt, these patients should be presumptively treated for sepsis and aggressively rewarmed.

Disposition

Otherwise healthy patients with mild hypothermia (32–35°C) due to cold exposure usually have no difficulty being rewarmed. Generally, they can be discharged safely unless they have associated injuries, including frostbite, which necessitate hospital admission. All other patients with hypothermia require admission. In some cases, patients may require transfer to a center with the capability to perform cardiopulmonary bypass.

Serum potassium levels greater than 10 meq/L may correlate with an inability to resuscitate the hypothermic patient. This degree of hyperkalemia is a marker of cell lysis, and although not proven in hypothermia, has been shown valid in cases of trauma or asphyxiation.

Pearls, pitfalls, and myths

Pearls

- Hypothermia can mask symptoms and signs of other diseases. It is crucial to measure core temperature and consider associated or alternative diagnoses. It can cause or mask an acute abdomen.
- Hypothermic patients can survive without cardiac activity. Contraindications to CPR include any sign of life, Do Not Resuscitate (DNR) status, or obvious lethal injuries. Dependent lividity, apparent rigor mortis, or fixed dilated pupils are not contraindications to CPR.
- A hypothermic patient with a normal hematocrit is likely anemic.
- Atrial dysrhythmias resolve with warming and do not require treatment.
- Insulin is ineffective at temperatures <30°C, as are most pharmacologic agents.
- IV fluids can be rewarmed in a microwave oven. The bag should be shaken before administration to prevent hot spots.
- Tympanic, oral, and bladder temperatures are unreliable.

Pitfalls

- Failure to diagnose hypothermia by failing to measure core temperature.
- Failure to handle the hypothermic patient gently, which may precipitate VF.
- Failure to prevent further heat loss by covering the patient, including the head and neck.
- Failure to diagnose traumatic injuries responsible for hypotension, tachycardia (relative to core temperature), or neurologic dysfunction.
- Being unaware that cardiac and other drugs are not absorbed well orally or intramuscularly, and are likely to remain inactive until rewarming occurs.
- Administration of room temperature or cold IV fluids or blood products.
- Administration of meperidine or phenothiazines, which abolish shivering.

Myths

- The axiom "No one is dead until they are warm and dead" is a myth. The truth is that some people are cold and dead.
- ABGs should be corrected for core temperature. In fact, uncorrected ABGs should be used to guide therapy.
- Hypothermia only occurs in cold climates. Hypothermia can occur under mild conditions both outdoors and indoors.

References

1. Auerbach PS. Some people are dead when they're cold and dead. *J Am Med Assoc* 1990;264:1856–1857.
2. Bessen HA. Hypothermia. In: Tintinalli JE (ed.). *Emergency Medicine: A Comprehensive Study Guide*, 5th ed., McGraw Hill: New York 2000. pp. 1231–1235.
3. Danzl D. Accidental hypothermia. In: Auerbach P (ed.). *Wilderness Medicine*. 4th ed., St. Louis: Mosby, 2001. pp. 135–177.
4. Danzl D. Accidental hypothermia. In: Marx JA (ed.). *Rosen's Emergency Medicine: Concepts and Clinical Practice*, 5th ed., St. Louis: Mosby, 2002. pp. 1979–1996.
5. Giesbrecht GG. Cold stress, near drowning and accidental hypothermia: a review. *Aviation Space Env Med* 2000;71:733–752.
6. Kornberger E, et al. Forced air surface rewarming in patients with severe accidental hypothermia. *Resuscitation* 1999;105–111.
7. State of Alaska Cold Injuries and Cold Water Near Drowning Guidelines. Section of Community Health and EMS, Juneau, AK, 2003.
8. Walpoth BH, et al. Outcome of survivors of accidental deep hypothermia and circulatory arrest treated with extracorporeal circulation. *New Engl J Med* 1997;337:1500–1505.

LIGHTNING INJURIES

Ken Zafren, MD

Scope of the problem

Lightning has been estimated to kill over 1000 people worldwide every year, although the number of fatalities in developed countries has been decreasing for the last 70–80 years. The death rate in the US decreased from over 6 per million to 0.4 per million annually during the twentieth century. At least 70% of lightning strikes are not fatal, but the majority of survivors experience significant sequelae.

Pathophysiology

Lightning is a direct current that produces extremely high voltage for very brief durations. Unlike alternating current, the direct current of lightning often flows over the exterior of the body, referred to as *flashover*. However, it may enter the body with devastating results.

Lightning produces injury by a number of different mechanisms:

1. Lightning may strike a person directly, which is often fatal.
2. More frequently, current splashes from nearby objects or people standing nearby; this is known as *side flash*.
3. Contact injury is produced when a person is in direct contact with an object that is hit or splashed by lightning.
4. Step voltage or ground current causes injury by flowing between two parts of the body in contact with the ground at different distances from the lightning strike, due to the voltage difference between these two points of contact.
5. Lightning can enter the body through the mouth, ears, or orbits.
6. Blunt injury can occur from the shock wave produced by lightning and the muscle contractions due to the current.

Victims can be thrown a significant distance or can lose balance and fall. Pressure injuries, including tympanic membrane rupture, frequently occur. Blunt injury occurs when falling or thrown objects hit the victim.

Direct lightning injuries are due to high voltage; the secondary effects are due to heat production and explosive force. Death is most commonly due to cardiorespiratory arrest. Respiratory arrest is often prolonged due to paralysis of the respiratory center in the medulla; this may lead to hypoxic cardiac arrest if not treated with ventilatory support. High-voltage brain injury or blunt head trauma may also cause death. Other direct injuries include contusions, tympanic membrane rupture, hematologic abnormalities such as disseminated intravascular coagulation (DIC), burns, and a variety of neurologic conditions.

In a lightning strike, the heart may stop instantly during myocardial depolarization, resulting in asystole. Cardiac activity usually resumes promptly, although it may be in jeopardy because of prolonged respiratory arrest. Various ECG changes can be seen in lightning strikes, and myocardial infarction occasionally occurs. Hypertension is common, although it generally resolves within a few hours without treatment. Hypotension may result from traumatic hemorrhage.

Neurologic injuries are often transient. Immediate injuries are typically transient, although they may be fixed and severe. Temporary neurologic symptoms include seizures, paralysis, deafness, blindness, confusion, amnesia, and coma. Temporary paralysis of the extremities is called *keraunoparalysis*. It is due to intense vasospasm and usually clears within hours. Delayed injuries, which are likely progressive, include seizures, neuromuscular disorders, ataxia, extremity weakness, paralysis, or chronic pain.

All organ systems may be affected. Pulmonary, gastrointestinal, and renal injuries may be immediate or delayed, and may be due to hypotension or other injuries. About half of lightning victims will have eye injuries, most commonly cataracts. These may be immediate or appear as long as 2 years later. Pupillary findings, including fixed, dilated pupils, are common and often transient. Hearing loss, vertigo, and damage to the auditory system is also seen. Over half of victims have tympanic membrane rupture, which usually heals without intervention. Psychiatric sequelae are common.

Burns are common. Burns are caused by the direct effects of lightning or by secondary heat production. Most direct burns are superficial, resulting from the rapid flashover effect. Burns also occur from vaporization of sweat or moisture in clothing, from melted synthetic clothing, and from heated metal objects. The terms *feathering* and *Lichtenberg figures* are synonymous; these refer not to burns but to skin markings caused by electron shower, and are pathognomonic of lightning injury (Figure 42.2). Entry and exit burns rarely occur.

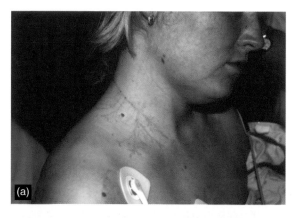

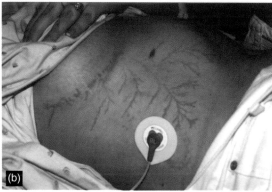

Figure 42.2
Feathering following lightning strike. (a) *Lichtenberg figures* originating from 14K gold necklace being worn by the victim at the time of the lightning strike. The necklace was melted into 3 sections. (b) *Lichtenberg figures* radiating caudally following area of skin in contact with cloth-covered wire from an underwire bra. *Courtesy:* Sheryl Olson, RN, BSN.

History

The history in lightning injury is variable. On one hand, the history may be straightforward when the strike is witnessed. On the other hand, lightning can strike "out of the blue," at great distance from a lightning storm, with the strike not witnessed. Victims are frequently amnestic of the event. History obtained from witnesses may prove helpful.

Was the patient found outdoors or in a building not protected from lightning? Was a known lightning storm in the vicinity? Was it a hot, humid day when lightning was likely?

In these circumstances, an unconscious or confused patient may have been a lightning strike victim.

If the event was witnessed, what was the mechanism of injury?

Was the patient struck directly, splashed, or affected by ground current? Did the patient fall, get struck by a falling object, or get thrown?

Did the patient require resuscitation at the scene?

If the patient required resuscitation from cardiorespiratory arrest, the prognosis is much worse.

Did the patient lose consciousness or have any neurologic deficits that have resolved?

The nature of the injuries and the time course of symptom resolution may provide clues to the severity of delayed injuries.

Past medical

This is as important as it would be for any patient with multiple injuries.

Physical examination

The main goal of the physical examination is to identify direct and indirect injuries caused by a lightning strike. In cases in which the mechanism of injury is uncertain, the physical examination may help identify lightning as the cause of the patient's presentation.

General appearance

Victims with minor injuries are usually alert and seldom have burns. Confusion, combativeness, or coma indicate a greater degree of injury. Paralysis, especially of the legs, may also be seen. The patient may be seizing. Severely injured victims may be in cardiac arrest. Signs of blunt trauma are common and should be identified.

Vital signs

Mildly injured victims will have normal vital signs or mild hypertension that resolves without treatment. Hypotension in a lightning victim should prompt search for traumatic hemorrhage.

Head, eyes, ears, nose, throat and neck

Burns on the head indicate severe injury. In addition to signs of blunt trauma, tympanic membrane rupture is a common finding. Blindness and deafness are common and are often temporary. Various eye and ear injuries, especially tympanic membrane rupture, are frequent and mandate more detailed examination. Hemotympanum and CSF otorrhea are signs of basilar skull fracture. If there is any question of cervical spine injury, the neck should be stabilized during the physical examination.

Skin

The presence of feathering (Lichtenberg figures) is pathognomonic for lightning injury. Linear and punctate burns also provide evidence of lightning injury. Partial thickness burns may become more evident with time. Full thickness burns may also occur.

Abdomen

Ileus may be present and may cause abdominal tenderness.

Neurologic

Mental status should be noted. It may be normal or the patient may be confused, combative, or comatose. Amnesia is common. Pupillary findings are an unreliable indicator of cranial nerve function. Autonomic dysfunction may cause nonreactive pupils, mydriasis, anisocoria, or Horner's syndrome. Lower extremity *keraunoparalysis* is found in two-thirds of severely injured patients; one-third have upper extremity keraunoparalysis. Paralysis of the extremities is the result of sympathetic stimulation with severe vasospasm. The affected limbs appear mottled and are cold to the touch. They may be numb and pulseless. Spinal paralysis, paresis, and cerebellar dysfunction may occur. Hemiplegia and aphasia have been reported, and simulate a cerebrovascular accident (CVA).

Differential diagnosis

Given a history of a lighting storm and witnesses to the strike, the diagnosis of lightning injury is straightforward. Victims with feathering, or punctate or linear burns should be treated for lightning injury. Victims found without appropriate

Table 42.3 Differential diagnosis of lightning injuries

Diagnosis	Symptoms	Signs	Work-up
Cardiac dysrhythmias	Variable	Variable	ECG, cardiac monitoring, cardiac markers
Central nervous system or spinal cord trauma, Cerebrovascular accident	Visual or hearing loss, amnesia, headache, paresthesias, extremity weakness	Altered level of consciousness, including coma. Confusion, localized weakness, paralysis	Appropriate imaging and specialty consultation
Multiple trauma, assault	Depends on injuries	Depends on injuries; scattering of clothing at scene may be due to lightning	Depends on injuries
Myocardial infarction	Chest pain, dyspnea, nausea/vomiting, diaphoresis	May be absent	ECG, cardiac markers, angiography
Seizure disorder	Amnesia of the event	Seizure or postictal state (altered level of consciousness or confusion); tongue injury, incontinence of urine or stool	Serial examination, CT head; may require EEG
Stokes–Adams attacks	None	Syncope without warning (drop attacks)	Echocardiography
Toxic ingestion, envenomation	Depends on the toxin or venom	Depends on the toxin or venom	Careful history and physical examination; laboratory testing as indicated

CT: computed tomography; ECG: electrocardiogram; EEG: elctroencephalograph.

historical or physical findings may represent other diagnoses. These injuries, however, may be the result of lightning even if a strike is not witnessed.

Diagnostic testing

Laboratory studies

Testing will depend on the severity of injury and on associated clinical factors.

Complete blood count

Obtain a CBC for all patients with moderate or severe injury. Its main use is in the evaluation of hemorrhage.

Basic metabolic panel

Obtain a BMP to assess renal injury or when electrolyte abnormalities are suspected.

Creatine kinase

Creatine kinase (CK), urinalysis (UA), and urine myoglobin are indicated to rule out rhabdomyolysis.

Cardiac markers

Cardiac markers are obtained in moderate to severe injury, when the ECG is abnormal, or the patient complains of chest pain.

Coagulation

Coagulation studies should be ordered in moderate to severe injury to assess for DIC.

Electrocardiogram

An ECG should be obtained to assess for possible cardiac injury. Prolongation of the QT interval is the most frequent rhythm abnormality. Atrial fibrillation, premature ventricular contractions, and ventricular tachycardia have been reported. Elevation of the ST segment and T wave changes may also be seen. Ischemic changes do not always reflect vascular distribution patterns in lightning strike victims; areas of focal necrosis may be found. ECG changes may be delayed 24 hours or more.

Radiologic studies

Plain Films

A chest X-ray (CXR) should be obtained to identify pulmonary injury or pneumothorax. Cervical spine X-rays should be obtained in patients whose neck cannot be clinically cleared. Other plain films should be obtained based on suspected injuries.

Computed tomography

Head CT is indicated in patients with altered consciousness or those with suspected head injury. CT of the cervical spine is the optimal study in unconscious or multiple-injured patients. CT angiography of the chest and CT of the abdomen and pelvis have the same indications as in other patients, including those with suspected trauma.

General treatment principles

As with all patients, treatment begins with the ABCs. Lightning victims should be treated according to cardiac and trauma care guidelines. Hypothermia, if present, should be addressed.

Cardiovascular care

Asystole and VF are seen more often in the field than in the ED. Atrial fibrillation, premature ventricular contractions, and ventricular tachycardia may occur. There is no evidence to differentiate treatment of dysrhythmias due to lightning injuries from those due to primary cardiac causes. Dysrhythmias may not occur until 24 hours after the injury. Premature ventricular contractions have been reported up to 1 week later. Most dysrhythmias resolve within days, but some may persist for months. Transient hypertension is the rule and does not usually require treatment. Delayed hypertension has been reported up to 72 hours after the injury. Persistent cases have been treated with beta-blockers and other antihypertensive agents.

Volume repletion

All patients require IV access, but volume resuscitation is seldom necessary. Hypotensive patients and those with extensive burns should receive appropriate volume resuscitation. Most lightning burns are superficial and do not require special treatment. The presence of hypotension should prompt a search for a source of bleeding.

Neurologic treatment

Neurologic injuries are treated as in any trauma patient (including appropriate consultation).

although some exceptions exist. Fixed, dilated pupils may be the result of local eye injury and do not necessarily reflect CNS injury. Paralyzed extremities that are cool, mottled, and pulseless may be observed, but the limb generally returns to normal in a few hours once the vasospasm resolves. Fasciotomies are almost never needed in these cases.

Miscellaneous injuries

Eye injuries may include immediate or delayed cataracts. Ear injuries, such as tympanic membrane rupture, usually heal spontaneously and do not require specific treatment. Any eye or ear injury resulting from lightning strike merits ophthalmology or ear, nose, and throat (ENT) consultation. Ileus can occur and may require treatment with NG tube decompression.

Special patients
Pregnant

Pregnant patients are not at increased risk for mortality from lightning exposures, but fetal death occurs in about half of cases due to the high conductivity of amniotic fluid. Fetal ultrasound and tocodynometry are mandatory after 20-weeks gestation. If the fetus is viable, the remainder of the pregnancy is considered high-risk.

Disposition

Most experts believe that asymptomatic patients with a normal ECG, including those with feathering, may be safely discharged after several hours of observation. These patients need close follow-up with neurology, ENT, and ophthalmology, as delayed sequelae are common.

Mildly injured patients who improve initially should be admitted for neurologic and cardiac monitoring, with consultation from specialty services as indicated.

Most lightning-injured patients should be admitted to a referral hospital with a full spectrum of consultative services. The trauma, neurosurgery, cardiology, neurology, ENT, and ophthalmology services are often consulted. Pregnant women beyond 20 weeks gestation will require admission for fetal ultrasound and a minimum of 4 hours of tocodynometric monitoring. The treatment for fetal demise is uterine evacuation.

Pearls, pitfalls, and myths
Pearls

- Apneic patients often survive without neurologic sequelae if ventilated adequately until spontaneous respirations resume. Cardiac activity usually resumes quickly if the patient is ventilated early and does not develop hypoxia.
- The amount of visible (external) damage does not always correlate well with the severity of internal injuries.
- Lightning current usually flows over the body, but can also enter through various orifices, including the eyes, ears, and mouth.
- Feathering (Lichtenberg figures) is pathognomonic of lightning injury. Punctate or linear burns suggest lightning injury.

Pitfalls

- Not resuscitating a lightning victim who has fixed, dilated pupils.
- Not treating keraunoparalysis expectantly.
- Not considering the diagnosis of lightning injury in a patient found comatose or confused, given the appropriate conditions.
- Not looking for a source of bleeding in a patient with hypotension following lightning injury.
- Not considering delayed and long-term sequelae, or providing appropriate specialty follow-up care.
- Treating a lightning victim like a patient with a high-voltage electrical injury. Large volume resuscitation, fasciotomies and other aggressive treatments common in high-voltage injuries are almost never necessary in lightning injuries.

Myths

- Most lightning strikes are fatal.
- Lightning cannot strike inside a building.
- It is dangerous to touch a lightning victim.
- "If you are not killed by lightning, you will be okay."
- Lightning injury causes few permanent sequelae.
- Lightning victims may recover after prolonged resuscitation because they are in suspended animation.

References

1. Andrews CJ, Colquhoun DM, Darveniza M. The QT interval in lightning injury with implications for the "cessation of metabolism" hypothesis. *J Wilderness Med* 1993:4(2):155–166.

2. Cooper MA. Lightning injuries: prognostic signs for death. *Ann Emerg Med* 1980;9(3):134–138.

3. Cooper MA, Andrews CJ, Holle RL, Lopez RE. Lightning injuries. In: Auerbach P (ed.). *Wilderness Medicine*, 4th ed., St. Louis: Mosby, 2001. pp. 73–110.

4. Price T, Cooper MA. Electrical and lightning injuries. In: Marx JA (ed.). *Rosen's Emergency Medicine: Concepts and Clinical Practice*, 5th ed., St. Louis, 2002. pp. 2010–2020.

5. Treat KN, Williams JM, Chinnis AS. Lightning injuries. In: Tintinalli JE (ed.). *Emergency Medicine: A Comprehensive Study Guide*, 5th ed., New York: McGraw Hill, 2000. pp. 1298–1302.

6. Zafren K, Thurman RJ, Storrow AB. Environmental conditions. In: Knoop KJ, Stack LB, Storrow AB (eds). *Atlas of Emergency Medicine*, 2nd ed., New York: McGraw-Hill, 2002. pp. 513–563.

NEAR-DROWNING

Ken Zafren, MD

Scope of the problem

Drowning is defined as death by suffocation after submersion in water (or in another liquid). Near-drowning refers to survival, at least temporarily, following submersion. There is less agreement about other terms, such as post-immersion syndrome or secondary drowning, which refer to complications or death after near-drowning.

Immersion syndrome is commonly used as a term for sudden death after submersion in very cold water. While this has traditionally been explained as being due to vagal stimulation causing dysrhythmia, another phenomenon termed "cold shock" has been recognized. This refers to an involuntary gasp and hyperventilation when a victim is suddenly plunged into cold water. This can lead to aspiration of water and to rapid submersion.

Drowning kills over 4500 people of all ages annually in the US, making it the fourth leading cause of accidental death. More drownings occur in home swimming pools than in any other place. Toddlers have the highest risk of drowning, followed by teenage boys.

Near-drowning is many times more common than drowning, but exact data are unavailable. One study estimated that there are 8000 hospitalizations and 31,000 ED visits annually for childhood near-drowning in the US.

Pathophysiology

After submersion, alert victims hold their breath and may struggle or panic. Soon, respiratory drive ("air hunger") causes an involuntary inspiration – gasping for breath. This results in aspiration of water, followed by convulsions and death due to hypoxemia. Some victims do not aspirate, but laryngospasm still causes hypoxemia and death. This has been termed *dry drowning*. In *wet drowning*, aspiration occurs.

Although aspiration of fresh water and sea water cause essentially opposite changes in blood volume and electrolytes, only a small percentage of victims aspirate sufficient quantities of either to cause clinically-significant effects. However, aspiration of any amount of fresh or sea water causes pulmonary damage, which may result in non-cardiogenic pulmonary edema. Pulmonary injury may be exacerbated by contaminants in the water, including bacteria, particulate matter, various chemicals, and vomitus. Cerebral hypoxia also may cause non-cardiogenic pulmonary edema.

Most patients will be acidemic. Initially, this is due to hypoventilation rather than lactic acidosis secondary to decreased tissue perfusion. Electrolyte abnormalities in near-drowning victims seldom require treatment.

Hypoxic-ischemic injury to the CNS may cause neurologic sequelae in a large percentage of near-drowning patients; fortunately, many patients recover without neurologic damage. Renal failure and coagulopathies, including DIC, may also occur.

History

History is important to establish the occurrence of near-drowning, to identify a precipitating event(s), and to provide clues to associated conditions and potential complications.

Did the patient have a coughing, choking, or vomiting episode near a pool or other body of water?

This may be the only clue to a near-drowning incident.

Is there a possible precipitating event that caused the near-drowning incident?

Alcohol or other drug intoxication, head or neck injury, cardiac arrest, CVA, seizures, and hypothermia are possible causes.

Is the patient suicidal or a victim of attempted homicide? Is there a possibility, in children, of neglect or non-accidental trauma?

This may be a clue to associated conditions and possible complications if the patient survives.

Was the patient diving into the water or surfing? Is there another mechanism for potential head or neck trauma?

If the history is unclear, the possibility of head and neck trauma should be considered.

Was the patient scuba diving?

This may be a clue to dysbaric injuries or cerebral air emboli.

What were the water temperature and duration of submersion?

This information will help guide resuscitation strategy. Submersion in water warmer than 20°C (68°F) and submersion longer than 5–10 minutes are predictors of increased mortality. Survival has not been reported in victims who have been submerged in warm water for over 30 minutes.

Was the water clean or dirty?

Near-drowning in dirty water has a worse prognosis and is more likely to lead to secondary infections.

Past medical

Underlying conditions such as a seizure disorder, psychiatric illness, medications, and alcohol or other drug use may complicate the management of the near-drowning victim.

Physical examination

General appearance

The patient may appear well or ill, and may be conscious or unconscious. The patient may appear dyspneic and may be using accessory muscles to breathe.

Vital signs

Core temperature should be measured. Tachypnea may provide a clue to pulmonary injury. Pulse and blood pressure, as well as respiratory rate, should be evaluated in relation to core temperature. Shock is uncommon in near-drowning victims; its presence mandates a search for other injuries.

Pulmonary

The chest may be clear or there may be wheezing or crackles. The absence of adventitial breath sounds does not rule out aspiration.

Neurologic

Patients arriving in the ED awake and alert have nearly 100% survival with normal neurologic status. Those with an altered level of consciousness yet arousable are also likely to survive without neurologic sequelae. Slightly less than half of comatose patients will survive without neurologic deficits, less than one-fourth will survive with neurologic damage and the remainder will die from hypoxic–ischemic brain injury or from pulmonary edema. Serial assessment of the Glasgow Coma Scale is mandatory. The remainder of the neurologic examination should be guided by suspected illness or injury.

Head-to-toe

A thorough examination, such as that performed in any trauma victim or medical patient, should be performed in order to identify associated injuries or conditions.

Differential diagnosis

Most cases of near-drowning will be clinically apparent by history and physical examination.

Table 42.4 Diagnostic possibilities in near-drowning

Diagnosis	Symptoms	Signs	Work-up
Hypoglycemia, CNS injury or infections, intoxication. Myocardial infarction, acute disturbances of cardiac rhythm, or an acute pulmonary event may result in a near-drowning	History of coughing, choking, or vomiting near water suggests near-drowning	Tachypnea is common in near-drowning; hypothermia may be present. Near-drowning victim may have wet skin, hair, or clothing. Toxidromes may be present if toxic exposure led to near-drowning	Look for other causes of decreased consciousness if history is unclear. Check fingerstick glucose, and response to naloxone and thiamine. Further studies may include head CT, lumbar puncture

Diagnostic testing

Diagnostic testing is not needed in asymptomatic near-drowning patients. All other patients should undergo laboratory, ECG, and radiographic studies as indicated by history and clinical findings.

Laboratory studies
Complete blood count

CBC is likely to be normal or show leukocytosis. It is unlikely to change initial treatment, but may be obtained as a baseline or as a clue to associated conditions. Hemolysis can occur.

Basic metabolic panel

Electrolytes are likely to be normal. Abnormalities may indicate aspiration of large volumes of water, and will guide treatment. Metabolic acidosis is a clue to tissue hypoxia. A low glucose may have caused an altered level of consciousness leading to near-drowning. Renal failure sometimes results from near-drowning.

Coagulation profile

This should be obtained in all patients with significant symptoms to rule out coagulopathies, especially DIC.

Arterial blood gas

Many authors advocate ABGs on all near-drowning patients. ABGs should be done on intubated patients, but their utility in spontaneously breathing patients is controversial. Most of the important information can be obtained from observation of the patient, pulse oximetry, and serum bicarbonate. The decision to intubate should be made on clinical grounds. With the increasing availability of end-tidal CO_2 monitoring and the universal availability of pulse oximetry, the use of ABGs is increasingly less justifiable.

Other studies

Ordering a CK should be considered to rule out rhabdomyolysis. A UA is also commonly obtained and may demonstrate myoglobinuria, although this is not usually important in initial management. A carbon monoxide level should be obtained if there is a history of possible exposure, such as swimming under a houseboat. Blood levels of aspirin, acetaminophen, and other medications may be indicated based on the history. Further laboratory testing should be dictated by the clinical situation and associated conditions that may be known or suspected.

Electrocardiogram

Most dysrhythmias will be clinically obvious and mandate an ECG. In a patient with significant dyspnea, chest pain, or history suggesting the possibility of cardiovascular disease, an ECG is indicated to identify ischemia. All patients requiring supplemental oxygen due to hypoxemia need an ECG.

Radiologic studies
Chest X-ray

A CXR should be obtained in all symptomatic near-drowning patients. The initial CXR may be normal, even in patients who later develop significant complications of aspiration.

Other plain films

Cervical spine films and other plain films should be obtained as indicated by the history or findings on physical examination.

Computed tomography

Head CT may be necessary if the possibility of head trauma exists. In near-drownings associated with traumatic injury, CT of the cervical spine, chest (CT angiography), and/or abdomen and pelvis may be indicated.

General treatment principles
Airway, Breathing, Circulation

As with all emergency patients, treatment begins with the ABCs. Ventilation should be initiated in apneic patients. If ventilation is inadequate and the airway is clear, the patient should be intubated. If the patient is conscious, non-invasive ventilatory support, such as nasal continuous positive airway pressure (CPAP) or bi-level positive airway pressure (BiPAP) are excellent alternatives. CPR should be performed if the patient is pulseless, and should be continued until core temperature is determined. If the core temperature is <35°C, the patient should be treated for hypothermia. In patients with core temperature 35°C or above, CPR is not likely to be successful if continued for >30 minutes. Dysrhythmias and other circulatory problems should be treated according to ACLS and hospital protocols.

Pulmonary management

If there is significant pulmonary involvement, positive airway pressure is generally necessary. Steroids and prophylactic antibiotics are not helpful after aspiration, although some authors recommend antibiotics if near-drowning occurred in highly contaminated water. Antibiotics are indicated for patients with signs of infection. Intubated patients should have a NG tube placed to decompress the stomach.

Neurologic management

Supportive care, with care to avoid hypotension and hypoxemia, is the key to managing patients with neurologic abnormalities.

Associated conditions

Associated injuries and conditions should be identified and treated appropriately as in other patients.

Special patients
Pediatric

Infants and children have demonstrated longer survival than adults in cold water near-drowning. The possibility of child abuse or neglect should be addressed with appropriate consultation and reporting, according to state law. The psychological effects on families should be considered when children experience near-drowning, with appropriate referrals given for mental health resources.

Disposition

Historically, all near-drowning victims were admitted and monitored. The current approach to admission for near-drowning is more selective. Patients clearly without significant symptoms prior to arrival do not require diagnostic studies and can generally be discharged after a brief period of observation. Family, social, and psychiatric

issues should be addressed prior to discharge. If there is any question about the history, if the patient has mild symptoms, or if the patient is a young child, pulse oximetry and a CXR are indicated. If these are normal, the patient should be observed for a minimum of 4 hours. These patients can be discharged if they remain asymptomatic, can be watched closely at home, and have the means to return if necessary. Patients with mild hypoxemia, those who remain symptomatic after observation, or those who develop respiratory symptoms should be admitted to a regular medical bed. Patients who are intubated and mechanically-ventilated require critical care unit admission.

Pearls, pitfalls, and myths
Pearls

- Near-drowning in cold water (<20°C) is associated with better survival than near-drowning in warm water.
- Patients in coma or who arrive in the ED without vital signs may survive neurologically intact.
- Initial CXR may be normal, even in patients with pulmonary injury.
- In near-drowning patients who are not hypothermic, CPR ongoing for >30 minutes is unlikely to result in successful resuscitation.

Pitfalls

- Failure to consider the cause of near-drowning, such as trauma (especially of the head or cervical spine), drug intoxication, hypoglycemia, cardiac arrest, or CVA.
- Failure to address the possibility of non-accidental causes, such as suicide, homicide, child abuse or neglect.
- Failure to rewarm a hypothermic near-drowning victim.

Myths

- Most drowning victims swallow large amounts of water leading to electrolyte abnormalities.
- The Heimlich maneuver is helpful in near-drowning victims without foreign body airway obstruction.
- All near-drowning victims require admission.

References

1. Feldhaus KM. Submersion. In: Marx JA (ed.). *Rosen's Emergency Medicine: Concepts and Clinical Practice*, 5th ed., St. Louis: Mosby, 2002. pp. 2050–2054.
2. Graf WD, Cummings P, Quan L, Brutocao D. Predicting outcome in pediatric submersion victims. *Ann Emerg Med* 1995;26(3):312–319.
3. Haynes BE. Near drowning. In: Tintinalli JE (ed.). *Emergency Medicine: A Comprehensive Study Guide*, 5th ed., McGraw Hill, 2000. 1278–1281.
4. Modell JH. Drowning. *New Engl J Med* 1993;328(4):253–256.
5. Newman AB. Submersion incidents. In: Auerbach P (ed.). *Wilderness Medicine*, 4th ed., St. Louis: Mosby, 2001. pp. 1340–1365.
6. State of Alaska Cold Injuries and Cold Water Near Drowning Guidelines. Section of Community Health and EMS, Juneau, AK, 2003.
7. Weinstein MD, Krieger BP. Near drowning: epidemiology, pathophysiology and initial treatment. *J Emerg Med* 1996; 14(4):461–467.

TERRESTRIAL VENOMOUS BITES AND STINGS

Robert L. Norris, MD

Scope of the problem

In 2001 there were >85,000 calls to US poison control centers regarding bites and stings. While the majority of these injuries can be handled with simple first aid alone, a number of victims will present to the emergency department (ED) for care. Presentations can be for acute systemic toxicity due to venom poisoning, local wounds apparently inflicted by a venomous creature, or anaphylactic reactions in a sensitized individual.

The venomous creatures exacting the greatest toll in terms of human injury include the arthropods, especially the hymenoptera or stinging insects (bees, wasps, hornets, yellow jackets, and fire ants), a handful of spider species, scorpions, and the venomous reptiles, particularly snakes.

The major impact of hymenoptera is seen in the 0.3–3.0% of the human population that is dangerously allergic to these insects and at risk of anaphylaxis if stung. The vast majority of deaths related to venomous creatures in the US are due to hymenoptera-induced anaphylaxis. The spiders of major consequence include the widow spiders (*Latrodectus* species) (Figure 42.3) which are found throughout much of the world, the brown spiders (*Loxosceles* species, the best

known of which is the brown recluse, *L. reclusa*) (Figure 42.4), and the Australian funnel-web spiders (*Atrax* and *Hadronyche* species). Scorpions are of limited medical importance in the US with only one potentially dangerous species (*Centruroides exilicauda*), but they are much more important in other regions of the world, particularly Central and South America, Africa and the Middle East. In Mexico, for example, scorpions take a higher toll in terms of human mortality than do venomous snakes. The most dangerously venomous scorpions fall into the genera *Centruroides*, *Tityus*, *Buthus*, *Buthacus*, *Androctonus*, *Leiurus*, *Mesobuthus*, and *Parabuthus*.

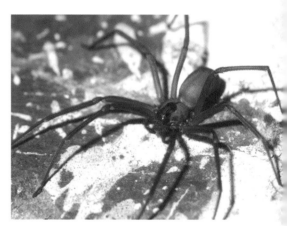

Figure 42.4
Brown recluse spider (*Loxosceles* species). Note the characteristic dorsal, violin-shaped marking. *Courtesy:* Michael Cardwell.

Venomous snakes fall into the families Viperidae (subfamilies Viperinae (vipers) and Crotalinae (pit vipers)) (Figure 42.5), Elapidae (including cobras, mambas, coral snakes, and all of the venomous snakes of Australia) and Hydrophidae (sea snakes). There are a few species of snakes in the family Colubridae that have salivary secretions that can be severely toxic to man (e.g., the boomslang (*Dispholidus typus*) and the twig snake (*Thelotornis kirtlandi*), both of Africa). The remainder of this family is largely harmless. There are two venomous species of lizards, the

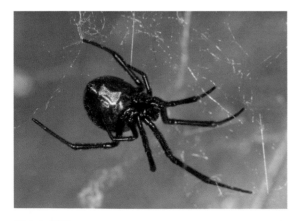

Figure 42.3
Black widow spider (*Latrodectus* species). Note the characteristic central hourglass. *Courtesy:* Michael Cardwell.

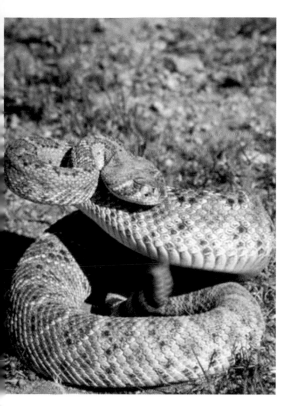

Figure 42.5
Rattlesnake (*C. Atrox*). *Courtesy:* Michael Cardwell.

Gila monster (*Heloderma suspectum*), and the Mexican beaded lizard (*H. horridum*), but bites by these species are quite rare unless an attempt is made to pick up the animal. Venomous lizards will not be discussed in this chapter.

Anatomic essentials

The venomous creatures discussed in this chapter all produce venoms in specialized glands, and deliver these venoms using sophisticated anatomic structures (such as fangs or stingers) to their victims or prey. These venoms are complex and lead to various local and/or systemic derangements depending on the species involved. A brief overview of the major venom types and characteristic clinical sequelae is found in Tables 42.5 and 42.6. One should keep in mind that venoms can vary not only between species, but also between individuals within a species, and that venoms affect different individuals in different ways. Therefore, a physician tasked with managing a victim of venomous bite or sting must be vigilant for atypical presentations and sequelae.

Table 42.5 Overview of venoms of major groups of terrestrial creatures

ARTHROPOD VENOMS
Hymenoptera
Bees, wasps, yellow jackets, hornets:
- Peptides such as melittin (which may be allergenic) and apamin
- Vasoactive amines (histamine, serotonin, acetylcholine, epinephrine, norepinephrine and dopamine)
- Enzymatic components (phospholipase A, hyaluronidase, and acid phosphatase) – major allergens
- Fire ant venom contains piperidine alkaloids and low-molecular weight polypeptides

Spiders
- Venoms of various spider species can be quite variable. While almost all groups of spiders are venomous, the vast majority of species have fangs too small to penetrate human skin and are, therefore, of no medical significance.

Brown spiders
- Sphingomyelinase D – may produce dermonecrosis and hemolysis

Widow spiders
- Alpha latrotoxin – a neurotoxin that stimulates the release of neurotransmitters from nerve terminals (epinephrine, norcpinephrine, and acetylcholine)

Australian funnel-web spider
- Atratoxin or robustoxin – neurotoxins found in different species

Scorpions
- These venoms are quite variable in different species
- Most toxic scorpions contain neurotoxic components
- Many species contain serotonin (increases pain)

Snake venoms
- Very complex

Viperids (vipers and pit vipers)
- Components can effect essentially any body system
- Among the most deleterious fractions are low-molecular weight components that cause cellular membrane and intercellular disruption (responsible for tissue destruction)
- Most viperid venoms contain components that can cause systemic coagulopathy (due to affects on the coagulation cascade at various sites)

Elapids
- Many of these venoms possess significant neurotoxicity, which can cause death due to respiratory depression
- Some species have components that cause severe tissue necrosis (e.g., most spitting cobras)

Hydrophids (sea snakes)
- Neurotoxicity
- Myotoxicity

Colubrids
- Most species in this family are completely harmless
- A few species can envenom humans with toxic secretions from a special salivary gland (Duvernoy's gland). These secretions are hemorrhagic

Table 42.6 Descriptions of clinical syndromes that can be anticipated after bites/stings of venomous terrestrial creatures

---

Hymenoptera stings
- Typical local reaction: initial pain, followed by itching wheal or hive limited to the sting site.
- Exaggerated local response: pain and itching that progress over many hours to days to involve the entire extremity.
- Anaphylaxis: a spectrum of diffuse hives, wheezing, laryngeal edema, hypotension, abdominal pain, vomiting, diarrhea, and possibly death.

Spider bites
- Species capable of inflicting a bite through human skin: pain, a local papule that may develop a small eschar which heals over a period of days.
- *Widow spiders*: bite felt as a pinprick, gradual onset of muscle pain and cramping in the involved extremity (which may spread to the trunk, resulting in respiratory distress or a rigid abdomen) which progress for several hours and may persist for 72 hours; associated nausea, vomiting, sweating, headache (possibly due to elevated blood pressure or intracranial bleeding), rapid heart rate or palpitations.
- *Brown spiders*: bite is usually painless; delayed onset of pain due to ischemia at the bite site; ischemic tissue develops an ulcer which may be progressive and, in rare cases, become severe, undermining normal skin and creating a necrotic "volcano lesion"; rarely, systemic poisoning can present with flu-like symptoms (fever, nausea, vomiting, etc.) with acute hemolysis and potential development of renal failure.
- *Funnel-web spiders*: severe pain, perioral tingling, muscle fasciculations, diaphoresis, lacrimation, hypertension, tachycardia, pulmonary edema, and respiratory distress.

Scorpion stings
- Non-neurotoxic scorpions (e.g., most US species): initial intense pain that passes quickly; possibly mild soft tissue swelling and local bruising; anaphylaxis is rare.
- Neurotoxic scorpions (e.g., *Centruroides exilicauda*): minimal local changes; restlessness, roving eye movements, salivation, respiratory distress, opisthotonus/emprosthotonus (may mimic seizures), elevated blood pressure.

Snakebites
- *Viperids*: most cause local soft tissue swelling and pain within minutes of the bite; pain may be severe and swelling may progress over hours to involve the entire extremity and even the trunk; ecchymosis; over time, necrosis of local tissues; systemic findings may include nausea, vomiting, muscle fasciculations, altered taste sensations, weakness, bleeding (from almost any anatomic site) and shock.
- *Elapids*: most can cause neurotoxicity with resulting muscle weakness (generally starting with the muscles of the head and neck innervated by cranial nerves – ptosis, diplopia, difficulty swallowing) that may progress to peripheral paralysis and respiratory failure; cardiovascular instability may also occur; onset of signs or symptoms of venom poisoning may be extremely rapid or may be delayed many hours.
- *Hydrophids*: primary findings included neurotoxic symptoms and signs similar to elapids as well as pain related to myotoxicity.
- *Colubrids*: most of these species are completely harmless and bites result in no more pain that would be expected from multiple tiny pinpricks; bites by the dangerous boomslang or twig snake can cause systemic hemorrhage.

History

What was the offending animal?

It is easiest to manage a victim of a venomous bite or sting if the animal that inflicted the injury can be identified. Often this is easy, particularly if the creature was seen and can be accurately described (or if it was killed and brought with the patient). More than 50% of venomous snakebites in the US occur to people who are intentionally handling the animal, making identification more straightforward in this situation. In some cases, identification of the offending animal can be difficult or impossible. A good example of this is the bite of the brown recluse spider, which is often initially painless and the victim does not present for hours or days until local ischemic pain begins or a necrotic lesion develops.

How long before presentation did the bite(s) or sting(s) occur?

Some bites, such as venomous snakebites, usually prompt the victim to seek medical care promptly. On the other hand, a victim of some spider bites may not present for hours to days after envenomation.

What prehospital management measures were tried?

A number of first aid techniques for venomous bites or stings may be instituted by well-meaning "rescuers." Many such measures are of no value. Some may even be worse than the bite or sting itself. For most arthropod envenomations, ice application to and elevation of the affected body part are adequate first-aid therapies. It is difficult, however, to make broad recommendations for snakebites beyond getting the victim to medical care as soon as possible. Little definitive research has been done on field management approaches for snakebite. Ice should be avoided in venomous snakebite, as additional cold injury can worsen local venom-induced tissue damage. One technique demonstrated to delay absorption of a number of snake venoms is the Australian pressure immobilization technique. The victim's entire bitten extremity is wrapped firmly (at pressures similar to those used for wrapping a sprained ankle), beginning at the bite site, and the limb is then splinted. Use of this technique in situations where necrosis is unlikely to occur following the bite, as with many elapid venoms, appears prudent. Use in situations where tissue loss may be compounded by limiting venom strictly to the site, as with most viperid venoms, may be unwise unless the victim is a great distance from medical care and has suffered a life-threatening bite. Techniques to avoid include application of electric shocks, incision and suction, use of tourniquets, and application of topical poultices, such as meat tenderizer.

What is the victim's tetanus status?

Since any bite or sting results in a break in the skin with concomitant tetanus risk, adequate immunization status should be ensured and updated as indicated.

Past medical

Co-morbid conditions such as heart or lung disease may make the overall envenomation syndrome worse. Prior history of a bite or sting by a similar creature may be important if the victim suffered an allergic reaction to the injury or if antivenom therapy was required. Victims suffering an anaphylactic reaction to a hymenoptera sting who are currently on beta-blocker therapy are much more difficult to treat, and may be refractory to epinephrine treatment (Chapter 11).

Physical examination

When approaching a victim of severe venom poisoning, it is best to conduct a rapid, focused initial examination while simultaneously beginning life-saving treatment (e.g., epinephrine administration to a victim of anaphylaxis). Once treatment is underway, a more thorough examination should be performed.

General appearance

Check for any evidence of cardiac or respiratory distress, including airway involvement.

Vital signs

These can be quite variable depending on the envenomation syndrome.

Hymenoptera sting with anaphylaxis: The victim may have a rapid heart rate, low blood pressure, and rapid respiratory rate. In a preterminal state, the heart rate may begin to fall and blood pressure may be unobtainable.

Spider bites and scorpion stings: When neurotoxic species are involved, blood pressure, heart rate, and respiratory rate may be elevated. Occasionally the temperature will also be mildly elevated. Following most arthropod poisonings, however, the vital signs will be normal.

Snakebite: Vital signs are variable. A victim of elapid or seasnake bite may present with a decreased respiratory rate (due to neurotoxic loss of respiratory muscle function). Viperid bite victims often have an elevation in respiratory rate, heart rate and blood pressure (often due to accompanying anxiety), but may present, in severe poisoning, with vital signs consistent with shock due to venous pooling, third spacing, and hemolysis.

Pulmonary

Listen for quality and regularity of cardiac sounds and for adventitial lung sounds. In severe scorpion, widow spider or snake envenomation, the victim may develop pulmonary edema with accompanying rales on lung examination.

Abdomen

The abdominal examination is rarely revealing. Occasionally, with widow spider bites, the victim will complain of severe abdominal pain and will have what appears to be severe guarding. This has led to negative exploratory laparotomies in cases where a history of spider bite was not available. Widow spider venom-induced rectus abdominis spasm can, however, be differentiated from peritonitis by the lack of rebound following spider bite and by the fact that these victims tend to be restless, unable to find a position of comfort, unlike patients with acute peritonitis who prefer to lie as still as possible. A rectal examination should be performed to assess for occult blood in the setting of viperid snakebite.

Neurologic

A careful examination focusing on cranial nerve (CN) function (particularly CNs II through VII) and motor function (including respiratory effort as well as peripheral muscle strength) is important when the patient has been bitten or stung by an organism with neurotoxic venom (e.g., elapid snakebite or neurotoxic scorpion sting).

Skin

A close evaluation of the bite/sting site is important. Any retained bee stings (commonly referred to as "stingers") can be scraped away. There may be diffuse urticaria if the victim is experiencing an allergic reaction to the venom. Spider bites may present with minimal local findings (e.g., widow spider bites) or may have significant necrosis (e.g., severe brown spider bites). Scorpion stings usually have few local findings (possibly some mild soft tissue swelling or bruising at the site following non-neurotoxic scorpion stings). For snakebites, the bitten extremity may demonstrate puncture wounds (though the bite pattern can be misleading), ecchymosis, and soft tissue swelling (Figure 42.6). The extremity should be marked at two or more sites proximal to the bite, and circumferences measured at these points every 15 minutes to help gauge progression of the poisoning until it is clear that the victim has stabilized.

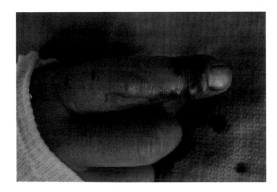

Figure 42.6
Rattlesnake bite to the distal index finger. Note the swelling, hemorrhagic blebs, and bloody discharge.

Lymphatic

Many arthropod and snake venoms are absorbed via the lymphatic system and may initiate an impressive lymphangitis. Regional lymph nodes draining a bitten extremity should be assessed for tenderness and lymphadenopathy.

Differential diagnosis

The differential diagnosis is usually straightforward in cases of venomous bites and stings. Often the victim will have witnessed the creature that inflicted the injury and be able to describe (or actually produce) it. If a snake is brought in with the patient, it should be evaluated cautiously, as even a dead snake or a decapitated snake head can have a bite reflex for up to 1 hour after being killed and can still render a serious bite.

Arriving at a diagnosis can be more difficult in cases of delayed presentation of possible spider bite when no spider was seen. In this scenario, the victim usually presents with a painful, swollen, red papule with or without an area of central necrosis. Such a lesion can indeed be caused by a spider, but is more likely the result of a bite from a flea, tick, bedbug or other arthropod. It also may be caused by a non-arthropod source, such as an infected plant puncture wound, or a local response to a systemic illness (e.g., toxic epidermal necrolysis, erythema nodosum, or diabetic ulcer).

Diagnostic testing
Laboratory studies

In most envenomation cases, laboratory studies are not necessary. There are very few diagnostic studies available to aid medical care providers treating victims of bites or stings. In Australia, an enzyme-linked immunosorbent assay kit is available to aid in identifying the offending species in suspected snakebites. These kits detect venom in wound aspirate, serum, or urine.

The following laboratory studies may be helpful in certain cases (Table 42.7).

Radiologic studies

Chest X-ray

A chest radiograph should be obtained in an envenomation syndrome whenever there are signs of respiratory distress, or if the victim has significant cardiorespiratory comorbidity.

Table 42.7 Laboratory testing for terrestrial venomous bites and stings

---

Complete blood count (CBC)
- *Suspected brown spider bite with systemic (flulike) symptoms*: to rule out hemolysis and thrombocytopenia.
- *Venomous snakebite*: to obtain a baseline hematocrit (in case the victim develops coagulopathy with systemic bleeding or hemolysis); the white blood cell (WBC) count is often elevated (without any secondary infection).

Electrolytes, renal function studies, and creatine kinase
- *Suspected brown spider bite with systemic symptoms or any abnormalities on the CBC*: to rule out renal dysfunction.
- *Venomous snakebite*: to rule out significant rhabdomyolysis or renal insufficiency. Sea snakes (and some viperids and elapids) can cause significant rhabdomyolysis with resulting hyperkalemia, myoglobinemia, myoglobinuria, and complicating renal failure. In these cases, a serum myoglobin and CK should also be measured.

Coagulation profile
- *Venomous snakebite and presumed brown spider bite with suspected systemic toxicity*: a serum sample should be sent for measurement of prothrombin time, partial thromboplastin time, International Normalized Ratio (INR), fibrinogen level, and fibrin degradation products to assess for possible consumptive coagulopathy.

Blood type and screen
- *Venomous snakebite*: to allow for cross-matching of blood in the rare event that coagulopathy or hemolysis mandates the need for transfusion. Both circulating snake venom and any administered antivenom can interfere with cross-matching as time progresses.
- *Presumed brown spider bite with suspected systemic toxicity*: to prepare for transfusion if needed to treat hemolysis or thrombocytopenia.

Urinalysis
- *Venomous snakebite or presumed brown spider bite*: point of care testing should be done on each voided specimen during the acute phase of poisoning to detect hematuria or myoglobinuria.

Electrocardiogram

An ECG should be obtained in an envenomation syndrome whenever the poisoning is severe, there are significant comorbidities, or the patient has chest pain or shortness of breath.

General treatment principles

Treatment may need to begin before a precise diagnosis is made, as in the case of a victim of arthropod-induced anaphylaxis. Any restrictive clothing or jewelry should be removed as soon as possible.

Patients presenting to an ED for evaluation of possible envenomation syndrome can be divided into two major groups. The first, and most common, is the clearly stable victim of a bite or sting who is concerned about possible complications (e.g., a victim who presents with a painful papule that might be a spider bite). The second is the potentially unstable victim of an acute envenomation that may be progressing (e.g., a venomous snakebite victim).

In the first type of patient, treatment is directed at trying to limit complications of the bite or sting. This involves supportive, conservative care including sound wound care (cleansing, dressing, splinting, and tetanus immunization as appropriate) and symptomatic treatment (e.g., antihistamines for itching). If signs or symptoms of secondary infection occur, the patient should receive appropriate antibiotics with good *Staphylococcus* coverage. If a brown spider bite is suspected, local ice treatment (every few hours over the course of 2–3 days) may be beneficial in slowing the action of venom enzymes. Ice should, however, be avoided in venomous snakebites due to the risk of compounding necrosis. If the victim has any systemic symptoms, laboratory studies should be obtained as outlined above (Table 42.7).

For potentially unstable patients (e.g., victim of serious widow spider bite, neurotoxic scorpion sting, or venomous snakebite), attention must first be directed at ensuring adequacy of the ABCs, in that order. Airway management must be aggressive if the patient was bitten by an elapid snake and presents with any evidence of respiratory depression or difficulty swallowing secretions. Oxygen should be started and cardiac and pulse oximetry monitoring instituted. Two large bore IV lines with normal saline should be started if there is any evidence of hemodynamic instability. If the blood pressure is low or the patient is significantly tachycardic, a bolus of IV fluid should be administered (20–40 ml/kg in a child; 500–1000 ml in an adult depending on the patient's cardiovascular reserve).

It must be determined whether an appropriate antivenom exists for the current envenomation syndrome, and whether or not it is necessary and available. Antivenoms exist for most of the world's venomous snakes, for widow spiders, and for some funnel-web spiders and scorpions. Antivenom choice is important, particularly when dealing with a venomous snakebite, as there is generally little benefit to using an antivenom produced for a remotely-related or unrelated species. For example, in North America, there would be no benefit in using a pit viper antivenom in treating a victim of coral snake bite. Conversely, widow spider antivenom is effective regardless of which *Latrodectus* species inflicted the bite. There are no commercially-available antivenoms outside of South America for brown spiders.

Antivenom is generally indicated if the victim demonstrates evidence of significant poisoning or evidence of progression. As not all hospitals carry all available antivenoms even against locally indigenous venomous creatures, a search for a source of the appropriate antiserum should begin early. Particularly in cases of bites by exotic species, poison control centers, or local or regional zoos may need to be consulted for assistance in locating antivenom.

Most antivenoms are produced by injecting horses or sheep with gradually increasing doses of the venom or venoms of interest. Once the animal has developed immunity to the venom(s), antibody laden serum is obtained, processed, purified (to variable degrees) and packaged, often in a lyophilized form. Many recently developed antivenoms are produced using technology to cleave the antibodies into the functional *Fab* fragments and the deleterious *Fc* fragments (which are discarded). These antibody fragment products tend to be more effective and safer to use than whole antibody products.

Administration of any antivenom (route, dose, timing) should be according to specific instructions in the package insert for the product chosen. The initial volume needed can vary from a single, 10-ml vial of widow spider antivenom, to six or more vials of rattlesnake antivenom. Additional doses may be required if signs, symptoms, or laboratory abnormalities progress or recur. Antivenoms should be administered in an unbitten extremity whenever possible in order to ensure adequate systemic distribution.

Since all antivenoms are currently derived from heterologous animal serums, they carry some risk of adverse reactions. These reactions can take the form of acute anaphylactic or anaphylactoid reactions, or delayed serum sickness (which generally presents 1–2 weeks following antivenom administration with symptoms such as hives, fever, myalgias, and arthralgias). Fortunately, with recent improvements in purification techniques, these reactions are becoming less common.

Antibiotics are usually not necessary for the treatment of venomous bites or stings, and should be reserved for cases with suspected secondary bacterial infection.

Additional treatment

Potential brown spider bites: If local necrosis is severe, these victims may require judicious debridement and/or skin grafting. Skin grafts should be delayed for 4–6 weeks to allow resolution of any ongoing venom effects. Some experts believe the use of dapsone (a polymorphonuclear leukocyte inhibitor) may reduce the extent of necrosis following these bites. While theoretically and anecdotally of value, dapsone is not approved for this purpose and has significant dose-dependent side effects, making its use controversial. Likewise, research results have been mixed on the use of hyperbaric oxygen (HBO) therapy to limit necrosis. If readily available and easily accessed, HBO can be tried for particularly severe wounds.

Widow spider bites: A combination of benzodiazepines and narcotic analgesics is useful in the management of severe pain, muscle spasms and agitation often seen with this envenomation syndrome. Calcium gluconate, while mentioned anecdotally by some authors, is of little or no benefit in the management of widow spider venom poisoning.

Venomous snakebites: Bites by viperid snakes often produce severe soft tissue swelling of the involved extremity. This swelling is usually restricted to the subcutaneous tissues, but, in rare cases, can occur within muscle compartments resulting in possible compartment syndrome. Differentiating a compartment syndrome from severe, subcutaneous swelling without vascular compromise requires direct intracompartmental pressure measurement using a wick catheter, needle and transducer, or a Stryker device. If pressures are found to be elevated (>30–40 mmHg), further antivenom should be administered while the limb is kept strictly elevated. If the victim's hemodynamic status is stable, a dose of IV mannitol (an osmotic diuretic) can be given in an effort to help reduce the intracompartmental pressure. If the pressure remains elevated over the next hour despite these treatments, a fasciotomy is required to ensure sustained blood flow to the muscles.

Special patients

As a general principle, victims at each end of the age spectrum may suffer more severe venom poisoning syndromes. Pediatric patients tend to receive the same venom load as an adult would when bitten or stung, yet they have less body mass and circulating volume to buffer the venom's effects. In situations where antivenom is required, pediatric doses meet or exceed those for adults due to this relatively greater venom load-to-body mass ratio. Elderly patients, likewise, may be more prone to severe venom effects in the face of comorbid conditions, and should be treated aggressively.

Disposition

Victims who are clearly stable following a bite or sting can usually be discharged from the ED after an appropriate period of observation (generally 6–8 hours). A symptomatic victim of hymenoptera sting who is worried about development of anaphylaxis (possibly due to a prior episode of anaphylaxis following bee sting), can be observed for at least 2 hours in the ED and discharged if asymptomatic. Victims of hymenoptera stings who experience a systemic reaction more severe than simple diffuse urticaria or mild bronchospasm should be admitted for observation, preferably to a monitored setting. Any patient who has experienced an anaphylactic reaction should, at the time of discharge from the hospital, receive a prescription for a self-administration epinephrine device, instructions to obtain a Medic-Alert medallion, and referral to an allergist for evaluation.

Patients who present with potential brown spider bites can be discharged for daily wound checks (for 3 days) if they have no systemic findings (fever, flu-like symptoms). If systemic abnormalities are present (as manifested by signs, symptoms, or laboratory abnormalities), these patients should be admitted for IV fluids and monitoring for development of severe hemolysis and potential renal failure.

Victims bitten by a venomous snake who have no evidence of venom poisoning should be observed for at least 6 hours. If they remain asymptomatic and have normal laboratory tests and vital signs at 6 hours, they can be safely discharged with instructions to return if delayed signs or symptoms of envenomation appear. An exception to this 6 hours guideline exists if the biting snake was an elapid, due to the potential delay in onset of findings of venom poisoning. In these cases, victims should be admitted for 24 hours of observation. Any snakebite victim with signs or symptoms of envenomation should be admitted to the hospital. The patient should be in a monitored setting during any antivenom administration.

Pearls, pitfalls, and myths

There are few topics in medicine as impacted by myths and folklore as the treatment of venomous bites and stings. Many anecdotal "remedies" still receive attention, particularly related to venomous snakebites. These include application of various poultices, use of extreme heat, incision and suction, electric shock therapy, and others.

The keys to managing any acute envenomation syndrome are to be a keen observer, anticipate multisystem involvement, and promptly request specialty consultation from a regional expert or poison control center.

The major pitfalls in managing envenomations lie in:

- performing an inadequate evaluation (particularly regarding the history and physical examination);
- failure to periodically reassess the victim for progression of venom poisoning;
- failing to recognize the importance of abnormal vital signs;
- failing to aggressively secure the airway in a patient developing respiratory insufficiency;
- failing to secure and administer antivenom, when indicated, in a timely fashion;
- premature discharge of a victim of venom poisoning when the onset of systemic findings may be delayed (e.g., a victim of elapid snake bite);

- diagnosing any lesion as a "brown (recluse) spider bite" in the absence of confirmatory evidence;
- failure to evaluate a victim of possible brown spider bite with systemic symptoms for hemolysis or renal insufficiency;
- discharging a patient without appropriate follow-up and after-care instructions (e.g., failure to prescribe an epinephrine self-administration kit and referral to an allergist for a victim of hymenoptera-induced anaphylaxis);
- failure to administer tetanus immunization when indicated, though these wounds can be considered to be at low risk for tetanus unless secondary infection occurs;
- failure to suspect compartment syndrome and objectively measure intracompartmental pressures in a victim of viperid bite with severe extremity swelling;
- failure to seek early specialty consultation when needed.

References

1. Bahna SL. Insect sting allergy: a matter of life and death. *Pediatr Ann* 2000;29(12):753–758.
2. Clark RF, Wethern-Kestner S, Vance MV, Gerkin R. Clinical presentation and treatment of black widow spider envenomation: a review of 163 cases. *Ann Emerg Med* 1992;21(7):782–787.
3. Gold BS, Dart RC, Barish RA. Bites of venomous snakes. *New Engl J Med* 2002;347(5):347–356.
4. Hartman LJ, Sutherland SK. Funnel-web spider (*Atrax robustus*) antivenom in the treatment of human envenomation. *Med J Australia* 1984;141:796–799.
5. Litovitz TL, Klein-Schwartz W, Rodgers GC, Cobaugh DJ, Youniss J, Omslaer JC, May ME, Woolf AD, Benson BE. 2001 annual report of the American Association of Poison Control Centers Toxic Exposure Surveillance System. *Am J Emerg Med* 2002;20(5):391–452.
6. Masters E. Loxoscelism. *New Engl J Med* 1998;339(6):379.
7. Moss HS, Binder LS. A retrospective review of black widow spider envenomation. *Ann Emerg Med* 1987;16(2):188–191.
8. Norris RL, Bush SP. North American venomous reptile bites. In: Auerbach PS (ed.). *Wilderness Medicine*, 4th ed., St. Louis: Mosby, 2001. pp. 896–926.
9. Norris RL, Minton SA. Non-North American venomous reptile bites. In: Auerbach PS (ed.). *Wilderness Medicine*, 4th ed., St. Louis: Mosby, 2001. pp. 927–951.
10. Polis GA (ed.). *The Biology of Scorpions*. Stanford, Stanford University Press, California, 1990.
11. Wasserman GS, Anderson PC. Loxoscelism and necrotic arachnidism. *J Toxicol Clin Toxicol* 1983–1984;21(4 and 5):451–472.

43   Ethics and end-of-life issues

Michael A. Gisondi, MD

Scope of the problem

Challenging ethical issues may suddenly arise when caring for critically-ill patients in the emergency department (ED). The rapid deterioration of such patients often prohibits lengthy deliberations about ethical dilemmas. Emergency physicians must possess a practical understanding of medical ethics in order to address these cases in a thorough and efficient manner.

Terminology

Modern philosophy links the definitions of morality and ethics. In the simplest forms, *morality* is the difference between right and wrong, while *ethics* represents the critical study of morality. Individuals choose from a variety of sources of moral authority, such as religion, cultural norms, politics, and law. As such, persons may regard situations or objects differently, based on the value systems espoused by their source of moral guidance. Ethics represents the cognitive evaluation of a principle or situation, acknowledging the fact that individuals possess different moral backgrounds. Ethical dilemmas arise when there is a conflict of values between persons arguing for competing moral imperatives – when people cannot agree on what is right and what is wrong.

Medical ethics is a discipline that studies differences in value systems as they apply to clinical situations. Medical ethics is most commonly taught through classroom discussion, as a means to familiarize providers with common ethical principles. *Applied health care ethics* is the practical extension of such discussion, recognizing that like all clinical decision-making, ethical dilemmas require action. The word "applied" then refers to the reality that physicians mediate ethical dilemmas and make tough decisions every day. They are not philosophers, but practitioners of medical philosophy.

Ethical theories

Most American physicians guide their ethical decision-making from duty-based concepts known as the "principles of biomedical ethics." These principles include respect for autonomy, non-malfeasance, beneficence and justice. *Respect for autonomy* is demonstrated when the patient is given the ability to exhibit self-governance, or self-determination. Patients should be allowed to make choices regarding their own health care. *Non-malfeasance* is loosely translated into the statement "do no harm." Physicians have an ethical obligation to limit the risks of poor outcomes that may result from diagnostic or therapeutic interventions. *Beneficence* in health care refers to the fundamental challenge to optimize a patient's condition and well-being; this may be through treatment of disease or provision of comfort care. *Justice* refers to the fair and equal treatment of patients, both in access to and quality of health care. Justice is also manifest through systems and institutional ethics, which in today's marketplace must respond to the reality of limited health care resources.

A competing, but no less valid ethical theory is that of virtue ethics. Defined in medieval times, the *virtues* were those character traits that shaped professional ethics in medicine for many centuries. Among the most critical markers of character for the virtuous physician were fidelity, trust, compassion, temperance, integrity, prudence, justice and self-effacement. For patients, the virtues of love (of something, such as health or life) and faith (that life can continue or health be restored) translate into the modernly accepted virtue of hope. These latter virtues serve as the basis of value systems employed by some critically-ill patients and their families, and as such, should be considered when making ethical decisions.

Making ethical decisions

As mentioned, the pace with which emergency physicians must make clinical and ethical decisions does not allow for extended discussions of ethical theory. Instead, physicians can benefit from a practiced, step-wise approach to ethical decision-making. First, one must recognize that an ethical dilemma exists. Next, the physician must choose an ethical framework to guide the deliberation process in an organized manner.

Finally, an action must be chosen and one's reasoning reflected in the medical record.

Recognizing the ethical dilemma

Ethical dilemmas must be recognized and characterized. They result from conflicts between values or the interpretation of values by patients, their families, physicians, staff, the hospital, society, the law and others. Once physicians recognize that tensions exist, the ethical conflict should be characterized as simply as possible. *"Mrs. X is in respiratory failure. Her daughter wants her intubated, despite a valid 'do-not-resuscitate' order in the patient's chart. The daughter's wishes (hope, beneficence) are at conflict with the physician's obligation to his patient (prudence, respect for autonomy)."*

Choosing an ethical framework

An ethical framework differs from a theory or Code of Conduct in that it represents a systematic, step-wise approach to addressing ethical dilemmas. It may be impractical for the physician to work through a detailed framework in an emergent situation, but familiarization with the steps of a given framework will make critical decisions proceed more smoothly. Two such ethical frameworks are included for consideration: Thomasma's "Ethical Workup Guide" and Iserson's "A Rapid Approach to Ethical Problems."

The ethical workup guide (David C. Thomasma, PhD. 1978)

Step 1: What are the facts in the case?

Mrs. X is in respiratory failure following a long progression of lung cancer. She has had ample time to consider the details of her living will, and apparently made an authentic choice to decline intubation. Her daughter has been estranged from her for many years, but now asks for "more time" in order to reconcile their differences.

Step 2: What are the values at risk in the case?

The daughter exhibits the virtue of hope. The physician realizes the futility of prolonging his patient's death. The daughter is also genuinely beneficent, in that she believes intubation is the optimal treatment for her dying mother. The physician has a duty to respect his patient's autonomous choice to decline life-saving procedures.

Step 3: Determine the conflicts between values and professional norms, and between ethical axioms, rules, and principles.

At conflict are the daughter's beneficent hope and the physician's prudence and duty to respect his patient's autonomy.

Step 4: Determine possible courses of action, and which values and ethical principles each course of action would protect or infringe.

Intubation might temporarily extend the patient's life, in accordance with the daughter's wishes. Non-invasive mechanical ventilation such as bilevel positive airway pressure (BiPAP) would be an option more respectful of the patient's wishes and the physician's obligation to his patient.

Step 5: Make a decision in the case.

Non-invasive ventilation instead of intubation.

Step 6: Defend this course of action. Why is "x" better than "y"?

Respect for patient autonomy is more important than the perceived beneficence of the daughter's wishes. One might also view the physician as being more beneficent to his patient, by honoring the patient's living will.

A rapid approach to ethical problems: to be used for decisions when there is insufficient time for detailed ethical analysis (Kenneth V. Iserson, MD. 1995)

Step 1: Is this a type of ethical problem for which you have already worked out a rule, or is it at least similar enough so that the rule could reasonably be extended?

- *Yes:* Follow the rule.
- *No:* Proceed to Step 2.

Step 2: Is there an option that will buy you time for deliberation without risk to the patient?

- *Yes*: Take that option.
- *No:* Apply the tests of impartiality, universalizability and interpersonal justifiability.
- *Test of impartiality*: Would you be willing to have this action performed if you were the patient?
- *Test of universalizability*: Are you willing to have this action performed in all relevantly similar circumstances?

– *Test of interpersonal justifiability*: Are you able to provide good reasons to justify your actions to others? Will peers, superiors, or the public be satisfied with the answers?

Choose an action and document thought process in the chart

Applied health care ethics expects that an ethical decision (action) will occur in parallel with other clinical decisions. Once the physician chooses a course of action, the thought process should be documented in the "medical decision making" section of the medical record. *"Given the patient's choice to decline intubation as described in her living will, I will support her respirations with non-invasive ventilatory methods (BiPAP), which appear to help her sense of dyspnea."*

End-of-life issues

Emergency physicians encounter patients who may quickly expire. One of the most meaningful expressions of the patient–physician relationship comes from the thoughtful and considerate treatment of dying patients. To respect patient autonomy during this process, physicians must quickly assess the patient's individual preferences for end-of-life care. Two issues are paramount: resuscitation wishes and naming of a surrogate decision-maker.

Resuscitation preferences

The term DNR is a poor descriptor of a patient's detailed preferences for end-of-life care (Table 43.1). For example, some patients may not wish to be maintained on a ventilator and therefore

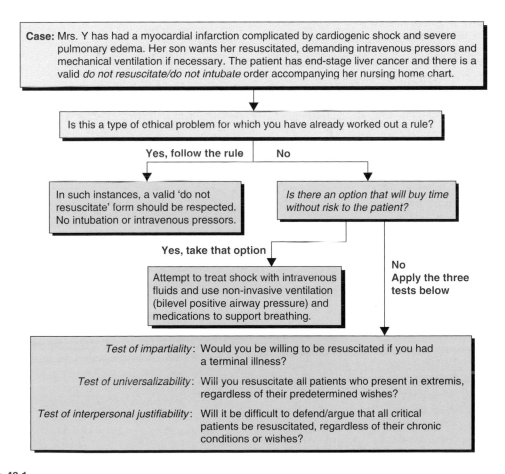

Figure 43.1
Using the rapid approach to ethical problems. Adapted from: Iserson KV: An approach to ethical problems in emergency medicine. In: Iserson KV, Sanders AB, Mathieu D (eds). *Ethics in Emergency Medicine*, 2nd ed., 1995. Tucson, AZ: Galen Press.

are labeled *do not intubate (DNI)*, but would want to be defibrillated if they developed ventricular fibrillation. Physicians should approach resuscitation preferences as separate questions and list the answers in the chart after the DNR phrase (DNR: no compressions, no intubation, no defibrillation; yes: pressors, intravenous (IV) fluid.

Table 43.1 Questions used to define resuscitation preferences

- If your heart was to stop beating, would you want chest compressions performed?
- If you were to stop breathing, would you want a breathing tube placed so that a ventilator could breathe for you?
- If your heart went into a life-threatening rhythm, would you want to be shocked out of it?
- If your blood pressure dropped, would you want medications that might make it normal again?
- Is it acceptable to give you intravenous fluid and antibiotic medications to treat your condition?

Identifying surrogate decision-makers

Surrogate decision-makers should be identified in the event a patient lacks capacity at a later time. Surrogates should have an appreciation of the patient's end-of-life preferences, so that they make future decisions in accordance with their wishes. Surrogates can be named in a number of ways. "Next-of-kin" is a common method that states use to legally identify surrogates, if one has not already been named in an advance directive. Advance directives are lengthy, descriptive statements that provide a detailed discussion of patient preferences, including the identification of a surrogate decision-maker. Advance directives are much more involved than DNR/DNI forms, which generally include answers only to specific resuscitation questions. "Living wills" can provide even more information, addressing preferences for the handling of the corpse and potential organ donation. A "health care proxy" form refers to the legal designation of a surrogate, only after prior consultation with an attorney. This proxy can be arranged alone, as part of an advance directive, or in conjunction with a living will.

Once resuscitation preferences and a surrogate decision-maker are known, the medical team can better plan for future decisions to escalate or withdraw life-sustaining care. When such information is unknown, society expects that physicians will fully resuscitate dying patients with two ultimate goals in mind: to save their life and to restore them

to a state in which they can make autonomous decisions. If patients are later found to have valid DNR/DNI orders, it is ethically justified to withdraw life-sustaining care in accordance to their previously identified wishes. Though withdrawal of care can be emotionally upsetting to health care providers, it represents a profound demonstration of one's respect for patient autonomy.

Death notification

As there is no "right" way to inform family members of a loved one's death, physicians can develop a method that fits their personality and bedside manner. It is important to keep in mind that while the primary objective is death notification, there is certain information that needs to be obtained from family members as well (Table 43.2). First, ask the names and relationships of everyone present and confirm that they would have had permission to know the medical details of the case. Always notify the surrogate decision-maker or next-of-kin before speaking to other family and friends. Briefly inquire about the details of events leading up to the patient's arrival in the ED, if these were unknown. Once loved ones begin grieving, they may not be capable of providing needed details. Next, explain exactly what you knew of the situation and what interventions were performed. Specifically state that the resuscitation was unsuccessful and that the patient *died*. Do not sugar coat the events with euphemisms for death, as it may be confusing to some family members. Use a sympathetic voice and offer physical gestures of comfort, such as handholding, if this seems appropriate. Acknowledge the efforts of the pre-hospital providers and nursing

Table 43.2 Important steps in death notification

- Notify only those individuals who have permission to hear about the details of the case.
- Identify next-of-kin and notify these individuals before addressing other family and friends.
- Briefly obtain any needed information about the pre-hospital events.
- Succinctly describe the emergency department course and interventions.
- State that the resuscitation was unsuccessful and that the patient *died*.
- Respond to grief with sympathetic gestures.
- Acknowledge efforts by pre-hospital staff, nurses and family members.
- Address the needs of those present.

staff, especially if they had interacted directly with family members. Reassure loved ones that they should not blame themselves, as many family members will feel that the outcome may have been different had they intervened earlier. If questions arise about other possible interventions or a more lengthy resuscitation, focus on the concept of brain anoxia using phrases such as "brain death" and "could not have been the same person given that length of time."

The discussion should end by addressing the needs of those present. Utilize your support staff and have them remain after the notification; never leave a family member alone when you exit the room. Ask if they would like a nurse or social worker to assist in contacting a funeral home and making arrangements for the corpse. Inquire about any spiritual needs that might be addressed by contacting a chaplain or spiritual advisor. Acknowledging cultural or religious needs may be the most comforting thing you can do for some families. Ask those present if they would like some time with the deceased. Prepare them for what they will see, and make certain someone from the healthcare team is available for them. Lastly, remember to ask if the surrogate requests an autopsy. This question is mandated by law in many states.

Special ethical issues in teaching hospitals

Unique ethical dilemmas arise in academic medical centers as a function of the training environment. The inherent nature of apprenticeship in medical education sometimes conflicts with patient expectations that their care be delivered by only the most well-trained individuals. Ethical issues arising from the teaching environment require special attention by both the instructor and learner.

Informed consent

Legal and ethical principles mandate that physicians obtain informed consent for all treatments delivered. Patients are generally asked to consent to treatment when they arrive at the ED, indicating that they agree to be examined by the physician and receive "routine" care (blood tests, radiographs and medications). While this initial consent implies that patients understand the benefits of such care, physicians should make every effort to review the risks of all significant interventions (i.e., new medications that may

cause adverse reactions). More "invasive" procedures require additional information before a patient can truly give informed consent. At many hospitals, this process includes separate consent forms which provide added documentation that a special discussion occurred.

There are four steps to obtaining informed consent:

1. The physician should assure that patients possess the capacity to make an informed choice. *Capacity*, which refers to the ability to understand one's options and make an authentic choice, differs from the legal term competence. *Competence* is a court-determined judgment of capacity; physicians may comment on a patient's decision-making capacity, but are not permitted to declare someone incompetent. If a patient cannot understand treatment options as a result of organic or psychiatric illness, a physician should describe them as "lacking decision-making capacity." Patients who lack capacity cannot consent to treatment, so a health care proxy should be identified (i.e., next-of-kin or predetermined surrogate decision-maker). Such patients may still be able to agree to treatment; however, both the consent and assent should be documented.
2. The risks and benefits of proposed interventions should be reviewed in detail. This need not be an exhaustive list of all possible outcomes, but rather a discussion of the most common and serious complications. Physicians should make every effort to provide an honest risk–benefit analysis, including alternative treatments and the choice to have no intervention whatsoever. This step is critically important in teaching hospitals. Students and residents should not obtain consent for a procedure or treatment if they are unable to provide detailed risk–benefit information. Additionally, patients should understand which team member will be performing an invasive procedure, as well as the designated attending physician available for supervision.
3. The patient must comprehend the information discussed. One way to assess such understanding is to ask the patient to repeat the salient points from the conversation, in his or her own words. They should not simply repeat medical jargon. Patient questions should be elicited and answered as well.

4. Patients should confirm that they feel comfortable with their decision, acknowledging that their choice was voluntary and without duress. Both medical staff and family members can unduly influence patients to provide consent that is neither authentic nor autonomous. It is acceptable and ethically responsible to ask patients if they felt that they made their decision without feeling pressured.

Research ethics and the emergency exception to consent

Teaching hospitals often conduct research activity as part of their academic mission. Patients identified as potential research subjects for studies must first provide informed consent prior to their participation. It is sometimes difficult to obtain consent for emergency medicine research projects, however, as patients often present gravely ill and alone. They may lack the decision-making capacity necessary for consent and have no surrogate available to speak on their behalf. This complicates emergency medicine research, as it limits the ability to enroll subjects and conduct studies. Additionally, patients who might benefit from novel interventions are sometimes precluded from receiving such care when they are unable to provide consent.

The Food and Drug Administration (FDA) recognized these limitations and defined a set of guidelines termed the "waiver of informed consent for emergency research." This waiver of consent can be granted by human subjects committees or institutional review boards if:

1. there is a necessity for such research (study subjects have a life-threatening condition for which current treatments are unsatisfactory); or
2. there is a prospect for direct benefit to the subjects (risks are reasonable given the critical nature of the medical condition); or
3. informed consent from patient representatives will be pursued (follow-up consent from surrogates or community notification of the ongoing study).

While these guidelines offer researchers a method by which to conduct emergency medicine studies, they provide important ethical assurance that research subjects will be protected and respected.

Procedures on the newly dead

Recently deceased patients are occasionally used to teach life-saving, invasive procedures to students and residents at teaching hospitals. An ethical dilemma exists between the need to respect the integrity and autonomy of patients and family members, and the need to train health care providers. In response to this issue, the American Medical Association's (AMA) Council on Ethical and Judicial Affairs created a set of guidelines to help institutions ensure ethically-responsible behavior in such learning environments. Prior to performing procedures on the newly deceased, the following considerations should be addressed:

1. The teaching of life-saving skills should be the culmination of a structured training sequence, performed under close supervision and in accordance with the wishes and values of all involved parties.
2. Physicians should attempt to assess if the deceased had expressed preferences for the handling of his or her body after death. If not, consent should be obtained from family members before proceeding. In the absence of expressed preferences or surrogate consent, physicians should <u>not</u> perform procedures for training purposes. These guidelines were incorporated into the 2003 AMA Code of Medical Ethics.

Pearls of wisdom: issues of professional ethics for physicians-in-training

- *Do not lie.* The pressure to perform well in training programs often leads students and residents to misrepresent their knowledge or actions. Patient well-being is the utmost concern. Avoid the trap of embellishing history and physical examination details in order to appear more complete to your evaluators.
- *Do not misrepresent yourself.* ED patients are acutely ill and vulnerable. They expect the best care possible and will assume that students or residents have more training than they actually do. Clearly describe your role on the health care team and be honest about your level of training. It is the attending physician's responsibility to supervise care and answer patient questions regarding the hierarchy of the teaching hospital.
- *Do not do procedures if you feel uncomfortable.* Busy EDs often afford too much autonomy and responsibility to their trainees. Learners

may be asked to perform procedures they have never seen or read about previously. Grades and evaluations are not as important as patient safety. Ask for supervision for procedures requiring skills you have not yet mastered, and refuse to perform them without assistance.

- *Do the right thing.* As a member of the health care team, you have an obligation to your patient. Sometimes you may feel that an ethical issue has arisen, but others on the team seem unaware or unconcerned. It is your duty to your patient to discuss such ethical issues with the team. It may result in a learning moment for you, as the attending physician may not have taken the time to explain his or her decision-making process. In other instances, you may feel it necessary to seek additional guidance elsewhere. Hospital ethics committees are available for consultation by any member of the health care team, including nurses, ancillary staff and physicians-in-training.

References

1. Adams JG, Wegener J. Acting without asking: an ethical analysis of the Food and Drug Administration waiver of informed consent for emergency research, *Ann Emerg Med* 1999;33(2):218–223.

2. Beauchamp TL, Childress JF. *Principles of Bioethics*, 3rd ed., New York: Oxford University Press, 1989.

3. Council on Ethical and Judicial Affairs, AMA. Performing procedures on the newly deceased, *Acad Med* 2002;77(12–1): 1212–1216.

4. Geiderman JM. Consent and refusal in an urban American emergency department: two case studies, *Acad Emerg Med* 2001;8(3): 278–281.

5. Iserson KV. An approach to ethical problems in emergency medicine. In: Iserson KV, Sanders AB, Mathieu D (eds). *Ethics in Emergency Medicine*, 2nd ed., Tucson, AZ: Galen Press, 1995.

6. Larkin GL, Marco CA, Abbott JT. Emergency determination of decision-making capacity, *Acad Emerg Med* 2001;8(3):282–284.

7. Pellegrino ED, Thomasma DC. *The Virtues in Medical Practice*, New York: Oxford University Press, 1993.

8. Pellegrino ED, Thomasma DC. *The Christian Virtues in Medical Practice*, Washington, DC: Georgetown University Press, 1996.

9. Thomasma DC, Marshall PA. *Clinical Medical Ethics Cases and Readings*, Lanham, MD: University Press of America, 1995.

44 Legal aspects of emergency care

Gregory Guldner, MD, MS and Amy Leinen, ESQ

Scope of the problem

Emergency physicians interact with various aspects of the legal system throughout their career. Along with a relatively high likelihood of malpractice claims, emergency physicians often interact with police as they assess and treat trauma patients. They must also routinely deal with complicated legal issues such as advance directives, informed consent, protection of minors, mandatory reporting to health authorities, involuntary confinement, and compliance with federal laws, such as the Emergency Medical Treatment and Active Labor Act (EMTALA).

This chapter introduces the most common legal concepts that arise in emergency medicine. It begins with a discussion of legal issues that develop during patient care, followed by a review of physician interactions with the criminal justice system, providing care under the EMTALA, and finally medical malpractice. The difficulty with any discussion of legal issues on a general level lies in the lack of consistency between the various legal systems. Broadly speaking, there are two main divisions – federal law and state law – and each of these divisions is further subdivided into criminal, civil, and administrative sections. The laws governing any particular issue may differ depending on the particular state involved (or the federal government) and whether criminal, civil, or administrative rules apply. This inconsistency results in a certain ambiguity when discussing legal issues in a general sense, and mandates that physicians understand the specific laws that govern in their practice location.

Patient care issues

Informed consent

Certain legal issues begin the moment any patient enters the emergency department (ED); consent to treatment will likely be the first encountered. Competent patients have the right to refuse medical care. Conversely, physicians must obtain consent prior to procedures and treatment or risk a charge of battery. Informed consent is a process whereby the physician and patient discuss the risks, benefits, and alternatives to a given procedure or treatment. Although a patient's signature on an informed consent document may be prudent, it does not by itself meet the legal requirement of this process. To give informed consent, a patient must have sufficient information on which to base a decision about treatment. The legal determination of whether the physician obtained informed consent varies from state to state, but relies on terms such as "appropriate" and "reasonable," thus leaving the issue far from clear in any given case.

Emergency exceptions to consent

Certain patients are unable to either consent to or refuse treatment based on their inability to participate meaningfully in the informed consent process. This typically occurs due to age, intoxication, underlying medical conditions, or acute changes in mental status. In documenting either informed consent or informed refusal, the physician should make a notation of the patient's mental status and ability to consent or refuse. Physicians should refrain from referring to a patient's *competence*, as this is a legal term determined by a court, not a physician. Rather, physicians should refer to a patient's *decision-making capacity*. When the patient cannot provide consent, all states have emergency exceptions to the consent process. Patients medically unable to express consent are presumed to consent to emergency stabilizing treatment. Intoxicated patients usually cannot provide consent, and fall under the emergency exception if the patient's decision-making capacity is impaired.

Treatment of minors

Although most children cannot provide legal consent, all states have exemptions for children presenting to the ED without a parent or legal guardian. In these situations, the physician can assume consent for any necessary stabilizing treatment. Additionally, federal law (EMTALA) requires that all children, whether accompanied by a consenting adult or not, receive a medical screening examination (MSE) and any necessary stabilizing treatment. In the rare case of a guardian or parent refusing to consent to life-saving treatment needed to stabilize a child, physicians should generally provide necessary treatment and obtain a court order after the fact. Note that age by itself does not necessarily preclude the ability to consent, as there are conditions that allow minors to make their own medical decisions. These conditions vary from state to state, but often include the ability to consent without parental knowledge to treatment for sexually transmitted illnesses, pregnancy, drug and alcohol dependency, rape, and mental health concerns. Emancipated minors, individuals who the law recognizes as adults despite their age, also can consent or refuse treatment without parental involvement. Circumstances that allow minors to apply for legal emancipation vary, but often include active duty in the armed forces, marriage, pregnancy, and parenthood.

Informed refusal

Patients with decision-making capacity may withdraw consent for treatment at any time. This may occur prior to the involvement of a physician, when patients leave the ED before being evaluated, or at some point thereafter when they either refuse treatment or leave against medical advice (AMA). When a patient withdraws consent, the physician must again determine his or her capacity to do so. Patients with impaired decision-making capacity cannot provide an informed refusal, and the physician has a duty to provide stabilizing treatment. The majority of patients who leave AMA do have the capacity to make that decision, but every effort should be made to uncover the underlying reason for deciding to leave. Occasionally, patients do not understand the various treatment options or the potential for deterioration of their condition. While a signature on an AMA form may be helpful defending against litigation, a note in the medical record detailing the patient's capacity and the process by which informed refusal occurred must supplement it. Ideally, a family member should witness this discussion and sign the AMA form as well.

Some patients will withdraw consent by simply leaving the ED, known as "eloping." These patients constitute a dilemma for the physician, as not all patients can "elope." For example, a 75-year-old patient with advanced Alzheimer's disease who wanders from the ED can neither "elope" nor provide informed refusal. Patients who "elope" should be discussed among involved care providers, including nursing and ancillary staff, to determine if the patient reasonably appeared to have the capacity to withdraw consent and leave. Patients who do not, such as the patient above, must be searched for and retrieved as soon as possible.

Advance directives

Often patients who do not have the capacity to consent have either a *do-not-resuscitate (DNR)* order or an *advance directive* that assists in determining their wishes. A DNR order usually relates only to the specific condition of cardiopulmonary arrest; that is, a patient does not wish intubation, chest compressions, or defibrillation should their heart stop. Unfortunately, unless these orders are explicit, it often remains unclear as to what exactly the patient would want for conditions less severe than cardiac arrest. If the patient displays signs of impending respiratory failure, should they be intubated? If they are hypotensive from unstable ventricular tachycardia, should they be cardioverted? Generally, a DNR order does not equal a "no care" or "comfort care only" order, and should be interpreted narrowly. The advance directive and *durable power of attorney for health care* can be more explicit than a general DNR, and may provide more direction to the emergency physician. One of the difficulties common in the ED arises when a patient is thought to have a DNR order by staff but no documentation exists. Unfortunately, the laws governing this situation vary from state to state, but written documentation or "actual knowledge" of DNR status must usually be present to withhold care. What constitutes "actual knowledge" may be debated in individual cases, but generally refers to situations in which a physician has personally seen the advance directive even though it is not currently present.

Involuntary detainment

Another situation in which patients may lose the ability to consent involves psychiatric conditions, such as severe depression resulting in a suicide attempt. In California, for example, patients who are suicidal, homicidal, or gravely disabled may be detained up to 72 hours for psychiatric evaluation. During this period, these patients may receive treatment necessary to stabilize a condition brought on by a suicide attempt, and they may be restrained by physical or chemical means necessary to protect themselves or others. The procedure for involuntarily detaining a patient is complex, and physicians should become thoroughly familiar with the laws in their area, carefully document the events that required detainment, and the methods of restraint implemented.

Privacy and confidentiality

Another common legal issue arising during patient care involves privacy and confidentiality issues. The Health Insurance Portability and Accountability Act (HIPAA) sets forth standards for hospitals with regard to both personal privacy and the confidentiality of medical records. While the medical records are typically owned by the hospital, the information within them is considered property of the patient. In general, medical information cannot be shared with a third party without the consent of the patient unless such information is necessary for medical treatment. This includes releasing information to other family members, insurance companies, and employers. Exceptions to this exist, as all states have mandatory reporting of victims of violence and of certain health conditions. Emergency physicians must be careful to obtain consent from patients prior to speaking with other family members, friends, or employers. The requirements of HIPAA do not apply to information shared between health care providers for the sole purpose of medical evaluation and treatment. Patients unable to consent due to medical conditions represent a special case that the courts have yet to fully explore. Generally, physicians should proceed with the assumption of what a reasonable person in a similar situation would want with regard to confidentiality. For example, refusing to update a spouse on the status of a critically-injured patient because the patient is unable to give consent for the release of medical information seems unreasonable. While the courts have yet to determine many issues in this area, they typically allow discretion when a physician acts in the best interest of an incapacitated patient. However, in cases of human immunodeficiency virus (HIV) infection, drug and alcohol intoxication, and mental illness, the risk of damage to the patient for a breach of confidentiality is often considered substantial, and the medical information of patients with these diagnoses should be shared cautiously, if at all. Similarly, certain medical information, such as drug or alcohol tests in the hands of civil authorities, may result in serious consequences to some patients. Physicians in most states may not provide the police medical information on a patient without that patient's consent or a court order (excluding mandatory reporting requirements).

The criminal justice system

Emergency physicians often interact with police, detectives, district attorneys, and criminal defense attorneys. Table 44.1 lists common interactions that may develop during these encounters.

Interacting with the criminal justice system is an inevitable part of emergency medicine, and

Table 44.1 Common legal issues involving the criminal justice system in emergency medicine

Encounter	Legal issues and practice suggestions
Police are searching for a suspect who may come to the ED.	Ensure that the ED has a mechanism to advise practitioners of criminal suspects.
Police bring injured suspect to ED for treatment prior to booking.	Those in custody retain their rights to refuse medical treatment (barring altered mental status).
Police request that ED obtains evidence through medical procedure (nasogastric tube, etc.).	Physician cannot force a medical procedure on a patient without the patient's consent, even at the request of police. A court order is necessary.
Police request medical information from physician (patient's blood alcohol level, etc.).	Laws vary from state to state. Usually, a patient must consent prior to releasing information to the police. Some states allow physicians to report intoxicated drivers. Most police agencies prefer to obtain their own blood or urine specimens for legal reasons.

(continued)

Table 44.1 Common legal issues involving the criminal justice system in emergency medicine (*cont*)

Encounter	Legal issues and practice suggestions
Physician evaluates patient who appears to be a victim of violence.	Physicians must report children and certain at-risk adults (elderly, cognitively-impaired, etc.) who are victims of violence or neglect. Many states require physicians to report victims of domestic violence or animal attacks. Some states require reporting all patients who sustain injuries from violence.
Physician receives a subpoena to testify as a witness.	Physician must either comply with subpoena or contact the party issuing the subpoena (usually prosecutor or defense attorney) and make alternative arrangements. Ignoring a subpoena may result in the court finding the physician in contempt.
Physician evaluates trauma patient prior to evidence collection (victim of gunshot wound, etc.).	Physician should avoid destroying evidence during treatment. Do not cut through bullet holes in clothing, destroy or discard personal belongings, or place chest tubes through gunshot or stab wounds. Refrain from describing wounds as "entry" or "exit" or speculating on bullet trajectory unless specifically trained to do so.
Patient presents with alleged sexual assault requesting evidentiary examination.	Physicians must provide a medical screening examination. In the medical record, use the term "alleged" because the physician has no direct knowledge of the events. Consider transferring to specialized sexual assault referral center if available after appropriate contacts have been made and safe transport is arranged.

developing an understanding of the laws that regulate interactions with victims, police, suspects, witnesses, and attorneys is essential.

EMTALA/COBRA

Prior to 1986, a critically-ill patient arriving in an ED faced the possibility of being refused care if he or she was unable to pay. These patients may have suffered significant injury or death due to delays in finding emergency care. To prevent such events, Congress passed the EMTALA in 1986 as part of the Consolidated Omnibus Budget Reconciliation Act (COBRA). EMTALA imposes several legal requirements on most EDs (Table 44.2).

EMTALA compels multiple other requirements, including that all persons who present to

Table 44.2 Major legal requirements mandated by Emergency Medical Treatment and Active Labor Act (EMTALA)

Requirement	Impact on emergency care providers
Medical screening	EDs must provide a MSE to any patient presenting to the ED to determine if an EMC exists. The MSE can neither be delayed to determine a patient's ability to pay, nor can the extent of the MSE differ from patient to patient based on his or her financial resources.
Stabilization	EDs must use any available resources, including consultation, to stabilize an EMC. They must neither delay stabilization to investigate financial resources, nor may they vary stabilizing management from patient to patient based on the patient's ability to pay.
Acceptance	If a patient has an EMC that cannot be stabilized at the initial ED, he or she should be transferred to an ED with the necessary capabilities. The receiving ED must accept the patient if they have the capacity to stabilize the EMC, regardless of the patient's financial resources, insurance status, or citizenship.
Penalties for violations	EDs that fail to comply with EMTALA's requirements face the loss of participation in medicare – a penalty that would financially devastate most hospitals. Individual physicians who violate the provisions of EMTALA face significant fines not covered by malpractice insurance.

MSE: medical screening examination; EMC: emergency medical condition.

the ED for evaluation be entered into a log book; that EDs post notices informing patients of their rights under EMTALA; that transfers for higher level of care need an accepting physician and must be accompanied by the appropriate medical records and necessary medical personnel; and that institutions having reason to believe another hospital violated EMTALA *must report* this violation to the Center for Medicare and Medicaid Services (CMS).

While EMTALA began as a way of protecting the medically-indigent, it has expanded significantly into an extremely complex network of legal mandates. Additionally, terms generally thought to have medical definitions, such as "emergency medical condition (EMC)," "screening examination," "stabilization," and "stable for transfer," now have legal definitions that may not parallel common medical parlance. Due to this, all physicians must know the duties this law mandates.

Medical malpractice

Many physicians think of medical malpractice as the primary medicolegal issue. Practitioners who ultimately face a malpractice claim usually see it as a personal attack on their character, and the process of defending against such a claim can result in significant emotional and financial stress. Unfortunately, medical malpractice litigation is an almost inevitable part of emergency medical practice, with the average emergency physician facing one claim for every 25,000 patients (one claim every 5–7 years depending on patient volume). Given that cases can last 3–5 years before resolution, many physicians find that litigation is an ongoing aspect of their professional lives.

Medical malpractice claims usually fall under the authority of *state* law, subject to *civil* rules and procedures (although federal lawsuits are possible). A lawsuit typically originates when the *plaintiff* believes that a treating physician failed in their *duty* to provide appropriate care. The most common allegations include: failure to diagnose (30%), negligent performance of a procedure (16%), misdiagnosis (10%), substandard treatment (6%), delay in diagnosis (6%), and delay in treatment (3%).

Once the plaintiff has retained an attorney, the attorney prepares an initial *pleading*, often called a *complaint*. These papers are then *served* on the defendant physician, a process that formally begins the lawsuit. The physician should then contact his or her malpractice insurance carrier, who assigns an attorney to the case. The physician's attorney then prepares a response to the complaint.

To prevail in a malpractice case, a plaintiff must demonstrate four elements:

1. The defendant physician had a *duty* to treat the plaintiff.
2. The defendant physician *breached* this duty.
3. This breach was the *cause* of the plaintiff's injury.
4. The plaintiff suffered actual *injury*.

One or more of these elements may be contested by the defense. The parties usually rely on expert witness testimony to establish or refute these elements. This often results in highly technical testimony that can be confusing to jury members. Additionally, the information on which these experts draw their conclusions comes primarily from the medical record, which may be illegible, incomprehensible, or incomplete. This frequently results in not only disagreements over issues of judgment, but also debates over issues of fact. For example, the plaintiff argues that peripheral pulses were not checked while the defense claims they were. The medical record provides the most persuasive evidence of who is more likely to be correct. This leads to the often-heard claim from those involved in risk management that "If it wasn't documented, it wasn't done."

Most medical malpractice claims do not end up in trial; they are settled. Settlement represents a risk reduction strategy in that the plaintiffs recover some award and the defendants prevent an unexpectedly high judgment against them. Of those cases that are decided by a jury, approximately 70–90% result in verdicts for the defense. Despite these favorable odds, most physicians involved in a malpractice claim report it as a distinctly unpleasant experience. This has resulted in substantial interest in methods to reduce the number of claims.

While many plaintiff's attorneys would assert that reducing malpractice claims simply requires practicing good medicine, there is evidence that many claims have little to do with negligence. Bad outcomes occur even with the best care. Despite the legal requirements to show both breach of duty and causation, more patients without evidence of negligence file suit than do those who suffered negligent care. This suggests that factors exist, other than excellent medical care, that can influence one's likelihood of being sued.

Perhaps the best known of these factors is the *interpersonal relationship* between the physician and patient. Patients and family members who believe that their physician showed genuine caring and excellent communication skills rarely contemplate a lawsuit, even in the face of a bad outcome or substandard care. Nearly half of the variance in patient satisfaction stems from patients' assessments of the physician's interpersonal skills and professional manner. When patients feel that their physician is open and honest, they more readily accept that medical care is not an exact science, and that clinical judgments can sometimes be wrong without claiming malpractice on the part of the physician. Conversely, when patients and/or families feel confused and ignored, they sometimes believe that the courtroom is the only venue in which they can learn the truth about what actually happened. A good bedside manner is critical in preventing the underlying emotional context that leads to this feeling of mistrust. Researchers compared the interpersonal skills of physicians with multiple malpractice claims to physicians without claims. They found that those who had never been sued spent more time with patients, told the patient what to expect, asked more questions to ascertain the patient's opinions and understanding, used more humor, and encouraged the patient to talk.

A second factor in reducing malpractice claims is the *quality of the medical record*. One of the first hurdles a potential plaintiff must negotiate is finding a plaintiff's attorney who believes the case will result in a favorable outcome. Often, the better the documentation, the more difficult successful litigation will be for the plaintiff. Many cases revolve around factual debates between the plaintiff and physician, and the medical record may provide the sole source of evidence for either side. The court often interprets an absence of a notation in the medical record as evidence that an act did not occur. One difficult task for a busy emergency physician is determining what exactly should be documented. Unfortunately, scant research on this topic exists. Common sense suggests that physicians should focus their efforts on high-risk areas, such as informed consent, informed refusal, and leaving AMA, as well as high-risk presentations, such as chest pain, abdominal pain, headache, fever, and trauma. In many cases, a mere word or two makes a tremendous difference. For example, consider the description of the onset of a headache as "gradual." A case of a missed subarachnoid hemorrhage may pivot on this one word.

Although a malpractice claim may originate from any patient and from any complaint, practitioners cannot be expected to invest substantial time and effort on the documentation and risk management issues for every patient they see. However, emergency physicians should be aware of the most common presentations among all cases resulting in litigation (Table 44.3).

Conclusion

Many physicians attempt to minimize their interactions with the law. Unfortunately, the nature of emergency medicine makes such interactions

Table 44.3 Common presenting complaints resulting in malpractice claims

Presenting complaint	Common unexpected outcomes	Percent of claims
Trauma	Missed foreign body Missed fracture Wound infection	20
Abdominal pain	Missed appendicitis Missed aortic aneurysm Missed myocardial infarction	14
Infections	Missed meningitis Missed pneumonia	10
Vaginal bleeding	Missed ectopic pregnancy	9
Chest pain	Missed myocardial infarction Missed pulmonary embolism	8

Adapted from the Risk Management Foundation of the Harvard Medical Institutions.

common. EDs represent the front line of medical care. The privilege of staffing these lines comes with inevitable legal duties and legal risks. Physicians must have substantial knowledge of the law as it pertains to emergency care and their practices, especially in their state.

Pearls, pitfalls, and myths

- Informed consent is not simply a signature on a release form. It is a process in which the physician and patient discuss risks, benefits, and alternatives. A signature without this process does not constitute legal informed consent.
- A patient with decision-making capacity can refuse care even if such refusal does not appear to be in their best interest. Performing procedures against a patient's wishes constitutes battery.
- Unaccompanied children presenting to the ED should receive any evaluation and treatment necessary to detect and stabilize an EMC even if parents or guardians are not present to provide consent.
- Unless needed for patient care, sharing an adult patient's personal health information with a third party, including other family members, requires their consent.
- Cooperate with law enforcement whenever possible, but be aware of the patient's rights and legal restrictions on sharing information with police.
- In treating victims of violence, emergency physicians must remember: (a) any legal requirements to report these events to authorities; and (b) to preserve and protect evidence, such as clothing or wounds on the victim.
- Most malpractice claims do not arise out of negligent care. They often stem from dissatisfaction with the interpersonal and professional relationship between the patient, family, and physician.
- Many malpractice claims can be avoided by: (a) improving the communication between physician, patients and family; and (b) careful documentation.

Referenes

1. Bisaillon D. *Overview of Emergency Department Claims*. Risk Management Foundation of the Harvard Medical Institutions, 1997. Available online at www.rmf.harvard.edu.
2. Bitterman RA. *Providing Emergency Care Under Federal Law: EMTALA*. Dallas, TX: ACEP, 2000.
3. Brennan TA, Sox CM, Burstin HR. Relation between negligent adverse events and the outcomes of medical-malpractice litigation. *New Engl J Med* 1996;335:1963–1967.
4. Doyle BJ, Ware Jr JE. Physician conduct and other factors that affect consumer satisfaction with medical care. *J Med Educ* 1977;52:793–801.
5. Hickson GB, et al. Obstetricians' prior malpractice experience and patients' satisfaction with care. *J Am Med Assoc* 1994;272:1583–1587.
6. Horn III C, Caldwell DH, Osborn DC. *Law for Physicians: An Overview of Medical Legal Issues*. Chicago, IL: American Medical Association, 2000.
7. Lee, NG. *Legal Concepts and Issues in Emergency Care*. Philadelphia: W.B. Saunders, 2001.
8. Levinson W, Roter DL, Mullooly JP, Dull VT, Frankel RM. Physician–patient communication: the relationship with malpractice claims among primary care physicians and surgeons. *J Am Med Assoc* 1997;277:553–559.
9. Richards EP, Rathbun KC. *Law and the Physician: A Practical Guide*. Boston: Little, Brown and Company, 1993.
10. Sanbar SS, Gibofsky A, Firestone MH, LeBlang TR, Liang BA, Snyder JW. *Legal Medicine*, 5th ed., Philadelphia: Mosby, 2001.

45 Occupational exposures in the emergency department

Stephen J. Playe, MD **and Cemil M. Erdem,** MD

Scope of the problem

Many health care providers are drawn to emergency medicine for the opportunity to treat a widely diverse population of undifferentiated patients. "Anyone could have anything" is one motto of the specialty. Although the exact percentage varies according to location, a substantial proportion of emergency department (ED) patients are actively infected or carriers of serious illnesses that can be transmitted to health care professionals. It is estimated that 75% of US emergency medicine residents sustain a needlestick injury during residency. In the US health care system, 60,000–800,000 needlesticks are reported each year, and an estimated 40–90% of these injuries are unreported. An accidental exposure can drastically transform a caregiver into a patient. This chapter's goal is to decrease the frequency of these events, and minimize their impact should they occur.

Pathophysiology

The chain of events can be conceptualized according to the following simple diagram.

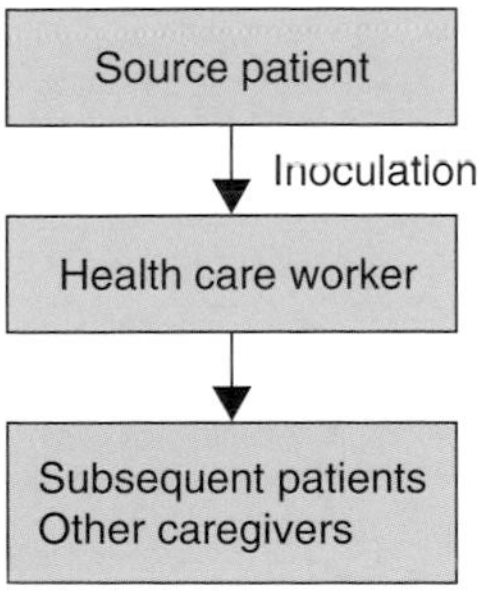

The source patient in the ED is not a factor that can be modified, given the diverse population presenting to the ED for care. The act of inoculation, however, may be prevented through behavior modification. Inoculation typically occurs in two fashions: directly and indirectly. *Direct inoculation* occurs when the surfaces of the source and the recipient come into primary contact, and the agent is transferred as a result of this contact. This includes skin contact, ingestion of an agent, direct spray of fluids onto mucous membranes, and droplet contact. Droplets arise from spitting, talking, and coughing, and rapidly settle out of the air in a matter of seconds. Generally speaking, droplets cannot traverse a distance >1 meter.

Indirect inoculation occurs by means of some intermediary. If this intermediary is living, it is called a *vector*; if inanimate, it is called a *vehicle*. A hypodermic needle or shard of glass would be considered a vehicle, as would an aerosol. An aerosol is a droplet, but of such minute proportions (1–3 μm) that it remains suspended in air and transported from one person to the next by air currents.

Regardless of route of inoculation, an exposed health care worker can become colonized or infected, and may cause infection to other patients, co-workers, or family members.

History

Once an exposure has occurred, a focused history allows one to best assess the risk and initiate an appropriate care plan.

What was the nature of the exposure? Was it percutaneous, direct contact, spray, or inhalation? If percutaneous, describe the exposure.

Certain factors have been correlated with increased risk of transmission in the case of a human immunodeficiency virus (HIV) needlestick. Deeper penetration, larger-bore needle, hollow versus solid needle, source blood readily apparent on device, and high viral load in the source blood are all associated with greater likelihood of infection transmission. These factors contribute to the delivery of a larger number of infectious particles, increasing the chance of infection.

Who is the source patient? What is the potential risk?

The source patient may know he or she is infected, and may volunteer this information. If a source patient is not known to have a communicable disease, certain factors increase the chance he or she may harbor occult, undocumented infection. Intravenous (IV) drug use, sexual promiscuity without barrier use, history of other sexually transmitted illnesses (STIs), and blood transfusion or organ transplantation are risks for bloodborne illnesses, such as HIV, hepatitis B (Hep B), or hepatitis C (Hep C).

Travel or residence in areas where tuberculosis is endemic (Africa, Asia except Japan, Middle East, South/Central America, Mexico, Eastern Europe, and the Caribbean), cohabiting infected family member, or residence in crowded settings such as prisons, drug rehabilitation facilities, and homeless shelters are risk factors for tuberculosis transmission.

What is your immunization status?

This question is applicable to the source patient as well as the health care worker. Documented Hep B vaccination is highly effective (80–95%) in preventing infection, and if antibody response is found adequate by assay, protection is essentially guaranteed. In the case of tuberculosis, skin-testing history in conjunction with chest X-ray is helpful in establishing disease activity. It should be emphasized that the long-term immunity conferred by the bacillus Calmette–Guérin (BCG) vaccine given in endemic areas is poor and unreliable, ranging from 0% to 80%, and should not be interpreted as proof of immunity. In contrast, 99% of persons who have received varicella immunization demonstrate a serologic response and immunity to occupational exposures to varicella and herpes zoster. A reliable, documented history of exposure to varicella is considered an adequate substitute for active vaccination, as the majority of previously infected individuals have lasting immunity. Tetanus vaccine should be readministered every 5 years to health care workers.

Physical examination

The physical examination of exposed health care workers is seldom helpful. In a percutaneous exposure, there may be a small puncture wound; in cases of inhalation, spray, or direct contact, meaningful physical evidence is unlikely to be found. This fact underscores the importance of a thorough history.

Examination of the source patient, if available, may be useful when fulminant disease is present. For example, a patient with thrush, fever, wasting, and pneumonia demonstrating a "bat-wing" appearance on chest X-ray raises concern for the risk of contagion. Most exposures, however, will not afford such a clear picture.

Selected agents

Table 45.1 provides a list of organisms causing commonly encountered clinically important exposures in the ED.

Table 45.1 Exposures in the ED

Organism and route of transmission	Vaccine exists?	Diagnostic testing	Diagnostic test: false-negative window period
Clostridium difficile: Fecal/oral contact	No	Stool culture. Rapid toxin assay.	Incubation period usually less than a week.
Coronavirus (SARS): Likely droplet	No	Enzyme immunoassay, reverse transcriptase PCR.	Incubation period of 2–7 days.
Hepatitis A and E virus: Fecal/oral	Hepatitis A – Yes Hepatitis E – No	Anti-hepatitis A virus antibody (not routinely performed in this self-limited disease).	Infected patient may not test positive for 15–50 days.

(continued)

Table 45.1 Exposures in the ED (*cont*)

Organism and route of transmission	Vaccine exists?	Diagnostic testing	Diagnostic test: false-negative window period
Hepatitis B virus: Blood-borne. Present in all body fluids.	Yes. Series of three shots required to build immunity Immunity can be measured by antibody level assay.	Hepatitis B surface antigen test is the first serum marker, to which the body responds with anti-Hepatitis B surface antibody.	Infected patient may not be positive for 4–12 weeks. As the immune system mobilizes, there is a "second window" when the only demonstrable marker of infection is the anti-Hepatitis B core protein antigen.
Hepatitis C virus: Blood-borne. Present in all body fluids.	No – in development	Anti-hepatitis C virus antibody. Qualitative or quantitative Hepatitis C virus RNA (PCR).	Infected patient may not test positive for 2 weeks – 6 months.
HIV: Blood-borne. Significant virus levels in cellular fluids only (blood, semen, vaginal secretions, CSF, synovial, pleural, peritoneal, pericardial, and amniotic fluids).	No – in development	ELISA or rapid HIV test as screen, Western blot confirmatory. Disease severity: estimated viral load via PCR.	Infected patient may not test positive for 12 weeks post-exposure.
Methicillin-resistant Staphylococcus aureus: Contact	No	Wound culture.	Incubation period of 4–10 days, presenting as typical *Staphylococcus* infection.
Mycobacterium tuberculosis: Droplet/aerosol	Not in the US. Bacillus Calmette–Guérin vaccine staves off fulminant pediatric pulmonary disease abroad.	Mantoux skin test. Sputum cultures for acid-fast bacilli. Chest X-ray.	Incubation period of 4–10 weeks, then purified protein derivative is expected to test positive in infected individuals.
Neisseria meningitidis: Droplet	Yes. Limited to travelers and high-risk populations. Poorly immunogenic in children.	CSF culture. Gram stain.	Incubation period of 2–10 days.
Varicella: Contact and airborne	Yes	ELISA and latex agglutination test available. Titer levels induced by vaccine as opposed to primary infection may fall below detection range of assay, which is why post-immunization testing is not routinely performed.	Incubation period of 7–21 days, majority manifest illness on days 14–17.

CSF: cerebrospinal fluid; ELISA: enzyme-linked immunosorbent assay; HIV: human immunodeficiency virus; PCR: polymerase chain reaction; RNA: ribonucleic acid; SARS: severe acute respiratory syndrome.

Prevention

As is often the case, prevention is more desirable than treatment. Effective prevention of occupational exposures in the ED requires many continuous and interrelated lines of defense (Figure 45.1).

Hand hygiene

Handwashing is often neglected in discussions of occupational exposure, and is often neglected in the modern practice of clinical medicine as well. Handwashing diminishes the carriage rates

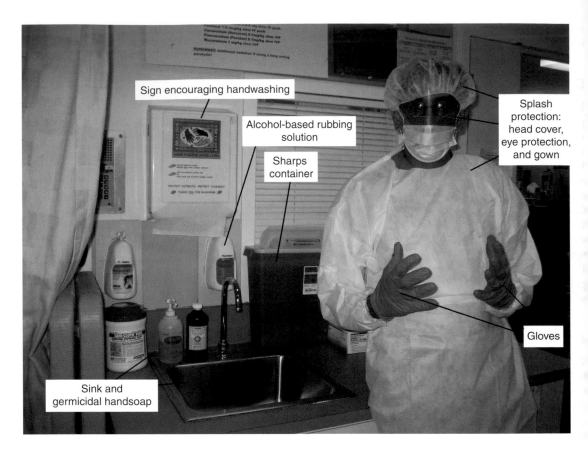

Figure 45.1
Health care worker with precautions in place. *Courtesy*: S.V. Mahadevan, MD.

of pathogens, and helps protect both physician and patient from infection. Poor compliance with handwashing has been repeatedly documented. Stated barriers to compliance include time requirements, irritation from soap and water, lack of access to sinks, and "being too busy." The advent of alcohol-based rubbing solutions overcomes many of these barriers. These solutions take only seconds to apply, dry without irritation, and have been found to be more effective than soap and water in killing pathogens. Handrubbing with these solutions is simple, fast, and significantly reduces exposure rates to contact pathogens in the ED.

Gloves

Gloves should be put on before contacting body fluids or open wounds, or for the general examination of patients when the health care worker's skin is not intact. Gloves are an adjunct to, not a substitute for, proper hand hygiene. They should be removed immediately after patient contact, so as not to contaminate other persons, charts, or equipment.

Contact precautions

These are an extension of standard precautions to all objects and surfaces in a patient's room who is thought by history, examination, or clinical suspicion to harbor a contact pathogen such as *Clostridium difficile*, methicillin-resistant *Staphylococcus aureus* (MRSA) or vancomycin-resistant *Enterococcus* (VRE). A sign reminding staff and announcing to visitors the necessity for gown and gloves may help increase adherence to standard precautions and prevent the spread of pathogens.

Splash protection

When the possibility of spray contamination exists, eye protection and gowns should be worn. Eyeglasses do not guard against side splash and are insufficient. Gowns should be disposed of immediately following a patient encounter.

Droplet precautions

Infections including influenza, streptococcal pharyngitis, meningitis, SARS-related coronavirus, mumps, rubella, pertussis, diphtheria, and most upper respiratory infections are transmitted by the projection of large particles of respiratory secretions that then can directly contact the eyes or the mucous membranes of the nose or mouth. Coughing, sneezing, talking, or singing can project these droplets approximately three feet. The droplets do not remain suspended in the air; thus, special air handling and ventilation is not required. Precautions include standard precautions plus eye protection and a standard surgical mask worn when working within three feet of the patient.

Aerosol protection

While treating patients with suspected tuberculosis or other aerosol-transmitted pathogens (e.g., tuberculosis, varicella or measles), a mask should be worn by both examiner and patient to minimize organism transmission. A negative-pressure isolation room limits spread to other ED patients. Given the prevalence of active tuberculosis in the homeless (1–5%) and HIV-infected populations (a third of HIV patients worldwide are co-infected with *Mycobacterium tuberculosis*), special vigilance is appropriate in both the triage and treatment of these patients to areas with appropriate aerosol precautions, especially if active coughing and respiratory symptoms are present.

Behavior modification

Often simple measures can drastically minimize the risk of exposure. Proper positioning, preparation, and control of procedures involving body fluids are essential. Asking for another set of hands in a busy ED may be a minor inconvenience to others, but is preferable to performing a procedure in an unsafe manner with potentially disastrous consequences. Another behavior which needs to change is that of recapping needles. Many health care workers, both new and seasoned, disregard warnings. Even the most dexterous among us will fail at this simple task eventually, or have a needle perforate the side of the cap. The only way we can avoid this mishap is to never attempt recapping needles in the first place.

System-based safeguards

The provision of accessible sharps containers that are emptied regularly, needleless IV systems, self-protecting needle systems, an effective and non-punitive exposure reporting system, and clear, consistent protocols for exposed health care workers are institutional-level measures that can help diminish exposure and risk of infection.

General treatment principles

Even with the best technique, preparation, and intentions, exposures are bound to occur. Once an exposure has occurred, and determined that the source patient represents a realistic likelihood of carrying one or more contagious diseases, post-exposure prophylaxis (PEP) should be initiated. Specific measures depend on the specific pathogen involved and the degree of exposure.

Human immunodeficiency virus

With a percutaneous exposure, the decision regarding PEP should be made as soon as possible. The optimum timing for beginning PEP in humans is unknown, but animal studies suggest the sooner it is started, the better. The current goal is that if anti-retroviral therapy is to be instituted, it should begin within 2 hours of exposure. The regimen can always be discontinued later.

The current Centers for Disease Control and Prevention (CDC-P) recommendations for PEP are presented (Figure 45.2). The aim of the algorithm is to assess the severity of both the exposure and likelihood that the source patient has HIV infection. The Exposure Code (EC) stratifies the risk of the exposure, including the relative risk for different exposure types. For example, a deep needlestick with a large-bore needle with visible blood at the tip is a more severe exposure than a patient coughing in one's unprotected eye. The EC reflects this difference in severity.

The HIV Status Code (HIV SC) represents the likelihood that the source patient in question in fact is HIV positive. A healthy 6-year old has a lower risk for carrying HIV than a man with track-marks and oral candidiasis; the HIV SC represents this relative risk of HIV infection.

Step 1: Determine the Exposure Code (EC)

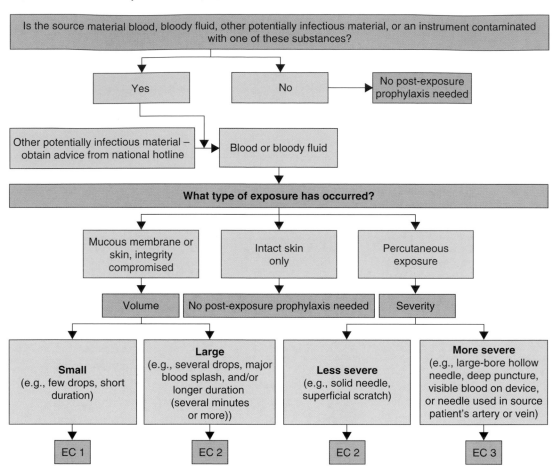

Step 2: Determine the HIV Status Code (HIV SC)

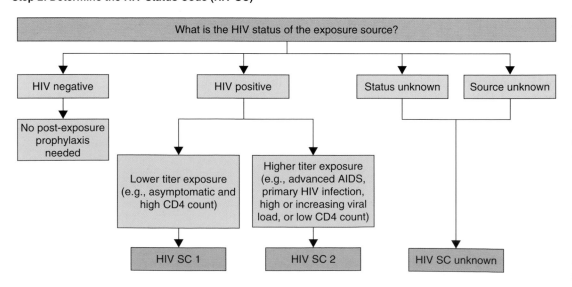

Figure 45.2
CDC-P recommendations for post-exposure prophylaxis.

Step 3: Determine the post-exposure prophylaxis recommendation

EC	HIV SC	PEP recommendation
1	1	*PEP may not be warranted.* Exposure type does not pose a known risk for HIV transmission. Whether the risk for drug toxicity outweighs the benefit of PEP should be decided by the exposed health care worker and treating clinician.
1	2	*Consider basic regimen.* Exposure type poses a negligible risk for HIV transmission. A high HIV titer in the source may justify consideration of PEP. Whether the risk for drug toxicity outweighs the benefit of PEP should be decided by the exposed health care worker and treating clinician.
2	1	*Recommend basic regimen.* Most HIV exposures are in this category; no increased risk for HIV transmission has been observed but use of PEP is appropriate.
2	2	*Recommend expanded regimen.* Exposure type represents an increased HIV transmission risk.
3	1 or 2	*Recommend expanded regimen.* Exposure type represents an increased HIV transmission risk.
2 or 3	Unknown	If the source or, in the case of an unknown source, the setting where the exposure occurred suggests a possible risk for HIV exposure and the Exposure Code is 2 or 3, *consider basic regimen.*

SC: status code; PEP: post-exposure prophylaxis; HIV: human immunodeficiency virus; AIDS: acquired immune deficiency syndrome.
Adapted from: Centers for Disease Control and Prevention. Public health service guidelines for the management of health care worker exposures to HIV and recommendations for post-exposure prophylaxis. *Morb Mortal Wkly Rep* 1998;47(RR-7).

Figure 45.2
CDC-P recommendations for post-exposure prophylaxis (*cont*)

Once the EC and HIV SC have been ascertained, the two are combined to assess overall risk, and determine the recommended PEP.*

The current *basic regimen* is 4 weeks of zidovudine (600 mg/day in two or three divided doses) and lamivudine (150 mg b.i.d. generally prescribed as Combivir, 1 tablet p.o. b.i.d.).

The *expanded regimen* is the basic regimen plus either indinavir (800 mg every 8 hours) or nelfinavir (750 mg t.i.d). Other regimens may be considered depending on local resistance patterns.

The rate of HIV infection following a needle-stick injury is estimated to be between 0.3% and 0.5%. This low incidence makes study of the efficacy of PEP challenging. Animal models and decreased maternal–fetal transmission of virus with prophylaxis suggest that these medications modify

* *Note*: These recommendations are described in the CDC-P public service guidelines for the management of health care worker exposures to HIV and recommendations for PEP (*Morb Mortal Wkly Rep* 2001;50(RR-11)) and are currently accepted as of February 2005. Medication recommendations and dosages are likely to change over time; current recommendations should be verified before instituting treatment.

transmission. A retrospective case–controlled study of exposed health care workers found that the use of zidovudine PEP was associated with a >80% reduction in HIV disease transmission.

The duration of required PEP is contested; pending definitive data, prophylaxis should continue for 28 days.

Follow-up surveillance of health care workers is imperative, and should be conducted for 12 months post-exposure, since late conversion has been reported.

Pending the outcome of serologic testing, patients should be counseled to avoid unprotected sex, and should not donate blood or tissues, share toothbrushes or razors, or breastfeed.

Consent for testing the source patient must be obtained before sending serology. Most patients are helpful and readily give consent when the situation is explained. If the patient is clinically unable to give consent, hospital policies based on state law should be followed.

Hepatitis B

Most health care workers in the US receive the Hep B vaccine. The vast majority of individuals

Vaccination treatment and antibody source response status of exposed workers[a]	Treatment		
	Source HBsAg positive	Source HBsAg negative	Source unknown or not available for testing
Unvaccinated	HBIG[b] × 1 and initiate Hep B vaccine series	Initiate Hep B vaccine series	Initiate Hep B vaccine series
Previously vaccinated			
Known responder[c]	No treatment	No treatment	No treatment
Known non-responder[d]	HBIG × 1 and initiate revaccination or HBIG × 2[e]	No treatment	If known high-risk source, treat as if source were HBsAg positive
Antibody response unknown	Test exposed person for anti-HBs[f]	No treatment	Test exposed person for anti-HBs
	1. If adequate,[c] no treatment is necessary		1. If adequate, no treatment is necessary
	2. If inadequate,[d] administer HBIG × 1 and vaccine booster		2. If inadequate, administer vaccine booster and recheck titer in 1–2 months

HBsAg: hepatitis B surface antigen; HBIG: hepatitis B immune globulin; HBV: hepatitis B virus; anti-HBs: anti-hepatitis B surface.

[a]Persons who have previously been infected with HBV are immune to re-infection and do not require PEP.
[b]Dose is 0.06 ml/kg intramuscular.
[c]A responder is a person with adequate levels of serum antibody to HBsAg (i.e., anti-HBs >10 mIU/ml).
[d]A non-responder is a person with inadequate response to vaccination (i.e., serum anti-HBs <10 mIU/ml).
[e]The option of giving one dose of HBIG and re-initiating the vaccine series is preferred for non-responders who have not completed a second three-dose vaccine series. For persons who previously completed a second vaccine series but failed to respond, two doses of HBIG are preferred.
[f]Antibody to HBsAg.

Figure 45.3
CDC-P guideline for hepatitis B post-exposure prophylaxis.
Source: Mikulich VJ, Schriger DL. Centers for Disease Control and Prevention. Abridged version of the updated US Public Health Service guidelines for the management of occupational exposures to hepatitis B virus, hepatitis C virus, and human immunodeficiency virus and recommendations for postexposure prophylaxis. *Ann Emerg Med* 2002;39(3):321–328.

mount an adequate response to the vaccine. Those demonstrating adequate antibody titers to the vaccine are essentially assured immunity. If the exposed individual is a documented antibody responder, no prophylaxis is required. If the health care worker is a known non-responder, or more commonly, if his or her response status is unverified, anti-HB immune globulin (anti-HBIG) is recommended *after* an antibody level is drawn. If the antibody is positive, suggesting successful immunization, treatment can be halted. Otherwise, the vaccine series should be repeated. Surveillance testing should follow, and proper aftercare instructions are similar to those for HIV, except that modification of sexual behavior and cessation of breastfeeding are not required.

There is no effective treatment for established Hep B infection.

The CDC-P guideline for Hep B PEP is given in Figure 45.3.

Hepatitis C

There is no vaccine or recommended PEP for Hep C.

Surveillance testing and counseling are important, and are similar to those for Hep B.

Tuberculosis

There is no immediate treatment required in the case of exposure to a patient with active tuberculosis. If subsequent Mantoux testing shows conversion, this is presumptive proof that infection has occurred. At this point pharmacotherapy is indicated. The travel history of the source patient is particularly important in this case, as high rates of resistance to standard therapies in some regions will guide therapy.

Meningococcal meningitis

Close household contacts of individuals with meningococcal meningitis should receive prophylactic antibiotics, as there is a 4/1000 incidence of secondary infection in the household of the index case. Close contact is defined as living in the same household as the index case for 4 or more hours in the past week, day care, dormitory or barracks contacts, and anyone with whom the patient has shared oral secretions (kissing, shared utensils, cigarettes).

Using this definition, most health care workers are spared chemoprophylaxis provided they exercise and maintain good precautions. Exceptions include mouth-to-mouth resuscitation, airway management, or inadvertent exposure to oral secretions without use of a protective mask.

Generally a one-time dose of ciprofloxacin is used as chemoprophylaxis when needed, but ceftriaxone, azithromycin, or rifampin are reasonable alternatives.

Varicella

Ideally, all health care workers should either receive immunization against varicella or have formal documentation of a prior infection. Both situations confer immunity in the vast majority of cases. Many adults without documented exposure are not susceptible, as the transmission rate in these individuals is only 5–15%. However, adult-onset varicella can be serious, with death rates as high as 50/100,000. Administration of varicella zoster immune globulin (VZIG) can avert or diminish the severity of a varicella zoster infection, and should be implemented in susceptible, exposed adults, especially those who are immunocompromised. It is important to note that indiscriminate use of VZIG would deplete the supply, which is used to treat high-risk neonates.

Exposed, susceptible health care workers should be temporarily relieved of patient care duty on days 10–21 following exposure, as this is typically when they might be infectious (even if the rash has not yet appeared). Should they contract the disease, they may return to work after the last crop of lesions has crusted over.

Special patients
Pregnant (or potentially-pregnant)

For HIV prophylaxis, there is little data regarding fetal risk. Current recommendations suggest that the best treatment for the fetus is the proper treatment of the mother. The basic and expanded regimens are used as in nonpregnant patients. One exception is that efavirenz (Sustiva) should not be used, as it has shown teratogenicity in primate models at doses biologically equivalent to the dose range in humans.

Additionally, pregnant caregivers in the ED should avoid occupational hazards unique to the hospital: inhalation anesthetic agents (particularly nitrous oxide), ethylene oxide (used in sterilizing equipment), anti-neoplastic drugs, ribavirin aerosol, radiation, rubella, Hep B, cytomegalovirus, varicella, HIV, herpes simplex, and human parvovirus B19.

Disposition

ED care following an exposure provides the first day of a long, stressful period for the exposed health care worker, during which he or she will likely agonize over having possibly contracted a life-threatening illness. It is important to ensure good follow-up, preferably by communicating its importance to the patient as well as notifying the patient's primary care physician directly. While it is important to communicate facts and get necessary blood work, it is equally important to understand that the patient's status as a health care professional does not insulate him or her from the angst of the situation, and to be sensitive to this.

Pre-printed information and instructions should be provided in the exposed person's preferred language.

Since recommendations change frequently, all clinicians are advised to consult on-line or telephone-accessed references (Figure 45.4).

Pitfalls

- Failure to have immunizations and screening tests up to date.
- Failure to consistently follow standard precautions.
- Inadequate hand hygiene.
- Failure to provide immediate copious irrigation of skin and mucous membrane exposures.

National Clinicians' Postexposure Prophylaxis
Hotline (PEPline)
www.ucsf.edu/hivcntr/resources/pep/index.html
Tel. (888)448-4911
Needlestick!
www.needlestick.mednet.ucla.edu/
Hepatitis Information Hotline
www.cdc.gov/hepatitis
Tel. (888)443-7232

Figure 45.4
Resources for occupational exposures.

- Failure to report and seek treatment following any occupational exposure.
- Failure to institute HIV PEP within 2 hours of exposure.
- Failure to consider and be sensitive to the stress and fear that an exposed health care worker might develop.

References

1. Alvarado-Ramy F, Beltrami EM. New exposure guidelines for occupational exposure to blood-borne viruses. *Clev Clin J Med* 2003;70(5):457–464.
2. Barclay III DM, Richardson JP, Fredman L. Tuberculosis in the homeless. *Arch Fam Med* 1995;4(6):541.
3. Cardo DM, Culver DH, Ciesielski CA, Srivastava PU, Marcus R, Abiteboul D, et al. A case–control study of HIV seroconversion in health care workers after percutaneous exposure. *New Engl J Med* 1997;337:1485–1490.
4. Diaz PS. The epidemiology and control of invasive meningococcal disease. Pediatr Infect Dis J 1999;18(7):633–634.
5. *Epidemiology and Prevention of Vaccine-Preventable Diseases*, 7th ed., Second printing. CDC Press. Available online. http://129.237.102.160/intlab/pinkbook/
6. Ferreiro RB, Sepkowitz KA. Management of needlestick injuries. Clin Obstet Gynecol 2001;44(2):276–288.
7. Fien PEM. The BCG story. Lessons from the past and implications for the future. *Rev Infect Dis* 1989;11(2):S353–S359.
8. Girou E, et al. Efficacy of handrubbing with alcohol based solution versus standard handwashing with antiseptic soap: randomised clinical trial. *Br Med J* 2002;325:36.
9. Ippolito G, Puro V, Heptonstall J, Jagger J, De Carli G, Petrosillo N. Occupational human immunodeficiency virus infection in health care workers: worldwide cases through September 1997. *Clin Infect Dis* 1999;28(2):365–383.
10. Larson E, Killien M. Factors influencing hand washing behavior of patient care personnel. *Am J Infect Cont* 1982;10:93–99.
11. Lee CH, Carter WA, Chiang WK, Williams CM, Asimos AW, Goldfrank LR. Occupational exposures to blood among emergency medicine residents. *Acad Emerg Med* 1999;6:1036–1043.
12. Moran GJ. Emergency department management of blood and body fluid exposures. *Ann Emerg Med* 2000;35(1):47–62.
13. *National Institute for Occupational Safety and Health, "NIOSH Alert: Preventing Needlestick Injuries in Health care Settings",* November 1999.
14. Rinnert K. Occupational exposures, infection control, and standard precautions. In: Tintinali (ed.). *Emergency Medicine*, 5th ed., New York: McGraw-Hill, Chapter 148, p. 1014.
15. Schriger DL, Mikulich VJ. Centers for Disease Control and Prevention. The management of occupational exposures to blood and body fluids: revised guidelines and new methods of implementation. Ann Emerg Med 2002;39(3):319–321.
16. Szmuness W, Stevens CE, Harley EJ, et al. Hepatitis B vaccine: demonstration of efficacy in a controlled clinical trial in a high-risk population in the United States. *New Engl J Med* 1980;303:833–841.

Appendices

Appendix A   Common emergency procedures

George Sternbach, MD

Introduction

Performing procedures in the emergency department is often a challenging process, as such activity may take place under less than ideal conditions. Time may be a consideration, as certain procedures are lifesaving or crucial to a patient's well-being. Circumstances may require that a procedure be performed without undue delay. The need to perform a procedure expeditiously should never lead one to rush the task, though, as the potential for error is magnified by haste. Attention must also always be paid to proper preparation and technique. Some procedures are time-consuming; adequate time should be budgeted for their completion.

Contraindications exist to most of the procedures in this section, and an effort should be made to elicit a patient history of illness or medications being taken that may constitute contraindications or precautions. In the unconscious, intoxicated or uncooperative patient, such medical history may be incomplete or difficult to obtain.

Some of the procedures described need to be performed utilizing sterile technique. It is very important that this be adhered to, because infection is always an undesirable and sometimes dangerous complication. In all instances, also assume that there is a risk of contracting infectious disease by contact with the patient's blood, secretions or other bodily fluids. Utilize precautions to avoid such contact, including gloves, eye protection, masks and surgical gowns, as appropriate.

Be aware what the complications of various procedures are, and assess the patient for signs of their appearance. Not all complications manifest immediately, but signs of some, such as pneumothorax consequent to central venipuncture, appear shortly after they are caused. In such instances, obtaining post-procedure diagnostic tests (e.g., a chest radiograph following subclavian or internal jugular cannulation) or instituting appropriate monitoring is imperative.

There are variations in the performance of some of the procedures described here, as well as "short cuts" known to experienced practitioners. Until you have mastered a particular procedure via standard technique, avoid the use of such alternate methods. When performing a procedure as a member of a resuscitation team, focus on the task and do not be distracted by other management activities being carried out simultaneously. Be aware of the materials required for the procedure and assemble these beforehand, so you do not have to break sterile technique or interrupt performance to ask an assistant for additional items.

Reference

Rosen P, Chan TC, Vilke GM, et al. *Atlas of Emergency Procedures*. St. Louis: Mosby, 2001.

Peripheral venous cannulation

Indications

The indications include the need for vascular access for the administration of intravenous (IV) fluids, blood products or medications. Even stable patients in whom such administration is anticipated are likely to benefit from having an IV line in place. For patients who require rapid volume resuscitation, short, large-bore peripheral IV catheters allow more rapid flow of fluids than do longer central venous catheters.

Contraindications

Whenever possible, avoid entry through skin that shows signs of infection or is burned. Do not use veins that have previously been involved with phlebitis or thrombosis, or extremities affected with lymphatic insufficiency. Insertion of a peripheral venous catheter may be difficult in patients who have venous collapse as a result of hypovolemia, who are obese, edematous or have a history of IV drug abuse.

Equipment

- Gloves
- Povidone–iodine antiseptic solution
- Tourniquet
- Over-the-needle venous catheter (angiocatheter)
- IV tubing set and fluid bag
- Sterile dressing
- Arm board
- Tape

Technique

This procedure is described on the arm, where it is most commonly performed, though the leg, scalp, or external jugular veins are sometimes utilized (Figure A.1). Prepare the IV setup by attaching IV tubing to the solution bag and running solution to fill the tubing. Place a tourniquet around the upper arm and search for a prominent vein. These are usually found in the antecubital fossa or the dorsum of the hand. If no prominent veins are apparent, apply a warm towel to the skin to induce venodilation. Tapping over a vein can also cause reflex dilation of the vascular wall. Having the patient open and close the fist will also distend the vein.

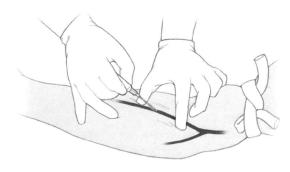

Figure A.1
Peripheral venous cannulation.

The tourniquet should be placed about 3–4 cm proximal to the puncture site. It should be tight enough to impede venous flow, but not so constricting as to curtail arterial circulation. Tie the tourniquet in a single loop in such a way that it can be released with one hand.

Prepare the site in sterile fashion. With the non-dominant hand, pull the skin taut and stabilize the vein. Puncture the skin with the needle/catheter unit, entering at about a 30° angle to the skin. Keep the bevel of the needle facing upward. Puncture the vein. When the vein is entered, blood will appear in the flash chamber of the angiocatheter. Holding the unit steady, advance the catheter over the needle and into the vein. Remove the needle, holding the catheter in place.

Attach the IV tubing to the catheter. Remove the tourniquet and simultaneously initiate flow by opening the valve on the tubing. Apply a sterile dressing and tape the catheter in place. Taping the tubing to the skin in a U-shaped loop will reduce the likelihood of the catheter being accidentally dislodged. It may be advisable to affix an arm board if the cannulation site overlies a joint.

Fluid should flow freely into the vein. If immediate subcutaneous swelling appears around the catheter site, it indicates the extravasation of fluid from the vein. In this instance, stop the infusion, withdraw the catheter and apply pressure over the area. Attempt cannulation at a different site.

Complications

Local bleeding is a common complication. Hematomas are usually produced when the posterior venous wall is punctured during cannulation. Such bleeding is almost always minor and can be controlled readily by application of pressure.

Accidental puncture of the posterior wall or displacement of the catheter will result in subcutaneous extravasation of IV fluid. This produces swelling and pain. The condition must be recognized early, and the infusion discontinued. Subcutaneous infiltration of certain high-osmolality solutions (e.g., potassium chloride, sodium bicarbonate) is particularly toxic to soft tissue and may lead to tissue necrosis.

Phlebitis, or inflammation of the vein, occurs frequently at IV sites utilized for several days or longer, but is not an immediate complication. Local subcutaneous infection is also a delayed complication, and its incidence can be diminished by careful skin preparation and technique.

Reference

Sweeney MN. Vascular access in trauma: options, risks, benefits and complications. *Anesthesiol Clin North Am* 1999;17:97–106.

Central venous cannulation

Indications

Catheterization of the central venous system may be performed for a number of reasons. One common reason is the inability to obtain peripheral venous access in a patient who requires urgent administration of IV fluid or medications. The need to infuse medications that are irritating to smaller peripheral veins also mandates cannulation of a central vein. Access to the central circulation is also necessary for measurement of central venous pressure, as well as for passage of a temporary transvenous pacemaker or pulmonary artery catheter.

Contraindications

There are no absolute contraindications to performing central vein cannulation. A relative contraindication is the presence of a coagulation disorder. This is particularly a factor in subclavian venipuncture. The presence of a markedly obese patient with poorly-defined anatomical landmarks, an uncooperative patient or the presence of overlying skin infection also constitute relative contraindications.

Equipment

- Sterile gloves
- Commercial central venous access kit, including the following:
  - povidone–iodine antiseptic solution
  - sterile drapes
  - anesthetic solution, syringe and needles
  - introducer needle
  - metal guide wire
  - catheter or sheath introducer
  - semi-rigid dilator catheter
  - gauze pads
  - scalpel with No. 11 blade
  - 5- and 10-ml syringes
  - 3- or 4-0 non-absorbable suture
  - antibiotic ointment
- IV solution and tubing

Technique

General

The Seldinger guide wire method (Figure A.2) is the recommended technique for insertion of a central venous catheter. This allows placement of a large-bore catheter over a wire inserted through a smaller bore needle. Identify the appropriate landmarks according to the vessel to be cannulated. Prepare the skin of the involved area with povidone–iodine solution. Surround the field with sterile drapes.

Infiltrate the skin and underlying subcutaneous tissue to be entered with about 5 ml of 1% lidocaine. Using the external landmarks to identify the puncture site, locate the vessel with an introducer needle (an 18-gauge, 2.5-inch needle) attached to a syringe. Aspirate while advancing the needle until blood flows freely into the syringe. This indicates that the vessel has been entered. If no blood is encountered, withdraw the needle to the skin edge and redirect.

Stabilizing the needle in place, remove the syringe and cover the hub of the needle with your thumb to prevent air from entering the vein. Pass the metal guide wire through the needle. The wire should pass smoothly through the needle into the vein. If you encounter resistance, withdraw the wire together with the needle and attempt the procedure again.

Once most of the wire been passed through the needle, withdraw the needle over the wire, leaving the wire in place. Be careful not to insert the entire length of the wire through the needle. Allow enough of the wire to protrude through the skin to allow passage of the catheter over it.

With a scalpel, make a small superficial incision of the skin at the point of entry of the guide wire. Pass the dilator over the wire with a twisting motion. This will create a passage in the subcutaneous tissue that will allow easier admittance of the catheter. Remove the dilator, leaving the wire in place. Be careful not to remove or lose the wire inadvertently.

Pass the catheter over the wire in a manner similar to passing the dilator. The catheter should advance smoothly, requiring no force to pass. Remove the guide wire through the catheter and attach the IV bag to the catheter via the tubing. As you withdraw the guide wire, be sure the catheter is not extracted inadvertently.

Suture the catheter to the skin, first injecting a wheal of anesthetic into the area into which the suture will be placed. Lower the IV bag below the level of the bed for a few seconds. Flow of

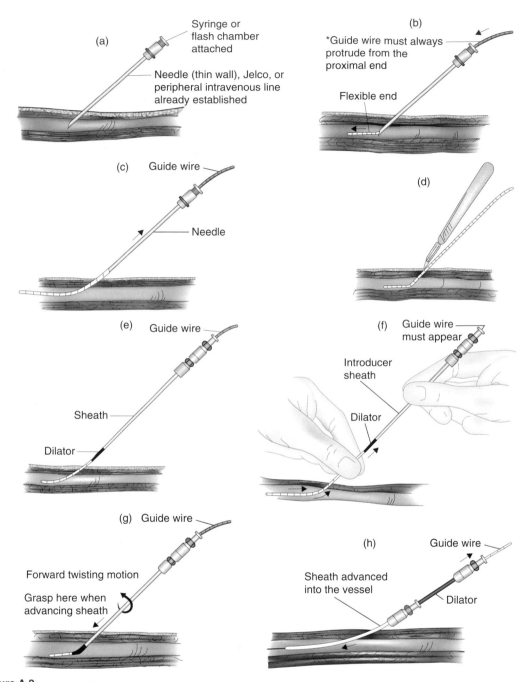

Figure A.2
Procedure for placement of Seldinger-type guidewire catheter. (a) The selected vessel is cannulated with a thin-walled needle, or an existing IV catheter is chosen to be changed with the wire technique. (b) The guidewire is threaded through the needle, with the flexible end first, into the lumen of the vessel. (c) The needle is removed so that only the wire now exists from the vessel. (d) The skin entry site is enlarged with a No. 11 scalpel. (e) The catheter sheath and the dilator are threaded over the wire and advanced to the skin. The wire must be visible through the back of the device. (f) If the proximal wire is not visible, it is pulled from the skin through the catheter until it appears at the back of the catheter. (g) The sheath and the dilator are advanced as a unit into the skin with a twisting motion. It is best to grasp the unit at the junction of sheath and dilator to prevent bunching up of the sheath. The wire (at the back of the catheter) must be held while the sheath and dilator are advanced as a unit. (h) Once the sheath and the dilator are well within the vessel, the guidewire and the dilator are removed. Reprinted from Clinical Procedures in Emergency Medicine, 4th ed., Roberts JR, Hedges J (eds). Copyright 2003, with permission from Elsevier.

blood into the tubing is an indication of intravascular location. Apply topical antibiotic ointment to the venipuncture site and a sterile dressing. When using the internal jugular or subclavian approaches, obtain a chest radiograph to ascertain that the catheter is in proper position and that no pneumothorax has been produced.

Internal jugular vein

Position the bed with the patient's head down at an angle of 10–15° (the Trendelenburg position). Turn the patient's head away from the side being used. The right side is preferred because of the straighter course of the vein to the superior vena cava. In critically-ill patients in whom simultaneous airway management is being performed, the subclavian or femoral approaches may be preferable.

There are several approaches to the internal jugular vein. A widely used one is entry in the triangle formed by the clavicle and the sternal and clavicular heads of the sternocleidomatoid muscle. The internal jugular vein runs lateral to the carotid artery in this triangle. Anesthetize the skin and soft tissue in the apex of the triangle. Insert the introducer needle at the apex at an angle of 30–45° to the skin and advance the needle toward the ipsilateral nipple (Figure A.3). Aspirate while advancing the needle. Brisk flow of blood into the syringe indicates entry into the internal jugular vein. Proceed with insertion of the guide wire and catheter using the Seldinger technique. Obtain a chest radiograph to verify correct catheter position and the presence of any complications.

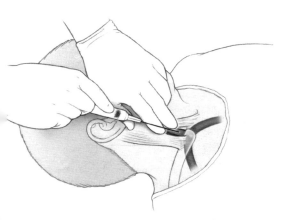

igure A.3
iternal jugular vein cannulation.

Subclavian vein

Position the bed in the Trendelenburg position as described for internal jugular cannulation (head down 10° to 15°). Prepare the skin overlying the clavicle, sternum and neck to the angle of the mandible. A rolled towel placed between the patient's shoulder blades to accentuate the sternoclavicular joint is helpful. Anesthetize the skin and soft tissue overlying and just inferior to the junction of the lateral and middle thirds of the clavicle.

Insert the introducer needle 1 cm inferior to the clavicle, at a point at the junction of the lateral and middle thirds of the clavicle. Direct the needle medially and cephalad, aiming for the suprasternal notch (Figure A.4). Use a shallow angle to the skin and advance the needle just posterior to the clavicle. Once the vein is entered, blood should flow briskly into the syringe. Proceed with insertion of the guide wire and catheter. Obtain a chest radiograph to verify correct catheter position and the presence of any complications.

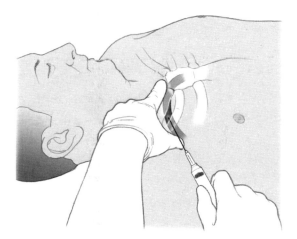

Figure A.4
Subclavian vein cannulation.

Femoral vein

Femoral vein cannulation has the advantage that this location is away from the neck and thorax, and may therefore be more accessible in the patient undergoing concurrent airway management or chest compressions. In addition, pneumothorax is not a concern as with the other two approaches. In cases of intra-abdominal injury, though, use of sites above the diaphragm is generally preferred to the femoral site.

Place the patient supine, with the hip slightly externally rotated. Feel the femoral arterial pulsation in the groin. The femoral vein lies just medial to the artery. When there is no palpable pulse, the artery can be expected to lie approximately at the midpoint of a line between the anterior–superior iliac crest and the pubic tubercle.

Prepare and drape the groin area in a sterile fashion. Anesthetize the skin and soft tissue in the area of the femoral pulsation. Insert the introducer needle approximately 2–3 cm distal to the inguinal crease and 1–2 cm medial to the femoral arterial pulsation (Figure A.5). The needle should be angled at 45° to the thigh. Aspirate as you advance the needle. Venous blood should flow briskly into the syringe when the femoral vein is entered. Reduce the angle to 20° and advance the needle an additional 2–3 mm to assure that the entire bevel lies within the femoral vein. Proceed with insertion of the guide wire and catheter as described previously.

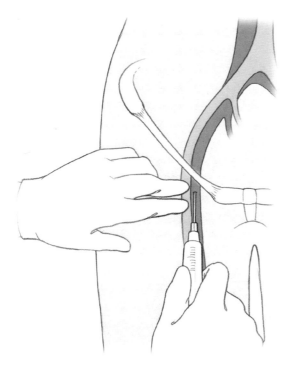

Figure A.5
Femoral vein cannulation with fingers on the pulse of the femoral artery.

Complications of central venous cannulation

Air embolism may occur if air enters the central circulation when the needle or catheter aperture is uncovered. The patient is particularly at risk to this occurrence when the syringe is removed for passage of the guide wire and when the catheter is attached to the IV apparatus. The risk of this complication can be reduced by occluding the hub of the needle and catheter with the thumb at these times.

Catheter position should be checked by obtaining a chest radiograph soon after performing the procedure. Malposition may consist of the catheter entering the wrong vein (e.g., the internal jugular vein rather than the superior vena cava in the subclavian technique), or knotting or kinking of the catheter.

Arterial puncture is probably the most common complication of central venous cannulation. This can be recognized by the appearance of bright red blood in the syringe and the presence of pulsatile flow. In puncture of the carotid artery during attempted internal jugular cannulation, a neck hematoma may be produced that can cause tracheal compression. However, when either the femoral or internal carotid artery is inadvertently punctured, the area around these vessels can be readily compressed. This is not true of the subclavian vessels, and bleeding from the subclavian artery or vein can therefore be particularly problematic, producing a hemothorax. If a subclavian catheter is inadvertently placed in the thoracic cavity, the fluid infused will extravasate into the thorax. Appropriate catheter location should therefore always be assured prior to beginning infusion of IV fluids.

If an insufficient length of guide wire is maintained outside the skin puncture site, the wire can migrate into the vessel and be lost in the venous system. The guide wire can also break especially if it is sheared against the needle when this is withdrawn. Insertion of the guide wire may irritate the right ventricle, especially with the internal jugular or subclavian vein approaches. This may provoke ventricular premature beats. If these appear on the cardiac monitor, the wire should be withdrawn a few centimeters until the ectopy ceases.

Pneumothorax is a hazard in the internal jugular and subclavian vein approaches. It is more likely to occur on the left side, because of the higher location of the left pleural dome. After performing the procedure, examine the patient for dyspnea, subcutaneous emphysema, tracheal shift or unilateral reduction of breath sounds. In addition, obtain a post-procedural chest radiograph. If an existing pneumothorax is known to be present, perform the procedure on the same side as this pneumothorax. Performing it on the opposite side places the patient at risk for bilateral pneumothoraces.

Infection is a possible complication of any venipuncture technique, but is more likely to lead to sepsis in central than peripheral venipuncture. Careful attention to sterile technique is therefore particularly important.

References

Agee KR, Balk RA. Central venous catheterization in the critically ill patient. *Crit Care Med* 1992;8:677–686.

Fitch JA. Central venous access in infants and children. *Crit Decis Emerg Med* 2002;17(1):1–7.

Reusch S, Walder B, Tramer MR. Complications of central venous catheters: internal jugular versus subclavian access – a systematic review. *Crit Care Med* 2002;30:454–460.

Tripathi M. Subclavian vein cannulation: an approach with definite landmarks. *Ann Thorac Surg* 1996;61:238–240.

Intraosseous infusion

Indications

Infusion of fluid or medications via an intraosseous (IO) line is usually reserved for acute life-threatening situations, such as cardiac arrest, especially in instances in which IV access cannot be obtained. Fluid that is infused into the bone marrow enters the systemic circulation via nutrient and emissary veins. Crystalloid solutions, blood products and many drugs can be infused with nearly immediate absorption into the circulation. All drugs typically administered in cardiac arrest can be delivered via the IO route.

The procedure is most often performed in children under 5 years of age, though it has been described as being used in adults as well. However, due to the nature of the mature marrow, infusion is not as effective in adults.

Equipment

Sterile gloves and drapes
Sandbag or rolled towel
Povidone–iodine solution
1% lidocaine local anesthetic, needles and syringe
Bone marrow aspiration needle (16- or 18-gauge) with trocar (if not available, use a lumbar puncture needle with stylet)
Tape and gauze pads
Clear medicine cup

- IV solution bag with tubing
- Pressure infusion pump

Technique

The procedure can be performed at a number of sites (distal femur, distal tibia, medial malleolus, iliac crest and sternum in adults), but is described here at the proximal tibia, the site most often used. The insertion site is 1–2 cm distal to the tibial tuberosity on the medial tibial surface. Prepare the skin in a sterile fashion with povidone–iodine solution. Support the leg by placing a sandbag or rolled towel behind the knee. If time and clinical conditions permit, anesthetize the skin with lidocaine solution.

Stabilize the leg with your non-dominant hand while holding the needle/trocar in the other. Insert the needle into the skin nearly perpendicular to the tibia but angled slightly away from the knee (Figure A.6). A commercial Jamshidi or other bone marrow needle is preferred, but 18- or 20-gauge lumbar puncture needles may be used in children younger than 18 months.

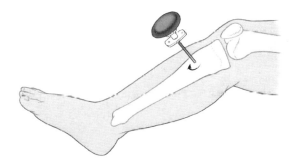

Figure A.6
Intraosseous cannulation proximal tibia.

Use a rotatory motion with constant pressure to advance the needle into the bone. There is a sudden release of resistance when the needle enters the marrow cavity. When the needle is in the marrow, it should stand perpendicularly without support. Remove the trocar and confirm the position of the needle by aspirating a small amount of marrow, or by injecting a small volume of saline to determine that there is minimal resistance and no subcutaneous extravasation. Occasionally, marrow may not return with aspiration, but placement is correct if fluid infuses without extravasation.

Attach the IV solution apparatus. Re-examine the area for signs of extravasation. Place gauze pads around the needle, tape these down and apply a clear medicine cup to protect the needle.

If necessary, apply a pressure pump to assist infusion.

Complications

There are few absolute contraindications to the procedure, but it should not be performed on patients with osteogenesis imperfecta, into a bone that has been fractured, or through infected skin. The most common complication is osteomyelitis, but even this is rare, being described in less than 1% of most series.

Other complications include sepsis, cellulitis, subcutaneous abscess, subcutaneous or subperiosteal infusion of fluid, bony fracture, and growth plate injury. The needle may be bent during insertion. There have been a few reported cases of compartment syndrome following IO infusion, but this appears to be a rare complication.

The likelihood of osteomyelitis can be reduced if the needle is left in place only long enough for resuscitation and stabilization, and by avoiding the procedure in bacteremic children. Subcutaneous infiltration (and the risk of subsequent compartment syndrome) can be minimized by careful observation of the infusion site. Infectious complications can be reduced by proper sterile technique. Adherence to bony landmarks avoids damage to the epiphyseal plate.

References

Orlowski JP. Emergency alternatives to intravenous access. *Pediatr Clin North Am* 1994;41:1183–1199.

Sawyer RW, Bodai BI, Blaisdell FW, McCourt MM. The current status of intraosseous infusion. *J Am Coll Sur* 1994;179:353–360.

Stovoroff M, Teague WG. Intravenous access in infants and children. *Pediatr Clin North Am* 1998;45:1373–1393.

Waisman M, Waisman D. Bone marrow infusion in adults. *J Trauma* 1997;42:288–293.

Arterial puncture

Indications

Arterial blood samples can provide important information regarding respiratory and acid–base status, including arterial pH, pCO_2, pO_2 and bicarbonate levels. Such information is often sought in patients to assess respiratory and metabolic status, in those with significant respiratory compromise, and in others who are severely ill.

Contraindications

Although there are no absolute contraindications, arterial puncture should be performed with extreme care in patients with the following: bleeding disorders or anticoagulation, severe arterial disease in the area, as evidenced by diminished pulse or audible bruit, evidence of absent collateral flow in areas where it normally exists, and previous vascular surgery in the area. Do not perform arterial puncture through skin that appears infected. When frequent blood sampling is anticipated, it may be preferable to insert an indwelling arterial catheter rather than performing repeated arterial punctures.

Equipment

- Prepackaged arterial blood gas kit including:
  – Antiseptic sponge or solution
  – Heparinized 5-ml syringe with 20- or 22-gauge needles
  – Syringe stopper
  – Gauze pads
- Syringe, and 25- or 27-gauge needles for anesthesia
- Local anesthetic solution

Technique

The blood sample is obtained with a 5-ml syringe, the barrel of which has been coated with heparin. If a prepackaged kit is used, the syringe already contains heparin. When preparing the syringe yourself, draw 2 ml of heparinized saline solution (1000 IU/ml) into the syringe. Draw back the plunger to coat the barrel and needle, and then eject the remaining heparin.

Select an arterial puncture site. Common sites are the radial, brachial and femoral arteries. The radial artery at the wrist is the most commonly used location (Figure A.7), though the femoral artery is often preferred in patients in circulatory shock. For the radial artery, palpate the pulse at the wrist, placing the hand in approximately 60° of dorsiflexion. Avoid hyperextending the wrist, as this may place excessive traction on the artery, making the pulse more difficult to feel. The brachial pulse can be felt on the flexor aspect of the elbow, just proximal to the antecubital fossa. The femoral artery enters the thigh after passing beneath the inguinal ligament; the pulse can be felt in the groin, midway between the anterior-superior iliac spine and the pubic symphysis.

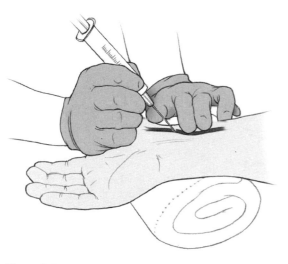

Figure A.7
Radial artery puncture at the wrist.

When the radial artery is considered, the *Allen test* should be performed to ascertain the adequacy of collateral ulnar flow. Perform the test as follows:

1. Palpate the radial and ulnar pulses at the wrist.
2. Compress both the arteries while having the patient repeatedly make a tight fist.
3. Instruct the patient to release the fist, and observe for blanching of the palm.
4. Release your compression of the ulnar artery, noting the time it takes for blanching to resolve. This should normally occur within 5–10 seconds.

When return of normal color to the palm is delayed, the adequacy of ulnar collateral flow can be questioned, and radial artery puncture should not be performed. The Allen test requires a cooperative patient. Moreover, even a normal Allen test does not guarantee the adequacy of collateral circulation.

Prepare the skin overlying the puncture area with antiseptic solution. In the awake patient, you may elect to anesthetize the skin by introducing a small volume of 1% plain lidocaine via a 25- or 27-gauge needle to make a small wheal. A large wheal may obscure the pulse.

Palpate the pulse with the index and middle fingers of the non-dominant hand. Puncture the skin over the artery between these two fingers. Advance the needle at approximately a 45° angle to the skin, parallel to the vessel. When the artery is entered, allow the syringe to fill with the force of arterial pressure. Obtain at least 3 ml of blood

for analysis. If no blood is encountered or the blood does not readily advance the syringe's piston, withdraw the needle and redirect it.

Once blood sampling is completed, withdraw the needle and apply pressure over the puncture site for at least 5 minutes. If the patient has a coagulopathy or is on anticoagulation therapy, apply pressure for 10–15 minutes. Expel any air bubbles present in the sample through the needle holding it upright, then plug the needle or cap the syringe to maintain anaerobic conditions.

Complications

Hematoma formation is the most common complication. This can be avoided by conscientious application of pressure after the procedure is completed. In any event, such bleeding is usually minor.

Infection at the site is another potential complication. Serious infections, however, are uncommon. Although it has been postulated that the femoral site is at particular risk to infection because of proximity to the groin and perineum, no studies substantiate this.

Puncture may induce arterial spasm, which in turn can produce ischemia and thrombus formation. Such spasm usually causes transient ischemia, without significant sequelae in most cases.

Nerve or venous injury from the needle is a potential complication. The femoral vein and nerve lie immediately to the medial and lateral sides of the artery, respectively. The median nerve lies just to the ulnar side of the brachial artery at the antecubital crease.

Reference

Clark VL, Kruse JA. Arterial catheterization. *Crit Care Clin* 1992;8:687–697.

Nasogastric intubation

Indications

Passage of a nasogastric (NG) tube is performed for a variety of indications. A common reason is for the purpose of evacuating the stomach of air (e.g., in gastric distention), gastric contents (intestinal obstruction, pancreatitis), blood (gastrointestinal hemorrhage) or ingested material (certain toxic ingestions). An NG tube should be placed to decompress the stomach of the trauma patient prior to performing a diagnostic peritoneal lavage. The tube may also be utilized as a conduit for administration of medication to the patient who is unable to swallow. An example is the obtunded poisoned patient to whom activated charcoal or an antidote needs to be administered.

A 16- or 18-French tube is appropriate for most purposes in adults. A larger tube may be needed for evacuation of particulate material or blood clots, but it may be necessary to pass such a tube via the oral rather than the nasal route.

Levine and Salem sump tubes are most commonly used. The Levine tube has a single lumen at the tip, and is adequate for instillation of material into the stomach or diagnostic aspiration. The Salem sump has a second vent lumen that attaches to a blue pigtail extension. This vent allows outside air to be drawn into the stomach, thereby permitting continuous flow through the tube. The Salem sump is preferred for continued suction or lavage.

Contraindications

The presence of injury to the mid-face, with possible fracture of the cribriform plate, constitutes an absolute contraindication to attempting passage of an NG tube. This condition creates the danger of passage of the tube into the cranium (Figure 6.20). Use of an orogastric tube should be considered in this setting. Do not attempt passage of an NG tube in a comatose patient with an unprotected airway, as this risks aspiration. Coagulopathy and severe thrombocytopenia are relative contraindications, as significant nasal hemorrhage can be induced in these patients.

Equipment

- Gloves, gown and mask
- NG tube
- Topical anesthetic/vasoconstricting liquid
- Lubricant jelly
- Water and a flexible drinking straw
- 50-ml plain-tipped syringe
- Surgical tape
- 5-in-1 tapered adapter

Technique

Wear gloves, a gown and facial mask when performing the procedure. Position the patient in the sitting position when feasible, and elevate the back of the bed so that the patient does not withdraw the head during insertion. Flex the neck slightly.

Estimate the distance that the tube will have to traverse as follows: measure the distance from the tip of the nose to the earlobe and add the distance from the earlobe to the xiphoid process. The tube has graduated markings at various distances from the distal end. Make note of the distance you have estimated relative to these markings. This distance is approximately 50–60 cm in the typical adult. Underestimating the distance will result in failure to pass the tube past the gastro-esophageal junction.

Check the nostrils for patency by inspection and by asking the patient to inhale while occluding each nostril in turn. When time permits, you may anesthetize and constrict the nostril by applying a topical liquid agent (e.g., 4% cocaine solution) to the nasal mucous membrane. You may also spray a topical anesthetic (e.g., benzocaine spray) into the posterior oropharynx to diminish gagging. Lubricate the most patent naris by injecting 5–10 ml of water-soluble lubricant jelly via a syringe. Coat the tip of the NG tube with this lubricant to a distance of about 6 cm from the tip.

Insert the tip of the tube into the inferior portion of the nostril and aim it directly backward, perpendicular to the axis of the face (Figure A.8a). Slide the tube along the nasal floor beneath the inferior turbinate. Do not direct it upward. Apply gentle pressure to advance the tube. Slight resistance may be encountered at the posterior nasopharynx. Have the patient sip some water through a straw to facilitate the tube's passage through the esophagus. If the tube twists or kinks in the mouth, withdraw it to the level of the nasopharynx to reattempt passage. Do not remove it entirely.

Once you have advanced the tube to the distance previously determined, confirm its appropriate position in the stomach. Rapidly insufflate 20–50 ml of air into the tube via a syringe, simultaneously listening with a stethoscope over the epigastrium (Figure A.8b). A rush of air will be audible as the air bolus enters the stomach. The egress of gastric contents through the tube is also an indication that the stomach has been intubated.

Once the tube's appropriate position has been ascertained, anchor the tube in place by wrapping adhesive tape around it and securing it to the nose. Apply a tapered 5-in-1 adapter and attach the tube to suction, if indicated.

Complications

An NG tube can be inadvertently passed through a fracture of the cribriform plate into the cranium. This is the reason that mid-facial trauma constitutes a contraindication to the procedure. The

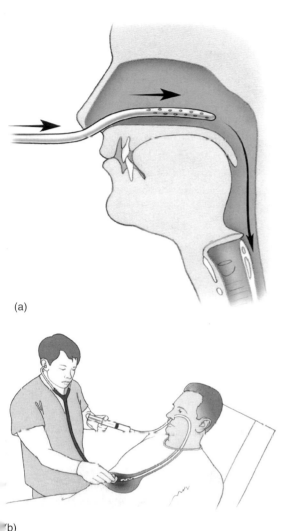

(a)

(b)

Figure A.8
Nasogastric intubation.

tube can also enter the trachea rather than the esophagus. This usually causes profound coughing and misting of the tube with respiration. When this occurs, withdraw the tube immediately and reattempt its passage.

Rather than advancing into the esophagus, the tube may coil in the oropharynx. This is a particularly common occurrence in the unconscious or uncooperative patient. The likelihood of this is greater with smaller caliber tubes, and can be diminished by using a larger tube or by cooling the tube in ice water prior to insertion, thereby rendering it stiffer.

Injury to the nasopharynx is a relatively common complication, producing a small amount of

bleeding. This is not cause for alarm. However, to avoid significant injury to the nasal mucosa, oropharynx or esophagus, only moderate pressure should be applied while advancing the tube. If nasal bleeding occurs, apply direct pressure to the nose until this stops.

Reference

Boyes RJ, Kruse JA. Nasogastric and nasoenteric intubation. *Crit Care Clin* 1992;8:865–878.

Bladder catheterization

Indications

Passage of a catheter into the bladder via the urethra may be necessary for a variety of reasons. Catheter placement may be required to relieve acute urinary retention due to mechanical obstruction or neurologic disease. Similarly, post-voiding residual urine volume is assessed by passage of a *urinary catheter* in patients with incomplete bladder evacuation. An uncontaminated sample of urine for diagnostic analysis can be obtained via catheterization.

In some situations in which a diagnostic pelvic ultrasound is performed, fluid will need to be instilled into the bladder via a catheter to provide an acoustic window for viewing pelvic contents. Prior to performance of diagnostic peritoneal lavage, it is recommended that (absent contraindications) the bladder be decompressed with a catheter to avoid inadvertent injury.

In some cases in which catheterization is performed for diagnostic urinalysis or urinary residual, a straight catheter can be inserted and promptly removed. In most other instances, a balloon-tipped (Foley) catheter is used, with the balloon inflated by injecting saline into the balloon port once the catheter is in the bladder and free flow of urine occurs. Foley catheters of 14-, 16- or 18-French sizes are most commonly used in adults. An indwelling urinary catheter is imperative for monitoring the urine output in seriously ill patients. Core body temperature can be assessed continuously with catheters equipped with temperature probes.

Contraindications

The most important contraindication is the presence of acute urethral injury. Signs suggesting this include the presence of a perineal hematoma, blood at the urethral meatus or a high-riding prostate gland.

Equipment

- Commercially-packaged catheter set of the following:
  - povidone–iodine antiseptic solution
  - cotton balls
  - forceps
  - lubricant jelly
  - sterile drapes
  - sterile gloves
  - urinary catheter
  - 10-ml syringe
  - sterile saline solution
  - urine collection system (tubing and bag)
  - surgical tape

Technique

The female patient

Place the patient in the lithotomy position, with the knees flexed and the hips flexed and abducted. Apply sterile gloves. Drape the perineum. Soak the cotton balls with the antiseptic solution. Spread the patient's labia with the non-dominant hand, exposing the urethra. Grasping a cotton ball with the forceps, prepare the peri-urethral area by applying the povidone–iodine solution over the meatus in an anterior to posterior direction. Repeat several times.

Coat the tip of the catheter with lubricant. Gently introduce the catheter into the meatus and quickly advance it until about half its length has been inserted. Urine should flow through the catheter. Inflate the balloon with 10 ml of saline solution. Pull the catheter back until the balloon is snug against the bladder. Attach the urine collection tubing and bag. Secure the catheter to the leg with tape.

The male patient

Place the patient in the supine position. Apply sterile gloves. Drape around the penis. Soak the cotton balls with the antiseptic solution. If the patient is uncircumcised, retract the foreskin. Grasp the penis with the non-dominant hand, holding it perpendicular to the perineum. Grasping a cotton ball with the forceps, prepare the periurethral area by applying the povidone–iodine solution over the meatus. Repeat several times.

Coat the tip of the catheter with lubricant, and lubricate the urethra. Lidocaine jelly can be used as a lubricant to lessen the discomfort of catheterization. Introduce the catheter into the meatus and quickly advance it until about half its length has been inserted (Figure A.9). Urine should flow through the catheter. Inflate the balloon with 10 ml of saline solution. Pull the catheter back until the balloon is snug against the bladder. Attach the urine collection tubing and bag. Secure the catheter to the leg with tape.

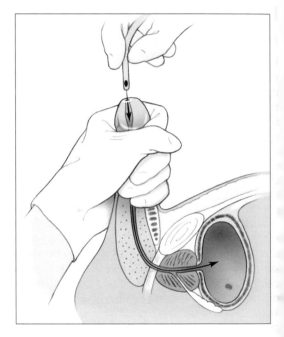

Figure A.9
Bladder catheterization.

Complications

Attempts to pass a catheter via a urethra that has been partially torn by a traumatic injury may result in complete urethral transection. For this reason, the clinical findings of urethral trauma must be sought, as their presence constitute contraindications to catheterization.

Microscopic and rarely gross hematuria may be produced by passage of a urinary catheter. Such bleeding is generally self-limited and requires no treatment. Urinary tract infection can be introduced if sterile procedure is not followed.

Occasionally it is difficult to pass a catheter into the bladder. This is most commonly the case in the male patient with an enlarged prostate. Use of a J-tipped coude catheter or more advanced urologic techniques may be necessary in such cases.

References

Boon TA, Van der Werken C. Urethral injuries revisited. *Injury* 1996;27:533–537.

Curtis LA, Dolan TS, Cespedes RD. Acute urinary retention and urinary incontinence. *Emerg Clin North Am* 2001;19:591–619.

Watnick NF, Coburn M, Goldberger M. Urologic injuries in pelvic ring disruption. *Clin Orthop Rel Res* 1996;329:37–45.

Lumbar puncture

Indications

Lumbar puncture (LP) is used in emergency medicine primarily as a diagnostic tool for meningo-encephalitis and subarachnoid hemorrhage. Although cerebrospinal fluid (CSF) findings obtained through this procedure may be useful in assessing a number of other neurologic diseases (e.g., multiple sclerosis, Guillain–Barre syndrome, neurosyphilis, pseudotumor cerebri or benign intracranial hypertension), these entities are not commonly encountered in emergency practice.

Indications for LP vary according to the clinical setting. Although cranial computed tomography (CT) is extremely useful in the diagnosis of subarachnoid hemorrhage and various other conditions, there is no alternative diagnostic technique to LP for detecting meningitis. A strong suspicion of the presence of meningitis calls for confirmation or exclusion of the diagnosis by this means. LP is frequently used to exclude meningitis in infants with fever or following febrile convulsions. The indications for LP in these settings are not standardized, and vary depending on the clinical presentation.

Contraindications

The procedure is contraindicated in the presence of skin or soft tissue infection overlying the puncture site because of the possibility of introducing infection into the CSF. Due to the risk of hemorrhage, the procedure is also relatively contraindicated in patients with severe bleeding diathesis, thrombocytopenia (platelet counts of less than 50,000/µl), and those who are anticoagulated. Spinal epidural or subdural hematomas are rare complications in such patients. If indications for LP are compelling, though, the procedure may be performed after efforts are made to reverse the coagulopathy.

The suspected presence of an intracranial mass (on the basis of clinical or CT findings) stands as a contraindication to the performance of lumbar puncture. Removing CSF in such cases may reduce lumbar pressure, causing a gradient that leads to rostro-caudal displacement of cerebral structures. Rapid neurologic deterioration may follow.

Equipment

Prepackaged LP kits are available that generally contain the following:

- A 5-ml syringe with a 25-gauge needle
- 1% lidocaine
- Spinal needle with stylet
- Four tubes for collection of CSF
- Povidone–iodine antiseptic solution
- Pressure manometer with three-way stopcock
- Sterile drapes
- Gauze pads
- Adhesive bandage

Technique

Proper positioning is essential for successful LP. The procedure is generally performed with the patient in the lateral position at the edge of the bed with the knees, hips and neck flexed and the lower back arched outward. The shoulders and hips are positioned perpendicular to the bed. An assistant is usually needed to maintain the patient in this position. Avoid excessive flexion of the head, as this can lead to airway obstruction or impede the flow of CSF, especially in neonates.

If LP is unsuccessful in the lateral position, it may be attempted with the patient seated. This may be the most efficacious position for obese patients. Have the patient lean forward, with the arms resting on a table or Mayo stand. CSF pressure in the seated position, however, is gravity-dependent, so the measurement of opening and closing pressures is not clinically useful when the procedure is done in the sitting position.

Under sterile conditions, prepare the back with povidone–iodine solution and apply sterile drapes. Infiltrate the skin and soft tissue overlying the entry spot with 2–3 ml of 1% lidocaine local anesthetic. Entry may be through the L 3–4 or L 4–5 interspace. The L 3–4 interspace can be located as being on a line connecting the posterior iliac crests. Use a styletted spinal needle of appropriate size. This is usually a 20- or 22-gauge needle 3½ inches in length in adults and 25-gauge needle 1½ inches in length in small children. Introduce the spinal needle through an anesthetic wheal in the midline of the back, midway between the spinous processes. Always ascertain the midline by palpation rather than inspection.

Advance the needle slowly with its bevel oriented horizontally and at a cephalad angle of 20–30° (Figure A.10). Direct the needle in the approximate direction of the umbilicus. If bony resistance is encountered, withdraw the needle and redirect it at a slightly different angle in the

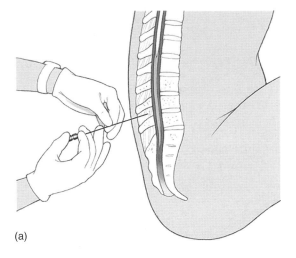

(a)

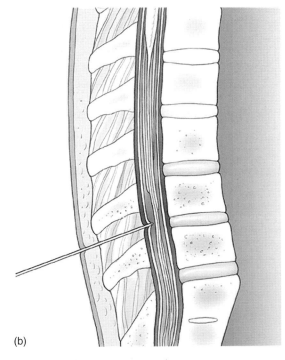

(b)

Figure A.10
Lumbar puncture.

cephalo-caudad direction. A slight "pop" or "give" may be felt when the arachnoid space is entered. Once this occurs, advance the needle a few millimeters further to ensure that the entire bevel lies within the subarachnoid space. Remove the stylet and observe if CSF flows from the needle. If it does not, rotate the needle 90° to overcome a possible obstruction by a nerve root abutting against the aperture. If no fluid returns, withdraw the needle almost to the skin edge and redirect it. If the patient complains of a sharp pain radiating to the leg, the needle may have struck one of the roots of the cauda equina. If this occurs, withdraw the needle and redirect it.

If blood returns through the needle and does not clear, remove the needle and repeat the procedure at another interspace. If the initial fluid is blood-tinged but subsequently clears, this is likely to represent a traumatic tap, with the origin of blood being the peridural venous plexus. This is not generally a dangerous complication, and no treatment is required.

When CSF appears in the hub of the needle, attach a three-way stopcock and manometer and measure the opening pressure. Straighten the patient's legs and advise him to relax when this is being done. Straining will increase intraabdominal pressure, which in turn will spuriously elevate intracranial pressure. The fluid level in the manometer should fluctuate slightly with respirations. Normal CSF opening pressure is 80–180 mmHg. If the opening pressure is extremely high (greater than 350 mmHg), additional fluid should not be withdrawn, unless that was the purpose of the procedure. Remove the needle, and use the fluid already in the manometer for analysis.

In all other cases, allow fluid to drip sequentially into four tubes, with 1–2 ml of fluid in each tube. Specific analytic tests performed on the CSF depend to a degree on the clinical condition being considered. However, analysis for cell count, glucose and protein level, Gram's stain, bacterial culture and xanthochromia should be done in all cases. *Xanthochromia*, a reddish or yellowish discoloration of CSF due to red cell lysis, is present in most cases of subarachnoid hemorrhage. Fluid in the first and fourth tubes should be used for cell count, the second for culture, and the third for glucose and protein levels.

Once sufficient fluid is collected, reinsert the stylet into the needle and withdraw the needle. Cover the puncture site with a sterile dressing. Maintain the patient in the recumbent position for the next 4 hours.

Complications

The most serious complication is precipitating uncal or cerebellar tonsillar herniation in patients with intracranial mass lesions. If signs of a herniation syndrome with neurologic deterioration appear following LP, immediate measures should be taken to lower intracranial pressure. LP may also precipitate neurologic deterioration in patients with spinal cord mass lesions.

The most common complication of lumbar puncture is post-procedure headache, occurring in approximately 10–15% of patients in whom the procedure is done. The etiology relates to persistent leakage of CSF through the dural puncture site. This produces CSF hypotension, with resultant traction on the meninges, vessels, and other pain-sensitive structures at the base of the brain. The most characteristic feature is pain that is present in the upright position and relieved by lying down.

Reference

Sternbach GL. Lumbar puncture. *Top Emerg Med* 1988;10.1 7.

Slit lamp examination

Indications

The slit lamp is a valuable instrument for examining the anterior segment of the eye. It provides positional stabilization of the patient's head, with projection of a light beam onto the eye. The examiner can evaluate each eye individually by binocular inspection through the microscope eyepieces.

Slit lamp examination allows a magnified evaluation of the cornea, conjunctiva and the anterior ocular chamber. It is useful for evaluation of injury to the eye, particularly for the diagnosis of corneal abrasion, iritis, ocular foreign bodies and hyphema. Foreign body removal from the cornea and conjunctiva can be done more precisely through the use of the slit lamp.

Contraindications

There are no contraindications to use of the instrument, but the examination cannot be done if the patient is unable to sit upright.

Equipment

- Slit lamp
- Fluorescein strips

Technique

Seat the patient with the chin in the chin rest and the forehead braced against the headrest. You may accommodate the patient's comfort by adjusting the table and chin rest heights appropriately. Turn the slit lamp on with the beam initially directed over the bridge of the nose, to reduce patient discomfort. Swing the light source to the lateral side of the eye to be examined, positioning it at a 45° angle to the eye. Use a vertically-aligned light beam.

Using the white light, set the light beam to the maximum height and minimum width. Focus the beam of white light on the cornea by moving the base of the slit lamp forward and backward with the joystick until the beam is sharpest on the patient's cornea. Adjust the focus of the eyepieces as you would for a regular microscope while viewing with each eye individually. Move the base left and right to scan across the cornea and conjunctiva. The cornea can be evaluated for abrasions by instilling fluorescein onto the eye and using the blue light filter. Widen the beam to 3–4 mm for this use.

Focus on the center of the cornea and then push the base slightly forward to focus on the anterior surface of the lens. The depth of the anterior chamber can be assessed in this way. Pull back on the joystick to focus midway between the cornea and the lens. The height of the light beam should be 3–4 mm and as narrow as possible for this portion of the examination. Cells may be identified in the anterior chamber – inflammatory white blood cells in iritis, red blood cells in microscopic hyphema. Inflammatory cells will look like specks of dust; red blood cells will look like brown particles.

Intraocular pressure may be measured using the applanation tonometer device found on most slit lamp microscopes. This technique requires a cooperative patient and the use of a topical anesthetic and fluoroscein stain. It is advised to compare pressure measurements between eyes, provided no contraindications exist (infection, ruptured globe).

Complications

None.

References

Harlan JB, Pieramichi DJ. Evaluation of patients with ocular trauma. *Ophthalmol Clin North Am* 2002;15:153–161.

Juang PSC, Rosen P. Ocular examination techniques for the emergency department. *J Emerg Med* 1997; 15:793–810.

Reduction of dislocations

Shoulder

Indications

The indication for this procedure is the presence of a dislocation of the glenohumeral joint of the shoulder. This is a common dislocation, often the result of athletic injury or falls. The reason for the frequency of this injury is the lack of intrinsic bony stability of the glenohumeral joint, as well as its wide range of motion.

The diagnosis is usually obvious on clinical grounds. The arm is held in slight abduction and external rotation, and range of motion is absent or severely limited. There is a loss of the normal rounded appearance of the shoulder, with a step-off deformity and squared appearance revealing the prominence of the acromion process. Though there is some controversy as to whether radiographs should be done in atraumatic shoulder dislocations, they should be performed in all traumatic injuries resulting in dislocation.

Contraindications

None.

Equipment

- Sheets to use for countertraction
- Medication and equipment for IV analgesia and sedation

Technique

There are a number of techniques for reduction of shoulder dislocations. Each has its advocates, and practitioners should be familiar with several methods. Administration of parenteral analgesia, muscle relaxants or procedural sedation is necessary in many cases.

The traction–countertraction technique is a frequently utilized method (Figure A.11). Position the patient supine with a folded sheet wrapped around the chest and under the axilla. Have an assistant apply countertraction with this sheet, and apply steady traction along the axis of the humerus with the shoulder abducted slightly. It may take several minutes of continued traction for the reduction to be effective.

In the external rotation method, place the patient supine and support the elbow with one

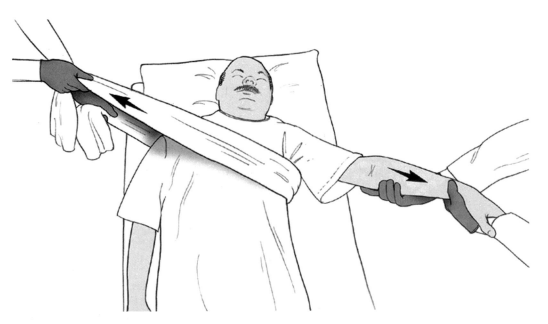

Figure A.11
Traction–countertraction technique for shoulder reduction.

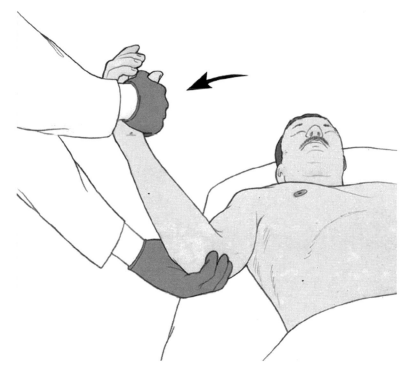

Figure A.12
External rotation method of shoulder reduction.

hand (Figure A.12). Adduct the shoulder and apply longitudinal traction. Slowly and gently externally rotate the shoulder. Once the shoulder is externally rotated to 90°, slowly abduct the shoulder until reduction occurs.

For the scapular manipulation technique, place the patient prone, with the arm hanging off the bed (Figure A.13). Apply downward traction to the arm. Push the inferior tip of scapula medially while stabilizing the superior portion of the scapula. Unlike other methods, this approach attempts reduction by reorienting the glenoid fossa rather than repositioning the humeral head.

Following reduction, ascertain the proper position of the shoulder through post-reduction radiographs. Immobilize the patient in a sling and swath or shoulder immobilizer. Repeat a neurovascular examination and document the results in the medical record.

Complications

Injury to the axillary nerve occurs in approximately 10% of cases of shoulder dislocation. This usually represents a traction neuropraxia, which has favorable prognosis for recovery of nerve function. To assure that the nerve has not been injured during the reduction process, it is important to test for its function prior to attempts at reduction, and to document the results of this examination in the medical record. The sensory portion of the nerve provides sensation over the lateral portion of the shoulder (the "military patch" distribution). Test sharp sensation over this area with a pin. The motor portion of the axillary nerve innervates the deltoid muscle. Have the patient attempt shoulder abduction. Feel the contraction of the deltoid muscle by placing your hand over it.

Fracture of the humeral head may occur as a consequence of reduction.

Radial head subluxation

Indications

Indication for this procedure is the presence of an acute radial head subluxation in a child. This is a very common childhood injury, seen most often between the ages of 1 and 5 years, with a peak incidence between ages 2–3 years. It is usually the result of sudden traction being applied to a

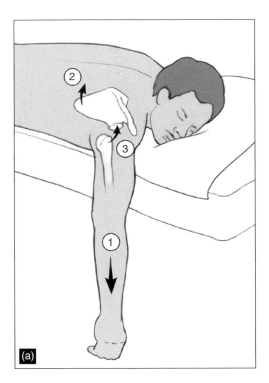

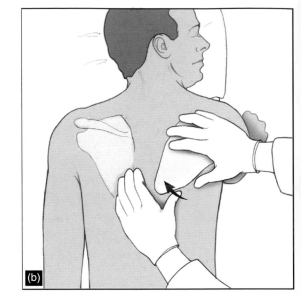

Figure A.13
Scapular manipulation.

child's hand or forearm. This typically occurs when a parent pulls a child up by the arm during play or to prevent a fall. This condition is also referred to as "nursemaid's elbow." It results in the pulling of the annular ligament over the radial head, with the interposition of this ligament (which maintains the radius in its normal relationship relative to the humerus and ulna) between the radius and the humeral capitellum.

The result is usually acute pain and unwillingness by the child to move the arm. The arm is held in slight flexion and pronation. Any attempt at motion is resisted by the child.

Contraindications

None.

Equipment

None.

Technique

Support the elbow and forearm with one hand, and place the thumb of the other hand over the area of the radial head. Simultaneously, slowly flex

the elbow and supinate the forearm. An audible or palpable click may be perceived with reduction. The child usually becomes pain-free and moves the arm normally shortly after reduction. Given the appropriate mechanism and successful reduction, neither radiographs nor immobilization is necessary.

Complications

Recurrence of the subluxation occasionally occurs.

Phalangeal

Indications

Dislocations of the interphalanageal and metacarpophalangeal joints are common injuries, often occurring during sports activities or falls. Bayonet-shaped or angulated deformities of the fingers are usually readily identified, and constitute indication for reduction. When a skin laceration accompanies the injury, irrigation of the wound and debridement of devitalized tissue may have to follow reduction. Such lacerations may need to be sutured after reduction is completed, and require antibiotics.

Contraindications

None.

Equipment

- Local anesthetic
- Syringe and 27-gauge needle

Technique

Reduction may require a digital nerve block, though it may be accomplished without anesthesia if the patient is stoic and not too much time has elapsed since the injury. Apply longitudinal traction with slight hyperextension (exaggerating the deformity) (Figure A.14). Reduction is accompanied by a palpable "click" and resolution of the deformity. Apply an immobilizing splint.

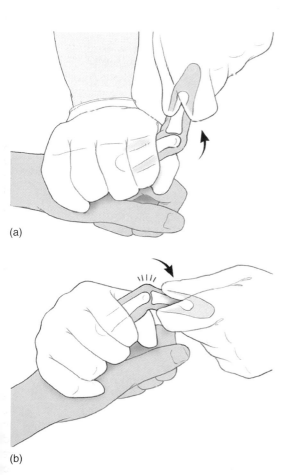

(a)

(b)

Figure A.14
Reduction of phalangeal dislocation.

Complications

Some dislocations, especially those of the metacarpophalangeal joints, may involve the interposition of soft tissue between the dislocated bones. Such dislocations resist the usual methods of reduction, and require operative management. Repeated attempts at closed reduction may produce damage to the soft tissues.

Patella

Indications

Dislocation of the patella usually results from a laterally-directed force applied to the medial side of the kneecap. The knee is often partially flexed at the time of injury. The displacement of the patella on the lateral aspect of the knee produces a dramatic deformity. The presence of dislocation constitutes an indication for reduction. Neurovascular impairment is rarely a feature of this injury.

Contraindications

None.

Equipment

None.

Technique

Although parenteral sedation may be helpful in reducing muscular spasm and pain, the reduction can often be achieved without administration of any medication. Apply medially-directed pressure over the lateral border of the patella combined with extension of the knee (Figure A.15). The patella can be felt to snap into place as reduction occurs. Following reduction, immobilize the knee using a knee immobilizer or a posterior plaster splint.

Complications

Though there are rarely any complications from the procedure itself, a traumatic joint effusion may follow this injury. Damage to the medial supporting ligaments of the patella may occur, leading to a predisposition for recurrent dislocation.

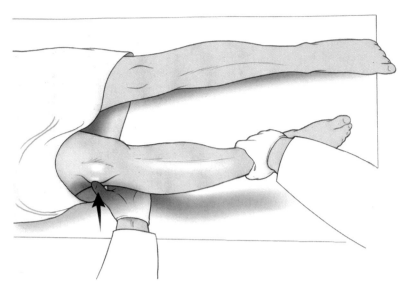

Figure A.15
Reduction of dislocated patella.

References

Aronen JG, Chronister RD. Anterior shoulder dislocations: easing reduction by using linear traction techniques. *Phys Sport Med* 1995;23:65–69.

Beeeson M. Complications of shoulder dislocation. *Am J Emerg Med* 1999;17:288–295.

Brady WJ, Perron AD. Dislocation of the glenohumeral joint. *Crit Decis Emerg Med* 2002;17(1):8–16.

Hossfeld GE, Uehara DT. Acute joint injuries of the hand. *Emerg Med Clin North Am* 1993;11:781–796.

Schunk JE. Radial head subluxation: epidemiology and treatment of 87 episodes. *Ann Emerg Med* 1990;19:1019–1023.

Tube thoracostomy

Indications

Tube thoracostomy (chest tube) is performed to remove blood (hemothorax), fluid (pleural effusion or empyema) or air (pneumothorax) from the pleural space. The clinical circumstances must be assessed in each case, though, as not all patients with a pneumothorax or pleural effusion require evacuation with a chest tube.

Thoracostomy tubes come in various sizes. Larger tubes (30–40 French) are needed for evacuation of a hemothorax, whereas relatively smaller ones (12–22 French) are likely to be adequate in the treatment of pneumothorax. The usual placement site for a thoracostomy tube is the fifth or sixth intercostal space in the mid-axillary line. For pneumothorax, a small tube is sometimes placed in the mid-clavicular line in the second intercostal space.

Contraindications

There are no absolute contraindications to insertion of a chest tube, provided the appropriate indications are present. Some relative contraindications exist. Coagulopathy is one of these, and the patient with a prolonged prothrombin time or thrombocytopenia should have these abnormalities corrected prior to chest tube insertion.

In massive hemothorax, pleural blood may act to tamponade a site of bleeding. Insertion of a thoracostomy tube in such circumstances may precipitate massive hemorrhage once the tamponade effect is removed. Such patients should be considered for open thoracotomy to control bleeding prior to chest tube insertion.

Equipment

- Sterile gloves and drapes
- Povidone–iodine antiseptic solution

- Lidocaine 1% local anesthetic with epinephrine
- Syringe and needles
- Scalpel with No. 10 blade
- Large curved scissors
- Large and medium Kelly clamps
- Chest tubes
- Water seal drainage apparatus (Pleuravac®) with tubing and serrated connector
- Needle holder
- Silk 1-0 suture
- Vaseline-impregnated gauze
- Gauze pads (4 × 4)
- Adhesive tape

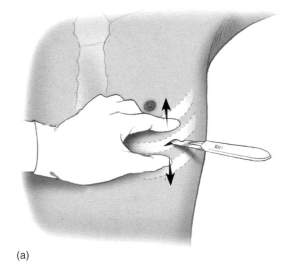

(a)

Technique

Prior to initiating the procedure, fill the drainage apparatus with water to the indicated levels. Place the patient in the supine or semi-upright position. In the awake and hemodynamically stable patient, consider administering IV analgesics and sedatives to make the procedure less painful. Raise the patient's arm above the head on the side used. Put on sterile gloves. Prepare the skin with povidone–iodine solution and drape in a sterile fashion. Anesthetize the skin over the insertion site by injecting lidocaine with epinephrine anesthetic. Infiltrate deeper using a long 25-gauge needle to infiltrate the subcutaneous tissue, muscle and parietal pleura. As much as 20–40 ml of local anesthetic may be required.

Make a 2–3 cm incision over the rib, with the axis of the incision parallel to the rib (Figure A.16a). Bluntly dissect the subcutaneous tissues, using the Kelly clamp or large scissors to separate the tissue by opening and spreading the instrument. Perform the dissection over the top of the rib to avoid the subcostal neurovascular bundle. The dissection tunnel should be large enough to admit your index finger. Direct the dissection in a caudad direction. Penetrate the parietal pleura with a clamp (Figure A.16b). After penetrating the pleura, open the clamp to expand the opening, and then remove the clamp in the open position. Insert your index finger through the pleural opening to assure the absence of adhesions and abdominal organs, and so as not to "lose" the hole's location (Figure A.16c).

Clamp the end of the chest tube with a large clamp and guide the tube through the dissected tunnel into the pleural space (Figure A.16d). Direct it cephalad and posteriorly, and advance until all the side holes over the distal portion are

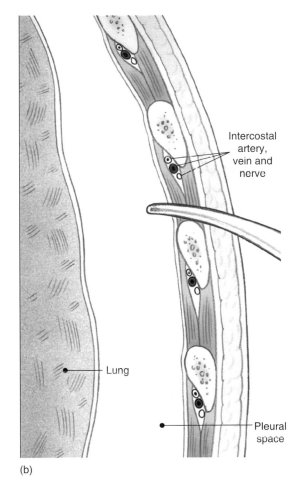

(b)

Figure A.16
The thoracostomy (a) incision, (b) clamp penetration.

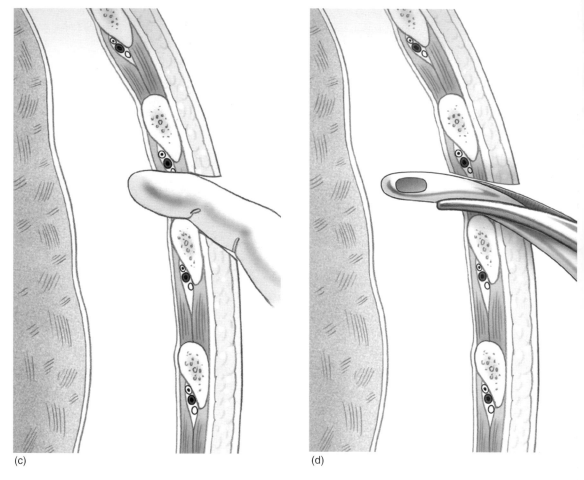

(c)   (d)

Figure A.16 (*cont*)
(c) insertion of finger and (d) insertion of chest tube using curved clamp.

within the thoracic cavity. Remove the clamp. Fluid (pleural effusion) or blood (hemothorax) should now enter the tube. In the case of pneumothorax, condensation of air will be seen on the walls of the tube coincident with respiration. Connect the tube to the water seal drainage apparatus. Tape the junction of the tube and the serrated connector.

Secure the tube to the skin with a purse-string suture, wrapping the suture around the end of the tube before cutting the ends. Cover the insertion site with Vaseline-impregnated gauze. Apply a dressing of 4 × 4 gauze pads. Tape the dressing and also tape a section of the tube in place to the skin. Obtain a post-procedure chest radiograph to assess for the proper position and function of the tube. The chest tube has a radioopaque stripe along its side to aid in radiographic identification.

Complications

Patients with severe chronic obstructive pulmonary disease may have large pulmonary bullae that may be mistaken for pneumothoraces. Insertion of a chest tube in this instance can worsen pulmonary function.

Failure to suture and tape the tube to the chest may result in accidental extrusion of the tube. Failure to tape the connections may cause separation of the chest tube from the water seal drainage apparatus, resulting in recurrence of the pneumothorax.

Failure to assure that all of the side holes of the thoracostomy tube are positioned within the pleural space causes aspiration of air from a pneumothorax into the soft tissue of the chest, producing subcutaneous emphysema. Passage of the tube into the subcutaneous tissue rather than the pleural space will fail to evacuate the space of fluid or air.

Bleeding may occur if an intercostal artery or vein is lacerated during the procedure. The lower border of the rib should be avoided as a site of incision to avoid these vessels. Intercostal nerves can be injured in similar fashion. Other intrathoracic vessels can be injured during insertion of the tube, and the tube should not be forced through the subcutaneous tunnel or into the pleural space. Laceration of lung adherent to the pleura, liver and other abdominal organs can occur. The entry site through the pleura should be palpated prior to insertion of the tube to avert such complications.

References

Iberti TJ, Stern PM. Chest tube thoracostomy. *Crit Care Clin* 1992;8:879–895.

Quigley RL. Thoracentesis and chest tube drainage. *Crit Care Clin* 1995;11:111–126.

Cervical spine clearance

Indications

Evaluating the patient for evidence of injury to the cervical spine is an important part of clinical trauma assessment. As spinal injury can produce catastrophic neurologic consequences, radiographs of the spine are commonly ordered for injured patients. The determination that a patient is at minimal risk of spinal injury, and does not require radiographic assessment involves a clinical determination to "clear" the spine of further immobilization and imaging.

Contraindications

Due to the clinical importance of this procedure, it must always be done by an experienced practitioner. To be recognized as being at low risk for cervical spine injury, the patient must meet all of the following criteria:

* There is no tenderness to palpation of the bones of the cervical spine.
* The patient has no deficit on neurologic examination or complaint of such deficit by history.
* The patient shows no evidence of being intoxicated with alcohol or other drugs that can affect level of consciousness.

* There is a normal level of alertness allowing the patient to fully comprehend and co-operate with the examination. The patient should be oriented to person, place and time, and should not exhibit inappropriate or delayed responses to external stimuli.
* There are no painful injuries elsewhere on the body that could distract the patient from recognizing the pain associated with a neck injury.

Equipment

None.

Technique

Assure that the above conditions are met. Palpate the midline of the neck posteriorly from the nuchal ridge to the prominence of the first thoracic vertebra. If the patient complains of any pain on this palpation, cervical radiographs are indicated.

If there is no such tenderness and the patient meets all the other conditions, remove any cervical immobilization devices without having the patient move his or her neck. Instruct the patient to very slowly flex the neck to the greatest degree possible, instructing him to stop if any pain occurs. If the patient can do this, have him extend the neck as much as possible, again instructing him to terminate efforts with any discomfort. Repeat the procedure with the patient themselves turning the head to the right and then the left. In each instance, movement should be stopped if any discomfort is produced. If the patient can perform full range of motion maneuvers painlessly in the absence of the above mitigating criteria, the presence of cervical spine injury can be excluded on clinical grounds.

Complications

Exacerbating cervical injury by allowing neck movement is the major complication. Whenever any doubt exists to the possibility of spinal injury, it should be assessed through radiographic imaging.

References

Hoffman JR, Mower WR, Wolfson AB, et al. Validity of a set of clinical criteria to rule out injury to the cervical spine in patients with blunt trauma. *New Engl J Med* 2000;343:94–99.

Mahadevan S, Mower WR, Hoffman JR, et al. Interrater reliability of cervical spine injury criterial in patients with blunt trauma. *Ann Emerg Med* 1998;31:197–201.

Panacek EA, Mower WR, Holmes JF, et al. Test performance of the individual NEXUS low-risk clinical screening criteria for cervical spine injury. *Ann Emerg Med* 2001;38:22–25.

Abscess incision and drainage

Indications

Indication for this procedure is the presence of a cutaneous or subcutaneous abscess (a collection of inflammatory and infectious products encapsulated by granulation tissue). The clinical hallmark is a tender mass that shows fluctuance – the liquid nature of the contents can be palpated through the skin. In most patients, a cutaneous abscess constitutes a local infection caused by skin flora.

Contraindications

There are no absolute contraindications to performing incision and drainage of an abscess. If there is evidence of local infection (e.g., redness, swelling), but no fluctuance, the procedure may be delayed until after a trial of antibiotic therapy. In the face and other areas where a scar is undesirable, repeated aspiration may be an alternative to incision and drainage. In the septic or severely immune compromised patient, the procedure may have to be delayed until after antibiotic therapy is initiated.

Equipment

- Sterile gloves
- Local anesthetic solution, syringe and needles
- Eutectic mixture of local anesthetics (EMLA) gel
- Sterile drapes
- Povidone–iodine antiseptic solution
- Irrigating syringe (30 ml)
- Saline irrigating solution
- Ribbon packing tape (¼ or ½-inch width)
- Scalpel with No. 11 blade
- Hemostat
- Scissors
- Gauze pads

Technique

Prepare and drape the area in sterile fashion. Performing incision and drainage is an extremely painful procedure, and it may be difficult to achieve adequate local anesthesia. Apply a layer of EMLA gel over the area of fluctuance. Cover this with a patch of Tegaderm or clear plastic wrap. After a period of 30–60 minutes, inject subcutaneous local anesthetic across the dome of the abscess (Figure A.17a). Using a scalpel with a No. 11 blade, make an incision over the area of maximal fluctuance and extend it into the abscess cavity (Figure A.17b).

Gently probe the cavity with a hemostat to free all loculated tissue (Figure A.17c). This may be the most painful portion of the procedure, as skin infiltration will not provide anesthesia in the depths of the cavity. Irrigate the abscess cavity with saline

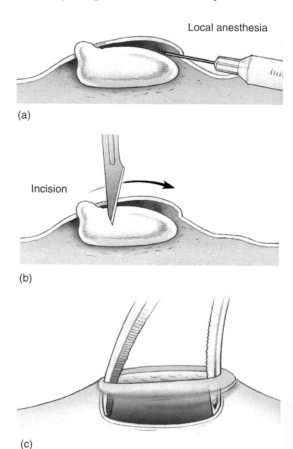

(a)

(b)

(c)

Figure A.17
Abscess infiltration, incision and drainage.

solution. Pack the wound with ribbon tape. Do not pack the cavity tightly, as this may trap purulent material. Apply a gauze dressing.

Complications

Whenever an incision is made in skin, there is risk of injury to surrounding tissue.

Infection can be spread into adjacent tissue or the bloodstream by abscess drainage. Inadequately probing the interior of the abscess cavity may result in the reaccumulation of infectious fluid and return of symptoms.

Reference

Bisno AL, Stevens DL. Streptococcal infections of the skin and soft tissues. *New Engl J Med* 1996;334:311–317.

Common emergency procedures

Appendix B   Wound preparation

Michelle Lin, MD

Overview

Management of a laceration before and after wound closure plays as important a role as the actual act of wound repair itself. Wound infection, which occurs in approximately 3–7% of all traumatic wounds, wound dehiscence, and poor cosmesis directly relate to the adequacy of wound preparation. The approach to proper wound management can be categorized into the following steps: setup, anesthesia, wound cleaning, local wound preparation, and post-closure wound care.

Setup

Preparation of both the patient and provider is essential in any case requiring wound management. Patient preparation includes:

1. Establishing sufficient lighting for good wound visualization.
2. Placing the patient in a reclined or semi-reclined position to anticipate a possible vasovagal event from pain or anxiety.
3. Positioning the patient so that the wound is most accessible to the provider, such as raising the patient's gurney to the provider's waist level.

Provider preparation primarily involves using universal precautions, including a gown, face or eye protection, and gloves. This becomes especially important during wound irrigation, when high-pressure irrigation fluid may splash blood-borne products unpredictably.

Anesthesia

After a complete neurovascular examination distal to the wound, the next step is anesthetizing the wound. This allows the provider to meticulously irrigate, explore, and examine tendon function before closure now that patient discomfort is no longer a limiting factor. According to a large American College of Emergency Physicians' study of medicolegal claims from the emergency department (ED), missing retained foreign bodies in wounds is the fifth leading cause of lawsuits.

Lidocaine and the longer-acting bupivacaine are the two most commonly used anesthetic agents. Both share onset of pain relief in 2–5 minutes. Lidocaine lasts for approximately 1–2 hours, bupivacaine lasts 4–8 hours. For the pediatric population, seemingly small volumes of an anesthetic may be toxic for the patient. It is therefore important to calculate the toxic anesthetic dose prior to administration (Table B.1). Lidocaine and bupivacaine toxicity can cause seizures, dysrhythmias, and cardiac arrest. The concurrent use of epinephrine improves hemostasis and reduces systemic anesthetic absorption by the mechanism of local vasoconstriction. Traditionally, epinephrine should not be used for end-circulation anatomic areas, including the fingers, toes, ears, nose, and penis.

Table B.1 Local anesthetic toxicity

Adult example		
	Toxic dose	Toxic volume for typical 70 kg adult patient
Bupivacaine	3 mg/kg	Using 0.25% bupivacaine: (3 mg/kg)(70 kg) % (2.5 mg/ml) = 84 ml
Lidocaine	4.5 mg/kg	Using 1% lidocaine: (4.5 mg/kg)(70 kg) % (10 mg/ml) = 31.5 ml
Lidocaine + epinephrine	7 mg/kg	Using 1% lidocaine + epinephrine: (7 mg/kg)(70 kg) % (10 mg/ml) = 49 ml
Pediatric example		
	Toxic dose	Toxic volume for a 2-year-old child (12 kg) with a leg laceration
Lidocaine	4.5 mg/kg	Using 1% lidocaine: (4.5 mg/kg)(12 kg) % (10 mg/ml) = 5.4 ml. Note: The provider should not use more than 5.4 ml, or 54 mg of lidocaine.

A study by Whilhelmi et al. demonstrated that digits injected with lidocaine + epinephrine had no added complications compared to lidocaine alone, suggesting that this dictum may be overconservative. For those "allergic" to these anesthetics, cardiac lidocaine, which is preservative-free, may be used. If a true lidocaine allergy exists, 1% diphenhydramine can serve as an effective alternative agent, although it causes relatively more pain on administration.

There are four different approaches to achieve wound anesthesia.

Topical

Topical anesthesia can be used as the sole means of anesthetizing a wound, or it may be used in conjunction with local infiltration. Due to the high vascularity of the face and scalp, topical anesthetics are most effective in this area. Two commercially-prepared agents are TAC (a mixture of tetracaine, adrenaline/epinephrine, and cocaine) and LET (a mixture of lidocaine, epinephrine, and tetracaine). TAC has been associated with several case reports of seizures and death from inadvertent mucosal absorption of cocaine; as a result, it is unavailable in most EDs.

A cotton ball soaked with approximately 3–5 ml of the anesthetic agent is applied to the open wound for at least 10 minutes. To maximize absorption, apply firm pressure with a strong adhesive tape. Alternatively, for the frightened pediatric patient, a family member can wear gloves and apply the cotton ball to the patient's laceration. The presence of blanched wound edges marks successful absorption of anesthetic, as absorption of epinephrine from TAC or LET causes local wound vasoconstriction. Caution should be taken with application around the eyes, to prevent inadvertent corneal exposure.

Local infiltration

Local infiltration, the most common approach to anesthesia in wound care, involves injecting an anesthetic into both wound edges at the dermal-subcutaneous layer. Starting at one apex, deposit a small amount of anesthetic in the subcutaneous tissue within the wound. This is not done through intact epidermal skin, as penetrating intact skin is more painful. Be sure to check for inadvertent vascular cannulation by aspirating for blood before instilling anesthetic. Advance the needle to its full length along one wound edge. Deposit

anesthesia while retracting the needle out of the skin. Reinsert the needle at the leading edge of anesthesia and continue this process circumferentially around the wound (Figure B.1).

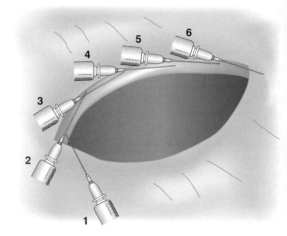

Figure B.1 Local anesthetic infiltration technique. Local infiltration first starts with a subcutaneous wheal of anesthetic at one apex from within the wound (Syringe 1 on bottom left). Subsequent injections (Syringe 2–6) along the wound edge start at the leading edge of anesthesia. The process should be continued for the other side of the wound for complete anesthesia.

Five different techniques can reduce the pain of anesthetic infiltration.

1. Premedicate the wound with a topical anesthetic (described above) or ice. This partially anesthetizes the wound edges before injecting with the needle.
2. As local anesthetics such as lidocaine and bupivacaine are weak acids, mixing the medication with bicarbonate produces a more neutral pH and less painful anesthetic. For 1% lidocaine, mix 1 ml of 8.4% bicarbonate with 9 ml of the anesthetic. For bupivacaine, mix 0.1 ml of 8.4% bicarbonate with 9.9 ml of the anesthetic. Excess bicarbonate added to bupivacaine may cause solute precipitation.
3. Warm the anesthetic syringe in your hand for several minutes to room temperature to reduce the pain of infiltration.
4. Inject the local anesthetic with the smallest diameter needle. A 30-gauge needle is preferred.
5. Slow the rate of medication injection, as pain results when the soft tissue stretches.

Regional block

A more elegant technique in wound anesthesia is a regional nerve block, where anesthesia is administered proximal to the wound site to block sensory innervation to the affected area. The primary advantage of this approach is the preservation of wound edges. Comparatively, local anesthetic infiltration often distorts landmarks. This factor is especially crucial when wound edges are under tension or poorly approximated. The most commonly used regional block is the digital block. Other regional blocks anesthetize the supraorbital, infraorbital, mental, median, ulnar, radial, saphenous, deep peroneal, superficial peroneal, posterior tibial, and sural nerves. The key to successful regional anesthesia is familiarity with the anatomy and proper technique.

The digital block anesthetizes an entire digit distal to the metacarpal–phalangeal or metatarsal–phalangeal joint. Each finger has an ulnar and radial digital nerve, located along the ulnar and radial volar (palmar) aspect of the digit, respectively. Each toe has a similar medial and lateral digital nerve located along the plantar aspect of the digit. In cross-section, these nerves lie at approximately the 4 and 8 o'clock positions of a digit with the surface of the fingernail or toenail at 12 o'clock. As a consequence, two injections are required for adequate anesthesia. First, after positioning the patient's hand or foot on a flat surface with the dorsal aspect facing up, insert the needle at the level of the web space. At a 45° angle aiming volarly, insert the needle along the proximal phalanx bone to reach the first digital nerve. After aspirating to check for inadvertent vascular cannulation, slowly inject 1–2 ml of the anesthetic. Remember to avoid using epinephrine. Repeat this process for the opposite digital nerve. For the thumb and great toe, a subcutaneous line of anesthesia should also be deposited to block the superficial branches supplying the dorsal part of the digit (Figure B.2).

Procedural sedation

Although the topic of procedural sedation exceeds beyond the scope of this section, it provides another option for wound closure. This option is primarily reserved for pediatric patients who cannot tolerate local or regional anesthesia because of emotional distress or concerns of anesthetic toxicity. Common agents include ketamine (for children less than 10 years old), propofol, etomidate, or a combination of fentanyl and midazolam.

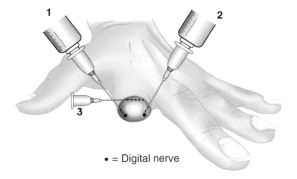

• = Digital nerve

Figure B.2 Regional anesthesia: digital nerve block. A digital nerve block can be achieved with injections at Sites 1 and 2. For the thumb and great toe, a third subcutaneous line of anesthesia (Site 3) is necessary to block superficial dorsal sensory nerves.

While the patient is sedated, a local or regional anesthetic may be administered for pain relief during the procedure and after the patient awakens.

Despite improved cosmetics from patient immobilization and decreased psychologic trauma, procedural sedation does not come without risks. One disadvantage is a longer ED stay for the patient, because the patient must have had nothing by mouth for 4–6 hours prior to the sedation, and usually requires time for the sedation to wear off following the procedure. Depending on the procedural sedation agent used, risks include agitation, vomiting, respiratory depression and apnea. A complete discussion of procedural sedation can be found in Appendix D.

Wound cleaning

Cleaning the wound prior to wound closure reduces the incidence of infection. Although a variety of irrigation solutions have been studied to minimize wound infection, the current standard is sterile normal saline with high-pressure irrigation. The type of solution used for irrigation may not be important; several studies have shown equal efficacy using tap water versus sterile normal saline. However, high pressure irrigation is the cornerstone of wound cleaning. By applying at least a 7 psi force to the wound, the irrigation fluid dislodges foreign bodies, contaminants, and bacteria. Although many commercially available kits can provide high-pressure irrigation, a simple device can be made by using a 30 ml syringe and an 18-gauge angiocatheter. Irrigation with this setup delivers over 7 psi of pressure (Figure B.3). Low-pressure irrigation,

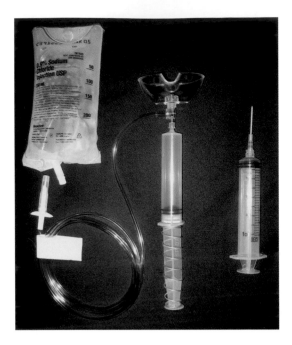

Figure B.3 Wound irrigation equipment.
A commercially-available unit (middle) or a syringe with
an 18-gauge angiocatheter (right) can deliver high-
pressure irrigation to a wound.

such as squeezing fluid out of a puncture hole made in a saline bottle, is inadequate. Although no studies have looked at the ideal irrigation volume, a common practice is to irrigate about 100 ml for every 1 cm of wound length. Slightly more irrigant may be used for distal extremity or contaminated wounds, which have a higher incidence of infection, and slightly less for facial and scalp wounds, which have a much lower incidence. Hollander et al. suggest that facial and scalp wounds require minimal, if any, irrigation prior to wound closure because the high vascularity of these areas significantly reduces the incidence of wound infection. There was also added benefit of improved cosmesis without irrigation because high-pressure irrigation caused unnecessary soft tissue swelling and damage.

There are two common misconceptions in wound cleaning. The first error is swabbing povidone–iodine or chlorhexidine into the wound for further sterilization. Studies have shown that although they impede bacterial growth, they are also cytotoxic and impair wound defenses. Thus, if using these agents, be sure to swab only the intact skin adjacent to the wound but not in the wound itself. A second error is to scrub the wound vigorously before wound closure. This injures underlying viable soft tissue and impairs optimal wound healing. Unless there are multiple small foreign bodies embedded in the skin, such as gravel, scrubbing is not recommended.

Local wound preparation

After anesthesia and irrigation, the wound should be examined under sterile conditions to maintain sterility and to reduce the risk of wound infection. Careful wound exploration should check for the presence of foreign bodies and involvement of more complex structures, such as tendon, muscle, joint capsule, and bone.

Three problems commonly arise during wound preparation. The first is bleeding, especially after wound irrigation. This is when early clots may become dislodged, and ongoing venous or arterial bleeding prevents adequate visualization of the wound. Hemostasis can usually be achieved by applying direct external pressure for several minutes. Persistent bleeding despite direct pressure can be approached by applying a tourniquet on an extremity proximal to the wound for no more than 60 minutes. The cuff pressure should be above the patient's systolic blood pressure. Patients often will not tolerate this tight tourniquet for more than 20–30 minutes. Additionally, in wounds that ooze slowly, an anesthetic with epinephrine can be used to wash over the wound and achieve transient vasoconstrictive hemostasis before wound closure. Following thorough exploration, wound repair and closure itself will generally stop further bleeding.

Another common problem with wound preparation is the proximity of hair to the wound. Hair strands should not become trapped in the wound during closure, to avoid a foreign body reaction. Hair should not be shaved, because this increases the rate of wound infection, providing a portal for bacterial entry. Eyebrow hair should never be cut or shaved because it grows slowly and irregularly after being cut, causing cosmetic asymmetry for the patient. Furthermore, eyebrows assist with wound edge approximation by serving as a landmark for skin edges. Instead, for lacerations near hair, apply a thin coat of a sterile petroleum-based jelly in the hair, such as neosporin or bacitracin, and mat the hair away from the wound edges.

A third problem frequently encountered in wound preparation is the presence of devitalized tissue along a wound edge. Nonviable tissue along wound edges impairs wound healing, because it can provide a nidus for infection. Excisional debridement of devitalized tissue can also allow more precise reapproximation of wound edges. Be careful of over-debridement, which may create excessive wound tension upon closure. Debridement near tendons and peripheral nerves may cause additional iatrogenic injuries.

Post-closure wound care

Continued care after wound closure plays an integral role in optimal wound healing. In order to prevent contamination and limit scab formation of the wound, apply a dressing consisting of a topical antibiotic ointment underneath a dry sterile gauze. For tissue adhesives, petroleum-based products should not be applied because they can degrade the adhesive and cause wound dehiscence. When applying a circumferential wound dressing, wrap the site loosely to avoid a tourniquet-like effect from inevitable soft tissue swelling. For wounds overlying joint surfaces, which may dehisce when the joint is flexed or extended, a splint should be applied to prevent range of motion of the joint.

Providers should not prescribe prophylactic systemic antibiotics for simple lacerations and wounds. The primary means of reducing wound infection is sterile irrigation, scrupulous wound exploration, and meticulous wound closure, not antibiotics. However, antibiotics are indicated in special high-risk cases (Table B.2).

Table B.2 Indications for systemic antibiotics for traumatic wounds

- Injury >6 hours old on the extremities
- Injury >24 hours old on the face and scalp
- Tendon, joint, or bony involvement
- Cartilage involvement
- Mammalian bite
- Co-morbid disease (diabetes mellitus, extremes of age, steroid use, morbid obesity)
- Puncture wound
- Complex intraoral wound

Discharge paperwork for the patient should include explicit instructions on wound care management, as well as specific comments about the possibility of wound infection (Table B.3). For the wound at higher risk of infection, such as a contaminated laceration of a finger, a human bite of an extremity, or a traumatic wound with devitalized tissue, a scheduled wound check within 48 hours is prudent to look for early signs of infection.

Table B.3 Sample patient discharge instructions

- Keep your wound elevated above the level of your heart to reduce tissue swelling.
- *For sutures*: Keep the wound dressing on and dry for 24 hours to prevent wound contamination. Afterward, change the dressing using dry gauze or a bandage. Gently clean the wound edges with mild soap and water. Keep the wound covered and dry as much as possible.
- *For tissue adhesives*: Keep the tissue adhesive completely dry until it spontaneously peels off in 7–10 days. Do not apply topical antibiotic ointment.
- Follow-up with your primary care physician in _____ days for suture removal.
- Return to the ED if you experience a fever (temperature > 100.4°F), or your wound becomes red around the edges, breaks open, or releases pus. Your wound may be infected and require antibiotics.
- After your sutures are removed (or your tissue adhesive falls off), the wound is not completely healed. Therefore, treat it gently. Apply sunscreen to sun-exposed wounds to prevent increased pigment uptake and darker scarring as a result of ultraviolet light. Continue this practice for the next 6–12 months.

Pitfalls in wound care

- Although wound irrigation may be time-consuming, it plays a significant role in minimizing infection. Do not underestimate the importance of high-pressure irrigation and meticulous wound exploration before wound closure.
- Regional blocks are vastly underutilized in providing anesthesia prior to wound closure. When compared to local infiltration of anesthesia, these offer the significant advantages of preserving landmarks and not increasing wound tension.
- Efforts should be taken not to shave hair adjacent to a wound. Instead, splay hair tufts away from the wound edges using a sterile petroleum-based product.
- Povidone–iodine and chlorhexidine swabbing for wound sterilization should occur only over intact skin. If applied into the wound itself, these may cause tissue damage and delay wound healing.
- Systemic antibiotics are not routinely indicated and frequently over-prescribed for simple lacerations.
- Careful discharge instructions to the patient should warn about the possibility of wound infection and scarring. They should also

provide clear instructions regarding wound care and all return visits necessary.

References

1. Bartfield JM, Gennis P, Barbera J, et al. Buffered versus plain lidocaine as a local anesthetic for simple laceration repair. *Ann Emerg Med* 1990;19:1387.

2. Chrintz H, Vibits H, Cordtz TO, et al. Need for surgical wound dressing. *Br J Surg* 1989;76:204–205.

3. Coventry DM. Alkalinisation of bupivicaine for sciatic nerve blockade. *Anaesthesia* 1989;44:467–470.

4. Cruse PJE, Foord R. A five-year prospective study of 23,649 surgical wounds. *Arch Surg* 1973;107:206–209.

5. Cummings P, Dec Beccaro MA. Antibiotics to prevent infection of simple wounds: a meta-analysis of randomized studies. *Am J Emerg Med* 1995;13:396–400.

6. Dailey RH. Fatality secondary to misuse of TAC solution. *Ann Emerg Med* 1988;17:159–160.

7. Edlich RF, Kenney JG, Morgan RF, et al. Antimicrobial treatment of minor soft tissue lacerations: a critical review. *Emerg Med Clin North Am* 1986;4:561–580.

8. Edlich RF, Rodeheaver GT, Morgan RF, et al. Principles of emergency wound management. *Ann Emerg Med* 1988;17:1284–1302.

9. Henry G, George JE. Specific high-risk clinical presentations. In: Henry G, Sullivan DJ (eds). *Emergency Medicine Risk Management: A Comprehensive Review*, 2nd ed., Dallas: American College of Emergency Physicians, 1997.

10. Hollander JE, Richman PB, Werblud M, et al. Irrigation in facial and scalp lacerations: does it alter outcome? *Ann Emerg Med* 1998;31:73–77.

11. Hollander JE, Singer AJ, Valentine, SM, et al. Risk factors for infection in patients with traumatic lacerations. *Acad Emerg Med* 2001;8:716–720.

12. Kelly AM, Cohen M, Richards D. Minimizing the pain of local infiltration anesthesia for wounds by injection into the wound edges. *J Emerg Med* 1994;12:593–595.

13. Noe JM, Keller M. Can stitches get wet? *Plast Reconstr Surg* 1988;81:82–84.

14. Seropian R, Reynolds BM. Wound infections after preoperative depilation versus razor preparation. *Am J Surg* 1971;121:251–254.

15. Ship AG, Weiss PR. Pigmentation after dermabrasion: an avoidable complication. *Plast Reconstr Surg* 1985;75:528–532.

16. Singer AJ, Hollander JE (eds). *Lacerations and Acute Wounds: An Evidence-Based Guide*, Philadelphia: F.A. Davis Company, 2003.

17. Singer AJ, Hollander JE, Quinn JV. Evaluation and management of traumatic lacerations. *New Engl J Med* 1997;337:1142–1148.

18. Steele MT, Sainsbury CR, Robinson WA, et al. Prophylactic penicillin for intraoral wounds. *Ann Emerg Med* 1989;18:847–852.

19. Stevenson TR, Thacker JG, Rodeheaver GT, et al. Cleansing the traumatic wound with high pressure syringe irrigation. *J Am Coll Emerg Phys* 1976;5:17–21.

20. Terndrup TE, Walls WC, Mariani PJ, et al. Plasma cocaine and tetracaine levels following application of topical anesthesia in children. *Ann Emerg Med* 1992; 21:162–166.

21. Whilhelmi BJ, Blackwell SJ, Miller JH, et al. Do not use epinephrine in digital blocks: myth or truth? *Plast Reconstr Surg* 2001;107:393–397.

Appendix C Laceration repair

F.C. von Trampe, MD, MPH and Wendy C. Coates, MD

Scope of the problem

Emergency physicians evaluate over 12 million patients with wounds in emergency departments (EDs) each year. They provide a wide spectrum of wound care, including laceration repair. This chapter addresses wound assessment and modalities of laceration repair.

Anatomic essentials

As the body's largest and the most exposed organ, the skin is subject to a variety of external forces encountered in daily activities. The skin's anatomic structure and layers must be considered when planning a repair (Figure C.1).

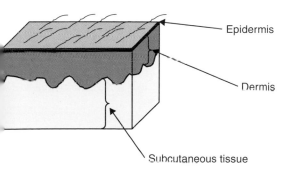

Figure C.1
Cross section of skin with associated structures.

Lacerations penetrating only the epidermis are minor and may not warrant major repair. The underlying dermis is one to several millimeters thick depending on its location on the body. The repair of this layer provides structural integrity for a healing wound. In some cases, especially wounds under tension, a separate deep dermal layer of closure may be required. The dermis rests on subcutaneous tissue which contains adipose and other loose connective tissue. The repair of subcutaneous tissue does not contribute to final wound strength. Re-approximation of subcutaneous tissue can eliminate potential spaces,

thereby decreasing risk of infection in selected wounds.

Wound healing and the final cosmetic outcome of a laceration repair depend on many factors, including dynamic and static tension. Static tension is determined by intrinsic skin factors such as collagen concentration. Anatomic determinants such as underlying bone, tendon, muscle and location over a joint space impact the dynamic tension of the repaired laceration. Natural lines of tension exist all over the body (Figure C.2). Wounds oriented along these lines are under less stress, and often lead to more favorable cosmetic outcomes. Lacerations that are oriented perpendicular to these lines are under higher tension; therefore, the method selected for closure may require more tensile support. In addition, these latter wounds may leave more noticeable scars.

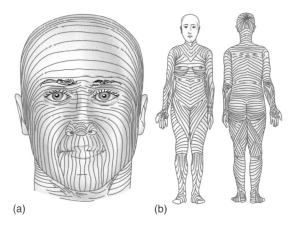

(a)   (b)

Figure C.2
The natural lines of tension are perpendicular to the longitudinal orientation of the underlying muscles. Wounds occurring along these lines generally have a more favorable cosmetic outcome.

History

When did it happen?

Time from injury to cleansing and closure affects the ability of the wound to be closed primarily

Table C.1 Wound closure in relation to time

Primary closure	Physical re-approximation of wound edges soon after injury.
Healing by secondary intention	Allowing a wound to granulate in from the edges with no wound edge re-approximation.
Delayed primary closure (healing by tertiary intention)	Physical re-approximation of wound edges after debridement, packing, and antibiotic prophylaxis for 3–4 days.

and its likelihood of becoming infected (Table C.1). Lacerations on the head and face can generally be closed up to 24 hours after injury, whereas injuries on the hands, feet, and trunk are considered to be at high risk for infection after 12 hours delay. Wounds that occurred more than 24 hours prior to evaluation may be considered for delayed primary closure (Table C.2).

What was the mechanism of injury?

Crush injuries, puncture wounds, burns, and contaminated wounds (human or animal saliva, feces, soil, organic material) warrant special consideration. Some of these wounds should not be considered for immediate repair in the ED, while others may need prophylactic antibiotics to decrease the chance of infection. In addition, circumstance and mechanism of injury (e.g., wound sustained on broken glass) may suggest the presence of foreign body contamination which would warrant imaging and exploration to detect and remove debris. Patients sometimes sense the presence of a foreign body, and the clinician can often palpate one underneath the skin surface.

A comprehensive history may uncover related conditions which can be more important than the laceration. For example, syncope leading to a minor forehead laceration obligates an extensive work-up and likely hospital admission, compared to a mechanical fall leading to a laceration in the same area. Wounds to the face should arouse suspicion for intimate partner violence (Table C.3).

Do you have any allergies to medications?

It is important to know medication allergies before giving tetanus prophylaxis, analgesics, wound anesthesia, antibiotics, or using latex products.

What is your tetanus immunization status?

An assessment of tetanus immunization status and subsequent immunization with tetanus immune globulin (TIG) or tetanus toxoid (most often as tetanus and diphtheria, Td) is important. Table C.4 provides guidelines for administering tetanus immunization according to current Centers for Disease Control and Prevention (CDC-P) guidelines.

Past medical

Information regarding pre-existing patient illnesses and comorbidities may impact disposition

Table C.2 Delayed primary closure technique

Wound characteristics	Day of evaluation (day 1)	Re-evaluation (day 3)
• Sustained >12 hours prior to evaluation (>24 hours on face) • "Dirty" wound, for example animal or human bite, infected wound	• Assess wound • Anesthetize • Detailed examination • Irrigate wound • Non-adherent gauze between wound edges • Sterile dressing • 5–7 days of antibiotics (e.g., cephalexin)	• Reevaluate wound for infection, maceration, necrotic tissue • Repair according to standards, or • Healing by secondary intention (referral may be indicated) • Finish antibiotic course

Table C.3 Medical history which may impact care of a patient with a wound

Immunocompromised

Diabetes	Extremity injuries often lead to infection because of poor circulation and immune system dysfunction. There can be relative tissue hypoxia. Have a low threshold for antibiotics and early wound reevaluation.
HIV/AIDS	Lower threshold for using appropriate antibiotics in wounds that are high risk for infection.
Steroid/immunosuppressant use	These medications cause prolonged healing time and weaken the immune system. These patients may need a prolonged period of healing prior to suture removal. These patients are also at high risk for infection.

Vascular

Bleeding disorder	Obtain impeccable hemostasis before closing these wounds. Prolonged bleeding may necessitate hematocrit assessment for anemia. Hematoma can serve as culture medium for wound infection.
Peripheral vascular disease	Poor peripheral circulation increases predisposition for infection. Carefully assess neurovascular status before repair of extremity injuries.

Other

Cardiac disease	Make sure that the wound resulted from a mechanical and not cardiac etiology.
Domestic/child/elder abuse	The key is to suspect these situations. Have a low threshold for suspicion and reporting when the story does not match the injury.

Table C.4 CDC-P guidelines for tetanus prophylaxis (Summary guide to tetanus prophylaxis in routine wound management, 1991.)

History of adsorbed tetanus toxoid (doses)	Clean, minor wounds		All other wounds[a]	
	Td[b]	TIG	Td[b]	TIG
Unknown or <3	Yes	No	Yes	Yes
≥3[c]	No[d]	No	No[e]	No

see Ref. [11] in reference section.

TIG: tetanus immune globulin.

[a] Such as, but not limited to, wounds contaminated with dirt, feces, soil, and saliva; puncture wounds; avulsions; and wounds resulting from missiles, crush, burns and frostbite.

[b] For children <7 years old; diphtheria, tetanus, and pertussis (DTP) (Td, if pertussis vaccine is contraindicated) is preferred to tetanus toxoid alone. For persons ≥7 years of age, tetanus and diphtheria (Td) is preferred to tetanus toxoid alone.

[c] If only three doses of fluid toxoid have been received, then a fourth dose of toxoid, preferably an adsorbed toxoid, should be given.

[d] Yes, if >10 years since last dose.

[e] Yes, if >5 years since last dose (more frequent boosters are not needed and can accentuate side effects).

decisions. This information may help guide decisions whether to use prophylactic antibiotics, and may predict which patients are prone to impaired wound healing (Table C.3).

Physical examination

The physical examination should take place in a well-lit area with the patient as comfortable as possible. Assess the wound in relation to the history provided by the patient to identify other possible injuries (e.g., retained foreign bodies). When focusing on the wound itself, there are several important principles to help guide your examination.

Description of the wound

Describe the anatomic location, length, and depth of the wound. The health of the wound margins and degree of tension should be noted. The different types of wounds should be considered in the description (Table C.5).

Table C.5 Types of wounds and characteristics

Type of wound	Characteristics	Treatment considerations
Abrasions	Superficial	Clean and dress.
Avulsions	Tissue is missing	Clean, complex repair, or referral.
Burns	1st, 2nd, or 3rd degree	Local wound care and possible resuscitation.
Crush injuries	Caused by blunt forces, may have significant tissue edema. Wound infection occurs at a lower bacterial load.	Address underlying trauma life support considerations, then attend to standard wound care techniques.
Lacerations	Sharply demarcated borders. Usually have good healing.	Follow standard wound care techniques.
Puncture wounds	May be small but indeterminate depth.	Evaluate for presence of foreign body and underlying injury. Surface cleaning and dressing.

Distal neurologic integrity

Examine for motor *and* sensory deficits prior to anesthetizing the wound. The remainder of the examination should be performed after the wound has been anesthetized. Nerves can be partially lacerated. Sensory information is carried peripherally in nerve bundles; loss of sensation may be the only manifestation of a partial nerve injury.

Distal vascular integrity

Assess and document signs of adequate or inadequate perfusion using a combination of pulses, capillary refill, and skin color. Vascular bruits may suggest pseudoaneurysms, vascular lacerations, or fistulas. Ankle brachial indices (ABIs) can be measured when there is concern for an arterial injury. Signs of poor perfusion should be explained and addressed before laceration repair. Determine and document neurovascular status following repair to ensure iatrogenic injuries did not occur during the repair.

Tendon integrity

Lacerated tendons are at risk for rupture. Many specialists advise tendon repair if there is greater than 50% disruption. Extensor tendons of the hand and foot can often be repaired by emergency physicians. Flexor tendons should be repaired by a trained specialist in the operating room. The tendon must be examined throughout its entire range of motion over the involved joint. Tendon lacerations in the position of injury may not be visible in the position of examination.

Joint space involvement

Laceration extension into a joint space portends morbidity for the patient and may require operative washout of the affected joint. Maintain a high suspicion for joint capsule disruption with wounds located over joints, mechanisms suggesting deep penetration, debris visualized on X-ray over a joint space, or the presence of a radio-opaque foreign body in the joint space itself (seen on two views of plain film radiography). These wounds may need to be assessed by a specialist.

Bone involvement

Obtain plain film radiography in any laceration with exposed bone to assess for the presence of fracture or retained foreign bodies. Cortical disruption of bone with proximity to a laceration is classified and treated as an open fracture. These wounds usually require antibiotics to prevent osteomyelitis.

Foreign bodies and wound contamination

Discovery of contamination in a wound obligates a thorough cleansing, careful assessment of whether or not to close the wound primarily (Table C.1), and careful exploration for other foreign bodies in the wound. Imaging modalities used to detect foreign bodies include: plain X-ray films, xerography, ultrasound (US), computed tomography (CT), and magnetic resonance imaging (MRI). MRI should not be chosen if a metallic foreign body is suspected.

Devitalized tissue

Crush, blast, or high speed missile injuries impart large forces to tissues and can cause necrosis of dermal and subcutaneous structures. Necrotic tissue can serve as a nidus for infection and impede normal tissue healing. Devitalized tissue should be debrided conservatively to preserve as much viable tissue as possible. This places the healing wound under less tension, and affords a cosmetic surgeon the most flexibility if subsequent wound revision is necessary.

Referral and consultation guidelines

When the history and physical examination is complete, the provider should determine if she or he possesses the skill necessary to proceed with the repair. Adequate wound preparation should take place prior to the referral, and a clean, dry dressing should be applied. Wound characteristics that should be considered for consultation and referral are noted in Table C.6.

Table C.6 Wounds appropriate for consultation/referral

- Primary provider is unable to perform optimal repair
  - Skill level does not match complexity of wound
  - Practice setting is too busy to allow adequate time for repair
- Underlying injury
  - Tendon
  - Nerve
  - Vascular
- Joint involvement or underlying fracture
- Eyelid: tarsal plate or lacrimal duct involvement
- Patient requests specialist
- Operative repair necessary
  - Skin grafting
  - Flap creation or rotation

Wound preparation

For details see Appendix B.

Diagnostic testing

Patients with lacerations rarely require an extensive diagnostic work-up. Radiologic imaging may be indicated for suspicion of a foreign body, joint space involvement, osteomyelitis, fracture, or underlying injury (e.g., CT of the brain). In patients presenting with a laceration as a minor part of their overall condition (e.g., a multiple trauma victim or patient with syncope), the work-up should focus on the primary event in addition to repairing the laceration.

General treatment principles

Methods of wound closure

There are multiple methods available for repair once the wound has been adequately assessed and the decision to repair has been made. The most commonly used method is reapproximation by suturing.

Suturing

Basic suturing supplies consist of needle drivers, tissue forceps (or skin hook), scissors, sterile drapes, sterile gloves, suture materials (Table C.7), and sterile gauze.

Numerous methods of suturing can be used to repair a laceration. Some approaches have specific advantages which may benefit certain laceration types. To begin the suturing process, the needle is attached to the needle driver which is placed in the palm of the dominant hand. The index finger is extended along the arms of the closed needle driver. The palm may be used for opening and closing the needle driver's locking mechanism (Figure C.3). In this position, the needle can be rotated along an imaginary axis, and optimal operator ergonomics are possible. An alternate method is to place the tips of the thumb and ring digits into the rings of the handle. The needle should always enter and exit at 90° to the skin surface for minimal tissue damage. Edge eversion is needed for vertical tissue alignment along dermal layers to optimize wound cosmesis.

Simple interrupted

The simple interrupted is the most frequently used stitch in wound approximation (Figure C.4). With

Table C.7 Types of sutures and their characteristics

Type	Sub-type	Strength	Reactivity	Infection risk	Comment
Absorbable	Chromic gut	++	+++	+	Often used for intraoral repairs
	Monofilament	++++	+	+	Very workable, also good for deep sutures
	Braided co-polymer	++++	+	+++	Useful for deep sutures requiring strength and absorbability
Non-absorbable	Silk	+	++++	++	Very reactive substance with few applications in ED
	Monofilament	+++	+	+	Use for most external closures

Suture size	Anatomic location
6–0	Face
5–0	Hands
4–0	Most extremity, scalp, and trunk wounds
3–0	Large wounds in non-cosmetic areas (not used in routine wound repair)
2–0 and larger	Emergent, life-saving closures (e.g., post-thoracotomy, scalping injury)
Staples	Scalp, non-cosmetic areas

Needle type	Characteristics and applications
Conventional cutting	Sharp point; useful for skin
Reverse cutting	Extra sharp point; minimal tissue trauma, useful for skin, tendons
Taper (round edged)	Pierces tissue; useful in peritoneum, viscera, myocardium
3/8 circle shape	Most common for routine repairs
Half-circle shape	Confined spaces (oral, nasal cavity, fascia)

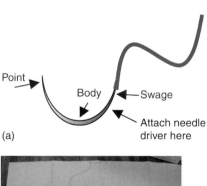

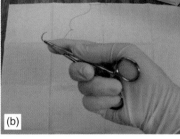

Figure C.3
(a) The needle is grasped at the proximal one-third of the body. (b) The needle driver rests in the palm of the hand.

the needle at a 90° angle to the skin surface, the dermis is penetrated. The needle is then driven through the opposing side of the laceration with extreme care to meticulously approximate each level of tissue. To secure the stitch, an instrument tie is generally done using a surgeon's knot (a flat double throw) followed by single throws tied sequentially in opposite directions (Figure C.5).

Five knots are needed to secure nylon sutures while three throws are generally adequate for braided, soft sutures. Wound edges should be gently approximated (not strangulated). When the knot is finished, it should be gently retracted to one side of the wound. This is to keep the knot from serving as a nidus of contamination, or from impinging on the healing wound tissue, making an unsightly divot in the final scar (Figure C.6). Suture placement should be symmetric. Cosmetically important areas may require a smaller suture interval for better appearance. There should be a consistent relationship between needle entry point and suture interval.

Horizontal mattress

The horizontal mattress suture is used to close a wound under mild to moderate tension. It is an especially useful alternative to two-layer closure in a patient who is at high risk for developing a wound infection. Its proper placement disperses tensile forces over a larger area, providing better perfusion of healing wound edges (Figure C.8).

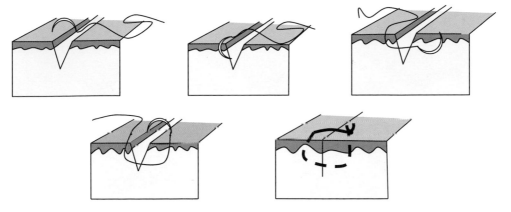

Figure C.4
Sequence illustrating the placement of a simple interrupted suture.

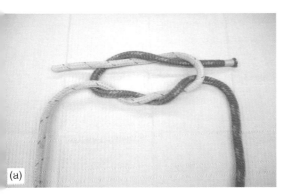

(a)

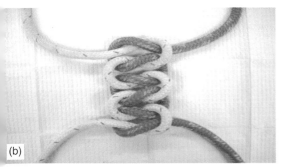

(b)

Figure C.5
(a) Initial knot used to secure a suture. Notice that the initial knot has two throws on the bottom and a single throw on top. This facilitates keeping tension in the suture in order to keep the wound margins together. (b) Picture illustrating sequential knots with throws in opposite directions.

Deep (intradermal) sutures

In a laceration of substantial depth and/or tension, the deeper tissues should be approximated. This helps relieve tension along the upper wound margins and improves healing and cosmesis.

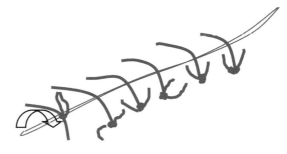

Figure C.6
Placing all suture knots off the wound and on one side improves cosmesis and facilitates suture removal.

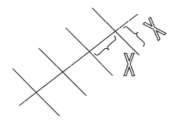

Figure C.7
The relationship of distance between sutures and the wound edges.

Placing absorbable stitches in the deeper structures requires "burying the knot" by entering the wound margin deeply on one side and reversing needle entry on the opposite side. Tying the knot as shown in Figure C.9 places the knot at the bottom of the laceration and prevents it from disrupting the surface appearance by "spitting" through the wound site. A superficial layer of closure can then be applied to re-approximate the epidermis. This can be done with simple interrupted sutures,

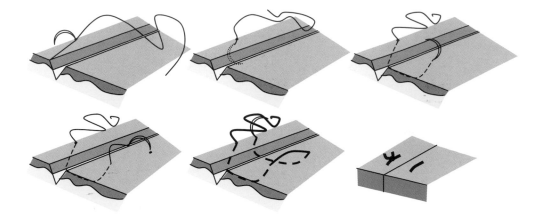

Figure C.8
Horizontal mattress sutures alleviate some of the "strangulation" effect of placing simple interrupted sutures along the margin of a wound under high tension.

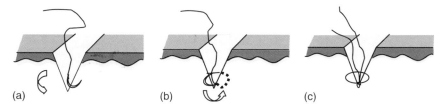

(a)   (b)   (c)

Figure C.9
Placing intradermal sutures increases the risk of infection in a wound. However, deep sutures can remove "potential" spaces where fluid collection may distort tissue anatomy and/or predispose to infection. In addition, deep sutures facilitate closure of wounds which are widely open at the surface. This sequence demonstrates burying the knot.

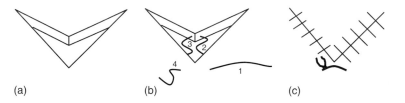

(a)   (b)   (c)

Figure C.10
Corner sutures with a half-buried mattress stitch may avoid necrosis of the distal tip of the flap.

wound approximation strips, or tissue adhesives. Placing a deep layer of absorbable sutures can increase the wound infection rate, especially in patients with dirty wounds (human or animal bites) or underlying medical conditions such as diabetes mellitus or poor circulation.

Corner stitch

"V"-shaped lacerations result in a small apical flap of tissue which can be friable and poorly perfused. Placing stitches directly through this tissue may cause necrosis and a poor cosmetic outcome. The half-buried mattress suture can help preserve distal perfusion and spreads tension along the distal flap. Care must be taken to assure that the suture is at the same tissue depth in each side of the laceration (Figure C.10).

Staples

Some wounds have less cosmetic importance, and require rapid closure. As a definitive or temporizing measure, stapling a laceration is an

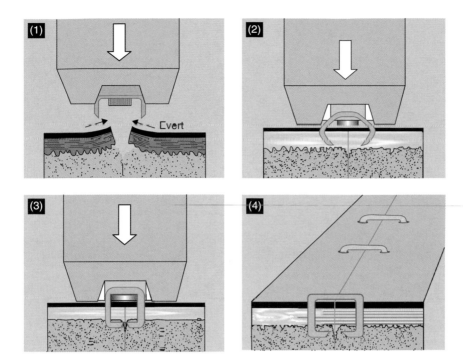

Figure C.11
A sequence illustrating wound stapling.

effective means for closing such wounds. Wounds appropriate for staples are linear, without ragged edges, and under minimal tension (edges need to align well without the use of tissue forceps when working alone). Although staples are most often used for scalp lacerations in the ED, it is imperative to remember that most men will have some balding, and a scar which was initially covered by hair may become a cosmetic problem with a receding hairline. To place staples, the stapling device is placed at the skin surface, and the staple is brought forward with a smooth motion using the trigger mechanism (Figure C.11). It is important not to indent the skin surface as this may cause improper vertical alignment of wound edges. Removal of staples in a timely manner will improve cosmetic outcome since staples are larger in diameter than most sutures. Commercial staple removers should be used to properly (and painlessly) remove staples. After staple removal, many physicians place tissue adhesive strips to augment the tensile strength of the closure for an additional time period.

Tissue adhesives

Tissue adhesives are recent additions to the armamentarium for laceration repair. Lacerations appropriate for tissue adhesives are clean, linear, and under little or no tension. Wounds are assessed and prepared in the same way as any other wound prior to closure (Appendix B). Impeccable hemostasis and dry overlying skin are required for successful closure. Wound edges are held together with finger tips or a commercially-available device as the liquid adhesive is stroked across the tissue defect, taking care to avoid getting adhesive within the wound or on the application device. Avoid use around the eyes to prevent corneal or lid adhesion. Tissue adhesives are not indicated for use on mucous membranes. There is no need for a wound dressing. The wound should be kept dry; ointment (including antibacterial) should not be used since it may dissolve the adhesive and cause the wound to prematurely dehisce. The use of these ointments can be helpful in removing unintended applications of tissue adhesive. In particular, ophthalmic ointments can aid in removing tissue adhesive from the eyes. Routine evaluation and treatment for corneal abrasions should follow if this occurs.

Tissue adhesives are well tolerated by pediatric patients. They provide a painless alternative to suturing. Some patients experience a warm sensation as the bonding process occurs.

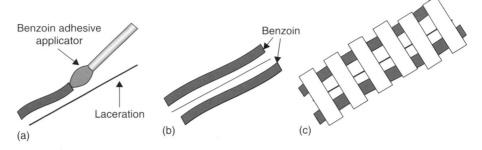

Figure C.12
(a) The application of wound adhesive strips. (b) Benzoin is applied as an adjunct for the tape strips. (c) Tape strips placed in a symmetric fashion to close a wound.

Choosing a topical anesthetic with vasoconstrictive properties is consistent with the overall reduction of pain in this repair modality.

Wound taping (butterfly closure)

The wound is assessed and prepared in the usual manner. Wounds appropriate for this technique are linear or curvilinear, clean, and under minimal tension. Pediatric patients tend to pick, soak, or pull at these tape, which may cause a wound to prematurely dehisce. Taping can be used in conjunction with a layer of deep sutures in order to keep the overlying skin closely approximated. To place the tape, wound edges are cleaned and tincture of benzoin adhesive is applied to both sides of the wound margin (taking care not to place inside wound). After several seconds of air drying, adhesive strips are placed at appropriate intervals to approximate the skin edges. One part of a laceration may require more strips than another part (Figure C.12). Wound adhesive strips generally fall of within a week of application. It is advisable to prevent these wounds and tapes from getting wet.

Wound care and patient disposition

When a laceration repair is complete, the patient's overall medical condition should be considered when planning disposition. Wound checks, use of antibiotics or analgesics, and tetanus or rabies prophylaxis are tailored to the individual patient. Wound care instructions and suture removal guidelines should be given to the patient (and family member or friend, if appropriate), both

Table C.8 Suture removal guidelines

Anatomic location	Days (average)
Face	3–5
Trunk	7–10
Arm (not joint)	7–10
Leg	10–14
Joint (splint)	14
Scalp	10–14

verbally and in writing (Tables B.3, C.8). The duration of suture placement and wound tension are proportional to increased scarring. However, sutures must remain long enough to allow the healing process to begin. Cosmetically important areas, such as the face, should have sutures in place for a shorter amount of time to reduce scarring. Fortunately, these wounds usually heal rapidly. Scars that are exposed to sunlight should have sunscreen applied for 6 months after injury. Routine use of antibiotics is not necessary for most wounds. Use of antibiotics for contaminated lacerations, such as human or animal bites, or in wounds selected for delayed primary closure is recommended.

Pearls, pitfalls, and myths

- Routine use of antibiotics is not necessary when adequate wound preparation occurs. Antibiotics are indicated in bite wounds and in wounds selected for delayed primary closure. They are often used in high-risk wounds in patients at increased risk of infection.

- Wound edges should be approximated meticulously, with gentle wound edge eversion.
- Devitalized tissue should be debrided conservatively.
- Foreign bodies should be considered prior to closure.
- Tissue adhesives are excellent alternatives for repairing clean wounds that are not under tension.
- Careful attention to proper technique makes a good cosmetic outcome more likely. The dermis provides the strength necessary for healing.

References

1. Harwood-Nuss A (ed.). *The Clinical Practice of Emergency Medicine*, 3rd ed., Philadelphia, PA: Lippincott Williams & Wilkins, 2001.
2. Hollander JE, Singer AJ. Laceration management. *Ann Emerg Med* 1999;34:356–367.
3. Markovchik V. Suture materials and mechanical aftercare. *Emerg Med Clin North Am* 1992;10:673–688.
4. Marx JA (ed.). *Rosen's Emergency Medicine: Concepts and Clinical Practice*, 5th ed., St. Louis, MO: Mosby, 2002.
5. Quinn JV, Wells GA. Tissue adhesive vs. suture wound repair at one year: randomized clinical trial correlating early, three month, and one year cosmetic outcome. *Ann Emerg Med* 1998;32:645–649
6. Ritchie AJ, Rocke LG. Staples versus sutures in the closure of scalp wounds: a prospective double blind, randomized trial. *Injury* 1989;20:217–218.
7. Rockwell BW, Butler PN. Extensor tendon: anatomy, injury, and reconstruction. *Plast Reconst Surg* 2000;106(7):1592–1603.
8. Simon HK, Zempsky WT. Lacerations against Langer's lines: to glue or suture? *J Emerg Med* 1998;16:185–189.
9. Singer AJ, Hollander JE (eds). *Lacerations and Acute Wounds an Evidence-Based Guide.* F.A. Davis Company, 2003.
10. Tintinalli JE (ed.). *Emergency Medicine: A Comprehensive Study Guide*, 5th ed., New York, NY: McGraw Hill, 2000.
11. Trott AT. *Wounds and Lacerations*, 2nd ed., St. Louis, MO: Mosby, 1997.

Appendix D   Procedural sedation and analgesia

Eustacia (Jo) Su, MD and Robert L. Cloutier, MD

Scope of the problem

Procedural sedation and analgesia (PSA) represents one of the great advances in emergency medicine's maturation as a specialty. It has become a routine part of emergency medical practice, encompassing many fundamental clinical skills including airway assessment and management and critical resuscitation skills. PSA is very safe in the hands of a properly-trained practitioner in the correct setting with appropriate monitoring and resuscitation equipment.

Older terminology attempted to describe the state of sedation and analgesia in static terms, such as *conscious sedation*. This definition required that patients given agents providing both sedation and analgesia remained conscious, and were still able to reflexively protect their airways. The terminology has evolved to reflect the continuum upon which sedation and analgesia occur, ranging from anxiolysis to analgesia and light sedation through deep sedation and general anesthesia. All of these levels may be applied to the emergency department (ED) setting with the exception of general anesthesia; this implies a complete loss of consciousness and protective airway reflexes.

Certain ED procedures and studies commonly require PSA (Table D.1).

Table D.1 Indications for procedural sedation and analgesia

- Incision and drainage of large abscesses
- Wound debridement
- Reduction of fractures, dislocations and prolapsed viscera (hernias)
- Tube thoracostomy
- Repair of complicated lacerations, especially in children
- Diagnostic studies (CT or MRI)
- Lumbar puncture in selected cases
- Cardioversion
- Removal of embedded foreign bodies
- Painful or anxiety-inducing procedures (e.g., pelvic examination in a young rape victim)

General treatment principles

The major considerations in selecting drugs for PSA include sedation, amnesia, analgesia and muscle relaxation. The first step is to determine the desired depth of sedation. A toddler who has sustained a minor head injury and is undergoing a computed tomography (CT) of the head requires much less sedation and essentially no analgesia when compared to a child who is having a burn debrided or a long bone fracture reduced.

Agents should be selected that provide adequate analgesia. Most sedatives provide little, if any, analgesia. While many analgesics provide some sedation, the level of sedation only becomes adequate when the patient develops significant respiratory depression from the amount of analgesic given. Duration of the procedure also influences the choice of drug and the route of delivery.

Individuals respond differently to drugs, even when the dose is calculated according to their weight. Careful titration produces the optimal response. This is best done using intravenous (IV) administration, since repeated oral doses are unpredictable and usually slow to onset, and repeated intramuscular (IM) injections are not acceptable.

Patient assessment and selection

If a patient needs a procedure that requires sedation and/or analgesia, first determine whether the patient is able to tolerate PSA (Table D.2). Candidates for procedural sedation in the ED *must* fall into either ASA class I or II. Patients with higher classifications are better served in a more controlled environment, such as the operating room (OR) or intensive care unit (ICU).

Next, select a target level of sedation and the duration required. Determine the drug and dosage range that will most likely produce the desired

Table D.2 American Society of Anesthesiologists' classifications for risk stratification

Class	Patient status
I	Normally healthy patient. The pathologic process for which the procedure is to be performed is localized and not a systemic disturbance.
II	Mild systemic disease under control (e.g., asthma).
III	Severe systemic disease from any cause.
IV	Severe systemic disease that is a constant life-threat, not always correctable by the operative procedure.
V	Moribund patient who is not expected to survive without the operation.

Table D.3 Nulla per os (NPO) status for children

Children <6 months old
- 2 hours fast for clear liquids
- 4 hours fast for milk, solids

Children 6 months–3 years
- 3 hours fast for clear liquids
- 6 hours fast for milk, solids

Children >3 years old
- 3 hours fast for clear liquids
- 6–8 hours fast for milk, solids

Adults
- 2 hours fast for clear liquids
- 6 hours fast for milk, solids

results and will adequately control the patient's pain for the duration of the procedure.

The time since the patient's last oral intake is the next risk factor to be considered. Loss of the airway protective reflexes increases the risk of aspiration of stomach contents. Gastric emptying time is variable, even among patients of similar ages. The American Academy of Pediatrics (AAP), American College of Emergency Physicians (ACEP), and the American Society of Anesthesiologists (ASA) all have separate guidelines for nulla per os (NPO) times, ranging from 4 to 6 hours. Some distinctions are made between NPO times depending on whether the food consumed was solid, full liquid or clear liquid, with solid food consumption pushing NPO times toward the 6-hour mark. These distinctions may vary between institutions. It is important to remember, however, that preservation of life or limb takes precedence over NPO status. NPO status for young children and toddlers is slightly more complex (Table D.3).

A pre-sedation history and physical examination, beyond a general medical screening examination, should focus on issues pertaining directly to the sedation procedure. The history should elicit factors that might increase the direct risks of medications and symptoms that suggest underlying upper respiratory tract illness or abnormality (i.e., asthma exacerbation or viral syndrome). Patients must also be asked about allergies, past experiences with sedation or general anesthesia, and time of last food or liquid intake.

The physical examination should focus on baseline vital signs, the oral cavity and the cardiorespiratory system, in particular, noting any potential impediments to endotracheal intubation and ventilation (see Chapter 2). Underlying reactive airway disease or upper respiratory tract infection should be ruled out with a careful examination of the pulmonary system. If the patient has an upper respiratory tract infection, a higher risk of developing laryngospasm occurs with some PSA agents. Evaluate the heart for the presence of murmurs or dysrhythmias.

Drug selection

Consider the following variables when choosing the PSA agents for a particular patient and procedure: patient comfort, how still the patient has to remain, degree of procedural invasiveness, degree of muscle relaxation, amount of pain, and duration of procedure. The ideal drug for PSA would have predictable dosing, instantaneous onset, easily adjustable duration of action, short recovery time, and both amnestic and analgesic properties. It would also have minimal hemodynamic effects, no respiratory depression, and would preserve protective airway reflexes (Table D.4).

The combination of a benzodiazepine (midazolam or valium) and a narcotic (morphine or fentanyl) has been, and continues to be, a mainstay of procedural sedation. The combination of these agents has been applied widely across many procedures performed in emergency medical practice. Important side effects include respiratory depression and hypotension. The recovery time for the combination of midazolam and fentanyl is generally longer than that for ketamine, propofol or etomidate. Table D.5 provides a list of reversal agents should they be needed.

Table D.4 Procedural sedation and analgesia medications

Medication	Recommended dosages	Route	Onset	Duration	Additional instructions/ mode of action	Precautions/contraindications
Etomidate	0.1–0.3 mg/kg	IV over period of 30 sec	60 sec	10 min	Considered a general anesthetic. Cardiac, respiratory and blood pressure monitoring required. Question of adrenal suppression (probably clinically insignificant). Not approved for children <12 years of age. However, much evidence supports its safe use in children <12.	May cause myoclonic jerks and pain at injection site. Avoid if seizure disorder, nausea, vomiting.
Fentanyl	1–3 mcg/kg	IV	1–2 min	Peak 10 min duration	Potent rapidly-acting analgesic. Hemodynamically stable but may cause respiratory depression and apnea. Dose can be titrated. Should not exceed a maximum dose of 5 mcg/kg. Synergistic action with concomitant benzodiazepine administration.	Push and flush slowly; monitor closely for respiratory depression, bradycardia, apnea. *Rigid chest syndrome* associated with large doses administered rapidly. Appears to be an idiosyncratic reaction. May not be reversible with naloxone.
	1–2 mcg/kg	IM	7–15 min	30–45 min		
Ketamine	1–2 mg/kg	IV – repeat 1 mg/kg as needed every 20 min	1–3 min	10–20 min	Dissociative agent provides analgesia, anxiolysis and amnesia. Dissociation is a binary process (patients either are or are not dissociated) and not a dose-dependent phenomenon (patients are not more dissociated with increasing doses). Use with benzodiazepine potentially reduces emergence reactions. May be combined with glycopyrrolate at 0.01 (mg/kg) or atropine at 0.01 (mg/kg) to decrease secretions. Combine with anti-sialagogue in single syringe for single IM injection. Positive cardiac inotrope.	Hallucinatory emergence reactions common in adults but uncommon in children. Potential for laryngospasm (1 : 250) so avoid in patients with active pulmonary or upper respiratory tract infection. Also avoid intraoral procedures; do not use in patients with increased intraocular or intracranial pressure.
	2–5 mg/kg	IM	2–3 min	30–60 min		
Methohexital (Brevital)	1 mg/kg	IV	1 min	10 min	Ultra-short barbiturate. Provides significant muscle relaxation. May cause hemodynamic instability, apnea.	Discontinue immediately if extravasation occurs to minimize tissue necrosis. If given intra-arterially, thrombosis and gangrene possible. Contraindicated in severe hepatic dysfunction or porphyria.
	25 mg/kg	PR	2–5 min	45 min		

(continued)

Procedural sedation and analgesia

Table D.4 Procedural sedation and analgesia medications (*cont*)

Medication	Recommended dosages	Route	Onset	Duration	Additional instructions/ mode of action	Precautions/contraindications
Midazolam (Versed)	0.05–0.1 mg/kg 0.1 mg/kg *Suggested pediatrics combination: 0.1 mg/kg IV when used with 1–2 mcg/kg IV fentanyl*	IV IM	1–3 min 2–5 min	1 hour 1–2 hours	Potent amnestic and muscle relaxant. No analgesic property. May repeat IV dose 0.1 mg/kg by giving increments of 0.05 mg/kg until adequately sedated. Must be given slowly over 30 seconds. With IM route use 5 mg/ml concentration to reduce volume.	Can cause respiratory depression if given rapidly or in addition to barbiturate therapy. Paradoxical hyperactivity possible. Will obtain faster onset with higher doses. PO route useful for anxiolysis. PR and intranasal routes advocated by some but not these authors.
Morphine sulfate	0.1 mg/kg	IV/IM	3 min peak effect	15–30 min	Opioid narcotic. Successful use dependent on appropriate dosing. Titration above 0.1 mg/kg dose may be required. Extremely painful injuries (i.e., femur fractures) are examples of severe injuries requiring judicious titration to achieve appropriate levels of pain relief. Dosing in infants 0.05 mg/kg due to decreased hepatic clearance.	Respiratory depression, apnea, histamine release, hypotension, prolonged sedation, bradycardia.
Nitrous oxide	Colorless gas mixed 50% with oxygen	Demand valve mask	3–5 min	3–5 min on withdrawal	Provides mild analgesia, anxiolysis and detached attitude toward pain and surroundings. Patient must be old enough to cooperate with face mask (approx. 5 years). Must washout with 100% oxygen for 5 min post-procedure.	Adverse effects include nausea, vomiting, disorientation, agitation and expansion of air-filled cavities.
Pentobarbital (Nembutal)	0.5–2 mg/kg 2–6 mg/kg	IV IM	30–60 sec 10–15 min	15+ min	Barbiturate with no analgesic properties. Titrate dosage based on the child's response; not to exceed a maximum dose of 6 mg/kg *or* 150 mg total dose.	Monitor carefully for respiratory depression. Contraindicated in patients suffering from acute intermittent porphyria, liver failure.
Propofol (Diprivan)	1–2 mg/kg IV Maintain infusion rate 67–200 mcg/kg/min	IV	5–7 sec	8–11 min per bolus dose or upon withdrawal of infusion.	Potent non-benzodiazepine non-barbiturate sedative hypnotic with no analgesic properties. Ideal for short painful procedures when used with analgesic adjunct.	Induces very deep levels of sedation and may cause respiratory depression, apnea and rarely hypotension. Pain frequently noted on injection, may be attenuated by adding lidocaine 1.0 mg/kg (maximum 20 mg) to initial bolus syringe.

IV: intravenous; IM: intramuscular; PO: per os; PR: per rectum.

Table D.5 Reversal agents

Medication	Recommended dosages	Route	Onset	Duration	Additional instructions/ mode of action	Precautions/ contraindications
Flumazenil (Mazicon)	*Adult:* 0.2 mg May repeat 60 sec × 3 Maximum dose 1 mg	IV	1–2 min	20 min	Used for the reversal of benzodiazepine-induced sedation. Administer slowly to avoid the adverse consequences of abrupt awakening, such as dysphoria and agitation. Repeat doses of flumazenil may be given at 20 minute intervals as needed to reverse sedation. Maximum dose of 1 mg at any one time; not >3 mg in 1 hour. A 1-mg dose sustains antagonism for 48 min.	Seizures may occur as reversal of sedative effects performed. Do not administer if myoclonic jerking noted. Duration of action shorter than midazolam and other benzodiazepines. Re-sedation may occur following initial reversal; monitoring must be performed for an appropriate period after initial reversal. Contraindicated in status epilepticus, increased intracranial pressure, tricyclic antidepressant overdose and chronic benzodiazepine use (>2 weeks).
	Pediatric: 0.01 mg/kg	IV				
Naloxone (Narcan)	*Adult:* 5–10 mcg/kg *Titrate to desired effect.* (Standard historical dose for OD 0.4–2 mg)	IV/ET/IM	1–2 min	Dependent upon the dose and route of administration; 30–60 min typical.	A narcotic antagonist preventing or reversing the effects of opioids, including respiratory depression, sedation and hypotension. *Titration preferred to rapid bolus.* Maximum dose of 10 mg. Dose conservatively to avoid acute withdrawal and agitation.	The patient responding satisfactorily to naloxone should be kept under continuous surveillance; repeated doses may be required since the duration of action of some narcotics may exceed that of naloxone. May use IV drip. Excessive use beyond the recommended dosage may actually potentiate respiratory depression in an already depressed patient.
	Pediatric: 5–10 mcg/kg *Titrate to desired effect.* Common starting dose 0.2 mg	IV/ET/IM				

ET: endotracheal; IM: intramuscular; IV: intravenous.

Importance of monitoring

Most EDs have written policies on sedation which outline staffing requirements, monitoring guidelines, approved medications, post-procedure observation, and discharge criteria. These should be reviewed carefully before attempting PSA. Obtain informed consent and discuss risks and benefits of PSA with every patient before proceeding.

Almost all of the agents used for PSA diminish respiratory drive. All of them produce varying degrees of loss of airway protective reflexes. Any combination of sedative and analgesic drugs will result in at least additive, if not synergistic, depression of both respiratory drive and airway protective reflexes.

Prepare for apnea and hemodynamic collapse ahead of time (Table D.6). Move the crash cart to the bedside in preparation for possible respiratory or cardiac arrest. Place the patient on cardiac and pulse oximetry monitors. Place towels or pillows nearby to help keep the patient's airway open during the procedure. Assign a provider to watch the patient, especially the respiratory frequency and depth. End-tidal capnography, if available, is a very useful adjunct, but is not a substitute for human vigilance. Closely monitor all vitals signs at least every 5 minutes during the sedation period, more frequently if mandated by hospital policy or the procedure.

Table D.6 Advance preparation for PSA

Pre-procedure checklist
- High-flow oxygen*
- Suction with large-bore catheter and appropriately-sized tip for patient*
- Vascular access equipment*
- Airway equipment*
- Monitoring
  - Capnography, if available
  - Pulse oximetry*
  - Cardiac and blood pressure monitors*
- Crash cart*
- Reversal agents (specific for procedural sedation and analgesia agents used)*
- Adequate staff for monitoring and documentation*
- Informed consent*

* Suggested minimum equipment.

Ensure that oxygen is immediately available, both by nasal cannula and bag-valve-mask. Most practitioners prefer to administer oxygen to the patient before starting and throughout PSA, to minimize the likelihood and duration of hypoxia.

Pre-oxygenation may delay the recognition of hypoventilation when pulse oximetry is used as the mainstay of monitoring. It is even more important to closely watch the patient's respirations if oxygen is already being administered.

Assemble the intubation equipment so that it is close at hand and ready for use. Turn on the suction and attach the appropriate tip to the tubing. Ensure that the suction apparatus is working properly prior to giving sedative or analgesic medications. Select the appropriate endotracheal tube sizes, stylet and laryngoscope blades, making sure that the handle and blades are functional. It is not necessary to open all the packaging, but you should be ready to do so quickly if the need arises.

If an IV is not already in place, assemble the necessary equipment so that one can be started quickly. If you are using drugs with known antidotes, make sure that these medications are at the bedside, ready to be drawn up. Post the calculated doses and volumes at the bedside, making sure that the team can easily see this information.

After completing all the preparations outlined above, document the pre-sedation history and physical examination, the PARQ (procedure, alternatives, risks and questions) discussion, and patient consent. Assemble the team, assigning one person to closely watch the patient's chest movement, skin color and level of sedation throughout the duration of the procedure and until the patient has fully recovered.

Recovery and discharge

The greatest risk of apnea or hypoxia is usually after the painful procedure is over but before the drugs have worn off. Do not leave a drowsy patient unattended. It is critical that a skilled health care provider continues to closely monitor the patient until adequate recovery from PSA has occurred (i.e., the patient is breathing normally, protecting his or her airway, and has returned to baseline cognitive and motor function). If an antidote (i.e., reversal agent) was used, continue to closely monitor the patient for at least another hour beyond the time the antidote was expected to wear off. This will ensure prompt identification of any potential recurrence of respiratory depression or sedation from the PSA agents.

Discuss discharge criteria with the patient and family/friends who will drive the patient home. Do not allow the patient to drive. Instruct the patient that subtle cognitive deficits and drowsiness may persist hours after PSA, and therefore s/he should neither drive nor operate heavy machinery for at least 24 hours after PSA. Patients and family or friends should fully understand instructions regarding the signs and symptoms which mandate immediate return to the ED.

Patients are considered safe for discharge when they are able to fulfill specific discharge criteria (Table D.7).

Table D.7 Criteria for safe discharge of patients after procedural sedation and analgesia

- No evidence of respiratory distress, hypoxia or hypoventilation
- No or minimal nausea, vomiting or dizziness
- Able to take fluids and medications by mouth
- Responsible person to accompany patient and monitor him/her at home: must be able to understand discharge instructions and criteria prompting emergent return to ED
- Vital signs stable for at least 30 minutes
- Baseline mental status achieved (alert, oriented, able to retain information or age-appropriate behavior)
- Return to pre-procedural sedation and analgesia or baseline motor function (age-appropriate behavior)

All patients must have a full understanding of late side effects that may occur as a result of their sedation. Vomiting may occur after discharge following the use of ketamine or narcotic analgesics. In rare cases, post-sedation hallucinations may occur with ketamine for a period of several weeks.

Special patients

Infants and toddlers have the most variable response to medications. Medications should be dosed according to a current and accurately measured weight whenever possible. Before starting PSA, select the appropriately-sized airway equipment and have it within easy reach at the bedside.

Patients on psychotropic medications may react unpredictably to some analgesics and sedatives, particularly ketamine.

The elderly often have diminished cardiorespiratory reserve and are often taking several medications which might interact with PSA agents. These patients require very careful, slow titration of medications and hypervigilance in monitoring their oxygenation and ventilation status.

IV drug users usually have a high tolerance to opiate analgesia, but not necessarily to the respiratory depression induced by the opiates. These patients require extra precaution.

The potentially hypovolemic patient should be optimally fluid resuscitated prior to giving sedative–analgesics in order to prevent hemodynamic compromise or even cardiovascular collapse.

Pearls, pitfalls, and myths

- Prior planning and careful preparation for the worst possible scenarios are the hallmarks of safe PSA. Begin with careful patient selection, proper monitoring procedures, availability of advanced airway management equipment, and close post-procedure and recovery observation.
- Pulse oximetry and capnography are essential for adequate monitoring but do not replace human vigilance. Assign a care provider to constantly monitor the patient's chest movement, color and mental status.
- Supplemental oxygen in a sedated, hypoventilating patient may improve oxygenation but will not improve ventilatory status. Manual stimulation and airway repositioning should be the first measures used to address decreasing oxygen saturation or increasing carbon dioxide levels.

References

1. American Academy of Pediatrics, Committee on Drugs. Guidelines for monitoring and management of pediatric patients during and after sedation for diagnostic and therapeutic procedures. *Pediatrics* 1992;89:1110–1115.
2. American Academy of Pediatrics, Committee on Drugs. Guidelines for monitoring and management of pediatric patients during and after sedation for diagnostic and therapeutic procedures: addendum. *Pediatrics* 2002;110:836–838.
3. American Society of Anesthesiologists. Task force on sedation and analgesia by non-anesthesiologists. Practice guidelines for sedation and analgesia by non-anesthesiologists. *Anesthesiology* 2002;96:1004–1017.
4. Cote CJ, Karl HW, Notterman DA, Weinberg JA, McCloskey C. Adverse

sedation events in pediatrics: analysis of medications used for sedation. *Pediatrics* 2000;106(4):633–644.

5. Green SM, Clark R, Hostetler MA, Cohen M, Carlson D, Rothrock SG. Inadvertent ketamine overdose in children: clinical manifestations and outcome. *Ann Emerg Med* 1999;34(4 Pt 1):492–497.

6. Green SM, Krauss B. Pulmonary aspiration risk during emergency department procedural sedation – an examination of the role of fasting and sedation depth. *Acad Emerg Med* 2002;9(1):35–42.

7. Green SM, Rothrock SG, Harris T, Hopkins GA, Garrett W, Sherwin T. Intravenous ketamine for pediatric sedation in the emergency department: safety profile with 156 cases. *Acad Emerg Med* 1998;5(10):971–976.

8. Green SM, Rothrock SG, Lynch EL, Ho M, Harris T, Hestdalen R, Hopkins GA, Garrett W, Westcott K. Intramuscular ketamine for pediatric sedation in the emergency department: safety profile in 1,022 cases (comment). *Ann Emerg Med* 1998;31(6):688–697.

9. Krauss B, Green SM. Sedation and analgesia for procedures in children. *New Engl J Med* 2000;342(13):938–945.

Appendix E   Focused assessment with sonography in trauma

Rita A. Sweeney, MD and Diku Mandavia, MD

Background

The focused assessment with sonography in trauma (FAST) is an important bedside examination used primarily by emergency physicians and trauma surgeons to identify free intraperitoneal, intrathoracic, or pericardial fluid. Physicians in Europe and Japan have been using bedside ultrasound (US) in the routine evaluation of trauma patients for over 30 years. The FAST exam has gained wide acceptance in the United States in the past decade. No other imaging modality has the ability to diagnose critical traumatic conditions as quickly or as accurately as bedside US. Ultrasonographic techniques are noninvasive, do not expose patients to radiation, and are performed with relatively inexpensive portable equipment. In the initial assessment of trauma patients, abdominal US is now replacing diagnostic peritoneal lavage (DPL), and echocardiography has replaced invasive subxiphoid pericardiotomy. With increasing numbers of emergency medicine residency programs incorporating formal US training into their curriculum, its role in emergency medicine practice is being further solidified.

Equipment

Essential components of US equipment are accessibility, portability, reliability and ease of use. Most trauma centers now have portable machines on site ready to be wheeled to the bedside at a moments notice. While most machines come with a variety of transducers, the most commonly-used transducer for the FAST examination is a 3.5 MHz microconvex transducer. The main advantage of the microconvex transducer is that the footprint can easily fit between the ribs when evaluating the upper quadrants and the heart. The need to rapidly evaluate and expedite care of trauma patients makes using different transducers for each view burdensome and inefficient. Since examinations should be recorded, printing, videotaping or digital storage capability is also necessary.

Ideal machine characteristics

- *Cost*: relatively low ($20,000–40,000).
- *Portability*: small, lightweight, easily movable.
- *Durability*: enclosed probe holders, flat "spill-proof" keyboard.
- *Image quality*: clear and sharp, with good resolution.
- *Probe selection*: electronic, multi-frequency, small "footprint."
- *Output*: thermal paper, videotape, digital storage, network capability.
- *Service*: on-site maintenance contract.

Procedure

FAST consists of multiple, focused ultrasonographic views of the abdomen and the pericardium. The primary objective of the FAST examination is to detect free intraperitoneal fluid. Used in this fashion, FAST has replaced DPL. Ultrasonographic evidence of hemoperitoneum strongly indicates that therapeutic laparotomy is required, whereas a "positive" DPL often does not. FAST is a useful screening test for hemoperitoneum despite its low specificity for injury location. Intestinal fluid and intraperitoneal urine can also produce positive FAST results, but like hemoperitoneum, both require surgical intervention. Ascites can confound the diagnosis but can be differentiated from hemoperitoneum by needle paracentesis. It is important to recognize that US will not reliably detect solid organ injury without hemoperitoneum; thus, high-risk stable patients should proceed to computed tomography (CT).

Clinical indications for the FAST exam

1. Blunt abdominal trauma.
2. Penetrating thoracic/abdominal trauma.
3. Unexplained hypotension in trauma.
4. Evaluation of the pregnant trauma patient.

The use of multiple views greatly increases the sensitivity of the FAST examination in the detection of hemoperitoneum. The paracolic gutter views have low sensitivity and have been eliminated from most protocols. Figure E.1 illustrates

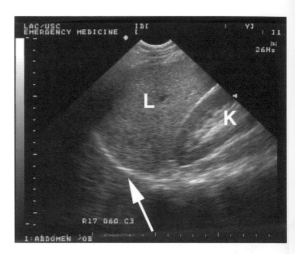

Figure E.2
Normal Morison's pouch. Arrow points to hyperechoic diaphragm (L: liver; K: kidney).

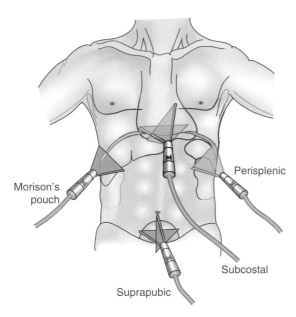

Figure E.1
Schematic of probe placement for the FAST examination (FAST: focused assessment with sonography in trauma). *Courtesy*: William Mallon, MD.

the basic views of the FAST examination. The important areas to be imaged are the following:

1. *Morison's pouch*: This area is the initial view for US evaluation of blunt trauma. As the landmarks are easy to find, this view is obtained within 10 seconds with the probe placed in the mid-posterior axillary line just below the nipple level at the 11th–12th intercostal space. The liver is seen as a solid homogeneous organ, with the kidney adjacent to it. The space between these organs, *Morison's pouch*, is a potential space that can fill with fluid (Figure E.2). Free fluid in this area appears as an anechoic (black) stripe (Figures E.3 and E.4). The amount of free fluid that may occupy Morison's pouch varies, but as little as 250 ml can be detected. Hyperechoic (white or gray) areas that surround the kidney represent normal perinephric fat and should not be confused with free fluid. In patients with smaller amounts of hemoperitoneum, placing the patient in reverse Trendelenburg can improve imaging sensitivity by making the upper quadrants of the abdomen more dependent. Following the examination of

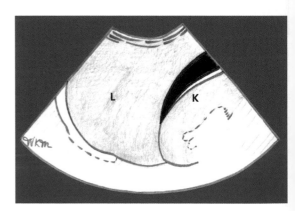

Figure E.3
Graphic representation of a positive Morison's pouch. L: liver; K: kidney. *Courtesy*: William Mallon, MD.

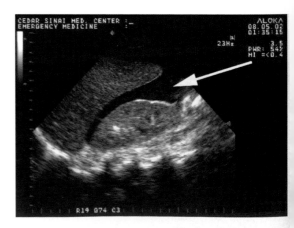

Figure E.4
Positive Morison's pouch. Arrow points to anechoic free intraperitoneal fluid.

Morison's pouch, angle the probe more cephalad and examine the diaphragm to look for fluid above or below it. Pleural fluid will appear anechoic or black above the diaphragm (Figure E.5). With practice, hemothoraces can be reliably detected.

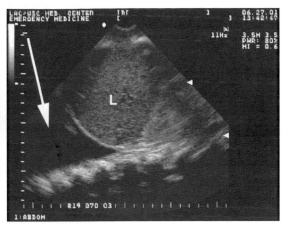

Figure E.5
Right pleural effusion seen as an anechoic area above the diaphragm (arrow) (L: liver).

2. *Perisplenic view*: To obtain this view, place the probe at the posterior axillary line at the 9th–11th intercostal space. A common mistake is not placing the probe posteriorly enough. Once the kidney is located, angle the probe slightly cephalad to visualize the spleen. Look carefully for free fluid surrounding it (Figures E.6 and E.7). Once the spleen and kidney are fully scanned, angle

the probe more cephalad to scan above and below the diaphragm, looking for fluid.

3. *Suprapubic view*: Ideally, this examination is conducted before the placement of a Foley catheter, as the full bladder provides an acoustic window for small amounts of free fluid posterior to the bladder. It is easily visualized with the probe positioned just cephalad to the pubis. The bladder is identified as a fluid collection that appears as a well-circumscribed anechoic area (Figure E.8). Having identified the bladder, look for free fluid anterior, posterior, and lateral to it (Figure E.9). In female patients, the uterus is seen posterior to the bladder. The rectouterine pouch (Pouch of Douglas) is a very dependent area of the peritoneal cavity and should be examined carefully for small amounts of free fluid.

4. *Pericardium*: It is especially important to evaluate the pericardium in patients with penetrating thoracic injuries, as it may harbor asymptomatic pericardial effusions. For this view, place the probe in the subcostal area just below the xiphisternum and angle it toward the patient's left shoulder. To view the heart adequately, increase the depth of ultrasonographic penetration in this view. A coronal section of the heart usually provides the examiner with a good four-chamber view of the heart (Figure E.10). The normal pericardium is seen as a hyperechoic (white) line intimately surrounding the heart.

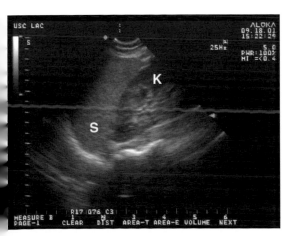

Figure E.6
Normal perisplenic view (S: spleen; K: kidney).

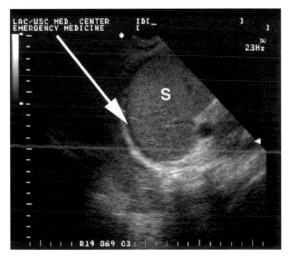

Figure E.7
Positive perisplenic view with free fluid between the spleen and diaphragm (arrow) (S: spleen).

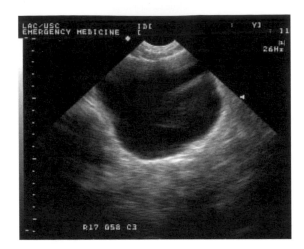

Figure E.8
Normal suprapubic view with full anechoic bladder.

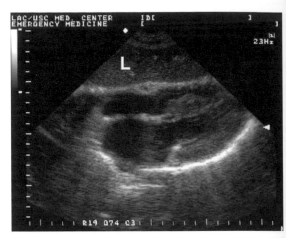

Figure E.10
Normal subxiphoid four-chamber view of the heart (L: liver).

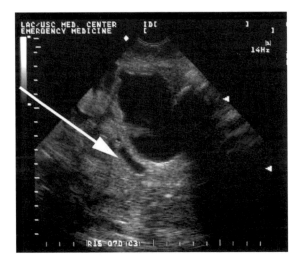

Figure E.9
Positive suprapubic view with fluid behind the bladder (arrow).

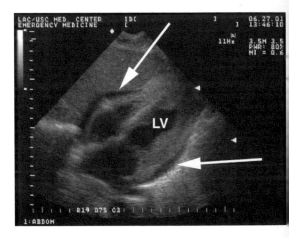

Figure E.11
Pericardial effusion seen on the subcostal view (arrows) (LV: left ventricle).

A pericardial effusion is identified as an anechoic area surrounding the heart within the pericardium (Figure E.11). Obtain a sagittal view for confirmation, since pulmonary effusions can be confused with pericardial effusions on this view. For patients with wounds in proximity to the heart, the FAST examination should begin with the pericardial view (focused echocardiography) to detect a possible life-threatening pericardial effusion resulting from a cardiac injury.

Summary

A summary of the FAST examination is given in Table E.1.

Limitations and pitfalls

To obtain the greatest clinical benefit from bedside US, the clinician must understand its technical limitations. The sensitivity of US in detecting free fluid varies between 80% and 98%; patient positioning can improve sensitivity. In addition, US is a real-time modality in which examination findings can change in a matter of minutes. Perform serial examinations in high-risk cases, when there is a change in vital signs or drop in hematocrit.

Table E.1 Focused assessment with sonography in trauma summary

View	Transducer position	Findings	Pitfalls
Morison's pouch	Between 11th and 12th ribs mid-axillary line with indicator toward right axilla (coronal plane)	Hemoperitoneum Hemothorax	Avoid excessive rib shadows by rotating probe so it is parallel to ribs
Perisplenic view	Between 10th and 11th ribs in posterior-axillary line with indicator toward left axilla (coronal plane)	Hemoperitoneum Hemothorax	Probe needs to be more cephalad and posterior than the right upper quadrant view; look above the spleen for fluid collections
Suprapubic view	Just superior to pubic bone and tilted caudally	Hemoperitoneum	Probe needs to be angled caudally, turn down gain which may obscure small amounts of fluid
Subxiphoid view	Subxiphoid region with probe under the xiphoid process and directed toward left shoulder (coronal plane)	Hemopericardium Pericardial tamponade	Increase US depth on this view, more pressure is often required; scan in the coronal plane

Table E.2 Common pitfalls in the focused assessment with sonography in trauma examination

Failure to perform multiple-view examination	Sensitivity is highly dependent on number of views obtained Morison's view is the most sensitive
Failure to consider other causes of fluid	Intestinal fluid 2° hollow viscus injury Intraperitoneal urine 2° bladder rupture Ascites (consider needle paracentesis to differentiate ascites from hemoperitoneum)
Failure to perform serial examinations	Clinical status of trauma patients very dynamic Consider serial examinations for patients with changing vital signs, decreasing hematocrit, high-risk mechanisms
Over-reliance on ultrasound	Interpret results in context with other important data elements, such as: • mechanism of injury • vital signs • hematocrit • radiographs • clinical suspicion Consider solid organ injury without hemoperitoneum in severe mechanisms Treat the patient, not the US

Solid organ injury without hemoperitoneum can occur and may not be appreciated by FAST. Thus, abdominal CT should be obtained in high-risk cases. In addition, US examination of extremely obese patients and patients with extensive subcutaneous emphysema is difficult. For such patients, a combination of procedures such as CT, DPL, and even pericardiotomy may be necessary to detect serious internal injury (Table E.2).

References

1. Jones RA, Welch RD. The FAST Exam. Ultrasonography in Trauma, The FAST Exam. D. Jehle and M. Heller. ACEP August 2003. pp. 15–38.
2. Ma J, Mateer J. Trauma. Emergency Ultrasound. OJ Ma and JR Mateer. McGraw-Hill 2003. pp. 67–88.

3. Mandavia D, Mallon WK. Using Bedside Ultrasonography to Evaluate Trauma Patients *J Critical Illness* 2000;15(7): 387–394.

4. Mandavia D, Kendall J. Pitfalls in Trauma Ultrasonography. Ultrasonography in Trauma, The FAST Exam. D. Jehle and M. Heller. ACEP August 2003. 87–106.

5. Mandavia D, Joseph A. Bedside Echocardiography in Chest Trauma *Emerg Med Clin North Am* – August 2004.

Appendix F   Interpretation of emergency laboratories

J. Michael Ballester, MD

The ability to diagnose and manage complex clinical scenarios seen in the daily practice of emergency medicine is dependent on correct laboratory ordering and interpretation. Emergency physicians are often faced with many patient presentations and a multitude of possible laboratory tests to aid diagnosis and treatment. Understanding the strengths and limitations of each individual test is crucial in applying the test in its correct clinical context. The emergency physician must make rational decisions about each laboratory test ordered and base each test ordered on the patient's clinical presentation. Using laboratory data in a "shotgun" mentality to hopefully "discover" a diagnosis often leads to inappropriate testing, unnecessary procedures, delays in care, and potential harm. This chapter will focus on interpretation of laboratory data that is routinely used in the emergency department (ED). It should be noted that normal reference values provided may vary between individual institutions, gender, and with age. It is recommended to refer to your institution's reference values.

Complete blood count with differential

Complete blood count (CBC) includes white blood cell (WBC) count, differential, hemoglobin (Hgb), hematocrit (HCT), platelet count, and red blood cell (RBC) indices.

Indications

1. Acute blood loss.
2. Evaluation of anemia.
3. Evaluation of thrombocytopenia.
4. Evaluation of serious infection.
5. Clinically suspected blood dyscrasia (i.e., leukemia or myelodysplastic syndrome).
6. Determination of neutropenia in the immunocompromised host.

Normal values

- WBC $4.3–10.8 \times 10^3 mm^3$
- Differential
  - Neutrophils 45–74%
  - Bands 0–4%
  - Lymphocytes 16–45%
  - Monocytes 4–10%
  - Eosinophils 0–7%
  - Basophils 0–2%
- Hemoglobin
  - Males 13–18 g/dl
  - Females 12–16 g/dl
- Hematocrit
  - Males 42–52%
  - Females 37–48%
- Platelets $130–450 \times 10^3$

Absolute neutrophil count (ANC) is calculated using the formula:

$$ANC = WBC \times \frac{polys + bands}{100}$$

If ANC < 1800, neutropenia is present.

Absolute lymphocyte count (ALC) is calculated using the formula:

$$ALC = WBC \times (\text{lymphocyte percentage})$$

The ALC can be used as a surrogate marker for the CD_4 count. Those patients with an ALC less than 1000 cells/mm^3 are at higher risk for opportunistic infections.

Abnormalities and causes

1. *Elevated WBC*: May be elevated in an acute infection, as well as stress, steroid use, and inflammatory states. Other causes include prolonged crying in infants, pain, vomiting, dysrhythmias, pregnancy, neoplasm, exercise, acute myocardial infarction (AMI), surgery, and seizures. Look for a "left shift" which indicates the presence of immature forms in the peripheral circulation (bands). This usually represents an infectious state.
2. *Decreased WBC*: May be decreased with infection, septicemia, viral illness, and immunocompromised states. Neutropenia, defined as ANC < 1800 cells/mm^3, places the patient at risk of infections from common and opportunistic organisms.
3. *Decreased HCT*: May be secondary to acute blood loss, hemolysis, or long-standing anemia. If suspecting acute loss, look for schistocytes on the peripheral blood smear. Pregnancy can also lower the HCT by 10%. Long-standing anemia can be evaluated by the RBC indices. Expect the HCT to drop from administration of fluids in hypovolemic shock or trauma resuscitation.
4. *Increased HCT*: An elevated HCT can be seen in hemoconcentrated states, high altitude, exercise, polycythemia vera, or chronic obstructive lung disease.
5. *Increased platelet count*: Thrombocytosis occurs when platelet counts are in excess of 1 million. Usually large and nonfunctioning, this condition is seen in myeloproliferative disorders or secondary to iron deficiency anemia, splenectomized states, chronic inflammatory disorders, or hemolytic anemia.
6. *Decreased platelet count*: Thrombocytopenia occurs when platelet counts are less than the normal range. It may be caused by bone marrow injury from drugs or chemicals, radiation, or infection. It can also be seen in bone marrow failure due to carcinoma,

leukemia, lymphoma, or fibrosis. Other causes include menses, or poor nutritional states such as iron, folate, and vitamin B_{12} deficiencies.

Pearls and pitfalls

1. Patients with serious infections may have completely normal or low WBC counts. Overreliance on normal WBC counts in the setting of acute infections may lead to misdiagnosis and delays in patient care.
2. Toxic granulations, Dohle bodies, and cytoplasmic vacuolization are remnants of phagocytosis found in neutrophils. These are indicative of more serious bacterial infections.
3. Acute hemorrhage will not be reflected in the Hgb or HCT early on.
4. Geriatric patients will more than likely demonstrate normal to low WBC counts in sepsis.

Serum chemistries

Serum chemistries, also known as serum electrolytes, include sodium, potassium, chloride, bicarbonate, blood urea nitrogen (BUN), creatinine, and glucose.

Indications

1. Evaluation of life-threatening hyper- or hypokalemic states.
2. Evaluation of mental status changes, coma, or new-onset seizure.
3. Evaluation of renal function, chronic hypertension, or diuretic use.
4. Evaluation of hyper- or hypoglycemia in the diabetic patient.
5. Assessing acid–base status by anion gap calculation and HCO_3^- measurement.
6. Evaluation of hydration and volume status, if poor oral intake, repeated vomiting, significant diarrhea, muscle weakness, or alcohol abuse.
7. Evaluation of hyperosmolar states.
8. Evaluation of upper gastrointestinal bleeding.

Normal values

- Sodium   135–145 mEq/L
- Potassium   3.5–5.0 mEq/L
- Chloride   95–110 mEq/L
- Bicarbonate   22–28 mEq/L
- BUN   8–22 mg/dL

- Creatinine   0.7–1.5 mg/dL
- Glucose   65–115 mg/dL
- Anion gap   10–15; sodium − (chloride + bicarbonate)

Abnormalities and causes

1. *Elevated sodium:* Hypernatremia is seen in hyperosmolar states, severe dehydration, and diabetes insipidus.
2. *Decreased sodium*: Hyponatremia is the most common electrolyte abnormality seen in hospitalized patients. It is further classified as *hypotonic* (diuretics, gastrointestinal losses, adrenal insufficiency, congestive heart failure (CHF), cirrhosis), *isotonic* (syndrome of inappropriate antidiuretic hormone (SIADH) secretion, psychogenic polydipsia), or *hypertonic* (hyperglycemia) based on plasma osmolality. Hyponatremia may also be factious due to hyperglycemia, hyperlipidemia, and hyperproteinemia.
3. *Elevated potassium*: Hyperkalemia is often the result of specimen hemolysis. True causes of hyperkalemia include acidosis, tissue damage, acute renal failure, drug-induced causes (potassium-sparing diuretics, non-steroidal anti-inflammatory drugs (NSAIDs), digoxin, ACE inhibitors), and oral and intravenous (IV) administration of potassium.
4. *Decreased potassium*: Hypokalemia is often from vomiting, diarrhea, diuretics, acute hyperventilation, insulin administration, or diabetic ketoacidosis (DKA).
5. *Increased chloride*: Metabolic acidosis, gastrointestinal bicarbonate loss, respiratory alkalosis, renal acidosis, or hyperparathyroidism.
6. *Decreased chloride*: Vomiting, gastric drainage, or diuretics.
7. *Increased bicarbonate*: Respiratory acidosis or metabolic alkalosis (Cushing's syndrome, vomiting, volume depletion).
8. *Decreased bicarbonate*: Respiratory alkalosis or metabolic acidosis (ketoacidosis, lactic acidosis, diarrhea, renal tubular acidosis, renal failure). Bicarbonate decreases by an average of 15% during pregnancy. May also lower by 5–8 mEq/L due to hyperventilation.
9. *Increased BUN*: Dehydration, high protein intake, exercise, renal failure, upper gastrointestinal bleeding, or CHF.
10. *Decreased BUN*: Low protein intake, high water intake, cirrhosis, or pregnancy.

11. *Increased creatinine*: Renal insufficiency, renal failure, rhabdomyolysis, dehydration, or strenuous exercise.
12. *Decreased creatinine*: Pregnancy, malnutrition, or water intoxication.
13. *Hyperglycemia*: Diabetes mellitus, hyperthyroidism, Cushing's disease, pheochromocytoma, acute illness, glucocorticoid use, lithium, or thiazides.
14. *Hypoglycemia*: Drugs, especially insulin, sulfonylureas, ethanol, insulinoma, sepsis, acute illness, starvation, adrenal insufficiency, growth hormone deficiency, renal failure, hypopituitarism, postprandial, after gastric surgery, or factitious (insulin/sulfonylurea misuse).

Pearls and pitfalls

1. Hyperglycemia causes pseudohyponatremia:

$$\text{sodium corrected} = \text{sodium} + \frac{\text{glucose} - 5}{3.5}$$

   General rule of thumb: for every 100 mg/dL increase in plasma glucose concentration, the plasma sodium concentration decreases by approximately 1.6 meq/L.
2. Most often hypo- or hypernatremia can be corrected by treating the underlying condition or by administration of normal saline; 3% saline is rarely needed and must be given very slowly to avoid *central pontine myelinosis*. Be sure to monitor urine output and check electrolytes frequently. Goal should be to correct the sodium gradually (maximum rate of 0.5 mEq/L/hour).
3. Serum potassium below 3 mEq/L indicates a total body deficit of 300–400 mEq of total body potassium. Each 10 mEq of potassium replaced will raise the serum potassium by roughly 0.1 mEq/L.
4. Hyperkalemia is often reflected in the electrocardiogram (ECG) with peaked T waves, followed by loss of the P wave, widening of the QRS complex, and sine wave-appearing tachycardia. Patients may complain of muscle cramps, weakness, paralysis, paresthesias, or tetany. Treatment includes close cardiovascular monitoring, immediate antagonism of potassium at the cardiac membrane with calcium chloride or calcium gluconate, lowering the serum potassium, and correcting the underlying cause. Serum potassium can be lowered by

administration of sodium bicarbonate, glucose and insulin, and nebulized beta-agonists. Definitive treatment to remove excess potassium from the body includes administration of oral/rectal exchange resins (i.e., polystyrene sulfonate) and hemodialysis.

5. Serum osmolality is calculated by the following equation:

$$\text{osmolality} = (2 \times \text{sodium}) + \frac{\text{glucose}}{18} + \frac{\text{BUN}}{3.8} + \frac{\text{EtOH}}{2.8}$$

An osmolal gap indicates the presence of millimolar amounts of an uncharged particle. If the osmolal gap is elevated, the patient's serum ethanol level should be measured. If the gap is greater than 10, then unaccounted osmols may represent methanol, ethylene glycol, isopropyl alcohol, acetone, acetylsalicylic acid, or paraldehyde.

6. An elevated anion gap usually indicates the presence of a metabolic acidosis. "MUDPILECATS" is a helpful mnemonic for an elevated anion gap metabolic acidosis:

M	methanol/metformin
U	uremia
D	diabetic ketoacidosis
P	paraldehyde/phenformin
I	iron/isoniazid
L	lactic acidosis
E	ethylene glycol
C	cyanide/carbon monoxide
A	alcoholic ketoacidosis
T	toluene
S	salicylates, seizure

7. Patients with severe acidosis tend to have elevated potassium levels. Even when a patient's total body potassium is severely depleted, the serum potassium will be high in acidotic states. This is commonly seen in DKA. As the patient is treated, serum potassium levels may fall precipitously if not closely monitored and corrected. Remember to correct the patient's potassium only after urine output has been established.

8. Use clinical judgment before ordering serum chemistries. Avoid using chemistry panels as screening tools.

9. Determining blood glucose is critical in the evaluation of any patient with mental status changes, stroke-like symptoms, coma, drug ingestion, or acute illness. If hypoglycemia is suspected, treat first with 1 amp of D_{50} prior to any delay in obtaining formal laboratory values. Bedside glucose determination using glucometers is very common and recommended as long as it does not cause significant delay in administering glucose.

10. Bedside glucometers are often inaccurate in patients with a low PO_2 or HCT, and are affected by an inadequate amount of blood, improper storage reagents, and machine calibration.

Other chemistries

Calcium

Indications

1. Altered mental status.
2. Recent thyroid and parathyroid surgery, neck trauma, or neck surgery.
3. Multiple myeloma, bone metastases.
4. New-onset renal failure, evaluation of weakness in a hemodialysis patient.
5. Acute pancreatitis.
6. Evaluation of tetany.

Normal values

- Calcium, free (ionized)   4.7–5.2 mg/dL
- Calcium, total   8.9–10.5 mg/dL

Abnormalities and causes

1. *Hypercalcemia*: Primary hyperparathyroidism, malignancies producing parathyroid-like protein, metastatic bone disease, sarcoidosis, acidosis and excessive ingestion of calcium-containing antacids.
2. *Hypocalcemia*: Acute pancreatitis, rhabdomyolysis, sepsis, malignancy, hepatic or renal insufficiency, tuberculosis, parathyroid adenoma resection, vascular or parathyroid injury during surgery or trauma, and malabsorptive states (pancreatectomy, small bowel resection) not allowing absorption of calcium from the small intestine.

Pearls and pitfalls

1. Hypocalcemia primarily causes neuromuscular (tetany, seizures, muscle cramps, weakness) and cardiovascular effects

(prolonged QT interval, dysrhythmias, cardiovascular collapse, refractory hypotension).

2. Calcium levels are most accurate when corrected for abnormal albumin:

   Corrected calcium (mg/dL) = 4 − [serum albumin (g/dL)] × 0.8 + serum calcium (mg/dL).

3. Classic peripheral neurologic findings of hypocalcemia include:
   - *Chvostek sign*: Tap over the facial nerve 2 cm anterior to the tragus of the ear. Twitching of the mouth, nose, eye, and facial muscles will occur.
   - *Trousseau sign*: Inflation of a blood pressure cuff above the systolic pressure causes local ulnar and median nerve ischemia, resulting in carpal spasm. Not recommended to perform this test; it is usually noted incidentally during vital sign measurement at triage.

Magnesium

Indications

1. Evaluation of ventricular dysrhythmias.
2. Neuromuscular weakness.
3. Poor nutrition, alcoholism, pancreatitis, malabsorptive syndromes.

Normal values

- Magnesium   1.4–2.5 mg/dL

Abnormalities and causes

1. *Elevated magnesium*: Dehydration, hemoconcentration, hypoglycemia, hemolyzed specimen, cell lysis syndromes, hemolytic anemia, renal failure, or DKA.
2. *Decreased magnesium*: Malabsorption, malnutrition, renal tubular injury, hypoparathyroidism, ethanol use, digoxin use, cyclosporines, or cisplatin use.

Pearls and pitfalls

Magnesium infusion is first-line treatment in torsades de pointes, eclamptic seizures; some use in severe asthma exacerbation (impending respiratory failure).

Magnesium should be infused slowly, to avoid complications such as a loss of reflexes, muscle weakness, hypotension, vasodilation, respiratory failure.

Liver function tests

Liver function tests (LFTs) include aspartate aminotransferase (AST), alanine aminotransferase (ALT), gamma-glutamyl transpeptidase (GGT), alkaline phosphate (ALK), bilirubin, and lactate dehydrogenase (LDH). Of note, AST was formerly known by SGOT; ALT by SGPT.

Indications

1. Evaluation of the synthetic, excretory, and metabolic function of the liver and biliary tract.
2. Evaluation of liver damage from toxic substances, drugs, autoimmune disorders, infectious processes, ecclampsia.

Normal values

- AST   8–40 IU/L
- ALT   Males 8–45 IU/L
               Females 6–38 IU/L
- GGT   Males 11–49 IU/L
               Females 7–32 IU/L
- ALK   30–130 IU/L
- Bilirubin   Total 0.3–1.1 mg/dL
               Direct 0–0.2 mg/dL
- LDH   100–212 IU/L

Abnormalities and causes

1. *Elevated AST*: Liver injury (acute and chronic hepatitis), obstructive jaundice, AMI (however seldom used due to its lack of specificity), skeletal muscle diseases, hemolytic anemia, gallstone pancreatitis, drug-induced liver or muscle injury.
2. *Decreased AST or ALT*: Pregnancy (both mg/dL) or chronic renal failure.
3. *Elevated ALT*: Hepatocellular injury, large myocardial damage, skeletal muscle disease, gallstone pancreatitis, or drugs inducing liver or muscle injury.
4. *Elevated GGT*: Obstructive jaundice, hepatitis, cirrhosis, metastatic liver disease, pancreatitis, prostate cancer, hyperthyroidism, or diabetes. Used by some as a general screen for liver disease. Elevated in approximately 70% of alcoholic liver disease.
5. *Decreased GGT*: Exercise, pregnancy, or hypothyroidism.

6. *Elevated ALK*: Biliary tract obstruction, metastatic liver lesions, primary biliary cirrhosis, drug-induced hepatitis, metastatic bone cancer, conditions that lead to increased bone turnover (osteomalacia, Paget's disease, osteosarcoma), or hyperthyroidism. Mainly used to detect and monitor liver or bone disease.
7. *Decreased ALK*: Pregnancy or blood transfusions.
8. *Elevated bilirubin*: Liver or biliary tract diseases, Dubin-Johnson syndrome, drug toxicity, or neonatal hyperbilirubinemia (may be normal).
9. *Decreased bilirubin*: Improper lab storage.
10. *Elevated LDH*: Hemolytic anemia, malignancies, acute hepatitis, MI, shock, strangulated bowel obstruction, amiodarone (chronic use), or hemolyzed specimens. Nonspecific marker of cell injury, seen with most types of cell damage.

Pearls and pitfalls

1. With most types of acute hepatitis, ALT is elevated to a higher degree than AST. Very high values occur with ischemic and toxic hepatitis. With muscle injury, AST is usually 3–5 times higher than ALT.
2. With alcoholic hepatitis, the AST:ALT ratio is about 3:1 because alcohol damages the mitochondria, a source of AST. With viral hepatitis, the ALT is usually greater than the AST because toxicity is more liver-specific.
3. During the course of common bile duct obstruction, the AST and ALT will be the first to rise, followed by the ALK and bilirubin.
4. The indirect bilirubin (unconjugated) can be measured by subtracting the direct bilirubin (conjugated) from the measured total bilirubin.

Amylase

Indications

Used in the diagnosis of pancreatitis.

Normal values

Amylase   60–110 IU/L

Abnormalities and causes

1. *Elevated amylase*: Acute pancreatitis, pancreatic pseudocyst, salivary gland inflammation, intestinal ischemia, DKA, choledocholithiasis, renal failure, cirrhosis, or ovarian cysts. It is also seen in ectopic pregnancy; however, it is not used as a screening test due to its lack of specificity.
2. *Decreased amylase*: Chronic pancreatitis, hypertrigliceridemia, pancreatic insufficiency, or malnutrition.

Pearls and pitfalls

1. May remain elevated in acute pancreatitis for only 36–48 hours after onset. Less specific than lipase in the diagnosis of pancreatitis.
2. May be normal in patients with chronic pancreatitis ("burnt-out" pancreas).

Lipase

Indications

Used to diagnose pancreatitis.

Normal values

Lipase   4–50 IU/dL

Abnormalities and causes

1. *Elevated lipase*: Pancreatitis, pancreatic pseudocyst, renal failure, heparin, or drugs causing pancreatic injury.
2. *Decreased lipase*: Hepatitis, falsely lowered in obstructive jaundice, pancreatic insufficiency.

Pearls and pitfalls

1. Testing for lipase is the most sensitive test for evaluating pancreatic injury. Will remain elevated for up to 7 days following pancreatic injury. Elevations of more than 3 times normal markedly increase the likelihood of pancreatitis.

Cardiac markers

Cardiac markers include creatine kinase (CK), CK isoenzymes MB (CK-MB), troponin, myoglobin.

Indications

1. Evaluation of patients with suspected acute coronary syndromes (ACS). Myoglobin, present in all muscle tissue, is generally

elevated within 2 hours of symptom onset. It is limited by its lack of specificity. Combining ECG interpretation with myoglobin within the first 4 hours of symptom onset has the best sensitivity for AMI. Between 4 and 12 hours of symptom onset, ECG, myoglobin, and CK-MB are the best predictors of AMI. Troponin levels have an advantage in that they remain elevated longer than CK-MB enzymes.

Normal values

- CK
  - Females   45–135 IU/L
  - Males   55–170 IU/L
- CK-MB   < 10 ng/mL (mass)
- Troponin-I   < 1.6 ng/mL
- Troponin-T   < 0.1 ng/mL
- Myoglobin   < 90 ng/mL

Abnormalities and causes

1. *Elevated CK*: CK is a muscle enzyme found in skeletal muscle, cardiac muscle, and brain tissue. It can be elevated after strenuous exercise, muscle damage, AMI, hypothyroidism, malignant hyperthermia, neuroleptic malignant syndrome, or intramuscular injection.
2. *Decreased CK*: Pregnancy, aging, malnutrition, or hyperthyroidism.
3. *Elevated CK-MB*: Myocardial infarction, myocarditis, cardiac contusion, or skeletal muscle injury (total CK-MB but not relative index).
4. *Troponins*: Troponins are small enzymes found in muscle tissue. Two of these enzymes (troponin-I and troponin-T) are found only in cardiac tissue. Troponin-I and Troponin-T may be elevated in myocardial infarction, unstable angina, and renal failure.
5. *Elevated myoglobin*: Skeletal muscle injury, myocardial infarction, renal failure, seizures, or exercise.

Pearls and pitfalls

- Myoglobin rises earliest with muscle injury (within 2–4 hours), peaks in 8–12 hours, and returns to normal within 24–40 hours. Lacks cardiospecificity since it is abundant in all muscle tissue.
- CK-MB is first detected by 3–4 hours in the blood, peaks by 12 hours and returns to

normal within 24–36 hours. With myocardial damage, CK-MB is greater than 10% of the total CK released. Values between 3% and 10% are indeterminate. A relative index is used to help by dividing CK-MB by total CK and multiplying by 100. A ratio less than 3 is indicative of skeletal muscle; a ratio greater than 5 indicates cardiac muscle injury.
3. Troponins rise in the blood 3–4 hours after injury and remain elevated for up to 10 days. A positive troponin in the setting of unstable angina or non-ST-segment elevation myocardial infarction is associated with a four times greater risk of death than patients without positive troponin values.
4. Normal cardiac markers within the first few hours after symptom onset does not rule out ACS and should not be used as a basis for discharging a patient.

B-type natriuretic peptide

Indications

1. Predominately secreted from the ventricular myocardium during myocardial pressure and stretching, B-type natriuretic peptide (BNP) is a diagnostic and prognostic marker in undifferentiated dyspnea and CHF.

Normal values

- Normal BNP: less than 100 pg/ml
- Intermediate: 100–400 pg/ml
- Elevated: greater than 400 pg/ml

Abnormalities and causes

1. A BNP level less than 100 pg/ml is highly accurate in excluding CHF as the cause of dyspnea. Increased levels need to be interpreted in the context of a patient's clinical status, as not every patient with an increased BNP level has decompensated CHF.

Pearls and pitfalls

1. The diagnosis of CHF can often be made on clinical and radiographic grounds, and a BNP level does not aid in diagnostic accuracy.
2. Intermediate levels may prove helpful in prognosis if a patient's baseline BNP level is known.

PT, PTT, INR

Definitions

1. *Prothrombin time (PT)*: Measure of the extrinsic (factor VII) and common (factor II, V, X) pathways, as well as coumadin monitoring.
2. *Activated partial thromboplastin time (PTT)*: Measure of the intrinsic (factors XI, IX, VIII) and common (factors II, V, X) pathways.
3. International normalized ratio (INR): Calculation based on a correction factor from a patient's and control's PT to normalize the PT, therefore facilitating accurate comparison among different laboratories.

Normal values

- PT: 9–15 seconds
- PTT: 22–33 seconds
- INR: Coumadin effective between 2 and 3 with low risk of bleeding.

Indications for obtaining PT

1. Warfarin (coumadin) therapy.
2. Suspected coagulopathy (disseminated intravascular coagulation, (DIC), hemophilia).
3. Active bleeding without obvious source.
4. Clinical evidence of liver disease.
5. History of abnormal, excessive, or spontaneous bleeding.
6. History of coagulopathy.
7. Before surgery or major vascular procedure if liver disease, malnutrition, or malabsorption exists or clinical history is not available.
8. Known or suspected warfarin overdose or excessive ingestion.

Indications for obtaining PTT

1. IV heparin therapy.
2. Suspected coagulopathy (DIC, hemophilia).
3. Active bleeding with or without obvious cause.
4. Clinical evidence of liver disease.
5. History of abnormal, excessive, or spontaneous bleeding.
6. History of coagulopathy.
7. Before surgery or major vascular procedure if liver disease, malnutrition, or malabsorption exists or clinical history is not available.

Abnormalities and causes

1. *Elevated (prolonged) PT*: Coumadin therapy, liver disease, vitamin K deficiency, antiphospholipid antibodies, congenital factor VII deficiencies, or antibiotics.
2. *Elevated (prolonged) PTT*: Heparin therapy, thrombolytic agents, drugs interfering with vitamin K, hemophilia A and B, DIC, moderate to severe Von Willebrand's disease, liver failure, antiphospholipid antibodies, or incompletely filled lab tubes.
3. *Decreased PTT*: Pregnancy, hemolysis, exercise, or anemia.

Pearls and pitfalls

1. Most common causes of prolonged PT and PTT include anticoagulant therapy, vitamin K deficiency (nutritional or secondary to broad-spectrum antibiotics and depletion of bowel flora), liver disease, and DIC.
2. Bleeding from excessive warfarin can be managed with 4–5 units of fresh frozen plasma for a short period. Vitamin K (5–10 mg) given orally, SQ or IV partially reverses the effect of warfarin.
3. Falsely elevated PTT times is seen if the plasma is excessively turbid or icteric.
4. A PT is *not* indicated before routine hospital admission, heparin therapy, routine preoperative testing, minor trauma, prior to initiation of heparin therapy if other co-morbid problems are ruled out, before low-dose subcutaneous heparin therapy, history of alcohol abuse without clinical evidence of liver disease or coagulopathy.
5. A PTT is *not* indicated in warfarin use, routine hospital admission, routine preoperative testing, minor trauma, before initiation of heparin therapy, low-dose subcutaneous heparin therapy, history of alcohol abuse without clinical evidence of liver disease or coagulopathy.

D-dimer (ELISA)

Indications

1. Evaluation of suspected venous thromboembolic disease.
2. Detecting fragments of cross-linked fibrin, mainly in DIC.

Normal values

D-dimer   <500 FEU

Abnormalities and causes

1. *Elevated D-dimer*: Venous thromboembolic disease, deep vein thrombosis (DVT), pulmonary embolism (PE), malignancy, DIC, pregnancy, or chronic inflammatory conditions.

Pearls and pitfalls

1. A patient with a negative D-dimer and a low pretest probability for PE is unlikely to have a significant PE.

Arterial blood gas

Arterial blood gas (ABG) includes blood pH, PCO_2, PO_2, bicarbonate.

Indications

1. Evaluation of respiratory and metabolic acid–base disturbances including poisonings, respiratory failure, or severe chronic obstructive pulmonary disease (COPD) exacerbations.
2. Undifferentiated shock.
3. Unexplained coma or confusion/obtundation.

Normal values

- Blood pH   7.38–7.42
- PCO_2 38–42 mmHg
- PO_2 83–108 mmHg
- HCO_3^- 22–26 mmol/L

Abnormalities and causes

1. *Elevated pH*: Vomiting, volume contraction, hyperaldosteronism, early CHF, drugs causing alkalosis, or anxiety.
2. *Decreased pH*: Ketoacidosis, lactic acidosis, renal failure, respiratory failure, chronic obstructive lung disease, drugs causing acidosis (isoniazid, iron, salicylates), or ethylene glycol.
3. *Increased PCO_2*: Respiratory failure, hypoventilation, COPD, CNS depression, metabolic alkalosis, or drugs depressing respiration (alcohol, barbiturates, opiates, benzodiazepines).

4. *Decreased PCO_2*: Hyperventilation, anxiety, interstitial lung disease, cirrhosis, metabolic acidosis, hyperthyroidism, PE, or aspirin.
5. *Increased PO_2*: Oxygen therapy, excessive air bubbles in specimen, hyperventilation, or aspirin.
6. *Decreased PO_2*: COPD, pneumonia, interstitial lung disease, PE, CHF, shock, CNS depression, right-to-left cardiac shunts, or drugs that depress respiration.
7. *Elevated HCO_3^-*: Respiratory acidosis, metabolic alkalosis (vomiting, Cushing's syndrome, volume depletion), diuretics, or glucocorticoids.
8. *Decreased HCO_3^-*: Respiratory alkalosis, metabolic acidosis (ketoacidosis, lactic acidosis, renal failure, diarrhea), carbonic anhydrase inhibitors, ethylene glycol, methanol, aspirin, or pregnancy.

Pearls and pitfalls

1. Prior to obtaining the sample, a patient must be evaluated for both radial and ulnar arterial blood supply. The *Allen's test* determines the presence of collateral flow from both the radial and ulnar artery in the hand. If abnormal, radial artery cannulation should be avoided to prevent possible ischemic injuries.
2. ABG specimens must be handled appropriately and run expeditiously. Errors arise from excess air bubbles in the sample, excess heparin in the syringe, and not immediately placing the sample on ice.
3. If a patient is hypoxemic, attempt to determine the etiology. Do not just treat with supplemental oxygen.
4. The ABG measurement in a patient with carbon monoxide poisoning will help by identifying the presence of a metabolic acidosis with a normal PO_2.
5. ABG samples are not necessary if pulse oximetry is sufficient to guide management.

Alveolar–arterial oxygen gradient

The alveolar–arterial (A–a) oxygen gradient can be used to differentiate between hypoxia caused by hypoventilation alone (i.e., neuromuscular diseases, overdoses) in which the A–a gradient is normal, and that caused by ventilation–perfusion mismatch, right-to-left shunting and diffusion abnormalities (i.e., PE, CHF, acute respiratory distress syndrome (ARDS), COPD) in which the A–a gradient is abnormal. The A–a gradient is calculated using the formula:

$$A\text{–a gradient} = (FiO_2 \times (\text{barometric pressure} - 47\,\text{mmHg})) - \left(PO_2 + \frac{PCO_2}{0.8}\right)$$

For an ABG drawn on room air at sea level, a more workable formula is:

$$A\text{–a gradient} = 150 - \left(PO_2 + \frac{PCO_2}{0.8}\right)$$

The A–a gradient is increased in smokers and patients with intrinsic lung disease. The A–a gradient increases as people age; a simple formula to take this variation into account is:

$$\text{normal A–a gradient} < \frac{\text{age}}{4} + 4$$

Pearls and pitfalls

1. The A–a gradient cannot be determined accurately in a patient who is receiving O_2 by nasal cannula, as the FiO_2 of the supplemental oxygen must be estimated.
2. Calculating the A–a gradient has clinical implications in that hypoxia in the presence of a normal gradient is treated by improving ventilation, whereas an increased A–a gradient should be treated with supplemental oxygen.
3. The A–a gradient is neither sensitive nor specific for the diagnosis of PE. A normal A–a gradient in a young, otherwise healthy patient does not exclude the diagnosis.

Urinalysis

Urinalysis includes specific gravity, pH, protein, glucose, ketones, blood, bilirubin, urobilinogen, nitrite, and leukocyte esterase. Microscopy includes crystals, epithelial cells, RBCs, WBCs, hyaline casts, granular casts, cellular casts, and organisms.

Indications

1. Evaluation of suspected asymptomatic bacteriuria, cystitis, urethritis, prostatitis, and pyelonephritis.
2. Evaluation of hydration status.
3. Evaluation of possible nephrolithiasis.
4. Evaluation for rhabdomyolysis.
5. Evaluation of acute renal failure and acute tubular necrosis.
6. Evaluation of DKA and ketonuria.

Normal values

Urine: Normally urine is sterile and transparent, with a specific gravity of 1.010 and normal pH. Urine is yellow due to urochrome pigment, with the degree of coloration related to urine concentration. Cloudiness indicates the presence of particulate matter such as crystals, RBCs or WBCs, mucus or bacteria.

Causes of abnormal color

- Red: Blood, Hgb, prophyrins, beets
- Brown: Hgb, myoglobin, bilirubin, nitrofurantoin
- Orange: Urates, pyridium, sulfasalazine
- Dark: Hgb, myoglobin, alkaptonuria

Abnormalities and causes

1. *Specific gravity*: May be variable due to disorders of urine-concentrating ability or changes in fluid status. Alkaline pH may lead to false results.
2. *pH*: Acid–base disorders affect the urine pH. Urinary tract infections (UTI) may produce alkaline pH.
3. *Protein*: Increased protein is seen in glomerular diseases, infections, tubular disorders, and exercise. Urine dipstick analysis is sensitive for albumin. Globulins are less easily detected. Other proteins such as Bence–Jones proteins may be missed entirely.
4. *Glucose*: May be elevated in patients with diabetes mellitus. Elevated glucose in the urine suggests a serum glucose $>170\,\text{mg/dl}$. Can be elevated in normal individuals after consuming a high-glucose beverage, as well as patients receiving dextrose infusions.
5. *Ketones*: Ketoacidosis will produce ketonuria. Dipstick urinalysis measures acetoacetic acid or acetone but not beta-hydroxybutyrate.
6. *Blood*: Any site of bleeding in the urinary tract will produce hematuria, including glomerulonephritis, tumors, stones, infection coagulopathy, hemolysis, or myoglobinuria with muscle damage.
7. *Bilirubin*: Most commonly seen in liver and biliary disease. Complete biliary obstruction

is suggested when the bilirubin is positive with a negative urobilinogen.

8. *Urobilinogen*: Seen in hemolysis or cirrhosis.
9. *Nitrites*: Positive in most Gram-negative organism infections. Based on organism's ability to convert urinary nitrates to nitrite.
10. *Leukocyte esterase*: Positive in the setting of most genitourinary tract infections.
11. *Crystals*: Uric acid and calcium oxalate, may be part of a normal urinalysis. Calcium oxalate is occasionally seen with nephrolithiasis.
12. *Epithelial cells*: Squamous or transitional cells are normal. An adequate specimen for analysis, either by mid-stream collection or urethral catheterization should have less than five epithelial cells per high-power field. *Clue cells* are vaginal epithelial cells to which bacteria have been attached.
13. *RBC*: Indicative of glomerular injury, nephrolithiasis, inflammation, or neoplasms.
14. *WBC*: Counts higher than five per high-power field indicate infections of the bladder, kidney, prostate, cervix or vagina.
15. *Hyaline casts*: Seen in causes of proteinuria (especially diabetes), dehydration, or exercise.
16. *Granular casts*: RBC casts seen in glomerulonephritis; WBC casts seen in pyelonephritis.
17. *Organisms*: Contaminated specimens, cystitis, pyelonephritis, or prostatitis.

Pearls and pitfalls

1. Accuracy of urine testing depends on the care with which specimens are collected and transported. Avoid specimen contamination with periurethral flora during collection. Use of sterile containers and prompt transport to the laboratory may prevent microbial growth.
2. Urine specimens with high numbers of leukocytes, RBC, presence of leukocyte esterase or nitrites, and culture colony counts of a single organism greater than 100,000 colony-forming units/ml (cfu/ml) are indicators of infection.
3. The presence of one organism per oil-immersion field of stained uncentrifuged urine is indicative of greater than 100,000 cfu/ml.
4. Urine dipsticks are often used in the ED setting. A positive leukocyte esterase test combined with positive nitrites is predictive of a UTI.
5. *Pyuria* (defined as greater than five WBCs per high-power field) does not always indicate

infection. *Sterile pyuria* can be found in inflammatory conditions such as appendicitis and pelvic inflammatory disease.

6. Urine cultures should be reserved for the following settings: children, pregnant women, immunocompromised patients, recently treated patients with clinical relapse, suspected neutropenia, known abnormalities of the urinary tract such as neurogenic bladder, pyelonephritis, diabetic patients, and renal dialysis patients.

Pregnancy tests

Tests of pregnancy include urine pregnancy tests, serum qualitative tests, and serum quantitative human chorionic gonadotropin (HCG) tests.

Indications

1. To identify or exclude the diagnosis of pregnancy in reproductive-aged females with vaginal bleeding, abdominal or pelvic pain, or sexual assault.
2. To determine a serum HCG for correlation with ultrasound diagnosis.
3. Diagnosis of ectopic pregnancy, monitoring of trophoblastic tumors, screening for fetal abnormalities.
4. Monitor the quantitative HCG in threatened abortions.

Normal values

Urine tests vary in the amount of HCG needed to produce a positive test. Assays using antibodies to the beta subunit (beta-HCG assays) will detect 25 mU/ml, recognizing pregnancy with 95% sensitivity by 1 week after the first missed menstrual cycle.

During pregnancy, plasma HCG levels increase predictably, except after 20 weeks.

Duration of pregnancy (weeks)	Plasma human chorionic gonadotropin (mU/ml)
1	5–50
2	50–500
3	100–10,000
4	1000–30,000
5	3500–115,000
6–8	12,000–270,000
8–12	15,000–220,000
20–40	3000–5000

Abnormalities and causes

1. *Elevated HCG*: In normal pregnancy, HCG becomes elevated 1–2 weeks after fertilization and doubles approximately every 2 days, reaching its peak at 8–10 weeks. In ectopic pregnancy, HCG levels rise more slowly. With trophoblastic tumors (molar pregnancy), HCG levels rise slowly at first, but continue to rise, reaching levels higher than expected in normal pregnancy. Spontaneous miscarriage and fetal nonviability are usually preceded by placental and fetal tissue death, causing failure of the expected normal rise in serum HCG.

Pearls and pitfalls

1. Beta-HCG of 2000 (around 35 days gestation) should have a visible uterine gestational sac on transvaginal ultrasound. Beta-HCG of 6000 (around 42 days gestation) should have a visible uterine gestational sac on transabdominal ultrasound.
2. Ectopic pregnancies often occur at very low HCG levels and should be aggressively sought if clinical signs or symptoms are suggestive. HCG levels tend to be higher in normal than abnormal pregnancy (ectopic, miscarriage).
3. A single quantitative HCG cannot be relied on to make decisions about a particular pregnancy; therefore serial HCGs and close follow-up should be assured.

Rh factor

Definition

Test of the presence or absence of antigens located on cell membranes. It is used in the context of measuring the ability of a woman to mount antibodies to antigens (that were obtained from the father) that may be present on fetal RBCs.

Abnormalities and causes

1. If a pregnant woman is Rh-negative, she can become sensitized to antigens and produce antibodies to fetal RBCs, causing severe fetal anemia and CHF (*hydrops fetalis*). In order to produce such an antibody response, blood must cross from the fetus to the mother. This usually occurs during delivery, spontaneous miscarriages, or previous transfusions (affecting subsequent pregnancies).
2. Any pregnant woman with threatened miscarriage or vaginal bleeding must have

Rh factor determination. Rh-negative women must be treated with an injection of anti-D immune globulin (RhoGAM).

3. RhoGAM can be given in both a mini-dose (50 mcg) or full-dose (300 mcg). Indications for the mini-dosing include ectopic pregnancy less than 12 weeks gestation, threatened miscarriage less than 12 weeks gestation, or complete miscarriage less than 12 weeks gestation. Full dosing should be given for ectopic, threatened or complete miscarriage greater than 12 weeks gestation, amniocentesis or fetomaternal transfusion from trauma.

Type and screen

Definition

A type and screen is the determination of different antigens present on a patient's RBC.

Indications

1. Anticipation of potential need for transfusion.
2. Determination of blood type for RhoGAM administration.

Type and crossmatch

Definition

A type and crossmatch is the laboratory actually identifying blood for transfusion to a patient and committing the number of units ordered for that particular patient.

Indications

1. Hemorrhagic shock.
2. HCT less than 21% without active bleeding or less than 30% with active bleeding.
3. Obvious upper or lower gastrointestinal bleeding.
4. Major vascular surgery, abruptio placenta or placenta previa.
5. Coagulation disorders.

Erythrocyte sedimentation rate

Definition

The erythrocyte sedimentation rate (ESR) is nonspecific measure of the level of systemi inflammation and the ability of RBCs to clump. RBC clumping increases with higher levels of fibrinogen.

Normal values

- Male   0–15 mm/hour
- Female   0–20 mm/hour

Abnormalities and causes

1. *Increased ESR*: Generally increased in any inflammatory, infectious, autoimmune, or malignant process. Striking elevations are seen in polymyalgia rheumatica and temporal arteritis.

Pearls and pitfalls

1. The ESR in many conditions is too non-specific to effectively rule in a particular disease process. It may be falsely elevated in conditions where cold agglutinins are present, such as mycoplasma or Epstein–Barr virus infections, and lymphoma. It is often elevated during the second trimester of pregnancy. ESR generally increases with age in males, and decreases with age in females.

Toxicology screen

Toxicology screens may identify the presence or absence of illegal or abused substances, such as amphetamines, barbiturates, benzodiazepines, cannabinoids, cocaine, methadone, opiates, and phencyclidine. Toxicology screens vary from institution to institution.

Indications

1. General screen for the presence of illegal or abused substances from the urine. Indicated in patients who are symptomatic and the diagnosis is unclear or questionable.

Normal values

Duration which certain drugs of abuse test positive:

- Amphetamines   2–3 days
- Barbiturates   Varies; up to several weeks
- Benzodiazepines Varies depending on half-life; most up to 2–3 days
- Cannabinoids   Up to 1 week in single use;
- Cocaine   8–12 hours after single use, 2–3 days in chronic users
- Methadone   2–3 days
- Opiates   1–2 days in single use; 2–4 weeks in chronic users
- Phencyclidine   5–7 days after single use; 1–2 weeks in chronic users

Pearls and pitfalls

1. A negative test does not necessarily exclude the presence of a drug. Many drugs are not detected by a toxicology screen (isoniazid, lithium, antihypertensives, anticoagulants, muscle relaxants, hallucinogens, newer antidepressants (SSRIs), cardiac medications, mushrooms, plants, beta-blockers, insect repellants, cyanide, solvents, antibiotics, hypoglycemics, pesticides, phenol, household products, herbicides, ethylene glycol, nitrates, nitrites, thyroid hormones, and H_2 antagonists).
2. Many false positive drug tests occur in compounds having similar chemical shape.
3. It is more appropriate to understand toxidromic presentations and narrow the scope of toxicologic screening by direct serum quantitative levels when appropriate.
4. Important specific serum drug levels can be ordered when clinically necessary, including acetaminophen, salicylic acid, ethanol, ethylene glycol, methanol, isopropyl alcohol, carbon monoxide, iron, tricyclic antidepressants, organophosphates, lithium, digoxin, dilantin, tegretol, and valproic acid.
5. A full serum toxicology screen may be useful in critically-ill patients in which an unsuspected toxin may dictate a change in management.

References

1. Aviles RJ, Arman TA, et al. Troponin T levels in patients with acute coronary syndromes, with or without renal dysfunction. *New Engl J Med* 2002;346(26):2047.
2. Cohen ME, et al. Prediction of bile duct stones and complications in gallstone pancreatitis using early laboratory trends. *Am J Gastroenterol* 2001;96(12):3305–3311.
3. Cost-Effective Diagnostic Testing in Emergency Medicine. *Guidelines for Appropriate Utilization of Clinical Laboratory*

and Radiology Studies, 2nd ed., Cantrill SV, Karas S (eds).

4. Dufor DR (ed.). *Clinical Use of Laboratory Data-A Practical Guide*, 1st ed., Baltimore: Lippincott Williams & Wilkins.

5. Kottke-Marchant K, Corcoran G. The laboratory diagnosisi of platelet disorders. *Arch Pathol Lab Med* 2002;126(February):133–145.

6. Morganroth ML. An analytic approach to diagnosing acid–base disorders. *J Crit Ill* 1990;5(7):138–150.

7. Morganroth ML. Six steps to acid–base analysis: clinical applications. *J Crit Ill* 1990;5(5):460–469.

8. Newby KL, Storrow AB, et al. Bedside multimarker testing for risk stratification in chest pain units. *Circulation* 2001;103:1832–1837.

9. Orebaugh SL. Normal amylase levels in the presentation of acute pancreatitis. *Am J Emerg Med* 1994;12:21–24.

10. Sucov A, et al. Test ordering guidelines can alter ordering patterns in an academic emergency department. *J Emerg Med* 1999;17(3):391.

11. Van Walraven C, Goel V, et al. Effect of population-based interventions on laboratory utilization. *J Am Med Assoc* 1998;280(23):2028–2033.

Index